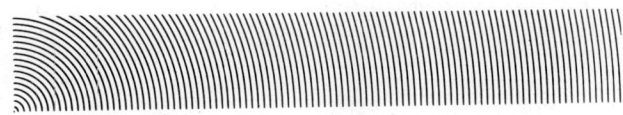

Maternal-Newborn Nursing
Care of the Growing Family

Maternal-Newborn Nursing
Care of the Growing Family
Second Edition

ADELE PILLITTERI, R.N., B.S.N., M.S.N., P.N.A.
Associate Professor of Nursing,
Niagara University,
Niagara Falls, New York

Little, Brown and Company, Boston

Copyright © 1981 by Little, Brown and Company (Inc.)
Second Edition
Second Printing

Previous edition copyright © 1976 by Little, Brown and Company (Inc.)

All rights reserved. No part of this book may be reproduced in any form or by any electronic or mechanical means, including information storage and retrieval systems, without permission in writing from the publisher, except by a reviewer who may quote brief passages in a review.

Library of Congress Catalog Card No. 80-83673

ISBN 0-316-70792-9

Printed in the United States of America

HAL

Cover design by Herb Rogalski

To Joe, with love

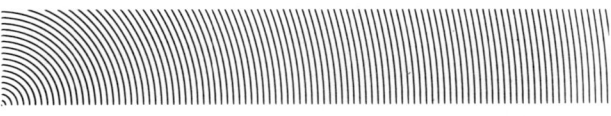

Preface

The demand by consumers for better health care and the expansion of the limits of practice by the nursing profession pose a dual challenge for students of nursing and educators alike. Scientific and technical knowledge is increasing at a rate faster than ever before; yet this rapid increase in nursing knowledge means that there is less time available in nursing programs to cover every aspect of care.

Care of the Growing Family was written with this challenge in mind. It is a two-volume set applicable for use with a standard course in maternal-child nursing or a curriculum in which concepts of maternal-child care are integrated throughout the program. These books would also be useful for a graduate nurse who is interested in reviewing or expanding her knowledge in this area. This volume, *Maternal-Newborn Nursing*, covers the nursing care of the mother and family from the planning of pregnancy through the child's first weeks. The second volume, *Child Health Nursing*, follows the child and family from the child's birth through adolescence. The two books may be used either singly or together.

New chapters on nursing process, problem-oriented recording, and legal aspects of maternal-newborn nursing have been added to this second edition. Other content has been rearranged to make it easier to locate in the text. No separate glossary is included, as a student of nursing should learn to refer to a medical dictionary for clarification of terms just as she/he refers to a pharmacology or nutrition book for additional information. Questions for study follow each unit so that a student can check progress in learning. Plans for care have been presented in a problem-oriented format, as this is the recording system students today will need to utilize tomorrow. This format was also chosen to demonstrate that plans of care are always individualized rather than there being a set plan of care for every instance.

Deciding what to term the person whom nurses care for is always a problem in textbook writing. Such a person in this text is termed a patient or, more directly, a woman, a mother, a fetus, an infant, a father, or a family.

I would like to thank the Children's Hospital of Buffalo for the release of photographs; Robert J. Ford, R.B.P., and Brian S. Smistek, Department of Medical Photography, Children's Hospital of Buffalo, for much of the photography; and Eileen Walsh, Department of Graphic Design, Niagara University, for her beautiful illustrations. Maureen and James Burgio were extremely helpful in supplying photographs of their children.

I am grateful to Julie Stillman and Debra Corman of Little, Brown and Company for their editorial guidance and support in producing the book.

A. P.

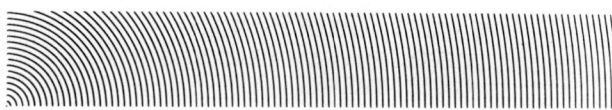

Contents

Preface vii

I. Maternal-Newborn Nursing 1

1. A FRAMEWORK FOR MATERNAL-NEWBORN NURSING 3

Definition of Maternal-Newborn Nursing 4 Pregnancy and Delivery as a Crisis Period 4 Problem Solving 6 Successful Crisis Intervention 9 The Maternal-Newborn Nurse 9 Standards of Maternal-Child Health Nursing Practice 10 References 14

2. TRENDS IN MATERNAL-NEWBORN NURSING 15

The Statistics of Maternal-Newborn Health 15 Steps Toward Reducing Maternal and Infant Mortality 19 Defining High-Risk Mothers and Infants 25 Expanding Roles for Nurses 25 Interpregnancy Care 25 References 26

3. THE NURSING PROCESS IN MATERNAL-NEWBORN CARE 27

The Roots of Maternal-Newborn Nursing 28 Steps of the Nursing Process 29 The Nursing Process and Problem Solving 35 References 36

4. PROBLEM-ORIENTED RECORDING — APPLICATION FOR NURSING 37

The Data Base 38 The Problem List 38 Problem-oriented Recording: Problem List 39 Problem-oriented Recording: Pregnancy Problem List 40 Progress Notes 40 Problem-oriented Recording: Progress Notes 42 Nursing and Problem-oriented Recording 42 References 42

5. LEGAL ASPECTS OF MATERNAL-NEWBORN NURSING 45

Sources of Law 45 Types of Law 45 Negligence 46 Malpractice 46 Standards of Care 46 The Nurse-Patient Relationship 47 Criteria for Establishing Malpractice 48 Incident Reports 49 Statute of Limitations 49 High-Risk Health Care Areas 49 The Suit-prone Nurse 50 The Suit-prone Patient 51 Informed Consent 51 References 51

Unit I. Utilizing Nursing Process: Questions for Review 53

II. The Interpartal Period 55

6. DEVELOPMENTAL READINESS FOR CHILD REARING 57

Infancy: A Sense of Trust 57   The Toddler Period: A Sense of Autonomy 58   The Preschool Period: A Sense of Initiative 59   School Age: A Sense of Industry 59   Adolescence: A Sense of Identity 60   Young Adulthood: A Sense of Intimacy 61   The Middle Years: A Sense of Generativity 62   Older Age: A Sense of Integrity 62   The Process of Achieving Maturity 63   Problem-oriented Recording: Progress Notes 65   References 66

7. PHYSICAL READINESS FOR CHILDBEARING 67

Development at Puberty 67   Female Internal Reproductive Organs 68   Female External Genitalia 76   The Pelvic Floor 77   Male External Genitalia 78   Male Internal Reproductive Organs 79   Mammary Glands 79   Pituitary-Hypothalamus Maturity 80   Pelvic Bony Growth 80   Knowledge of Reproductive Organs 80   Problem-oriented Recording: Progress Notes 80   References 82

8. THE PHYSIOLOGY OF REPRODUCTION 83

The Menstrual Cycle 83   Education for Menstruation 87   Menstrual Disorders 87   Menopause 88   Terminology of Menstruation 89   References 89

9. HUMAN SEXUALITY 91

Sex Roles at Life Stages 91   Sex Roles and Parenting 92   Sexual Responses 93   Influence of the Menstrual Cycle on Sexual Response 93   Influence of Pregnancy on Sexual Response 94   Peak Sexual Response 94   Contraceptives and Sexuality 94   Sexuality Problems 94   Nursing Responsibility and Human Sexuality 95   References 96

10. FAMILY PLANNING 97

Birth Control Methods 97   Future Family Planning Methods 109   Problem-oriented Recording: Progress Notes 109   References 109

11. INFERTILITY AND STERILITY 111

Fertility Studies 112   Causes of Male Infertility 112   Assessment of Male Infertility 113   Plans and Interventions in

Male Infertility 114 Causes of Female Infertility 115 Assessment of Female Infertility 119 Plans and Interventions in Female Infertility 119 Support During Fertility Studies 120 Problem-oriented Recording: Progress Notes 121 References 121

Unit II. Utilizing Nursing Process: Questions for Review 123

III. The Prepartal Period: Preparing for Parenthood 125

12. PSYCHOSOCIAL ASPECTS OF PREGNANCY 127

The Pregnant Woman 127 The Psychological Tasks of Pregnancy 128 Emotional Responses to Pregnancy 132 The Practical Tasks of Pregnancy 134 The Pregnant Father 135 The Pregnant Family 136 The Unwed Pregnant Woman 137 The Unwed Expectant Father 139 Problem-oriented Recording: Progress Notes 140 References 143

13. GROWTH AND DEVELOPMENT OF THE FETUS 145

Fertilization: The Beginning of Pregnancy 145 Implantation 146 The Decidua 146 Chorionic Villi 147 The Placenta 148 The Umbilical Cord 150 The Membranes and Amniotic Fluid 151 Origin and Development of Organ Systems 152 Monthly Estimates of Fetal Growth and Development 157 Teratogens 162 Assessing Fetal Well-Being and Maturity 170 Problem-oriented Recording: Progress Notes 179 References 181

14. PHYSIOLOGICAL CHANGES IN PREGNANCY 183

Local Changes 183 Systemic Changes 186 Weight Gain 191 Effects of Physiological Changes 192 References 193

15. THE DIAGNOSIS OF PREGNANCY 195

Presumptive Signs 195 Probable Signs 196 Positive Signs 199 Problem-oriented Recording: Progress Notes 200 References 201

16. THE FIRST PRENATAL VISIT 203

Conducting an Initial Interview 204 Parts of an Interview 206 The Husband's Role in an Initial Interview 209 The

Physical Examination 210 Expected Date of Confinement 219 Risk Assessment 219 Open Communication—Key to Nursing Care 219 References 220

17. HEALTH MAINTENANCE DURING PREGNANCY — 221

Assessment of Minor Symptoms of Early Pregnancy 221 Personal Care During Pregnancy 226 Danger Signs of Pregnancy 229 Nursing Interventions at Prenatal Visits 230 Assessment of Minor Symptoms of Mid or Late Pregnancy 231 Personal Care Update 233 Preparation-for-Childbirth Classes 233 Signals of Beginning Labor 233 Preparation for the Baby's Care 234 Arrangements for Labor and Delivery 235 Open Communication—Key to Nursing Care 236 Problem-oriented Recording: Progress Notes 236 References 237

18. NUTRITION AND PREGNANCY — 239

Nutritional Requirements 239 Daily Needs 246 Nutritional Problems in Pregnancy 247 Cultural Influences 251 Fad Diets 252 Nutritional Counseling 253 Problem-oriented Recording: Progress Notes 255 References 256

19. PREPARATION FOR PARENTHOOD — 259

Expectant Parents' Classes 259 Preparation-for-Childbirth Classes 263 Problem-oriented Recording: Progress Notes 272 References 273

Unit III. Utilizing Nursing Process: Questions for Review   275

IV. Period of Parturition: Becoming a Parent — 277

20. PSYCHOSOCIAL ASPECTS OF LABOR — 279

Readiness for Labor 279 The Stress of Labor 280 Reducing Stress in Labor 280 Stages of Labor 282 The Father and Labor 284 The Unmarried Woman in Labor 285 The Unmarried Man and Labor 285 Home Births 286 Problem-oriented Recording: Progress Notes 286 References 288

21. THE LABOR PROCESS — 289

Fetal Cranial Determinations 289 Fetal Presentation and Position 291 Theories of Labor Onset 297 Signs of Labor 300 Divisions of Labor 303 Danger Signals of Labor 311 References 314

22. **THE LABOR EXPERIENCE: NURSING INTERVENTIONS** 315

Assessment on Admission to the Hospital 315 Nursing Interventions: Preparatory Division of Labor 324 Nursing Interventions: Pelvic Division of Labor 332 Nursing Interventions: Placental Stage 337 Emergency Delivery of an Infant 338 Problem-oriented Recording: Progress Notes 339 References 341

23. **ANALGESIA AND ANESTHESIA IN LABOR AND DELIVERY** 343

Nursing Interventions to Minimize Discomfort 344 Prepared Childbirth Exercises 346 Medication for Pain Relief During Labor 346 Hypnosis 351 Medication for Pain Relief During Delivery 352 Preparation for the Safe Administration of Anesthetics 354 The Risk of Anesthesia 358 Problem-oriented Recording: Progress Notes 359 References 362

Unit IV. Utilizing Nursing Process: Questions for Review 363

V. The Postpartal Period: Parenthood   365

24. **PSYCHOSOCIAL ASPECTS OF THE POSTPARTAL PERIOD** 367

Parental Love 367 The Neonatal Perception Inventory 370 Phases of the Puerperium 373 Rooming-In 374 Concerns of the Postpartal Period 375 The Unwed Mother 376 The Unwed Father 377 The Mother Who Chooses Not To Keep Her Child 377 Sibling Visitation 378 Problem-oriented Recording: Progress Notes 378 References 379

25. **PHYSIOLOGY OF THE POSTPARTAL PERIOD** 381

Involution 381 Systemic Changes 384 Progressive Changes 385 References 386

26. **THE POSTPARTAL EXPERIENCE: NURSING INTERVENTIONS** 387

Immediate Postpartal Care 387 Continued Interventions During Hospital Stay 390 Preparation for Discharge 400 Problem-oriented Recording: Progress Notes 403 References 404

Unit V. Utilizing Nursing Process: Questions for Review 405

VI. The Newborn — 407

27. PERSONALITY DEVELOPMENT IN THE NEWBORN — 409

Newborn Tasks 409 Developmental Task: Trust Versus Mistrust 410 Classes on Mothering 411 Sensory Stimulation 411 Infant Development 412 Temperament 412 References 414

28. PHYSIOLOGICAL DEVELOPMENT IN THE NEWBORN — 417

A Newborn Profile 418 Vital Signs 419 Cardiovascular System 421 Respiratory System 423 Gastrointestinal System 424 Urinary System 425 Autoimmune System 425 Neuromuscular System 425 Appearance of the Newborn 429 Physiological Adjustment to Extrauterine Life 441 References 441

29. HEALTH ASSESSMENT OF THE NEWBORN — 443

History Taking 443 Physical Assessment of the Newborn 444 Assessment of Gestation Age 450 Assessment of the Maternal-Newborn Interaction 459 Problem-oriented Recording: Progress Notes 460 References 460

30. NUTRITIONAL NEEDS OF THE NEWBORN — 461

Nutritional Allowances for the Newborn 461 Breast-Feeding 463 Formula-Feeding 477 Introducing Solid Food 483 Problem-oriented Recording: Progress Notes 484 References 485

31. NEWBORN CARE: NURSING INTERVENTIONS — 487

Delivery Room Care 487 Care of the Newborn in the Hospital 493 Care of the Newborn at Home 501 Health Problems in the Newborn 503 Health Maintenance at Home 508 Newborn Safety 508 Problem-oriented Recording: Progress Notes 511 References 511

Unit VI. Utilizing Nursing Process: Questions for Review 513

VII. The High-Risk Pregnancy — 515

32. THE IMPACT OF A HIGH-RISK PREGNANCY — 517

Defining the Concept "High-Risk" 517 Accepting the Pregnancy 518 Accepting the Child 518 Identifying Coping

Abilities 518   Immobilizing Reactions to High-Risk Pregnancy 519   The High-Risk Father 522   References 522

33. DEVIATIONS FROM THE NORMAL IN PREGNANCY: NURSING INTERVENTIONS 523

Bleeding During Pregnancy 523 Premature Rupture of Membranes 545 Pregnancy-induced Hypertension 545 Chronic Hypertensive Vascular Disease 553   Diabetes and Pregnancy 554   Heart Disease and Pregnancy 558   Anemia 561 Urinary Tract Disorders 562   Respiratory Disorders 563   Venereal Disease 564 Collagen Disorders 568   Gastrointestinal Diseases and Pregnancy 568 Neurological Conditions 569   Multiple Gestation 570   Hydramnios 572   The Postmature Pregnancy 573   The Elderly Primpara 573   The Pregnant Adolescent 573   Hyperemesis Gravidarum 575 Pseudocyesis 576   Drug Dependence 576 The Battered Woman 578 Problem-oriented Recording: Progress Notes 579   References 580

34. GENETIC DISORDERS AND PREGNANCY 583

Mendelian Inheritance: Dominant and Recessive Genes 583   Division Defects 585   Familial Tendencies 588   Genetic Counseling 588   Legal Aspects of Genetic Screening 591   Rh Incompatibility 591   Commonly Inherited Disorders 593   References 597

35. DEVIATIONS FROM THE NORMAL IN LABOR AND DELIVERY: NURSING INTERVENTIONS 599

Dystocia 599   Uterine Dysfunction: Difficulty with the Force 599   The Fetus: Difficulty with the Passenger 603   The Birth Canal: Difficulty with the Passageway 612   Cesarean Section 613 Induction of Labor 616   Forceps Delivery 618   Vacuum Extraction 618 Anomalies of the Placenta and Cord 618 Problem-oriented Recording: Progress Notes 619   References 620

36. DEVIATIONS FROM THE NORMAL DURING THE PUERPERIUM: NURSING INTERVENTIONS 621

Hemorrhage 621   Puerperal Infection 625   Postpartal Pregnancy-induced Hypertension 630   The Woman Whose Child Is Delivered by Cesarean Section

630 The Mother Whose Child Is Born Handicapped 631 The Mother Whose Child Is Born Prematurely 632 The Woman Whose Child Has Died 633 Postpartal Psychosis 633 Problem-oriented Recording: Progress Notes 633 References 634

Unit VII. Utilizing Nursing Process: Questions for Review 635

VIII. The High-Risk Infant 637

37. IDENTIFYING THE HIGH-RISK INFANT 639

Regionalization 639 Transport of High-Risk Infants 639 Mother-Child Bonding 642 Following High-Risk Infants at Home 644 References 644

38. THE INFANT WITH A CONGENITAL ANOMALY OR NEONATAL ILLNESS 647

Priorities in First Days of Life 647 Initiation and Maintenance of Respirations 647 Establishment of Extrauterine Circulation 655 Temperature Regulation 656 Nutrition 657 Prevention of Infection 662 The Infant with Congenital Anomalies 664 Illness in Newborns 679 Problem-oriented Recording: Progress Notes 693 References 693

39. THE INFANT WITH ABNORMAL GESTATION AGE OR BIRTH WEIGHT 695

Infants Small for Gestation Age 695 Infants Large for Gestation Age 696 The Low-Birth-Weight Infant 697 The Postmature Infant 711 Problem-oriented Recording: Progress Notes 711 References 712

Unit VIII. Utilizing Nursing Process: Questions for Review 713

Appendixes 715

Appendix A. The Pregnant Patient's Bill of Rights 717

Appendix B. Conversion of Pounds and Ounces to Grams for Newborn Weights 719

Answers to Unit Questions 721
Index 723

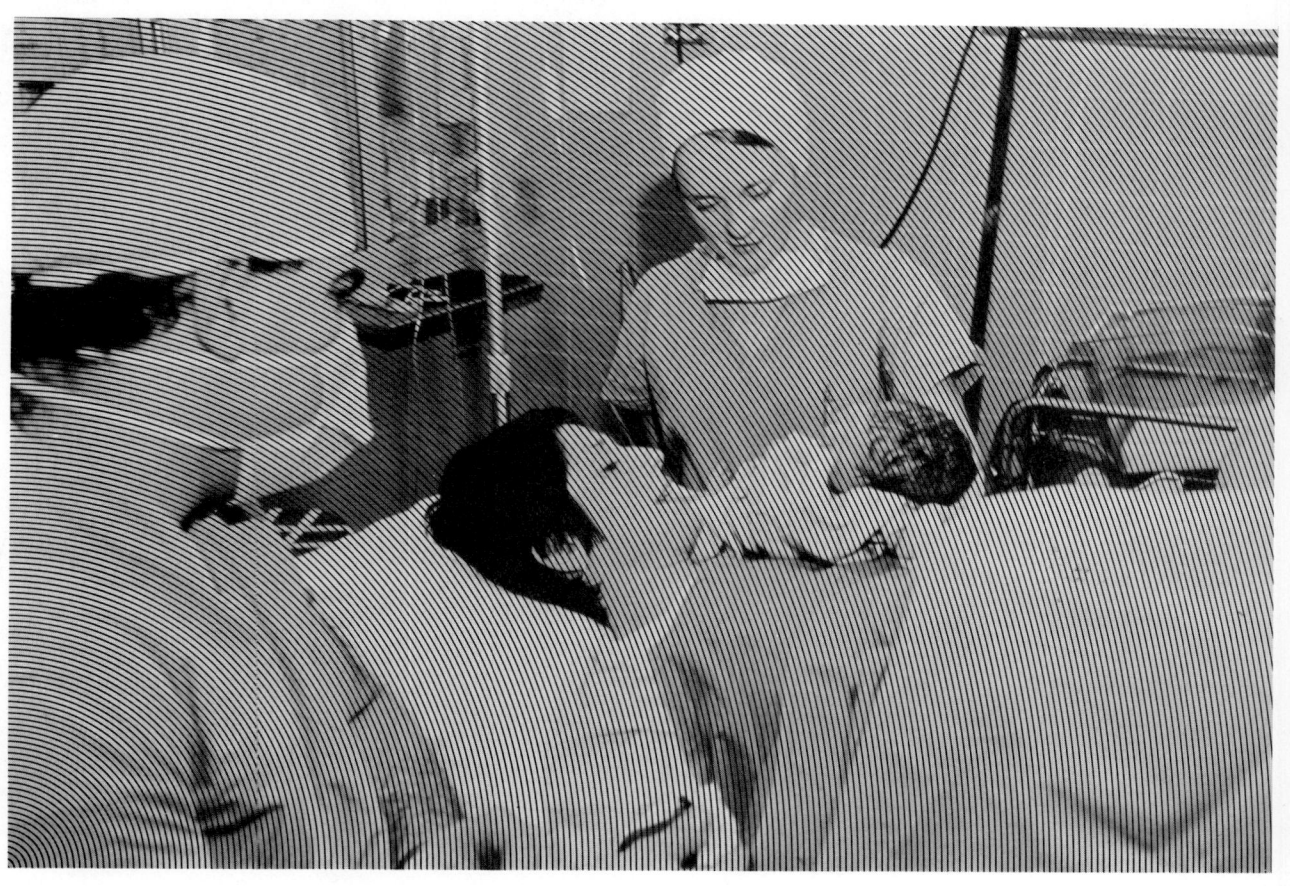

I. Maternal-Newborn Nursing

Notice
The indications and dosages of all drugs in this book have been recommended in the medical literature and conform to the practices of the general medical community. The medications described do not necessarily have specific approval by the Food and Drug Administration for use in the diseases and dosages for which they are recommended. The package insert for each drug should be consulted for use and dosage as approved by the FDA. Because standards for usage change, it is advisable to keep abreast of revised recommendations, particularly those concerning new drugs.

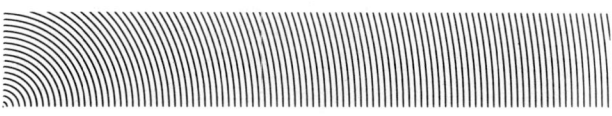

1. A Framework for Maternal-Newborn Nursing

A sperm and an ovum meet in the velvety softness of a fallopian tube. They fuse. A pregnancy begins. Subtle changes begin in the woman's body.

She wakes in the morning sick to her stomach. She looks in a mirror and notices a fine glow to her face. She worries. She hopes. She dreams. She finds herself humming while she is doing dishes one morning. She visits a physician. He tells her that what she has suspected is true: she is pregnant. He shows her a calendar and circles a date. On that day, a Monday in March, seven months away, she will give birth.

She tells no one but her husband about her pregnancy, yet everyone who knows her seems to guess. Her walk, her preoccupation with herself, and finally her growing abdomen betray her.

One afternoon she feels a flutter inside her abdomen. She wonders what is happening, then laughs as she realizes this strange new feeling inside her is one she has been waiting to feel: the feel of life. She begins to visualize and plan for this life that is to be. She contemplates the life she has lived, her readiness to care for a new life. She questions her ability to be a mother, her ability to deliver the child, her ability to be a wife. She sews. She waits. She shops. She waits. She reads. She waits. She prepares. She waits.

She grows impatient and angry with waiting. She grows uncomfortable and angry with her pregnant body.

Finally, when it seems as if she cannot wait any longer, she wakes at night to contractions, announcing that the child inside her is as ready as she for birth. The contractions increase. She goes to a hospital. The contractions strengthen and change. She pushes. Her child is born.

He cries. She holds him.

She cries with exhilaration. Because she has just participated in an experience that only half the population of the world can ever experience. Because she has come through a crisis period in her life with new self-esteem and confidence in herself to be able to face whatever will come after.

It is a fallacy to believe that all children are wanted or will be given good care after they are born. It is equally foolish to believe that all women should be or need to be mothers to find fulfillment. For the woman who chooses this life-style, however, the moment of delivery of her firstborn can be an unmatched fulfillment. And being with a woman through a pregnancy and delivery in a nursing role can be unmatched job satisfaction.

Definition of Maternal-Newborn Nursing

Obstetrics is the branch of medicine that deals with the management of pregnancy, parturition (labor and delivery), and the puerperium (the six weeks following childbirth). The word *obstetrics* is derived from the Latin word *obstetrix*, meaning "midwife," or the person who "stands by" (*obstare*) a woman during childbirth. In light of the range of responsibilities and concerns now involved in the care of a woman throughout pregnancy and childbirth, the older term *obstetrical nursing* has been replaced by the newer and more descriptive term *maternal-newborn nursing*.

Maternal-newborn nursing is directly concerned with the care of the woman during pregnancy, parturition, and the puerperium, as well as with the care of the child prenatally, intrapartally, and during the neonatal period, the 28 days following birth. Because pregnancy and care of the newborn are events that occur as part of family interaction, maternal-newborn nursing deals indirectly with the woman before and after her pregnancies and with the interactions among her and her new child and other family members. The all-pervading goal of maternal-newborn nursing is to assure that children be not only physically, mentally, and emotionally well born but also born well.

Pregnancy and Delivery as a Crisis Period

Although they are planned for and often joyfully anticipated, pregnancy and childbirth are always stressful and represent a crisis to some degree because of the role change that is intrinsic to pregnancy. A second, third, or even a ninth pregnancy is no less stressful than the first, because it is the woman's first experience with that particular pregnancy.

Stress in life may be situational (death of a loved one, ill health, loss of wealth or love) or developmental (toddlerhood, with its increasing independence; adolescence, with its new body functions and changes; pregnancy; adulthood, with new responsibility). A true crisis state occurs with the stress if the person experiencing the stress does not have or cannot utilize previously developed coping mechanisms to deal with the stress. A period of disorganization or disturbance will occur, and the person may make various unsuccessful attempts at solution. Eventually, some kind of resolution is achieved—one that may or may not be in the best interests of that person or the people around him.

If the resolution is reality-oriented, that is, indicates acceptance of the inevitable, strengthens interpersonal ties, and restores equilibrium, it is an adaptive resolution. The person has not only resolved a crisis but has also enriched his ability to cope with future crises. If the resolution is not reality-oriented, that is, results in lasting interpersonal disturbances or in newly formed neurotic or psychotic syndromes, it is a maladaptive resolution [6]. Preventing maladaptive resolutions of crises is essential for the promotion of mental health.

CRISIS INTERVENTION

Specifically, whether an individual can manage crisis situations or needs help in handling life events has to do with three main variables: the individual's perception of the event, the type and availability of support people she has to call upon, and the ways of coping or managing stressful events she has found successful in the past [1].

Perception of the Event

Families involved in childbearing usually consist of young adults. By young adulthood most persons have had experience with both success (they have completed a school experience) and lack of success (somewhere along the line they have been refused a loan or a job they especially wanted). They have achieved a degree of responsibility for their own care and possibly that of another if they have chosen to marry. They have had opportunities to make decisions. They are at a time in life when they are ready for children.

The woman who is only a teenager when she becomes pregnant has had much less experience in decision making. The biggest decision an eighth-grader or a high school freshman may have made is whether to wear her hair long or short or whether to take English or math in the last period of her school day. She has had little experience with real responsibility (occasional baby-sitting is not the same as 24-hour-a-day care of an infant). In the light of her background, she may perceive her pregnancy as a tragedy rather than as an anticipated event.

A woman who is past young adulthood when she becomes pregnant has the advantage of being experienced in decision making and responsibility, but she also may be enjoying the freedom and the absence of responsibility from infant care that is currently her circumstance. The stage of life, therefore, that a woman and her family are in at the time pregnancy occurs can cause a pregnancy to be viewed as a major crisis, an adjustable manageable crisis, or not a crisis at all.

Whether a woman is married or not, has other

children or not, has career plans or not, has adequate financial resources or not, all are other factors that influence her perception of the event.

Support Persons
Support persons are those who play a significant part in giving counsel or guidance in times of stress. In order to be effective they must be the right kind of persons—capable of offering support—and they must be available when needed. A husband is the traditional support person for a woman, parents for a young girl. For pregnancy, however, a close girl friend or a neighbor who has had children may be a stronger support person than a husband who knows little about children or parents who are angry that their daughter is pregnant. The father of the child of an unmarried pregnant woman may or may not be supportive, depending on what the coming event means to him.

Some persons who ordinarily would be supportive may not be available because of physical distance. On the other hand, some families separated by great distance maintain close contact by mail or phone. Husbands who are separated from their wives by work (salesmen, military personnel, truck drivers) may be very supportive throughout a pregnancy, more supportive perhaps than a husband who is home every evening but who does not perceive the coming child in the same way that his wife does. During labor, the actual presence of the support person is important. A husband's absence at this time can be deeply disappointing to a woman. When families were extended, that is, contained grandparents, aunts, and uncles in addition to the nuclear family of father, mother, and children, a woman received her main support and intervention from the family group during pregnancy. Preparing the family cradle ("Four generations of the family have slept in it.") and polishing a family baby spoon ("This is the spoon you ate from when you were small.") are activities that give a woman proof that childbirth is a positive, endurable, continuing, generation-to-generation process.

Some of the support the woman received from the extended family was in the form of old wives' tales: "Don't reach up during pregnancy, or you'll twist the baby's cord." "Don't eat strawberries, or your child will be born with a birthmark." "Don't sew on Sunday, or the baby's cord will knot." As unfounded as these warnings were, they nonetheless provided a sense of continuity, of security that the women who handed down these tales had successfully passed through the birth process.

Many young couples today do not have the support of an extended family, since families today are largely nuclear in structure. Further, more and more women are unmarried when they have a child (single-unit families). Nuclear families, for the most part, live in apartments or suburban communities where they may know their neighbors only well enough to say "hello" on the elevator or across the backyard fence. For support during health crises they turn to health care personnel. During pregnancy, they rely on health care personnel for reassurance that they are well, that they will be adequate parents, that their babies will be healthy.

The adaptive resolution the woman achieves handling the stress and crises of pregnancy and birth—whether she becomes more able to cope with stress, more aware of her family's support, more attuned to and appreciative of life than she was before; or becomes bitter and disappointed in her life and less able to cope with stress—depends a great deal on the amount and kind of support or crisis intervention she receives from the health personnel who care for her during pregnancy, labor, delivery, and the days following birth.

Having a child is never accomplished alone. It involves interaction with family members and friends and, most importantly, the father of the child. How the woman manages during pregnancy depends also on how these people around her cope with crisis; in turn, how well they cope with crisis may depend on the amount and kind of support they receive from health care personnel (Fig. 1-1).

Fig. 1-1. Having a baby is a family affair. If ready support people are not available at this time, health personnel need to fulfill this role. (Courtesy of the Department of Medical Photography, Children's Hospital, Buffalo, N.Y.)

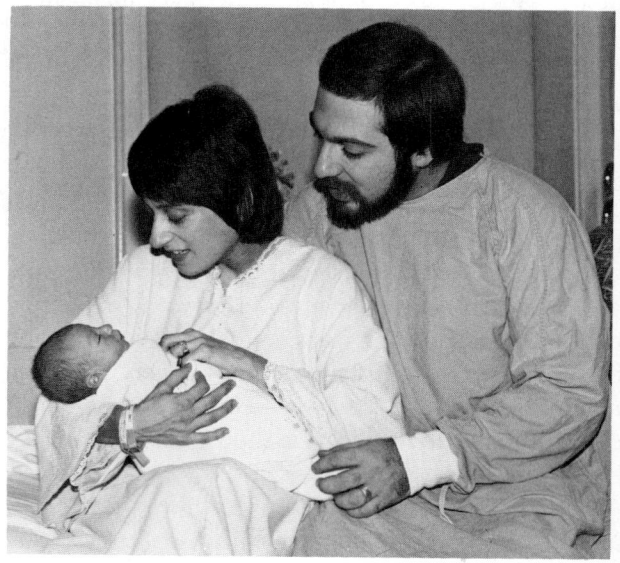

Besides family and health personnel support people, individuals have a network of additional support such as church groups, community organizations, or social clubs. Some women join a specific group for the support they can receive from it (the woman who joins Alcoholics Anonymous). Others originate support groups to meet their needs (Parents of Retarded Children or the La Leche League for Breast Feeding Mothers). During a complication of pregnancy, such groups may become primary support sources because of the specific need they serve and help they can offer.

Coping Mechanisms

A person copes with a new stress situation in the same manner she has coped with past situations. Because a coping mechanism worked once, however, is no guarantee that it will work again, even under similar circumstances.

A 2-year-old, for example, uses temper tantrums as a coping mechanism. This type of behavior is not likely to be effective for a woman trying to resolve a dispute with an insurance company or one who has just learned that she is pregnant. Some coping mechanisms such as crying or aggression are effective for short-term resolutions. They force other people to change the degree of stress in order to stop the crying or the anger. These methods are ineffective during a long-term crisis—a pregnancy, for example. No one can cry for nine months; no one will listen to someone crying for nine months.

Ignoring the situation is another ineffective coping mechanism to use in pregnancy because a pregnancy cannot be ignored. It continues to exist whether the person wills it or not.

The components of effective crisis resolution are shown in Fig. 1-2A. Figure 1-2B shows ineffective crisis resolution.

When a person is first faced with a stress situation—something unexpected has happened—she reacts with the most familiar mechanism she knows. In many instances, the coping mechanism is adequate for the situation; the stress is resolved and the crisis is over. An example of this is a woman who knows that her charge account bill is overdue but chooses to ignore it. Her husband pays it to maintain their credit rating. The crisis is resolved even though her coping mechanism was one of a very limiting nature: ignoring the situation. This type of primary coping intervention success is shown diagramatically in Fig. 1-3.

Suppose the husband is out of town, however. Now the woman's coping mechanism does not work. The crisis continues. The woman must use a coping mechanism other than her most familiar one. In this instance, she calls the store and accuses the store computer of making an error and asks for a new account statement. The store manager agrees to do nothing about her overdue account until a new computer scan can be run. Although ineffective at her first try at resolution, the woman has now successfully reduced the crisis (at least for another month). The use of secondary coping mechanisms is shown diagrammatically in Fig. 1-4.

But suppose the store manager does not respond to the woman's demands for a new statement. Now neither her usual coping mechanism nor her new coping mechanism has been effective. The crisis continues. She has used all the resources at her disposal. The crisis will continue until someone from outside intervenes to help her solve the conflict. It is important that some outside intervention occur in crisis situations or the stress eventually becomes overwhelming for the individual. Mental health cannot be maintained in the face of constant unresolved crisis.

Problem Solving

The most effective coping mechanism in any situation is problem solving. Problem solving is superior to crying, fainting, ignoring, or anger; such mechanisms only postpone facing the problem, a temporary measure. Problem solving ends the crisis.

Helping a person learn to solve problems, then, not only helps her through a present crisis but adds problem solving to her repertoire of coping mechanisms and prepares her to be better able to end crisis situations within the scope of mental health in the future. This has important implications when working with pregnant women because soon they will be responsible for not only those disturbances that touch their own lives but also those that touch the life of a new individual.

Problem solving consists of five steps: identifying the problem, planning alternatives for action, selecting one action to try, implementing the action, and evaluating the outcome of the action and whether further action is needed. These steps are shown in Fig. 1-5.

IDENTIFYING THE PROBLEM

Helping someone identify a problem is often more difficult than it appears because your own values of what is or is not a problem tend to interfere. If you find a woman moaning in labor, for example, it is

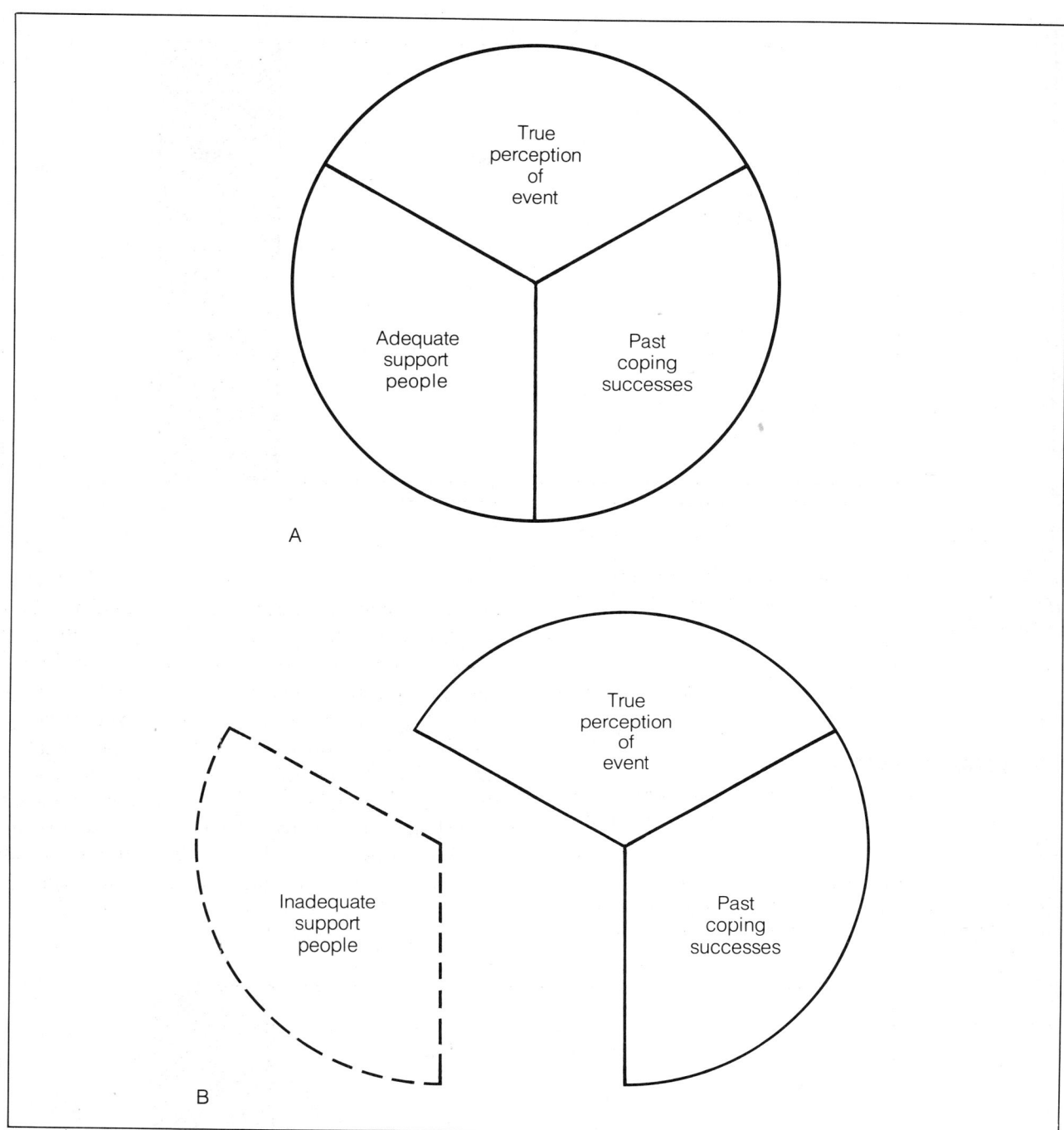

Fig. 1-2. A. Effective crisis resolution. Without all three components, crisis resolution will be ineffective. B. Ineffective crisis resolution. With a missing component, crisis resolution cannot be completed.

natural to assume that her labor contractions are beginning to hurt and that is why she is uncomfortable. You give her something for pain. She does not appear to grow any less uncomfortable. Her problem was not the discomfort of labor contractions but that of extreme thirst. You failed to solve her problem because her problem was not clearly identified.

A 17-year-old comes into a prenatal clinic stating that she is constantly nauseated and wonders if she might be pregnant. The clinic doctor suggests a menstrual extraction to abort a possible pregnancy. The girl does not return. She wanted only the nausea aborted; the pregnancy was fine with her.

No problem can be solved until everyone concerned is certain what the problem is. Ask, What out of everything wrong concerns or worries you the most? If I could do only one thing for you, what would that thing be? Once a person is sure in her

A Framework for Maternal-Newborn Nursing 7

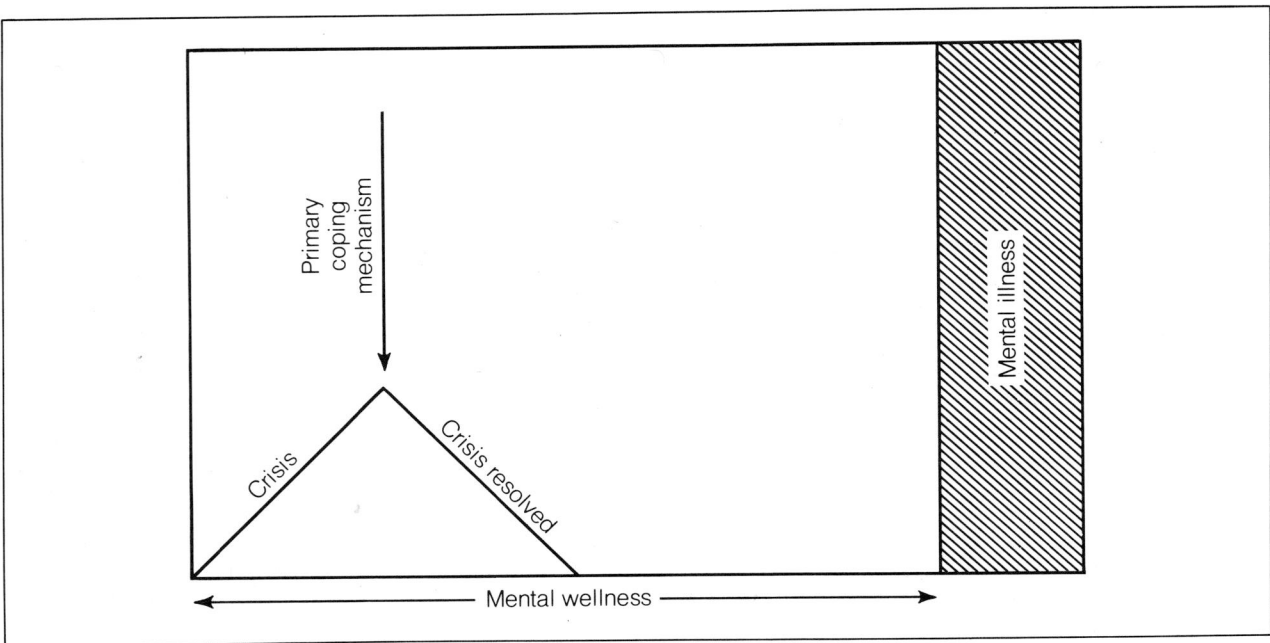

Fig. 1-3. Primary coping mechanism. For a simple problem, a primary coping mechanism is adequate to achieve crisis resolution.

mind what her problem is, solutions begin to be possible.

PLANNING ALTERNATIVES

The only alternatives that people can choose in any situation are those they know. A major function in problem solving for health care personnel is letting people know all the alternatives available to them. A 17-year-old who cannot stand being nauseated every day during early pregnancy, for example, has a number of alternatives: taking medication, eating dry crackers (the time-honored treatment for nausea of pregnancy), eating nothing each day until noon, ending the pregnancy, killing herself. It is always distressing to hear people who have attempted suicide explain that they chose suicide because they simply did not know any other way to end their upsetting situation.

Fig. 1-4. Secondary coping mechanism. The primary coping mechanism used was not adequate. The crisis required a secondary coping mechanism for resolution.

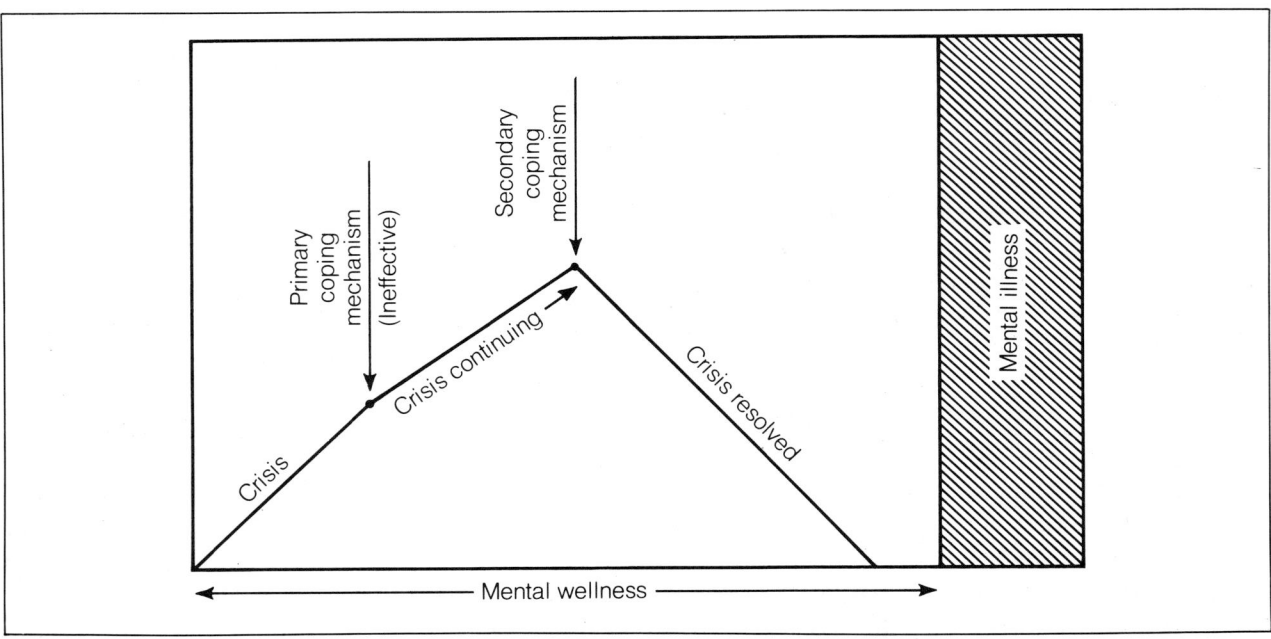

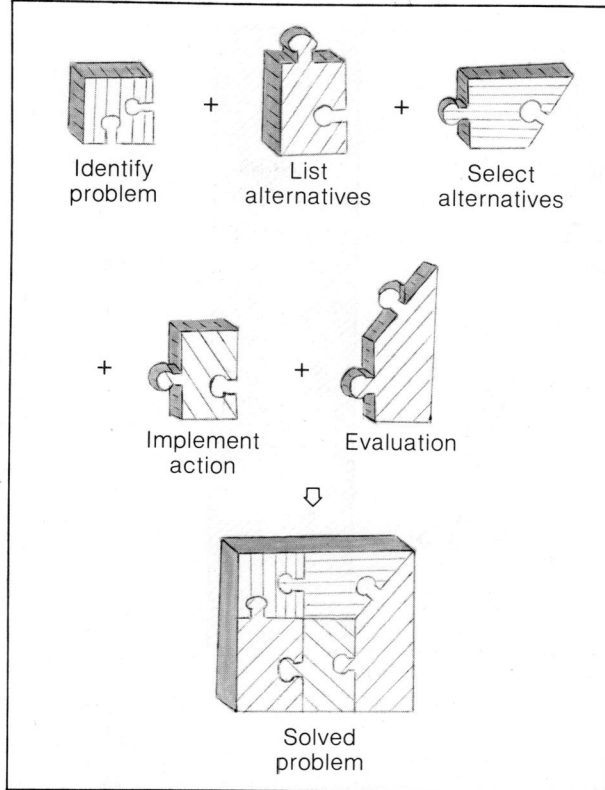

Fig. 1-5. Steps in problem solving.

CHOOSING FROM AMONG ALTERNATIVES

Most people do not have much difficulty choosing among alternatives once they are aware of the ones available to them. Before they choose, they must be sure that they have thought through "what would happen if" they chose that alternative. If the 17-year-old with morning sickness, for instance, chooses to take medication daily for her nausea, she will have no more nausea during her pregnancy. If she chooses to eat nothing until noon each day, she may also not have nausea, but she may be unable to take in an adequate diet and the baby inside her may suffer. The alternatives people choose to try in situations differ greatly from person to person depending on their values and what is or is not important to them.

IMPLEMENTING THE PLAN

Some people are talkers, some are talkers and doers, some are doers. People who can solve problems up through the point of selecting alternatives but then cannot carry them out well do not handle stress well. (In many instances, however, talking about what they should do is so therapeutic that it becomes an action.) People who are doers (without planning) invariably do not handle stress situations well either; although they expend a great deal of energy in problem solving, they are stabbing in the dark, so their energy is wasted.

Some people need urging to carry out the plan they have decided is most effective. Others need urging to think one more time before they act, to find a balance between planning and implementation in problem solving.

EVALUATION

Evaluation is a step often forgotten in problem solving. Let us return to the young girl who is concerned with the nausea of early pregnancy. A medication is prescribed for her. Unfortunately, the nausea does not improve. If there is no evaluation as to whether the intervention was effective in solving her problem, health care personnel will proceed as if everything is now all right; the girl, disappointed with the lack of help she has received, will not return for further care. Nine months of pregnancy will pass unsupervised.

Evaluation is necessary because it sets the stage for further problem solving, for identifying or reidentifying the problem and beginning the cycle over again until the person seeking help is at least temporarily crisis-free.

Successful Crisis Intervention

During crisis periods, people do not need outside intervention as long as their primary or secondary coping mechanisms are working. Once their known coping mechanisms have failed, however, they need some form of help. At this point they are susceptible to suggestion.

Pregnancy is an extremely vulnerable time in life because it is the announcement of a major life change (not for another 18 years will the woman sleep soundly at night) and of a major accomplishment (men build bridges and companies but nothing that smiles back at you). Because it is a sustained crisis, it may exhaust usual coping mechanisms before it runs its nine-month course. As you monitor the course of a pregnancy, your offers of support and suggestions for problem solving can be influential in ensuring an adaptive fulfilling outcome to pregnancy.

The use of outside intervention to reduce crisis in contrast to the outcome of unresolved crisis is depicted in Figs. 1-6 and 1-7.

The Maternal-Newborn Nurse

It is often said that no one can be a good maternal-newborn nurse unless she has given birth herself; until she has lain in a hospital bed and heard thoughtless

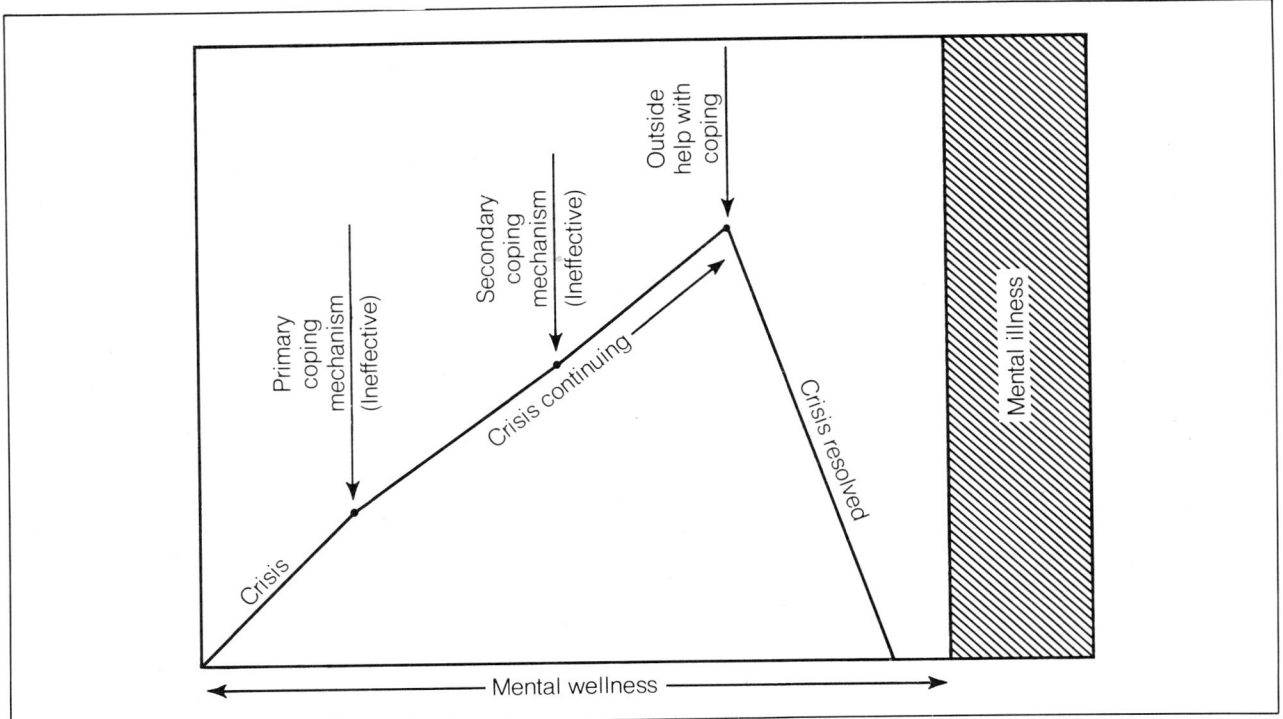

Fig. 1-6. Tertiary coping mechanism. The person's primary and secondary coping mechanisms were both inadequate to effect crisis resolution. Outside intervention was necessary to bring about resolution and keep the person within bounds of mental wellness.

comments of health personnel (who are watching perhaps their thousandth delivery) float down to her, asking questions about her "pains" and urging her to "breathe with contractions" (as if she intended to stop breathing); until she has felt the force and the overwhelming helplessness that comes with labor contractions. Such criteria would necessarily restrict the number of persons who could become maternal-newborn nurses and are thus impractical. It is more important that a nurse caring for a pregnant woman and her family be able to empathize with feelings of joy, pain, fear, threat, hope, achievement, disappointment, satisfaction, and terror, for all these emotions occur with pregnancy and childbirth. If you can anticipate the feeling that comes with planning and hoping against hope for something, yet constantly being steeled for instant, devastating disappointment, come. You are ready to learn the skills that a nurse in maternal and newborn care must have.

Standards of Maternal-Child Health Nursing Practice

Every nurse is responsible for practicing with a level of care that will provide optimal protection and safety to a woman and her unborn and newborn child. In order that there be consistency of care among nurses, various organizations in nursing have developed standards of nursing practice as guidelines. Individual health care agencies supplement these guidelines with particular policies for actions and care in that setting based on the specific woman or child or current circumstances.

In 1973 the Executive Committee and the Standards Committee of the Division of Maternal-Child Health Nursing Practice of the American Nurses' Association [2] developed 13 process standards for maternal-child health nursing practice (reprinted with permission of the American Nurses' Association):

STANDARD I

Maternal and child health nursing practice is characterized by the continual questioning of the assumptions upon which practice is based, retaining those which are valid and searching for and using new knowledge.

Rationale: Since knowledge is not static, all assumptions are subject to change. Assumptions are derived from knowledge of findings of research which are subject to additional testing and revision. They are carefully selected and tested and reflect utilization of present and new knowledge. Effective utilization of these knowledges stimulates more astute observations and

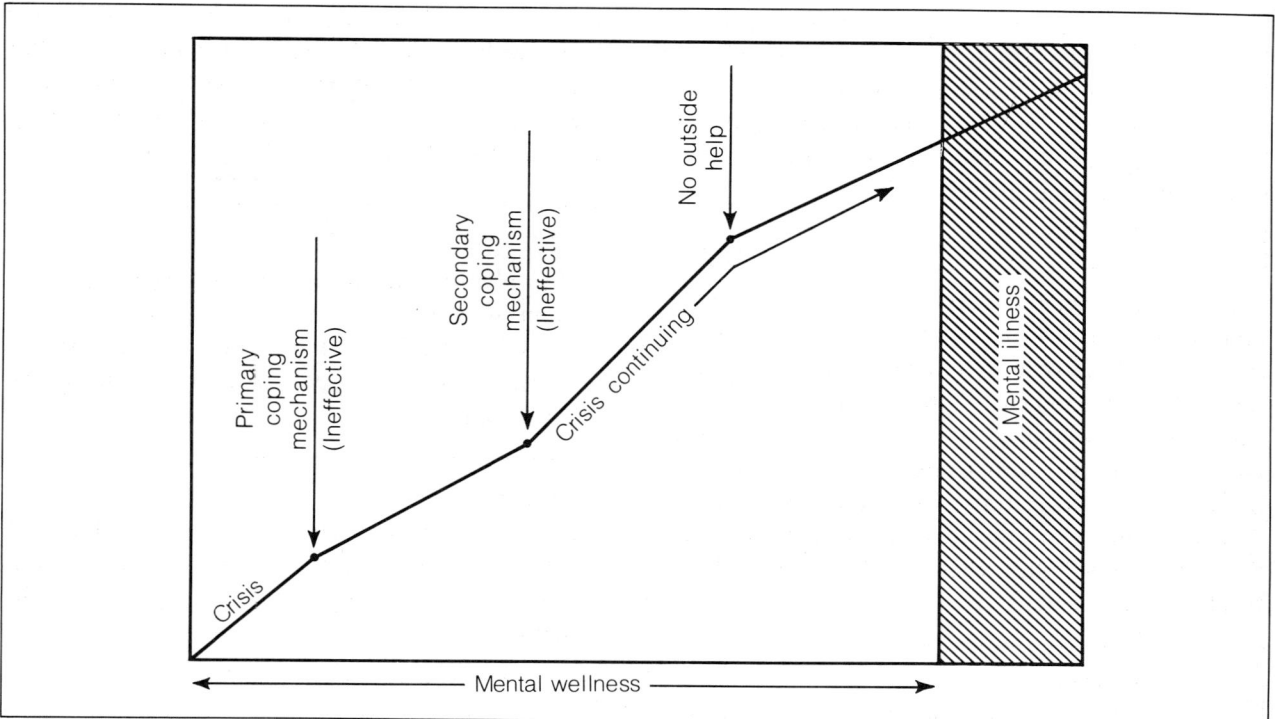

Fig. 1-7. Unresolved crisis. The person sought no help (or was offered no help) after primary and secondary coping mechanisms failed. The crisis situation proceeds unchecked; the outcome will be continued inability to cope with life situations.

provides new insights into the effects of nursing upon the individual and family. To question assumptions implies that nursing practice is not based on stereotyped or ritualistic procedures or methods of intervention; rather, practice exemplifies an objective, systematic and logical investigation of a phenomenon or problem.

An example of how nurses have met this standard in maternal-newborn nursing is seen in the increased interest they have shown in helping mothers learn to breast-feed their newborn infants. Twenty years ago, new mothers were taught that bottle-feeding was safest and most nutritious for newborns. Now, almost all health care personnel accept the philosophy that human milk is best for human infants. A basic assumption—infants should be fed in the best way possible—has been retained; new appreciation of the components of breast milk has led to new practices.

STANDARD II
Maternal and child health nursing practice is based upon knowledge of the biophysical and psychosocial development of individuals from conception through the childrearing phase of development and upon knowledge of the basic needs for optimum development.

Rationale: A knowledge and understanding of the principles and normal ranges in human growth, development and behavior are essential to Maternal and Child Health Nursing Practice. Concomitant with this knowledge is the recognition and consideration of the psychosocial, environmental, nutritional, spiritual and cognitive factors that enhance or deter the biophysical and psychological maturation of the individual and his family.

That nurses are meeting this standard is reflected in the increased interest in health screening tests as part of routine nursing assessment in the newborn period so that newborns with less than optimal development potential can be identified early and be provided with those special services or care needed. Helping women to learn more about their body functions at all stages of pregnancy and parturition helps them to maintain better health practices all the years of their lives.

STANDARD III
The collection of data about the health status of the client/patient is systematic and continuous. The data are accessible, communicated and recorded.

> Rationale: Comprehensive care requires complete and ongoing collection of data about the client/patient to determine the nursing care needs and other health care needs of the client/patient. All health status data about the client/patient must be available for all members of the health care team.

As nurses meet this standard, they become more and more involved in problem-oriented recording systems, as these systems allow data collected during prenatal months to be easily transmitted to the health care personnel who are with the woman at the time of labor and delivery. Participating in problem-oriented recording systems lets nurses share their expertise and their concerns with other health care persons. Thus the nurse can be both a teacher and a learner of better health care practices.

> STANDARD IV
> *Nursing diagnoses are derived from data about the health status of the client/patient.*
> Rationale: The health status of the client/patient is the basis for determining the nursing care needs. The data are analyzed and compared to norms.

As nurses initiate more independent nursing functions, making nursing diagnoses becomes more and more an intrinsic part of optimal care and practice. Utilizing scales that identify women as high risk for having a child born with some form of difficulty is an example of independent nursing action that helps to safeguard women and their unborn children in everyday practice.

> STANDARD V
> *Maternal and child health nursing practice recognizes deviations from expected patterns of physiologic activity and anatomic and psychosocial development.*
> Rationale: Early detection of deviations and therapeutic intervention are essential to the prevention of illness, to facilitating growth and developmental potential, and to the promotion of optimal health for the individual and the family.

Nurses in prenatal, natal, and postnatal areas are in first-line positions to identify deviations from the normal that will affect either the woman or her child. Because many of the problems that occur during pregnancy, such as pregnancy-induced hypertension, begin with subtle symptoms, the continuity of care that a nurse offers to women and their families enables her to detect small changes before they become irreversible and compromise the pregnancy.

> STANDARD VI
> *The plan of nursing care includes goals derived from the nursing diagnoses.*
> Rationale: The determination of the desired results from nursing actions is an essential part of planning care.

Because pregnancy is a time of crisis, pregnant women are easily influenced and are "ripe" for health teaching. Establishing goals specific for each woman allows this to be done most effectively and with far-reaching results.

> STANDARD VII
> *The plan of nursing care includes priorities and the prescribed nursing approaches or measures to achieve the goals derived from the nursing diagnoses.*
> Rationale: Nursing actions are planned to promote, maintain, and restore the client/patient's well-being.

In an area in which health care practices always affect not one but two individuals (and equally often an entire family) it is easy for secondary goals and plans to "slip through the cracks" unless nursing care plans detail priorities of action.

> STANDARD VIII
> *Nursing actions provide for client/patient participation in health promotion, maintenance and restoration.*
> Rationale: The client/patient and family are provided the opportunity to participate in the nursing care. Such provision is made based upon theoretical and experiential evidence that participation of client/patient and family may foster growth.

In no other area of nursing are patients allowed to participate more fully in their care than in the area of maternal-newborn nursing. Teaching women to care for their own health during pregnancy and that of their newborn child is an intrinsic part of maternal-newborn nursing.

> ### STANDARD IX
> *Maternal and child health nursing practice provides for the use and coordination of all services that assist individuals to prepare for responsible sexual roles.*
>
> Rationale: People are prepared for sexual roles through a process of socialization that takes place from birth to adulthood. This process of socialization, to a large extent, is carried out within the family structure. Social control over child care increases in importance as humans become increasingly dependent on the culture rather than upon the family unit. The culture of any society is maintained by the transmission of its specific values, attitudes and behaviors from generation to generation. Attitudes and values concerning male and female roles develop as part of the socialization process. Attitudes toward self, the opposite sex and parents will influence the roles each individual assumes in adulthood and the responsibilities accepted.

Nurses in maternal-newborn nursing have at their disposal knowledge of methods of birth control or family planning so that people can assume responsible sexual roles. They are a source of information for understanding responses that are sexual in nature and helping people to view childbearing as an extension of their sexual roles. Young mothers look to nurses for role models of female or male adult roles.

> ### STANDARD X
> *Nursing actions assist the client/patient to maximize his health capabilities.*
>
> Rationale: Nursing actions are designed to promote, maintain and restore health. A knowledge and understanding of the principles and normal ranges in human growth, development and behavior are essential to Maternal and Child Health Nursing Practice.

Helping the woman with heart disease, diabetes mellitus, or a kidney disorder maintain a long-hoped-for pregnancy, or helping a mother or father touch and accept an ill newborn with an understanding of the child's strengths as well as the extent of his handicap, is reflected in this standard.

> ### STANDARD XI
> *The client's/patient's progress or lack of progress toward goal achievement is determined by the client/patient and the nurse.*
>
> Rationale: The quality of nursing care depends upon comprehensive and intelligent determination of the impact of nursing upon the health status of the client/patient. The client/patient is an essential part of this determination.

Some women set unrealistic standards for themselves or their children. Couples who are seen for infertility problems need guidance in setting appropriate goals for themselves and evaluating progress toward their goals. Only by evaluation are people able to assess what is happening at the present time and make plans for the future.

> ### STANDARD XII
> *The client's/patient's progress or lack of progress toward goal achievement directs reassessment, reordering of priorities, new goal setting and revision of the plan of nursing care.*
>
> Rationale: The nursing process remains the same, but the input of new information may dictate new or revised approaches.

Because pregnancy is such a major life change for women, goals that are applicable at the beginning of pregnancy may not be applicable at a later point in pregnancy; if a complication occurs, goals may need to be revised to meet new demands; if a newborn's health is compromised at birth, goals may need to be revised again and again in the first few years of life.

> ### STANDARD XIII
> *Maternal and child health nursing practice evidences active participation with others in evaluating the availability, accessibility and acceptability of services for parents and children and cooperating and/or taking leadership in extending and developing needed services in the community.*
>
> Rationale: Knowledge of services presently offered parents and children is the first step in determining the effectiveness of health care to all in the community. When it is recognized that needed services are not available, accessible or acceptable, the nurse takes leadership in working with consumers, other health disciplines,

> the community and governmental agencies in extending and/or developing these services. Services must be continually evaluated, expanded and changed if they are to improve the health and well-being of all parents and children within our society.

Maternal-newborn nursing is a rapidly growing field of nursing. Where once nurses interacted with obstetricians, anesthesiologists, and occasionally dieticians in order to coordinate health care for women and their newborns, they must now interact with perinatologists, geneticists and genetic counselors, respiratory therapists, neonatologists, pediatric nurse practitioners, clinical nurse specialists, endocrinologists, internists, cardiac surgeons, community health nurses, orthopedists, nurse midwives—as many specialties as exist. Nurses are responsible for providing many of the education services needed by women during pregnancy (preparation for childbirth classes, child-rearing classes).

Standards serve as guidelines for planning quality practice. They are important as criteria for assessment of nursing practice in an area of health care delivery that is expanding as rapidly as is the area of maternal-newborn nursing.

References

1. Aguilera, D., and Messick, J. *Crisis Intervention: Theory and Methodology*. St. Louis: Mosby, 1974.
2. American Nurses' Association. *Standards of Maternal-Child Health Nursing Practices*. Kansas City, Mo.: The Association, 1973.
3. Baird, S. F. Crisis intervention theory in maternal-infant nursing. *J.O.G.N. Nurs.* 5:30, 1976.
4. Brandwein, R. A. Women and children last: Divorced mothers and their families. *Nurs. Digest* 4:39, 1976.
5. Brink, P. (Ed.). *Transcultural Nursing*. Englewood Cliffs, N.J.: Prentice-Hall, 1976.
6. Caplan, G. *Principles of Preventive Psychiatry*. New York: Basic Books, 1964.
7. Gray, A. The courts, the government, and the obstetric care consumer: An inventory. *Birth Family J.* 6:227, 1979.
8. Horowitz, J. A., and Perdue, B. J. Single-parent families. *Nurs. Clin. North Am.* 12:503, 1977.
9. Kreutner, A. K., and Hollingsworth, D. R. *Adolescent Obstetrics and Gynecology*. Chicago: Year Book, 1978.
10. Lubic, R. W., and Ernst, E. K. The childbearing center: An alternative to conventional care. *Nurs. Outlook* 26:754, 1978.
11. Scully, R. Stress in the nurse. *Am. J. Nurs.* 80:911, 1980.
12. Snow, L. F., et al. The behavioral implications of some old wives' tales. *Obstet. Gynecol.* 51:727, 1978.
13. Stichler, J. F., et al. Pregnancy: A shared emotional experience. *M.C.N.* 3:153, 1978.

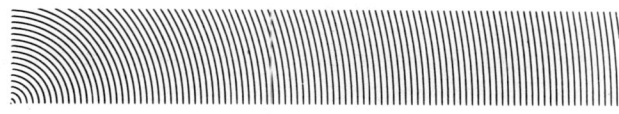

2. Trends in Maternal-Newborn Nursing

Each year in the United States about 3.3 million women give birth.

How safe is it for women to have babies today? How safe is it to be born today? Do women still die in childbirth? Do infants die? How many infants die shortly after birth? Before 1 year of age? What can be done to make pregnancy and childbirth safer for both women and infants? More satisfying for women and their families?

The Statistics of Maternal-Newborn Health

A number of statistical terms are used internationally in expressing the outcome of pregnancies and deliveries so that statistics reported from different countries can be compared readily:

> *Birth rate:* The number of births per 1,000 population
> *Divorce rate:* The number of divorces per 1,000 population
> *Fetal death rate:* The number of fetal deaths (over 500 gm) per 1,000 live births
> *Infant mortality:* The number of deaths per 1,000 live births occurring at birth or in the first 12 months of life
> *Maternal mortality:* The number of maternal deaths per 100,000 live births that occur as a direct result of the reproductive process
> *Neonatal death rate:* The number of deaths per 1,000 live births occurring at birth or in the first 28 days of life
> *Perinatal death rate:* The number of deaths occurring in fetuses over 500 gm and in the first 28 days of life per 1,000 live births

BIRTH RATE

The *birth rate* is the number of births per 1,000 population. The birth rate in the United States started to decline about 1955. It hit a low of 14.8 per 1,000 in 1976, then began to rise again slightly because of the increasing number of women of childbearing age (15 to 44 years of age). That the birth rate today is still much lower than before 1955 is due to an accelerated trend toward voluntary reduction in family size through family planning and the use of contraceptive measures.

The average size of the completed family in the United States today is 1.5 children. This low birth rate is threatening to some persons involved in maternal or newborn care, who wonder what will happen to their jobs if fewer and fewer children are conceived and born. The answer will be, it is hoped, that all children born in the near future will receive the kind of health care that is advocated but not always available today. The decline in birth rate will perhaps allow the reality of maternal-newborn care to approximate the theoretical standards more closely. Using a broad definition, one of every seven pregnancies today is in some way a high-risk pregnancy. One child in every seven, therefore, requires some form of special concern or care at birth.

FETAL DEATH RATE

Fetal death rate is the number of fetal deaths per 1,000 live births. A fetal death is defined as the death in utero of a child (fetus) weighing 500 gm or more, roughly the weight of a fetus of 20 weeks or more gestation. Fetal deaths may occur because of maternal factors (maternal disease, incompetent uterus, maternal malnutrition) or fetal factors (fetal disease, chromosome abnormality, poor uterine attachment). A large number of fetal deaths still occur for reasons yet unknown.

Fetal death rate is important because it reflects to a degree the overall quality of maternity care.

NEONATAL DEATH RATE

The first 28 days of life comprise the *neonatal period*. The child during this time is known as a *neonate*. *Neonatal death rate* is the number of deaths per 1,000 live births occurring at birth or in the first 28 days of life. The neonatal death rate reflects not only the quality of care available to women during pregnancy and childbirth but also the quality of care available to infants during the first month of life.

Immaturity of the infant is the chief cause of these early deaths. Approximately 80 percent of infants who die within 48 hours after birth weigh less than 2,500 gm (5½ pounds).

PERINATAL DEATH RATE

The *perinatal period* is a time beginning when the fetus reaches 500 gm (about the 20th week of pregnancy) and ending about four weeks after birth. The *perinatal death rate* is the sum of the fetal and neonatal rates.

INFANT MORTALITY

Infant mortality is the number of deaths per 1,000 live births occurring at birth or in the first 12 months of life. It includes the neonatal death rate. This rate is the traditional standard used to compare one country's overall conditions of health and health care with those of other countries.

Thanks to medical advances and improvements in child care, infant mortality in the United States is falling. The decline since 1960 is shown in Table 2-1.

Notice the inconsistency between white mortality and that of all other groups, namely, 12.4 versus 21.0. The Native American population is included in the "all other" category, and its high infant mortality is one of the reasons our national rate is so high. Many, if not most, reservation Native Americans live in abject poverty. The women cannot afford an adequate diet during pregnancy, nor do they necessarily receive adequate prenatal care. More and more children of Native American women are being delivered in hospitals, so mortality in the immediate neonatal period is the same as it is for whites. The many infant deaths occur after the children are taken home, into the poverty situation. The Native American infant mortality is improving markedly, however, because of improved overall health care.

Low birth weight is a continuing problem of black Americans. The high number of low-birth-weight infants born to black women adds greatly to infant mortality in the United States. It has been assumed in the past that low birth weight was a genetically prevalent trait in blacks and that little could be done to change it. With better prenatal nutrition, however, birth weight in black infants increases. The problem, then, appears to be not so much genetic as nutritional. Therefore, it is attributable to poverty and, with proper guidance and improved living conditions, can be corrected.

The steady drop in total infant mortality in the United States is certainly encouraging. Figure 2-1 shows death rates per 100,000 population by age and sex for the years 1950 through 1977. Note that death is more likely to occur during the first year of life than at any other age under 65.

Table 2-2 shows the infant mortality in the United States compared to other countries. One would expect that the United States, which has the highest gross national product in the world and is capable of landing men on the moon, would have the lowest infant mortality. In fact, in 1976 (the most recent year for which world statistics are currently available) our infant mortality was higher than that of 12 other countries.

Why is infant mortality higher in some countries than in others? One factor may be different systems of health care delivery. In Sweden, for example, a comprehensive health care program provides free maternal and child health care to all residents. Women who attend prenatal clinics early in pregnancy receive

Table 2-1. Infant Mortality Rates (per 1,000 Live Births) by Color: United States, 1960–1978

	White			All Other			Total		
	Under 1 Year	Under 28 Days	28 Days to 11 Months	Under 1 Year	Under 28 Days	28 Days to 11 Months	Under 1 Year	Under 28 Days	28 Days to 11 Months
1960	22.9	17.2	5.7	43.2	26.9	16.4	26.0	18.7	7.3
1961	22.4	16.9	5.5	40.7	26.2	14.5	25.3	18.4	6.9
1962	22.3	16.9	5.5	41.4	26.1	15.3	25.3	18.3	7.0
1963	22.2	16.7	5.5	41.5	26.1	15.4	25.2	18.2	7.0
1964	21.6	16.2	5.4	41.1	26.5	14.6	24.8	17.9	6.9
1965	21.5	16.1	5.4	40.3	25.4	14.9	24.7	17.1	7.0
1966	20.6	15.6	5.0	38.8	24.8	13.9	23.7	17.2	6.5
1967	19.7	15.0	4.7	35.9	23.8	12.1	22.4	16.5	5.9
1968	19.2	14.7	4.5	34.5	23.0	11.6	21.8	16.1	5.7
1969	18.4	14.2	4.2	32.9	22.5	10.4	20.9	15.6	5.3
1970	17.8	13.8	4.0	30.9	21.4	9.5	20.0	15.1	4.9
1971	17.1	13.0	4.0	28.5	19.6	8.9	19.1	14.2	4.9
1972	16.4	12.4	4.0	27.7	19.2	8.5	18.5	13.6	4.8
1973	15.8	11.8	3.9	26.2	17.9	8.3	17.7	13.0	4.8
1974	14.8	11.1	3.7	24.9	17.2	7.7	16.7	12.3	4.4
1975	14.2	10.4	3.8	24.2	16.8	7.5	16.1	11.6	4.5
1976	13.3	9.7	3.6	23.5	16.3	7.2	15.2	10.9	4.3
1977	12.4	8.7	3.7	21.0	14.5	6.5	14.1	9.9	4.2
1978	—	—	—	—	—	—	13.6	9.4	4.2

Source: Vital Statistics Report, Provisional Statistics, 27:13, 1979. U.S. Department of Health, Education, and Welfare, Public Health Service, National Center for Health Statistics, Hyattsville, Md.

a monetary award. Sweden's infant mortality is the lowest of any country tabulated.

Methods of delivering infants may also play a part in mortality. In The Netherlands, for instance, cesarean sections are performed in only a small percentage of all deliveries. In the United States the number of cesarean sections being performed is growing yearly. About 5 percent of all infants delivered by cesarean section have some respiratory difficulty for a day or two after birth. One cesarean section often leads to another, so that the number of such procedures performed tends to pyramid, constantly increasing the risk to newborns.

In the United States, infant mortality varies from state to state (Table 2-3). Note that in the District of Columbia, which has the questionable distinction of having higher infant mortality than any state in the country, the rate is almost three times what it is in New Hampshire, the state with the lowest infant mortality.

MATERNAL MORTALITY

Maternal mortality is the number of maternal deaths per 100,000 live births that occur as the direct result of the reproductive process. As with infant mortality, there has been a consistent decline in maternal mortality since approximately 1940 (Table 2-4). It has declined so much that since 1960 it has been compiled on the basis of 100,000 live births, not on the 1,000 base ordinarily used.

Three causes are responsible for 70 percent of all maternal deaths. These are hemorrhage, infection, and pregnancy-induced hypertension. Hemorrhage can occur for a number of different reasons, including placenta previa, premature separation of the placenta, and blood dyscrasias, all of which are discussed in detail in later chapters. Infections may occur any time following rupture of the fetal membranes until the uterus returns to its prepregnant state. Infection may be associated with poor technique by hospital personnel in caring for the mother in labor, at delivery, or during the days following childbirth when the placental site in the uterus is prone to infection because of its denuded surface. Pregnancy-induced hypertension, a condition peculiar to pregnancy, is manifested by vasoconstriction, increased blood pressure, proteinuria, edema, and, sometimes, convulsions. The first signs of pregnancy-induced hypertension may occur during pregnancy, labor, delivery, or immediately following birth.

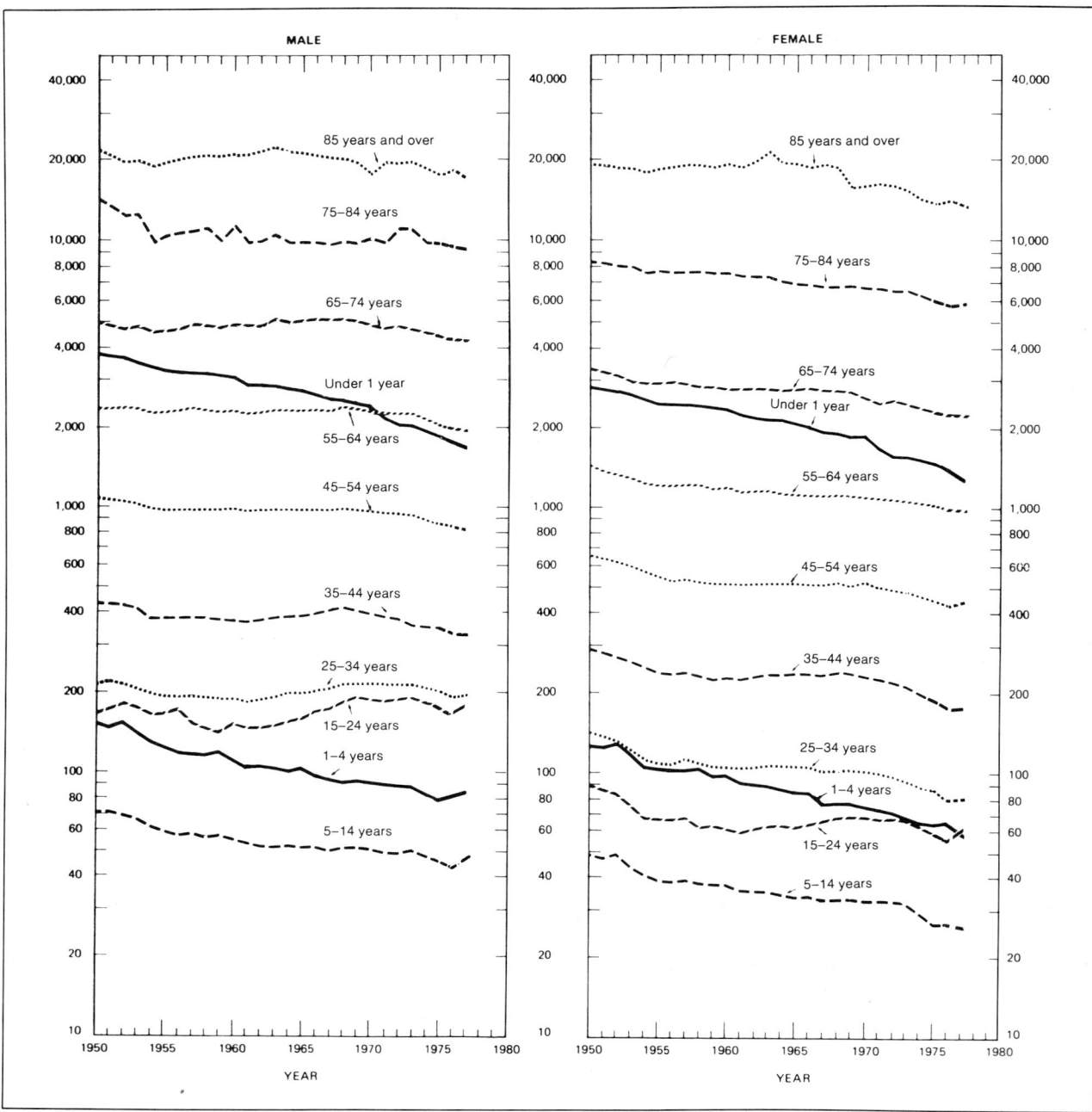

Fig. 2-1. Death rates per 100,000 population in the United States, 1950–1977. (From Vital Statistics Report, Provisional Statistics 26:4, 1978. U.S. Department of Health, Education, and Welfare, Public Health Service, National Center for Health Statistics, Hyattsville, Md.)

Nurses giving maternal-newborn care should impress on their minds the three main causes of maternal mortality so strongly that they flicker like neon signs every time they care for a woman during pregnancy, in childbirth, or during the puerperium. These conditions are for the most part preventable, and nurses who are alert to the signs and symptoms of hemorrhage, infection, and beginning hypertension are invaluable guardians of the health of pregnant and postpartum women.

DIVORCE RATES

Because maternal mortality is falling, it seems as if more children are being reared in intact families than ever before. Because the divorce rate is steadily increasing, however, this is not the case. The divorce rate for the United States for the years 1960 through 1978 is shown in Table 2-5. The rate in 1978 was 5.2 per 1,000 population, or a total of 1,128,000 divorces a year. In some areas of the country the divorce rate is 1 in 4. In many instances, then, the woman is single

Table 2-2. Infant Mortality Rates (per 1,000 Live Births) for Selected Countries, 1976

Rank	Country	Rate
1	Sweden	8.3
2	Japan	9.3
3	Denmark	10.3
4	Netherlands	10.6
5	Switzerland	10.7
6	Finland	11.0
7	Norway	11.1
8	England and Wales	14.2
9	France	14.7
10	Scotland	14.8
11	Hong Kong	14.9
12	Canada	15.0
13	United States	15.2

Source: *Health in the United States Chartbook*, 1978. U.S. Department of Health, Education, and Welfare, Public Health Service, National Center for Health Statistics, Hyattsville, Md.

Table 2-3. Infant Mortality Rate (per 1,000 Live Births) by State, 1978

State	Rate	State	Rate
New Hampshire	8.3	Virginia	13.3
Wyoming	9.0	Michigan	13.4
Maine	9.2	Nebraska	13.8
Wisconsin	9.2	Oklahoma	13.8
Connecticut	9.6	Texas	13.8
Idaho	9.7	Florida	14.2
Massachusetts	9.7	Arkansas	14.3
Montana	10.0	Maryland	14.4
Nevada	11.3	New Mexico	14.5
Vermont	11.4	Georgia	14.7
Kansas	11.5	Illinois	14.7
Washington	11.5	Pennsylvania	14.8
California	11.6	Arizona	15.0
Hawaii	11.8	West Virginia	15.1
Iowa	11.8	Rhode Island	15.7
New Jersey	11.8	Missouri	16.0
Colorado	11.9	Tennessee	16.1
Delaware	12.0	Alaska	16.3
Kentucky	12.0	New York	16.3
South Dakota	12.0	North Carolina	16.3
Utah	12.0	Alabama	16.4
Indiana	12.2	Mississippi	17.1
Minnesota	12.3	Louisiana	17.8
Ohio	13.0	South Carolina	18.5
North Dakota	13.1	District of Columbia	23.1
Oregon	13.2		

Source: *Vital Statistics Report, Provisional Statistics* 27:13, 1979. U.S. Department of Health, Education, and Welfare, Public Health Service, National Center for Health Statistics, Hyattsville, Md.

Table 2-4. Maternal Mortality Rate per 100,000 Live Births, 1960 to 1978

Year	Rate	Year	Rate
1960	37.1	1969	22.2
1961	36.9	1970	21.5
1962	35.2	1971	18.8
1963	35.8	1972	18.8
1964	33.3	1973	15.2
1965	31.6	1974	14.6
1966	29.1	1975	12.8
1967	28.0	1976	12.3
1968	24.5	1977	11.2
		1978	9.9

Source: *Vital Statistics Report, Provisional Statistics* 27:13, 1979. U.S. Department of Health, Education, and Welfare, Public Health Service, National Center for Health Statistics, Hyattsville, Md.

Table 2-5. Divorce Rate in the United States, 1960 to 1978

Year	Rate	Year	Rate
1960	2.2	1969	3.2
1961	2.3	1970	3.5
1962	2.2	1971	3.7
1963	2.3	1972	4.1
1964	2.4	1973	4.4
1965	2.5	1974	4.6
1966	2.5	1975	4.9
1967	2.6	1976	5.0
1968	2.9	1977	5.0
		1978	5.2

Source: *Vital Statistics Report, Provisional Statistics* 27:13, 1979. U.S. Department of Health, Education, and Welfare, Public Health Service, National Center for Health Statistics, Hyattsville, Md.

and has had a recent loss of a support person during a pregnancy and the postpartum period.

Steps Toward Reducing Maternal and Infant Mortality

The availability of skilled professional prenatal care and women's recognition of the importance of such care are important steps in safeguarding the health of women and children. Women today usually either see an obstetrician or a family physician or attend a community clinic early in pregnancy. Fewer low-birth-weight babies are born to women who begin prenatal care early in pregnancy than to those who do not. Many health problems of pregnancy are correctable if recognized when they first appear, uncorrectable later. Pregnancy-induced hypertension (the third leading cause of maternal mortality) is an example of a disorder that if recognized early can easily be controlled and will not be detrimental to the woman or her child; if allowed to continue unchecked, it can lead to death of the mother and the infant.

The areas of pregnancy care and perinatal and neonatal care are expanding rapidly today as the overall emphasis of health care in the United States shifts from the treatment of illness to the prevention of illness, from the concept of treating ill newborns to that of preventing illness in newborns.

PERSONAL CONCERN FOR THE PATIENT

Health care consumers are growing more discriminating in what they demand from health personnel. Changes in both private offices and clinics will have to be made if women are to continue to accept prenatal care. Waiting in line, being called by a number, and being treated as a punched data card, with little regard for privacy, were once accepted fatalistically. Today, women are asking why they must be treated so indifferently and protest such treatment by their poor attendance at health care facilities. Many groups are so distressed by the mechanical way in which women are treated during labor that they are advocating home births.

Personnel in health care facilities may offer excuses for these conditions, claiming, for instance, that there is no money to make improvements. The items that women are most concerned with, however, do not cost money. Being addressed by name, being interviewed as if they were important, not just as a repository of wanted facts, having people knock on examining room doors before entering, having examining tables turned so women are not unnecessarily exposed—these courtesies are all free. During and after labor and delivery, being allowed to have a support person with them, being allowed to have their other children visit, being able to care for the newborn in their room rather than having the child taken away to a central nursery—these, too, are free.

Nurses have a great deal to do with creating the atmosphere, conveying the feeling that although a woman is the eighty-sixth patient to be examined in this clinic or seen in this labor unit this week she is still important. She counts. The child inside her counts. Such concern costs nothing.

Nurses are the people who dispense or fail to dispense these amenities. Consequently, nurses bear a great deal of the responsibility for clinic and office attendance and for keeping childbirth in hospital surroundings, where safety for the woman and her child can be maintained.

COMPREHENSIVE PRENATAL CARE

During the last two decades maternal and infant care projects have been designed as one way of reducing maternal and infant mortality and morbidity caused by complications of pregnancy and childbirth. These projects provide women of low income with the services of allied health care personnel, such as social workers, nutritionists, and home health aides, as well as nurses and physicians. Great differences have been demonstrated in the outcome of pregnancy in women who make use of the projects, as opposed to nonproject women. In a project in Chicago, involving women 15 years of age or younger at the time of conception, neonatal mortality was 36.8 for 4,400 nonproject women and 19.0 for those who participated in the project. In New York City, neonatal mortality was reported as 13 percent lower for infants born to women in the program than for the city as a whole [11].

These projects demonstrate what can be accomplished toward reducing infant and maternal mortality. More comprehensive measures such as these are needed if all the infants delivered to women at the poverty level (about 20 percent of all infants delivered) are to be included in such programs.

ROLE OF THE COMMUNITY HEALTH NURSE

As important as the monthly visits to a private or clinic physician are the home visits of community health nurses. A mother who may feel too embarrassed to admit at the clinic that she rarely eats may talk about the problem and be receptive to nutrition suggestions in her own home. A mother who feels she will be told she is foolish if she admits to fears while at a busy clinic may feel free to talk about such fears while she is at home. Talking about her fears may put them in a perspective, so that she can start to handle them. Knowing that a person has been concerned enough about her health to visit her home may be motivation enough for her to make the extra effort to get to the clinic or the physician's office and so receive the benefits of prenatal care.

Whether or not the visits of a community health nurse are successful depends on the same factors that determine a woman's acceptance of prenatal care in the clinic or physician's office, on whether or not the nurse's attitudes and actions convey a personal, concerned interest.

IMPROVING NUTRITION

It is well documented that the nutrition a woman receives before and during a pregnancy strongly influences the course of pregnancy and the health of the baby. The father's nutrition before conception may also have a bearing on the infant's health. According to Antonov [3], of children born during the siege of Leningrad in 1942 during a period when the little food available was of poor quality, 41.2 percent were premature births. When food was not so scarce, the premature birth rate was only 6.5 percent. In another classic study, Burke [6] reported that all stillborn infants, all infants (except one) who died within a few days of birth, all premature infants, all functionally immature infants, and the majority of infants with congenital malformations were born to women on inadequate diets.

Good nutrition is an area of health teaching in which school nurses can be effective, since the nutritional patterns a person learns as a child tend to persist throughout his life. Unfortunately, many children are taught nutrition in such a technical way that they are "turned off" by the subject ever afterward. It is a challenge to maternal-newborn nurses to "turn on" women to good health.

SOCIOECONOMIC FACTORS

A number of socioeconomic factors influence infant mortality. The more siblings a mother has, for example, the more likely she is to have a stillborn child. In middle-class women, there is a sharp rise in the number of stillbirths among those who have four or more siblings. Among women whose fathers were unskilled manual laborers, there is a sharp rise in stillbirths between women with no siblings and those with one sibling, and again between women with one sibling and those with two or three. The difference probably occurs at the point at which a scarcity of resources began to have an effect on growth in childhood and thus on the woman's reproductive efficiency.

If stillbirths are related to depletion of resources in the mother's family, family planning or limiting the number of children to those who can be economically and emotionally cared for should reduce infant mortality in future generations. Family planning is an area of health supervision in which the maternal-newborn nurse should develop expertise, since she may be the person with whom the woman feels she can best talk about such subjects.

Child spacing can have a direct influence on perinatal mortality. Data from the Maternity and Infant Care Project in New York City [11] show that when deliveries occur a year or less apart, the neonatal death rate is 35 per 1,000. If the interval following delivery is one to two years, the neonatal death rate drops to 17 per 1,000. After a two- to three-year interval, the rate drops to 7 per 1,000.

In infants 2,500 gm or more (normal-birth-weight infants) the morbidity is considerably higher during the first year of life for those whose family income is less than $8,000 than for those whose family income is in the middle range ($8,000 to $14,999). This is shown in Table 2-6.

Another important factor in planning health care for women in the childbearing age is the number of women in this age range who work in order to bring their family income into the middle range—about 45

Table 2-6. Infant Morbidity by Family Income

Birth Weight	Family Income	Severe Impairment (%)	Moderate Congenital Anomalies (%)	Significant Other Illness (%)	Brief or No Illness (%)
2,500 gm or less	Less than $8,000	4.0	17.0	21	58
	$8,000–$14,999	5.2	16.3	16	62
	$15,000 and more	5.2	14.8	14	66
Over 2,500 gm	Less than $8,000	2.4	12.6	16	69
	$8,000–$14,999	1.5	11.5	13	74
	$15,000 and more	2.2	14.8	15	68

Source: *Special Report*, No. 2, 1978. The Robert Wood Johnson Foundation, Princeton, N.J. Based on data compiled by The Johns Hopkins University Health Services Research and Development Center.

percent. This means that many of the old instructions for pregnancy such as "Get lots of rest" have to be modified to "Try and get a period of rest each day."

HOSPITALIZATION FOR CHILDBIRTH

A factor strongly influencing maternal and infant mortality and related to the current decline in these rates is the trend for women to be hospitalized for childbirth. In 1940 only about 40 percent of live births occurred in hospitals; today the figure is between 96 and 100 percent.

A growing number of persons now advocate childbirth at home, in "natural" surroundings, free from the cold, structured hospital environment. They believe that childbirth at home is more enjoyable and may be experienced as the truly exciting event that it should be.

Rather than promote the practice of having babies at home, it would be much better to center the operations of labor and delivery units more around concern for the individuality of patients than concern for rules, to make childbirth as enjoyable in a hospital as it is at home. How quickly the laughter stops at home when a mother hemorrhages, 30 minutes away from medical help! How long the heartache lasts when a baby never breathes, 30 minutes away from resuscitation equipment!

The Committee of the Fetus and Newborn of the American Academy of Pediatrics and the American College of Obstetricians and Gynecologists issued the following joint statement in 1979 (*Pediatrics* 63:166, 1979):

> Labor and delivery, while a physiologic process, clearly presents potential hazards to both mother and fetus before and after birth. These hazards require standards of safety which are provided in the hospital setting and cannot be matched in the home situation.
>
> We recognize, however, the legitimacy of the concern of many that the events surrounding birth be an emotionally satisfying experience for the family. We support those actions that improve the experience of the family while continuing to provide the mother and her infant with accepted standards of safety available only in hospitals which conform to standards as outlined by the American Academy of Pediatrics and the American College of Obstetricians and Gynecologists.

Because nurses control the atmosphere of hospitals, making them either friendly or cold places in which to be a patient, they can be instrumental in keeping childbirth in hospitals.

BIRTHING ROOMS

One way of making hospital births more like those at home is the use of birthing rooms in hospitals. A *birthing room* is a room furnished with colorful curtains, a comfortable chair for a support person, and a bed that much more resembles a home one than a hospital one. Supplies for labor and delivery are in readiness but are concealed in wall cabinets, so the room has a comfortable, nonclinical atmosphere.

Following labor, the woman is not moved to a delivery room for the birth of her child, but the bed is converted into a delivery table or the woman is allowed to deliver without the use of stirrups (the traditional delivery position with a delivery table). Following birth, the infant is cared for in the same room; he remains with the mother and accompanies her to her postpartum rooming-in suite.

Each birthing room must be a self-contained labor and delivery room (Fig. 2-2). Thus if a hospital has six labor rooms and one delivery room, it has to purchase equipment for only one delivery room. If it converts its facilities to six birthing rooms, it must have six complete delivery room setups. Obviously this change entails additional expense.

In order to minimize the duplication of equipment such as radiant heat warmers and anesthetic equipment, many hospitals limit the use of birthing rooms to women who wish to deliver without any anesthetic and who appear to be as free from potential delivery difficulties as can be predicted. As satisfaction with such rooms grows, however, on the part of both women and their physicians, even women with complications may use them.

Women appreciate birthing rooms because they do

Fig. 2-2. A mother and father share a close moment together in a birthing room. The baby is 30 minutes old. (Courtesy of the Department of Medical Photography, Children's Hospital, Buffalo, N.Y.)

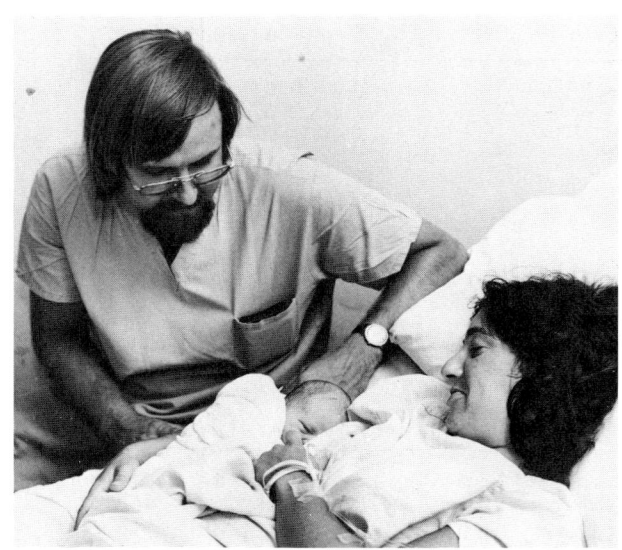

not have to be moved to a cart and transferred to a strange room (possibly away from their support person) at the time labor is becoming hardest for them; husbands are welcome in birthing rooms for the delivery as well as for labor. Husbands do not feel intimidated, as they do by the surgical atmosphere of a delivery room, so they can truly function as support persons.

Use of birthing rooms separates women physically more than traditional labor rooms might, so that detailed observation by nurses on progress in labor is necessary in order to help a physician coordinate care among so many settings.

ALTERNATIVE BIRTH CENTERS
Another way of making birth more homelike, yet offering the protection of medical or skilled nursing personnel, is the development of alternative birth centers. In such a center, a woman is observed on an ambulatory basis throughout her pregnancy. She delivers at the center in an attractive birthing room, stays only about 24 hours, and then is discharged with clear follow-up care and supervision determined.

A woman is generally ineligible for care at a birth center if she has a high-risk factor such as previous cesarean section, is an elderly primipara, or has an accompanying physical illness such as diabetes or a cardiac disease.

One drawback to alternative birth centers is the cost of delivery if the woman's health insurance does not cover this type of health service.

Nurse-midwives play a big role in supervising the health and welfare of women who use alternative birth centers and in protecting the health of their newborns.

OBSERVATION AND RECOVERY ROOMS FOR NEWBORNS AND MOTHERS
Even though recovery rooms for surgical patients have been available in hospitals for decades, some hospitals still do not utilize a recovery room for women or newborns after childbirth.

A great many mothers still receive some anesthesia during delivery, and they have the same problems of anesthesia recovery as do all surgical patients. In addition, all new mothers need careful observation for determination of the amount of bleeding and for signs of postpartum hypertension.

A woman who stays in a birthing room under the watchful eye of a nurse who is responsible for such observation is far safer than one returned immediately to a postpartum unit, where her needs can be overlooked because of the needs of other patients. Mothers who would like a water pitcher filled or ask for medication for suture pain voice their requests strongly and loudly, but hemorrhage, infection, and hypertension are silent killers.

Because of placental transfer, an infant whose mother receives a general anesthetic during delivery also receives the anesthetic. He is in just as much need of an anesthesia recovery room as is any postoperative patient. All infants need the protection of a careful watch period following birth because independent respirations are a new experience for them; the change from fetal to extrauterine circulation does not always happen quickly or surely; they may have some mucus or fluid in the lungs that can lead to obstruction of the airway. Maintaining body temperature at the proper level also poses some difficulty. Heart failure, respiratory obstruction, and hypothermia, like maternal complications, are silent killers. They can be missed in a nursery of crying, hungry infants.

INTENSIVE CARE NURSERIES
It is generally assumed that newborns with a good birth weight (over 2,500 gm, or 5½ pounds) will thrive at birth. In a survey of statistics from high-risk intensive care facilities [13], it was discovered that close to 30 percent of infants of normal birth weight experience significant health problems in the first year of life. These findings are summarized in Table 2-7.

Infants who can be categorized as high risk should be transferred to a neonatal intensive care unit or intensive care nursery (ICN). In nine hospitals throughout the United States and Canada, the introduction of neonatal intensive care units resulted in decreased neonatal mortality of up to 42 percent [13].

It is sometimes argued that saving small babies from dying at birth is not necessarily good health care, as some small babies then develop such neurological abnormalities that they cannot function effectively as adults. A team of pediatricians at the University of Southern California has studied infants born weighing less than 3 pounds, 5 ounces (1,500 gm) and reports that the most striking change in end results today is, along with an increase in survival rate (more than 30 percent improvement), a decrease in definitely abnormal infants [17].

The number of intensive care nurseries in hospitals has risen greatly in recent years. They have tended to become status symbols for hospitals. If such a unit is called an intensive care nursery but lacks the laboratory facilities, equipment, and skilled personnel needed to maintain a high level of quality care, it may be more of a hazard than no unit at all, because its

Table 2-7. Morbidity in Infants to 1 Year of Age

Birth Weight	Severe Impairment (%)	Moderate to Mild Congenital Anomalies (%)	Significant Other Illness (%)	Brief or No Illness (%)
1,500 gm or less	13.0	29.0	15	43
1,501–2,000 gm	5.3	20.7	17	57
2,001–2,500 gm	3.4	14.6	19	63
Over 2,500 gm	2.0	12.0	15	71

Source: *Special Report*, No. 2, 1978. The Robert Wood Johnson Foundation, Princeton, N.J. Based on data compiled by The Johns Hopkins University Health Services Research and Development Center.

mere presence may prevent an infant from being transferred to a nearby center where effective care is available.

The cost of keeping an infant in a neonatal intensive care unit is about $500 a day. Costs of $20,000 to $50,000 are not rare for care during a high-risk pregnancy and care for a high-risk infant. Almost all states have adopted guidelines for health insurance companies that prevent the companies from excluding coverage of intensive newborn care, so the cost of such high-risk care does not preclude infants from having it. When infants are hospitalized in regional centers for care (Fig. 2-3) the mother who is left behind in a small community hospital needs a great deal of support. She has "lost" her infant as surely as the mother whose child dies unless health care personnel help her maintain contact with the infant through telephone calls or snapshots and encourage her to visit as soon as she is able.

CONSOLIDATION OF CARE

In view of the falling birth rate, no single hospital may be able to afford a corps of highly skilled health care personnel to be available at all times to care for women and newborns (it is impossible to limit births to a 9-to-5 schedule, so it is impossible to limit quality care to only those hours) and the best equipment obtainable to safeguard both mother and child. Thus, concepts of consolidation or regionalization are being explored.

When travel was by horse and buggy and roads were rough, small community hospitals at frequently spaced intervals were the answer to health care. With the highways and emergency vehicles now available, the scope of the "community" can be much larger, enabling enough deliveries in one place to justify the cost of the equipment necessary for optimum maternal and infant care.

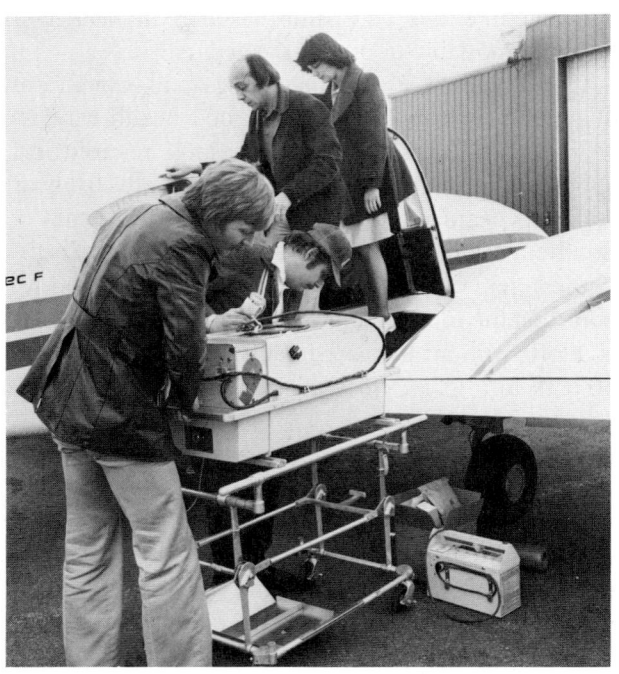

Fig. 2-3. An infant transport unit is moved from the transporting airplane to a transport van. Safe movement of ill newborns to regional centers is a new nursing responsibility. (Courtesy of the Department of Medical Photography, Children's Hospital, Buffalo, N.Y.)

TRANSPORTING HIGH-RISK PATIENTS

When regionalization concepts of newborn care first began, transporting the ill or premature infant was the method chosen. Now, both obstetricians and neonatologists are looking at the subject in a new light. Instead of transporting the infant, it may be safer to transport the mother, the uterus having advantages as a transport incubator far exceeding any commercial incubator yet designed.

Unfortunately, transporting of mothers has several problems that have yet to be solved. The referring hospital loses a patient and so may lose revenue. Removing a woman from her community upsets her family; it also limits her own doctor's participation in her care. Certainly, women who are transported distances for perinatal care need strong support from nursing personnel or they will feel that they are lost in the system.

It is difficult for many people to relinquish the community concept, to accept a van staffed by a physician and maternal nursing practitioners and traveling from community to community as giving as good prenatal care as that dispensed in a red brick community hospital that has been standing in one spot for 50 years. People find it hard to believe that transporting a woman to a consolidated health care facility for childbirth can be an improvement over the traditional wild dash in the family car to the local community hospital. Nurses, like other people, tend to resist change. On the other hand, because nurses are mainly women, they should be the prime innovators in changing concepts of maternal-newborn care.

Defining High-Risk Mothers and Infants

Serious attempts to identify a woman who may have difficulty in pregnancy are being made, usually by means of standardized record systems in which point scores are assigned to various criteria such as high blood pressure or previous pregnancy loss. By adding the total risk score, one can identify a high-risk woman. Some scoring systems have identified more than 150 factors that might affect the woman or the fetus or both, as many as 30 factors that might affect the mother after birth, and an additional 150 items that might affect the newborn infant.

Some factors that place a woman at risk are (1) age less than 17 years or more than 35 years, (2) hypertension, (3) diabetes, (4) previous premature birth or stillbirth, and (5) abnormal duration of labor or delivery. Some factors that place the newborn at risk are (1) prematurity, (2) difficulty establishing respirations at birth, and (3) congenital anomalies.

Expanding Roles for Nurses

Although birth rates are declining, it does not follow automatically that women in the future will have more physician time and care at their disposal during pregnancy and childbirth. It has been estimated that in the near future, 40 percent of the infants born in the United States will be delivered in municipal and community hospitals, in which there is currently an insufficient number of physicians. With the decrease in the number of physicians choosing obstetrics as a career, it is unlikely that in the foreseeable future there will be an adequate number of physicians to deliver infants or even to supervise obstetrical care in these hospitals. The gap in care must be filled by paramedical personnel or nurses prepared for expanded roles as either maternal-newborn practitioners, pediatric nurse associates, or nurse-midwives.

A maternal-newborn practitioner would be able to interview and examine women during pregnancy and so assess their physical and psychological health; obtain pelvic measurements, so that the type of delivery could be predicted; teach women self-care during pregnancy; and prepare them for labor, delivery, and care of the infant. She would be able to evaluate the woman in labor, including assessment of her stage of labor and the health of the fetus. Following delivery, she would assess the health of the newborn, teach self-care to the mother, and help her with feeding and caring for her infant. She would promote interpregnancy health and provide information for family planning or child spacing as requested.

The pediatric nurse associate, working with a pediatrician, would assess the health of newborns by examination and advise the mother on the infant's care. She might make a home visit a week after the mother goes home with the infant to catch the small problems that arise with new babies before the problems become magnified. She would be available by telephone for future consultation. She would see the child during his years of growing up for well-child care and preventive health care measures such as immunizations. She would offer advice and counsel on the expected crises of childhood and manage minor illness in children in consultation with a pediatrician. Such a role allows the physicians or pediatricians to devote more time to ill children and thereby to improve the quality of their practice.

A nurse-midwife working with a team directed by an obstetrician might assume full responsibility for the care and management of women with uncomplicated pregnancies. A nurse who is capable of taking over these functions enables the obstetrician with whom she works to devote the bulk of his time to high-risk mothers or to women in whom complications develop during pregnancy or delivery, thereby improving the quality of his practice. In Sweden, a country with a low infant mortality (8.3, versus 15.2 for the United States), nurse-midwives play a much larger role in maternity care than they do in the United States.

Interpregnancy Care

It is becoming more and more evident that the state of the mother's health at the time pregnancy begins is as important as the health she maintains during pregnancy. Women should be urged to have a health assessment prior to conception, so that any existing medical problems, including malnutrition, can be corrected before a pregnancy begins. They should be encouraged to maintain good health practices throughout their childbearing years in preparation for a future child.

Nurses can be instrumental in supervising health practices at all ages and helping women to enter pregnancy in optimum states of health.

References

1. Adamsons, K. Centralizing care of high-risk OB patients. *Perinat./Neonatol.* 3:14, 1979.
2. Allgaier, A. Alternative birth centers offer family-centered care. *Hospitals* 52:97, 1978.
3. Antonov, A. N. Children born during the siege of Leningrad in 1942. *J. Pediatr.* 30:250, 1947.
4. Baldwin, W., and Cain, V. S. The children of teenage parents. *Fam. Plann. Perspect.* 12:34, 1980.
5. Brandwein, R. A. Women and children last: Divorced mothers and their families. *Nurs. Digest* 4:39, 1976.
6. Burke, B. S., et al. Nutrition studies during pregnancy. *Am. J. Obstet. Gynecol.* 46:38, 1943.
7. Franklin, J. Home-like deliveries in the hospital. *Birth Fam. J.* 5:235, 1978.
8. Garant, C. A. The process of effecting change in nursing. *Nurs. Forum* 17:152, 1978.
9. Mauksch, I. G. Critical issues of the nurse practitioner movement. *Nurse Pract.* 3:15, 1978.
10. Notelowitz, M. The single-unit delivery system—a safe alternative to home deliveries. *Am. J. Obstet. Gynecol.* 132:889, 1978.
11. Pearse, W. H. The maternity and infant care program. *Obstet. Gynecol.* 35:114, 1970.
12. Pomerance, J. J., et al. Cost of living for infants weighing 1,000 grams or less at birth. *Pediatrics* 61:908, 1978.
13. *Special Report*, No. 2, 1978. The Robert Wood Johnson Foundation, Princeton, N.J.
14. Rooks, J. B. Are we making an impact? *J. Nurse Midwifery* 23:15, 1978.
15. Sugarman, M. Regionalization of maternal and newborn care—how can we make a good thing better? *Perinat. Neonatol.* 2:39, 1978.
16. Sweeney, W. J., and Caplan, R. M. *Advances in Obstetrics and Gynecology*. Baltimore: Williams & Wilkins, 1978.
17. Teberg, A., et al. Recent improvements in outcomes for the small premature infant. *Clin. Pediatr.* (Phila.) 16:307, 1977.
18. Thompson, T., et al. The results of intensive care therapy for neonates. *J. Perinat. Med.* 5:59, 1977.
19. Trandel-Korenchuk, D. M., et al. How state laws recognize advanced nursing practice. *Nurs. Outlook* 26:713, 1978.

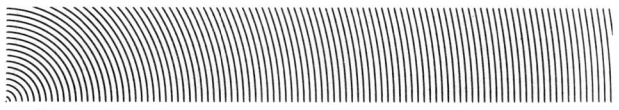

3. The Nursing Process in Maternal-Newborn Care

If they have done their work well, all nurses, during the ages, have done nursing by a process. Only in recent years, however, has the nature of the process been investigated and the steps of the process labeled so that all nurses can have an understanding of the steps necessary to carry out and achieve quality nursing care.

It takes two people to make the nursing process happen: a person who is a nurse (or who is learning to be one) and a person with whom this nurse interacts. The actual interaction may consist of physical ministrations, counseling to improve health, teaching to prevent illness, or even an agreement between the two parties that no intervention is necessary.

A person who enters a purposeful relationship with a nurse has traditionally been called a patient. A *patient* is usually defined as a person under medical care.

Because the modern nurse may give nursing care to people not under medical supervision at the time, the term *patient* is viewed today as old-fashioned by many theorists in nursing. The term *client* is used instead. A client is a person who actively participates in a relationship, such as a lawyer-client relationship. *Client,* however, is identified by Webster as a word that stems from a vassal or serf or one who must give service to a master, or whose participation is less than willing, actually forced. This is not the relationship implied or desired in a nursing relationship.

In this text, therefore, persons with whom nurses interact are termed *patients* or, more specifically, *women, newborns, mothers, fathers, parents,* or *families* (Fig. 3-1). This puts the responsibility on nurses to establish and maintain the relationship. Patients who are ill or under stress (the reason they are in need of nursing services) can be free to act ill and under stress and not have to put on a false front to please the nurse who takes care of them.

In most instances, a nurse-patient relationship is a one-to-one relationship. The person involved in the relationship changes during maternal-newborn nursing, depending on the stage of the pregnancy, the health of the newborn, and the circumstances of the individual situation. The relationship is established with a woman alone when she always comes for prenatal care by herself, with a husband singly at such visits if he has concerns he wants to voice separately from those of his wife. Sometimes the relationship is established with the husband and wife together when they are interacting as a unit (during labor or at the time a couple is told that their child has been born with a health problem). Sometimes the relationship is established with an entire family (at a time when a

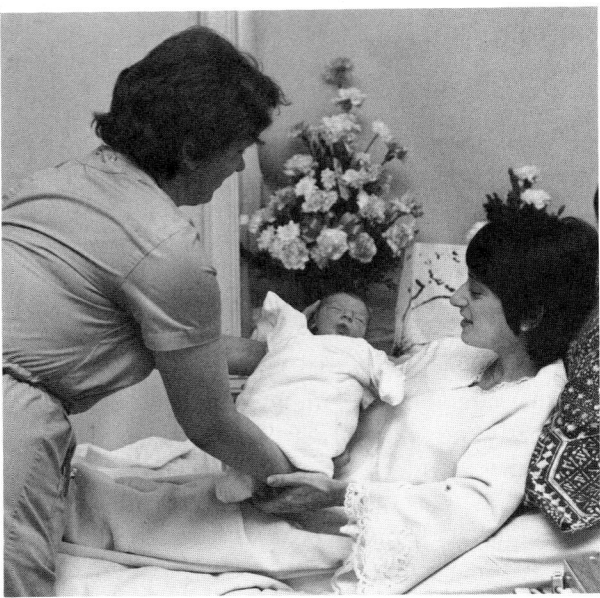

Fig. 3-1. Nurse-patient relationships in maternal-newborn nursing invariably involve more than one patient. (Courtesy of the Department of Medical Photography, Children's Hospital, Buffalo, N.Y.)

family—parents, brothers, and sisters—are told that their new family member is going to die or when they are first getting acquainted with their new family member). Even when the relationship involves a nurse and a single person, it is influenced by other people around that person (family centered), because childbearing and child rearing are influenced by social and cultural factors.

The Roots of Maternal-Newborn Nursing

In order to understand the practice and process of maternal-newborn nursing today, it is helpful to look at the ways it has been practiced in the past.

In all early civilizations, formal prenatal care was nonexistent. Advice for a pregnant woman came from her mother or friends. Women who had experience in helping with childbirth passed their knowledge on to other women in the community, until an informal core of such knowledge was gradually established. Such women came to be known as *midwives*, a word derived from *mid* meaning "with" and *wif*, or "wife" (a person who was with the wife).

Childbirth was so totally women's business that as late as 1522 a Doctor Weitt in England was burned alive for dressing as a woman and observing a delivery. By the 1800s, that trend had reversed, and childbirth became a physician's concern (and, because most physicians of the time were men, a man's concern). Home deliveries with midwives were discarded in preference to hospital deliveries. In large hospital wards, however, a physician completed a vaginal examination on one woman in labor, then walked immediately to the next bed and examined the woman there without any means of discouraging cross-contamination or infection. Physicians even came directly from autopsy rooms, where they had handled grossly infected internal organs, and, without washing their hands, examined women and delivered children. The rate of puerperal sepsis or childbed fever was epidemic.

In 1847, before the germ theory had been recognized, Ignaz Philipp Semmelweis determined that some agent was being spread from woman to woman, causing the fatal illness. He insisted that physicians in his section of the hospital disinfect their hands before attending any labor patient. Although his intervention significantly reduced infections, he was ridiculed, and after he was no longer able clinically to supervise hand-washing, people returned to old ways and infection rates rose again.

Semmelweis's deduction that something he could not see was causing infection in his hospital wards (when other physicians were saying that puerperal fever was caused by such things as phases of the moon) is an example of scientific problem solving at its best. It is an example of how anyone, using a scientific process or performing nursing based on a process, can improve health care.

Nurse-midwives (really the forerunner of nurse practitioners or nurses functioning in expanded roles) have throughout history supervised care during pregnancy and childbirth, but after childbirth became a physician's responsibility in the 1800s, nurses assumed a lesser role. Recently, however, they have stepped again into the part they originally played—that of patient advocate, a person to see that pregnancy, childbirth, and the postpartal period is a rewarding time in life, not one filled with concern and loneliness, and often, in the past, extreme terror.

After Pasteur showed in the late 1800s that streptococci are the usual cause of puerperal sepsis, steps to isolate women in labor began. By the 1930s and 1940s, the concept of labor as a wellness, not an illness, event was almost lost in the attempts to keep the mother in labor isolated from outside people (especially her husband) who might carry germs to her. It was mandated that her newborn infant be separated from her as well lest she transmit organisms to the child. (Streptococcal infections, spreading through large nurseries, killed as many newborns as they did mothers.)

When the concept of rooming-in was introduced in the 1950s, a return to breast-feeding and delivery by prepared childbirth was advocated in the 1960s, and humanizing labor and delivery suites were advanced in the 1970s, nurses, having given these innovations close scrutiny (nurses, like everyone else, are not always comfortable with change), at the end of the 1970s became proponents of these attempts to make pregnancy and childbirth as fulfilling an experience as it can be. They have a right to be proud. A great deal of the increased responsibility they have assumed is due to their taking a scientific look at what was happening to women during pregnancy and childbirth and initiating nursing intervention that could improve the experience.

Steps of the Nursing Process

The nursing process consists of four steps: assessment, planning, implementation, and evaluation. These steps are of a circular nature. If evaluation shows that a problem has not been solved or a need has not been met, the process of assessing and replanning with new intervention will begin again. It is not a static process, one in which once patient problems have been identified and brought to a resolution the job is done. Because nurses and patients do not live in vacuums, patient needs one day may not be needs the next; plans made one day may not work out the next.

Cultural, religious, environmental, and situational influences and health problems that are becoming better or worse affect everyone and change their needs. Thus the nursing process, if it is to be effective, is forced to be a fluid process.

The interaction between outside influences and the nursing process in maternal-newborn nursing is shown in Fig. 3-2.

ASSESSMENT

Assessment is another word for studying or gathering enough information to make a conclusion as to whether nursing intervention is necessary. Methods used to gather data are interviewing, physical assessment, and studying laboratory or ancillary data for pertinent findings.

Interviewing

Because pregnancy is highly visible, a pregnant woman finds that wherever she goes—a party, the grocery store, the beauty shop—people's conversations with her always drift around to her pregnancy. It is easy for health care people to fall into the same trap—to talk about the obvious, or to assume that because a woman is pregnant all her worries or problems are concerned with the pregnancy.

Generally, her chief concerns *are* those of the pregnancy. Pregnancy is such an all-pervading state that everywhere she is she acts differently because of it. At a party she no longer accepts alcoholic drinks; at the grocery store she buys more high-protein foods; at the beauty shop she asks to have her hair cut simply because she is fatigued easily and wants something easy to manage. At a health care facility her response to questions about any concerns she may have will invariably be pregnancy-related. Many physicians appear to be so busy (and are very busy) that, unless she is strongly assertive, the woman declines to voice the second or third or fourth question she has.

A nurse who is a skilled health interviewer can add a great deal to the quality of health care offered by identifying and helping to manage the second concerns of women. Specific content of health histories is discussed in chapters on antepartal, partal, and postpartal care.

Physical Assessment

Physical assessment is a skill that is being learned by more and more nurses. What aspects of physical assessment are used in various settings depends on the setting and the circumstances. At any phase in pregnancy, labor and delivery, or the postpartal period, using skills of physical assessment can be invaluable in helping to differentiate the symptoms a woman is describing as normal variations of pregnancy from serious happenings that need immediate attention. For example, all pregnant women begin to feel short of breath toward the end of pregnancy. When you are listening to fetal heart sounds, if you also listened to a woman's chest and heard rales—the sound of fluid in lung alveoli, an almost certain indication of pneumonia—you would know at once that the woman should not wait her turn to be seen in this busy clinic today. Pneumonia interferes with oxygen exchange at the alveola-blood interface. The fetal oxygen supply will be compromised if the pneumonia and the lack of oxygen exchange become acute. Physical assessment used this way helps to establish priorities of care and to safeguard the health of both woman and fetus.

Physical assessment involves four basic steps: inspection, palpation, percussion, and auscultation.

INSPECTION. Inspection is observation, or assessment by means of the eyes. Many of the minor discomforts of pregnancy are detected by simple observation: The woman has dark circles under her eyes (fatigue); she presses a hand against her back as she

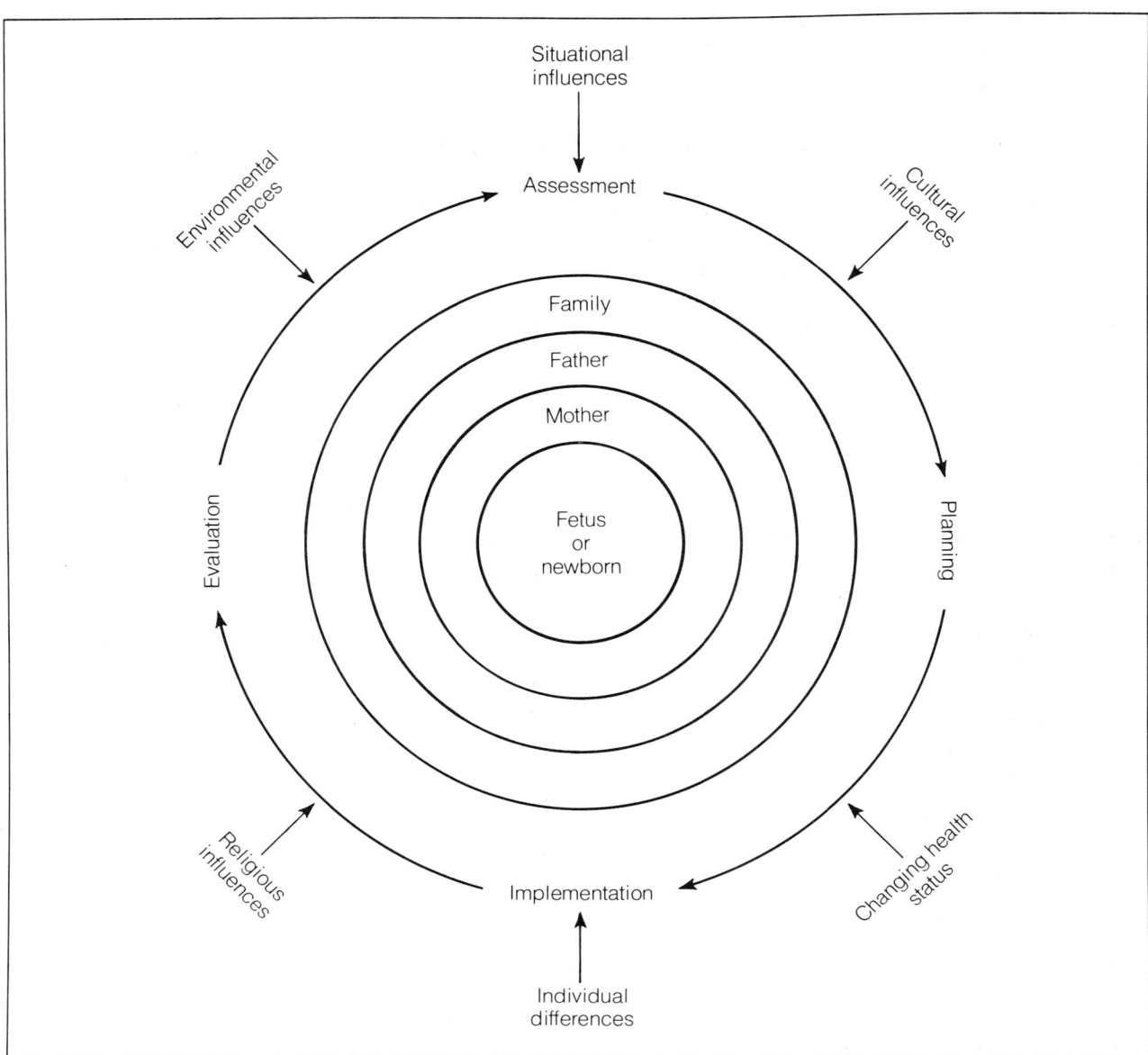

Fig. 3-2. The nursing process and outside influences.

walks (back pain); she asks to use the bathroom while she is waiting to be seen (frequency of urination); she presses a hand against the top of her uterus as she walks (shortness of breath). Toward the end of pregnancy, observing her profile will reveal that *lightening*, or the settling of the fetal head into the pelvis preparatory to delivery, has occurred.

Because inspection involves no instruments or even touching, it is easy to dismiss it as an unimportant assessment tool. In evaluating the health of pregnant women and their newborns, however, it is an extremely helpful one.

PALPATION. Palpation is assessment by using the hand to feel or touch. Temperature is best felt by the back of the hand; the fingertips can generally discriminate small details most accurately. Palpation is used at every pregnancy visit to assess whether the uterus is growing or not, at the time of labor to determine the position and presentation of the baby, and during the postpartal period to assess uterine contraction. It is useful in estimating the extent of edema, one of the danger signs of pregnancy.

PERCUSSION. Percussion is the act of determining the density of body parts by evaluating the sound made by those parts when they are struck by the finger. To percuss, place the middle finger of your left hand on the surface to be percussed. Keep the remainder of your left hand up away from the surface so your hand does not deaden the sound you will elicit. Strike the first knuckle of your left hand with the flexed tip of the middle finger on your right hand (Fig. 3-3). If you are over a dense body part (a bone),

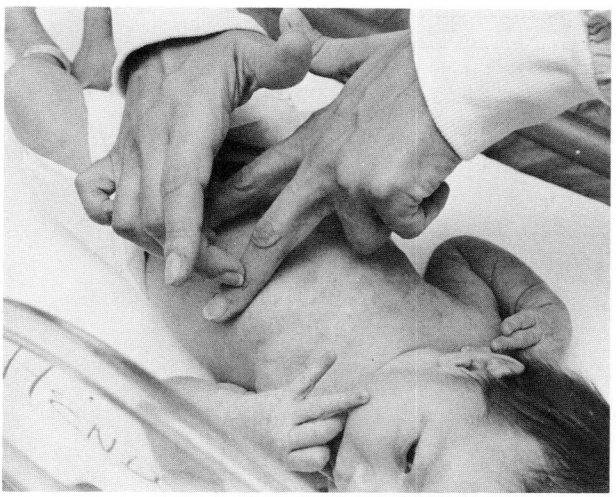

Fig. 3-3. Percussion, an assessment technique to determine the density of body parts done by striking the first knuckle of the left hand with the flexed tip of the middle finger on the right hand. (Courtesy of the Department of Medical Photography, Children's Hospital, Buffalo, N.Y.)

the sound heard is dull or flat. If you are over a gas-filled area such as the stomach, the sound is tympanic. Over fluid-filled spaces the sound is resonant (echoing). Percussion is helpful in detecting whether a woman is emptying her bladder or whether a large quantity of urine is always being retained. An empty bladder sounds dull, a full one is resonant, an over-extended one is hyperresonant.

AUSCULTATION. Auscultation is assessment by means of the ear. When you listen to the sounds of the fetal heartbeat at every prenatal visit and in labor, you are using the technique of auscultation.

Physical assessment is a useful assessment tool at all phases of childbearing. Its specific utilization is discussed in the chapters on pregnancy, labor, and the postpartal period.

Laboratory Determinations

A third aspect of assessment is the study of laboratory or other ancillary data. As some laboratory values change during pregnancy, analysis of results must always be made in the light of the knowledge of the pregnancy. Normal values of common tests are discussed in later chapters along with the reasons for and value of the tests. Many new laboratory or clinical tests such as the oxytocin challenge test or the use of fetal heart monitors are supervised by nurses. As a nurse, you are the first person to know that the fetus is in difficulty, because of your assessment procedure.

Analysis

After the gathering of data, the next step in assessment is to list patient needs or to establish any discrepancies between the state of health of the patient and optimum health and well-being. Some discrepancies that might exist in a pregnant woman are obesity (women should enter a pregnancy neither overweight nor underweight), lack of support people (pregnancy is a stress; women need support people around them during it), and lack of knowledge of proper nutrition (good nutrition will provide an optimal growth environment for the fetus).

Determining a person's needs is not easy because some needs arise from a physiological basis, some from a psychosocial basis, and some from an environmental or a cultural basis. During pregnancy, some needs are specific to the pregnancy and some stem from health problems or psychosocial pressures of the age group. Every patient has needs that are due to his or her own individuality.

There are many ways of looking at patient needs. With a systems theory approach, needs are identified according to body systems. With a self-care nursing model, health is defined as the ability to perform self-care, and needs are determined to the extent that the person is unable to fulfill self-care. If an adaptation approach is utilized, needs are assessed in terms of the inability of the patient to adapt to or cope with life situations or illness. If a format such as Abdellah's 21 Functions of Nursing [1] is used, needs are listed according to, for example, those of inadequate elimination and ingestion.

MASLOW'S HIERARCHY OF NEEDS. Most classification systems of needs depend to some extent on Maslow's hierarchy of needs (Fig. 3-4) [14]. In this system, a need is viewed as an internal tension caused by some change in the individual or his surroundings. The tension results in goal-directed behavior that will persist until reduction of the tension (meeting of the need) has been achieved. A woman develops a headache. She takes some aspirin with no relief. She talks to a neighbor and borrows some Darvon, still with no relief. She makes an appointment with a physician, who refers her to an ophthamologist, who prescribes glasses. The headache continues. She sees a neurologist. She will persist in tension-reducing behavior until she has achieved tension reduction or has exhausted all her resources in that area. This explains why people sometimes "doctor-shop" or visit one physician after another, why they sometimes do not take medication prescribed for them, why they do not follow orders explained to them. Despite the seemingly right intervention, the needs were not truly met

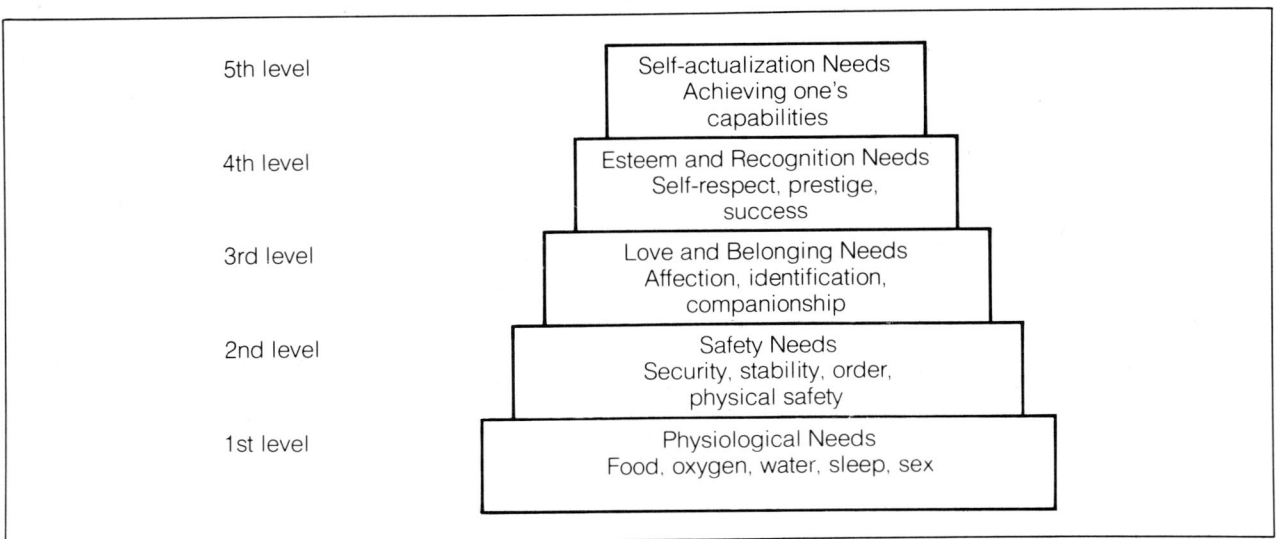

Fig. 3-4. Maslow's theory of the hierarchy of needs. (Data based on Hierarchy of Needs in "A Theory of Human Motivation" from Motivation and Personality, *2nd Edition, by Abraham H. Maslow. Copyright © 1970 by Abraham H. Maslow. By permission of Harper & Row, Publishers, Inc.)*

(probably because they were not truly identified) and the patients continue to seek resolution of the problem from other sources.

Maslow's first-level needs are those that people wish to have met first—needs for air, food, water, sleep, and activity. Sex is often included in this level as well. A great deal of pregnancy counseling is geared toward making certain that a woman meets these needs so that her child can have adequate nutrition and growth potential.

Second-level needs are needs for safety, such as protection, freedom from fear and anxiety, and security. These needs emerge as basic physical lifesaving needs are met. Safety needs are felt strongly by a pregnant woman; the very size of her abdomen late in pregnancy makes her less able to protect herself. She may have to stop work outside her home. Financial insecurity then becomes a problem for her.

Third-level needs are those for love and belonging. All people desire to have friends, to have a feeling of being loved. During pregnancy, when a woman may not feel as physically attractive as she did before, a woman may need people around her to reinforce their love for her. She is very aware that things inside her are changing (she begins to change from thinking of herself as a daughter to thinking of herself as a mother); she needs reassurance that the people around her can accept this change and will continue to love her in a new role.

Fourth-level needs center around self-esteem or a feeling of liking oneself and thinking of oneself as a worthwhile person. Because pregnancy changes a woman's physical appearance and her role in life forever after, the woman spends a great deal of time during pregnancy questioning what type of person she is and whether she is capable of dealing with this major change. When she first sees her newborn, she has little self-confidence that she will be a good mother or can even learn all the things she will need to know to mother.

The final need, reached only after all others have been fulfilled, is self-actualization. Self-actualization is knowing that one is doing and being what one was meant to do and be in life. For many women, childbirth fulfills this need, and only after that event do they reach this fifth level of achievement.

It is important in analyzing needs according to Maslow's hierarchy of needs to remember that environmental or situational influences change the order of importance of needs. A person who has just been deserted by a loved one may seek love (a third-level need) over eating (a first-level need) because her situational influences are so strong at that time. All during pregnancy, needs may be temporarily misplaced by the stress of the pregnancy and this unusual happening in life. In all circumstances, people are assessed individually and their needs determined not only by guidelines such as Maslow's but by their own individual values and preferences.

In stating needs it is helpful to list both those things that a person lacks (knowledge of nutrition, financial security) and strengths the person possesses (a concerned, caring personality, strong support people) so that the latter can be reinforced and maintained. Also, not just present needs but future problems that could occur if preventive measures are not taken have to be identified. An example of this type of need in pregnancy is knowledge of preparation for childbirth or reduction of obesity. The woman does not need knowledge of exercises for childbirth at her first prenatal visit, but in nine months she will need a knowledge of childbirth. She will be advised not to try to diet during pregnancy, but for years to come she will need to consider the possibility of reducing the obesity to prevent heart disease.

Planning nursing interventions, then, depends on strengths and needs of the patient, on the individuality of the patient, and on both future and present factors.

NURSING DIAGNOSIS. Stating problems or needs of patients is part of the process of making a nursing diagnosis. In the best form, a nursing diagnosis is not only a statement of a problem but a projection of what has led to the problem. That is, not "anxiety," but "anxiety due to facing childbirth alone because of work pattern of husband"; not "hypertension," but "hypertension due to chronic kidney disease."

Assessment, then, the first step in the nursing process, has two major divisions: data gathering and analyzing needs and stating these needs as a nursing diagnosis. Assessment is the foundation of the nursing process and gives guidelines and substance to the three steps that follow.

PLANNING AND NURSING PROCESS

The second step in the nursing process is planning. The nursing process often goes wrong because of inadequate data gathering (so that one is not truly aware of the nature of the problem) or inadequate planning (people plan what would solve the problem for *them*, not for the patient).

Good planning begins with setting short-term and long-term goals for solving the problem in collaboration with the patient. If "fear of having more pain in labor than she will be able to tolerate due to lack of knowledge of labor and a belief in old wives' tales" is a nursing diagnosis, an expected outcome or goal of nursing intervention would be to reduce the fear to a level that is not incapacitating to the patient and can be managed with a minimum of analgesia and anesthesia in labor. Elimination of all fear about labor would be an unattainable goal. Labor is an unknown, and fear of the unknown is always strong. Elimination of all pain in labor is also an unattainable goal because of the very nature of labor. Sometimes nursing interventions seem ineffective and working as a nurse is discouraging, not because progress is not occurring, but because the goal for the intervention was set too high to be attained.

Reduction of fear of childbirth is a short-term goal. Recognition of health persons as better sources of information concerning health phenomena (rather than old wives' tales) would be a long-term goal. This will help the woman in the future—on a day she is told that she will have to have gallbladder surgery, on a day her baby is ill—to ask questions of factual sources and therefore be able to handle these events better than she does with her present reliance on unfactual sources.

Setting patient goals without patient input is ineffective planning. A goal such as "Patient will lose 10 pounds by next visit" will not be achieved if the patient does not see a *need* to lose weight. "Patient will take iron supplement daily" will not be achieved unless the patient views taking the iron supplement as important and something that she should do. After discussing this need with the patient and realizing that she does not perceive an iron supplement as necessary for health, you might have to restate your goal as "Patient to attend class on nutrition during pregnancy." Later, after the patient is more knowledgeable, you might be able to move your goal up to where you originally wanted it to be: "Patient will take iron supplement daily."

After establishing a goal, you need to select the alternative ways of reaching it. For a woman who is afraid of pain in childbirth, there are a number of possible solutions: Provide facts about childbirth, help her enroll in a preparation-for-childbirth class, stay with her in labor, make certain her physician discusses pain relief for labor with her, or have her talk to a mother who has just delivered a baby about the little pain she experienced.

In order to pick the best alternative from this list, you need to be aware of facilities for health provision in the community and the capabilities of yourself and the health providers with whom you work. For example, suggesting a formal preparation-for-labor class is ineffective planning if such a class is not available in the woman's community. There would be no reason for *both* doctor and nurse to discuss the possibilities of pain relief in labor if both do it well. That is overkill and might lead to a feeling of, "Whom are they trying to convince?" Knowing the capabilities of the health personnel with whom you work eliminates this type of situation. If a physician enjoys talking about what pain relief in labor is available, and does it well and reassuringly, your role might be limited to writing a note to the physician to remind him that the woman has a lot of anxiety in this area, and asking her after a doctor-patient discussion whether she has any questions or feels any differently about labor. If the physician with whom you work always shrugs off the issue of pain in labor with a nonchalant "Don't worry about that until you're in labor," your nursing plans would have to include this as something you should do.

As what you hope to accomplish must be discussed with a patient, so must the methods by which you propose to accomplish it.

In the example given of the woman for whom the goal was to be "Takes iron supplement daily," you might discover when you discuss how this will be carried out (fill prescription, take daily) that an iron preparation tends to give her extreme constipation and so she will not take it. Your plan will have to change to an agreement with her to use an iron supplement for a trial period of one week and see whether constipation occurs; ask the physician for a prescription for a stool softener for the woman to take in addition to the iron pill; plan with her a diet rich in naturally occurring iron sources so that the iron supplement is needed only every other day, or some other alternative that is acceptable to her.

Medical and nursing literature is full of articles on noncompliant patients, as if these are special types of people. In reality, noncompliant patients are usually the outcome of poor health care planning. The alternatives chosen for them were solutions acceptable to the health care team but not to the patients.

Thorough planning, listing all the solutions to a problem that might be carried out (brainstorming), then selecting the one that will be most workable or most realistic to the patient situation helps to improve nursing practice. If time and again you must cross off an alternative such as "Suggest formal preparation for childbirth classes" from your list because no such classes are available in the community, sooner or later you will ask why such classes are not available and you will begin to arrange for you or someone else to teach them, improving health care in your community.

The second step in the nursing process, then, like the first, is actually a combination of steps: (1) realistic goal setting (in terms of the circumstances and acceptable to the patient) and (2) selection of acceptable solutions to problems (equally realistic and acceptable to the patient).

IMPLEMENTATION

Implementation is the carrying out of the planning phase completed as step 2. If planning was done realistically, the implementation step flows easily, readily, enjoyably, and successfully.

In all phases of maternal-newborn nursing, teaching is a major method of intervention. Principles of teaching-learning are shown in Table 3-1.

Table 3-1. Teaching-Learning Principles

1. Learning does not take place until there is a readiness or felt need for learning.
2. People under stress do not learn as easily as those who are not under stress (their readiness is affected).
3. The speed and ability with which different people learn vary widely.
4. The methods by which people like to be taught (structured or unstructured) vary widely.
5. People learn only at the level at which they are. If material is presented at a level too easy for them, they are bored; at a level too difficult, frustrated.
6. Readiness for learning is most likely to occur when it is seen that the new knowledge will have a direct impact on the learner's life.
7. People continue to learn best when they are given praise or a reward for correct learning.

Pregnancy, labor and delivery, and the postpartal period, when the responsibility for a new life is so keenly felt, are times of stress. Teaching during these times, therefore, must always be done with consideration that people do not learn effectively under stress. The woman who is concerned that her newborn is going to die does not hear postpartal instructions on suture line care. The husband of a woman admitted in active labor does not hear that smoking is not allowed in labor rooms. A statement such as "I know I told you that" reveals more about the teacher (unaware of the effect of stress) than the learner (overwhelmed by the stress of an ill newborn).

Women who are not yet sure they want to be pregnant (or hoping or fearful that a positive pregnancy test is wrong) are not ready for health teaching concerning their pregnancies. Only later, when they know that this pregnancy is for certain, are they able to listen to instructions on how they should change their eating patterns or plan a rest period every day.

On the first day post partum, many women are not interested in learning about such things as bathing their babies or changing diapers because the baby is not real to them yet. By the second or third day, when they have realized that the pregnancy is over, that this baby is not just their imagination but someone they will be taking home the next day to care for, forever after, interest in how to care for a baby jumps dramatically (learning takes place only when there is a felt need).

Because the things important for women to understand about pregnancy, childbirth, or child care are not taught in formal school classes, people vary widely in the amount they know about such things as body anatomy and feeding babies. It is important to assess what level women are at before you begin teaching so you do not insult them (explaining what foods are rich in vitamin C to a woman who is a dietitian) or present material at so difficult a level that the person cannot comprehend it (trying to explain uterine contractions to a woman who does not know where or what her uterus is).

In teaching, it is always easier to find fault with a learner than to praise her. Pregnancy is a nine-month process. In order to continue learning over that long a time frame, women need reinforcement that you are pleased with how they have responded to your suggestions and the effort they have made to try to do things correctly even if perfection has not been achieved. A simple statement such as "I can tell you're really trying" or "You've learned to do that very well" inspires people to attack new areas of knowledge and continue to learn more and more.

Some teaching in maternal-newborn nursing is done best in groups (parent classes), some individually (helping a woman learn to breast-feed). Some is structured (formal classes), some spontaneous (a woman asks at a routine office visit why babies do not drown in utero). In order to be an effective teacher, you must be prepared with information that can be offered in both formal and informal settings. Learning takes place best when a moment of readiness is realized. That moment may occur early in the morning at the time you are ready to teach, but it may not occur until you are less ready at the end of a long day.

Implementation, the third step in the nursing process, must, like all steps, be done with patient input or it will not be successful.

EVALUATION

Evaluation is the means whereby the first three steps of the nursing process (assessment, planning, and implementation) are measured in terms of whether they are effective or not. It should be a rewarding step; if not, at least a revealing one, because if evaluation shows that the interventions proposed have not been effective (no measurable change has taken place) it leads into a new cycle of assessment, planning, implementation, and evaluation.

If nursing care is not effective, it may be because the assessment was inadequate (the problem was not fully recognized), planning was inadequate (inappropriate goals were established), implementation was inadequate (plans were never carried out), or evaluation was inadequate (everyone was so sure change would occur that no one looked closely to see that change really did occur). It is easy to assume, especially in areas of teaching, that because the teaching was well done, learning will take place, and no more intervention is necessary.

Asking women to repeat the instructions that they have just been given often reveals that, although the timing for instructions seemed right and the person seemed to be listening, nothing has been comprehended. Discharge from the hospital is such a big step (how exciting it is to see the baby dressed in real clothing, not just a hospital gown) that instructions given at the time of discharge are often unheard. Evaluating whether nursing intervention is effective may be disappointing in these instances (although you feel you did a beautiful job, you feel you should have done more) but leads to more constructive interventions (at a time of discharge, women need written as well as oral instructions so that later they have a reference source for the information). The step of evaluation, then, becomes a means of quality control.

The Nursing Process and Problem Solving

The nursing process is a problem-solving format. It can be pictured as the same as basic problem solving (Fig. 3-5). Learning takes place on a number of different levels, from signal learning (the simplest) through

Fig. 3-5. The nursing process as problem solving.

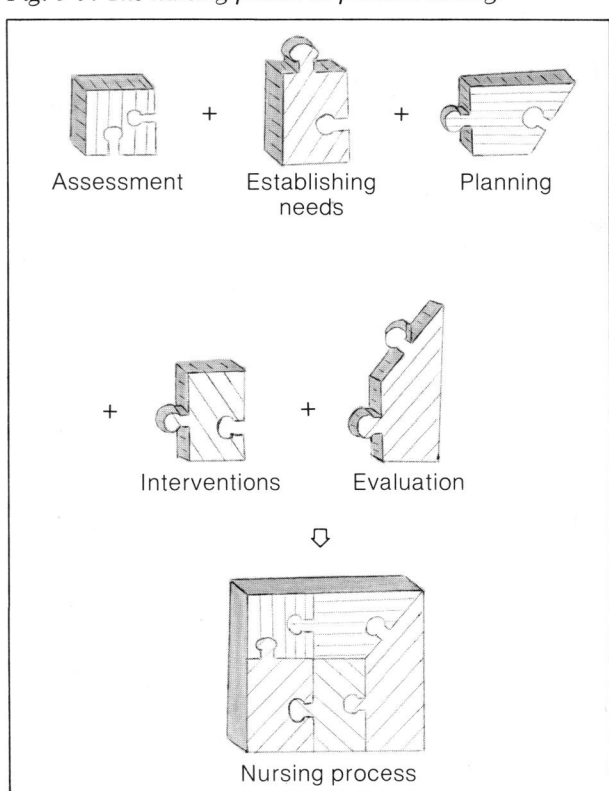

multiple discrimination to problem solving (the most difficult). Because problem solving is an advanced form of thought, it is the form that is applicable in all situations and at all levels of difficulty.

Because pregnancy, labor and delivery, and care of a newborn are new processes for those involved, problems will arise. It is reassuring for people to realize that the nurses who offer them care do so by a process that is aimed directly at meeting their needs through problem solving.

References

1. Abdellah, F. G. The nature of nursing science. *Nurs. Res.* 18:390, 1969.
2. Aspinall, M. J. Nursing diagnosis—the weak link. *Nurs. Outlook* 24:433, 1976.
3. Aspinall, M.J. The why and how of nursing diagnosis. *M.C.N.* 2:354, 1977.
4. Binzley, V. State: Overlooked factor in newborn nursing. *Am. J. Nurs.* 77:102, 1977.
5. Bishop, B. A guide to assessing parenting capabilities. *Am. J. Nurs.* 76:1784, 1976.
6. Branch, M. F., and Paxton, P. P. (Eds.). *Providing Safe Nursing Care for Ethnic People of Color.* New York: Appleton-Century-Crofts, 1976.
7. Gebbie, K. M., and Lavin, M. A. *Classification of Nursing Diagnoses.* St. Louis: Mosby, 1975.
8. Gordon, M., et al. Nursing diagnosis: Looking at its use in the clinical area. *Am. J. Nurs.* 80:672, 1980.
9. Grier, M. Decision making about patient care. *Nurs. Res.* 25:105, 1976.
10. Gulbrandsen, M. W. Guide to health assessment. *Am. J. Nurs.* 76:1276, 1976.
11. Hefferin, E. A., and Hunter, R. E. Nursing assessment and care plan statements. *Nurs. Res.* 24:360, 1975.
12. Lamonica, E. L. *The Nursing Process: A Humanistic Approach.* Reading, Mass.: Addison-Wesley, 1979.
13. Maloney, E., et al. *How to Collect and Record a Health History.* Philadelphia: Lippincott, 1976.
14. Maslow, A. H. *Motivation and Personality* (2nd ed.). New York: Harper & Row, 1970.
15. Mundinger, M. O., and Jauron, G. D. Developing a nursing diagnosis. *Nurs. Outlook* 23:94, 1975.
16. Murray, R., and Zentner, J. *Nursing Assessment and Health Promotion Through the Life Span.* Englewood Cliffs, N.J.: Prentice-Hall, 1975.
17. Paterson, J. G., and Zderad, L. T. *Humanistic Nursing.* New York: Wiley, 1976.
18. Price, M. R. Nursing diagnosis: Making a concept come alive. *Am. J. Nurs.* 80:668, 1980.
19. Roy, Sr. C. A diagnostic classification system for nursing. *Nurs. Outlook* 23:90, 1975.
20. Turnbull, S. J. Shifting the focus to health. *Am. J. Nurs.* 76:1985, 1976.
21. Winslow, E. H. The role of the nurse in patient education. *Nurs. Clin North Am.* 11:2, 1976.
22. Yura, H., and Walsh, M. B. *The Nursing Process.* New York: Appleton-Century-Crofts, 1978.

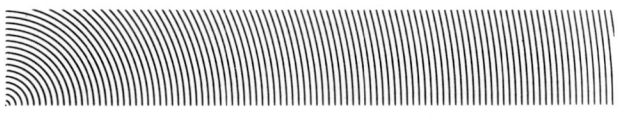

4. Problem-oriented Recording — Application for Nursing

In order to improve the quality of medical recording, in 1969 Lawrence Weed suggested a new form of recording medical information [12]. Because the system he proposed was originally designed to improve physician charting, it was termed *problem-oriented medical recording* (POMR). The system had so many advantages for all health care providers, however, that it was quickly adopted in all areas of health care. It is therefore now more commonly known as simply *problem-oriented recording,* or POR. A system that provides for documentation of patient concerns, it could as easily be called *patient-oriented recording.*

In POR charting, all health care providers record information on one section of the chart, eliminating separate pages for physicians' progress notes, nurses' notes, physical therapists' consultation notes, and so on. The advantage of this arrangement is that it allows easy sharing of information among health care personnel. Health care providers—physicians, nurses, dietitians, specialists—all have complementary but different bodies of knowledge. When different disciplines record their observations and plans on separate pages in a chart, questions can be asked of a patient two or three times, tests can be duplicated because one caregiver did not realize that another was doing that test, and a problem can be overlooked because everyone assumes that someone else is aware of the problem and managing it when no one is taking responsibility for it.

POR charting also allows health personnel to teach and help one another, because everyone's thoughts and plans of care are recorded in one place.

Some nurses feel threatened at the prospect of recording on the same page as other caregivers, afraid that their notes will sound superficial next to those of a physician or their analysis of a patient's motor function scant next to that of a physical therapist. This will indeed be the case, but a nurse is not expected to record at the level of a physician in the area of medical expertise or at the level of a physical therapist in the area of motor function. In assessing total family interaction, ability of a family to utilize health information, mothering ability, or response to a medication administered, the nurse's note is the most informed. A physician's or a physical therapist's note would seem shallow in those areas next to a nurse's. Nursing has a strong primary body of knowledge, and no one can match a nurse's expertise when she is recording observations drawn from it. In addition, POR recording is not a competitive exercise. It is a communication system to measure the level of health of individuals who rely on health care personnel for guidance and help. As nurses form a major part of the health care system they need to participate in the system. POR charting can help everyone move toward one of nursing's goals—to look at whole patients rather than at bits and pieces of people at sporadic intervals.

POR charting is compatible with the steps of the nursing process. By means of the POR system, information is gathered by history, physical examination, and laboratory analysis to establish a data base (Fig. 4-1). From this base of knowledge, problems (both real and potential) are identified. Interventions for problems are then formulated.

The Data Base

To establish a comprehensive base of knowledge, a thorough history must be taken from patients the first time they are seen at a health care facility. Such a comprehensive body of information from women during pregnancy includes chief concern, family profile, past health history, gynecological and obstetrical history, family history, and a review of systems.

A complete physical assessment must be done to establish baseline values. At the first visit in pregnancy, laboratory data such as blood type, hemoglobin and hematocrit levels, and urine tests for glucose and protein are gathered.

From this store of information, patient problems are identified. As additional data become available at later dates, additional problems are identified.

The Problem List

All problems of patients (and a problem is defined widely as an *area of need*) are listed and numbered on a central problem list. It is kept in a conspicuous place in the front of the patient record so as to be readily available to everyone concerned. The date the problem is first recognized is recorded. As long as a problem is in existence, it is an active problem. When total resolution of the problem has been achieved, it is moved to another space on the problem list under a column titled Resolved.

Fig. 4-1. The physical examination and rate of fetal heart tones are information incorporated into a patient data base in problem-oriented recording. (Courtesy of the Department of Medical Photography, Children's Hospital, Buffalo, N.Y.)

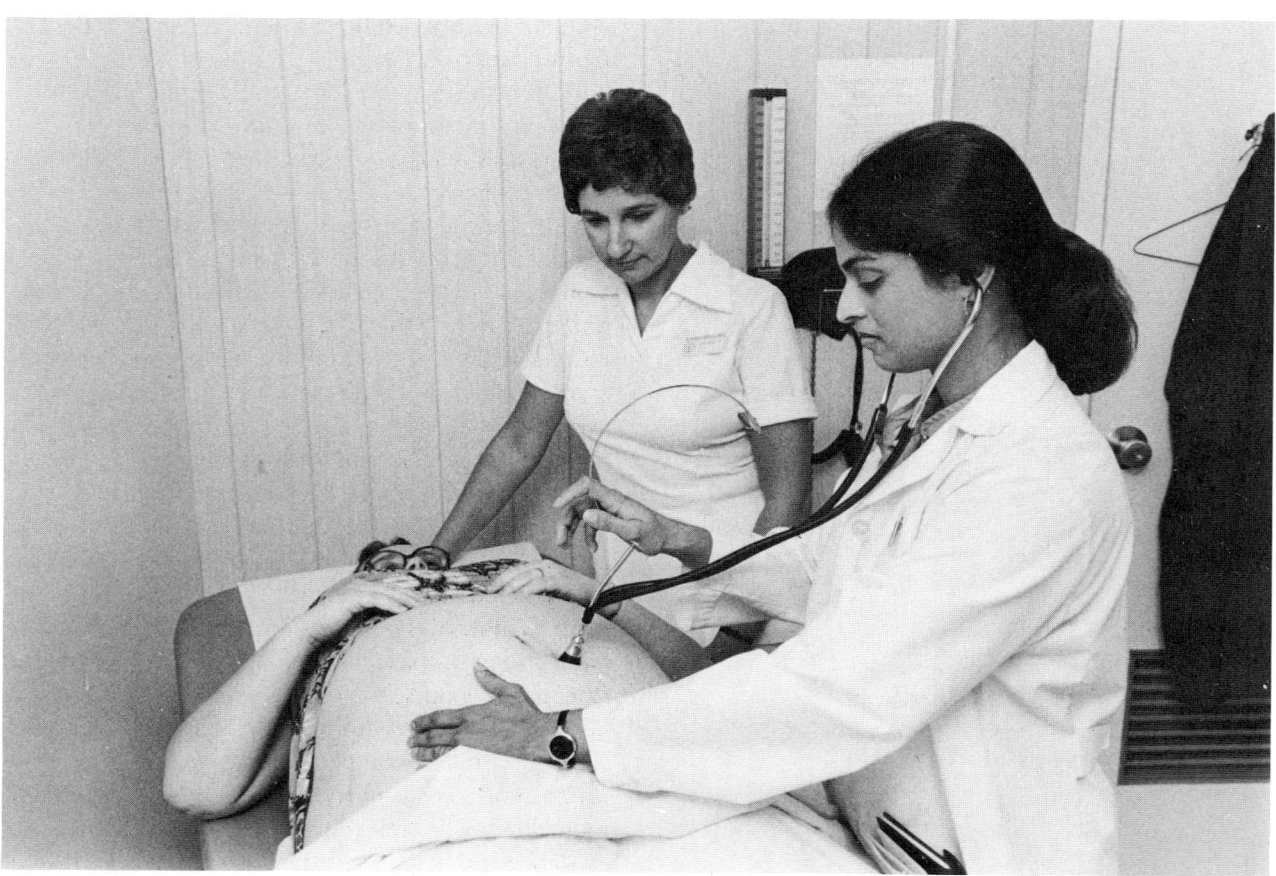

Numbers are not reused. If an individual had tuberculosis as a child and this was given the number 2, when the initial lesions healed the problem would be moved to the resolved column. The number 2 is not reused, because if at some later time that problem again becomes active, tuberculosis will be changed back to the active column and carried again under the number 2.

Potential problems, such as heavy smoking or working in an environment in which there is exposure to a compound such as asbestos that is known to be carcinogenic, are listed as well as immediate problems. Health care providers can thus be alerted to watch for problems due to these threats in the future.

Problems might be identified in any of the following areas:

A specific diagnosis, e.g., pregnancy-induced hypertension
A symptom, e.g., nausea
A sign, e.g., edema
A syndrome, e.g., failure to thrive
A psychological problem, e.g., anxiety
A social problem, e.g., lack of support persons
An abnormal laboratory finding, e.g., low hemoglobin
A demographic problem, e.g., exposure to toxic substances
A risk factor, e.g., heavy alcohol usage

Keeping track of problems on a numbered list allows better continuity of care to be offered to patients. It prevents concerns from "slipping through the cracks" when the person is seen by different caregivers in different locations.

Mary Kraft is a 23-year-old woman seen at a prenatal clinic. She has been followed by a family-centered practice since birth. Her POR problem list is shown below.

Problem-oriented Recording: Problem List

Name: Mary Kraft
Age: 23

Date of Problem	Number	Active	Resolved
3-14-57	1	Newborn	4-14-57
3-17-57	2	Jaundice (ABO incomp.)	9-7-59
4-14-57	3	Health maintenance	
1-22-64	4	Varicella (chickenpox)	1-29-64
8-20-73	5	Auto accident with facial lacerations	11-6-73
9-4-75	6	Heavy smoker	
2-14-77	7	Pregnancy (3-month abortion)	5-5-77
6-28-78	8	Infertility	9-1-80
9-1-80	9	Pregnancy	

Most people consider the newborn period a time of particular hazard in terms of potential health problems. This was problem 1 for Mary. Mary had more jaundice than usual at birth, due to a blood incompatibility. This was her second problem. Problem 1 was moved to the resolved list at the end of the newborn period (the first 28 days of life). Jaundice was carried as an active problem until she was 2 years of age, at which time she was evaluated and found to have no sequelae.

Health maintenance was listed as problem 3 when Mary was brought in for her first well-child checkup. Because health maintenance is a concern throughout life, it is never a closed problem. At 6 years of age Mary had chickenpox. In high school she was in an automobile accident. Both these events had no long-term sequelae and so are closed. Heavy smoking was identified as a potential problem when Mary was 18. Because she has not changed her smoking habits, this is still an active problem. Mary had a pregnancy that led to a miscarriage when she was 20 (problem 7). That is a closed problem. Mary had difficulty getting pregnant after the miscarriage and was seen for some preliminary infertility testing (problem 8). That became a closed problem with her new pregnancy (problem 9).

Mary's problem list from her birth to the present supplies important information in connection with the current pregnancy. Although Mary is not likely to have a blood incompatibility problem with this pregnancy, the fact that she had one as a newborn should alert you to her probable concern about the possibility. She will undoubtedly have some anxiety that she may miscarry again. Her heavy smoking may affect this pregnancy's outcome because of the detrimental influence of smoking on fetal growth.

NEEDS OF PREGNANCY

During every pregnancy, women have needs that require specific consideration and intervention. Some common ones are education for childbirth, nutritional counseling, and education for child rearing. Problems of a specific pregnancy might include vaginitis, hypertension, or lack of a support person.

In order to keep a central problem list to a workable size, problems that arise as part of a primary health problem can be referred to in progress notes as subdivisions of the primary health problem—9a, 9b, and so on. If a subproblem will have long-term sequelae, however, it should not remain a subproblem but at the end of the pregnancy should be given a primary number. Most women who develop hypertension during pregnancy return to having normal blood pressure readings at the end of pregnancy. Hypertension would be carried only as a subproblem. A woman whose blood pressure remained elevated following pregnancy would have hypertension listed as a major problem on her problem list as this would now warrant continued monitoring and care. Some women develop pseudo diabetes mellitus during pregnancy. Although it fades at the end of pregnancy (gestational diabetes), the chances are comparatively high that the woman will develop true diabetes mellitus later in life, so this occurrence would be given a primary number.

PREGNANCY PROBLEM LIST

Mary and her husband live in a two-bedroom apartment. They owe payments on their furniture and on their car. In order to pay these monthly expenses, Mary works as an admissions clerk at the hospital. She has a high school education. She went a year to a business school but did not graduate and so cannot work as the legal secretary that she originally planned to be. In order to be on duty at 7:00 A.M., she drinks only coffee for breakfast. To save money, she eats no lunch. On the two evenings a week that her husband attends night school (he is working toward a master's degree) she eats very little dinner as she does not like to cook just for herself.

Mary's husband is an English teacher at the high school. He is the only black teacher on the faculty. Mary is self-conscious at faculty functions because she is the only black woman there. In the apartment complex in which they live, they are the only black family. Their neighbors are friendly, but the women near Mary do not invite her to share coffee or "woman talk" with them.

Mary has been so nauseated for the past week that she has been unable to go to work. She looks exhausted and thin at her first prenatal visit.

Problems relating to this pregnancy that could be identified from just this scant data base are shown below.

Problem-oriented Recording: Pregnancy Problem List (Problem 9)

Name: Mary Kraft
Age: 23

Date of Problem	Number	Active	Resolved
9-1-80	9a	Nausea	
9-1-80	9b	Inadequate nutrition	
9-1-80	9c	Lack of extended support people	
9-1-80	9d	Fetal growth evaluation (heavy smoker)	
9-1-80	9e	Limited financial resources	

Progress Notes

Using a POR format, a progress note is written on each problem that has been identified. Included are Subjective data, Objective data, an Assessment of the problem, and a Plan of intervention. Because the first letters of these four categories spell the word SOAP, writing progress notes is sometimes referred to as "soaping."

Data the patient gives that you cannot document (a woman states that her ankles swell each evening) are *subjective* data. Data that can be documented because you see the condition or you have a laboratory test proving it (the woman's ankles are swollen; a laboratory report shows that she has 4+ protein in her urine) are *objective* data. Data in these categories should include both positive and negative findings. A *positive* finding is one that is abnormal. A *negative* finding is one that is normal.

The assessment statement is the same as a nursing diagnosis, or a statement as to what you think the problem is. The plans for intervention should include information in three categories: diagnostic steps that are still necessary, therapeutic steps that need to be carried out, and educational steps that need to be taken in order to help the person return to wellness or to prevent illness in the future.

Most physicians utilizing POR formats do not list a

goal or expected outcome of their plans; the goal of medical care is almost always directed toward only one end: saving life and restoring health. Because nurses deal with broader and often less tangible patient concerns, it is helpful for nurses using POR charting to list the goals or expected outcomes of the proposed interventions.

Stating the expected outcomes of interventions is particularly useful if complete restoration of health cannot realistically be accomplished. For example, Mrs. G. is seen at a prenatal visit. She is the mother of five boys. She expresses her individuality and creativity by cooking; she has won awards for baking. Although setting a goal of limiting weight gain during pregnancy to 30 pounds is a typical goal for most women, it may not be a realistic one to expect for someone like Mrs. G., who must continue to cook for a large family who like rich desserts and pastries. You and the physician with whom you work agree that (although she is already slightly obese) because she has a normal blood pressure a weight gain of up to 50 pounds will be all right for her. This should be stated conspicuously on her chart so everyone who comes in contact with her during her pregnancy will be aware of it. The information will prevent a nurse who weighs her at a visit when you are not there from scolding her for gaining too much weight. It is difficult for people to maintain confidence in health care providers who are inconsistent in demands. It is frightening when one is pregnant (if people cannot agree on something as simple as weight gain, how can one be sure that they will agree on what is needed for safe delivery?).

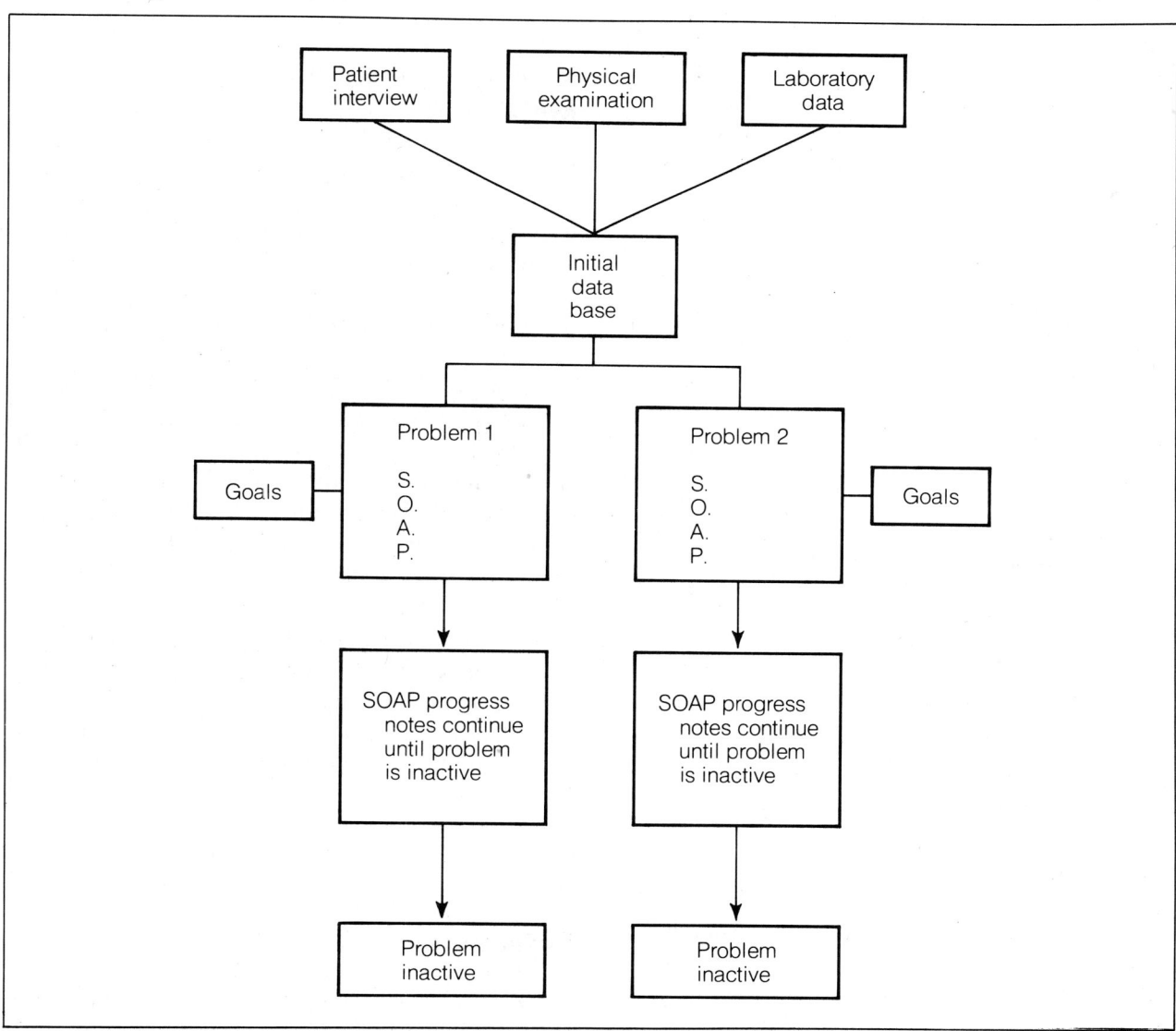

Fig. 4-2. Problem-oriented recording format.

A diagram of POR charting steps is shown in Fig. 4-2. Progress notes written on one of the problems identified from Mary's pregnancy problem list are shown below.

Problem-oriented Recording: Progress Notes

9-1-80
6 weeks from last menstrual period

Problem: 9a Nausea

> S. States she vomits 1× q day; not able to eat anything until noon, then appetite okay. No abdominal pain, no diarrhea, no fever. Takes sodium bicarbonate for nausea.
> O. Looks tired, thin, uncomfortable.
> A. Nausea due to early pregnancy.
>
> Goals: a. Patient's nausea will be reduced to a point where pregnancy can be enjoyed and intake will be nutritious and adequate.
> b. Nausea will not persist beyond 12 weeks of pregnancy.
>
> P. 1. Ask M.D. for prescription for medicine for nausea (nausea interfering with nutrition).
> 2. Assure that nausea is normal in early pregnancy.
> 3. Caution not to take over-the-counter drugs.
> 4. Nutrition counseling done; review next visit when nausea is decreased.
> 5. Patient to call if nausea lasts longer than 1 week with medication.

9-27-80
10 weeks from last menstrual period

Problem: 9a Nausea

> S. Taking Bendectin t.i.d.; no nausea now, eating 3 meals a day.
> O. Looks more cheerful; has gained 2 pounds.
> A. Nausea decreased due to Bendectin therapy.
> P. 1. Reassured that nausea in early pregnancy is normal.
> 2. Instructed to take Bendectin 2 more weeks, then taper dose.
> 3. Nutrition for pregnancy reviewed.
> 4. To call if nausea returns after Bendectin is stopped.

10-26-80
14 weeks from last menstrual period

Problem: 9a Nausea

> S. Nausea faded at 12th week of pregnancy; none now; taking no medication for nausea; no difficulty with eating.
> O. Weight gain 3 pounds.
> A. Nausea limited to 12th week of pregnancy; normal course.
> P. Problem moved to inactive problem list.

Nursing and Problem-oriented Recording

Nurses as a group have been slow in accepting the POR format of charting, persisting in using a standard time-oriented format—what they did at 9 o'clock, what they did at 10 o'clock, and so forth—a record which, if not carefully written, actually lists more actions and concerns of the nurse than of the patient. Most nurses have chosen to continue to keep nursing care plans separate from charts, secreting the goals and rationale for their nursing care rather than sharing them with other caregivers.

POR charting can be the answer to this dilemma. It lets you include the goals and rationale of what you are doing in daily charting. POR charting allows nursing care planning to be read by other health care providers, so that other members of the health profession can see the amount of planning that goes into quality nursing care. It urges all health care providers to look at patients in the holistic method, which is typical of nursing's approach to patient care. Most importantly, it makes nursing care planning the ongoing and fluid concept it should be, best meeting patient needs.

References

1. Ademoware, A. S., and Meyers, E. Use of the problem-oriented record by nurses caring for high-risk antepartum patients. J.O.G.N. Nurs. 6:17, 1977.

2. Blair, E. M., et al. Instrument development: Measuring quality outcomes in ambulatory maternal-newborn nursing. *Nurs. Adm. Q.* 2:81, 1978.
3. Green, R. B. Nursing care plans for the special care nursery. *Superv. Nurse* 10:23, 1979.
4. Harris, R. J. Facilitating change to the problem-oriented medical record system. *J. Nurs. Adm.* 8:35, 1978.
5. Kleinbeck, S. V. SOAPing the preoperative interview. *A.O.R.N. J.* 28:1031, 1978.
6. Lamonica, E. L. Problem-oriented Records. In *The Nursing Process: A Humanistic Approach*. Reading, Mass.: Addison-Wesley, 1979.
7. Larkin, P. D., and Backer, B. A. *Problem-oriented Nursing Assessment*. New York: McGraw-Hill, 1977.
8. Malloy, J. L. Taking exception to problem-oriented nursing care. *Am. J. Nurs.* 76:582, 1976.
9. McCloskey, J. C. The problem-oriented record vs the nursing care plan: A proposal. *Nurs. Outlook* 23:492, 1975.
10. McGugan, M. B., et al. An androgynal approach to teaching the problem-oriented method of charting. *J. Contin. Educ. Nurs.* 10:7, 1979.
11. Snyder, P. Goal setting. *Superv. Nurse* 9:61, 1978.
12. Weed, L. L. *Medical Records, Medical Education and Patient Care*. Cleveland: Case University Press, 1969.
13. Wiley, L. The nursing care plan: A communication system that really works. *Nursing 78* 8:28, 1978.
14. Wooley, F. R., and Kane, R. L. Improving Patient Care Through the Interdisciplinary Record. In A. M. Reinhardt and M. D. Quinn (Eds.), *Current Practice in Family-centered Community Nursing*. St. Louis: Mosby, 1977.

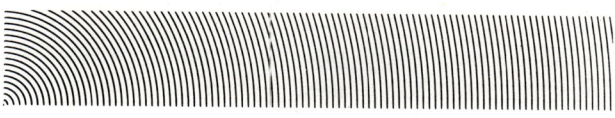

5. Legal Aspects of Maternal-Newborn Nursing

As nursing becomes more complex, the legal responsibilities of nurses become more complex. Legal obligations must be considered.

Sources of Law

A law can be defined as a *man-made rule* that regulates human social conduct in a formally prescribed and legally binding manner. In the United States, laws are derived from two separate sources: statutory law and common law.

STATUTORY LAW

A statutory law is a *legislated law* or rule made by a governing body. It is equally binding on all citizens in that jurisdiction. Laws that set speed limits or prohibit robbery or littering are examples. Nurse practice acts, because they are laws formulated by state legislatures, are examples of legislative (statutory) laws pertinent to nursing.

COMMON LAW

Common law is a *judicial decision*. Legislative bodies cannot anticipate all the situations that can arise or all the different ways people will break laws. Thus, when a situation occurs that has never happened before (someone discovers how to transfer funds from other bank accounts to his bank account by computer), a judge examines the circumstances and makes a decision as to the nature of the act. He asks, if someone robs a bank by this method, is it the same as robbing a bank by showing a gun to a teller or is it different? Once a circumstance has been considered by a judge (that bank robbing is bank robbing no matter how it is done), there is a *precedent* as to the nature of that kind of act. When the same circumstances arise again, the second person will probably find himself held as liable as was the person who was involved when the precedent was set. Common law is often called the *law of precedents*.

Types of Law

In the United States there are two major divisions, or types, of law: criminal and civil law.

CRIMINAL LAW

A *crime* is an offense against the government or against society as a whole. A person who commits a crime has charges brought against him by the governing body. Embezzlement, murder, and forgery are examples of crimes. If a money penalty is involved as punishment, the money is paid to the governing body (paying a speeding ticket or paying a fine for embezzlement).

CIVIL LAW

A *civil offense* is an offense against an individual. If a money penalty is involved as punishment, the money is paid to the injured individual. Nurses may be guilty of either criminal or civil actions or both. Practicing without a nursing license, for example, is a crime or a criminal law offense. It is in violation of a state law; it has the potential of endangering a large number of people. Negligence and malpractice harm individuals; they are, therefore, civil offenses. Any money to be paid because of a negligence or malpractice suit is paid to the individual harmed by the error.

Negligence

All adults are responsible for conducting themselves at all times so as not to bring harm to others. Negligence is omitting to do something that a reasonable person would do under the same circumstances or doing something that a reasonable person under those circumstances would *not* do.

On a slippery, icy day, for example, the reasonable man shovels his front walk so that people, such as the mailman, who must walk on it will not slip and be injured. If a man did not shovel his walk and the mailman slipped, fell, and broke a leg, the man might be found guilty of negligence, or of not doing what the average person does.

Malpractice

Malpractice is professional negligence, either the omission of something that a reasonable nurse would do in the circumstances or the commission of something that a reasonable nurse would not do in those circumstances.

Taking vital signs frequently for the first hour following childbirth, for example, is an activity that the average nurse appreciates is important and does conscientiously. Not taking vital signs during that time could be interpreted as malpractice if injury happened to the patient during that time. The term *prudent* is often used in legal documents to denote reasonableness; legal phraseology considers what the prudent nurse would do.

Standards of Care

Whether a nurse has acted in a reasonable or prudent manner in a situation is often not an easy decision to make; in every situation there is always more than one way to do something. A number of sources are used to determine standards of nursing practice.

LEGISLATIVE SOURCES

Nurses are responsible for observing legislative law. The chief legislated laws that concern nurses are the nurse practice acts. You should be familiar with the wording of the Nurse Practice Act of your state so you can be certain that you are not only practicing within the scope of it but practicing to the full extent allowed by the Act. Nurses who take it upon themselves to make a medical diagnosis are at that point practicing medicine and functioning outside the standard level of nursing in the state.

COMMON LAW SOURCES

Common law sources are many. Which source would be used in any given instance depends on the circumstances and specific issues involved.

Health Agency Policies

You should be familiar with the policies and procedures of the health agency with which you work, as working in compliance with them is what the average nurse does. If a procedure is written poorly or wrongly, attempting to have it changed through the agency policy committee is more professional than just ignoring it. If the policies and procedures of an agency are such that you cannot work within them and still practice quality nursing, you will probably be wise to work elsewhere.

Job Descriptions

The average nurse works under the job description of her nursing position. If a job description is too limiting or "just not you," you are best advised to bend your efforts toward having the job description changed or obtaining a different position. It is difficult to justify performing functions outside your job description in the eyes of the law.

Voluntary Standards

Nursing organizations such as the National League of Nursing and the American Nurses' Association are concerned with setting practice standards. Standards for maternal-newborn nursing are discussed in Chap. 1. A nurse who does not meet these standards of care is not practicing at the level of the reasonable or average nurse.

Bills of Rights

The American Hospital Organization has devised a bill of rights for the hospitalized patient. Specialty groups have listed rights for the handicapped, the child, and the mentally retarded. The Pregnant Patient's Bill of Rights is shown in Appendix A. Such a list of rights has implications in the determination of average practice standards.

Level of Knowledge

The more background and experience a nurse has, the higher the standard of care she is expected to provide. This places a responsibility on nurses to use all their knowledge every time they give patient care. For example, a new graduate would be expected to pick up changes on a fetal heart monitor strip when they first become evident. A nurse who has had experience working with fetal heart monitors or has taken an advanced course in fetal heart monitoring would be expected to pick up subtle changes even before they become truly definitive on the fetal monitor strip. This philosophy, that nurses must perform at the highest level they have attained, ensures patients the best care possible.

Average Practice Criteria

In order to lay a groundwork of what is average care, any nurse might be asked to come to court and testify on the standard level of care in her community or agency. In this role, she is called an expert witness. Expert witnesses are often asked to assess whether or not the nurse in question used suitable judgment in determining her course of action.

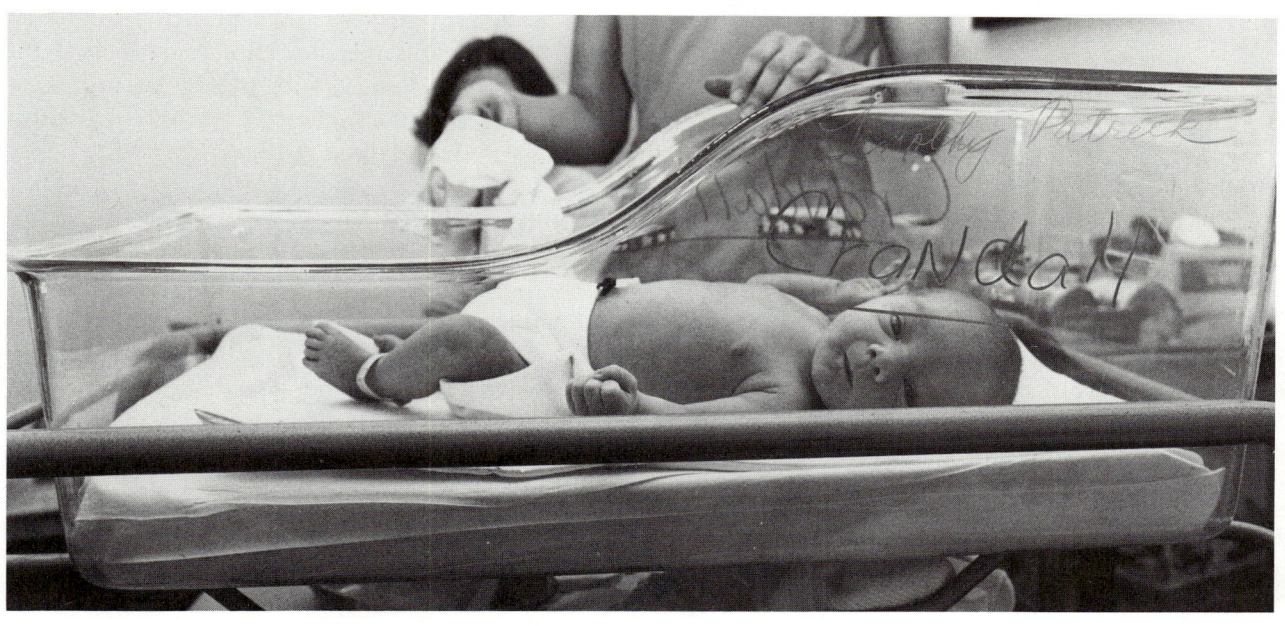

Fig. 5-1. A nurse owes a special duty of care to all patients, especially those who are not able to voice their concerns well. (Courtesy of the Department of Medical Photography, Children's Hospital, Buffalo, N.Y.)

It is assumed that nurses will use judgment in delivering nursing care. For example, a physician orders "vital signs [VS] every 15 minutes for 1 hour" for a woman who has just delivered a child. In actuality he means far more than that. He not only means that you should take vital signs but assumes that you will *compare* the present readings with those previously taken to see whether a descreasing or increasing trend is occurring, make a decision as to whether the readings are normal or not, record the readings so they become part of the permanent record, and, if they are abnormal, alert him to that. An expert witness might testify that the order, VS q15min for 1 hour, denotes all those activities, and not doing them all is not consistent with the standard of nursing care in that community.

Textbooks and Professional Journals

Nursing textbooks are compilations of nursing knowledge. If a textbook states that women in labor should be asked to void every 4 hours, for example, this becomes a standard for care in labor against which nursing actions and safe practice can be measured.

The Nurse-Patient Relationship

In the eyes of the law a nurse-patient relationship is a very special, binding one. A nurse owes a special duty of care to a patient over and above that duty she owes to other people, and she must continue to give care and guard the safety of the patient until she is relieved appropriately (Fig. 5-1).

Initiating a nurse-patient relationship involves no

more action than beginning nursing care with that patient. No statement such as "Hello, I'm Miss Smith; I'm going to be your nurse for the day" is even necessary. Thus the relationship can be initiated as fully with an unconscious or anesthetized patient or a newborn who has no comprehension of legal aspects as with a legal-age consenting adult.

Whether a nurse-patient relationship exists or not has legal implications because of the special duty of care owed by a nurse to a patient.

ABANDONMENT

If a nurse initiates a nurse-patient relationship, she must maintain it until she is relieved appropriately. If you begin to care for a woman in labor, for example, then go to lunch without asking anyone to continue your care while you are gone and something detrimental happens during your unsupervised absence, you might be held liable for abandonment. A patient has the right to expect continuity of supervision from professional people whether you are physically present every minute or not.

In maternal-newborn nursing it is important to determine what procedures (abortion, perhaps) you ethically do not want to assist with. If you are asked to help with an abortion, for example, and you begin care, you must continue care until you are properly relieved despite any ethical conviction you have about assisting with abortions. The time to decide what you ethically want to do or not do is before your initiation of a nurse-patient relationship.

Criteria for Establishing Malpractice

In order for malpractice to be proved, three criteria must be present:

1. The nurse must have omitted doing something that a reasonable nurse would do under the circumstances or have done something that a reasonable nurse would not do under the circumstances.
2. Patient injury must have occurred.
3. There must be proximal cause between the action of the nurse and the injury.

For example, Mrs. K. has a urinary tract infection following delivery of her infant, and you are asked to administer ampicillin 250 mg to her. You make an error in calculating the dose and administer 500 mg of ampicillin instead. You have made an error; the first criterion is present. Because safe ampicillin doses vary widely, however, no harm occurs to the patient; the second criterion does not exist.

In another instance, a physician orders penicillin to be given to a woman in her sixth month of pregnancy to treat a urinary tract infection. You ask her whether she is allergic to penicillin and you check her records to see that she has no previous allergy to penicillin. A few minutes after you inject the medication, however, the woman becomes extremely short of breath and undergoes an anaphylactic reaction. This leads to a spontaneous abortion. The woman brings suit against you for administering an unsafe drug to her. Although there is patient injury and the administration of the drug led directly to the injury, because you did what the average nurse does before administering penicillin (asked about allergies, checked the chart for allergies) not all three of the criteria necessary for malpractice are present. It is very unlikely these circumstances would result in a successful legal action.

In a third example, you make an error and give an injection of ampicillin meant for Mrs. A. to Mrs. B. Although there was no medical reason for Mrs. B. to receive the ampicillin, ampicillin is not contraindicated during pregnancy so no harm results. A month later, the woman begins vaginal spotting and aborts. She brings suit against you for the medication error. Two criteria for malpractice are present: an error on your part and an injury (she has aborted). Since there is no proximal cause between an injection of ampicillin and abortion, however, the third criterion for malpractice is still not present.

RES IPSA LOQUITUR

Ordinarily, proving that a nurse has made an error is the responsibility of the patient. In certain instances, the proof of error is not difficult. If a patient should receive a burn on her arm, for example, in the shape of a heating pad after you applied such a pad to her arm, it is obvious that the burn resulted from the heating pad. *Res ipsa loquitur,* freely translated, is the Latin phrase for "the thing speaks for itself," or proof that an error has been made speaks for itself.

CONTRIBUTORY NEGLIGENCE

Contributory negligence occurs when a patient plays a part in his own injury. For example, you tell a woman after delivery of her baby that she should not get out of bed without your help because she will feel light-headed following her anesthetic. She ignores your instructions and walks to the bathroom by herself and falls and injures herself. She has contributed to her injury. Contributory negligence would not apply if at the time you gave the instruction she was too sleepy or in some other way could not understand or comprehend the importance of your message.

RESPONDEAT SUPERIOR

Every nurse is responsible for her own actions. She is also responsible for the personnel she supervises. As an everyday example of the application of this doctrine, if you take your car in to be repaired, you can expect to have it repaired at the level that you discuss with the owner of the repair shop, whether he actually repairs it or has a helper do it. If you are team leader and ask a practical nurse to pass medications for the day to help out (something ordinarily a registered nurse's duty) and she makes an error, you are responsible for her error by the doctrine of *respondeat superior* (literally, "let the master answer"). A patient has the right to expect that you will coordinate a level of care for him equal to that you would give yourself.

Incident Reports

One of the criteria for evaluating whether an action constitutes malpractice is whether you did what the average nurse would do *in those circumstances*. An incident report is your avenue to explain what the circumstances were. The three topics that you want to comment on are whether an error occurred or not, whether an injury occurred or not, and any connection between the two (proximal cause).

THE ERROR

State exactly what happened as you know it. You asked a woman her name to be certain that she was Mrs. Smith; she said yes. Unfortunately, there were two women in clinic named Mrs. Smith; you gave ampicillin to the wrong woman.

Incident reports are not the place for apologizing ("I'm sorry I did this but I learned a lot from it; I'll be a better nurse in the future"). In many states, incident reports are admissible evidence in court. It is a constitutional right that you do not have to testify against yourself. Self-incriminating statements on incident reports are a form of testifying against yourself.

Angry statements—"This is an example of why this policy is stupid"—are inappropriate on incident reports. They do not evidence sound thinking and they interfere with demonstrating that although you have made an error you are overall a responsible person.

THE INJURY

Some nurses are reluctant to describe a patient's injury thoroughly on a report because the description will reveal that an injury did indeed occur. In actuality, the description serves to show the limitation of the injury. A statement such as "There was an elevated, reddened area 2 cm by 1 cm on Mrs. J.'s right elbow after she fell, but she moved the joint readily without evidencing pain" shows that certainly the woman did bump her elbow when she fell. It also shows that the elbow must not have been broken; that is, it defines the extent of the injury.

THE PROXIMAL CAUSE

If you make an error in administering nursing care, it is imperative to include in your report the response of the patient to that error. If you gave an excessive dose of insulin to Mrs. J., who is pregnant and diabetic, for example, it would be important to document that, despite your error, at the time the insulin reached its maximum effect her blood sugar fell only to 80 mg per 100 ml. If her child is born later with a congenital anomaly, you have documented that, although you made an error, there is probably little connection between your error and the pregnancy's poor outcome.

Statute of Limitations

If you commit an error in nursing practice today, it is difficult to feel completely free of having a suit brought against you until it is no longer possible for a malpractice suit to be instituted against you. All states have statutes of limitations, or time spans, in which people can bring suit. After that period of time has passed, the threat of lawsuit is over. In most states the time span is three to five years. The exception is involved in the maternal-child health area of nursing. If parents choose not to bring a lawsuit against health personnel concerning a child's injury, there are instances in which the child was allowed to bring the suit himself when he reached legal age. This has implications for detailed charting. No one can remember what she did or what she was thinking three or five years ago, much less 20 years ago.

High-Risk Health Care Areas

All of maternal-newborn care is a high-risk area because you always care for two persons when you are caring for a pregnant woman; you care for individuals unable to protest or guide you into safe practice when you care for newborn infants. Within the maternal-newborn area some situations have higher risk for potential incidents than others. High-risk factors are:

New equipment (with which you are unfamiliar)
Electrical equipment (the possibility of burns or electrical shock always exists)

- Medication (individual differences may affect safe dosage)
- Heating and cooling devices (the possibility of burn always exists)
- Controversial areas such as research or new procedures (misunderstandings of the procedure may result)
- Emergency situations (action may be undertaken too swiftly, before all safety factors are considered)

NEW EQUIPMENT

Any time you are dealing with new equipment you must be certain that you thoroughly understand the purpose of the equipment and how to operate it. Ignorance, because you did not understand how to operate a piece of equipment, is no excuse for causing patient injury. Get proper instructions before beginning care.

ELECTRICAL EQUIPMENT

Electrical equipment is always a high-risk factor because of the inherent dangers of injury from electrical shock. Modern intensive care nurseries are built with a minimum of 12 electrical outlet plugs for each baby. This reflects, in a 30-bed nursery, 360 chances for electrical injury. It is a nursing responsibility to see that frayed or broken cords are not used, that outlets are not overloaded, and that electrical cords or plugs are not allowed to come in contact with water sources.

MEDICATIONS

Medicine giving is an area that is ripe for error due to the constantly increasing number of medicines for which a nurse is responsible. You have an added responsibility not to administer a drug that has teratogenic (capable of causing fetal injury) properties to pregnant women.

HEATING AND COOLING DEVICES

Whenever you work with equipment that has the potential to heat or cool, you are working with equipment that has the potential to burn. Postpartum women often have sitz baths, K-pads, or heat lamp treatments ordered for them to encourage perineal healing. Infants of low birth weight are often placed in incubators or under radiant heat sources or phototherapy lights. You must be aware of proper use of such equipment. Be meticulous about temperature settings, time limits, distance required, and specific precautions such as shielding the baby's eyes from phototherapy lights.

CONTROVERSIAL AREAS

In previous generations, childbearing was regarded as a process so unique that few interventions to interfere with or even assist it were attempted. Today, pregnancy may be initiated by artificial insemination; it may be ended by abortion. The fetus may be viewed by a fetoscope and even have a blood transfusion given to it in utero. Most of the controversy that arises over new procedures is concerned with ethical considerations, but there may be legal dimensions as well. Be certain that no procedure is carried out until informed consent has been obtained to ensure that there are no misunderstandings of the procedure later.

EMERGENCY SITUATIONS

In emergencies, steps of care must be taken quickly, but basic safety rules never change. A woman has the right to expect that additional complications will not happen to her due to someone's carelessness in an emergency situation.

Good Samaritan Laws

Many states have Good Samaritan laws or statutes that govern the actions of professional people in emergencies. Before Good Samaritan laws were passed, a nurse might have stopped at the scene of a car accident and found a pregnant woman bleeding heavily from a neck vein. She might have torn off the bottom of her skirt to make a compress to apply pressure to the wound. Later, after the woman was removed to the hospital, the wound site became infected and the woman developed septicemia and had an extended hospital stay. The woman might have initiated a lawsuit because a nurse should have known that with an open wound nothing but a sterile compress should have been applied.

In an emergency, perfect conditions, such as having a source of sterile compresses, do not apply. Good Samaritan laws state that the criterion against which a person in an emergency should be judged is not that of ideal conditions but what existed at the scene and time of the accident. In the example given, therefore, using a clean compress to halt extreme bleeding would be proper. If the nurse had used a greasy rag from the car trunk or had let the extreme bleeding go unchecked, then the care could be questioned.

The Suit-prone Nurse

Some nurses practice as if to attract lawsuits. People in general bring lawsuits against health personnel because they are unhappy with the quality or outcome of care. The concern or attitude of those who give that care has a great deal to do with this unhappiness. A nurse who practices impersonally—not extending to women the courtesy of calling them by name or of remembering their names, not explaining procedures before they are carried out, not explaining what medications are being given and how they will work, not explaining what a woman can expect from a treatment or laboratory test—is asking for people to be unhappy with her. Obviously, a nurse who practices on the edge of safety—knowing a little but not a lot about the danger signs of pregnancy, the drugs she administers, or the equipment she works with—is a nurse who is suit-prone. More importantly, she is a poor model as a nurse.

The Suit-prone Patient

Pregnancy, labor and delivery, and the first days of the postpartum period are stressful. People under stress may not "hear" instructions given to them or may interpret them wrongly. During all phases of maternal-newborn nursing, therefore, instructions should be given with the appreciation that they are being offered to people under stress and that they may have to be repeated before they are comprehended. People under stress need support persons around them to serve as buffers. If they do not have them, they turn to health care personnel. If they do not receive support from health care personnel, they may turn to lawyers.

A major role of a nurse in maternal-newborn care is to serve as a supportive, concerned person for anyone who needs this type of interaction during a particularly important time.

A patient who understands what is going to happen to her because she has had adequate health teaching about pregnancy will not be surprised by what she is going through; she is less likely to be angry and upset because it is not a surprise. Health teaching, therefore, is a function of maternal-newborn nursing not only because not being surprised by events helps to encourage mother-infant bonding but also because it has legal aspects.

A woman who has a complication of pregnancy that results in death or morbidity of her infant loses a great deal. Sometimes she loses not only the child but future childbearing potential. A woman who is feeling loss is under enormous stress. She may seek a source of blame for what has happened to her. Unless she has very good explanations and feels trust and confidence in the people who care for her, she may bring a lawsuit. This type of lawsuit, initiated out of anger, helplessness, or a feeling of doing something even though it will not bring back the child, is generally groundless. It can be prevented if health care personnel appreciate what the loss of a child means to people and offer more constructive ways to deal with the frustration they face.

Informed Consent

In order for a person's signature on a consent form to be legal, the consent must be informed. That is, the person must be aware of what he is signing and understand the risks and expected outcome of the procedure and the risks and expected outcome if he does not consent to the procedure.

Many times you are asked to witness patients' signatures on consent forms. You must be certain that you are witnessing the signature of a person who has been informed, or you must have listened to the explanation of the procedure.

The term *informed* has special meaning for pregnant women in that the explanation must include not only any risk for the woman but risk for the fetus as well. If you did not hear the explanation or do not feel it was given accurately, you should not witness the form, or, if you witness it, you should add after your name, "witnessed signature only."

In many states, a pregnant teenager who is living away from home or is the parent of a child is considered an "emancipated minor." Although she cannot vote, an emancipated minor can sign consent for her own health care and that of her child. States have differing rules as to whether a teenager may sign consent for treatment for venereal disease or contraceptives. Federal law stipulates that a girl may consent to an abortion in early pregnancy without her parent's consent.

You should be familiar with the rules governing emancipated minors in your state. These rules are made because parents often do not accompany teenagers into health care facilities, and unless the minor's signature is accepted as legal in these instances, she would not be able to receive health care.

References

1. Bentz, J. M. Missed meanings in nurse-patient communications. *M.C.N.* 5:55, 1980.
2. Bernstein, A. H. Liability of hospitals—a continuing challenge. *Hospitals* 51:163, 1977.
3. Creighton, H. Legal concerns of nursing research. *Nurs. Res.* 26:337, 1977.
4. Creighton, H. Liability of a nurse for negligence. *Superv. Nurse* 9:53, 1978.

5. Creighton, H. Slander. *Superv. Nurse* 9:64, 1978.
6. Creighton, H. More about informed consent. *Superv. Nurse* 9:84, 1978.
7. Fox, J. G., et al. Innovations in family and community health practice and the law. *Fam. Community Health* 1:19, 1978.
8. Hollowell, E. E. What every nurse should know about tort liability. *Hospitals* 51:97, 1977.
9. Hurt, T. The status of Good Samaritan statutes. *Health Educ.* 8:4, 1977.
10. Hysterectomies: Clinical necessity and consent. *Regan Rep. Nurs. Law* 18:2, 1977.
11. Kelly, L. S. The rights of young people in health care. *Nurse Pract.* 2:10, 1977.
12. Leitch, C. J., et al. A state by state report: The legal accommodation of nurses practicing expanded roles. *Nurse Pract.* 2:19, 1977.
13. Mancini, M. Nursing, minors and the law. *Am. J. Nurs.* 78:124, 1978.
14. Mumme, J. L. Seven surefire ways to lose a malpractice case. *R.N.* 40:60, 1977.
15. Newton, M., et al. Guidelines for handling drug errors. *Nursing 77* 7:62, 1977.
16. Nursing mistakes at patient's bedside: No M.D. liability. *Regan Rep. Nurs. Law* 17:2, 1977.
17. Paul, E. W., et al. Teenagers and pregnancy: The law in 1979. *Fam. Plann. Perspect.* 11:297, 1979.
18. Piazza, D. S., et al. Clinical nurse specialists: Issues, power and freedom. *Superv. Nurse* 9:47, 1978.
19. Rothman, D. A., et al. The nurse and informed consent. *J. Nurs. Adm.* 7:7, 1977.
20. Rozovsky, L. E. Answers to the 15 legal questions nurses usually ask. *Nursing 78* 8:73, 1978.
21. Sheffield, R. Complex medicolegal issues surround modern nursing practice. *Hospitals* 52:105, 1978.
22. Trendel-Korenchuk, D. M., et al. How state laws recognize advanced nursing practice. *Nurs. Outlook* 26:713, 1978.

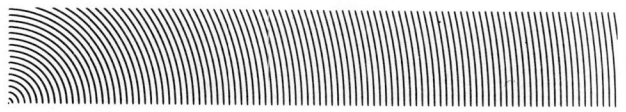

Unit I. Utilizing Nursing Process: Questions for Review

1. Standards of maternal-newborn nursing help to establish
   a. A body of nursing knowledge
   b. Consistency among nurses as to ways to practice
   c. Legal criteria for nursing practice
   d. All of the above

2. Steps of the nursing process are generally accepted as
   a. Assessment, goal setting, planning, evaluation
   b. Observation, planning, criteria setting, evaluation
   c. Planning, reassessment, operations, evaluation
   d. Assessment, planning, implementation, evaluation

3. In Maslow's hierarchy of needs, security (an important need during pregnancy) is what level need?
   a. First
   b. Second
   c. Third
   d. Fourth

4. A pregnant woman's ability to manage the crisis of pregnancy depends on
   a. Her perception of the event
   b. Her support people
   c. Her ways of coping in the past
   d. All of the above

5. The trend in health care delivery in relation to newborn care is toward
   a. Preventing illness in newborns
   b. Treating illness as quickly and forcefully as possible
   c. Treating illness only if the potential outcome for the baby is favorable
   d. None of the above

6. Transporting newborns to intensive care centers is done best by
   a. Transport incubator in the first hour of life
   b. Transport incubator after 24 hours of stabilization
   c. Transporting the mother prenatally
   d. Transporting both mother and infant within 48 hours of birth

7. Separation of infants and mothers at birth was proposed in the past *mainly* to
   a. Decrease maternal-newborn interaction at birth
   b. Prevent spread of infection
   c. Create more nursing positions due to large nurseries
   d. Allow mothers to rest after childbirth

8. Mrs. Smith is seen in a prenatal clinic. She states that she is worried because she is constantly tired. If you recorded this information in a problem-oriented format, you would record it as
   a. Objective data
   b. Assessment
   c. Subjective data
   d. Initial plan

9. You test Mrs. Smith's urine and discover that she has 3+ protein in the urine. In a POR format, you would record this finding as
   a. Objective data
   b. Assessment
   c. Subjective data
   d. Progress note

10. According to a POR format, a plan for nursing care should include information in what three areas?
    a. Diagnostic, educational, and follow-up
    b. Rehabilitation, prevention of illness, and maintenance of health
    c. Therapeutic, diagnostic, and educational
    d. Educational, physical, and psychological interventions

11. Mrs. Smith asks you if she can deliver her baby in a birthing room. Birthing rooms in labor units of hospitals allow for
    a. Less need for expensive delivery room equipment
    b. Less nursing staff because no delivery room nurse is needed
    c. A more home-like atmosphere
    d. A structured formal atmosphere that will reduce anxiety

12. Teaching prenatal care is an important nursing intervention in maternal-newborn nursing. Which of the following is true of teaching-learning during pregnancy?
    a. Pregnancy is a nonstressful time, so learning takes place readily.
    b. Teaching about child care in early pregnancy is successful because it offers the information before the woman is even ready for it.
    c. Pregnant women learn best in groups.
    d. When a woman voices a concern, she is probably ready for information on that topic.

13. In the United States, infant mortality is
    a. Falling, but still higher than that of some other countries
    b. The lowest possible rate it can be
    c. Increasing because of home deliveries
    d. Increasing because of initial resuscitation measures

14. Infant mortality is defined as
    a. Death of all infants under 500 gm per 1,000 population
    b. Death of fetuses over 500 gm per 100 live births
    c. Death of infants at birth and during the first year of life per 1,000 live births
    d. Death of infants during the first year of life from causes other than birth

15. The infant period of life is
    a. The least hazardous period of life
    b. More hazardous than any other period under age 65
    c. Hazardous only if prenatal care is not available
    d. Equal in hazard to the school-age period

16. Neonatal mortality is defined as
    a. The sum of the fetal and infant mortality rates
    b. The death of infants during the first 28 days of life per 1,000 live births
    c. The death of any fetus over 500 gm and under 9 pounds per 1,000 live births
    d. The incidence of babies who die at birth

17. You are using a new resuscitator with Mrs. Smith's newborn. You realize after a few minutes that it is causing damage to the baby's lungs because you are using it improperly. Legally
    a. You cannot be held liable for damage to the baby as use of new equipment exempts you from blame.
    b. The hospital, not you, is liable, because it is their equipment.
    c. You are liable for your own actions as a nurse.
    d. You are liable only if you have used the equipment before.

18. The statute of limitations in terms of law refers to
    a. The time limit you have to file an incident report after a patient care error
    b. The limit of the amount of money for which a nurse can be sued
    c. The time an injured patient has to bring legal suit against you
    d. The limit of the number of times you can be sued in a lifetime

19. You begin care for Mrs. Smith at 3:00 P.M. At 3:30 P.M. your nursing shift is over but no evening nurse has yet arrived. If you leave without providing adequate supervision for Mrs. Smith
    a. You can be held liable for abandonment if harm results from your actions.
    b. You owe Mrs. Smith no legal obligation at the time your nursing shift ends.
    c. You owe her no legal obligation as you had not yet cared for her one full hour.
    d. None of the above.

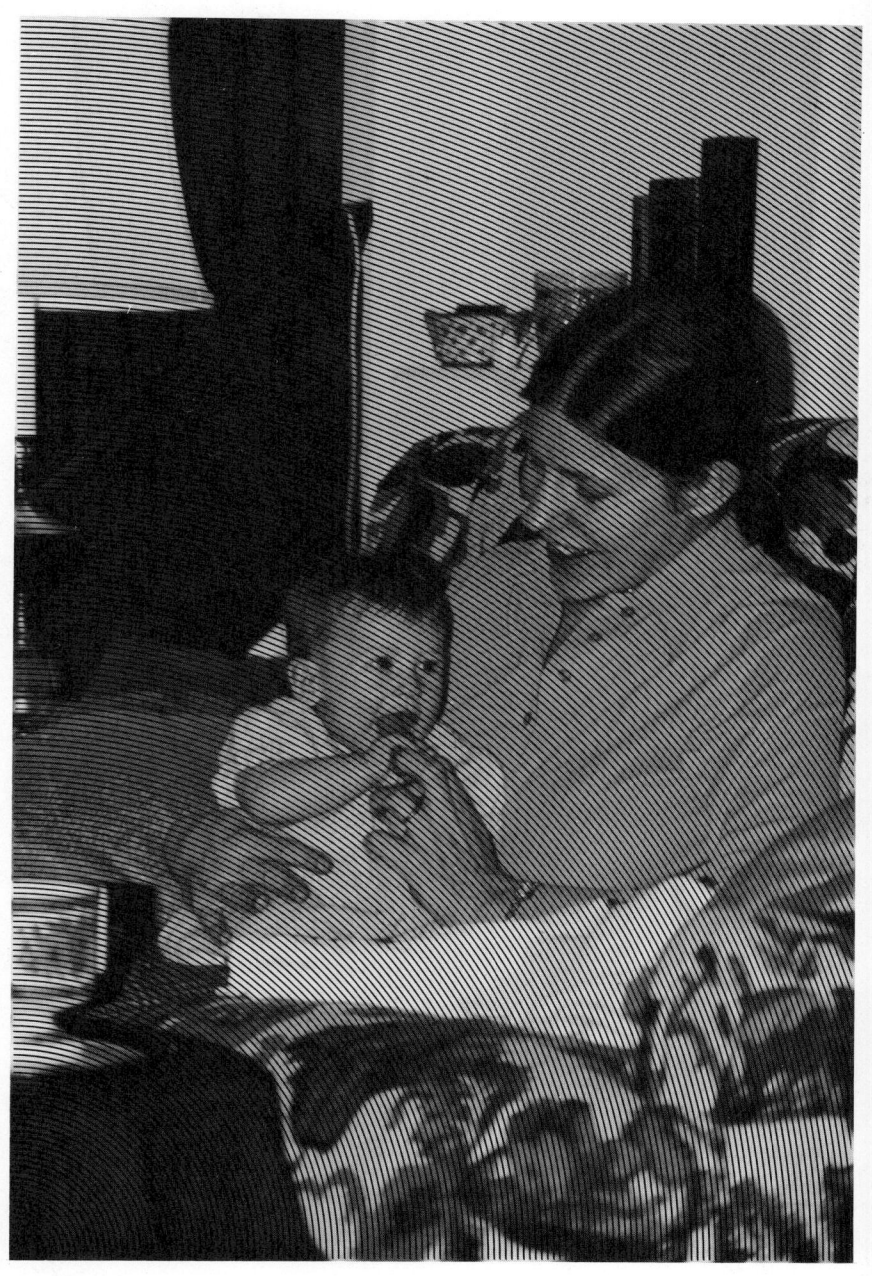

II. The Interpartal Period

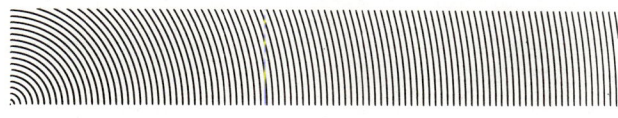

6. Developmental Readiness for Child Rearing

Being ready to be a parent is more than being physically capable of conceiving and producing children. It involves being mature enough emotionally to have another individual dependent on you, being able to sacrifice your own needs when they conflict with those of a child. It means having the maturity to maintain some form of employment so that financial resources are available for child rearing.

Erikson [5] has described eight stages of man and the psychosocial or developmental steps toward maturity that people take at each stage (Table 6-1). People pass from one developmental stage in life to another, depending not so much on chronological age but on whether they have completed the developmental task of the earlier stage. In order to be effective parents, men and women need to have completed at least the developmental tasks (sometimes called developmental crises) up through adolescence.

Infancy: A Sense of Trust

The developmental task of infancy (birth to 1 year) is that of learning to trust or learning to love. The infant whose needs are met when they arise, whose discomforts are quickly removed, who is cuddled, fondled, played with, and talked to, learns to accept the world as a safe place and people as helpful and dependable.

If infant care is inconsistent, inadequate, or rejecting, however, the opposite of a sense of trust (mistrust) develops in the child. He can become fearful and suspicious of people and the world around him.

People give love to others most freely when they are assured that they will receive love in return. An infant will offer to love the adults who care for him, but if his love is rejected time and again, as happens to a child who is moved from one foster home to another foster home, he will stop trying. After a while he loses the ability to reach out and offer love. Like the burnt child who avoids fire, the emotionally burnt child avoids the pain of emotional attachment.

Although he continues to grow and learn new motor skills and, on the surface, appears to be progressing normally, emotionally he becomes "stuck" at the infant stage. He may live his life as a "loner," making few close friends. He may have difficulty establishing heterosexual relationships (it is too great a risk to reach out to a partner, to offer love, because he may be rejected again and he has been hurt enough). He will not leave himself that vulnerable again—better to keep to himself and be lonely than be hurt.

Having a sense of trust is vital to being a good parent. It is the cornerstone on which parenthood is built. A parent is asked to give a great deal of time and

Table 6-1. Periods of Developmental Crises

Age Period	Developmental Task	Developmental Outcome
Infancy (1 to 12 months)	Trust	Learns to love
Toddlerhood (1 to 3 years)	Autonomy	Learns to make decisions, to be independent
Preschool age (3 to 5 years)	Initiative	Learns to solve problems, to do things
School age (5 to 12 years)	Industry	Learns to do things well
Adolescence (13 to 18 years)	Identity	Learns who she is and what she wants to do in life; is independent from parents
Young adulthood (19 to 30 years)	Intimacy	Learns to relate effectively on deeper planes
Middle age (30 to 60 years)	Generativity	Learns to look beyond herself at community and world needs
Older age	Integrity	Learns to be content with what she has achieved, to feel fulfilled in life

Source: Adapted from *Childhood and Society* (2nd ed.), Revised, by Erik H. Erikson, with the permission of W. W. Norton & Company, Inc. Copyright 1950, © 1963 by W. W. Norton & Company, Inc.

attention in the early weeks of a newborn's life without getting a great deal of interaction in return. People who have a sense of trust view the early weeks of a newborn's life as enjoyable because giving care is an activity that is enjoyable. People without a sense of trust may interpret the child's inability to follow their finger well, not yet smiling back at their smile, falling asleep instead of listening to them (typical newborn behavior) as rejection. They withdraw into themselves and initiate their protective mechanism—not reaching out to the child any more—and begin another cycle of what happened to them, creating another child who has difficulty loving because he is not loved.

The infant's sense of trust is learned through consistent mother-child interaction. When an infant is hungry, his mother feeds him and takes away his discomfort. When he is wet, his mother changes him and again takes away his discomfort. When he is lonely, his mother comes and holds and talks to him and takes away his discomfort. By this process he learns to trust that when he has a need, someone will come and care for him.

Following some schedule of care goes a long way toward helping an infant form a sense of trust. This does not mean that mothers should plan a rigid schedule of care; but some order to a day (breakfast, then bath, then playtime, then nap) offers direction as to what is coming next. That infants thrive on a routine is shown by their love of nursery rhymes. Even though a rhyme makes no sense, the sound of the same thing said over and over (patty-cake, patty-cake, baker's man . . .) is reassuring.

The mother who works needs to make plans so that her child has consistency when she is not with him. She needs to discuss with the baby-sitter or day-care center the routine she wants the child to follow so that whether she is present or not consistency will still be there. She needs to choose a day-care center where the child will have as few different caregivers as possible.

Fortunately, although developmental tasks are mastered easiest at that stage of life in which the person seems "ripe" for the task, if the person does not master the task at that age he can achieve it later in life. A child who reaches school age without a firm sense of trust can have it strengthened at school by a teacher who is worthy of trust. A person may enter adulthood without a firm sense of trust but be lucky to find a marriage partner who is so trustworthy and caring he is able to help his partner develop a sense of trust.

At the same time, a child who has developed a strong sense of trust may have it destroyed by the separation or death of a parent or a disastrous marriage relationship. Battered wives, because they are treated so badly by one they trusted, may have this happen to them.

The Toddler Period: A Sense of Autonomy

The developmental task of the toddler years (12 months to 3 years) is that of gaining a sense of autonomy or independence. It is shown clearly in toddler actions—temper tantrums, foot stomping, shouting "no"—actions that show the child has just glimpsed himself as a person independent of his parent, able to do things for himself.

Just as people do not learn to do many new tasks without practice, toddlers cannot learn to be independent without practice or making some mistakes. They insist on putting on their own clothes and get their shoes on the wrong feet. They insist on winding a toy themselves and break it. They insist they do not need a nap and fall asleep at the dinner table with their food half eaten.

It takes patience to be the parent of a toddler, but if a child is given opportunities to try new things, he learns to be comfortable in his ability to go and do. If he is constantly stopped from doing, he learns, instead of autonomy, a feeling of doubt, or little confidence in his ability to do things.

A sense of autonomy is necessary for a person to parent; rearing children calls for making many decisions every day. Being able to make a decision is part of being independent; being able to stand by a decision is part of being independent. Standing by decisions leads to consistency and helping children to learn trust in the infant period.

Taking care of a new baby means doing tasks never attempted before. A sense of autonomy allows a mother to try things she has never done before. Without it, she can become overwhelmed by new responsibility.

During a child's growing years, a father may find that he has to change his place of employment. A sense of autonomy allows him to take on a new job, even in a new city or country, without being overwhelmed.

Children learn a sense of autonomy by being permitted to make decisions. A sense of autonomy is strengthened at any point in life by exposure to decision making. Many new parents need help with decision making about their baby's care in the first few days of the child's life or help strengthening a sense of autonomy at this critical point.

The Preschool Period: A Sense of Initiative

The developmental task of the preschool period (3 to 5 years) is that of developing a sense of initiative or of learning how to do things. The child requires ample opportunity to try new things. He needs play materials that can be arranged or molded into many different shapes and forms. Just as decision making is learned as part of learning independence, problem solving is learned as part of a sense of initiative. At no other time in a child's life is his imagination at a higher peak than during these years. At no other time in life is he able to suggest so many ways of completing a task.

The ability to solve problems is an excellent prerequisite for parenthood. It allows a parent to adapt to changes in the child as he grows from an infant who likes to be held and rocked to a toddler who would much rather be down and doing things on his own, from a preschooler who enjoys new experiences to a school-age child who likes to follow rules.

A parent with a poor sense of initiative may be upset by the number of problems any one day of child rearing poses. The newborn period, when everything is new and different from what she is used to, may be extremely difficult if she does not have a strong sense of initiative or an ability to discover alternative routes or solutions to problems.

Pregnancy, because it involves so many changes, may be very difficult for the parent who cannot solve problems.

School Age: A Sense of Industry

A sense of industry or accomplishment is the developmental goal of the school-age period. Learning a sense of initiative is learning how to do things; learning a sense of industry is learning how to do things well.

A 3- or 4-year-old tackles a project energetically and enthusiastically, but his finished product may look little like what he said in the beginning he was going to make. The edges are raw and unfinished. He does not care. He has created. A school-age child is much more concerned that his project look as he projected. He asks, "Is it all right?" and often adds despairingly, "I do sloppy work."

Achieving a sense of industry is also the ability to learn how to stick with a task until it is done. A parent needs a sense of industry because what he has undertaken—child rearing—is not a transient task but one of the longest he will ever assume, one that lasts 18 to 21 years. That takes a lot of "sticking-to-it."

Having a strong sense of industry is what allows parents to achieve in the working world. Achieving at an occupation gives the parent a strong financial base, and at least some financial base is necessary for child rearing.

Parents without a strong sense of industry may be unable to hold steady jobs and so may move frequently during the child's growing years, creating a potential source of insecurity in the child. They may be ineffective parents in teaching responsibility to a child, enthusiastic about their child's making a hockey team, for example, but not willing to follow through with driving the child to practice. Many of the things a child learns during his growing years are learned by watching the people who are important to him and imitating and adopting what they think is important. It takes an independent person to teach independence, a creative one to teach creativity, a steady, dependable person to teach how to stay with a job until it is finished. Role modeling on how to complete jobs (a sense of industry) is significant in preparing children for their own adult roles in life.

Adolescence: A Sense of Identity

The developmental task of the adolescent period is that of learning a sense of identity (Fig. 6-1) or of knowing who you are. This is a particularly difficult task to achieve because the adolescent's body is changing rapidly. He literally is not the same person one week that he was the week before.

An adolescent is able to list the many people he is—a son, a student, a scout, a paperboy, a grandchild, a club member—and he has to learn how to integrate all these roles into one person.

He begins a day thinking that he is quite handsome, only to look in a mirror and discover that his face is covered with red papules. A girl thinks of herself as petite, only to find when she lines up in gym class that her rapid growth over the summer has made her one of the tallest girls in the class. She thinks of herself as almost mature, but her parents insist on making her decisions, such as whether she should go on vacation with the family or not. How, out of all the contradictions around her, can she find out who she is?

There are four main areas in which an adolescent must make gains in order to achieve a sense of identity: accepting a changed body image, establishing what kind of person to be, making a career decision, and gaining emancipation from parents.

BODY IMAGE

The child who has a strong sense of trust, autonomy, initiative, and industry (is able to trust people, be independent, solve problems, and concentrate on a task) is best equipped to deal with the change in body image that occurs with puberty.

A sense of trust allows a girl to believe that even if she is "ugly" and ungainly she will still be loved for what is inside her. A sense of autonomy helps her to function without total dependence on what her peers are telling her about herself. Ability to solve problems allows her to select clothing or activities that complement rather than distract from her new growth.

Girls may have difficulty accepting breast development if they have been led to believe that "nice girls don't do conspicuous things." They may limit their social contacts or attempt to slouch continually to hide what is happening to them. Their self-esteem is low. Girls who have late development or little breast development have the same low self-esteem. It is hard to trust yourself to say the right things if one part of your body has betrayed you, because other parts may also betray you.

A girl who has trouble living with her new body because it has changed from the way it was in childhood will have an even more difficult time with body image if she becomes pregnant. That accepting the changing body image in pregnancy is a problem for any woman is reflected in pregnant women's frequent questions about the weight they are gaining and their concern in the postpartal period with losing weight and attempting to fit back into prepregnancy clothing.

WHAT KIND OF PERSON?

Deciding who you are or what kind of person you will be (a miser, a philanthropist, a creator, a destroyer, a religious person, a nonreligious person, a caring person, a noncaring person) is an internal development. Adolescents spend a lot of time talking with each other about how people reacted in a situation and how they would have reacted differently to see if the reaction of the person they are describing "fits" them, if they are that kind of person.

A preliminary step to discovering who you are is

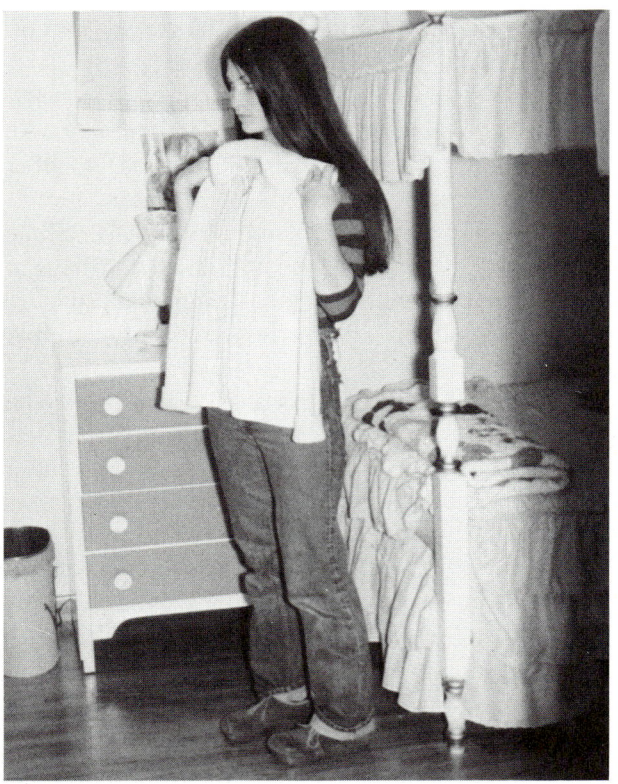

Fig. 6-1. Readiness for childbearing means thinking of oneself as a woman and no longer as a child.

that of discovering who you are *not*. Adolescent girls typically form cliques—groups of girls who talk alike, dress alike, think alike—and exclude anyone who talks differently, thinks differently, or dresses differently. This action appears cruel, and many adults remember their adolescence as years of nothing but heartbreak because they were always excluded. It is not so much cruel, however, as developmental, part of knowing who you are. You are like the girls who dress like you; you are *not* like those who dress differently.

Some adolescents are forced into joining boys or girls they really would not have chosen to associate with, except that they are excluded from other associations. Some evidence acting-out or delinquent behavior because being known as the terror of the block is better than not being known at all (having no identity).

In order to be a parent and guide a child into deciding who he or she is, a person first needs to know who *he or she* is. Pregnancy is difficult to accept if a girl and boy are still adolescents. Suddenly, on top of trying to decide what kind of persons they are, they are expecting a baby. These people have had an identity thrust upon them—that of a parent. For an adolescent, this identity often carries suggestions of being a bad person, or at least an immoral one, and on top of their other problems, it creates a role that is very difficult to handle.

MAKING A CAREER DECISION

Part of deciding what kind of person you are is deciding what type of job you want to do in life. People identify strongly with their occupations. To the question "What are you?" people rarely answer, "A good person, a mother, a conscientious person"; they answer, "A nurse, an accountant, a housewife."

Because career decisions must be made from such a wide range of choices today, career choice becomes more and more difficult. Because most occupations require education, decision making about a career has to be done in the adolescent years. Parents of children are not very helpful about giving guidance in this area. In a world so changed since they were adolescents the advice that was sound then may no longer be relevant.

Before a person becomes a parent, it is helpful if he or she has made a career decision. This lays the foundation for when and how he is going to live and adds stability to a family unit.

Although pregnant adolescents cannot be excluded from school because of their condition, pregnancy is certain to have some influence on their education. Many girls drop out of school once they are pregnant (they are excluded from their group because they are different). With little education, their income potential will be severely limited just at a time when they need more income than the average person their age because they have a child.

EMANCIPATION FROM PARENTS

Gaining independence from parents is often difficult from two standpoints: Parents may not be willing to grant independence yet, and the child is not really sure that he wants to be totally independent. Part of adolescent struggle is related not so much to doing adult things but to struggling for the right to do them. An adolescent, for example, may fight for the right to stay out until midnight on school nights, then, having won the privilege, never use it. Winning the battle is more important than what the battle is about.

Adolescents who are pregnant may do the same thing in prenatal visits. They may fight for the right to weigh themselves, then ask to have their weight rechecked.

As a rule, the closer the parent-child relationship, the more intense will be the struggle to gain independence. A child who has no close ties to his parents can merely walk away. The adolescent who loves his parents has difficulty severing the bond between them.

An adolescent may need some help in understanding that being independent from parents does not mean having to stop loving them; it simply means he must stop depending on them to meet all his needs. Relationships formed as equals can be more lasting and deeper than those of daughter and parent or son and parent.

Before people become parents, it helps if they have gained independence from their own parents. One of the mental tasks of pregnancy for a woman is making a mental switch from thinking of herself as a daughter at the beginning of pregnancy to thinking of herself as a mother at the end. If she is still a daughter, living at home, it may take longer than the nine months of pregnancy to complete this task, so she may not be ready for child rearing at the end of the pregnancy.

Young Adulthood: A Sense of Intimacy

With young adulthood comes the developmental task of achieving a sense of intimacy. The ability to form intimate relationships is strongly correlated with the sense of trust built in the infancy period. If an infant is unable to form a sense of trust, he may be unable to interact with others or develop deep enough connec-

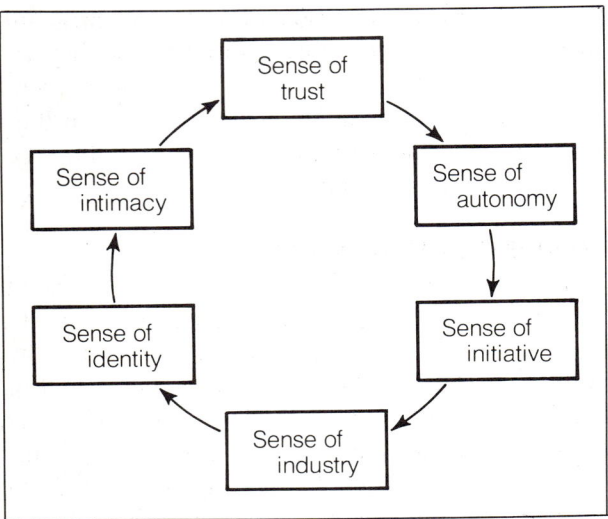

Fig. 6-2. Developmental tasks as the basis for lasting relationships.

tions with them to serve as the basis for lasting relationships. The relationship of developmental tasks is shown in Fig. 6-2.

Most sexual relationships between adolescents are built not on a sense of intimacy but on sexual attraction. Those built on sexual attraction (puppy love) are searing in their intensity and in the hurt that occurs when the relationship crumbles. It takes adolescents a number of such relationships before they learn that other values, such as kindness, companionship, and common interests, have to be involved in a relationship to make it last.

Acquiring a sense of intimacy means also being able to form lasting relationships with members of the same sex. Anticipating others' needs at a particular time is part of a sense of intimacy. People who have achieved this ability have many close friends or support people. This is important for beginning child rearing, as everything at that point is so new and different that support is necessary.

It is unfortunate when adolescents become parents before a sense of intimacy is achieved. A relationship built on less than that will not be able to stand the rigors of child rearing. A parent needs support people derived from firm relationships at the time of the birth of a child, when a child is ill or hurt, and during many of the expected crises of everyday developmental happenings with children.

The Middle Years: A Sense of Generativity

Although many young couples begin having children while they are adolescents still struggling with a sense of identity, others begin having children while they are struggling to achieve a sense of intimacy in young adulthood. Still others wait until closer to middle adult years to start their families. Many women have their last child as middle-aged adults.

Some people assume that, once they have reached adulthood, the way they are is the way they will always be. They are surprised to see their bodies change (men become bald; women and men both gain weight); they are unprepared for the developmental task of middle adult life, that of achieving a sense of generativity. *Generativity* means moving away from oneself to become involved with the world or community. The activities of middle-aged adults reflect generativity: being members of committees and clubs, supporting Little League teams, being block parents.

Peck and Berkowitz [10] have enumerated four subdevelopmental steps that must be taken by the middle-aged adult, not unlike those of the adolescent: increasing self-esteem through self-awareness, separating from parents and children, reviewing his or her value system and changing or reinforcing it, and initiating plans for the future that take into consideration the aging process.

The woman who finds herself pregnant during her middle adult years may have a hard time adjusting to the pregnancy because she has difficulty completing these steps. Her self-esteem may be lowered (she worries that she looks foolish being pregnant "at her age"). She has to face the fact that she will soon be separated from her parents (parents die) but she cannot even begin to consider separating from this child for another 18 years. It is difficult for her to review her value system and change it because it cannot change. She is still a mother, her husband a father. Nothing is changing for them. It is difficult to initiate new plans for the future. The future will go on much like the past in diapers, school plays, high-school proms.

To other women, having a baby at midlife is a joyous event, a last chance to remain young, to have what they thought was over. Each mother's reaction to having a baby during her middle adult years needs to be evaluated individually so that it can be determined whether she accepts the pregnancy as a positive or a negative step in her life.

Older Age: A Sense of Integrity

Few people in the older age category are seen in maternal-newborn settings, as they are past their childbearing years. Many couples have parents or grandparents, however, who are in this age group, so this age group's influence is felt strongly in maternal-newborn settings.

The developmental task of older age is to achieve a sense of satisfaction with what you are. Most people are able to do this by looking back over their lives and realizing that they made some mistakes (they should have bought a house sooner in life; they should have finished college) but overall they have accomplished a great deal (have made a marriage partner happy for forty or more years, have parented children who are responsible adults).

For some older people, having a grandchild or a great-grandchild is the final assurance they need that they have been successful in life. A grandmother's suggestions to a granddaughter (bathe the baby in oil, not water; protect the umbilical cord with a binder) is information a grandmother offers not only to ensure the safety and well-being of the child but also to make the event real to herself, to bring herself to a final life step, or to form a sense of integrity. Rejecting this type of information in the light of this situation is very difficult for granddaughters to do, even after you have pointed out that the advice is old-fashioned and no longer considered appropriate.

The Process of Achieving Maturity

When civilizations were simpler, physical maturity and developmental maturity occurred close together. Today, when many young people stay in school until they are at least 21 years old and therefore are dependent on parents until that age, they may achieve physical maturity five years or more before they have the necessary developmental maturity to use their physical readiness wisely.

Just as physical maturity occurs at different ages (some girls have their first menstrual period as early as 9, some as late as 17, yet both groups are normal), so developmental maturity occurs at different ages. Everyone knows a person who, although chronologically mature, still functions as an adolescent.

It is difficult to plan interventions that are constructive in helping people reach physical milestones more quickly. There *are* interventions to facilitate developmental maturity and readiness to be effective parents. Assessing whether people are developmentally ready to be parents, therefore, is a nursing function in pregnancy. Being certain that people are ready to be parents protects both the physical and the mental health of the next generation. Because each generation lays the groundwork for the next generation, no other nursing intervention may be so far-reaching as that aimed at helping people to be better parents.

STEPS OF INTERVENTION

If parents seem to be lacking in a developmental stage of growth, some constructive intervention can be accomplished during pregnancy or the days immediately post partum.

A Sense of Trust

Helping women to strengthen a sense of trust is important during pregnancy because only by having a sense of trust can one effectively transmit it to others. Being a trustworthy person—that is, being certain that if you tell a woman in labor that you are going to leave her for a few minutes and then coming back after only a few minutes, promising a woman in a prenatal clinic that you will see her at the next visit and then making every effort to be there, telling a woman after delivery that you will review her prenatal instructions with her the next day and making sure that you remember to do it—means acting in ways that demonstrate trustworthiness. Explaining procedures to patients, anticipating events so there are no surprises, taking the time to reassure—all are good examples of trustworthiness.

Rubin [13] stresses that if a woman is touched in labor and has her needs met the first few days post partum she is more likely to handle her infant kindly and attempt to meet his needs than if she is left alone in labor and advanced to total independence too quickly after delivery.

A Sense of Autonomy

Some new parents are exceedingly anxious in the newborn period. They worry that their sense of autonomy or their ability to make decisions, in relation to caring for their child, is inadequate. They fear that they will not know whether the child has had enough to eat or whether he is sick. Letting parents make decisions in the first few days after birth (allow some time for just resting and reassurance) helps to strengthen their confidence in their ability to make decisions. Asking "Do you think it's warm enough for the baby to be without a blanket?" is asking for a small decision but it helps to build practice in making choices about baby care.

Women need to be reassured when they have made a good decision. Many women call prenatal clinics or offices reporting minor discomforts of pregnancy. The statement "That always happens during pregnancy; don't worry about it" is correct, but not as therapeutic as "That is something that often happens in pregnancy; it's nothing to worry about but you were wise to call and check because you weren't certain." The second response reinforces the woman's ability to make decisions even if the decision she made (she was ill) was wrong.

Some women make poor decisions during pregnancy about their own health and in the newborn period about their child because they are not knowledgeable enough about changes in pregnancy or newborns to make good decisions. Providing women with information through classes or one-to-one discussion goes a long way toward making decision making easier.

A Sense of Initiative

People cannot solve problems unless they know the options available to them. Patient education, therefore, is important in helping people to strengthen a sense of initiative.

It is usually helpful to women during pregnancy to review with them some problems you can anticipate they will be facing as pregnancy progresses: How are finances to be reallocated when the woman stops work? Where is a baby going to sleep in a one-bedroom apartment? How is a mother of six children, having her seventh, going to find time for a rest period each day? After the birth of the child, it is advisable to review with women their plans for the first days at home. Does the woman have anyone to help her to keep her from becoming exhausted? If she lives in a two-story house and is not supposed to go up and down stairs more than once a day for the first week, how is she going to manage? In times of stress, thinking through problems is one of the most difficult things to do. Some women find themselves frozen in front of the refrigerator, unable to make even the simplest of choices, such as what meat to defrost for dinner. Having someone to listen to their plans and assure them that the plans sound sensible is always helpful. In many instances, the actual problem solving is not difficult. It is the step before that, getting to a concrete stage of thinking about the problem or realizing that there is one, that poses the obstacle.

Since a great deal of child rearing involves successful problem solving under stress, any practice in this area is helpful.

A Sense of Industry

It is often hard for women to feel that they are doing things well (sense of industry) during pregnancy because things change so from the beginning to the end of pregnancy that everything is always new; they barely feel comfortable with their body when it changes still more. Parents need reassurance in the newborn period that they are doing things well because, again, everything seems so new and unpracticed. Even women having their second, third, or fourth child have feelings of uncertainty with their newborn because this is their first experience with this child. Everyone, in his eagerness to teach, can easily find himself criticizing the things people are doing wrong and forgetting to comment on the things that are being done right. Being praised for things done right strengthens a sense of industry.

A Sense of Identity

Keeping a firm hold on a sense of identity can be very difficult during pregnancy as a woman evolves from one person at the beginning of pregnancy (a woman with no children or one or two children) to another person at the end of pregnancy (a mother of a child or two or three children).

Knowing what is likely to happen during pregnancy and in labor or delivery, knowing what a newborn will look like beforehand, is information that helps the woman anticipate change and adapt to it more readily. Patient education, again, becomes an important part of yet another developmental crisis.

Some young women develop a sense of identity for the first time during pregnancy. They did not know who they were before; now at least they know they are about to be mothers. Statements such as "I hope I can manage with three under three," or "I can't believe that in just three more weeks I'll be a mother" show that the woman is role-playing her new identity. They need to be recognized and discussed so that the sense of identity can be strengthened during pregnancy.

A Sense of Intimacy

Women do not feel instinctive rushes of affection toward newborn babies in many instances. They need assurance that emotions labeled "a strange feeling" or "scared" are much more common in women in the first few days of their child's life.

A great deal of learning how to hold a newborn securely, how to do the "motherly" motions of jiggling, rocking, or stroking is the result of role modeling or watching others. Handling the woman's baby in front of her, therefore, and pointing out positive characteristics of the child (his nose is cute, her hair is curly) help a woman strengthen a sense of intimacy.

A Sense of Generativity

Many women resent a child born to them late in life because they view the child as totally changing their life-style or forcing them to continue a life-style they were ready to change. Exploring with a woman ways she can continue a career or community service and still be pregnant or care for a newborn can help her to realize that at this time in life she can achieve the best of two worlds, that it might be possible for her to participate actively in her club by addressing envelopes or making phone calls at home as her activity rather than spending days as a volunteer away from home. This type of planning is sensible and will strengthen her sense of generativity or the developmental phase the older woman may be entering as she has her last child.

Assessing Readiness for Child Rearing

Assessment of a couple's readiness for child rearing is an important nursing assessment during pregnancy. Examples of SOAP progress notes written on three women who might be seen in prenatal settings follow.

Problem-oriented Recording: Progress Notes

Christine McFadden
15 years
First prenatal visit (LMP 16 weeks ago)

Problem: Developmental readiness for childbearing

> S. 15 years old; junior in high school. Maintains a B average; swims on girls' varsity team. Has taken responsibility for 5-year-old sister after school since she was 12 (parents own delicatessen and both work). States, "I didn't mean to get pregnant but having a baby will be more fun to take care of than a 5-year-old." Has not told father of child (a high school senior) or her own parents of possibility of pregnancy yet. States, "Parents will be wild." No plans for abortion: "I couldn't hurt a baby."
> O. Appears older than 15; adult conversation patterns.
> A. Developmental immaturity due to age 15 and current status as a student in school.
>
> Goals: a. Able to discuss how child will change her life other than being "fun."
> b. To remain in school throughout pregnancy; return to school after delivery.
> c. Establish workable relationship with parents.
> d. Clarify the relationship she wants to have with father of child.
>
> P. 1. Discuss how pregnancy may cause changes in friends and family.
> 2. Discuss how pregnancy may change dietary or social life-style.
> 3. Urge to tell father of child and parents about pregnancy.
> 4. Later in pregnancy after adaptation is improved, discuss child rearing plans and need for help with baby care.

Problem-oriented Recording: Progress Notes

Mary Kraft
22 years
First prenatal visit (LMP 9 weeks ago)

Problem: Developmental readiness for childbearing

> S. Lives with husband in 2-bedroom apartment. Husband has full-time job as high school English teacher; she works part-time in the public library. Has been planning on being pregnant since spontaneous loss of a pregnancy at 3 months, 2 years ago. Hasn't mentioned possibility of pregnancy to husband. States, "I can't believe I'm really pregnant." Finances adequate even without her job.
> O. Mature-mannered.
> A. Developmentally ready for childbearing and rearing.
>
> Goal: Discuss pregnancy with husband and family so that adaptation can begin (difficult until 3 months or time of previous miscarriage has passed).
>
> P. 1. Give reassurance that pregnancy is real if M.D. confirms.
> 2. Continue to assure that pregnancy is going well (as appropriate) at continued visits.

3. Provide discussion time at visits for worry over loss of last pregnancy to be voiced.
4. Discuss preparation for baby later in pregnancy after she is ready to accept pregnancy as real.

2. Observe for signs of depression, increased stress due to inappropriateness of childbearing for her now.
3. Later in pregnancy when adaptation is better, discuss plans for baby (physical space and finances may be problems).

Problem-oriented Recording: Progress Notes

Angie Baco
42 years
First prenatal visit (LMP 12 weeks ago)

Problem: Developmental readiness for childbearing

S. Lives with husband and 4 children (19, 17, 15, and 7). Seven-year-old has learning disability; special classroom at school. Husband has full-time job as construction worker. Finances "okay, but not great." Patient wasn't planning on becoming pregnant (contraception failure). States, "I'm too old for diapers again. My daughter just had a baby." Husband states, "I'll be retiring and this kid will still be in high school." Children's reactions vary from pleasure (the 17-year-old) to disbelief (the 15- and 7-year-olds) to disapproval (the 19-year-old). Religion precludes abortion as an option. States, "I'll just have it, that's all."
O. Appears tired; nervous mannerisms during interview.
A. Has passed developmental readiness for childbearing.

Goals: a. Discuss with family the reality of pregnancy and how this will affect family members.
b. Clarify in own mind what pregnancy means to her.

P. 1. Allow discussion time at visits for talk about how life is going to change.

References

1. Baldwin, W., and Cain, V. S. The children of teenage parents. *Fam. Plann. Perspect.* 12:34, 1980.
2. Cronenwett, L. R. Transition to Parenthood. In L. K. McNall and J. T. Galeener (Eds.). *Current Practice in Obstetric and Gynecologic Nursing*. St. Louis: Mosby, 1976.
3. Davis, B. O., and Flaherty, P. (Eds.). *Human Diversity: Its Causes and Social Significance*. Cambridge, Mass.: Ballinger, 1976.
4. Diekelmann, N. L. *Primary Health Care of the Well Adult*. New York: McGraw-Hill, 1977.
5. Erikson, E. *Childhood and Society* (2nd ed.). New York: Norton, 1964.
6. Hurlock, E. B. *Developmental Psychology* (4th ed.). New York: McGraw-Hill, 1975.
7. Johnson, N. L. Parenting education. *Health Educ.* 9:5, 1978.
8. Maclachlan, E. A., et al. Learning about children and family life. *Child. Today* 7:7, 1978.
9. Murphy, N. Training professionals to support and increase the competence of young parents. *J. Nurs. Educ.* 17:41, 1978.
10. Peck, R. F., and Berkowitz, H. Personality and Adjustment in Middle Age. In B. L. Neugarten (Ed.). *Personality in Middle and Late Life*. Englewood Cliffs, N.J.: Prentice-Hall, 1964.
11. Peters, E. N., and Hoekelman, R. A. A measure of maternal competence. *Health Serv. Res.*, 88:523, 1973.
12. Romney, S. L., et al. *Gynecology and Obstetrics: The Health Care of Women*. New York: McGraw-Hill, 1975.
13. Rubin, R. Maternal touch. *Nurs. Outlook* 11:828, 1963.
14. Sheehy, G. *Passages: Predictable Crises of Adult Life*. New York: Dutton, 1974.
15. Smith, D., et al. Toward improvements in parenting. *J.O.G.N. Nurs.* 7:22, 1978.
16. Stranik, M. K., et al. Transition into parenthood. *Am. J. Nurs.* 79:90, 1979.

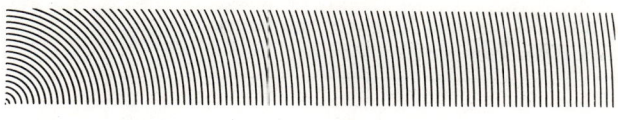

7. Physical Readiness for Childbearing

Readiness for childbearing has both physical and psychosocial aspects. Physically, a woman must have mature endocrine function, ovaries and a uterus mature enough to initiate ovulation and sustain a pregnancy, and pelvic formation large enough to provide a sufficient-sized birth canal. If she wishes to breast-feed she must have mature breast development.

Men must have endocrine and organ maturity enough to cause formation of spermatozoa, and they must have ejaculatory ability.

Development at Puberty

In early life, the uterus is extremely small, about the size of an olive, and its proportions are reversed from what they are later on; the cervix is the largest portion of the organ. At about 8 years of age, an increase in the size of the uterus begins. The maximum increase in size does not occur until about 17 years of age, a fact that probably helps account for the low-birth-weight babies typically born to adolescent girls.

The mechanism that initiates sexual development is not well understood. One theory is that a girl must reach a critical weight of about 95 pounds before the hypothalamus is "triggered" to send initial stimulation to the anterior pituitary gland to begin gonadotrophic hormone formation [4].

THE ROLE OF ANDROGEN

In males, androgenic hormones are produced by both the adrenal cortex and the testes; in the female, by the adrenal cortex and possibly the ovaries. It is difficult to distinguish male from female fetuses in the early days of development. It is the production of testosterone, an androgenic hormone secreted by the male testes, that appears to make the difference in whether male or female sex characteristics develop.

At puberty, the androgenic hormones are responsible for muscular development, physical growth, and an increase in sebaceous gland secretions causing typical acne in both boys and girls. The level of testosterone is low in males until puberty (about 11 to 13 years), when it rises to influence the development of testes, scrotum, penis, prostate, and seminal vesicles, the appearance of male pubic, axillary, and facial hair, laryngeal enlargement and its accompanying voice change, and maturation of spermatozoa.

In girls, testosterone influences enlargement of the labia majora and clitoris and formation of axillary and pubic hair.

The end products of androgenic hormones are excreted in urine as 17-ketosteroids. Testing for urinary 17-ketosteroids is therefore an often ordered test of sexual maturity. Under 10 years of age, there is usually little present in urine. Twelve-year-olds excrete about 1 mg of 17-ketosteroids a day; adolescent females 5 to 14 mg per day; adolescent males 8 to 22 mg per day.

THE ROLE OF ESTROGEN

At puberty, the hypothalamus stimulates the anterior pituitary gland to begin secreting gonadotropic hormones, chief of which is follicle-stimulating hormone (FSH). FSH causes maturation of ovarian follicles in females. Ovarian follicles secrete a high level of estrogen, which is actually not one substance but several compounds (chiefly B-estradiol and estrone). It can be considered a single substance, however, in terms of action.

The increase in estrogen level in the female at puberty influences the development of the uterus, fallopian tubes, and vagina, typical female fat distribution and hair patterns, breast development, and an end to growth as it closes epiphyseal lines of long bones.

In the male, estrogen initiates the production of spermatozoa.

SECONDARY SEX CHARACTERISTICS

The stage of sexual development that an adolescent has reached has been categorized by Tanner [8, 9]. A description of Tanner stages is shown in Table 7-1.

There is a wide variation of times that adolescents move through these developmental stages. Any schoolroom reveals a wide difference in the amount of maturity evident in the children.

In girls, pubertal changes typically occur in the following order: (1) growth spurt, (2) increase in the transverse diameter of the pelvis, (3) breast development, (4) growth of pubic and axillary hair, and (5) vaginal secretions. Menstruation usually begins between the time a girl develops pubic hair and the time she develops axillary hair. Menarche (the first menstrual period) may occur as early as age 9 or as late as age 17 and still be within a normal age range. Pubertal changes in girls are shown in Fig. 7-1.

In boys, pubertal changes typically take place in the order of (1) growth spurt, (2) increase in size of genitalia, (3) hypertrophy of breast tissue, (4) growth of pubic, axillary, facial, and chest hair, (5) deepening voice, and (6) production of spermatozoa. Puberty changes, as a whole, occur later in boys than in girls, the age range being about 12 to 16 years.

Time sequences for developmental changes are shown in Fig. 7-2.

Some girls seen at prenatal clinics are afraid they are pregnant because their menstrual periods started

Table 7-1. Tanner Stages of Secondary Sex Characteristic Development

Boys	
Stage I	Genital size the same as childhood; no distinction between the hair on penis and over the abdomen.
Stage II	Initial enlargement of scrotum and testes; there is reddening and beginning rugae of scrotal skin; there is sparse growth of long, straight, slightly pigmented hair at base of penis.
Stage III	Penis begins to enlarge in length; scrotum becomes more rugated; hair is darker and coarser and curly.
Stage IV	There is increased size of penis; pubic hair is adult in type.
Stage V	Penis, testes, and scrotum are adult in size and shape; facial and axillary hair as well as pubic hair is present.
Girls	
Stage I	Only slight elevation of the nipple; no distinction between pubic and abdominal hair.
Stage II	Breast bud is present; areola is noticeable; there is sparse growth of long, straight hair at pubic area.
Stage III	The breast nipple and areola further increase in size and pigmentation of the areola is obvious; pubic hair is darker, coarser, and curly.
Stage IV	There is projection of breast areola and nipple to form a secondary mound; pubic hair is adult in type.
Stage V	Breasts and pubic hair are adult in type; axillary and some facial hair is present.

Source: J. M. Tanner, *Growth at Adolescence* (2nd ed.). Oxford, England: Blackwell, 1962.

regularly for two or three months, then became irregular or appeared to have stopped. If they are sexually active, they need to have a pregnancy test done to rule out pregnancy, but irregular menstrual periods are the rule rather than the exception for the first year. The reason is that menstrual periods tend to be anovulatory for the first year.

Female Internal Reproductive Organs

Female internal reproductive organs are shown in Fig. 7-3. They are the ovaries, the fallopian tubes, the uterus, and the vagina.

THE OVARIES

The ovaries (the female gonads) are about 4 by 2 cm and are the size and shape of almonds. They are grayish white in color and appear pitted on the surface.

They are suspended in the pelvis by two ligaments, the utero-ovarian and the infundibulopelvic ligaments. The first of these two ligaments attaches the ovary loosely to the body of the uterus; the second attaches it to the pelvic sidewall. The ovary is further held in its suspended position by lying in close contact with the fimbriated end of the fallopian tube and the posterior surface of the broad ligament. The ovaries are unique among pelvic structures in that they are not covered by a layer of peritoneum. Because they are not encased this way, ova can escape from them and enter the uterus by way of the fallopian tubes.

Ovaries have two principal divisions: a layer of surface epithelium and the inner cortex filled with connective tissue. It is in the cortex that immature (primordial) follicles which will mature into ova grow. This layer of tissue contains a rich supply of nerve fibers and blood vessels to supply the growing cells.

The function of the ovaries is to produce, mature, and discharge ova. In the process, estrogen and progesterone are produced. If ovaries are removed prior to puberty (or are nonfunctional), the uterus and breasts will not mature at puberty and hair distribution will assume a more male pattern than is normal. After menopause, or cessation of ovarian function, the uterus and breasts undergo atrophy. Ovarian function, therefore, is necessary for maturation and maintenance of secondary sex characteristics in females.

THE FALLOPIAN TUBES

A fallopian tube arises from each corner of the uterus and extends outward and backward so that each open distal end lies next to the broad ligament and an ovary. Fallopian tubes are about 10 cm in length in a mature woman.

Although a fallopian tube is one smooth hollow tunnel, it can be anatomically divided into four separate parts.

The *interstitial* portion is that part of the tube that lies within the uterine wall. This portion is only about 1 cm in length; the lumen of the tube is only about 1 mm in diameter at this point.

The *isthmus* is the next distal portion. It is, like the interstitial tube, extremely narrow. This segment is about 2 cm in length.

The *ampulla* is the longest portion of the tube. It is about 5 cm in length. It is in the ampullar portion that fertilization of an ovum usually takes place.

The *infundibular* portion is the most distal part of the tube. It is about 2 cm long and is funnel-shaped. The rim of the funnel is covered by fimbriated cells that help guide the ova into the fallopian tube.

The lining of the entire fallopian tube is comprised of mucous membrane, which contains both mucus secreting and ciliated cells. Beneath the mucous lining are connective tissue and a muscle layer supplied by blood from the ovarian artery and vein. The muscle of the tube helps produce peristaltic motions that conduct the ova the length of the tube. This migration of the ova is further aided by the action of the ciliated lining and the mucus, which acts as a lubricant. The mucus produced may also act as a source of nourishment for the fertilized egg; the mucus contains protein, water, and salts.

Because the fallopian tubes are open at the distal end, they provide a connection between the outside of the body and the peritoneum. That this protential pathway exists makes childbirth possible. It also leads to pelvic inflammatory disease if disease spreads from the external genital organs through the vagina and uterus to the tubes and the peritoneum.

The function of the fallopian tubes is to convey the ova from the ovaries to the uterus and to provide a place for fertilization of the ova by sperm.

THE UTERUS

The uterus is a hollow, muscular, pear-shaped organ located in the pelvis, posterior to the bladder and anterior to the rectum. It is about 5 to 7 cm long, 5 cm wide, and in its widest upper part 2.5 cm deep. A nonpregnant uterus weighs about 60 gm.

The uterus consists of three parts: the body, the isthmus, and the cervix (Fig. 7-4). The body of the uterus, or its uppermost part, forms the bulk of the uterus. The lining of the cavity is continuous with that of the fallopian tubes, which fuse at the upper aspects (the cornua). The portion of the uterus between the points of attachment of the fallopian tubes is the *fundus*. During pregnancy, the body of the uterus is the portion of the structure that contains the growing fetus.

The isthmus is a short segment between the body and the cervix. In the nonpregnant uterus it is only 1 to 2 mm in length. During pregnancy this portion enlarges greatly to aid in accommodating the growing fetus.

The cervix is the lowest portion of the uterus. It is 2 to 5 cm long. About half the cervix lies above the vagina; about half extends into the vagina. The cavity of the cervix is the cervical canal. The point where the canal begins at the isthmus is the *internal cervical os*; the distal opening is the *external cervical os*.

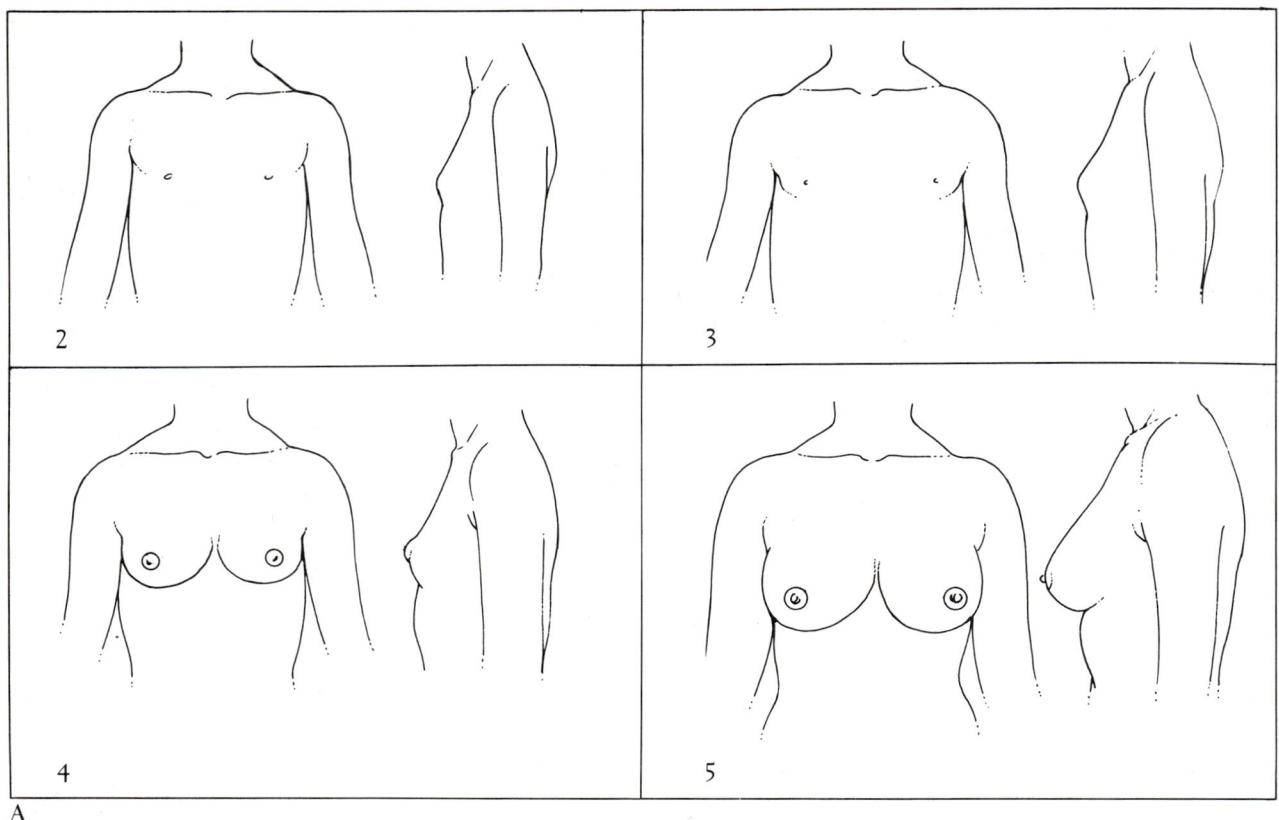

Uterine and Cervical Coats

The uterine wall is composed of three separate coats: an inner one of mucous membrane, a middle muscular layer, and a peritoneal sheath (Fig. 7-4). The mucous membrane lining the cervix is the *endocervix*; that lining the uterus is the *endometrium* (endothelium).

The endometrial layer of the uterus is important in terms of menstrual function and childbearing. It is composed of two layers of cells. The innermost layer, the basal layer, is not much influenced by hormones. The glandular layer is greatly influenced by the hormones estrogen and progesterone and is the layer that grows and becomes so thick and responsive that it is capable of supporting a pregnancy. If pregnancy does not occur, both layers are shed as the menstrual flow.

The endocervix, although continuous with the endometrium, is not affected in the same way by hormones. It provides a lubricated surface so that spermatozoa can readily enter the cervix. Because it secretes an alkaline fluid, it decreases the acidity of the upper vagina, ensuring sperm survival. During pregnancy the endocervix becomes plugged with mucus, which forms a seal to keep out ascending infections.

The lower third of the cervical canal is lined not with mucous membrane but with stratified squamous epithelium similar to that lining the vagina. Locating the point at which the tissue differentiates is important when one is helping with Papanicolaou smears (tests for cervical cancer) because this tissue interface is the most frequent place for cervical cancer to begin.

The *myometrium*, or muscle layer, is composed of three interwoven layers of smooth muscle. The muscle fibers run in longitudinal, transverse, and oblique directions. When the uterus contracts at the end of pregnancy to expel the fetus, equal pressure is exerted at all points throughout the cavity. Following childbirth, this interlacing network of muscle fibers constricts blood vessels coursing through the layers and limits loss of blood.

The parietal peritoneum serves as the outermost layer of the uterus. The function of the uterus is to receive the ovum from the fallopian tubes and provide a place for its growth should it be fertilized.

Uterine Supports

The uterus is suspended in the pelvic cavity by a number of ligaments. A single sheet of fascia (the *anterior* or *pubocervical ligament*) passes from the anterior surface of the cervix to fuse with the fascia covering the symphysis pubis. This anterior segment of fascia also supports the bladder. If it is overstretched

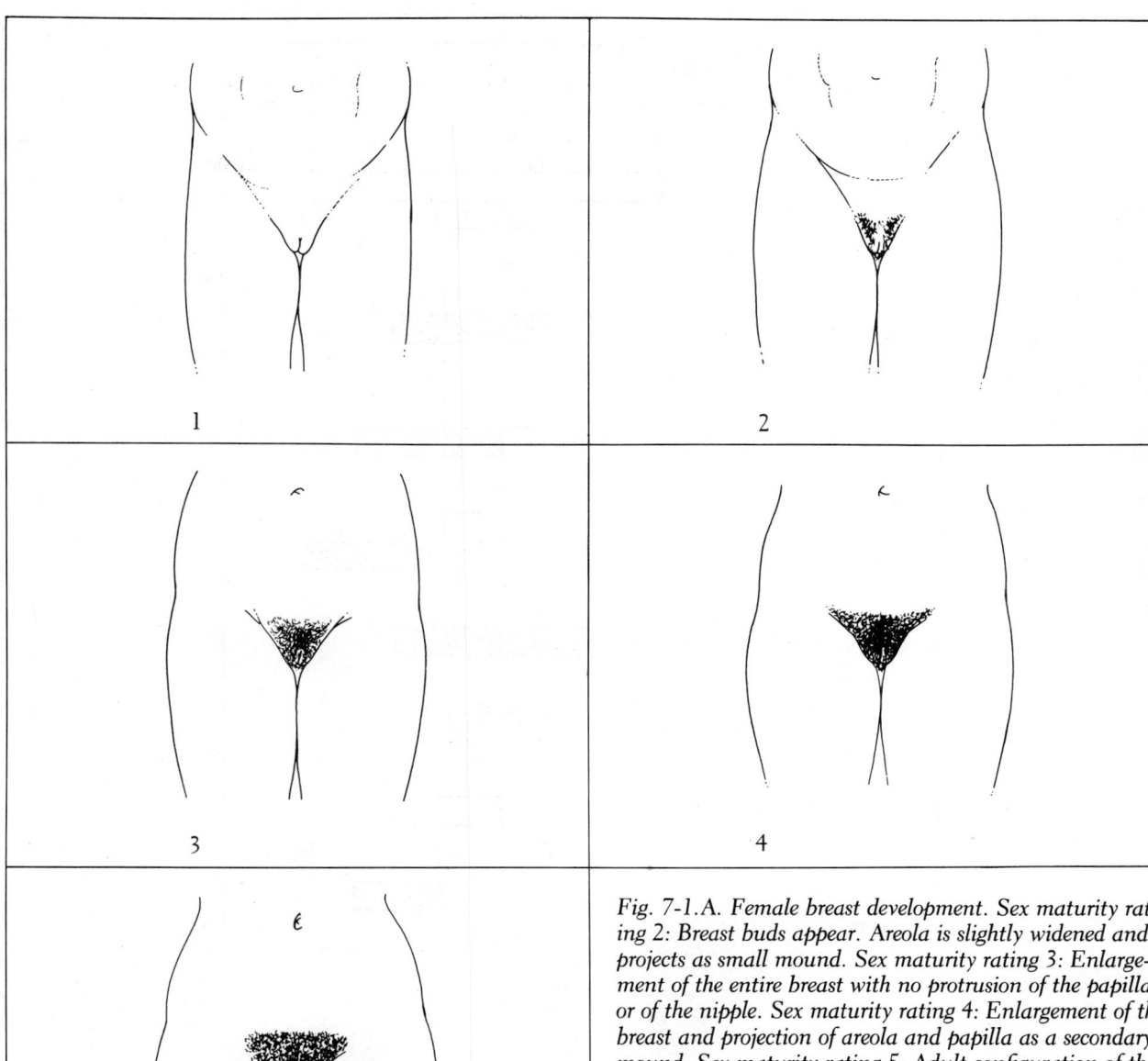

Fig. 7-1. A. Female breast development. Sex maturity rating 2: Breast buds appear. Areola is slightly widened and projects as small mound. Sex maturity rating 3: Enlargement of the entire breast with no protrusion of the papilla or of the nipple. Sex maturity rating 4: Enlargement of the breast and projection of areola and papilla as a secondary mound. Sex maturity rating 5: Adult configuration of the breast with protrusion of the nipple. Areola no longer projects separately from remainder of breast. B. Female pubic hair development. Sex maturity rating 1: Prepubertal. No pubic hair. Sex maturity rating 2: Straight hair is extending along the labia and between rating 2 and 3 begins on the pubis. Sex maturity rating 3: Pubic hair has increased in quantity, is darker and is present in the typical female triangle but in smaller quantity. Sex maturity rating 4: Pubic hair is more dense, curled, and adult in distribution but is less abundant. Sex maturity rating 5: Abundant, adult-type pattern. Hair may extend onto the medial aspect of the thighs. (From E. Fuller, A physician's guide to sexual maturity. Patient Care 13:122, 1979. Copyright © 1979, Patient Care Publications, Inc., Darien, Ct. All rights reserved.)

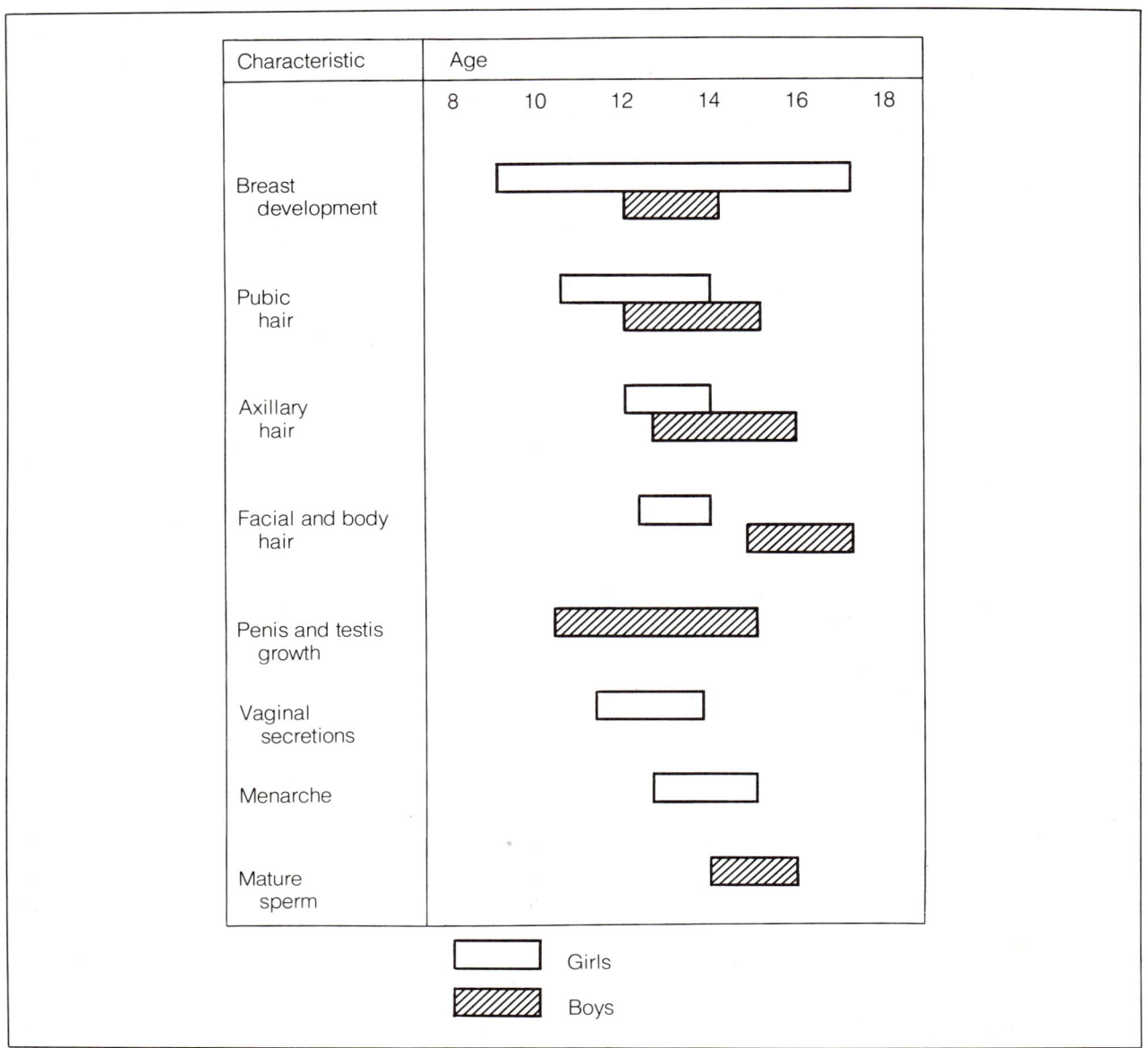

Fig. 7-2. Time sequences for developmental change.

during pregnancy, it may not support the bladder afterward and the bladder may sink into the anterior vagina (a cystocele) (Fig. 7-5A).

A fold of peritoneum behind the uterus is the *posterior ligament.* The posterior ligament forms a pouch (the cul-de-sac of Douglas) between the rectum and uterus. As this is the lowest point of the pelvis, pus or blood in the pelvis tends to collect in this space. The space can be examined for the presence of pus or blood by insertion of a culdoscope through the posterior vaginal wall (culdoscopy). Damage to support posterior to the uterus through childbearing may lead to a pouching of the rectum through the posterior vaginal wall (a rectocele) (Fig. 7-5B).

The broad ligaments are two folds of peritoneum, one covering the uterus at the front and one at the back and extending to the pelvic sides. The lower third of each ligament is composed of dense connective tissue. These are known as the cardinal ligaments because they form the main support for the uterus and, in addition, support blood vessels and nerves.

The round ligaments are two fibrous muscular cords that pass from the body of the uterus near the attachments of the fallopian tubes through the broad ligaments into the inguinal canal and insert into the fascia of the vulva. The round ligaments act as "stays" to steady the uterus. If a pregnant woman moves quickly, she may pull one of these ligaments and feel a quick, sharp pain that is frightening in its intensity.

The uterosacral ligament passes from the upper

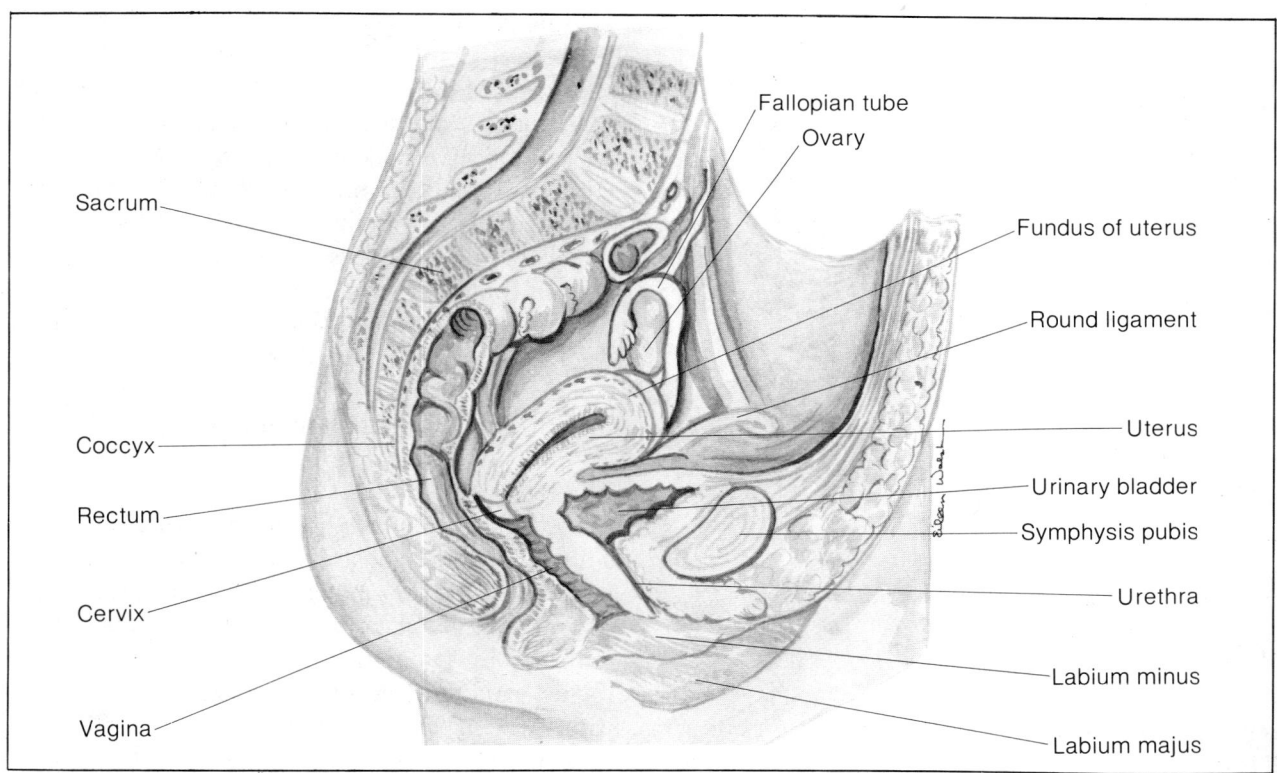

Fig. 7-3. Female internal reproductive organs.

Fig. 7-4. Anterior view of female reproductive organs showing relationship of fallopian tube and body of the uterus.

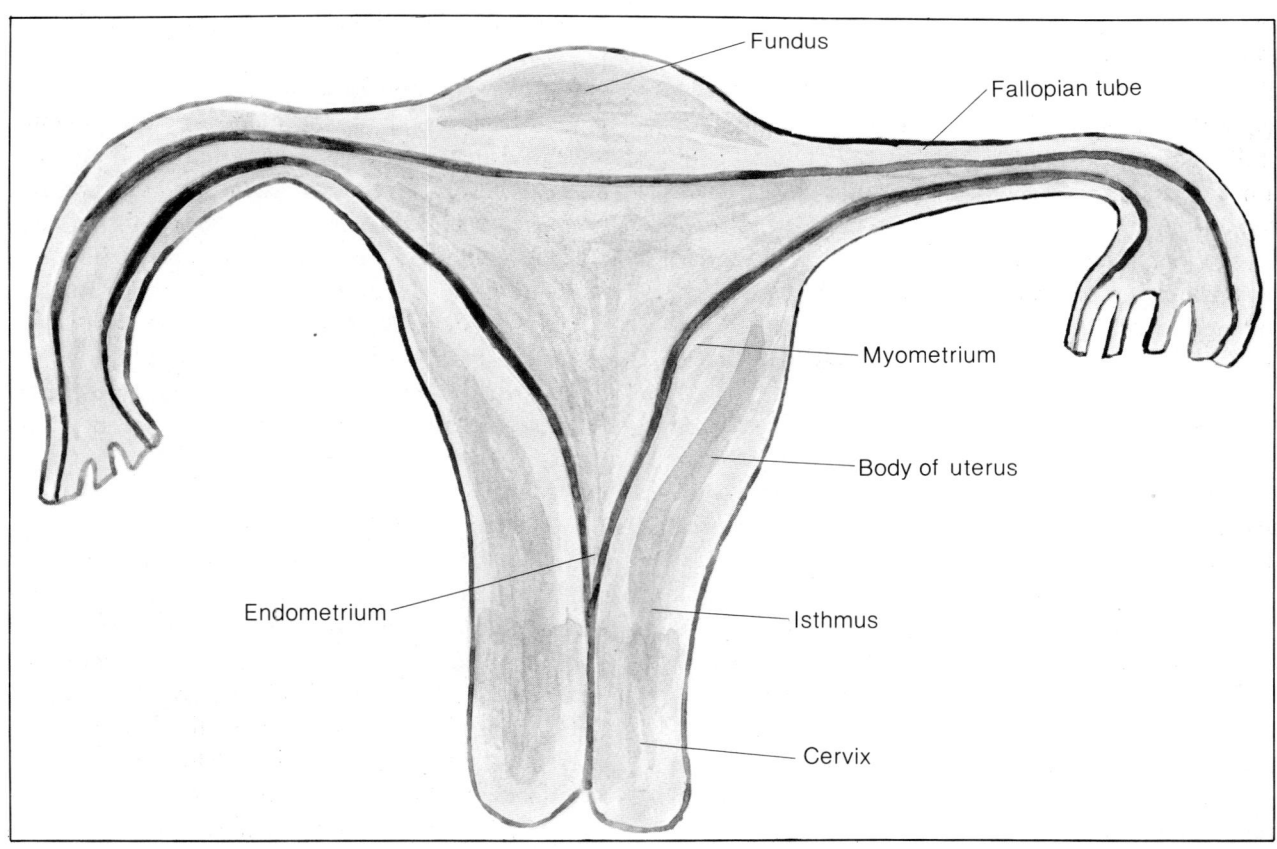

Physical Readiness for Childbearing 73

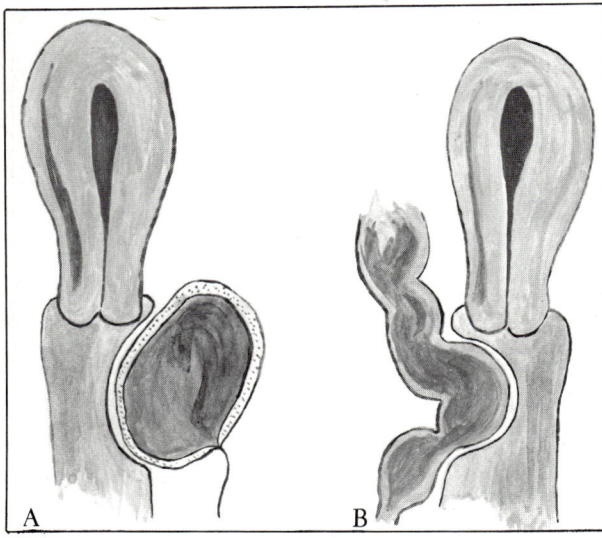

Fig. 7-5. A. Cystocele. The bladder has herniated into the anterior wall of the vagina. B. Rectocele. The posterior wall of the vagina is herniated.

cervix backward to fuse with the fascia of the sacrum. It counteracts the forward pull of the round ligaments.

That a uterus is a suspended, not a fixed, organ is important in childbearing. Because it is not fixed in one position, the uterus is free to enlarge without discomfort during pregnancy.

Uterine Blood Supply

The large abdominal aorta divides to form the two iliac arteries; main divisions of the iliac arteries are the hypogastric arteries. The uterine arteries are a division of the hypogastric arteries. Because the uterine blood supply is not far removed from the aorta, it is copious and adequate to supply the growing needs of a fetus. The ovarian artery is a direct subdivision of the aorta. After supplying the ovary with blood, the vessel joins the uterine artery, a fail-safe system to ensure that the uterus will have an adequate blood supply. The blood vessels that supply the cells and lining of the uterus are tortuous in nonpregnant women. As a uterus enlarges with pregnancy, the vessels "unwind" and so can stretch to maintain an adequate blood supply as the organ enlarges. The uterine veins follow the course of the arteries; they empty into the internal iliac veins.

The ureters from the kidneys pass directly in back of the ovarian vessels near the fallopian tubes; as shown in Fig. 7-6, they cross just beneath the uterine vessels before they enter the bladder. This close anatomical relationship has implications in surgery such as tubal ligations and hysterectomies because the ureter may be injured if bleeding must be controlled by clamping the uterine or ovarian vessels.

Uterine Nerve Supply

The uterus is affected by both afferent (sensory) and efferent (motor) nerves. The efferent (motor) nerves arise from T5 through T10 spinal ganglia. The afferent (sensory nerves) join the hypogastric plexus and enter the spinal column at T11 and T12. That sensory innervation from the uterus registers lower in the spinal column than does motor control has implications in controlling pain in labor. If an anesthetic solution is injected into the spinal column at a low point (L3 or L4), it will rise and stop the pain of uterine contractions (T11 and T12 level) without stopping motor control or contractions (the T5 to T10 level).

The Bicornuate Uterus

In the fetus, the uterus first forms with a septum or a fibrous division, longitudinally separating it into two portions. As the fetus matures, this septum disappears, so that typically at birth no remnant of the divison remains. In some women, the septum never atrophies, and the uterus remains as two smaller compartments. In others, half of the septum is still present. Still other women have oddly shaped "horns" at the junction of the fallopian tubes, a remnant of incomplete formation. All these malformations will decrease the ability to conceive to some extent and to carry a pregnancy to term. Some variations of uterine formation are shown in Fig. 7-7. The exact effects of these deviations are discussed in later chapters.

Uterine Version and Flexion

Ordinarily, the body of the uterus is tipped slightly forward. *Anteversion* is a condition in which the fundus is tipped very far forward. *Retroversion* means that the fundus is tipped back. *Anteflexion* means that the body of the uterus is bent sharply forward at the junction with the cervix. *Retroflexion* means that the body is bent sharply back. Extreme abnormal flexion or version positions may interfere with fertility as they may block the deposition or migration of sperm. Examples of abnormal uterine positions are shown in Fig. 7-8.

THE VAGINA

The vagina is a hollow muscular-membranous canal located posterior to the bladder and anterior to the rectum. It extends from the cervix of the uterus to the external vulva. When a woman is lying on her back, the course of the vagina is backward and downward.

Because of this downward slant, the length of the anterior wall of the vagina is about 6 to 7 cm long, the posterior wall 8 to 9 cm long. At the cervix end of the structure, there are recesses on all sides of the cervix.

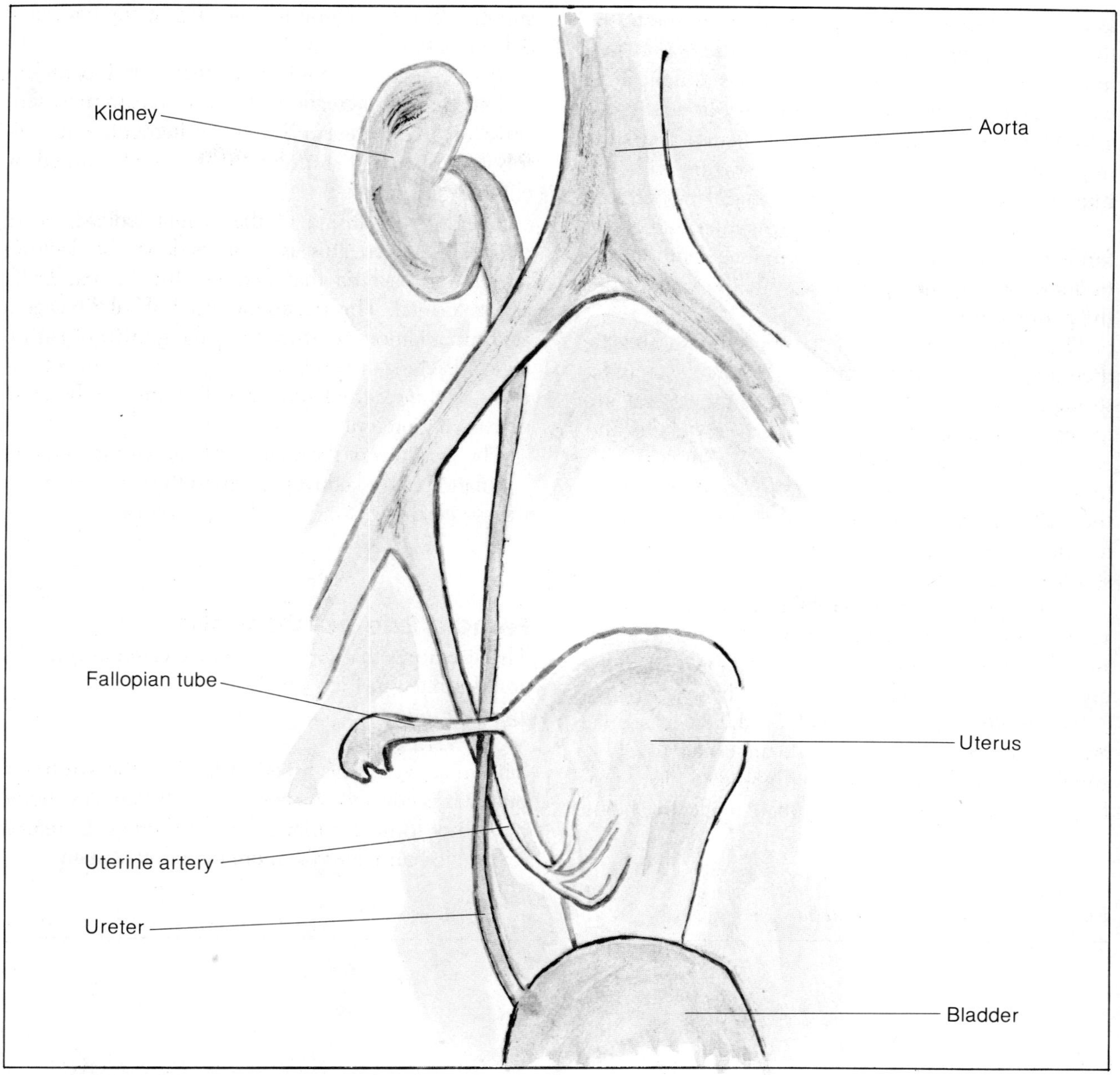

Fig. 7-6. Blood supply to the uterus.

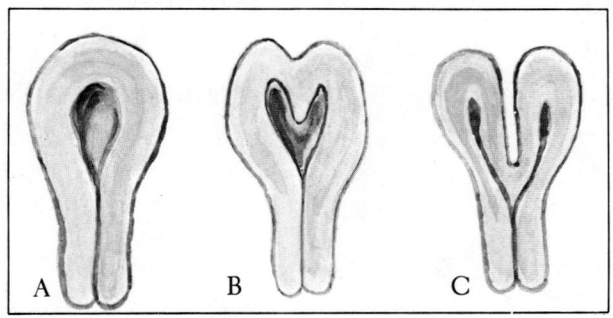

Fig. 7-7. A. Normal uterus. B. Bicornuate uterus. Abnormal shape of uterus allows less placenta implantation space. C. Septum dividing uterus.

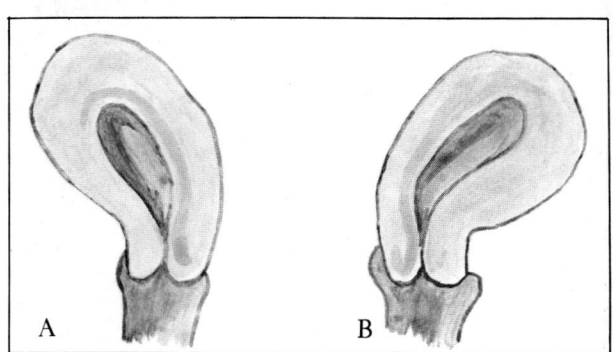

Fig. 7-8. Uterine flexion and version. A. Anteversion. B. Retroflexion.

Physical Readiness for Childbearing 75

Behind the cervix is the posterior fornix, at the front, the anterior fornix, and at the sides, the lateral fornices. That these recesses exist has implication whenever a woman is seen in a health care setting for self-induced abortion. An instrument such as a knitting needle, when pushed into the vagina with the intention of inserting it into the cervical os and disrupting a pregnancy, invariably penetrates one of the fornices instead and, rather than induce abortion, introduces pathogenic organisms from the vagina into the peritoneum.

The vagina is lined with stratified squamous epithelium. It has a middle connective tissue layer and a strong muscular wall. The walls of the vagina are folded, with rugae. Thus the vagina is very elastic and can expand at the end of pregnancy to allow a full-term baby to pass without tearing. A circular muscle, the bulbocavernosus muscle at the external opening to the vagina (the introitus), acts as a voluntary sphincter to the vagina.

As one preparation for childbirth, women are advised to relax and tense the external vaginal sphincter muscle periodically to make it more supple for delivery and to help maintain tone after delivery.

The vaginal artery, a branch of the internal iliac artery, provides the vagina with an excellent blood supply. Vaginal tears at childbirth tend to bleed profusely because of this blood supply. An effective blood supply is also the reason that healing of any trauma at delivery takes place rapidly.

The vagina has both sympathetic and parasympathetic nerve innervations. It is not an extremely sensitive organ, however, Sexual excitement, often attributed to vaginal stimulation, is actually caused by clitoral stimulation.

The internal lining of the vagina tends to store glycogen. When this is broken down by lactose-fermenting bacteria that frequent the vagina, lactic acid is formed. This makes the usual pH of the vagina acid, a condition detrimental to the growth of pathological bacteria. Even though the vagina connects directly to the external surface, infections are therefore not usually present.

The function of the vagina is to act as the organ of copulation and to convey sperm to the cervix so it can meet with the ovum in the fallopian tube.

Female External Genitalia

The structures that form the female external genitalia are illustrated in Fig. 7-9.

MONS VENERIS

The mons veneris is a pad of fat over the symphysis pubis. It is covered by coarse hairs. In females, pubic hair tends to have a triangular distribution. In males, the pubic hair pattern is more diamond-shaped.

Fig. 7-9. Female external genitalia.

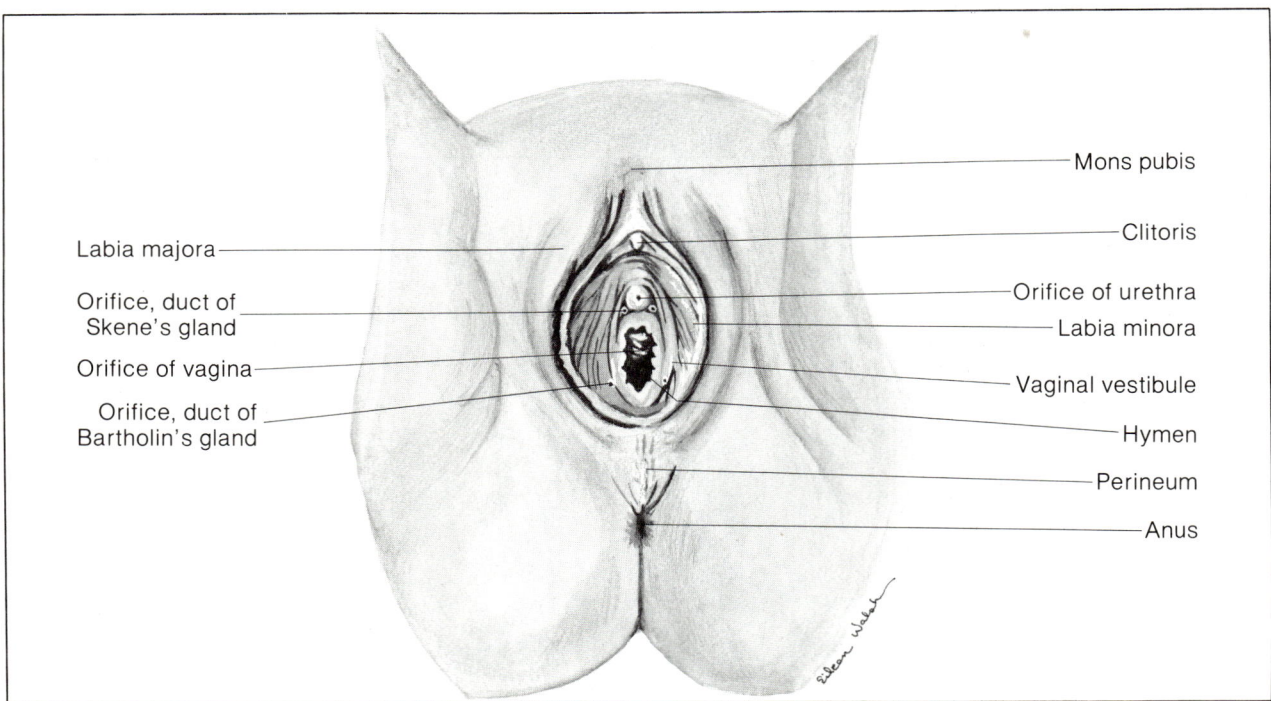

76 The Interpartal Period

LABIA MINORA
Just posterior to the mons veneris spread the folds of the labia minora. Prior to menarche (the first menstrual period) the folds of the labia minora are fairly small; at childbearing age they are firm and full; after menopause (the last menstrual cycle) they atrophy and again become much smaller. Normally, the folds of the labia minora are pink; the internal surface is covered with mucous membrane, the external surface with skin.

LABIA MAJORA
The labia majora are folds of fatty tissue lateral to the labia minora. Covered by pubic hair, the labia majora serve as protection for the external genitalia, the opening to the bladder, and the uterus.

VESTIBULE
The vestibule is the flattened, smooth area inside the labia. The opening to the bladder (the urethra) and the uterus (the vagina) both rise from the vestibule.

CLITORIS
The clitoris is a small (about 1 to 2 cm) rounded organ of erectile tissue at the forward junction of the labia minora. The clitoris is sensitve to touch and temperature and is the center of sexual arousal and orgasm in the female. When the ischiocavernosus muscle contracts with sexual arousal, the venous outflow for the clitoris is blocked. Venous congestion from this blockage leads to erection.

SKENE'S GLANDS
Skene's glands are located just lateral to the urinary meatus.

BARTHOLIN'S GLANDS
Bartholin's glands are located just lateral to the vaginal opening. Both sets of these glands lubricate the external vulva during coitus. Both sets of glands may become infected and produce a discharge and pain.

THE FOURCHETTE
The fourchette is the ridge of tissue formed by the posterior joining of the two labia minora and the labia majora. This is the area cut (episiotomy) prior to delivery of a child to enlarge the vaginal opening.

THE PERINEAL BODY
Posterior to the fourchette is the perineal muscle or the perineal body. Because this is a muscular area, it is easily stretched during childbirth to allow for enlargement of the vagina and passage of the fetal head. Many exercises suggested for pregnancy are aimed at making the perineal muscle more relaxed and more expandable so easy expansion during delivery can occur.

THE HYMEN
The hymen is a tough but elastic semicircle of tissue covering the opening to the vagina in childhood. Due to the use of menstrual tampons and active sports participation even many virginal girls do not have intact hymens at the time of their first pelvic examination. Occasionally a girl will have an imperforate hymen, or a hymen so large it does not allow passage of menstrual blood from the vagina or allow for sexual intercourse.

BLOOD SUPPLY
The blood supply of the external genitalia is mainly from the pudendal artery and a portion of the inferior rectus artery. Because of the good blood supply, trauma to this area following childbirth heals quickly.

NERVE SUPPLY
The anterior portion of the vulva derives its nerve supply from the ilioinguinal and genitofemoral nerves. The posterior portion of the vulva and vagina is supplied by the pudendal nerve. Much of anesthesia for childbirth is concerned with blocking the pudendal nerve to eliminate pain sensation at the perineum during delivery.

The Pelvic Floor
The pelvic floor is composed of both superficial and deep muscle layers. The slope of the pelvic floor is downward and forward, so that at delivery, when the presenting portion of the fetus touches the pelvic floor, it is pushed forward to be delivered under the pubic arch.

SUPERFICIAL MUSCLE LAYERS
The bulbocavernosus muscle fibers have their origin in the perineal body. They pass anteriorly, surrounding the vaginal orifice, to insert at the undersurface of the symphysis pubis. It is this muscle that acts as a voluntary vaginal sphincter.

The transverse perineal muscle fibers originate at the ischial tuberosities and pass medially to insert at the perineal body. The transverse perineal muscles are strong. They support the anal canal during defecation and the lower parts of the vagina during delivery.

The ischiocavernosus fibers originate at the ischial

tuberosities and pass obliquely to insert beside the bulbocavernosus muscle fibers at the symphysis pubis. By contraction, they cause erection of the clitoris.

The external anal sphincter fibers arise from the coccyx and pass on either side of the anus. They fuse and insert into the tranverse perineal muscles.

DEEP MUSCLE LAYERS

Although there are three deep muscles of the pelvic floor, they fuse together to form one continuous sheet of muscle, the levator ani. Intactness of the levator ani is necessary for urinary continence and for defecation. This is an important muscle in the second stage of labor as it is the major muscle used to push the fetus through the birth canal.

Male External Genitalia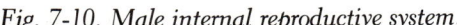

The sex of an individual is determined at the moment of conception by the chromosome formation of the particular ovum and sperm that join to create the embryo. In early uterine life, male and female embryos appear similar, and it is difficult to determine from gross inspection whether the individual will be male or female. Although males and females look grossly different by the time of birth, the reproductive structures they possess are analogues of each other.

External genital organs of the male are the penis and testes. Male reproductive anatomy is shown in Fig. 7-10.

TESTES

Testes are ovoid glands that lie in a rugated, skin-covered pouch, the scrotum. Each testis is encased by a protective white fibrous capsule and is composed of a number of lobules, each lobule containing interstitial cells (Leydig cells) and a seminiferous tubule.

Leydig cells are responsible for the production of testosterone, an androgenic hormone, which is in turn responsible for the development of secondary male characteristics such as distribution of pubic hair (a diamond shape in contrast to the triangular shape of a woman's pubic hair). The presence of testosterone at puberty leads to bone growth and muscle development. When the level of testosterone is at an adult level, it causes closure of the epiphyseal lines in long bones or the end of growth in height in males. The circulating level of testosterone in blood influences the production of gonadotropic hormones by the pituitary gland. Production of gonadotropic pituitary hormones stimulates the production of spermatozoa.

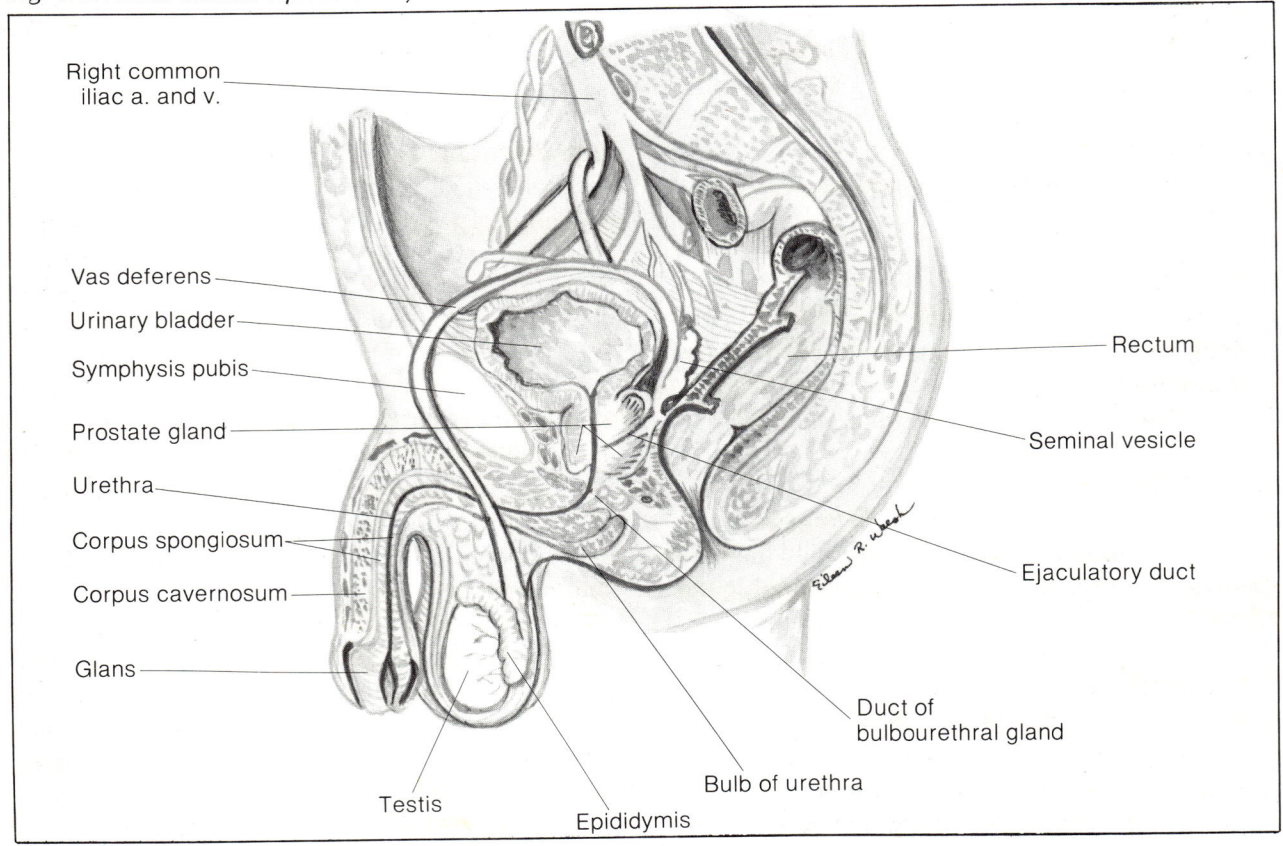

Fig. 7-10. Male internal reproductive system.

Spermatozoa are produced by the seminiferous tubules.

In most males one testis is slightly larger than the other and is suspended slightly lower in the scrotum than the other. Thus they tend to slide past each other more readily on sitting or muscular activity and there is less possibility of trauma. Most body structures of importance are more protected than are the testes (the heart, kidneys, and lungs are surrounded by ribs of hard bone). Since spermatozoa do not survive at body temperature, however, the testes are suspended outside the body where the temperature is about 1° lower than body temperature and sperm survival is ensured.

THE SCROTUM

The scrotum is a rugated skin-covered pouch suspended from the perineum. It contains the testes, epididymis, and the lower portion of the spermatic cord.

THE PENIS

Three cylindrical masses of erectile tissue and the urethra are contained in the shaft of the penis. With sexual excitement, there is venous congestion in the erectile tissue; this causes distention or erection of the penis. At the distal end of the organ is a bulging ridge of tissue, the *glans*. A retractable casing of skin or prepuce protects the nerve-sensitive glans at birth. In the United States, most male children are circumcised at birth and have the prepuce removed. The urethra passing through the penis serves as the outlet for both the urinary and the reproductive tracts in men.

Male Internal Reproductive Organs

THE EPIDIDYMIS

The seminiferous tubules of the male testes lead to a single tightly coiled tube, the *epididymis*. Because the epididymis is so tightly coiled, its length is deceptive; it totals about 20 feet. It is extremely narrow in diameter, so infection (epididymitis) can lead to easy scarring of the lumen and prohibit passage of sperm beyond the scarred point.

The epididymis is responsible for conduction of sperm from the testes to the vas deferens, the next step in the passage to the outside. Some sperm are stored in the epididymis. A small part of the fluid that surrounds sperm (semen, or seminal fluid) is produced by the epididymis.

THE VAS DEFERENS

The vas deferens carries sperm from the epididymis through the inguinal canal into the abdominal cavity. It is surrounded by arteries and veins and protected by a thick fibrous coating. All together, these structures are the *spermatic cord*. The cord passes over the top of the bladder and at its distal end joins the seminal vesicle and the ejaculatory duct. Vasectomy, or severing of the vas deferens, is a popular means of male birth control.

EJACULATORY DUCTS

The two ejaculatory ducts pass through the prostate gland and join the urethra.

THE URETHRA

The *urethra* is a hollow tube leading from the base of the bladder to the outside through the shaft and glands of the penis. It is about 8 inches long. Directly below the bladder it passes through the prostate gland. The urethra is lined with mucous membrane.

SEMINAL VESICLES

The seminal vesicles are two convoluted pouches that lie along the lower portion of the posterior surface of the bladder and empty into the urethra. These glands secrete the viscous portion of the semen.

PROSTATE GLAND

The prostate gland lies just below the bladder. The urethra passes through the center of it, like the hole in a doughnut. The prostate secretes a thin alkaline fluid that, when added to the secretion from the seminal vesicles and that already accompanying sperm from the epididymis, protects sperm from being immobilized by the naturally low pH level of the urethra due to the passage of urine through the same lumen.

BULBOURETHRAL GLANDS

Two bulbourethral, or Cowper's, glands lie beside the prostate. They empty into the urethra. Like the prostate gland, they secrete an alkaline fluid that helps counteract the acid secretion of the urethra and ensure the safe passage of spermatozoa. The content of semen is derived from the prostate (60 percent), the seminal vesicles (30 percent), the epididymis (5 percent), and the bulbourethral glands (5 percent).

Mammary Glands

The rise in estrogen formation at puberty begins breast maturation in girls. Boys often have a transient increase in breast size at puberty from estrogen stimulation. This is most evident in obese boys.

The increase in breast tissue in both sexes is due to an increase in connective tissue and deposition of fat.

The glandular tissue of the breasts, necessary for successful breast-feeding, remains undeveloped until a pregnancy begins.

Breasts are composed of glands divided by connective tissue partitions into about 20 lobes. All the glands in each lobe produce milk and deliver it to the nipple by a milk duct. The blood supply to the breasts is profuse, blood being supplied by thoracic branches of the axillary, internal mammary, and intercostal arteries. This effective blood supply is important in bringing nutrients to the milk glands when milk for feeding a newborn becomes necessary.

A diagram of breast anatomy—prepregnant, pregnant, and during lactation—is shown in Chap. 30 (Fig. 30-1).

Pituitary-Hypothalamus Maturity

In order for a person to be able to initiate ova or sperm formation, her or his pituitary-hypothalamic control of gonadotropic hormones must have reached a point of maturity. The initiation and effect of these hormones are discussed in Chap. 8, with the physiology of reproduction.

Pelvic Bony Growth

In order for a baby to be delivered vaginally, it must be able to pass through the ring of pelvic bone. Pelvic bone growth must be sufficient, therefore, or the infant will be too large to be born except by cesarean section. This is often a problem for the girl under 14 years of age. Diagrams of the pelvic bone and the methods by which the diameter of the bone are measured are shown in Chap. 16.

Knowledge of Reproductive Organs

Most women have little knowledge about the reproductive organs. They speak vaguely about ovaries, "tubes," and "the womb," or "private organs" or "private parts." The fact that some women refer to reproductive organs as "private parts" almost implies that it is more proper for them to know little about the function of these organs than to know a lot about them.

In order to understand why conception occurs, why some pregnancies are lost on account of anatomical factors (incompetent cervix), why conception cannot occur in the presence of illness (endometriosis), or what happens during labor and delivery, women (and their male partners) need basic knowledge of where organs are located and what their primary functions are.

Women who attend preparation-for-childbirth classes are taught about their reproductive anatomy so they can use their bodies effectively in childbirth and not struggle against natural processes. Nurses are called on more and more to be informed sources of information about the anatomy and physiology of childbearing and to have a working knowledge of what physical readiness for childbearing requires.

Three examples of assessments for physical readiness for childbearing follow.

Problem-oriented Recording: Progress Notes

Christine McFadden
15 years
First prenatal visit (LMP 16 weeks ago)

Problem: Physical readiness for childbearing

S. Menarche at 12 years; menstrual periods q 28–35 days, 5 days' duration, mod. heavy. Cramping enough to keep her home from school 1 day/month.
Active in school sports; member of swimming team.
Good health; no known kidney, heart, diabetes, tuberculosis, venereal disease; no abdominal surgery; no previous pregnancies (para 0, gravida 1).
Will be quitting school sports because of pregnancy. States, "I won't miss it. It was constant stretching until you hurt."

O. Pelvic measurements:
Diagonal conjugate: 12 cm.
True conjugate, therefore: 10–10.5 cm.
Ischial tuberosities: 11 cm.
Blood pressure: 110/80; P: 80, R: 22.
Weight 122.

A. Questionable physical readiness because of small pelvic measurements (T.C. only 10–10.5 cm).

Goals: a. Maintain an active physical program during pregnancy despite loss of formal program.
b. Complete pregnancy without reten-

tion of extra weight or varicosities in postpartal period.
c. Remain in school during pregnancy.
d. Describe reason that vaginal delivery may not be possible on account of pelvic measurements.

P. 1. Mark chart for M.D. evaluation of pelvic measurements.
2. Discuss exercise program for pregnancy:
   a. Walk with 5-year-old sister daily after school.
   b. Maintain routine gym program in school with minor considerations.
3. Mark chart for postpartal discussion of menstrual cramps so they don't interfere with activities so much.
4. Mark chart for discussion of cesarean section by 28th week of pregnancy if M.D. confirms possible need.

Problem-oriented Recording: Progress Notes

Mary Kraft
22 years
First prenatal visit (LMP 9 weeks ago)

Problem: Physical readiness for childbearing.

S. Menarche at 13 years; menstrual periods now 30–32 days, 6 days' duration, heavy; painful cramping. Had infertility work-up during last year. Diagnosis of endometriosis and conservative abdominal surgery for removal of endometriosis implants done 2 months ago. Fully recovered in terms of energy and activity.
Overall health good although she is often "dead tired." No known kidney, heart, diabetes, tuberculosis, venereal disease. Had surgery for appendicitis (no sequelae) at 12 years. 1 previous pregnancy ending in spont. abortion at 3 months two years ago (no known cause). Para 0, gravida 2. No formal sports or exercises; a "little tennis."
Wants to continue work and wonders if she will be able to.

O. Pelvic measurements (from old record of previous pregnancy)
   Diagonal conjugate: 13.5 cm.
   True conjugate, therefore: 12–11.5 cm.
   Ischial tuberosities: 11 cm.
Blood pressure: 100/78; P: 76, R: 20.
Weight: 111 (prepregnancy wgt. 10 lb under desirable wgt.).
Recent abdominal surgical scar appears well healed.

A. Pelvic measurements adequate.
Physical readiness for childbearing.

Goals: a. Maintain a physical exercise program during pregnancy.
b. Continue part-time job, as desired.
c. Complete pregnancy without retention of extra weight or other physical complications such as varicosities.
d. Deliver vaginally.

P. 1. Observe recent abdominal incision for stress at visits.
2. Discuss exercise program for pregnancy:
   a. Walk to work on nice days rather than drive (two blocks away).
   b. Continue tennis but not to point of fatigue.
   c. Break up periods of sitting at library desk every hour by stretch and short walk.
3. Ask M.D. to stress physical capacity for normal pregnancy because of previous pregnancy loss.

Problem-oriented Recording: Progress Notes

Angie Baco
42 years
First prenatal visit (LMP 12 weeks ago)

Problem: Physical readiness for childbearing

S. Menarche at 10 years; menstrual periods now 26–30 days, 5 days' duration, light; no cramping or discomfort.
Works as housewife; participates in no sports

other than "driving children to school activities." Family does some weekend camping.

Overall health good with exception of varicosities in right leg that are painful on standing.

No known kidney or heart disease; no tuberculosis. No abdominal surgery or venereal disease. 6 previous vaginal deliveries. B.W.'s: 6-12, 7, 7-5, 7-6, 8-2, 9-13. Had "touch of diabetes with last pregnancy," controlled by diet. No abortions, stillbirth, premature. 5th child died at birth of congenital heart disease; 6th child has learning disability (para 6; gravida 7).

O. Pelvic measurements not repeated; 6 previous vaginal deliveries. No pelvic injury since last child.

Blood pressure: 124/84, P: 90, R: 24.
Weight: 150 (30 lb over desirable weight).
Urine neg. for sugar and acetone.

A. Guarded physical readiness for childbearing due to: gestational diabetes by history in last pregnancy, obesity, and varicosities.

Goals:
a. Early detection of gestational diabetes by glucose tolerance test and urine testing.
b. Complete pregnancy in optimum health with as little advancement of varicosities as possible.
c. Maintain a preventive exercise program for varicosity and hemorrhoid formation.
d. Maintain an exercise program for overall health.
e. Deliver vaginally.

P. 1. Schedule glucose tolerance test if M.D. confirms need.
2. Review urine testing procedure used in last pregnancy if M.D. confirms need.
3. Discuss measures to prevent varicosities and hemorrhoids:
   a. Shoes off, feet up for ½ hour 2 × day.
   b. Knee-chest position for 15 minutes 2 × day.
   c. Put on support hose before rising in A.M.
   d. Limit time standing in one place (cooking, ironing, etc.) to 1 hour.
   e. Ask 19-year-old son or husband to drive children to activities if driving time is long.
4. Discuss routine exercise program: Walk to park daily in nice weather (3 blocks)
5. Mark chart for close observation for development of gestational diabetes and thrombophlebitis due to varicosities.

References

1. Brown, M. S., and Alexander, M. M. Physical examination: Female genitalia. *Nursing 76* 6:39, 1976.
2. Cohen, M. I. The process of adolescence: Its psychologic and physiologic basis. *Pediatr. Nurs.* 4:27, 1978.
3. Dayani, E. Concepts of wellness. *Nurse Pract.* 4:31, 1979.
4. Frisch, R. E., and Reville, R. Height and weight at menarche and a hypothesis of critical body weight and adolescent events. *Science* 169:397, 1970.
5. Fuller, S. S. Holistic man and the science and practice of nursing. *Nurs. Outlook* 26:700, 1978.
6. Hogan, M. Prenatal care training. *J. Sch. Health* 48:486, 1978.
7. Marks, A. Health screening of the adolescent. *Pediatr. Nurs.* 4:37, 1978.
8. Marshall, W. A., and Tanner, J. M. Variations in the pattern of pubertal changes in girls. *Arch. Dis. Child.* 44:291, 1969.
9. Marshall, W. A., and Tanner, J. M. Variations in the pattern of pubertal changes in boys. *Arch. Dis. Child.* 45:13, 1970.
10. Meyer, M. R. Adolescent gynecology: Problems and ponderings. *Pediatr. Nurs.* 4:43, 1978.
11. Russo, J. R. Adolescent menstrual disorders. *Female Patient* 5:19, 1980.

8. The Physiology of Reproduction

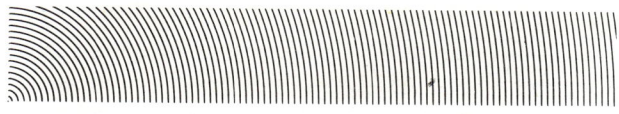

In order to understand how fertilization and growth of a new human being take place, it is necessary to understand the physiology of a normal menstrual cycle, or the process that precedes fertilization.

The Menstrual Cycle
MENARCHE

Menarche is the term applied to the first menstruation in girls. First menstruation occurs as one of a number of maturational changes that are associated with puberty: growth of axillary and pubic hair, broadening of the hips, breast development, and changes in endocrine functions. Although the average age for menarche is 12 to 13 years, it may occur as early as age 9 or as late as age 17 and still be within the range of normal. Because it may occur as early as age 9, school nurses or nurses working in pediatric clinics or pediatricians' offices who are responsible for sex education of girls should include information on menstruation as early as the fourth grade. It is a poor introduction to sexuality and womanhood for a girl to begin menstruation unwarned and unprepared for the important internal function it represents.

Menopause is the cessation of menstrual cycles. The age range at which this occurs is wide, between 40 and 55 years. Both the age of menarche and the age of menopause tend to be familial (if menarche occurred early in a mother, it will probably occur early in her daughter; if menopause began early in a mother, it may begin early in her daughter).

The length of a menstrual cycle differs from woman to woman, but the accepted average length is 28 days (from the beginning of one menstrual flow to the beginning of the next). However, it is not unusual for cycles to be as short as 20 days or as long as 45.

The length of the average menstrual flow is 5 to 7 days although some women have periods as short as 1 day or as long as 9 days. Because there is such variation in the times that menarche and menopause occur and such variation in length, frequency, and amount of menstrual flow, many women have questions as to what is "normal." Contact with health personnel during a pregnancy is often the first opportunity they have to find answers to questions they have had in mind for some time. When you ask a possibly pregnant woman, "When was your last menstrual period?" her answer may be, "I'm awfully irregular," or, "I wish my body did things like the books say," instead of a date. Pregnancy will be an opportunity for this woman to learn more about her body and to be more comfortable with herself and the way her life is subtly influenced by periodic surges and declines of hormones.

Four body structures are involved in the physiology of the menstrual cycle: the hypothalamus, the pituitary gland, the ovaries, and the uterus.

THE HYPOTHALAMUS

Beginning with puberty, every month a *releasing factor* is transmitted from the hypothalamus to the anterior pituitary gland to begin production of gonadotropic hormones. Diseases of the hypothalamus causing deficiency of this factor result in delayed adolescence. Diseases causing early activation of the releasing factor lead to abnormally early sexual development, or precocious puberty.

PITUITARY HORMONES

The anterior pituitary gland produces two hormones that act on the ovaries to initiate or influence the menstrual cycle: the *follicle-stimulating hormone*, a hormone that is active early in a cycle and is responsible for maturation of the ovum, and *luteinizing hormone* (also called interstitial cell-stimulating hormone), which becomes most active at the midpoint of the cycle. Luteinizing hormone initiates ovulation or release of the mature egg cell from the ovary and growth of the uterine lining during the second half of the menstrual cycle.

OVARIAN CHANGES

Under the influence of follicle-stimulating hormone and luteinizing hormone—called gonadotropic hormones because they cause growth (trophia) in the gonads (ovaries)—one ovum matures and is discharged from the ovary.

Division of Reproductive Cells

At birth, each ovary contains about 2 million immature ova (*oocytes*), which were formed during the first five months of intrauterine life. These cells have the usual cell components: a cell membrane, an area of clear cytoplasm, and a nucleus containing chromosomes.

Reproductive cells differ from all other human body cells in the number of chromosomes they contain. All the other cells have 46 chromosomes, consisting of 22 pairs of autosomes and one pair of sex chromosomes. Female body cells contain two X sex chromosomes (XX); male body cells contain an X and a Y sex chromosome. Ova and spermatozoa have only half the usual number of chromosomes because of the difference in the way reproductive cells divide.

Cells in the body, such as skin cells, undergo cell division by *mitosis*, or daughter cell division. In this type of division, all the chromosomes are reduplicated in each new cell. Oocytes and immature spermatozoa (spermatocytes) divide in intrauterine life by one *mitotic* division. Activity then appears to halt until at least puberty, when a second type of cell division, *meiosis* (cell reduction), occurs. In meiosis, the new cells contain only half the number of chromosomes of the parent cell. In the male, this occurs just before the spermatozoa mature. In the female, it occurs just before ovulation. Ova therefore have 22 autosomes and an X sex chromosome; a spermatozoon has 22 autosomes and either an X or a Y sex chromosome.

Maturation of Oocytes

Each oocyte lies in the ovary surrounded by a protective sac, or thin layer of cells, called *follicle cells*. The oocyte in this underdeveloped state is called a *primordial follicle*. The maturation of these primitive follicles appears to stop about the fifth month of intrauterine life. The majority never develop beyond the primitive state and actually atrophy, so that by 7 years of age there are only about 500,000 present in each ovary; by 22 years there are about 300,000; by menopause, or the end of the fertile period in females, none are left (all have either matured or atrophied). "The point at which no functioning oocytes remain in the ovaries" is one definition of menopause (change of life).

Ovulation

During the fertile period of a woman's life (from menarche to menopause), each month, activated by follicle-stimulating hormone from the anterior pituitary, one of the primordial follicles begins to grow and mature. Its follicle cells produce a clear fluid containing a high content of estrogen and some progesterone. The fluid is termed *follicular liquor* or *follicular fluid*. The structure grows in size and propels itself toward the surface of the ovary. It is visible on the surface as a clear water blister about ¼ to ½ inch across. At this stage of maturation the small ovum (barely visible to the naked eye, about the size of a printed period) with its surrounding follicle cells and fluid is termed a *graafian follicle*.

The ovum is at first attached to the edge of the graafian follicle by a thin strand of cells; later, it floats free in the fluid. By the midpoint of a menstrual cycle (the 14th day of a typical 28-day cycle) the ovum has divided by a mitotic division into two separate bodies: a primary oocyte, which contains the bulk of the cytoplasm, and a secondary oocyte, which contains so little cytoplasm it is not functional. The structure also has accomplished a meiotic division and has reduced its number of chromosomes to its haploid number of 23 (*haploid* means "having only one member of a pair").

At the midpoint in the menstrual cycle, perhaps as early as the 8th or as late as the 20th day of the cycle (few women have an exact 28-day cycle), following an upsurge of luteinizing hormone from the pituitary, the graafian follicle ruptures. The ovum is set free from the surface of the ovary, a process termed *ovulation*. It is swept into the open end of a fallopian tube.

After the ovum and the follicular fluid have been discharged from the ovary, the cells of the follicle still remain in the form of a hollow, empty pit. The follicle-stimulating hormone has done its work at this point and now decreases in amount. The second pituitary hormone now begins its work. Luteinizing hormone acts on the follicle cells of the ovary, causing them to produce, instead of follicular fluid, which was high in estrogen with some progesterone, a bright yellow fluid, *lutein*, which is high in progesterone with some estrogen. This yellow fluid fills the empty follicle, which is then termed the *corpus luteum* (yellow body).

The basal body temperature of a woman drops slightly (1°F) just before the day of ovulation, because of the extremely low level of progesterone present at that time. It rises at least 1°F the day following ovulation, because of the concentration of progesterone that is present at that time. The woman's temperature remains at this increased level until about the 24th day of the menstrual cycle, when progesterone level again decreases.

If conception (fertilization by a spermatozoon) occurs as the ovum proceeds down a fallopian tube, and the fertilized ovum is implanted on the endometrium of the uterus, the corpus luteum will remain throughout the major portion of the pregnancy, reaching peak activity at about the 16th to 20th week. If conception does not occur, the unfertilized ovum atrophies after four or five days, and the corpus luteum (called "false") will then remain for only about eight to ten days. As the corpus luteum regresses, it is, in both cases, gradually replaced by white fibrous tissue, and the resulting structure is termed a *corpus albicans* (white body).

UTERINE CHANGES
First Phase of Menstrual Cycle
Each month, changes take place in the uterus as well as in the pituitary gland and the ovaries. Immediately following a menstrual flow (the first four or five days of a cycle), the endometrium, or lining, of the uterus is very thin, about one cell layer in depth. As the ovary begins to form estrogen (in the follicular fluid, under the direction of the pituitary follicle-stimulating hormone), the endometrium begins to proliferate, or grow very rapidly, increasing in thickness about eightfold. This increase continues for the first half of the menstrual cycle (from about the 5th to the 14th day). This half of a menstrual cycle is the proliferative, estrogenic, follicular, or postmenstrual phase.

Second Phase of Menstrual Cycle
At the midpoint of the cycle, the formation of progesterone in the corpus luteum (under the direction of the luteinizing hormone) causes the glands of the uterine endometrium to become corkscrew or twisted in appearance and dilated with quantities of glycogen and mucin, an elementary sugar and protein. The capillaries of the endometrium increase in amount until the lining takes on the appearance of rich, spongy velvet. This second phase of the menstrual cycle is the progestational, luteal, premenstrual, or secretory phase.

Final Phase of Menstrual Cycle
What occurs next depends on whether the released ovum meets and is fertilized by a spermatozoon. As indicated, if fertilization does not take place, the corpus luteum in the ovary begins to regress. As it regresses, the production of progesterone and estrogen decreases. With the withdrawal of progesterone stimulation, the endometrium of the uterus begins to degenerate (at about the 24th to 25th day of the cycle). The capillaries rupture, with minute hemorrhages, and the endometrium sloughs off. Blood from the ruptured capillaries, along with mucin from the glands, fragments of endothelium tissue, and the microscopic, atrophied, and unfertilized ovum, is discharged from the uterus (the menstrual flow). This is the end of the arbitrarily defined menstrual cycle, but because it is the only external marker of the cycle, the first day of menstrual flow is used to mark the beginning day of a new menstrual cycle. A typical 28-day menstrual cycle and the times when hormones are secreted at peak levels are shown diagrammatically in Fig. 8-1.

The menstrual flow contains only about 25 to 50 ml of blood; it seems more because of the accompanying mucus and endometrial shreds. It does not clot, because when the capillaries of the endometrium first rupture the blood clots almost immediately and is then liquefied by fibrinolytic activity. Once blood has clotted and liquefied, it will not clot again. The iron loss in a menstrual flow is about 12 mg.

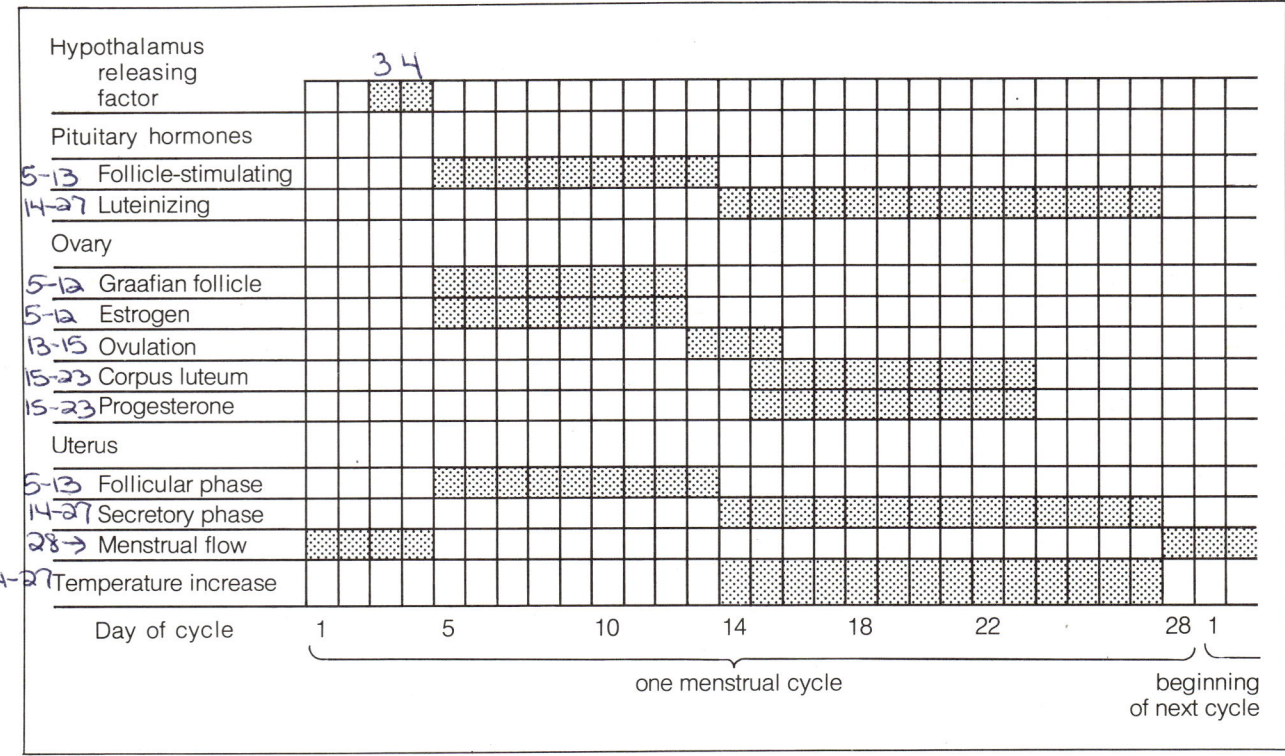

Fig. 8-1. Twenty-eight-day menstrual cycle.

Characteristics of the menstrual cycle and flow are summarized in Table 8-1.

CERVICAL CHANGES

The mucus of the uterine cervix changes each month during the menstrual cycle. The changes are helpful in establishing fertility. (Mucus changes in consistency at the time of ovulation; if no change in cervical mucus occurs, it implies that ovulation has not occurred.) The awareness that such changes take place with ovulation allows women to plan sexual relations so that they coincide with ovulation, assuring that pregnancy will occur, or to avoid sexual relations at the time of ovulation, to prevent pregnancy (the rhythm method of birth control).

During the first half of the cycle, when hormone secretion from the ovary is low, cervical mucus is thick and scant. If you place a drop of it between your finger and thumb and then draw them apart, the mucus will not form a thread but will break at only about 1 cm. If a drop of mucus is placed on a slide, allowed to dry, and then examined under a microscope, it reveals a nondescript pattern. Cervical mucus during the first half of the menstrual cycle contains many leukocytes; sperm survival in this type of mucus is poor.

At the time of ovulation, cervical mucus becomes thin and copious. It can be compared to the feel of fresh egg white. The ability to thread or spin is called *spinnbarkeit*. The quality of spinnbarkeit is so great at this time that it will thread a distance of 13 to 15 cm. If mucus is dried and examined under a microscope, it forms a fern-like pattern resembling miniature fossilized ferns. This is due to sodium and water concentrations that high estrogen levels have caused to be retained. No leukocytes are present; sperm penetration and survival at the time of ovulation in this thin mucus is excellent.

As progesterone becomes the major influencing

Table 8-1. Characteristics of Normal Menstrual Cycles

Beginning (menarche)	Average age of onset 12 or 13 years; average range of age 9 to 17 years
Interval between cycles	Average 28 days; cycles of 20 to 45 days not unusual
Duration of menstrual flow	Average flow 3 to 7 days; ranges of 1 to 9 days not abnormal
Amount of menstrual flow	Difficult to estimate; average 25 to 50 ml per menstrual period; saturating a pad or tampon in less than an hour is heavy bleeding
Color of menstrual flow	Dark red; a combination of blood, mucus, and endometrial cells

hormone during the second half of the cycle, cervical mucus again becomes thick. It looses its property of spinnbarkeit and its ability to fern. Leukocytes are again present; sperm survival is again poor.

These cervical changes are summarized in Table 8-2.

Education for Menstruation

Early preparation for menstruation is important preparation for future childbearing and for a girl's concept of herself as a woman. A girl who is told that menstruation is a normal function, which occurs every month in all healthy women, has a better attitude toward menstruation and toward herself than a girl who wakes up one morning to find blood on her pajamas and receives an explanation, "You'd better get used to that. You're going to have to put up with it for the rest of your life." In the first instance, the girl can trust her body; it is doing what every woman's body does. In the second instance, her body is out of control. How can she accept and enjoy growing up if it involves something so unpredictable? In the first instance, menstruation is a mark of pride, of growing up. In the second it is bothersome and bad; being a woman, who menstruates, is being second-rate to a man, who does not.

Girls who are well prepared for menstruation and view it as a positive happening tend to have fewer episodes of painful cramps and missed school days than those who view it as an ill time.

Menstrual Disorders

Concerns about menstruation generally fall into two categories: concern about cycles that are either too frequent or too far apart and concern about painful or uncomfortable menstruation.

MITTELSCHMERZ

In some women, either the release of the ovum from its follicle at the midpoint of the cycle or perhaps irritation caused by a drop or two of follicular fluid or blood in the abdominal cavity causes abdominal pain. For many women this pain is only a few sharp cramps; other women experience a few hours of full discomfort. It occurs typically as one-sided pain in one of the lower quadrants of the abdomen (near an ovary).

Young girls may be worried that when this occurs in the right lower quadrant it is a symptom of appendicitis. However, the lack of associated symptoms (such as nausea, vomiting, and fever), the coincidental timing at the midpoint of a menstrual cycle, and its short limited duration all help to differentiate mittelschmerz from other types of abdominal pain.

PREMENSTRUAL TENSION

The high level of progesterone secreted by the corpus luteum just prior to menstruation causes many women to have one or two days of irritability or fatigue before their menstrual flow begins. Some women experience accompanying feelings of fullness, or "bloating," as significant edema occurs in tissues as a result of the high levels of salt-retaining estrogen at this time. These sensations diminish after the first day of the menstrual flow and generally need no treatment.

It is important that women recognize whether or not premenstrual tension occurs with them so that they can keep a perspective on things. They can learn to recognize that such a thing as a broken washing machine is just a broken washing machine; it only seems to be a catastrophe because they are about to have their menstrual period.

DYSMENORRHEA

Dysmenorrhea is painful menstruation. There is an attitude among many physicians that dysmenorrhea

Table 8-2. Cervical Changes During the Menstrual Cycle

Assessment Criteria	48 Hours Preovulation	Day of Ovulation	48 Hours Postovulation
Cervical mucus			
Viscosity	High (thick)	Low (thin)	High (thick)
Quantity	Scant	Copious	Scant
Spinnbarkeit	Little (1 cm)	Extreme (15 cm)	Limited (3 cm)
Leukocytes	Many	None	Moderate
Sperm survival	Little	Excellent	Limited
Fern test	Atypical pattern	Ferning pattern	Negative for ferning
pH	Acid (under 7.0)	Alkaline (7.5)	Acid (under 7.0)

"will go away" or "is all psychological" and so needs no treatment. Bad experiences with menstruation, however, do not help a woman to accept her body or to enjoy being a woman. In addition, dysmenorrhea can be a symptom of underlying illness such as pelvic inflammatory disease, uterine fibroid tumor, or endometriosis (abnormal formation of endometrial tissue). It is advisable, therefore, that women with dysmenorrhea be referred to physicians who are sympathetic to the reality of their discomfort.

Simple dysmenorrhea is usually experienced as abdominal cramping or as "aching, pulling" sensations of the vulva and inner thighs or as both. Some women have mild diarrhea with the abdominal cramping. These painful symptoms can generally be controlled by common analgesics such as aspirin. Abdominal breathing (breathing in and out slowly, allowing the abdominal wall to rise with each inhalation) may be helpful.

During the first one or two years after menarche, dysmenorrhea rarely occurs, probably because early menstrual cycles may be anovulatory. As ovulation begins, typical menstrual discomfort begins. If there is some consolation in dysmenorrhea, then, it is that it usually signifies the occurrence of ovulation.

The pain is probably from the release of prostaglandins at the time of ovulation. Women with extreme menstrual pain may be treated with mefenamic acid, an antiprostaglandin inhibitor. Low dose oral contraceptives to prevent ovulation may also be effective.

MENORRHAGIA

Menorrhagia is abnormally heavy menstrual flow. It is difficult to determine what a heavy flow is, but asking a woman to estimate how long it takes her to saturate a sanitary napkin or tampon during her menstrual flow provides a gross estimate of the amount of flow. A sanitary napkin or tampon holds about 25 ml of fluid. Saturating a pad or tampon in less than an hour means a heavy flow, which should not continue at that rate for more than the first 2 hours of a menstrual flow.

Menorrhagia may indicate a systemic disease (anemia), a blood dyscrasia, or a uterine abnormality such as a fibroid tumor. It can lead to excessive iron loss, and women with heavy menstrual flows may need to be maintained on iron supplements to achieve sufficient hemoglobin levels.

METRORRHAGIA

Metrorrhagia is bleeding between menstrual periods. It can occur as a normal process in some women, who have spotting at the time of ovulation (mittelstaining). It may occur in women on birth control pills (breakthrough bleeding). Vaginal irritation from infection might lead to midcycle spotting. Spotting may also represent a temporary low level of progesterone production and endometrial sloughing (dysfunctional uterine bleeding).

If metrorrhagia occurs for more than one period and the woman is not on birth control pills, she should be referred to a physician for examination, particularly if she is over 30 years of age, as vaginal bleeding is also an early sign of uterine cancer.

ENDOMETRIOSIS

Endometriosis is the presence of uterine endometrial cells outside the uterus, often in the cul-de-sac of the abdominal cavity, the uterine ligaments, and the ovaries. This abnormal implantation of tissue is probably due to excessive endometrial production and a reflux of menstrual blood and tissue through the fallopian tubes at the time of the menstrual flow.

The excessive production of the tissue is related to estrogen secretion. Many women with endometriosis do not ovulate, and estrogen secretion continues through the cycle rather than becoming secondary in production to progesterone late in the cycle, as happens in ovulating women.

Endometriosis can lead to dysmenorrhea because at the time of menstruation the displaced uterine tissue responds in the same way as that inside the uterus (causing even greater release of prostaglandins). It may lead to dyspareunia (painful sexual intercourse) if there is tissue present in the pelvic cul-de-sac, putting pressure on the posterior vagina. It may cause infertility due to fallopian tube blockage by implants.

Endometriosis may be either a cause or a symptom of infertility in women. It is a perplexing disorder. It is always difficult to explain to women why overproduction of uterine tissue leads to infertility; it seems as if overproduction should make them more fertile. Diagnosis and treatment of this menstrual cycle abnormality are discussed in Chap. 11.

AMENORRHEA

Absence of a menstrual flow, or amenorrhea, suggests pregnancy but is by no means diagnostic of pregnancy. Amenorrhea may occur as the result of tension, anxiety, fatigue, or chronic illness. Signs and symptoms of pregnancy and how amenorrhea is considered in the light of these are discussed in Chap. 14.

Menopause

Menopause, or the cessation of menstruation, is an event marked by ambivalence in most women. Although they do not feel too badly about being finished with menstrual periods and free of the concern of unexpectedly becoming pregnant, they also may feel "old" at the loss of a function that so dramatically marked their coming of age.

Menopause occurs as the ovaries become less and less influenced by the stimulation of the pituitary hormones. The level of estrogen production by the ovaries decreases. The decline in estrogen production leads to the physical symptoms that many women feel at "change of life." Since estrogen production by the adrenal glands continues after that of the ovaries drops, the woman is not without estrogen; she merely has declining levels of it.

Typical symptoms are "hot flashes," or sweating or flushing of the face. The uterus and vagina reduce in size, and vaginal secretions diminish. The woman may be aware of this change as sexual relations may become painful for her at this time because of vaginal dryness. Just as estrogen added to fat deposition at puberty, the loss of estrogen causes fat deposits to be reabsorbed, leading to loss of breast firmness and generally reduced tone. Estrogen at puberty aids bone growth; lowered amounts of estrogen may lead to osteoporosis, or bone demineralization.

In the past, women at menopause were given estrogen supplements to limit or reduce the body changes they experienced. Now, long-term administration of estrogen has been implicated in the development of uterine cancer. Estrogen is not administered routinely, therefore, to postmenopausal women. However, some women have such extreme symptoms that they need short-term therapy, more gradually tapered, than their own systems can achieve.

Terminology of Menstruation

A woman's overall outlook on menstruation and whether she views it as a healthy function are often reflected by the terms she uses to describe it.

"The curse" tends to have a negative connotation, certainly. Inability even to put a name on the happening—"when 'you know' happens . . ."—may indicate a feeling of dirtiness or uncleanliness (something ladies don't talk about any more than they do dust under beds). Listening to the names used to describe menstrual happenings may give you a clue as to how the woman will be able to discuss problems related to her pregnancy (she can not describe vaginal discharge if she thinks it is improper to use the term vaginal). If she views menstrual flows negatively, how

Table 8-3. Terms of Menstrual Physiology

Amenorrhea	Absence of menstruation
Menarche	The first menstrual period; initiation of ovarian function
Menopause	Cessation of ovarian function; the last menstrual period
Menorrhagia	Excessively heavy menstrual flow
Menstruation	Periodic discharge of bloody fluid representing the sloughing of the uterine lining from a nonpregnant uterus
Menses	Menstruation
Metrorrhagia	Vaginal bleeding between menstrual flow periods
Mittelschmerz	Lower-quadrant pain in the mid-menstrual cycle at the time of ovulation

is she going to regard the vaginal discharge she has after a baby is born?

Terms related to menstruation are summarized in Table 8-3.

References

1. Atunes, C. M., et al. Endometrial cancer and estrogen use. *N. Engl. J. Med.* 300:9, 1979.
2. Ballard, P. Menstrual disorders in adolescence. *Compr. Pediatr. Nurs.* 2:21, 1978.
3. Barber, H. R., et al. Dysmenorrhea. *Female Patient* 5:81, 1980.
4. Boston Women's Health Book Collective. *Our Bodies Ourselves* (2nd ed.). New York: Simon & Schuster, 1976.
5. Evans, E. D., and McCandless, B. R. *Children and Youth: Psychosocial Development* (2nd ed.). New York: Holt, Rinehart & Winston, 1978.
6. Field, P. A., et al. The premenstrual syndrome: Current findings, treatment, and implication for nurses. *J.O.G.N. Nurs.* 5:23, 1976.
7. Katzman, E. M. Common disorders of female genitalia from birth to older years: Implications for nursing interventions. *J.O.G.N. Nurs.* 6:19, 1977.
8. Kreutner, A. K., and Hollingsworth, D. R. *Adolescent Obstetrics and Gynecology.* Chicago: Year Book, 1978.
9. Loevsky, J. Menstruation: Alternatives to pharmacological therapy for menstrual distress. *J. Nurse Midwifery* 23:34, 1978.
10. Martin, L. L. *Health Care of Women.* Philadelphia: Lippincott, 1978.
11. McDonough, P. G., et al. Managing menstrual disorders in adolescents. *Contemp. Obstet. Gynecol.* 8:27, 1976.
12. Tyson, M. C. Let's talk about menopause. *Nursing 78* 8:34, 1978.

13. Weideger, P. *Menstruation and Menopause: The Physiology and Psychology, the Myth and Reality.* New York: Knopf, 1976.
14. Weiss, G. Secondary amenorrhea: Step by step to diagnosis. *Consultant* 18:95, 1978.
15. Whisnant, L., et al. White middle-class adolescent girls' attitudes toward menarche. *Nurs. Digest* 4:52, 1976.
16. Whisnant, L., et al. Implicit messages concerning menstruation in commercial educational materials prepared for young adolescent girls. *Nurs. Digest* 6:58, 1978.
17. Williams, J. *Psychology of Women: Behavior in a Biosocial Context.* New York: Norton, 1977.
18. Witty, K. T. Quelling severe menstrual cramps. *Patient Care* 12:198, 1978.

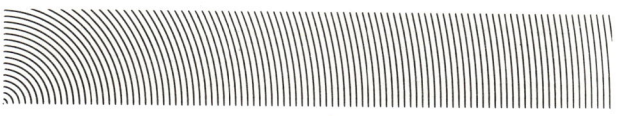

9. Human Sexuality

It is difficult for women to identify their place in society today because the traditional role of a woman (that of a passive, accepting person who receives the sexual act) overlaps with a more modern view of woman (that of an active, initiative person). It is equally difficult for many men, if they are nurturing, sharing people, to fit into the traditional male dominant, demanding role.

Discussing views on sexuality is often hard because women do not always regard sexuality as something that should be discussed or even consider it in a way concrete enough to discuss it.

In the 1950s, Kinsey and his associates [7] were the first group of researchers to describe sexual practices and the state of human sexuality. In 1966, Masters and Johnson [10] elaborated on common sexual needs. Their research documented the physiological responses of both men and women to sexual stimulation. They gathered a great deal of data on sexual responses during pregnancy and the postpartal period.

Sex Roles at Life Stages
PRENATAL SEX ROLES

Biological sex determination is established with the fusing of an ovum and a sperm in the first moment of conception. Until about the 12th week of intrauterine life, it is difficult to tell by gross inspection whether the fetus is male or female. At 12 weeks, the wolffian duct has become the dominant tract and male external genitalia are apparent, or the müllerian ducts have become dominant and female external genitalia are prominent. Occasionally, children who are chromosomally female are born looking more like males than females and infants who are chromosomally male are born appearing as female infants because of influences on the fetus in utero.

SEX ROLES IN INFANCY

From the day of birth, female babies are treated differently from male babies. They are wrapped in pink blankets, not blue ones; people bring them petite rattles or dresses with ruffles; on the whole they are treated more gently by parents than male babies; they are held and cuddled more. Male babies are wrapped in blue; people tend to buy bigger rattles and present them with miniature jogging suits or terry cloth shirts that say COACH across the front. Admonitions given babies are often different. A girl is told "Don't cry. You don't look pretty when you cry." A boy might be told, "You've got to learn to be tougher than that if you're ever going to make it in this world."

By the end of the first year, differences are usually strongly evident. Girls play for longer times with quiet toys, checking back with mother frequently; boys spend more time in gross motor activity, away from mother for longer periods of time than girls.

PRESCHOOL SEX ROLES

Children can point out the difference between men and women (Aunt Sally and Mommy are women; Uncle Jimmy and Daddy are men) as early as 2 years of age. By age 3 or 4 they know for certain what sex they are and that sex is a permanent differentiation. Along with the knowledge of which sex they are they have absorbed cultural expectations of that sex role. Watching preschool children at play demonstrates this fact strongly. Girls role-play being mothers. They imitate cooking, washing dishes, cleaning. Boys are fathers and go to work with pretend lunch pails or briefcases. The reason children assume one outward sex role or another is partly the basic chromosomal structure and partly the influence of their family members (who are influenced by their friends, the community, and the total culture). Comments such as "Is that how a lady sits?" "What kind of mommy are you going to be, treating a doll that way?" or, "Boys will be boys" express approval or disapproval for their actions, and the action is strengthened as apparently right for them or discarded in favor of actions that will bring approval. A great deal of current knowledge of sex roles comes also from the constant bombardment of family-situation programs on television.

If the child lives in a home where both mother and father are kind, loving people, sex role identification progresses smoothly; it is easy to want to be like someone who treats you well and with whom you feel secure. If one parent does not have a high nurturing capacity, however, it may be hard for the child of the same sex to identify with that person, or the identification may occur, but because the adult is not a good role model the child perpetuates the poor role.

A man who views the masculine role as aggressive, abrupt, and rough may notice in later years that his son is rougher with and less caring about a younger sibling than he likes to see. A man who maintains a passive role in a marriage, relinquishing authority to a more assertive wife, may find that his son has difficulty identifying with him, because the female role in this instance, that of the aggressive, decision-making person, is more appealing. Although the true cause of homosexuality is not known, difficulty with establishing early sex role identification appears to have a direct relationship.

SCHOOL-AGE SEX ROLES

As children move into the school-age period, the differences between boys and girls in terms of sex roles become wider and wider. There are definitely girl games and boy games and girl activities and boy activities to do after school. Teachers often contribute to this division by expecting boys to be poorer readers, to act rougher in the hallways; they accept less neat work from them.

Today girls are beginning to move into many male-dominated areas such as the Little League or shop or auto repair courses, and many activities of the school-age period are now unisex activities.

ADOLESCENT SEX ROLES

At puberty, as the adolescent begins the process of establishing a sense of identity, or a certain understanding of who he is and what kind of person he wants to be, the problem of final sex role identification surfaces again. Most early adolescents maintain strong ties to their gender group, boys with boys, girls with girls. Some adolescents choose a child of their own sex a few years older than themselves to use as their model of sex role behavior. Parents often worry about this type of attachment and express concerns that the relationship has homosexual connotations. Ordinarily, however, teenagers are just being certain that they understand who they are before they are ready to interact with members of the opposite sex.

Sex Roles and Parenting

People tend to parent as their parents parented. Those who come from intact homes have rather firmly fixed notions by the age of parenthood what their roles in the care of children will be. They may believe, for example, that fathers should play with babies—toss them in the air, play patty-cake with them—but should not be asked to change diapers. Fathers should be in charge of discipline; mothers should be in charge of nutrition and manners and proper grammar. Conflicts in parenting can occur if parents-to-be do not take time to discuss some of the views they have on parenting and see whether they are in agreement as to male and female roles and their relationship with their children.

People raised in single-parent homes may have more difficulty with parenting than those who had constant role models or they may, because they did not have a firm example of one of the parenting roles, be more flexible and therefore more able to adapt to the expectations of their marriage partner. A man who saw his father only on weekends, so each experience with him was something special, may have trouble being that enthusiastic every day relating with his children and feel that he is failing in his role.

Trying to live up to television role models of parenting (the house is always neat, the children are always well behaved, and all problems can be solved by clever one-liners) is also very difficult.

One sad finding that has emerged from studying sex role identification in relation to parenting is the finding of Kempe and Helfer [6]: Children who are battered by their parents grow up to imitate that role model and become battering parents themselves. They assume the role their parents exemplified for them even though objectively they can voice the fact that it is not a good role model, that theirs was not a happy childhood and they would have liked it otherwise.

It is important for young couples to talk to each other about sex roles before they involve a third person in their lives. Many women view their bodies as distasteful, see themselves and all women as less than men. Conflicts in the role they have chosen often come to light for the first time during pregnancy as they worry about what type of parent they are going to be. Being able to talk to health personnel about the sex role they have adopted in life is helpful.

Sexual Responses

It was believed since the nineteenth century that sex was a male desire, that the average female was not interested. Recent research reveals that women enjoy sexual relations as much as men and that both men and women have typical reactions to sexual stimulation.

According to Masters and Johnson [10], four stages occur in response to sexual stimulation: an excitement stage, a plateau stage, a stage of orgasm, and a stage of resolution.

EXCITEMENT STAGE

The excitement stage is a time of vasocongestion and increasing muscular tension as sexual arousal occurs. In women, vasocongestion causes the clitoris to increase in size and mucoid fluid to appear on vaginal walls as lubrication. The vagina widens in diameter and increases in length. The breast nipples become erect.

In men, erection occurs; there is scrotal thickening and elevation of the testes.

In both sexes, there is an increase in heart rate, respiratory rate, and blood pressure.

PLATEAU STAGE

The plateau stage is reached just prior to orgasm. In the woman, the clitoris is drawn forward and retracts under the clitoral prepuce; the lower part of the vagina becomes extremely congested (formation of the orgasmic platform). There is increased nipple engorgement.

In men, the vasocongestion has led to full distention of the penis. Heart rate has increased to 100 to 175 beats per minute; respiratory rate to about 40 per minute.

ORGASM

Orgasm is a vigorous contraction of muscles in the pelvic area. This violent contraction expels or dissipates blood and fluid from the area of congestion. The average woman has 8 to 15 contractions at intervals of one every 0.8 second.

In men, muscle contractions surrounding the seminal vessels and prostate first project semen into the proximal urethra. They are followed immediately by three to seven propulsive ejaculatory contractions, occurring at the same time interval as in the woman, that force semen from the penis.

STAGE OF RESOLUTION

The stage of resolution is the period during which the external and internal genital organs return to a quiet state. This takes about 30 minutes in both men and women.

Statistics on whether women achieve a stage of orgasm from coitus alone vary from early reports by Freud that women were neurotic if they did not always achieve orgasm through intercourse to findings of Hite [4] that only 30 percent of women regularly experience orgasm from intercourse alone. About 90 percent of women are capable of achieving orgasm if manual or direct clitoral stimulation is used in conjunction with coitus.

Influence of the Menstrual Cycle on Sexual Response

During the second half of the menstrual cycle—the luteal phase—there is increased fluid retention and vasocongestion in the woman's lower pelvis. Because some vasocongestion is already present at the beginning of the excitement stage of sexual response, women appear to reach the plateau stage more quickly and achieve orgasm more readily. Women also seem to be more interested in initiating sexual relations at this time.

Influence of Pregnancy on Sexual Response

Pregnancy is another time in life when, because of the rapidly growing fetus in the lower pelvic area, vasocongestion of the area occurs. Some women experience their first orgasm during the first pregnancy. Following a pregnancy, many women experience increased sexual capacity as the new growth of blood vessels during pregnancy lasts for some time and continues to facilitate pelvic vasocongestion. This is why discussing sexual relationships is a part of health teaching during pregnancy. At a time when a woman may want a sexual contact very much she needs to be free of old wives' tales, such as that orgasm will cause a miscarriage.

Peak Sexual Response

The peak sexual response of men appears to take place in late teen years. The peak response in women, however, tends to be much more delayed, occurring more frequently during the late 30s. This difference in peak age of response probably stems from the fact that men are taught early in life (boys will be boys) that sexual activity is expected of them. Girls, on the other hand, are still taught that sexual activity is not expected of them until after marriage. It may take women until their 30s, therefore, to overcome this inhibition against enjoying or wanting sex. The discrepancy in the age of peak sexual response may account for a number of husbands who find sexual partners other than their wives during pregnancy. Pregnancy, with its sexual restrictions due to awkward body size and possible prohibition of sexual intercourse (to lessen the possibility of introducing infection) during the last month of pregnancy, occurs at a time in life before the highest point of sexual response in women, at the peak of sexual response in men.

Contraceptives and Sexuality

Because birth control pills contain estrogen, and excess estrogen decreases the desire for sex, some women on birth control pills express a lowered interest in sex. This may be enough to make this method of birth control unacceptable for the woman since it interferes with her relationship with her sexual partner. Other women find that feeling confidence they will not become pregnant while taking birth control measures make sexual relations more pleasurable for them.

Sexuality Problems

People seen in offices or clinics for infertility problems may have sexual problems as the basis for their infertility. A woman who is seen for pregnancy may comment that she feels lucky to be pregnant because she or her sexual partner has a problem in this area.

PHYSICAL ILLNESS

Men who have had spinal cord injuries may or may not be capable of erection, depending on the level of the cord injury. Following a heart attack, many men forgo sexual activity, afraid that the stimulation of the activity will cause them to have a second heart attack. Obese men may have difficulty achieving deep penetration because of the bulk of their abdomens. Chronic diseases, such as peptic ulcer or severe allergy, that cause frequent pain or discomfort may interfere with the man's overall well-being and his interest in sexual activity.

Obese women may have difficulty with sexual relations, again on account of the bulk of their abdomens. Women who have had a mastectomy may feel embarrassed about exposing their bodies. People with ostomies may feel uncomfortable about exposing their abdomens.

Education to help people deal with body image or physical illness problems is necessary to make these people more at ease with themselves.

IMPOTENCE

Impotence is the inability to achieve or maintain an erection. Some reasons impotence occurs are physical, such as debilitating disease or drug dependence. In many instances, the problem appears to be psychological. Doubts about ability to perform or overall masculinity might be the cause. Excessive stress at home or at work might be a cause. The treatment of impotence depends on the factors involved. Surgical implants to aid erection are possible. If the cause is psychological, sexual counseling may be helpful.

PREMATURE EJACULATION

Premature ejaculation is ejaculation prior to penile-vaginal contact. The term is often used to mean ejaculation prior to the sexual partner's satisfaction. Premature ejaculation is unsatisfactory for both partners: for the woman, because she cannot achieve orgasm on account of loss of the man's erection, and for the man, because he has failed to help her achieve orgasm.

The cause of premature ejaculation, like that of impotence, appears to be most often psychologically based. Masturbating to orgasm (where orgasm is achieved quickly owing to lack of time) may play a role. Other reasons suggested are doubt about masculinity and fear of impregnating. Sexual counseling to help the female partner put less pressure on the male (and he on himself) to achieve may be helpful in alleviating the problem.

VAGINISMUS

Vaginismus is involuntary contraction of the muscles at the outlet of the vagina when sexual intercourse is attempted. This muscle contraction prohibits penile penetration.

Vaginismus may occur in women who have had unfortunate sexual experiences such as rape. It can also be the result of early learning patterns, in which sexual relations were viewed as "bad" or "sinful." As with other sexual problems, sexual or psychological counseling to reduce this response may be necessary.

DYSPAREUNIA

Dyspareunia is pain during intercourse. It can be due to endometriosis, vaginal infection, or hormonal changes such as those that occur with menopause. It can be psychological. Treatment is aimed at the underlying cause.

FAILURE TO ACHIEVE ORGASM

The failure of a woman to achieve orgasm can be due to poor sexual technique, concentrating too hard on achieving orgasm, underlying fear, or negative attitudes toward sexual relationships. Treatment is aimed at relieving the underlying cause; it consists of instruction for both partners in better sexual techniques and counseling as to basic feelings about sexuality.

Nursing Responsibility and Human Sexuality

Because the sexual role and people's concepts of sexuality influence the ways they think, feel, plan—truly all activities of life—the sex role or concept of sexuality that parents-to-be have chosen for themselves has a great deal to do with the type of parents they will become (Fig. 9-1).

During crisis periods (and pregnancy is a crisis) people often question their life-styles and beliefs. For this reason, questions about human sexuality or sex roles may be asked at prenatal health visits. The nurse's largest contribution in this area is to make it clear that such questions can be discussed. Thus problems of sexuality are brought out of the closet and made as solvable as other health problems.

Fig. 9-1. Human sexuality and its effects on childbearing.

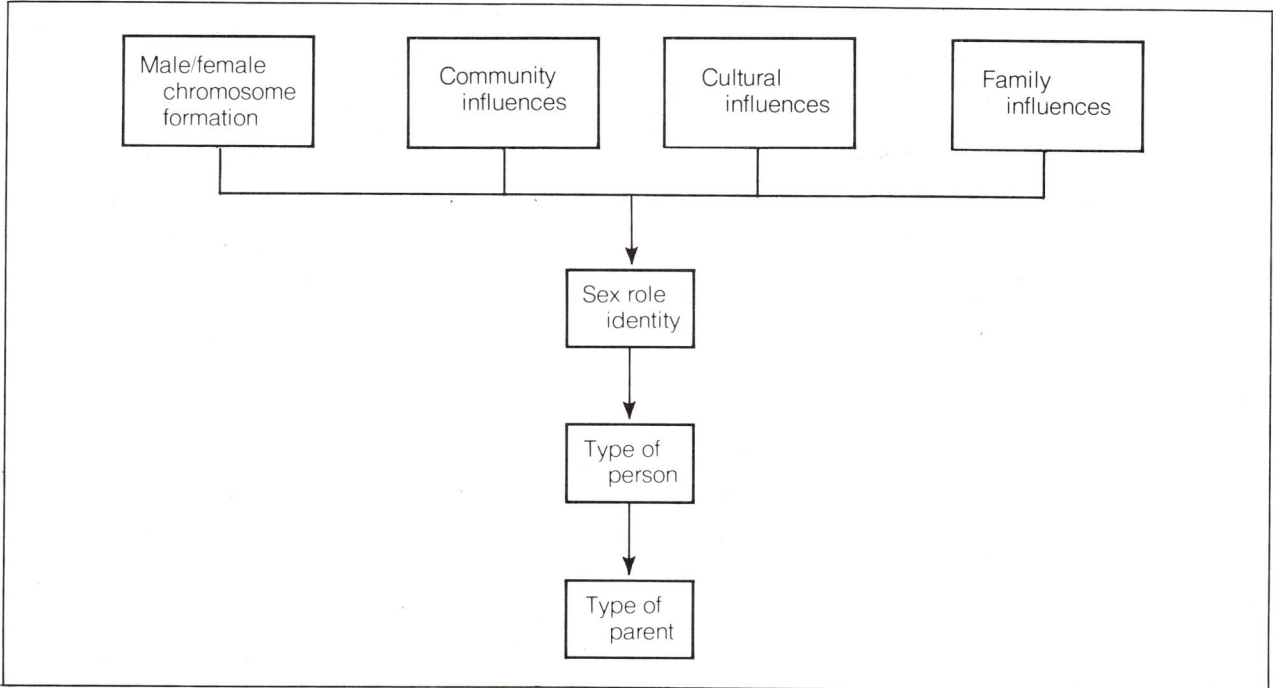

References

1. Dorin, A. Adolescent sexuality, adolescent depression: The nurse practitioner as counselor. *Pediatr. Nurs.* 4:49, 1978.
2. Dresen, S. Sexuality. In N. Diekelmann (Ed.). *Primary Health Care of the Well Adult.* New York: McGraw-Hill, 1977.
3. Goldstein, B. *Human Sexuality.* New York: McGraw-Hill, 1976.
4. Hite, S. *The Hite Report.* New York: Macmillan, 1976.
5. Holdsworth, A. V. Sex problems in marriage—the nurse's role in a marital and sexual difficulty clinic. *Nurs. Mirror* 147:23, 1978.
6. Kempe, C. H., and Helfer, R. (Eds.). *Helping the Battered Child and His Family.* Philadelphia: Lippincott, 1972.
7. Kinsey, A., et al. *Sexual Behavior in the Human Female.* Philadelphia: Saunders, 1953.
8. Krozy, R. Becoming comfortable with sexual assessment. *Am. J. Nurs.* 78:1036, 1978.
9. Malinowski, J. S. Sex during pregnancy: What can you say? *R.N.* 41:48, 1978.
10. Masters, W. H., and Johnson, V. E. *Human Sexual Response.* Boston: Little, Brown, 1966.
11. Mims, F. H. Human sexuality workshop: A continuing education program. *J. Contin. Educ. Nurs.* 9:29, 1978.
12. Paksta, N.S. All about sex . . . after a coronary. *Am. J. Nurs.* 77:602, 1977.
13. Renshaw, D. C. Adolescent sexuality: How to deal with it effectively. *Consultant* 18:72, 1978.
14. Sedwick, R. Myths in human sexuality. *Nurs. Clin. North Am.* 10:539, 1975.
15. Stanford, D. All about sex . . . after middle age. *Am. J. Nurs.* 77:608, 1977.
16. Stephens, G. T. Creative contraries: A theory of sexuality. *Am. J. Nurs.* 78:70, 1978.
17. Taylor, R. B. Physical origins of sexual dysfunction. *Female Patient* 5:61, 1980.
18. Watts, R. J. The physical interrelationships between depression, drugs and sexuality. *Nurs. Forum* 17:168, 1978.
19. Whitney, N. The first coital experience of one hundred women. *J.O.G.N. Nurs.* 7:41, 1978.
20. Wood, R. Y., and Rose, K. Penile implants for impotence. *Am. J. Nurs.* 78:234, 1978.

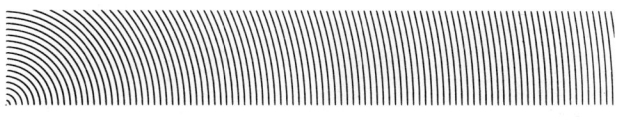

10. Family Planning

Family planning is a broad term that includes active intervention for couples who are having difficulty conceiving children, helping couples space children so they have time to enjoy each child, counseling couples who have the potential for conceiving children with genetic abnormalities as to their best course of action, and helping couples and individuals who do not want to have children to avoid conception.

That a woman has the right to control the size of her family is a recent philosophy. Prior to introduction of "the pill," the methods of family planning available were so limited that, aside from abstinence from sexual relations, planning and spacing for those who were concerned was difficult.

As women become aware in other areas of their lives that they do not have to accept events passively but can change and influence them, the ability to prevent unwanted children or to delay having children until a more appropriate time in life becomes both a desire and a concern of women.

As men begin to view having children as "family centered," not merely "woman's business," they begin to participate more actively in family planning.

As early as 1966, the Board of Directors of the American Nurses' Association issued the following resolution (*Am. J. Nurs.* 66:2376, 1966):*

It is the responsibility of registered nurses:
1. To recognize the right of individuals and families to select and use such methods as are consistent with their own creed and mores.
2. To recognize the right of individuals and families to receive information about family planning if they wish.
3. To be responsive to the need for family planning.
4. To be knowledgeable about state laws regarding family planning and the resources available.
5. To assist in informing individuals and families of the existence of approved family planning resources.
6. To assist in directing individuals and families to sources of such aid.

Birth Control Methods

In order to be ideal as a method of family planning a contraceptive should be completely safe and effective, free of side effects, easily obtainable, inexpensive, and acceptable to the user. The effectiveness of various contraceptive measures is shown in Table 10-1.

ORAL CONTRACEPTIVES

Oral contraceptives, commonly known as "the pill," are most frequently composed of synthetic estrogen combined with a small amount of synthetic proges-

---

*Copyright 1966, American Journal of Nursing Company. Reproduced with permission from the *American Journal of Nursing*, November, Vol. 66, No. 11.

Table 10-1. Effectiveness of Common Methods of Contraception

Method	Approximate Effectiveness (%)
Male sterilization	99
Female sterilization	99
Oral contraceptive	96
Intrauterine device	95
Condom and spermicide	94
Diaphragm	90
Condom	85
Spermicide	80
Rhythm method	75

Source. C. R. Garcia, Contraception at the crossroads. *Contemp. Obstet. Gynecol.* 13:81, 1979. Used by permission from *Contemp. Obstet. Gynecol.*, Medical Economics Co.

terone. The estrogen content acts to suppress the gonadotropic hormones of the pituitary and therefore to halt ovulation. The progesterone fraction may increase the viscosity of cervical mucus, limiting sperm motility and access to ova. Progesterone also interferes with endometrial maturation to such a degree that implantation is unlikely.

Oral contraceptives must be prescribed by a physician. When used correctly, they are 100 percent effective in preventing conception. Because women occasionally forget to take them, their actual effectiveness is between 96 and 100 percent.

Most pills contain estrogen and progesterone components in a combination form. A former sequential pattern, whereby during the first part of a cycle the pills contained only estrogen and later pills contained progesterone, is no longer available. Women who take a combination often report scant menstrual periods; some worry that they are pregnant because their menstrual flow is so atypical. The progesterone contained in the last pills of the sequential type caused more endometrial sloughing to occur and a woman's menstrual period was more nearly normal. Unfortunately, sequential forms were suspected of causing an increased rate of endocervical cancer and for this reason are no longer available.

A pelvic examination and a Papanicolaou smear are done before oral contraceptives are prescribed. The instructions for taking pills are roughly similar for all brands. Generally, a pill is taken daily for 21 days, beginning on the 5th day after the start of the menstrual flow. Three or four days following discontinuance of the pill, a new menstrual flow will begin. This cycle is then repeated. If menstrual bleeding does not take place, the woman begins the new cycle of pills on the 8th day after she stopped the previous cycle. Days that a woman should take pills are shown in Fig. 10-1.

Notice that in the first month of the hypothetical situation the woman's menstrual period (shown by the shaded bar) began on the 3rd day after she completed her 21-day period of taking pills. She began taking pills again on the 8th day after she stopped, regardless of the length or start of the menstrual period. The next month, no menstrual period occurred. On the 8th day, the woman restarted a 21-day pill cycle, nevertheless.

In order for birth control pills to be effective, they must be taken consistently and conscientiously. Many women leave them in plain sight on the bathroom counter or kitchen counter so as to be easily reminded to take them. Women with young children in the house need to be cautioned, however, that this is a dangerous practice from the standpoint of childhood poisoning. Women who have difficulty remembering to take a contraceptive in the morning, because of a busy schedule of getting ready for work or getting children or husband off to school or work, may find it easier to remember to take a pill a day if they do it at bedtime. It makes no difference what time of day the pill is taken; the key word is *daily*.

In order to help women remember the pattern of pill taking (and to eliminate having to count days between pill cycles) certain brands of oral contraceptives are packaged with 28 pills in a circular dial dispenser. The woman begins to take pills on the 1st day of her menstrual period. The first five pills are placebos; the next 20 are the real pills. She starts a second dispenser of pills the day after finishing the first dispenser. There is no need to skip days because, again, the first five pills of the new dispenser are placebo tablets.

Still newer brands of pills stipulate that the woman should begin to take pills on a chosen day and continue for three weeks daily, then skip a week, and begin a new dispenser of pills on the same day of the week that she originally started. This pattern helps her to remember when it is time to start a new dispenser. It also allows her to schedule the time of her menstrual period to some extent (if she starts taking pills on a Monday, she will begin her period four days after she ends a three-week cycle or on a Thursday; if she starts her three-week cycle on a Friday, she will begin her menstrual period on a Monday or avoid having menstrual periods on weekends).

Side Effects

Some women dislike taking oral contraceptives because of side effects they experience. The main side

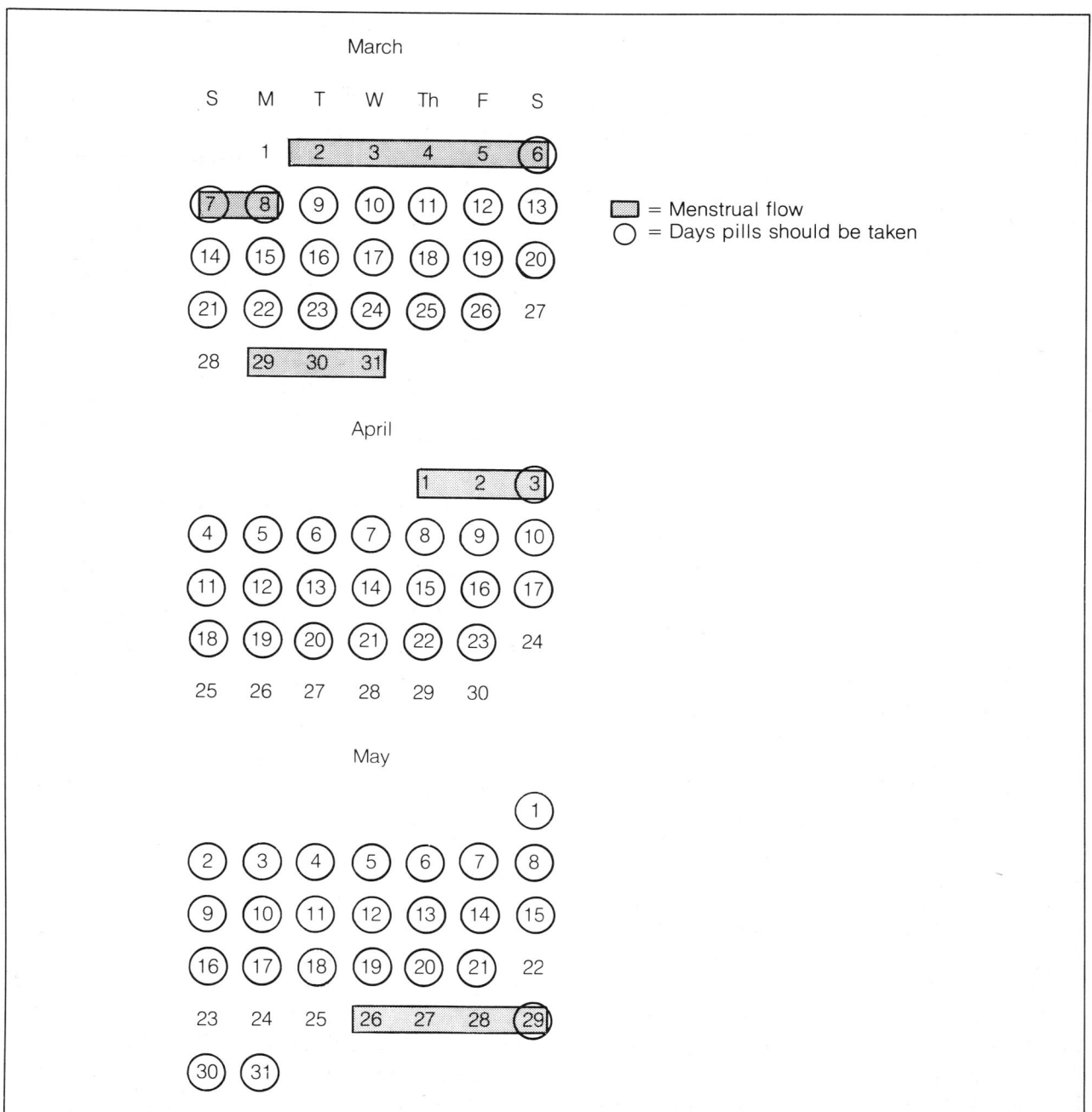

Fig. 10-1. Timetable for oral contraceptive use.

effects are nausea, weight gain, headache, breast tenderness, breakthrough bleeding (spotting outside the menstrual period), acne, and monilial vaginal infections.

Breast-fed infants have lower weight gains when the mother is on oral contraceptives during lactation, since the mother's milk supply is decreased. Women who are breast-feeding, therefore, should probably not be taking oral contraceptives.

Because of the increased tendency toward clotting in the presence of estrogen, mothers with a history of thromboembolic disease or a family history of cerebral or cardiovascular accident should not be placed on the pill routinely. Women who smoke, are over 35 years of age, are obese, or have high blood pressure, high serum cholesterol levels, or pulmonary disease are particularly at risk for heart attack if they are taking oral contraceptives.

Estrogen tends to interfere with sugar metabolism. Women with diabetes mellitus or a history of liver disease, including hepatitis, should also be considered individually before being placed on the pill. Other instances in which oral contraceptives may be contraindicated are breast or reproductive tract malignancy, undiagnosed vaginal bleeding, migraines, epilepsy, or sickle cell disease.

The risk of oral contraceptives plotted against the risk of pregnancy and childbirth is shown in Table 10-2. Newer forms of birth control pills containing only progesterone are available for women who cannot tolerate estrogen therapy. The advantage of this type of pill is that it is taken every day, even through the menstrual flow, so that planning when to take the pills is minimal. Unfortunately, these pills are not as dependable in preventing pregnancy as the estrogen-based forms.

The cost of oral contraceptives and the woman's ability to follow instructions faithfully must both be considered before such contraceptives are prescribed. The woman on oral contraceptives should return for a pelvic examination yearly, and it is generally advised that once a year she discontinue taking them for a month to allow a month of normal ovarian function. During that month she would need to use another method of contraception.

Effect on Sexual Enjoyment

For the most part, not having to worry about pregnancy because the contraceptive being used is reliable makes sexual relations more enjoyable for couples using birth control pills.

Some women appear to lose interest in sex after taking the pill for about 18 months, possibly because of the long-term effect of altered hormones in their body. Sexual interest increases again after they are changed to another form of contraception. Some women find the nausea they experience on the pill interferes with sexual enjoyment as well as with other activities. Women who have been reared to think that sex is permissible only if it is engaged in to produce children may find little enjoyment in the act when they use a birth control method. Some women use the fear of pregnancy to discourage sexual encounters and are unhappy when their ploy is no longer acceptable. They may find so many "side effects" with any method of contraception tried that they discontinue it. Women taking birth control pills should be told that there are now many different forms and strengths of pills. If they are having side effects with one brand, then, they might be able to take another brand involving a different strength of estrogen without problems.

Effect on Future Pregnancy

After a woman discontinues an oral contraceptive, she should expect that she may not become pregnant for

Table 10-2. Mortality of Women Associated with Pregnancy and Childbirth Compared to Use of Oral Contraceptives

Age (Years)	Pregnancy and Childbirth[a]	Oral Contraceptives[b]	
		Nonsmokers	Smokers
15–19	11.1	1.2	1.4
20–24	10.0	1.2	1.4
25–29	12.5	1.2	1.4
30–34	24.9	1.8	10.4
35–39	44.0	3.9	12.8
40–44	71.4	6.6	58.4

[a] Per 100,000 live births, U.S.A., 1972–1974.
[b] Per 100,000 users per year.
Source. C. Tietze, What price fertility control? *Contemp. Obstet. Gynecol.* 12:32, 1978. Used by permission from *Contemp. Obstet. Gynecol.*, Medical Economics Co.

six to eight months. In one study, premature births and infants with congenital anomalies occurred less frequently in women who had been on the pill before conceiving than in women not using oral contraceptives [21]. This may be the result of the phenomenon that neonatal mortality in children spaced two to three years apart tends to be lower than in children who are spaced one year apart.

If the woman suspects that she has become pregnant she should discontinue taking the pill if she intends to continue the pregnancy. High levels of estrogen or progesterone might be teratogenic to a growing fetus (not so great a worry now that birth control pills contain very low doses of hormones in contrast to the original doses of estrogen in pills).

The Adolescent Girl

Because estrogen causes epiphyseal lines of long bones to close and growth to halt, girls under 16 years of age are not usually placed on the pill. Another reason for not prescribing oral contraceptives for adolescent girls is that a well-established menstrual cycle of at least two years' duration should probably also be required. This reduces the chance that the oral contraceptive will cause permanent suppression of pituitary regulating activity. Adolescent girls may not take pills reliably enough to make them effective (adolescent compliance to any form of medicine taking is low). In addition, the cost of a continuing supply of pills may make this a prohibitive method of birth control for the girl who has a limited money supply.

INTRAUTERINE DEVICES

A plastic (recently, copper-coated) spiral, loop, T-shape, 7-shape, or ring inserted into the uterus can act as a means of contraception. The mechanism of its contraceptive action is not fully understood. Possibly, the presence of a foreign substance in the uterus so hastens the journey of the fertilized zygote through the fallopian tube that the zygote arrives in the uterine cavity before the uterine endometrium is ripe for implantation. Without good implantation, the zygote will not survive. Another possibility is that the endometrium forms cytotoxins that attack and destroy a blastocyst in the presence of a foreign body. Although intrauterine devices (IUDs) have been used in women only in recent years, this ancient method of contraception was used in camels as long ago as the time of Christ (a stone was inserted into the camel's uterus).

An intrauterine device must be fitted by a physician, who first performs a pelvic examination and takes a smear for a Papanicolaou test. The device is inserted either during the menstrual flow or before the patient has had intercourse following the menstrual flow. The physician is thus assured that the woman is not pregnant at the time of insertion. Insertion is done in the physician's office. The woman may feel a sharp cramp as the device is passed through the internal cervical os. It is inserted in a collapsed position, then enlarged to its spiral or T-shape form in the uterus when the inserter is withdrawn. Properly fitted, the device is contained wholly within the uterus, although a string attached to it protrudes through the cervix into the vagina (Fig. 10-2).

Intrauterine devices have several advantages over oral contraceptives. Usually only one insertion is necessary, and no further attention is needed. Thus, although the initial insertion involves the cost of a visit to a doctor, there is no continued expense. The patient may notice some spotting or uterine cramps the first two or three weeks after insertion; some women have a heavier than usual menstrual flow for two or three months. Occasionally, a woman continues to have cramping and spotting and is likely, in these instances, to expel the device spontaneously. After each menstrual flow, the woman should examine with a finger the string attached to the IUD to make certain that the device is still in place. Some physicians suggest that the woman not use tampons with an intrauterine device, to prevent the possibility of the two strings becoming entangled or to prevent her from pulling the wrong string. She should have a yearly pelvic examination and Pap test.

Intrauterine devices are contraindicated in women with cervicitis, endometritis, salpingitis, or pelvic inflammatory disease and in the woman whose uterus is known to be distorted in shape (the IUD might cause increased irritation and spread of infection; it might perforate an abnormally shaped uterus).

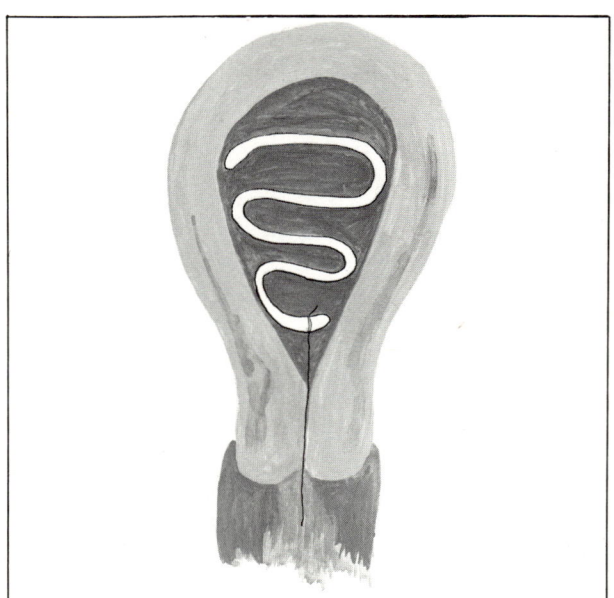

Fig. 10-2. An intrauterine device: here, a Lippes Loop in place.

Effect on Sexual Enjoyment
Women are unable to feel an IUD if it is properly fitted, even during sexual relations, so it does not interfere with sexual enjoyment. The spotting that occurs the first few weeks after insertion is bothersome. Women can be assured that this is a temporary problem and will pass. For the occasional woman who continues to have cramping and spotting, another method of contraception is usually recommended. *Actinomyces* infections may occur with IUD use, requiring treatment.

Effect on Future Pregnancy
If a woman should become pregnant while using an IUD, the device is generally removed vaginally to prevent infection and septic abortion during the pregnancy, although instances of finding the device outside the membranes at the time of delivery, with no damage to the fetus, have been reported. At the time of removal of the device during pregnancy, there is some risk that the intactness of the pregnancy will be disrupted. In some instances, IUDs may cause ectopic (tubal) pregnancy due to delay of the zygote in the fallopian tube.

The Adolescent Girl
It is now possible for nulliparous women (those who have never had children) to be fitted with IUDs. A T-shape or 7-shape (copper coated) device is usually chosen. Girls need a review of reproductive anatomy before they have IUDs inserted so that they understand exactly where the device is being positioned;

Family Planning

otherwise, they worry that it is somehow free-floating in their abdominal cavity and might become misplaced into stomach or intestines.

DIAPHRAGMS

A diaphragm is a circular rubber disk that fits over the cervix and forms a barricade against the entrance of spermatozoa. It is prescribed and fitted initially by a physician or nurse practitioner to ensure a correct fit. Since the shape of the cervix changes with pregnancy, miscarriage, cervical surgery (D&C), or therapeutic abortion, a woman must return for a fitting after any of these occurrences. Gaining or losing more than 20 pounds in weight may change pelvic and vaginal contours to such an extent that having the diaphragm competency checked after weight gain or loss is advisable.

Before intercourse, the woman coats the diaphragm with a contraceptive jelly and then inserts it into the vagina. Spermatozoa remain viable in the vagina for 6 hours. Thus, a diaphragm should remain in place for at least 6 hours following intercourse, and it may be left in place for as long as 24 hours. If it is left in longer, however, the stasis of fluid may cause cervical infection.

If the woman inspects the diaphragm periodically to see that the rubber is not deteriorating and checks it with a finger after insertion to be certain it is fitted well up over the cervix (Fig. 10-3), its efficiency as a contraceptive is very high.

Diaphragms may not be competent if the uterus is prolapsed, retroflexed, or anteflexed to such a degree that the cervix is also displaced in relation to the vagina. Intrusion on the vagina by a cystocele or retrocele (walls of the vagina are displaced by bladder or bowel) may make inserting a diaphragm difficult. Diaphragms should not be used in the presence of acute cervicitis as the close contact of the rubber may cause additional irritation.

Effect on Sexual Enjoyment

Some women dislike using diaphragms because they must insert them prior to intercourse (although they may be inserted up to 2 hours beforehand, minimizing this problem). Frequent penile insertion during intercourse may dislodge the diaphragm, so it may not be the contraceptive of choice for some couples. If intercourse is repeated before 6 hours, the diaphragm should not be removed and replaced, but more spermicidal jelly should be added. Some couples may find this precaution restricting.

Effect on Future Pregnancy

If a woman should become pregnant while using a diaphragm, there is no risk to the fetus. People tell bad jokes about babies looking as if they had been strained through diaphragms, and some women may need help identifying them as merely bad jokes and not reality.

The Adolescent Girl

Adolescents may be fitted for diaphragms, although because an adolescent's vagina varies in size, as she matures and starts sexual relations, the device may not remain as effective as with older women. Adolescents may need to be reminded that diaphragms must be individually fitted; otherwise they may borrow a friend's, or a group of girls will pool their money to pay for one.

VAGINALLY INSERTED SPERMICIDAL PRODUCTS

Spermicidal jellies or creams, when inserted into the vagina, cause the death of spermatozoa before they can enter the cervix. These jellies are actively spermicidal and change the vaginal pH to a strong acid level, a condition not conducive to sperm survival.

With an applicator supplied with each product, the woman inserts the jelly or cream into the vagina before intercourse (Fig. 10-4). She should do this no more than 1 hour prior to intercourse for most effective results. She must be certain to insert the product far back in the vagina. She should not douche for 6 hours following coitus to ensure that the cream or jelly has completed its spermicidal action. Since no prescription is necessary for the purchase of such creams or jellies, they offer an independent method of birth control.

A newer form of spermicidal product is the vaginal

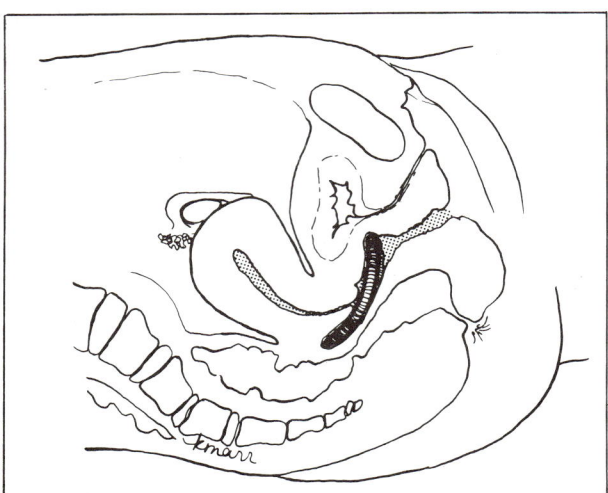

Fig. 10-3. Proper placement of contraceptive diaphragm. (From K. R. Niswander, Obstetric and Gynecologic Disorders: A Practitioner's Guide. Flushing, N.Y.: Medical Examination Publishing Co., 1975.)

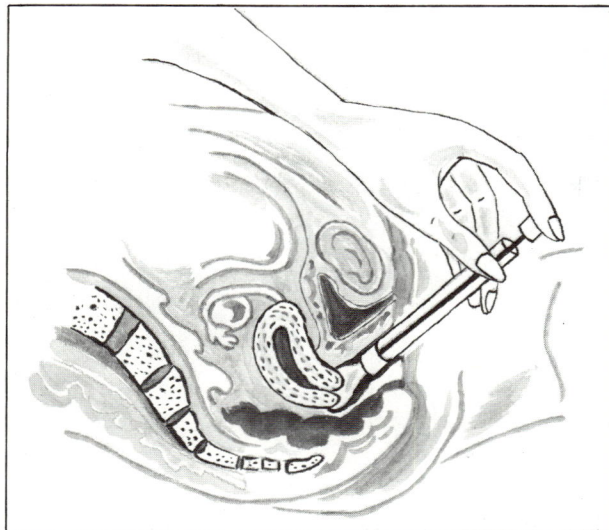

Fig. 10-4. Application of a spermicidal preparation.

tablet. The tablet is small and can be inserted into the vagina easily; on contact with vaginal secretions or precoital penile emissions, it dissolves and a carbon dioxide foam that protects the cervix against invading spermatozoa forms. Another newer method is a foam-impregnated sponge which is inserted vaginally. Moisture, again, creates an internal foaming action and contraception protection. Also available are cocoa-butter and glycerin-based vaginal suppositories. Inserted vaginally, the suppository dissolves and frees the spermicidal ingredients. Because it may take about 15 minutes for the suppository to dissolve, it must be inserted 15 minutes prior to coitus.

Vaginally inserted spermicidal products are contraindicated in women with acute cervicitis because they further irritate the cervix. They are generally inappropriate for couples who *must* prevent conception (perhaps the woman is taking a drug which is teratogenic or the couple absolutely does not want the responsibility of children) because the effectiveness of all forms of these products is only about 80 percent, compared to the higher 95 to 100 percent effectiveness rate of diaphragms, IUDs, and oral contraceptives. Women nearing menopause should be advised not to use a type of contraceptive that depends on vaginal moisture to be activated; they may have less vaginal secretion at this time of life than they did previously. Some women find the vaginal "leakage" they have after use of these products bothersome. Vaginal suppositories, because of the cocoa-butter and glycerin bases, are most bothersome.

Effect on Sexual Enjoyment

Although spermicidal products must be inserted fairly close to coitus, they also are so easily purchased (no prescription, no physician appointment necessary) that many couples find the inconvenience of insertion only a minor problem. If a couple is concerned that the method does not offer enough protection, worry about becoming pregnant may interfere with sexual enjoyment. Some women and even their partners find the foam or moisture irritating to vaginal and penile tissue.

Effect on Future Pregnancy

If contraception should occur, there is no reason to think that the fetus will be affected. Some women worry that a sperm that survived the cream or foam must have been weakened by migrating through it and will produce a defective child. They can be assured that conception occurred because the product did not completely cover the cervical os; the sperm that reached the uterus was free of the product and unharmed.

The Adolescent Girl

Many adolescents use vaginal products as a method of birth control. There is little money involved because a physician appointment is not needed, and no parental permission is involved. Adolescents should be cautioned that this method has a high pregnancy rate (20 percent). All women need to be cautioned that preparations labeled "feminine hygiene" products are for vaginal cleanliness and are not spermicidal; they are not birth control products.

Because of the settings in which adolescents engage in sex (in cars or hurriedly on couches) some girls find having to insert the product awkward and consequently omit using it even though they have purchased it and intended to be more cautious.

THE RHYTHM METHOD

The rhythm method of family planning requires that a couple abstain from sexual intercourse on the days of a menstrual cycle when the woman is able to conceive (the period surrounding ovulation).

In order to have a framework on which to base calculations of safe times, a woman should keep a record of 12 menstrual cycles (a minimum of six). Her *first fertile day* is determined by subtracting 18 from the number of days in the shortest menstrual cycle she has had over the last 12 months. The last fertile day is determined by subtracting 11 days from the longest menstrual cycle during the 12-month period. For example, if she had menstrual cycles ranging from 26 to 32 days, her fertile period (the period during which she must abstain from intercourse) would be from the

8th day (26 − 18) to the 21st day (32 − 11). This schedule is shown in Fig. 10-5.

In this hypothetical situation, the woman has only nine days during the 1st month illustrated that are "safe days" for her. In the 2nd month, because her menstrual cycle was fairly short (27 days), there are only seven safe days available. This short period of safe days is the reason the rhythm method is not an acceptable form of birth control for some couples.

The numbers 18 and 11 are used because conception usually occurs between the 18th and 11th days from the end of the cycle. This method of contraception is about 85 percent effective if the woman has regular menstrual cycles and is motivated to maintain monthly records. In actual practice it is less effective than this because of irregular cycles and failure to keep records over a long period of time. The method will not work reliably if the woman's menstrual cycles are irregular or she does not accept the responsibility for calculating fertile days. It is unreliable in the postpartal period until regular periods are established again. It is inaccurate in the lactating woman, who may not have menstrual flows as markers for calculation.

Fig. 10-5. Timetable for using rhythm as a family planning method.

Unlike previously mentioned methods of birth control, the rhythm method depends on cooperation of the sexual partner. Some women find this a disadvantage; some couples enjoy this criterion as it makes family planning truly "family" planning.

Effect on Sexual Enjoyment

Because there is no prescription or medication involved, there is no cost involved. More spontaneity in sexual relations is possible than with methods that involve vaginal insertions. On the other hand, the required days of abstinence may make the method unsatisfactory and unenjoyable for a couple.

Effect on Future Pregnancy

No artificial methods of contraception are involved. Therefore, there are no effects on future pregnancies except the possibility that the child conceived is unwanted and the parents cannot adjust to the conception, pregnancy, and child.

The Adolescent Girl

As girls tend to have irregular menstrual cycles for several years after menarche, the rhythm method is often ineffective as a means of birth control for young adolescents. Also, it requires the girl to keep a calen-

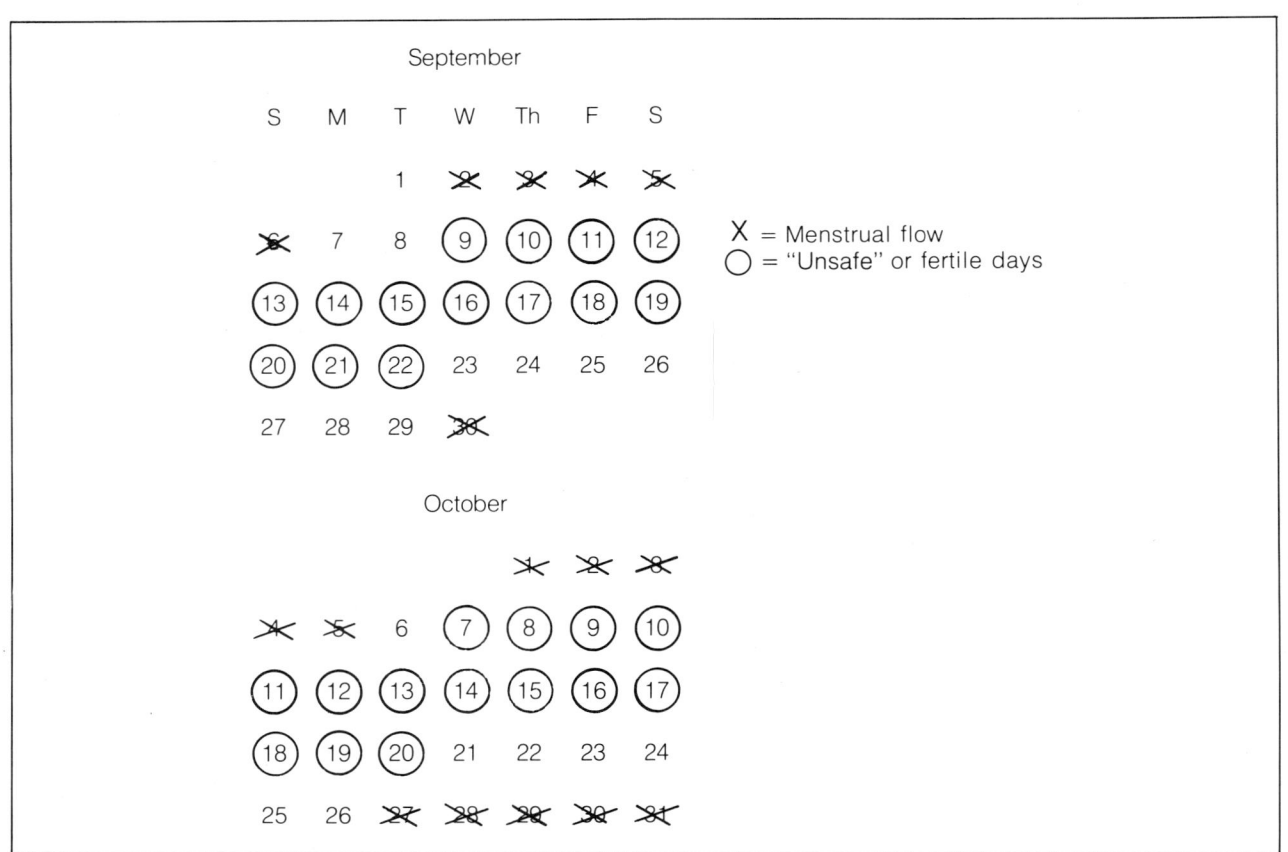

dar of safe and unsafe days and to be able to say "no" to encounters on unsafe days.

Rhythm and Basal Temperature

Just prior to the day of ovulation, the woman's basal body temperature will fall about half a degree. At the time of ovulation, the temperature will rise a full degree. This higher level will be maintained for the rest of the menstrual cycle.

To use this method of contraception, the woman should take and chart her rectal temperature each morning immediately after waking, before she undertakes any activity. This is her basal temperature. She should then calculate her first fertile day as in the rhythm method (i.e., shortest menstrual cycle minus 18). This will be her first day of abstinence (as with the rhythm method). As soon as she notices a slight dip in temperature followed by an increase, she knows that she has ovulated. She continues abstinence only until the third day of the sustained high temperature; thus the period of abstinence is usually shortened by three or four days (Fig. 10-6).

The danger of this method is that a temperature rise may be the result of illness rather than of ovulation.

Fig. 10-6. Timetable for using rhythm in conjunction with basal temperature as a family planning method.

The woman may interpret the increase in temperature wrongly and mistake a fertile day for a safe one.

Rhythm and Ovulation Determination

Prior to ovulation each month, cervical mucus is thick and does not stretch when pulled between the thumb and a finger (the property of spinnbarkeit). With ovulation and for two days afterward, the cervical mucus becomes thin and watery and stretches a distance of 12 to 15 cm before the strand breaks.

By making use of this knowledge, a woman can more accurately predict her day of ovulation than by the rhythm method alone.

To use this method, the woman establishes her first day of sexual abstinence the same as for the basic rhythm method (18 days subtracted from her shortest period). She then tests her vaginal secretions daily for the property of spinnbarkeit. She continues abstinence only three days after spinnbarkeit occurs, like the basal body temperature modification, allowing her possibly to shorten the total period of abstinence each month by three or four days.

The woman must be conscientious about assessing vaginal secretions daily or she will miss the phenomenon of changing cervical secretions. The feel of vaginal secretions following sexual relations is unreliable

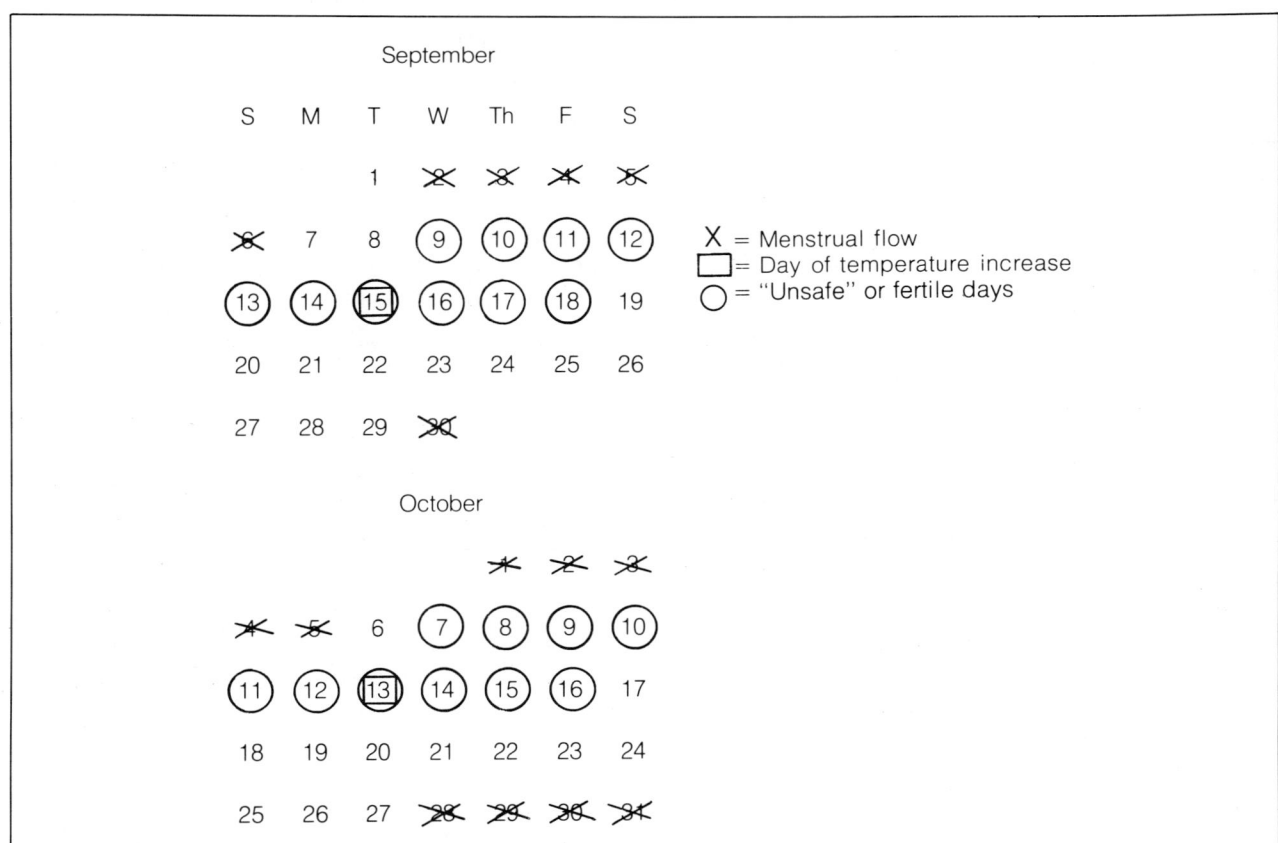

as seminal fluid (the fluid containing sperm from the male) has a watery, postovulatory consistency and can be confused with ovulatory mucus.

THE OVULATION METHOD

Women may use the naturally occurring changes in cervical mucus as a singular method of natural family planning. Used alone, this is often called the *Billings method*, after its originator [2]. To use cervical evaluation alone, the woman assesses her vaginal secretions daily following her menstrual flow. When the quality of secretions changes and they become wet and slippery and demonstrate spinnbarkeit properties, she begins to abstain from sexual relations. She continues abstinence until three days after the mucus has become sticky and unstretchable again. For most women, this limits the period of abstinence to a very short time, about five to seven days.

In order to acquaint herself with the feel of vaginal changes during a cycle, a woman should abstain from coitus for a full month. During following months, she should abstain from coitus every other day during the first part of each cycle so she can evaluate cervical mucus free of seminal fluid.

A woman must be highly motivated to use the ovulation method. It may be helpful to a woman who is lactating and therefore does not have menstrual flow markers for the rhythm method or for the woman who has such irregular periods that the rhythm method leaves her very few safe days.

CONDOMS

A *condom* is a rubber sheath (similar to a finger cot but larger in diameter) that is placed over the erect penis prior to coitus. It prevents pregnancy because spermatozoa are deposited not in the vagina but in the tip of the condom. The use of condoms has an efficiency rate of about 85 percent. This is one of the few "male-responsibility" birth control measures available. No prescription is needed for the purchase of these products. As well as being contraceptive, they have the added potential of lessening the chance of spreading venereal disease.

There are no contraindications to the use of condoms except for rare rubber sensitivity. As they are not as effective a means of contraception as other forms, they should be used with caution by couples who must for medical reasons delay conception.

Effect on Sexual Enjoyment

In order to be effective in use, condoms must be applied prior to any penile-vulvar contact because preejaculation fluid may contain some sperm. As soon as the penis begins to become flaccid following ejaculation, the penis (with the condom held carefully in place) must be withdrawn. If it is not withdrawn at this time, sperm may leak from the now loosely fitting sheath into the vagina. Some men find that condoms dull their enjoyment of sex; some women resent the fact that the man must withdraw promptly following ejaculation.

Some men enjoy the use of condoms because they put the responsibility for conception on their shoulders.

Effect on Future Pregnancy

There is no effect on children who are conceived while a condom is being used.

The Adolescent

Adolescents may need to be cautioned that condoms should not be reused as even a pinpoint hole can allow thousands of sperm to escape. Some adolescent boys have infrequent coitus and therefore use condoms that they have owned and stored for a long time. The efficiency of these old condoms, especially if they are carried in a warm pocket should be questioned. For many adolescent couples, use of a vaginally inserted preparation by the girl and a condom by her partner is the preferred method of birth control. Efficiency of these two methods of birth control, used in conjunction, becomes about 90 percent.

COITUS INTERRUPTUS

Coitus interruptus is one of the oldest known methods of contraception. The couple proceeds with coitus until the moment of ejaculation. Then the man withdraws and the emission of spermatozoa takes place outside the vagina. Unfortunately, ejaculation may occur before withdrawal is complete and, despite the care used, some spermatozoa may be deposited in the vagina. Since there are always a few spermatozoa in preejaculation seminal fluid, even though withdrawal seems controlled, fertilization from them may occur. For these reasons, coitus interruptus offers little protection against conception.

Effect on Sexual Enjoyment

Some couples obtain sexual satisfaction when using this method. Others find that it interferes with satisfaction.

Effect on Future Pregnancy

There are no effects on children conceived when the procedure is used.

The Adolescent

Adolescent boys often lack the control or experience to use coitus interruptus.

POSTCOITAL DOUCHE

Douching after sexual intercourse is also an old method of preventing conception, but a poor one. Spermatozoa enter the cervical canal within 90 seconds after ejaculation; they reach the site of the fallopian tubes within 5 minutes. Any douching that is done in the postcoital period is already after the fact, therefore, and actually may promote conception by washing sperm against the cervix.

Douching for any reason is contraindicated in women during the postpartal period until they have returned for a postpartal examination to be assured that the external cervical canal has closed and fluid will not enter the cervix. Because frequent douching may change the flora and acidity of the vagina, it may invite monilial or fungal infections.

MORNING-AFTER PILL

To prevent pregnancy from an unprotected act of sexual intercourse, diethylstilbestrol (DES), also known as stilbestrol, a synthetic estrogen, may be prescribed by a physician. To be effective, this oral medication must be started no later than 24 hours after the unprotected intercourse. The high level of estrogen interferes with the production of progesterone and therefore prohibits good implantation. It is a helpful method of eliminating pregnancy in women or girls who have been raped. The method should always be used cautiously, since high levels of estrogen in the body are associated with thromboembolism. If DES has been given during early pregnancy, vaginal carcinoma may occur in the child of the pregnancy when the child reaches puberty. Therefore, if DES is given to prevent conception and is ineffective, the child of the pregnancy should be monitored into puberty to see whether vaginal cancer is developing. This is only a possibility, not a certainty, particularly because such a short course of DES (5 days usually) is utilized.

Because DES carries such a high risk to the woman and to her fetus if it is unsuccessful, it is not a routine method of family planning.

STERILIZATION

Both men and women can use sterilization as a means of preventing conception.

In sterilization of a male, a small incision is made in each side of the scrotum. The vas deferens at that point is then cut and tied, blocking the passage of spermatozoa. The procedure is called *vasectomy* and can be done under local anesthesia in the physician's office. It is 100 percent effective, although spermatozoa that were present in the vas deferens at the time of surgery may remain viable for as long as six months. An additional birth control method should be used until six months have passed. The man should think of the procedure as irreversible, although newer techniques of microsurgery can make it reversible to a limited extent.

Some men resist the concept of vasectomy because they are not sufficiently aware of their anatomy to know exactly what the procedure involves. Vasectomy does not interfere with the production of sperm; the testes continue to produce sperm as always; the sperm simply do not pass beyond the severed vas deferens but are absorbed at that point. The man will still have full erection and ejaculation capacity. Because he also continues to form seminal fluid, he will ejaculate seminal fluid; it just has no sperm included in it.

The incision site for a vasectomy is shown in Fig. 10-7.

Following vasectomy, some men form antibodies against sperm. Even if reconstruction of the vas deferens is successful, then, the sperm they produce do not have good mobility and are incapable of fertilization. The actual ability to reverse vasectomy procedures is therefore low, about 30 percent [17].

Sterilization of women could include removal of the uterus (hysterectomy), but it generally refers to a surgical procedure, such as tubal ligation, that occludes the fallopian tubes and thereby prevents passage of the ova into the uterus.

The simplest operation for female sterilization is laparoscopy (Fig. 10-8). Under general anesthesia, an incision about an inch long is made just under the woman's umbilicus. A lighted laparoscope is inserted

Fig. 10-7. Placement of a vasectomy incision.

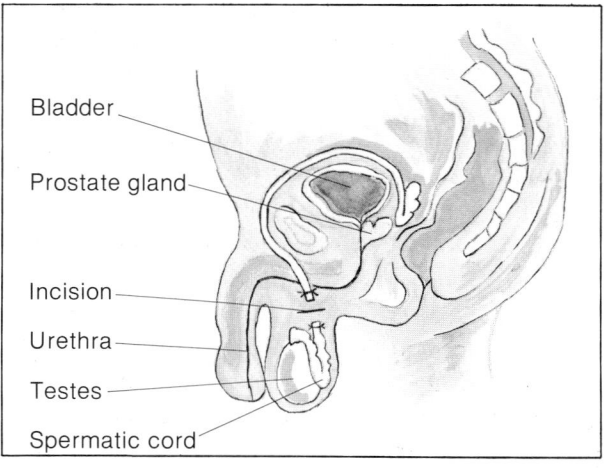

Family Planning

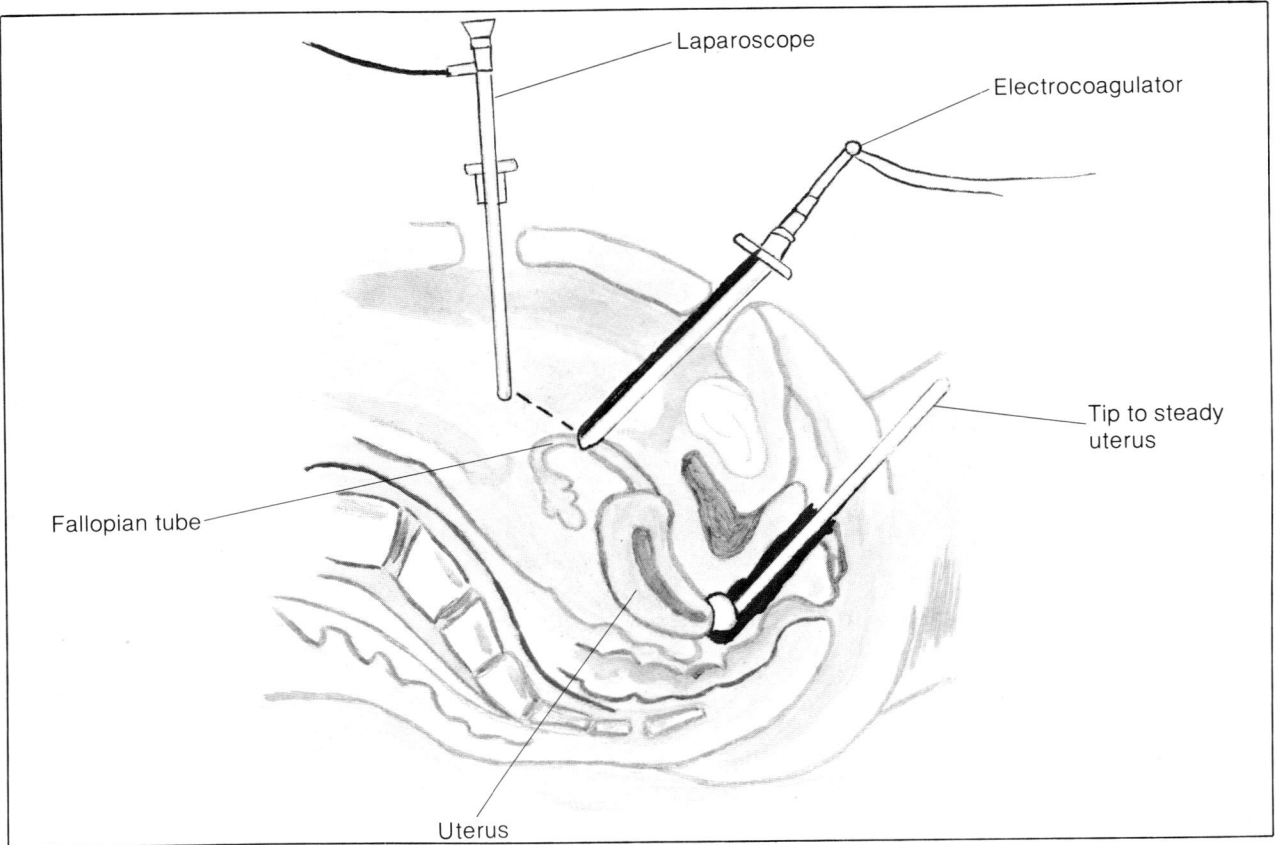

Fig. 10-8. Laparoscopy for tubal sterilization. The patency of the tubes is destroyed by application of an electrical current. Two small abdominal incisions are used here.

through the incision. Carbon dioxide is then pumped into the incision to lift the abdominal wall upward out of the line of vision. The surgeon locates the fallopian tubes by viewing the field through the laparoscope. He passes an electrical current through the instrument for about 3 to 5 seconds. This coagulates the tissue of the tube and seals it. The operation is quick, and the woman is either kept in the hospital overnight or discharged in a few hours. She may notice abdominal "bloating" following the procedure for the first 24 hours until the carbon dioxide is absorbed. She may notice sharp diaphragmatic or shoulder pain as some of the carbon dioxide escapes under the diaphragm.

Women need to be informed prior to the procedure that their menstrual cycle will be unaffected by the procedure. Otherwise they are disappointed or worried that, unlike hysterectomy, the operation allows them to still have menstrual periods.

It is difficult to reconstruct fallopian tubes after they have been cauterized. There is a possibility that the anastomosis site after such a repair, because it is irregular, will lead to ectopic (tubal) pregnancy. After reconstructive surgery of this type (salpingoplasty), the pregnancy rate is about 15 percent. Of that 15 percent, 10 percent of pregnancies will end as tubal pregnancies [17]. Tubal ligation or laparoscopy for sterilization, therefore, should not be undertaken lightly but only after the woman has decided firmly that she not only does not want children now but also will not want them at some future date.

Sterilization should not be undertaken in individuals, either male or female, who equate being fertile with being a full person. Such a person might feel little self-esteem afterward.

Effect on Sexual Enjoyment

Sterilization may lead to increased sexual enjoyment as it completely eliminates the possibility of pregnancy. If either partner changes his or her mind, however, about having children or additional children, the surgery may become an issue between them that interferes not only with sexual enjoyment but with other aspects of their relationship as well.

The Adolescent

Sterilization is not usually advised for adolescents. Their future goals may change so drastically that what they want at age 16 or 18 may not be what they want at all at age 30. Adolescents should be counseled to utilize more temporary forms of birth control. Later, if they still feel sterilization is the method of family planning for them, the option is still open.

ABORTION

Abortion is not a form of contraception in the usual sense. It does not prevent conception but interferes with an already established pregnancy. It is discussed in Chap. 33, with other interferences of pregnancy.

Future Family Planning Methods

Since estrogen is responsible for most of the side effects associated with oral contraceptives, studies are being made of extremely low-dose estrogen pills. Studies utilizing only progesterone are continuing. It is possible that a progesterone injection once a month or a progesterone-impregnated diaphragm will be used in the future. Progesterone could perhaps be implanted under the skin once a year in a slowly dissolving plastic capsule. Possibly a woman could be "vaccinated" with antibodies against spermatozoa. A male oral contraceptive may be developed. Until some method satisfies all the criteria for an ideal contraceptive—complete safety, no side effects, low cost, easy availability, and user acceptability—research in this field will continue.

Nursing progress notes in reference to family planning follow.

Problem-oriented Recording: Progress Notes

September 6
Christine McFadden
15 years

Problem: Family planning

> S. 15-year-old female seen for advice on contraception. Has been sexually active for 3 months; has not been using any form of birth control. Menarche at 12 years, menstrual cycle 28–35 days' duration, moderately heavy flow, cramping enough to keep her home from school 1 day/month. Last menstrual flow 1 week ago.
> No history of venereal disease, vaginal infections, pelvic inflammatory disease, uterine malformation.
> O. Height: 5'2"; development: Tanner 4.
> A. Candidate for contraceptive counseling because active sexually.
>
> Goals: a. Can voice contraceptive options available and her preference.
> b. Can explain how to use method of choice.
> c. Can explain any follow-up care necessary for method chosen.
>
> P. 1. Suggest IUD (at 5'2", growth may not be complete enough for oral contraceptive; adolescent poor compliance leaves other methods in doubt).
> 2. Routine VDRL, gonorrhea plate.
> 3. Discuss ability to say no to sexual relationships she does not want.
> 4. Discuss method and follow-up of contraceptive method chosen.

September 13
Christine McFadden
15 years

Problem: Family planning

> S. (Telephone call) Patient had IUD fitted 1 week ago (a CU-T). Has had spotting for 7 days, moderate cramping for last 2 days. Expelled IUD this A.M. No further vaginal bleeding or cramping. Device appears to be intact from her description.
> O. —
> A. Expulsion of complete IUD; further contraceptive assistance needed.
> P. 1. Schedule for appointment September 15.
> 2. Caution about danger of sexual relationships in the meantime.
> 3. Reassure that no harm results from expulsion of IUD.

References

1. Berkman, S. Late complications of tubal sterilization by laparoscopy. *Contemp. Obstet. Gynecol.* 9:118, 1977.
2. Billings, J. *Natural Family Planning: The Ovulation Method* (3rd ed.). Collegeville, Minn.: The Liturgical Press, 1975.

3. Bradbury, B. Preventing the diaphragm baby syndrome, a matter of technique, teaching and time. *J.O.G.N. Nurs.* 4:24, 1975.
4. Britt, S. Fertility awareness: Four methods of natural family planning. *J.O.G.N. Nurs.* 6:9, 1977.
5. Corner, G. W., and Harris, B. A. Sterilization by minilaparotomy. *Female Patient* 4:51, 1979.
6. Cowart, M., and Newton, D. Oral contraceptives: How best to explain the effects to patients. *Nursing 76* 6:44, 1976.
7. Diebel, P. Natural family planning: Different methods. *M.C.N.* 3:171, 1978.
8. Dryfoos, J. G., et al. Contraceptive services for adolescents. *Fam. Plann. Perspect.* 10:223, 1978.
9. Ford, K. Contraceptive use in the United States. *Fam. Plann. Perspect.* 10:264, 1978.
10. Freeman, E. W. Abortion: Subjective attitudes and feelings. *Fam. Plann. Perspect.* 10:150, 1978.
11. Garcia, C. R. Contraception at the crossroads. *Contemp. Obstet. Gynecol.* 13:81, 1979.
12. Hatcher, R. A., et al. *Contraceptive Technology 1976–1977* (8th ed.). New York: Halsted Press, 1976.
13. Hubbard, C. W. *Family Planning Education* (2nd ed.). St. Louis: Mosby, 1977.
14. Huxall, L. K. Today's pill and the individual woman. *M.C.N.* 2:359, 1977.
15. Huxall, L. K. Update on IUDs. *M.C.N.* 5:186, 1980.
16. Lieberman, E. J. Teenage sex and birth control. *J.A.M.A.* 240:275, 1978.
17. Martin, L. L. *Health Care of Women.* Philadelphia: Lippincott, 1978.
18. Moore, O. F., et al. Family planning clinic "dropouts." *Nurse Pract.* 3:14, 1978.
19. Murray, L. Searching for safe contraceptives. *Contemp. Obstet. Gynecol.* 9:37, 1977.
20. Palmer, R. J. Reversibility as a consideration in laparoscopic sterilization. *J. Reprod. Med.* 21:57, 1978.
21. Peterson, W. F. Pregnancy following oral contraceptive therapy. *Obstet. Gynecol.* 34:363, 1969.
22. Robbie, M. O. Health care for adolescents: Contraceptive counseling for younger adolescent women. *J.O.G.N. Nurs.* 7:29, 1978.
23. Scales, P., et al. Male involvement in contraceptive decision making. *J. Community Health* 3:54, 1977.
24. Segal, S. J. Contraceptives and the young: Present status and future prospects. *Pediatrics* 62:1211, 1978.
25. Shapiro, S. Oral contraceptives and myocardial infarction. *N. Engl. J. Med.* 293:195, 1975.
26. Silber, S. J. Vasectomy and vasectomy reversal. *Fertil. Steril.* 29:125, 1978.
27. Stern, M., et al. Cardiovascular risk and use of estrogens or estrogen-progesterone combinations. *J.A.M.A.* 234:811, 1976.
28. Tanis, J. L. Recognizing the reason for contraception non-use and abuse. *M.C.N.* 2:364, 1977.
29. Timby, B. Ovulation method of birth control. *Am. J. Nurs.* 76:928, 1976.
30. Westoff, C. F., and Jones, E. F. Contraception and sterilization in the United States, 1965–1975. *Fam. Plann. Perspect.* 9:153, 1977.
31. Zelnik, M., et al. Sexual and contraceptive experiences of young unmarried women in the United States. *Fam. Plann. Perspect.* 9:55, 1977.

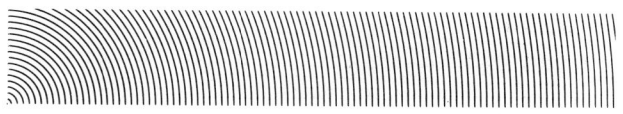

11. Infertility and Sterility

From the time a woman is told that she is pregnant until she holds her infant in her arms she worries that she may not be able to carry her child to term. In about 10 to 15 percent of American couples, the concern is an even greater one. They are fearful that they are not able to initiate a pregnancy, that one of them is infertile or perhaps even sterile.

It is important for the welfare of children, the physical health of the woman, and the mental health of the couple that couples have only as many children as they want or can care for. Not all couples want or should have children, but those who do want children should be able to conceive and bear them.

Infertility is said to exist when a pregnancy has not occurred after at least one year of effort. In *primary infertility*, there have been no previous conceptions; in *secondary infertility*, there has been a previous viable pregnancy but the couple seems unable to conceive now. In *sterility*, some definite factor prevents conception.

In 30 to 35 percent of couples with an infertility problem, the man is infertile. In 30 to 35 percent of instances of female infertility, the fallopian tubes are involved; in 20 percent, the cervix; and in 15 percent, a hormonal factor [2]. In 5 to 10 percent of couples, no known cause for the infertility can be discovered.

Many couples think they have a problem of infertility because they are unaware of the average length of time it takes for a couple to achieve a pregnancy. When participating in sexual intercourse an average of four times per week, 50 percent of couples take six months to conceive; after 12 months, 80 percent of couples will have done so. These times are longer if sexual relations are less frequent. If conception is not achieved by 12 months (which it is not in 20 percent of couples), a couple will begin to have serious doubts about their ability to conceive.

Many young couples today try to organize their lives into time blocks. The first two years of marriage, both partners will work and they will furnish their home; or they will both attend school and finish their educations. The third year of their marriage they will have their first child. Couples who program their lives this way grow apprehensive when conception does not occur according to plan. Sometimes simple counseling, with an explanation that conception is not as predictable as a degree after four years of college, will alleviate their apprehension. There is a general feeling that infertility tends to occur in couples who desperately want a baby. The woman is said to be "trying too hard." It is difficult to document which is the chicken and which the egg in such couples. Perhaps they want a child desperately because their plans have been frustrated, and it is not their desperation that is causing the infertility, but their infertility that is causing the desperation.

Women who have been taking oral contraceptives or using an intrauterine device (IUD) for birth control may have difficulty becoming pregnant for a number of months after discontinuing the pills or having the IUD removed. Couples should be counseled regarding this possibility.

Fertility Studies

The age of the couple and the degree of apprehension they seem to feel make a difference in determining when they should be referred for evaluation to a gynecologist or an obstetrician who does fertility studies. As a rule of thumb, if the woman is under 30, she should be referred after one year of infertility. If she is over 30, she should be referred after six months of infertility. The older the woman, the more quickly studies should be undertaken, since adoption, the alternative to childbearing, is also limited by age. It would be doubly unfortunate if a couple delayed fertility testing so long that by the time they discovered they were incapable of conception they would also be considered too old by an adoption agency. If the couple is extremely apprehensive over their apparent infertility, no matter what their ages, studies should never be delayed.

Although infertility is almost automatically assumed to be the woman's problem, fertility studies involve both partners. It may well be the man's problem, and it most assuredly is the couple's problem. Also, fertility testing in the male is relatively easy. It is a waste of health personnel's time and of the woman's time to conduct extensive fertility studies on her until the man has been demonstrated to be fertile.

Couples are in a vulnerable position when they call a clinic or physician's office to ask for help with infertility. They are admitting that they need help, a concession many people find difficult to make. To admit that they cannot conceive a child is, because of social and family pressure, demeaning to them. The couple may be worried about the future of their marriage. Each partner may wonder whether the other will be able to accept marriage with a person who is infertile. Some people would rather not know the exact reason for the infertility, on the theory that no news is at least not bad news.

Couples need to discuss at the first visit to the clinic or physician the reasons for their being interested in a fertility series. Those who seriously desire children because they love and want children should be differentiated from those who want children because of family or social pressure; from those who are attempting to strengthen a weak marriage with a child; from those who want to know for their own peace of mind that they are fertile, but who do not want children; and from those who want to know that they are indeed infertile so that they can discontinue contraceptive measures.

Not all couples know what motivations brought them to this visit. Encouraging them to take a look at their motivations helps them to learn more about themselves and will offer clues to their reactions to the outcome of the studies. Depending on their motivation for undertaking the studies, a couple's reaction to the results of the studies may vary from relief to stoic acceptance to grief for the children never to be born. They need the support of health personnel throughout the course of infertility studies, so that if the news is bad, it comes from people who have stood by them from the first day they steeled themselves to ask, "Exactly why are we childless?"

Infertility studies are time-consuming; at least 8 to 12 weeks is required for a minimum series. If the first tests reveal abnormalities, further studies may be necessary, extending the time to three or four months. After all this, the results may reveal no known cause for the apparent infertility. Couples should be prepared for both these eventualities at the first visit, so that they are not unnecessarily alarmed by the time the studies take, or do not feel cheated when the results are indeterminate.

Causes of Male Infertility

A number of factors may lead to male infertility: a disturbance in spermatogenesis (the production of sperm cells); an obstruction in the seminiferous tubules, ducts, or vessels that prevents movement of spermatozoa; qualitative or quantitative changes in the seminal fluid that again prevents motility of spermatozoa; and a problem in ejaculation or deposition that prevents spermatozoa from being placed close enough to the cervix to penetrate it and fertilize the ovum.

INADEQUATE SPERM COUNT

The minimal sperm count considered normal is 40 million per milliliter of seminal fluid, or a total of 125 million per ejaculation. At least 50 percent of sperm should be motile, and 70 percent should be normal in shape. Inadequate sperm counts may be caused by chronic infection such as tuberculosis or recurrent sinusitis. The decrease in sperm production occurs because of the slightly elevated temperature accompanying these diseases. Spermatozoa must be maintained at a temperature slightly less than body temperature (this is why the testes are suspended in the scrotal sac away from body heat) for the sperm cells to be normal and motile. Men who work at desk jobs, which increase scrotal heat, are likely to have lower sperm counts than men whose occupations allow them to be ambulatory at least part of each day. Men who drive a great deal each day (salesmen, motorcyclists) may be affected the same way.

Basic production of spermatozoa may be impaired by a disease such as the orchitis that follows mumps. This problem cannot be alleviated or treated at present but can be prevented in the future if every child receives mumps vaccine.

Exposure to excessive x-rays or radioactive substances may impair spermatozoa production. Men should have adequate protection from these substances if they are exposed to them in their employment. The testes of boys and men having pelvic x-rays should be covered by a protective shield.

Excessive use of alcohol or drugs may affect sperm production in that they cause general ill health and debilitation or malnutrition. Endocrine imbalance may be responsible for inhibition of spermatogenesis. Thyroid and pituitary imbalances are the two endocrine problems most often at fault.

Low vitamin intake may play a role in male infertility. Although vitamin E apparently aids fertility, the sexual prowess attributed to this vitamin at present is probably exaggerated.

Surgery on or near the testes (inguinal herniorrhaphy, for example) may impair circulation to the testes, with resultant reduction or absence of spermatogenesis. Trauma to testes such as may occur in a sports accident sometimes causes testicular damage. Cryptorchidism (undescended testes) at birth may lead to lowered sperm production if the repair to lower the testes into the scrotal sac was not completed until after puberty or the spermatic cord was twisted at the time of surgery.

OBSTRUCTION OF SPERM MOTILITY
Obstruction may occur at any point in the pathway that spermatozoa must travel to reach the outside: the seminiferous tubules, the epididymis, the vas deferens, the ejaculatory duct, and the urethra (see Fig. 7-10). Tubal infection, such as occurs with gonorrhea or ascending urethra infection, may result in adhesions and occlusions; congenital stricture of a spermatic duct is sometimes seen.

CHANGES IN SEMINAL FLUID
Infection of the prostate gland through which the seminal fluid passes, or infection of the seminal vesicles, where sperm is "pooled" waiting for ejaculation, will change the composition of the seminal fluid to such an extent that sperm motility may be reduced.

DIFFICULTY WITH EJACULATION
Too frequent intercourse may reduce sperm count. Anomalies of the penis, such as hypospadias (urethral opening on the ventral surface of the penis) or epispadias (urethral opening on the dorsal surface), may cause deposition of spermatozoa too far from the cervix to allow for cervical penetration. Obesity may interfere with penetration.

Psychological problems and debilitating diseases may result in an inability to achieve ejaculation (impotence). Impotence is primary if the man has never been able to achieve erection and ejaculation, secondary if at one time it was not a problem but now is. Impotence can be an easily solved problem if it is associated with stress such as work or home responsibility and this stress can be relieved. Impotence can also be a manifestation of an underlying psychological problem (the man tends to view sex as aggressive, attacking behavior and cannot participate in such behavior). If the impotence is caused by deep-seated psychological issues (psychogenic infertility), a solution to the problem will include psychological or sexual counseling and may involve long-term care.

Premature ejaculation may affect the proper deposition of sperm; the use of precoital lubricants may inhibit such deposition.

Assessment of Male Infertility
It is best to begin fertility testing with the man because the tests done in the male are simple and easy to carry out. However, many men cannot admit that they might be infertile. In such instances, testing may have to be initiated in the woman. The man can be tested when he has reconciled himself to the need.

HISTORY
As with any medical investigation, a male fertility study begins with a careful history. The history should cover general health, diet, alcohol, drug or tobacco use; congenital problems such as hypospadias or cryptorchidism; illnesses such as mumps, orchitis, urinary tract infection, or venereal disease; and operations such as herniorrhaphy. It should also cover present illnesses, particularly endocrine illness. The man's occupation and work habits now and in the past

(does his job involve sitting at a desk all day or exposure to x-rays or other forms of radiation?) are important. Other essential facts are the frequency of intercourse and masturbation, the occurrence of impotence or premature ejaculation, the coital positions used, whether or not lubricants are used, what contraceptive measures have been used, and whether or not the man has ever fathered children by a previous marriage or relationship.

PHYSICAL ASSESSMENT

The man needs a thorough physical assessment to rule out present illness. Of particular importance is the observation of secondary sexual characteristics and genital abnormalities, such as the absence of a vas deferens or undescended testes.

SEMEN ANALYSIS

For a semen analysis, after four days of sexual abstinence, the man ejaculates by masturbation into a clean, dry specimen jar, and the spermatozoa are examined under a microscope. They are counted, and their appearance and motility are noted. An average ejaculation should produce 2.5 to 5.0 ml of semen. As previously noted, it should contain a minimum of 40 million spermatozoa per milliliter of fluid, or a total of 125 million per ejaculation (the average normal sperm count is 50 to 200 million per milliliter). Two hours after ejaculation, 60 to 70 percent of sperm cells should still be vigorously active; 6 to 8 hours later, 25 to 40 percent should still evidence good motility. Liquefaction of the sample usually occurs within 10 to 30 minutes.

If the man is unwilling to submit to a semen analysis, a sperm analysis may be made at the same time one of the tests for female cervical mucus (the Sims-Huhner test) is done. If the results of the sperm count and semen analysis are substandard, two or three specimens should be examined for verification.

LABORATORY TESTS

In order to rule out poor health as a causative factor, the following laboratory tests are also usually included in the male studies: urinalysis, complete blood count, blood typing, including Rh factor, serological test for syphilis, and sometimes a sedimentation rate, protein-bound iodine test, and a cholesterol level determination. More extensive studies that might be required are bioassay of urine for 17-ketosteroids (the breakdown of androgen in urine). Testicular biopsy or x-ray study of the excretory portion of the genital tract using a contrast medium might rarely be indicated.

PSYCHOLOGICAL ASSESSMENT

The man needs an opportunity to discuss with the physician or nurse his overall attitude toward sexual relations, pregnancy, and raising children. It is good to explore with the man how he gained his knowledge of sexual relations. From the street gang or from a reliable source? What is his attitude toward coitus? What does he know about sexual technique?

How sexually active was he before marriage? Some men worry that because they were very active sexually when they were young they have spent all their viable sperm. They need to be assured that normally sperm is continually produced. Others may think that not having children now is punishment for early irresponsible encounters. They may worry that because they masturbate they will produce deformed children.

Some may worry that their wife may die in childbirth and so they really do not want her to be pregnant. Others are afraid that they will not be able to support a family or to be a good father and so would like things to remain as they are.

Some men need referral to a psychologist for counseling. Others benefit from a frank discussion, separating old wives' tales from reality, preparing their minds as well as their bodies for possible fatherhood.

Plans and Interventions in Male Infertility

The treatment of male infertility involves treating, if possible, the underlying cause of the infertility, such as chronic disease or current infection. If the vas deferens is obstructed, the obstruction is usually extensive and difficult or impossible to relieve by surgery. If spermatozoa are present but the count is low, a man might be advised to abstain from intercourse for seven to ten days at a time in order to increase the count. If the underlying cause cannot be corrected, which unfortunately often happens (e.g., the reason for infertility is a prior infection such as mumps orchitis), artificial insemination is a possible solution.

ARTIFICIAL INSEMINATION

To prepare for artificial insemination, the woman must take basal body temperatures for a number of months in order to be able to predict by the rise in temperature at the time of ovulation what day during her cycle ovulation usually occurs. Just before, on, and two days after the day of ovulation, the physician takes the seminal fluid of the husband's ejaculate and, using a syringe, places it at the opening to the cervix. The woman rests in a supine position for approximately 15 minutes in order to allow the spermatozoa ample opportunity to enter the cervix.

If the husband's sperm count is substandard, the couple may choose donor insemination. The procedure is the same, except that a donor's semen is used instead of the husband's or in addition to the husband's. Donors are traditionally medical students who have no history of disease and no family histories of possibly heritable disorders. The blood type, or at least the Rh factor, can be matched with the mother's, to prevent Rh incompatibility. Sperm banks, supplying frozen spermatozoa, are now available. Sperm from these sources is from screened donors and can be selected according to desired physical characteristics. It is available for insemination any day of the month.

Artificial insemination must be agreed on by both husband and wife. There are legal complications in some states that must be considered. Some couples have religious beliefs that deter them from using artificial insemination.

Artificial insemination is a discouraging process to some couples because, since the average couple takes six months to effect conception, so will the couple using artificial insemination. The six months are long and filled with the tension of having pregnancy so near and yet so elusive.

Causes of Female Infertility

The factors that cause infertility in women are analogous to those causing infertility in men: anovulation (faulty or inadequate production of ova); problems of ova transport through the fallopian tubes to the uterus; uterine factors such as tumors or poor endometrial development; and cervical and vaginal factors that immobilize spermatozoa.

ANOVULATION

Anovulation is the most serious cause of infertility in women because it is the one most difficult to correct. Pituitary or thyroid disturbances may be the root cause. Immaturity or disease of the ovaries may be a factor. Chronic or excessive exposure to x-rays or radioactive substances may be involved. General ill health or poor diet may contribute to poor ovarian function. There are several tests for ovulation.

Basal Body Temperature

Before getting out of bed each morning, the woman takes her rectal temperature. She must be certain to do this before moving around, since activity changes the basal level. She plots the daily temperatures on a monthly graph, noting conditions that might affect her basal temperature (colds, other infections, sleeplessness). At the time of ovulation, the basal temperature dips slightly, then rises a degree higher and stays at that level until three or four days before the next menstrual flow. The increase in basal body temperature marks the time of ovulation. Graphs of basal body temperature are shown in Fig. 11-1.

In Fig. 11-1A, the woman's temperature dips slightly at midpoint in her cycle, then rises sharply, an indication of ovulation. Toward the end of the cycle (the 24th day) her temperature begins to decline, indicating that progesterone levels are falling and that she did not conceive.

In Fig. 11-1B, the woman's temperature rises at midpoint in the cycle and remains at that elevated level past the time of her normal menstrual flow, suggesting that pregnancy has occurred.

In Fig. 11-1C, there is no preovulatory dip and no rise of temperature anywhere during the cycle. This is the typical pattern of a woman who does not ovulate.

Fern Test

When high levels of estrogen are present in the body, as they are just prior to ovulation, the cervical mucus forms fern-like patterns when it is smeared and dried on a glass slide. This is known as *arborization*, or ferning. When progesterone is the dominant hormone, as it is just after ovulation when the luteal phase of the menstrual cycle is beginning, a fern pattern is no longer discernible. Fern tests are usually done at midcycle and again before menstruation, so that both patterns can be demonstrated. Women who do not ovulate continue to show the fern pattern throughout the menstrual cycle (progesterone levels never become dominant), or they never demonstrate it because their estrogen levels never rise.

Spinnbarkeit Test

At the height of estrogen secretion, the cervical mucus becomes thin and watery and can be stretched into long strands. This stretchability (to a distance of 13 to 15 cm) is in contrast to its state when progesterone is the dominant hormone. Taking spinnbarkeit patterns at a midpoint and a late point in the menstrual cycle can demonstrate that progesterone is being produced and, by implication, that ovulation has occurred.

Uterine Endometrial Biopsy

Uterine endometrial biopsy may be used as a test for ovulation. A corkscrew-like appearance of the endometrium (a typical progesterone-dominated endometrium) suggests that ovulation has occurred.

Endometrial biopsy is done by introducing a thin probe and biopsy forceps through the cervix. It in-

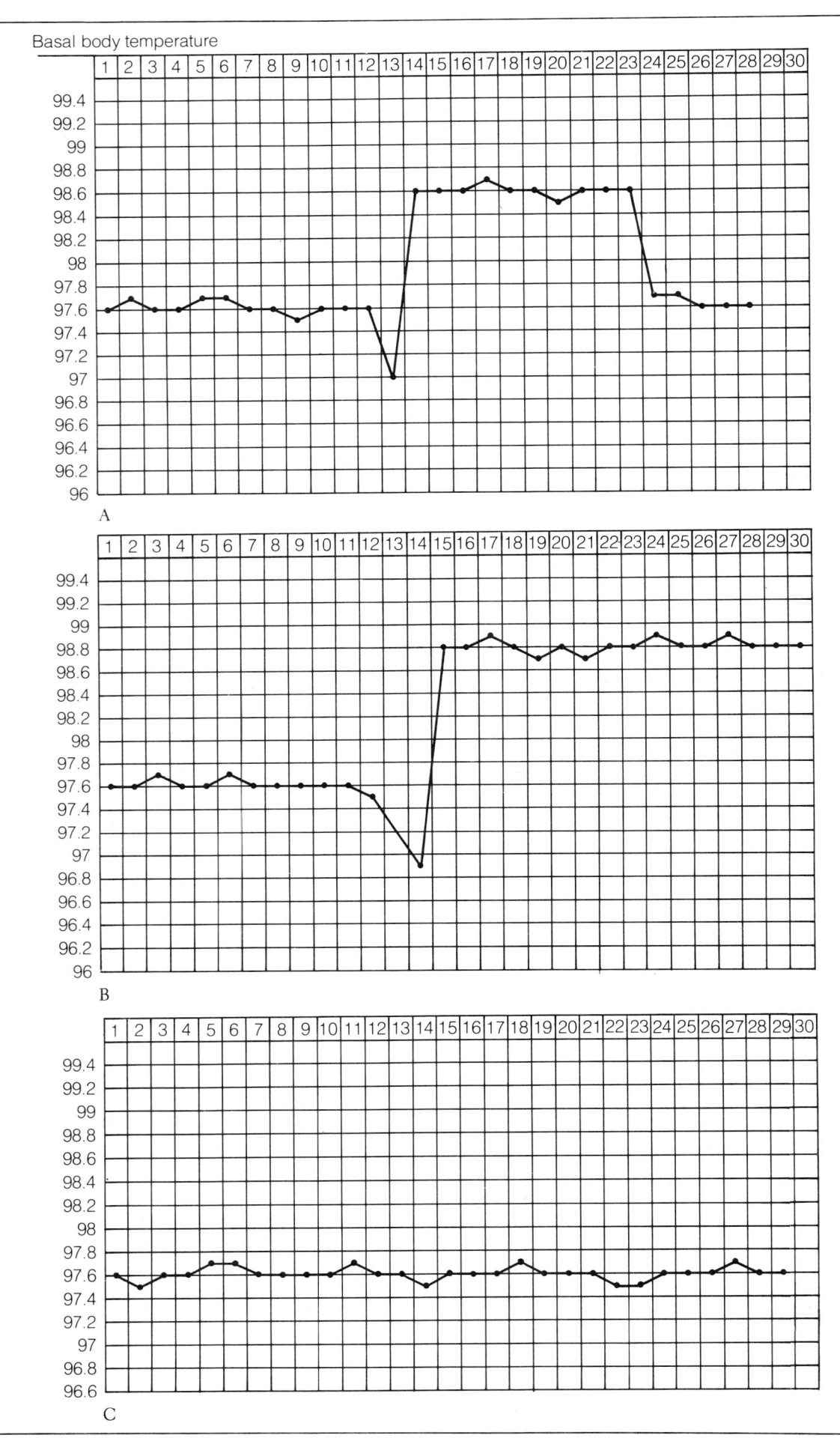

volves slight discomfort from the maneuvering of the instruments, and there is a moment of sharp pain as the biopsy specimen is taken. It is usually done during the 24th to 26th day of a typical menstrual cycle. It is contraindicated if pregnancy is suspected or if an infection such as acute pelvic inflammatory disease or cervicitis is present.

Culdoscopy and Laparoscopy

Culdoscopy is a sterile procedure that permits direct visualization of the organs of reproduction through a culdoscope inserted into the posterior fornix of the vaginal canal. A culdoscope is a thin, hollow metal tube with a small light at the distal end. With the culdoscope in place, both ovaries can be inspected grossly for the presence of a graafian follicle, corpus luteum, or corpus albicans, providing evidence of previous ovulation. Laparoscopy, or introducing a lighted tube through a small incision in the abdomen, can be used to examine ovaries the same way.

TUBAL FACTORS IN INFERTILITY

Difficulty with tubal transport usually occurs because of chronic salpingitis, which is most often due to chronic pelvic inflammatory disease (gonorrhea) but sometimes results from a ruptured appendix or abdominal surgery in which infection was involved and adhesions formed. Occasionally, congenital webbing or strictures of the fallopian tubes occur.

There are several tests of tubal patency.

Rubin Test

A Rubin test (Fig. 11-2), a traditional test for patency, is usually done on the third day following cessation of menstrual flow, before the ovum has entered the fallopian tube. The woman lies in a lithotomy position. Carbon dioxide is instilled into the cervix under pressure. It passes through the uterus and fallopian tubes into the pelvic cavity if the tubes are patent; with normal patency, carbon dioxide passes through when a pressure of under 100 mm Hg is used. When pressure over 100 mm Hg is necessary for passage, stricture is suggested. No passage whatsoever with a pressure of 200 mm Hg indicates occlusion.

Within a few hours after the test, as the carbon dioxide is diffused into the peritoneum and collects under the diaphragm, the woman experiences sharp, almost excruciating pain in one or both shoulders.

Fig. 11-1. Basal body temperature chart for determining ovulation. A. Ovulation without conception. B. Ovulation with conception. C. An anovulatory cycle.

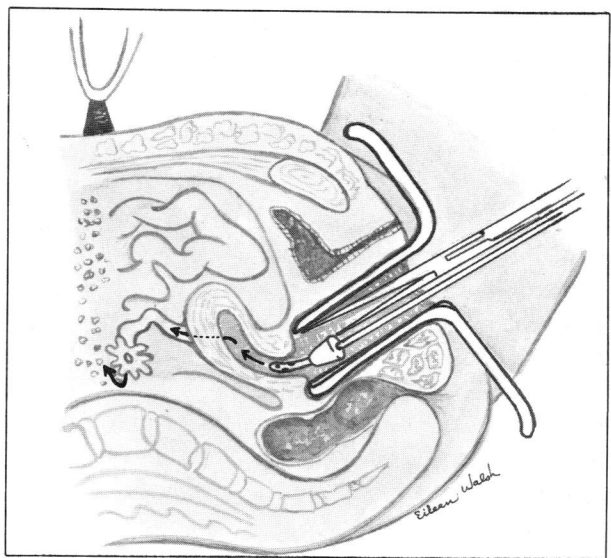

Fig. 11-2. Rubin test for tubal patency. Carbon dioxide injected into the uterus can be demonstrated moving through patent fallopian tubes.

She should be warned that this may happen or she may worry that she is having a heart attack or has torn a shoulder ligament. Ask the woman on her next visit whether she felt this pain. Its occurrence helps to demonstrate patency. (She will not have forgotten the pain, since it is sharp enough to be remembered for a long time.) Auscultating the abdomen with a stethoscope while the carbon dioxide is infusing may aid in establishing bilateral patency, since the passage of the carbon dioxide can be heard.

Rubin tests should not be done when uterine bleeding or infection is present. Infective organisms or blood might be forced up the tube into the abdominal cavity.

Uterosalpingography

Uterosalpingography (hysterosalpingography) is roentgenography of the fallopian tubes using a radiopaque medium. It is done at the same time of the month as the Rubin test is done, and the contraindications are the same. The radiopaque material is introduced into the cervix under pressure. It outlines the uterus and both tubes, provided the latter are patent. Because the medium is thick, it distends the uterus and tubes slightly, causing uterine cramping that is momentarily painful. Following the study, the contrast medium will drain out through the vagina.

The instillation of carbon dioxide and of radiopaque material may be therapeutic as well as diagnostic. The pressure of the gas or solution may actually break up adhesions as it passes through the fallopian tubes, thereby increasing their patency. It is important that tubal x-ray examinations be done just following menstruation so a growing zygote is not irradiated.

UTERINE FACTORS IN INFERTILITY

Tumors such as fibromas may be a cause of infertility in that they block fallopian tubes or limit the space available for effective implantation; many women with huge fibromas, however, become pregnant. A congenitally deformed uterine cavity may also limit implantation sites, but this is a rare occurrence. Inadequate endometrium formation resulting from poor secretion of estrogen or progesterone from the ovary is the main cause of infertility due to a uterine factor (the primary factor here is actually ovarian). Endometrial biopsy will reveal any inadequacies of the endometrium.

Endometriosis

Endometriosis is an implant of uterine endometrium outside the uterus. The most common sites of endometrium spread are the cul-de-sac of Douglas, the ovaries, the uterine ligaments, and the outer surface of the uterus and bowel.

The spread of endometrium is probably due to regurgitation through the fallopian tubes at the time of menstruation. Viable particles of endometrium regurgitated this way begin to proliferate and grow at the new sites. At laparotomy, the implants appear as ragged purplish growths. On the ovaries, cysts filled with old blood are often seen (brown or chocolate cysts).

ASSESSMENT. If endometriosis is minimal, the woman will not be aware of any symptoms related to it. If moderate or extensive, the woman may feel pain at the time of menstruation as patches of ectopic endometrium also undergo preflow breakdown and bleeding (blood is irritating to the peritoneal membrane). The woman may report dyspareunia (pain on penile-vaginal penetration) if the implants are in the cul-de-sac of Douglas.

Endometriosis tends to occur most often in white nulliparous women. Pelvic examination may show that the uterus is displaced by tender, fixed, palpable nodules. Nodules in the cul-de-sac or on an ovary may be palpable as well. Endometriosis leads to infertility as fallopian tube implants tend to cause fallopian tube obstruction; it may also reflect an endometrium that is more friable (adheres less well) than normally.

PLANNING AND INTERVENTION. Treatment for endometriosis can be either medical or surgical. Use of birth control pills may cause regression of the implants, due primarily to the extreme sloughing of tissue following progesterone administration. Danazol, an androgen, may cause shrinkage of the tissue. Laparotomy and excision of the implants is often more effective. A laparotomy is major surgery, however, so a course of conservative medical treatment may be undertaken first. It is difficult for a woman who wants to have children to understand why she is being asked to take birth control pills. It seems to be the exact opposite treatment that she needs. Be certain the woman has a good understanding of what is being attempted (she needs a diagram of uterine and tubal anatomy so she can understand what *regurgitation* means, an appreciation of how progesterone acts on endometrial tissue, and support to be patient for a minimum of six months).

EVALUATION. The best proof that treatment has been effective is that the woman becomes pregnant. Following birth of the child, the woman is usually advised to have a second child (provided she wants more than one child) as soon after the first child as possible rather than to wait the traditional two or three years between children, before endometrial implants have a chance to grow again. Be careful in the postpartal period that you do not give traditional advice (spacing children conserves maternal energy, produces healthier children, and encourages infant-parent bonding), advice that does not apply here.

Asherman's Syndrome

Trauma from uterine infection or repeated uterine surgery may lead to such uterine scarring that no implantation sites are available and so infertility occurs. This is *Asherman's syndrome.*

CERVICAL FACTORS IN INFERTILITY

Infection of the cervix (erosion) may cause such changes in the cervical mucus that spermatozoa do not penetrate it easily or cannot survive in it. A tight cervical os may compound infertility but is rarely enough of a problem to be the sole cause of it.

At the time of ovulation, cervical mucus becomes thin and watery and can be easily penetrated by spermatozoa for a period of 12 to 72 hours. If ovulation does not occur, or estrogen levels do not increase at the midpoint of the cycle, the cervical mucus does not become receptive to penetration. The Sims-Huhner test is used to determine whether or not this change has occurred.

The Sims-Huhner Test

In the Sims-Huhner test, the time of ovulation is taken from the woman's basal body temperature graph. The couple has intercourse at that time, using no precoital lubricants. Following intercourse, the woman lies on her back for at least 30 minutes to ensure that spermatozoa will reach the cervix. She uses no postcoital douches and reports to the clinic or physician's office within 2 to 8 hours following intercourse.

With the woman in a lithotomy position, the physician removes a specimen of cervical mucus and examines it grossly for ferning and the ability to form long strands. It is examined under the microscope for viable spermatozoa. At the time of ovulation, the amount of cervical mucus present should be moderately large to profuse. It should appear clear, thin (low viscosity), have few cells (under five leukocytes per high-power field), have an alkaline pH, and form strands (spinnbarkeit) 13 to 15 cm in length. If the male partner is fertile and there is little destruction of spermatozoa, spermatozoa will be present in the cervical mucus (over five per high-power field), more than 25 percent will be motile, and penetration will be at the rate of 1.5 to 2.0 mm per minute.

VAGINAL FACTORS IN INFERTILITY

Infection of the vagina may cause the pH of the vaginal secretions to change, limiting or destroying the motility of spermatozoa. Some women, particularly those with ABO blood incompatibility possibilities, appear to have sperm-immobilizing or sperm-agglutinating antibodies in the blood plasma which act to destroy sperm cells in the vagina. This is actually a systemic response to a local invasion.

Tests for vaginal adequacy usually include a pelvic examination for gross abnormalities and probably a vaginal secretion culture. Abnormal results from a Sims-Huhner test may suggest a sperm agglutination problem.

Assessment of Female Infertility
HISTORY

The woman's menstrual history should be obtained, including the age of menarche, the length and frequency of menstrual periods, the amount of flow, and any difficulties she experiences. She should be asked about present or past infections, her overall health, with a stress on endocrine problems, and abdominal or pelvic operations she might have had. How often does she use douches or intravaginal medication or sprays? (These may interfere with vaginal pH.) Is she exposed to occupational hazards such as x-rays or toxic substances? It is also important to obtain a history of previous pregnancies or abortions and to ask questions about her use of contraceptives.

PHYSICAL ASSESSMENT

A thorough physical assessment is necessary to rule out present illness. Of particular importance are secondary sex characteristics, since these are an indication of maturity and pituitary function. A complete pelvic examination is needed to rule out gross anatomical defects and infection.

LABORATORY TESTS

To determine the woman's general state of health, laboratory tests like those done on the man will be made: urinalysis, a complete blood count and possibly a sedimentation rate, a serological test for syphilis, and a T_3 and T_4 uptake determination. A basal metabolic rate may be taken. If the woman has a history of menstrual irregularities, the urine may be assayed for 17-ketosteroids, follicle-stimulating hormone, estriol, and pregnanediol.

PSYCHOLOGICAL ASSESSMENT

As with a man, a woman needs the opportunity to discuss with the physician or a nurse her overall attitudes toward sexual intercourse, pregnancy, and raising children.

It is good to explore with her how she was introduced to the phenomenon of menstruation. Was she prepared for it or not? Is her present husband her only sex partner? Did she have premarital coitus? Some women are afraid of pregnancy because they worry that old sperm from premarital encounters will be activated, and the resulting child will look like their previous sexual partner, not like their present one. Others are afraid of pregnancy because they think they may be punished for premarital affairs by giving birth to a defective child. Others are so frightened at the thought of labor and delivery that, although they are saying they want to have a child, they are actually petrified at the thought.

Some women need referral to a psychologist for counseling for such problems. Others benefit from a frank discussion, separating old wives' tales from reality, preparing their minds as well as their bodies for possible motherhood.

Plans and Interventions in Female Infertility

As with men, treatment of infertility in a woman is directed toward the underlying cause. If it appears to be a vaginal infection, the infection will be treated according to the causative organism. Some vaginal infections are obstinate and tend to recur, requiring close supervision and follow-up. The possibility that the sexual partner is reinfecting the woman needs to be considered. If the spermatozoa do not appear to survive in the vaginal secretions, artificial insemination may offer a solution.

If the cause is a uterine tumor, removal of the tumor by surgery may be necessary. If the problem is abnormal uterine formation, such as a septal uterus, surgery for this is now available. If the problem is tubal insufficiency, diathermy or steroid administration may be helpful. A Rubin test or a hysterosalpingography may be repeated to see whether it has a therapeutic effect. Plastic surgical repair is sometimes feasible.

If the problem appears to be a disturbance of ovulation, endocrine therapy may be necessary. In some instances, therapy with estrogen and progesterone is sufficient. In other women, ovulation can be stimulated by the administration of human menopausal gonadotropins (Pergonal) followed by administration of human chorionic gonadotropin. Human menopausal gonadotropins (derived from post-menopausal urine) are combinations of follicle-stimulating hormone and luteinizing hormone. Clomiphene citrate (Clomid), an estrogen antagonist may also be used to stimulate ovulation. The administration of clomiphene citrate and human menopausal gonadotropins may overstimulate the ovary, and multiple births may result. Women who are administered these compounds should be counseled that this is a possibility.

TEST-TUBE BABIES

The term *test-tube baby* brings to mind pictures of infants growing in giant test tubes the way they are pictured in science fiction books and films.

Theoretically the process of nurturing a fetus outside a uterus is possible. Much of the difficulty in structuring such a system lies with duplicating placental function, a formidable undertaking. There is still no adequate substitute that can supply the total needs of a growing fetus as well as they are met in utero.

Conception outside the human body is possible, however. Basically, this is what is meant today by the term *test-tube baby*.

Women who ovulate but have blocked fallopian tubes can have an ovum removed by laparotomy at the time ovulation would occur. Under sterile laboratory conditions, the ovum is exposed to spermatozoa taken from a donor or from the woman's husband. When it is evident that fertilization has occurred, and the first steps of growth have begun, the fertilized ovum (now a zygote) is removed from the laboratory medium and placed in the woman's uterus. If the timing is correct and the zygote is placed in the woman's uterus at the time it would normally have arrived there if it had traveled the usual fallopian tube route, it will implant. After that point, the remainder of the pregnancy will proceed as would any normal pregnancy.

Ethical considerations are involved in interfering with nature this much. There is a chance that an ovum might be injured in transfer and a defective child might result. There is danger that if bacteria are introduced at any point, maternal infection can occur.

It is unfortunate that the term test-tube baby is used for this process as it implies more manipulation than is actually done. Terms like *tubal bypass* or *extrauterine conception* best express the intent of the process and do not imply experimentation with human life but progress toward helping infertile women and couples achieve pregnancy and produce children.

Support During Fertility Studies

A couple's anxiety becomes more and more acute as fertility studies proceed. Some physicians give the results of each test as it is done; others prefer to wait until the basic series of tests is completed before the couple is told the outcome.

Since tubal insufficiency is a major cause of infertility (in 30 to 35 percent of cases) and gonorrheal infection is a prime cause of tubal insufficiency, infertility problems can be expected to increase in the future along with the currently rising incidence of gonorrhea. However, since the solutions to infertility are also increasing, more and more infertile couples will eventually conceive. At one time a woman who was anovulatory could not be helped. Now she not only can be stimulated to ovulate but may find herself the mother of twins, triplets, or even quintuplets.

A woman who has had to seek help for infertility is a woman with less confidence in her body than one who becomes pregnant with ease. She is likely to worry more during pregnancy than the average woman that she will not carry the pregnancy to term. Back pain, frequency of urination, heartburn—all normal occurrences of pregnancy—may be interpreted as ominous signs. She needs added support during pregnancy and added reassurance that her difficulty in conceiving is unrelated to the complications of pregnancy.

Couples who are unable to be helped in achieving fertility and conception need time and support to grieve. Adoption, once a ready alternative for infertile couples, is now more difficult to accomplish because of the reduced number of babies available for adoption. The couple needs continued follow-up and concern. Encouraging bonding with adopted children is discussed in Chap. 37.

Problem-oriented Recording: Progress Notes

Mary Kraft
22 years

Problem: Infertility

S. Had a spontaneous abortion 1½ years ago; unable to conceive since. Sexual relations about 2 × week. Keeps temperature chart daily; is aware of concept of fertile and infertile periods. Has temperature increase suggesting ovulation on 17th day of cycle as a rule. Menstrual cycle 30–32 days, 6 days' duration, heavy flow with painful cramping. No history of venereal disease, no chronic illness, normal activity level although she has a scanty diet pattern. Had abdominal surgery for appendicitis as 12-year-old, no Gyn surgery. Sometimes has dyspareunia.
Became pregnant first time after 3 months of sexual relations. Spont. abortion at 2½ months, no known cause, no apparent sequelae, no D&C performed.
Has slight vaginal discharge now, some pruritus.

O. Hemoglobin: 12 mg, normal urinalysis.
White, frothy vaginal discharge present.

A. Infertility by history.
Vaginal discharge (vaginal infection?)

Goals: a. To be free of vaginal discharge by 1 week.
b. Able to explain purpose of all fertility tests scheduled.
c. Able to explain results of tests, negative and positive findings.
d. Voice possibility of poor outcome from testing.

P. 1. Discuss treatment for vaginal discharge as outlined by M.D.
2. Schedule fertility testing pattern determined by M.D.
3. Discuss husband-wife relationship and coping ability in view of frustration and disappointment of infertility and possible length of testing period.

References

1. Behrman, S. J. Artificial insemination. *Clin. Obstet. Gynecol.* 22:245, 1979.
2. Behrman, S. J., and Kistner, R. W. A Rational Approach to the Evaluation of Infertility. In S. J. Behrman and R. W. Kistner (Eds.). *Progress in Infertility*. Boston: Little, Brown, 1975.
3. Gray, M. J. Sexual problems in infertility. *Female Patient* 5:21, 1980.
4. Kistner, R. W. Endometriosis and infertility. *Clin. Obstet. Gynecol.* 22:101, 1979.
5. Lowenstein, G. A Husband's Feelings About Not Being a Father. In L. K. McNall and J. T. Galeener (Eds.). *Current Practice in Obstetric and Gynecologic Nursing*. St. Louis: Mosby, 1976.
6. Manning, B. E. Resolve: A support group for infertile couples. *Am. J. Nurs.* 76:258, 1976.
7. Mocarski, V. The nurse's role in helping infertile couples. *M.C.N.* 2:264, 1977.
8. Moghissi, K. S. Basic workup and evaluation of infertile couples. *Clin. Obstet. Gynecol.* 22:9, 1979.
9. Rutledge, A. L. Psychomarital evaluation and treatment of the infertile couple. *Clin. Obstet. Gynecol.* 22:255, 1979.
10. Siegler, A. M. Evaluation of tubal factors in infertility and management of tubal abortion. *Clin. Obstet. Gynecol.* 22:81, 1979.
11. Speroff, L. Treating the patient who doesn't ovulate. *Contemp. Obstet. Gynecol.* 12:121, 1978.
12. Steinberger, E. Management of male reproductive dysfunction. *Clin. Obstet. Gynecol.* 22:187, 1979.
13. Taymor, M. L. Evaluation of anovulatory cycles and introduction of ovulation. *Clin. Obstet. Gynecol.* 22:145, 1979.
14. Trussell, J., et al. Early childbearing and subsequent fertility. *Fam. Plann. Perspect.* 10:209, 1978.
15. Wallach, E. E. Evaluation and management of uterine causes of infertility. *Clin. Obstet. Gynecol.* 22:43, 1979.
16. Wieke, V. R. Psychological reactions to infertility and implications for nurses in resolving feelings of disappointment and inadequacy. *J.O.G.N. Nurs.* 5:28, 1976.
17. Zimmerman, B. M. The exceptional stresses of adoptive parenthood. *M.C.N.* 2:191, 1977.

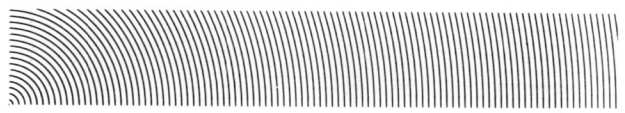

Unit II. Utilizing Nursing Process: Questions for Review

1. Wanda, 22 years old, is seen because she is possibly infertile. A Rubin test is ordered for her. This is a test of
   a. Tubal patency
   b. Cervical competency
   c. Sperm survival
   d. Thyroid function

2. You caution Wanda that shortly following the procedure she may experience
   a. Nausea and vomiting
   b. Abdominal cramps
   c. Faintness and dizziness
   d. Sharp shoulder pain

3. Wanda has been trying for a year to become pregnant. In a year, what proportion of couples usually do conceive?
   a. 40 percent
   b. 60 percent
   c. 80 percent
   d. 100 percent

4. Wanda has endometriosis and is placed on birth control pills. Which of the following would you explain to her?
   a. How progesterone acts on endometrial tissue
   b. That endometriosis is a mild infection
   c. How estrogen acts on the pituitary
   d. How sperm cannot survive with endometriosis

5. Mrs. Smith is 40 years old and a heavy smoker. She has very irregular menstrual cycles. Assuming that all the following methods of birth control are acceptable to her, which would you recommend to her?
   a. An oral contraceptive
   b. Vaginal foam for her; a condom for her partner
   c. The rhythm method
   d. An IUD

6. Linda is 15 years old. She hates the thought of an intrauterine device yet wants something for birth control with high reliability. Which of the following methods would you recommend to her?
   a. An oral contraceptive
   b. Vaginal foam for her; a condom for her partner
   c. Postcoital douching
   d. An IUD

7. Mrs. Jones uses a diaphragm for birth control. After which of the following occurrences should she have her diaphragm checked for competency?
   a. A weight loss of 20 pounds
   b. Abdominal surgery
   c. A weight gain of 5 pounds
   d. A cervical infection

8. To find her fertile days using the rhythm method, a woman should subtract
   a. 14 from 28
   b. 18 from her shortest period, 11 from her longest
   c. The length of her average period from the ideal of 28
   d. 18 from her longest period, 11 from her shortest

9. At ovulation, cervical mucus has the properties of
   a. High viscosity and alkalinity
   b. Acidity and ferning
   c. Low viscosity and spinnbarkeit
   d. Increased leukocytes and tackiness

10. During the second half of a typical menstrual cycle (days 14 to 28) the endometrium of the uterus becomes
    a. Thin and transparent, due to progesterone stimulation
    b. Twisted and rugated, due to follicle-stimulating hormone
    c. Thick and purple-hued, due to estrogen stimulation
    d. Corkscrew-like, due to progesterone stimulation

11. Ovulation is apparently initiated by a surge in
    a. Luteinizing hormone
    b. Progesterone
    c. Follicle-stimulating hormone
    d. Estrogen

12. A woman can use her basal temperature reading to detect her day of ovulation. A basal temperature should be taken
    a. First thing in the morning
    b. At noon after resting for an hour
    c. Before she has any high-calorie foods for breakfast
    d. The last thing at night before she falls asleep

13. A sense of autonomy is helpful for a parent to have as it strengthens his or her ability to
    a. Love warmly
    b. Make decisions
    c. Relate to the opposite sex
    d. Work diligently

14. Christine is 15 years old. She may have difficulty being a parent because she has not yet developed an adolescent sense of
    a. Holism
    b. Autonomy
    c. Generativity
    d. Identity

15. Janet is concerned because she does not regularly experience orgasm. Orgasm is mainly a result of
    a. Penile stimulation
    b. Vaginal stimulation
    c. Clitoral stimulation
    d. Sensory arousal

16. Many women find that they achieve orgasm easily during pregnancy, because of
    a. Increased pituitary hormone levels
    b. Pelvic vasocongestion
    c. Cervical dominance
    d. Vaginal vasoconstriction

17. Which of the following findings might lead you to suspect that a couple could have a problem of sexuality?
    a. The husband recently had a heart attack.
    b. The woman is older than the man.
    c. The woman uses an IUD.
    d. All of the above.

18. At puberty, which of the following statements is true of the action of testosterone in girls?
    a. It has no place in female reproductive development.
    b. It influences growth of axillary and pubic hair.
    c. It causes breast development.
    d. It initiates estrogen production.

19. Barbara is worried because she is 13 and does not yet menstruate. Menstruation in girls usually occurs
    a. Before 12
    b. Between the development of pubic and axillary hair
    c. Before breast development
    d. None of the above

20. In a supine position, the course of the vagina is
    a. Almost parallel with the bed surface
    b. Curved sharply downward
    c. Slanted downward and backward
    d. Slanted upward for 2 cm, then downward

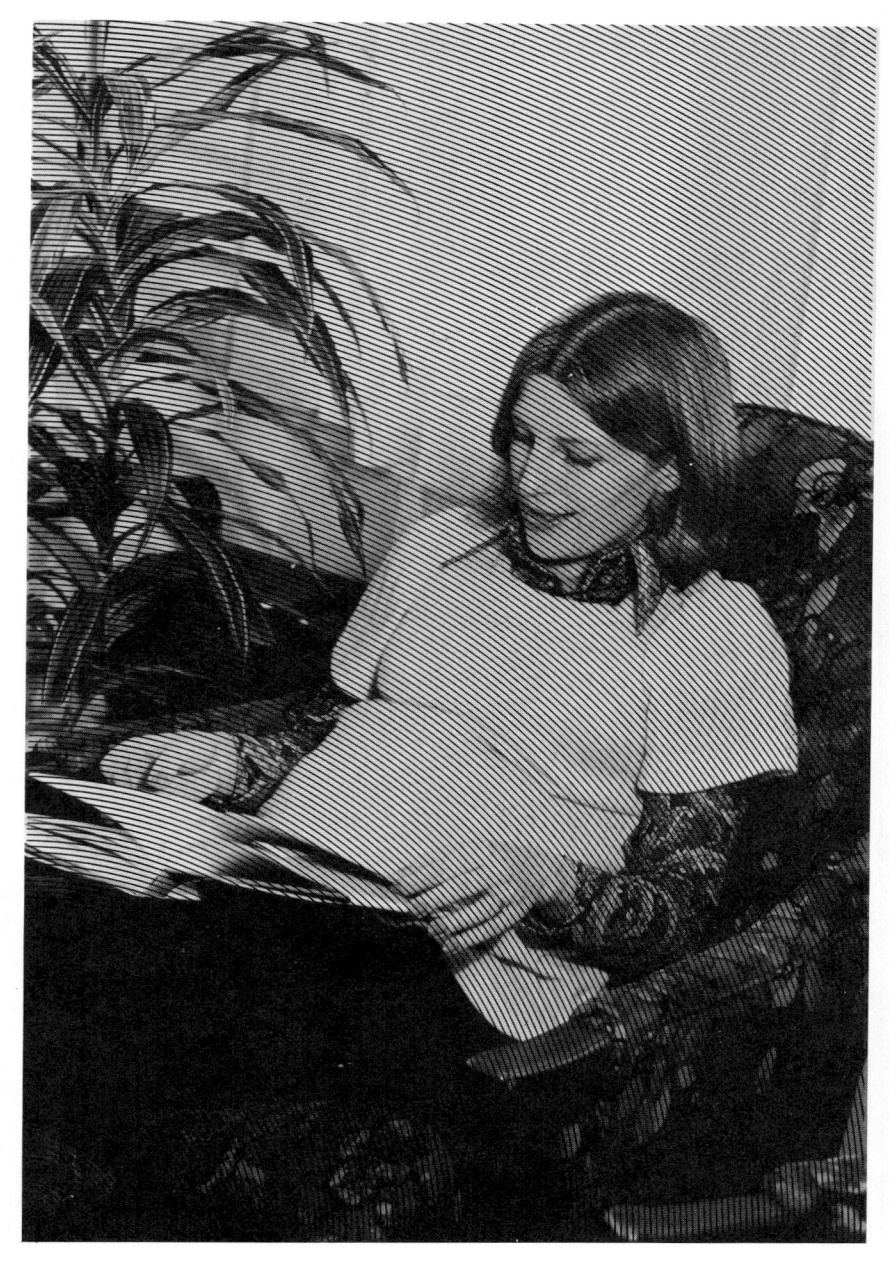

III. The Prepartal Period: Preparing for Parenthood

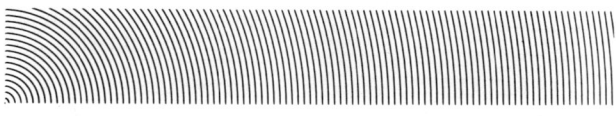

12. Psychosocial Aspects of Pregnancy

The psychological changes of pregnancy are a direct consequence of the child growing within the woman, the physical changes this pregnancy entails, and the increased responsibility and concern for the new family member resulting from the pregnancy. It is unrealistic to discuss the psychological aspects of pregnancy apart from its physiological aspects, or the development of the unborn child. In terms of nursing care, the psychological aspects are inseparable from the physiological. Both must be kept in mind during prenatal visits if a woman is to have an uncomplicated pregnancy and establish a healthy mother-child relationship, and if the family is to adjust adequately to its new member.

The Pregnant Woman

Because the first signs of pregnancy are subtle—nausea in the morning, a feeling of fatigue, the absence of a menstrual flow—the woman is the first to know or suspect that she is pregnant.

INITIAL REACTIONS TO PREGNANCY

A woman may run the gamut of emotions during pregnancy, from the surprise of finding herself pregnant (or wishing she were not) to pleasure and acceptance as she feels the child stir within her, to fear for herself and her child, to boredom with the process and wishing to get it all over with so that she can get on with the next step—rearing her child—to surprise again that the process is over and she really has given birth.

From a physiological standpoint, it is fortunate that a pregnancy is nine months long. This gives the fetus time to mature and to be prepared for life outside its protective uterine environment. Nine months of pregnancy are also needed for psychological reasons; it gives the family time to prepare psychologically for the coming of the child.

In view of the availability of birth control measures today, one would judge that few pregnancies would be a surprise. In reality, every pregnancy is a surprise [27]. The woman who was not planning on being pregnant will obviously be surprised. The woman who was looking forward to being pregnant is surprised that it has really happened (no woman is absolutely certain in advance that she can conceive whenever she wishes to) and that it happened this month instead of next month or the month before.

If pregnancy announced itself by more reliable signs, women could be more certain how they feel about being pregnant. It is strange that such an important life function is heralded by the absence of a body function rather than by the addition of something.

Along with the first feeling of surprise that they are pregnant, as many as 80 percent of women experience a feeling that is less than pleasure and may be disappointment or anxiety [26]. The reasons they give for their displeasure at the news are many: I don't want a baby. I don't want a baby *now*. I want a baby, but I don't want to be pregnant for the next nine months. I want a baby and I want to be pregnant, but I don't want any part of labor and delivery. I can't afford to give up my job. My husband doesn't want a baby. Fortunately, most of these women change their attitudes toward the pregnancy by the time they feel the child stir inside them.

CULTURAL INFLUENCES

A woman's attitude toward a pregnancy depends a great deal on the culture in which she was raised, the culture in which she lives now, and the individual experiences she had with pregnancy as a child.

As in most technologically advanced nations, childbearing in the United States is a medically oriented process. The woman goes to a physician during pregnancy; she is treated for morning sickness and other discomforts of pregnancy with a medical prescription; at the time of delivery, she is admitted to a hospital. Maternal and infant mortality figures attest to the value of this kind of care during pregnancy and delivery, but the emphasis on medical management also conveys a feeling that pregnancy is an illness. Some women therefore view being pregnant as being ill. When a woman perceives herself as ill, it is difficult to talk to her about getting enough exercise or eating sufficient nourishing food because ill people typically need to rest and to eat sparingly.

The pregnant woman often visits the physician's office alone. The implication is that childbearing is a woman's business, and a husband who believes this will be hard put to understand that his wife needs his emotional support during pregnancy.

In the United States, most women are made to feel that they are responsible for the health of the child growing within them. In many other cultures there is little stress on this responsibility, and the outcome of a pregnancy is felt to depend on some supernatural agency. It is difficult to teach a woman to take extra precautions during pregnancy, such as discontinuing the use of a potentially harmful medication, if she believes that the health of her newborn is ultimately out of her hands.

It is important to keep in mind when planning health instruction that the material taught must be based on its relevance to the patient, not on its relevance to you. If you believe that, ideally, parents should be over 21 before they have children, or that the best home is a shuttered cottage surrounded by a white picket fence, take a deep breath before you begin to talk to a pregnant, unmarried adolescent about her diet during pregnancy. If you believe strongly that families should be limited to two children for zero population growth, be careful of the tone of your voice when you talk to a woman who is pregnant with her tenth child. These are your beliefs, and they work for you, but they may mean little or nothing to the girl or woman in front of you because of the differences in your backgrounds.

The home in which the woman was raised is as important as the general culture from which she comes. If she was raised in a family where children were loved or viewed as pleasant outcomes of a marriage, she is more likely to have a positive attitude toward a pregnancy than is the woman who was reared in a home where children were felt to be in the way or were blamed for the breakup of a marriage. No matter how often a girl is told that pregnancy is natural and simple, if she has heard horror stories about excruciating pain and endless suffering in labor, she cannot be overjoyed to find herself pregnant. If her mother has constantly reminded her, "If you hadn't come along, I could have gone to college" or "I could have had a career," she is likely to think of pregnancy as a kind of disaster.

That people love as they have been loved is said so often now that it has become a cliché, but it has a great deal of relevance to whether pregnancy and childbirth are viewed positively or negatively. If a woman has difficulty loving, she will have difficulty accepting a fetus growing within her. In order to mother well (being a mother is a second adjustment step, over and above being pregnant) the woman must feel pleasurable anticipation at the prospect of rearing a child. The woman who views mothering as a positive activity because her mother was able to view it as a fulfilling life role is more likely to be pleased when she becomes pregnant than one who devalues mothering.

The Psychological Tasks of Pregnancy
ACCEPTING THE PREGNANCY

A number of developmental and psychological tasks must be accomplished by the woman during pregnancy. The first of these is accepting the pregnancy.

Nausea and vomiting, frequency of urination, tiredness, perhaps slight tingling in the breasts, and amenorrhea are the first indications of pregnancy.

However, they do not make pregnancy certain. A visit to a physician or clinic and a diagnosis of pregnancy is a major step in helping the woman to accomplish the task of accepting the pregnancy. The fetus may be only an hour older when the woman leaves the physician's office than when she entered it, but if a diagnosis of pregnancy was the outcome of the visit, she *feels* "more pregnant."

Our culture structures celebrations around the important life events. Christenings, bar mitzvahs, marriages, birthdays, deaths—all have a ritual to help those concerned take a step toward or accept the coming change in their lives. A diagnosis of pregnancy is the initiation ceremony of pregnancy. Think of a diagnosis visit as having special, hidden meaning, different from an ordinary visit to the physician.

A second ceremony of pregnancy is *quickening*, or the moment the woman first feels life. Until this time she tended to think of the life inside her as an integral part of herself. She knew it was there; she ate for it, she slept for it, but it was just a part of her body like her arms or legs. With quickening, the child becomes a separate entity, and the mother begins to give the child an identity. She imagines how she will feel in the delivery room when the physician announces, "It's a boy" or "It's a girl!" She imagines herself picking out baby clothes, selecting toys, mending little blue jeans, teaching her child the alphabet or how to cook. She pictures herself seeing a daughter off to college, watching a son play football. She sees herself as the mother of the bride, or groom, at a wedding. This anticipatory role playing is an important task for the woman to undertake in that it leads her to a larger concept of her condition. Not only is she pregnant, but she is going to have a child as well!

Most women can name a point during pregnancy when they knew they wanted their child. For some who carefully planned the pregnancy it is the moment after they recover from the surprise of suspecting they are pregnant. For others it is the day of diagnosis. In one woman it may be a personal moment: her father and mother expressing their joy, or a look of pride on her husband's face. It might be quickening, the moment she realized that the fetus inside her was not passive but active, when she suddenly knew the stranger she had lived with for five months. It might be a moment she first shopped for baby clothes and picked up a size 0 shirt. It might be the moment she set up the crib; seeing a crib in *her* house made the pregnancy, the coming baby, real and desired.

Accepting the pregnancy might not come until labor begins, or hours into labor. It might be the moment she is taken to the delivery room or be the moment she first hears the baby cry, or first touches or feeds the baby. The moment may come late, a week, or three weeks, after she takes the baby home. But at some point—the usual times tend to cluster around diagnosis and quickening—a woman will know that she and her baby are going to get along, that they will make a go of it.

How close the woman is to achieving acceptance is sometimes evident in her ability to follow prenatal instructions. Until she views the growing structure inside her as something of value, she will have difficulty following a proper diet. If she wants very much to be pregnant but is not yet convinced that she is, she may have difficulty eliminating excessively high-carbohydrate foods from her diet. After all, her weight gain may be the most certain proof she has that she is pregnant.

Preparations for a baby's coming imply that acceptance has been achieved. Thus, it is good to ask the woman what she is doing to get ready for her baby. Once she has accepted her pregnancy and that she is having a baby, she begins to "build the nest." Between the 5th and 7th months of pregnancy, most women begin to plan where the infant will sleep, what he will wear, how he will be fed, what his name will be.

It is easy to infer that a woman who uses the term *it* for the fetus inside her has not yet accepted her pregnancy. However, many women, although they have chosen a name for the child and are very sure which sex they want, continue to refer to the baby as *it* during pregnancy. They would deny being superstitious, but nonetheless they are worried that referring to the child as *she* will somehow turn the child into *he*, or vice versa.

Caplan [3] has documented several abnormal maternal fantasies about the pregnancy or child. The first of these is a conception of the fetus as an older child. A woman with such a fantasy may feel despondent in the newborn period, when she must care for a helpless, dependent infant rather than the older child she fantasized.

A second fantasy that may reveal nonacceptance of the pregnancy or of the reality that a child is to be born is that the baby is already an adult. "I hope she has her grandmother's tiny feet; she can be a dancer." "I hope she's as smart as my husband; I want her to go to college." "I want him to quarterback for Notre Dame." These are typical examples of this kind of fantasy. Such a woman may be attempting to fulfill her own ambitions through her child rather than accepting the child as having a life of his own.

A third woman who may have difficulty is the one

who knows exactly what her child will look or be like. She may not be able to accept her child as he is, but will expect him to measure up to her fantasy standards. Yet another woman who may have difficulty is the one who insists she can tell that she is having a boy or a girl. She may have a hard time mothering a child of the opposite sex.

Whether or not the woman feels secure in her relationship with the people around her, especially the father of her child, is important in her acceptance of a pregnancy. Pregnancy is easier to accept when a woman has confidence in the solidity of her marriage or, if she is not married, that the father of the child will be there to give her emotional support. She will be less comfortable when she learns she is pregnant if she has an unreliable partner who may shortly disappear, leaving her alone with the responsibility of child rearing.

The woman's ability to cope with or adapt to stress, to resolve conflict, and to adapt to new life contingencies plays a major role. Part of this ability to adapt (to be able to mother and no longer need mothering, to love a child as well as a husband, to be a mother of four, not just of three) involves the woman's basic temperament, that is, whether she always adapts quickly or slowly, whether she faces new situations with an intense or a low-key approach, and whether or not she has had past experience with change and stress.

Some women view a pregnancy as a threat. A woman who thinks of brides as young but mothers as old may believe that pregnancy will rob her of her youth. If she thinks of children as sticky-fingered and time-consuming, she may view the pregnancy as taking away her freedom. If she has heard that pregnancy will stretch her abdomen and breasts permanently, her concern may focus on losing her looks. She may feel that the pregnancy will rob her financially and ruin her chances for promotion on her job. These are very real feelings, and they must be taken seriously by you when you are working with pregnant women. They cannot be shrugged off by a cliché ("A door closes, another one opens") or repression ("You shouldn't think that way; you'll love having a baby in the house"). The woman needs an opportunity to express such feelings so she becomes aware of their intensity and can begin to work them through to resolution.

REWORKING DEVELOPMENTAL TASKS
Women work through previous life experiences during pregnancy as one of the tasks of pregnancy. Needs and wishes they have repressed for years surface to be studied and reworked, to such an extent that if the woman were not pregnant, such behavior might be called pathological.

Primary among those life experiences are the woman's relationship with her parents, particularly with her mother. For the first time she finds she can empathize with her mother's concern when she used to return late from high school dates. She herself is already worrying about her child if she feels no movement within her for a few hours, yet she is only five months pregnant!

Fear of dying is a common fear of childhood that is revived during pregnancy. Thinking about this is not unrealistic; women do die in childbirth.

In order for the woman to work through past fears and conflicts, she needs to think about them when she is alone and to talk about them with others. She "throws out comments" when talking to her husband or to health care personnel, to test their reactions. "I really hated my mother when I was a kid" is a typical opener for a woman during pregnancy. If you respond to that in a therapeutic way ("Would you like to talk about that?"), she will feel free to reveal the intensity of her conflict with her parents, how much she hated them at times, how she cannot bear to think of the child inside her feeling that way about her (it almost makes her dislike her child before he is born). If the response to her remark is less than therapeutic ("Oh really? Now where is the urine specimen you said you brought in?") or trite ("Don't worry; everyone feels the same way"), she will usually not repeat the comment at that visit or may try it out on other health care personnel.

Her cues to what she is thinking may be subtle. "Am I ever going to make it through this?" might mean that she is tired of her backache, but it might also be a plea for reassurance that she will survive this event.

A woman needs to have confidence in the health care personnel who care for her during pregnancy, so that she can express some of the thoughts that are bothering her. It is easier and less time-consuming to ignore the comments that pregnant women make about their relationships with their families or husbands or their fears about the baby. However, an aim of maternal-newborn nursing is to ensure the welfare of the baby, and helping a woman to verbalize her thoughts, to straighten out old conflicts or crises, contributes to the establishment of a good mother-child relationship, which is essential for the baby's well-being.

PREPARING FOR MOTHERHOOD

Preparing for motherhood is an extension of the phenomenon of accepting the pregnancy and the child. It is necessary, however, that it be completed during pregnancy or during the weeks afterward, or parenting cannot proceed.

Kempe and Helfer [16] relate the battered child syndrome to a poor mothering image. Poor mothering ability may also produce children who exhibit the syndrome of failure to thrive because of the parents' lack of attachment and emotional concern.

Rubin [27] has identified a number of steps through which a woman must pass before she is ready to be a mother. These steps are as important to the woman about to become a mother for the second, third, fourth, or sixth time as they are for the woman about to become a mother for the first time.

Mimicry

The process of mimicry in the pregnant woman is not so different from that of the preschooler who mimics parent roles. When a preschooler follows after her mother dusting the furniture, her parents may express approval. When she mimics the position in which her father stands to use the toilet, her parents may express disapproval. As a result, the child chooses to imitate her mother.

The pregnant woman begins to spend time with other pregnant women or acquaintances of hers who have young children. She may spend more time talking to her own mother; this may be the first time she has truly talked to her since the conflicts of adolescence set up a barrier. She imitates actions, words, tasks that exemplify mothering.

ROLE PLAYING

The second step in the process is role playing. The woman offers to babysit for a neighbor or relative who has a new baby. She imitates the way the mother deals with the child. She is role playing at "being a mother" (Fig. 12-1).

FANTASY

In fantasy, the woman performs much the same work she did in accepting the pregnancy. She fantasizes what it will be like to be the mother of a boy, the mother of a girl. She sees if she can find a "fit" that is comfortable for her. Hopefully, she sees herself as fitting both roles, because she has no way of knowing which motherly role she will be called on to assume.

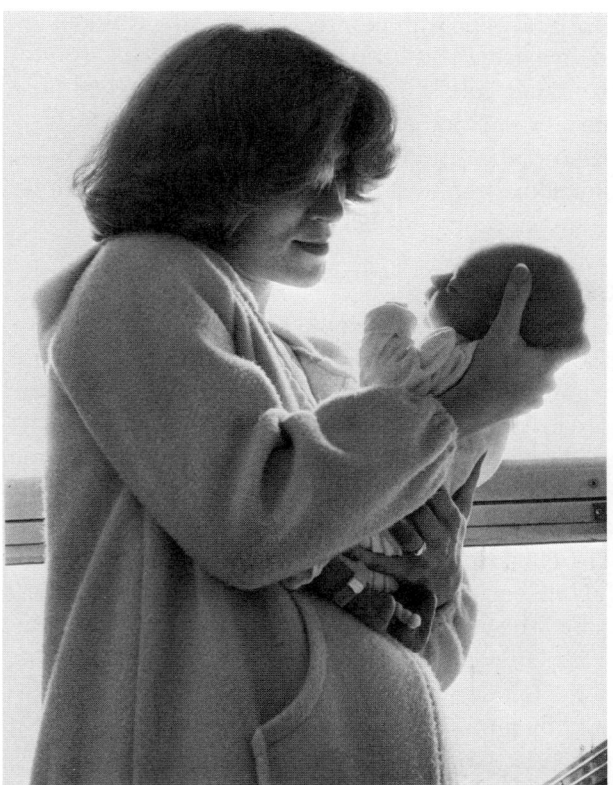

Fig. 12-1. *Psychological preparation for childbirth involves caring for babies or role playing what being a mother will be like. (Courtesy of the Department of Medical Photography, Children's Hospital, Buffalo, N.Y.)*

TAKING-IN

The fourth step is a taking-in. Rubin [26] refers to this step as introjection-projection-rejection. It is a continuation of actively acquiring a mother role "fit." The step begins with the woman becoming aware of her need to learn to mother (introjection). She then finds a role model of a mother among her friends or family (projection). The behavior of the role model is observed closely. The mother transposes herself into the model person's role. If the other woman's behavior seems to fit how the pregnant woman will be able to mother, then this woman adds to her existing knowledge and behavior repertoire. If the behavior does not seem to fit—the role model chosen was too rough with her children or too unconcerned—the woman will cast this model aside (rejection). She will then choose another role model and will continue this process until she finds one that is right for her.

This step is an important one in helping an adolescent girl to become a good mother. If the only role model she has are other girls her own age, who typically are not very interested in the commitment to mothering; if it is her own mother, and the mother is unable to cope with poverty, or too many children, or an ineffectual husband, the young girl will assume the same role. She needs exposure to good role models—in mothers' classes, at the clinic, in the physician's office, in a social agency—to be able to find a maternal role that will be worth copying and integrating into her own behavior.

GRIEF WORK

The thought that grief could be associated with such a positive process as childbirth is at first bizarre. But before a woman can firmly take on a mother role she has to "give up" present roles. She cannot be the mother of three and the mother of four at the same time; the mother-of-three image will have to go. She cannot be a child if she is to be an effective mother. The child in her will have to go. She cannot think of herself equally as a career woman and a mother. Either she will be a career woman who mothers in her spare time or a mother who squeezes in a career; one of the roles will have to be suppressed or perhaps temporarily put aside. This is grief work. The result of it will be a woman ready to accept a new role as a mother.

There are a number of life contingencies that may interfere with a woman's developing a relationship with her new child (accepting the pregnancy) or becoming a mother. Some of these are listed in Table 12-1. These life situations should be kept in mind when working with pregnant women. All too often, in both prenatal clinics and physicians' offices, considerable time is spent on taking a history on the initial visit, but on subsequent visits very few questions are asked. Thus, life contingencies may be overlooked that could have as great an effect on the newborn child as the physical things that have happened to the woman since she was last in the office.

It is easy to convince yourself that asking questions such as "How does your husband feel about your being pregnant?" or "Has anything changed in your home life since you were in the clinic last time?" is meddling. But such questions are not meddling to one who believes that mental health has as high a priority as physical health. Some nurses are reluctant to ask questions about these kinds of situations because they are aware that they cannot handle all the feelings that will be aroused. It is a fallacy to think that *any* person has the solutions to all the problems that people will pour out to health care personnel if they are given even the slightest opening to talk of things other than the swelling in their ankles or how much weight they have gained. You need the wisdom to recognize what you can handle, together with knowledge of the persons or social agencies who are equipped to deal with problems you cannot solve. This is a much more positive approach to mental health and one that is not very different from the way you handle medical problems. For example, you may or may not be in a position to correct beginning hypertension in a woman during pregnancy, but knowing that pregnancy-induced hypertension is a major cause of maternal mortality, you will not neglect to take a blood pressure simply because you will not be making the decision as to how to correct the problem.

Table 12-1. Life Contingencies Associated with Mothering Breakdown in the Perinatal Period

1. Multiple births
2. Children born within 10 to 12 months of each other
3. Dislocating moves in pregnancy or newborn period involving changing geographical areas and need to find new ties
4. Moving away from a family group or back to the group for economic reasons at a critical period for mother and child
5. Unexpected loss of security by reason of job losses, to husband; to the pregnant woman
6. Marital infidelity discovered in prenatal period
7. Illness in self, husband, or relative who must be cared for at a critical period
8. Loss of husband or of the infant's father close to prenatal period
9. Role reversals if a previously supporting person becomes dependent
10. Conception and course of pregnancy associated with loss of a person with whom there was a deeply significant tie
11. Previous abortions, sterility periods, traumatic past deliveries, loss of previous children
12. Pregnancy health complications
13. Experience with close friends or relatives who have had defective children
14. The juxtaposition of conception with a series of devaluing experiences

Source. J. Rose, The Prevention of Mothering Breakdown Associated with Physical Abnormalities of the Infant. Chapter XII in G. Caplan (Ed.), *Prevention of Mental Disorders in Children: Initial Explorations.* New York: Basic Books, Inc., Publishers, © 1961.

Emotional Responses to Pregnancy

Pregnancy is an intrusive process. A separate individual has invaded the woman's body and is growing inside it. She cannot ignore its presence any more than she can ignore that of a stranger who walked into her home and sat for nine months at her kitchen table. She might try to pretend no one was there, or when out of the house momentarily forget he was there. Sometimes, if he conversed with her or told amusing stories, she might be grateful he was there. But it would be virtually impossible not to have some feeling about his presence.

A great deal of a woman's reaction to pregnancy is similar—that is, ambivalent. She wants the pregnancy and yet she does not want it. She enjoys being pregnant and yet she does not enjoy it. Some nurses assume ambivalence means that the positive feelings counteract the negative feelings, the accepting feelings the rejecting feelings, so the woman is left feeling almost nothing toward her pregnancy, making pregnancy a calm, neutral period nine months long. This is not the case. No matter how neutral she wants to be, sooner or later she will have to walk into the kitchen. A stranger will be sitting at the kitchen table. She has to experience some emotion at his being there.

NARCISSISM

A woman's reaction to the intrusion of pregnancy can be manifested in a number of ways. Self-centeredness is generally an early reaction to pregnancy. A woman who previously was barely conscious of her body, who dressed in the morning with little thought about what to put on, who was unconcerned about her posture or her weight, suddenly begins to concentrate on these aspects of her life. She dresses so that her pregnancy will or will not show and dressing becomes a time-consuming, mirror-studying procedure. She makes a ceremony out of fixing her meals. Remember, there is a stranger in her life, someone coming to dinner, someone who is watching her (the stranger sitting in the kitchen).

A woman sometimes manifests narcissism by a change in her activities. She may stop playing tennis, even though her physician tells her it will do no harm in moderation. She criticizes her husband's driving when it never bothered her before. She is unconsciously "protecting" her body and thus her baby. She may be so unaware of what she is doing that she rationalizes her behavior. Tennis becomes "too tiring" or "boring." She describes her husband's driving as "reckless." What she means in both instances is that she feels threatened.

When working with a pregnant woman, it is important to remember that she feels a need to protect her body, that her *self* is important to her. She regards unnecessary nudity as a threat to her body (be sure to drape properly for pelvic and abdominal examinations). She resents casual, thoughtless remarks, such as "Oh, my, you're getting fat!" (a threat to her appearance) or "You don't like milk?" (a threat to her judgment).

There is a tendency to organize health instruction to pregnant women around the baby. "Now be sure to keep this appointment. You want to have a healthy baby." "You really ought to drink more milk for the baby." This approach is particularly inappropriate early in pregnancy, before the fetus stirs and before the woman is convinced not only that she is pregnant but that there is a baby inside her who is going to be born. At this stage she may be much more interested in doing things for herself, since it is her body, her tiredness, and her well-being that will be affected.

INTROVERSION VERSUS EXTROVERSION

Although introversion, or turning inward, to concentrate on oneself and one's body is common during pregnancy, some women react in an entirely opposite fashion and become more extroverted. They become active, appear healthier than ever before, and are more outgoing. Their faces glow, and they appear to "bloom" more and more with each month. Some women who undergo this change are just extremely happy to be pregnant. It tends to occur in women who are finding unexpected fulfillment in pregnancy, who had seriously doubted that they would be lucky enough or fertile enough to conceive. Such a woman regards her expanding abdomen as proof that she is equal to her sisters. In her eyes her pregnancy is a badge certifying equality. Although such a woman may become more interesting during her pregnancy, she is certain to confuse those around her, who may have regarded her as quiet and self-contained.

DECREASED DECISION MAKING

People who were dependent on a woman before pregnancy may feel hurt because now that she is pregnant she seems to have strength only for herself. A pregnant woman may lose interest in her job outside the home because the work seems alien to the events taking place in her body, which constantly remind her that a new round of life is beginning. She may have difficulty with decision making because she does not have enough interest to concentrate on a problem. This does not mean that a pregnant woman should not work. Pregnancy is not an illness; the outside interest and stimulation make the time go faster; the social contacts and the work she does are helpful to her and to her employer.

Decrease in responsibility taking is a reaction to the stress in pregnancy, not to the pregnancy itself. Nonpregnant women and many men function under just as much stress at work because of marital discord or illness or death of a loved one and have just as much difficulty with decision making in these circumstances. Pregnancy may be less stressful than these situations because of its predictable outcome.

EMOTIONAL LABILITY

Mood changes occur frequently in a pregnant woman, partly as a manifestation of narcissism (her feelings are easily hurt by remarks that would have been laughed off before) and partly because of hormonal changes, particularly the sustained increase in estrogen and progesterone. Mood swings are so common they make the woman's reaction to her family and to clinic or office routines unpredictable. What she found acceptable one week she may find intolerable the next. She may cry over her children's bad table manners at one meal and find the situation amusing and even charming at the next. A husband needs to be forewarned of these mood swings before his wife becomes pregnant, or at least very early in pregnancy, so that he will accept them as a part of a normal pregnancy. Otherwise, such changes in mood may cause him concern about his wife's mental health or about their relationship.

CHANGES IN SEXUAL DESIRE

Most women report that their sexual desires change, at least to some degree, during a pregnancy. For women who were always worried about becoming pregnant, sex during pregnancy may be truly enjoyed for the first time. Others may feel a loss of desire or may unconsciously view sexual relations as a threat to the body they must protect. Some may be frightened that sexual relations will bring on early labor.

Both wives and husbands should be warned early in pregnancy that such changes may occur, so that they will be interpreted in the correct light, that is, as differences, not as loss of interest in the sexual partner. The physiological changes due to the increase in estrogen and progesterone may well serve as a physical basis for these changes.

The Practical Tasks of Pregnancy

In addition to the main tasks of pregnancy, Duvall [8] has identified a number of practical adjustments that must be made during pregnancy before the woman is ready for her baby. Although some of these are housekeeping adjustments, such as preparing a sleeping space for the infant, some are psychological adjustments, such as those involved in the need for financial changes or changes in attitudes.

ARRANGING FOR THE INFANT'S PHYSICAL CARE

If the parents already have an extra bedroom and the additional equipment needed for a baby will be no financial burden, arranging for the baby's physical care may be a minor task. Frequently, however, providing space for a baby means moving to a larger apartment, or changing the older children's sleeping arrangements, or buying a new home. Purchasing a crib on a minimum income may require the sacrifice of some other item the couple very much wants. For these reasons, this task of pregnancy may be one of the most difficult.

DEVELOPING NEW ECONOMIC PATTERNS

About 50 percent of women work during their first pregnancy. Then, just at a time when the couple's expenses are increasing (medical expenses, clothing, food, more costly living arrangements), the woman takes a leave of absence or resigns, cutting the family income drastically. If the woman's income was counted on to maintain the family's style of living—and it generally is—adjustment to a lesser income will be difficult to make. The woman may also have some strong feelings about not contributing to the family income or may fear that she will have no control over how income is to be spent. This is a devaluing experience that may make accepting her pregnancy difficult for her or may interfere with her relationship with her newborn child.

REEVALUATION OF HOUSEHOLD ASSIGNMENTS

If the woman has intense nausea and vomiting early in pregnancy, or she tires easily in later pregnancy, the husband may, for the first time, find himself assuming chores in the home that he never imagined he would do. If he was raised to believe that household tasks are strictly women's work, he may find these new demands too devaluing to endure. If he is able to envision household chores not as sex-related but merely as jobs that must be done in order to ensure the smooth running of the home, he will be able to perform them and to give as his reason, "We are having a baby at our house."

ACQUISITION OF KNOWLEDGE ABOUT PREGNANCY, CHILDBIRTH, AND PARENTHOOD

A woman is more likely to acquire knowledge about pregnancy, childbirth, and child rearing than a man because as part of her role-playing behavior during pregnancy she is drawn into a world of talk about babies. It is helpful to most couples to attend education-for-childbirth or -parenthood classes during a pregnancy. Attending such classes helps the couple accept the pregnancy ("I must be going to have a baby, otherwise why would I be here?"), exposes the woman to role models of mothering, and provides information about pregnancy and child care to both parents. The content of such classes is discussed in Chap. 19.

The Pregnant Father

The father has traditionally been the forgotten person in the childbearing process. There are still many men who are raised to think of childbearing as a woman's concern. Thus, a man may expect that during pregnancy and at childbirth he will be relegated few tasks other than to "boil water" (with no idea what he is to do with the water once it is boiled!). He suspects that such tasks are merely busywork to keep him out of the mainstream of events. Fortunately, it is beginning to be recognized that men have an important role in childbirth and must take the same steps during pregnancy that women must take.

ACCEPTING THE PREGNANCY

For the husband, accepting the pregnancy means not only accepting the certainty of the pregnancy and the reality of the child to come but also accepting his wife in her changed state. As noted before, it is helpful to forewarn the husband of the changes he can expect in his wife. Otherwise, he will interpret her mood swings, change of sexual interest, introversion, or narcissism as loss of interest in him.

A man needs to give his wife emotional support while she is working through accepting a pregnancy, and she should reciprocate when he is going through the process in his turn. A husband may feel jealous of the growing baby, who, although not yet physically apparent, seems to be taking up a great deal of his wife's time and thought. He may feel as if he has been left standing in the wings, waiting to be asked to take part in the event. To compensate for this feeling he may become absorbed in his work, in producing something concrete, feeling that he must demonstrate that he, too, is capable of creativeness. This preoccupation with work may limit the amount of time he spends with his wife, just when she needs his emotional support most.

Whether or not he is able to accept the pregnancy and the coming child depends on the same factors that are crucial in women, namely, his cultural background, past experience, and relationships with family members. If he was raised to believe that men do not show emotion, he may not be able to say easily, "I want this baby; I'm glad," when his wife tells him of the diagnosis. He may not be able to say, "It's great to feel it kick. That's a reassuring feeling." He may be unable to say, "I love you. Looking fat, unhappy with yourself, stomach full of baby or not, I love you."

However, even though he is inarticulate, he may be able to convey such emotions by a touch or a caress—a reason his presence is always desired at a prenatal visit and certainly in a labor and delivery room. His wife will know that his hand on hers is as meaningful an expression of emotion as the spoken word.

Many men experience physical symptoms such as nausea, vomiting, and backache the same way as or more intensely than their wives experience these symptoms. As their wives' abdomens begin to grow and they begin to take up more body space, men may perceive themselves as taking up more body space as if they, not their wives, were the ones who were pregnant [10].

These are healthy happenings and show the interest and the depth with which the man is accepting the pregnancy.

REWORKING DEVELOPMENTAL TASKS

Men have to do the same reworking of old values and forgotten developmental tasks as do women. Many men obtain their sex education from other boys and so come into manhood believing in many old wives' tales, sometimes not even being certain in what part of the woman's body a fetus grows. A man may believe that breast-feeding will make his wife's breasts pendulous and no longer attractive to him. He may believe that childbirth will stretch his wife's vagina so much that sexual relations will no longer be enjoyable. He needs factual education to update his knowledge.

He has to rethink his relationship with his father and to come to a better understanding of the kind of father he is going to be.

PREPARING FOR FATHERHOOD

The man has role playing and grief work to do during pregnancy before he can be a father. He has to imagine himself as the father of a boy, the father of a girl. He has to cast aside a father-of-two image to accept a father-of-three image (difficult to do if he keeps concentrating on the cost of baby clothes or tuition or the loss of his wife's income during a maternity leave). If this is the first time he is to be a father, he has to relinquish the image of being "one of the boys" or a "carefree bachelor." These freedoms may not seem so precious if he examines them truthfully, but giving them up is difficult. A man does not seem thirsty until you tell him he cannot have any water; a man does not mind giving up a well-ordered, uncluttered life until a pregnancy compels it.

CONCERNS OF EXPECTANT FATHERS

Fathers-to-be may not voice their concerns well because they feel that the things they are concerned about are things they should somehow already know and so should not ask about, or they do not want to compound their wives' anxieties by appearing anxious themselves.

In one study [22], when fathers were asked after delivery of their child what things concerned them most about pregnancy, labor, or delivery, they showed that the matters fathers are supposed to worry about (getting to the hospital on time, infant care, and finances, for example) were not great worries. They were more concerned with their wives' physical health during pregnancy, with having sufficient knowledge about what was happening during labor, and with their ability to help their wives during labor. These findings are summarized in Table 12-2.

Although this study utilized a small sample of fathers, it shows the significance to fathers of a statement such as "Your wife is doing fine" at the end of a prenatal visit. A question like "Could I review what's going to happen in labor with you?" might be the most important question that the man is asked in nine months.

The Pregnant Family

Most parents today are aware that older children in a family need some warning that a new baby is on the way. However, knowing that such preparation is called for and being able to give it are two different matters. Many couples need suggestions from health care personnel as to how this task should be accomplished.

"How soon should I tell the older children?" is a common question. The answer depends on the ages and personalities of the older children and on the parents' ability to accept the pregnancy. School-age children should probably be told of the coming event when the parents know that it is definite. Parents are bound to discuss the pregnancy, and it is frightening for a child to walk into a room and hear the conversation suddenly halt. It is far more perplexing and worrisome to know that *something* is going on, *something* is happening, than to know *exactly* what is happening: that no matter how much you may dislike the prospect, a new baby is coming.

Preschoolers should be told at the time preparations for the coming infant begin. This is the point at which

Table 12-2. Concerns of Expectant Fathers

MUCH CONCERN
Feelings about being able to help wife in labor
Preference for boy or girl
Concerns about wife's physical health during pregnancy
Feelings about pain or discomfort that wife experienced during delivery
Feelings about not being with wife during delivery
Concerns about having sufficient knowledge or being kept informed about what was going on during the period of labor

SOME CONCERN
Concerns about the amount of time wife will have to spend with the baby at home
Feelings about change in wife's figure
Feelings regarding mood changes in wife
Concerns about sexual relations during pregnancy
Feelings about being able to ease wife's discomforts
Concerns about providing wife with emotional support and understanding
Concerns about health of unborn child, possibility of mental and physical defects
Concerns about being a father
Concerns about discipline of child
Temporary mood changes experienced by expectant fathers
Changes in feelings toward wife
Feelings about love and attention received from wife
Concerns about environmental effects of war, crime, drugs, and pollution on child's health and development
Feelings toward babies of friends or neighbors

NO CONCERN
Physical discomforts experienced by expectant fathers
Concerns about loss of freedom and less spare time
Feelings about attention that wife received from friends and neighbors
Concerns about the kind of mother the wife would be
Concerns about what to expect during pregnancy
Concerns about being able to maintain social and leisure-time activities once the baby was born
Concerns about medical care wife received during pregnancy
Concerns about providing for child's needs without depriving himself and his wife of their needs
Concerns about getting wife to hospital in time
Concerns about holding, feeding, and taking care of newborn
Concerns about role parents or parents-in-law played during wife's pregnancy
Concerns about finances
Difficulties deciding on name for child

Source. L. K. McNall, Concerns of Expectant Fathers. In L. K. McNall and J. T. Galeener (Eds.). *Current Practice in Obstetric and Gynecologic Nursing*, Vol. I. St. Louis: Mosby, 1976.

they become aware that something is happening. They need limits or boundaries put on the happening, so it does not loom so large in their minds that they cannot cope with it. "A baby is coming. Soon our family will be Mommy, Daddy, you, and a new baby. Four of us. That's what is happening."

It is important that parents prepare a preschool child for the initial helplessness of the infant. There is a tendency to say, "Soon you'll have a little brother or sister to play with." The child who is prepared by that explanation will be disappointed when his mother shows him a very small baby who does not respond at all to his favorite toys.

If a toddler is going to be moved from the crib to an adult bed, it is important that the parents make the change at least by the 6th month of pregnancy. It is a positive experience to be moved from a crib to a regular bed because "you are a big girl (or a big boy) now." It is a crushing experience that plants seeds of jealousy to be moved because "the new baby needs your bed."

The same principle applies to starting a toddler in nursery school or kindergarten. He should be started, if possible, during the pregnancy, or about six months afterward, but not in the period shortly after the new baby's birth. He will feel unloved and rejected if he is sent off to school just when the new baby comes home. Later, he will feel proud that *he* is old enough to go to school while the baby has to stay home.

Children ask many questions about a new baby. Where is he growing? What is he doing? Is he eating now? How does he get out? How did he get in? If these questions are answered one by one during the process of childbearing, easily and naturally as they occur, childbearing becomes once and for all a positive, miraculous aspect of life. Examples of answers to the above questions are: "A baby grows in a special place in Mommy's tummy." (It is important that the preschooler knows it is a special space so he does not envisage the new baby smothering in the food his mother eats.) "A baby doesn't seem to do much in his special place. He just grows and gets ready to be born." "He doesn't have to eat while he's inside Mommy. A special cord gives him food through his belly button. See where your special cord fed you when you were inside me?" "I'll go to the hospital when it's time for the baby to come and the doctor will help the new baby be born. Babies come out of a special opening between the mother's legs." "Babies begin to grow as a seed so tiny you can't even see it. When two people love each other, the father puts his penis inside the place in mother's body where babies are born. A seed from Daddy's penis mixes with a seed from Mommy's body, and that makes a baby start to grow."

These are simple explanations but enough to answer the child's questions truthfully. If his first question is answered responsibly and openly, he will feel free to ask a second if he wishes. There is no reason to tell the child any more than he asks. Remember the boy who came home from school and asked, "Where did I come from?" His mother spent a half hour explaining "the birds and the bees" to him. When she was finished, the child said, "Thanks, I wondered. The kid who sits behind me said he comes from Cleveland."

If parents feel uncomfortable answering questions about childbirth, it might be helpful if they arranged for the child to see a dog or cat in the neighborhood giving birth to a litter. He will be able to relate his observations to the birth of the new baby. Warn parents to stress, however, that although the puppies and kittens they see born are going to be given away, the new brother or sister will be here to stay.

Children under school age need to be prepared for the separation from their mother that childbirth will entail. Overnight stays with grandparents or at a neighbor's are a good way to accustom both children and mother to being apart briefly.

Both preschool and school-age children need to be reassured periodically during pregnancy that a new baby is *adding* to the family and will not replace anyone in either parent's affection.

The Unwed Pregnant Woman

Although the overall birth rate in the United States is decreasing, the birth rate among girls under 15 years of age is increasing, and the birth rate among girls between 15 and 19 is staying about the same. Along with the increase in out-of-wedlock pregnancies, acceptance of such pregnancies has grown—or if not acceptance, at least a recognition that they occur, that they occur frequently, and that health care personnel have the same obligation to meet the needs of these women during pregnancy and childbirth as they do to meet the needs of married women.

The day of the sheltered "secret" home for unmarried pregnant women, where they would stay for nine months, deliver, place the child for adoption, and return home as if nothing had happened, is almost over. Something did happen, and as much as the woman and her family wanted to pretend it did not, the psychological scars of starting to love a kicking stranger and then having to give him away (never to mention him again, to be safe) remained. Today, pregnant women who are unmarried usually attend prenatal clinics or come to physicians' offices as most married women do. They deliver at community hospitals, and a great many of them keep their babies.

Pregnant adolescent girls differ from pregnant adults in that they are more prone to the complications of pregnancy. Mortality is higher for infants of mothers in this age group than for infants of women 20 to 34 years of age. In addition to extra worry about her health and the physical outcome of a pregnancy, the unmarried adolescent has greater difficulty working through the psychological tasks of pregnancy.

ACCEPTING THE PREGNANCY
Pregnancy comes as a surprise to all women, and it should not necessarily be any more of a surprise to an unmarried woman than to a married one. Any woman who does not use a reliable contraceptive runs the risk of impregnation. Adolescent girls report, however, almost without exception, being surprised that they are pregnant. They were following the "it can't happen to me" philosophy, and now it is almost impossible for them to believe that it *has* happened to them. Occasionally, a young adolescent has a child because she was unaware that sexual intercourse leads to impregnation, or she believed an old wives' tale (e.g., that if her blood type is different from her boyfriend's she cannot conceive).

There are many reasons for the unmarried woman to want a baby. She may imagine that it will give her a hold on a boyfriend she does not want to lose (married women sometimes have children to hold on to a husband). She may want to show her parents that she is mature and does not have to follow directions (married women have children for the same reason). She is lonely and wants someone to love or to love her (again, married women have children for the same reason).

These are important concepts to keep in mind when mentioning the subject of adoption to unmarried women. They may have as great an attachment to the baby or as much of a desire to have the child as a married woman.

TELLING PARENTS ABOUT THE PREGNANCY
Many adolescent girls come to health care facilities late for prenatal care because they are having difficulty believing that they are pregnant and because a second, equally important problem is troubling them. They do not want to face telling their parents about the pregnancy. They anticipate that their parents' reaction to the news will be anger, rage, disappointment, or grief. It is important to remember that this is a major concern for an adolescent girl. She cannot listen to your explanation of good nutrition or the danger signals of pregnancy if her mind is filled with worry about how the people at home will react to this pregnancy.

Recognize the problem. Ask at a first visit, Have you told anyone yet that you might be pregnant? Have you told either of your parents? Are you worried about telling them? Talking this over with someone who understands her concern will not make the girl's problem go away but may make it possible for her to face it. Any problem that can be talked about almost spontaneously becomes a problem that has bounds and limits, that can be handled.

Most girls report at a second visit that their parents were not nearly so angry about the pregnancy as they had anticipated. Their parents, after all, knew their daughter and her boyfriend were going steady and knew they were being left unsupervised. Some parents react as if they had been waiting to hear this news, having accepted it as inevitable months before it happened.

Help the girl to remember other instances when she was afraid to tell her parents something: a time she stayed out too late, the time she broke her bicycle. She will probably tell you that her parents were more understanding on those occasions than she had anticipated. They realized that people do forget about time and that no bicycle is built to last forever or to withstand shock.

You cannot accompany the girl to help her tell her parents, but your support can go with her and will in most instances be enough to help her face this early task of a pregnancy out of wedlock. A married woman whose husband does not want any more children faces the same task and needs the same support to help her break the news. She needs to recall instances when her husband reacted in a calmer, more accepting way to bad news than she thought he would.

FACING A PREGNANCY ALONE
Pregnancy is a crisis situation. Almost automatically, the single woman has more difficulty adjusting to and accepting a pregnancy and a new child because she almost automatically has fewer support people around her than her married counterpart. She may feel acute loneliness during pregnancy. Acute loneliness brings with it depression, and a common symptom of depression is inability to function or make decisions.

Deciding whether to cook green beans or corn for dinner becomes a major problem for a depressed person. Whether to walk outside or not, whether the twinges she feels in her back are beginning labor contractions or just backache, whether she should phone a doctor or not—all are difficult decisions for someone depressed.

The single woman needs enough questions asked of her at prenatal visits so loneliness and depression can be revealed and evaluated. Talk time at prenatal visits also helps the woman improve or develop socializing skills, which will aid her in establishing more lasting relationships than the one that led to her pregnancy and has now left her alone.

Some women begin a pregnancy married and then, through trauma (a car accident, a work injury) or illness, separation or divorce, lose their husbands during pregnancy. These women need to be evaluated very carefully, as their loneliness is likely to be extremely acute during this time, when they feel the need stronger than ever before for someone around them to care about them.

REWORKING DEVELOPMENTAL TASKS

Pregnancy in an adolescent is particularly fraught with anxiety because the developmental tasks of pregnancy are superimposed on those of adolescence. Erikson [9] defines the tasks of adolescence as achieving a sense of identity, emancipating from parents, establishing a value system, and choosing a vocation.

A girl who is in the process of separating from her parents, of becoming independent, may be devastated by the knowledge that in nine months someone will be dependent on *her*. She is torn between being mothered and mothering. She may experience a great deal of difficulty establishing future intimate relationships once she realizes that her present relationship has led to a situation detrimental to her. The girl who drops out of school because she is pregnant has special difficulty selecting a vocation. Further, if health care personnel treat her as if she were shameless and irresponsible, she may become unable to think of herself as a worthwhile person or to establish a sound value system.

The adolescent is extremely concerned with body image as part of the task of establishing identity, that is, the kind of a person he or she is. Adolescent unwed mothers, therefore, may be less concerned about the future of the baby and planning for it than they are with their bodily changes, the possible permanence of these changes, and the disruption of their daily lives.

BECOMING A MOTHER

Role playing and fantasy may be hard for the young unmarried woman. It may be impossible for her to cast aside the role of daughter in her grief work because she is still so obviously a daughter.

She needs support from the father of the child. If he can talk about the pregnancy, if it seems real to him, then it will seem more real to her. Emotional support from the unwed partner has special significance—it is given absolutely voluntarily. Remember this when debating whether or not an unmarried father should be allowed in the examining room or in the labor or delivery room. If he is there, it is because of emotional ties, not marriage ties. He can be an important person for the young woman to have with her in a stress situation.

The major need of unwed women during pregnancy is additional talk time—time to voice their concerns and to begin to think through solutions. If this additional time and attention is not given, because of busy clinic or office schedules or nurses who think of patients as stereotypes rather than as persons with individual needs, the adolescent girl may reach the end of pregnancy with many of its tasks unresolved.

The Unwed Expectant Father

For generations, the unwed father has been dismissed as a person who had no interest in a pregnancy or further concern about the mother's or infant's health. Statements such as "It's always the woman who pays" or "Love 'em and leave 'em" reflect these societal values.

In the past, many men were forced into the role of disinterested observer, whether or not that was truly the role they wanted, for financial reasons. If they were still in school or were married and had another family to support, the only way they could be free of the expense of doctors and hospital bills was to disappear quietly into the background as soon as the diagnosis became certain.

Today, with health care costs and childbearing costs usually being covered by third-party payers rather than individuals, unmarried fathers are free to have an emotional interest in the pregnancy. Before, when the child was going to be placed for adoption, it was easier to pretend that nothing had happened, to dismiss the pregnancy as none of their concern. Now, with most young women choosing to keep their babies, the situation is less easy to ignore. Some couples plan on having children without ever marrying; they see having children but not marriage as their life-style. These unmarried fathers, although their last name is different from the woman's, are very much fathers and have exactly the same involvement and commitment to the pregnancy and child as their married counterparts.

ACCEPTING THE PREGNANCY

An unwed father may have a great deal of difficulty accepting the pregnancy if he has doubt whether the baby belongs to him or not. He tries to picture what the child will look like; doubts that the baby will look like him appear and dissolve the image. He tries to picture himself as a father, then realizes he will never play a father role to this child; the image disappears again. Because the unwed father can relate to some extent to being a father, however (and sometimes more easily than the woman can see herself as a mother), if the woman decides to have an abortion (and that is her decision, not one he needs to be consulted on) or the baby is born less than perfect, the man may be left with a deep sense of loss and may have few people around him for support who are even aware that he has lost anything.

REWORKING DEVELOPMENTAL TASKS

The unwed father has to rework developmental tasks the same as the married man—as difficult a problem for him as it is for his unmarried partner. It is hard to review his relationship with his parents if they insist that he handle this problem by ignoring it. It is equally hard to review a sense of identity because his identity is now so unclear. He is a father and yet he is not a father. People may tell him that the woman took advantage of him, that she became pregnant to trap him, that if she were really a nice woman she never would have let this happen. He may begin to doubt his ability to evaluate people. He loses self-esteem. He is in many ways a helpless, second-rate person in this situation.

GRIEF WORK

The unmarried father has very real grief work to do during pregnancy, grieving not only for life the way it was before but possibly for the loss of his child's mother (angry with him because she is pregnant, told by her parents to stay away from him, so introverted by her own pregnancy work that she is unable to meet any of his needs) and for loss of the child (it will be placed for adoption, or the woman will keep it but he doubts that he will be allowed to visit).

Unmarried fathers need time during pregnancy to talk about how it feels to be a father when they have little outward connection with the pregnancy yet have deep emotional ties with the woman or the growing fetus that are stronger than even they may realize.

Nursing assessments of psychological adjustment to pregnancy follow.

Problem-oriented Recording: Progress Notes

Christine McFadden
15 years
First prenatal visit: LMP about 16 weeks

Problem: Psychological adjustment to pregnancy

S. Pregnancy unplanned although not using any contraceptive method at time. Parents are angry with her, not supportive. Father of child now ignores her. "He's a popular guy in school. Popular guys don't get girls pregnant; it puts him down." Swimming coach (formerly an important support person) seems angry with her for "letting the team down." Close girl friends "don't care one way or the other."
Doesn't want abortion—"I couldn't hurt a baby."
Plans for caring for baby involve "having a baby of my own will be fun."

O. Eyes are tear-filled when discussing reactions of father of child; appears angry at parents' reaction.

A. Unplanned pregnancy, but apparently not unwelcome.
No active support people at present.

Goals: a. Establish adequate support people either in family, friends, or health personnel.
b. Reestablish a workable relationship with parents and possibly father of child.
c. Explain impact of having child on life situation in more realistic terms.
d. Accept and view self as mother by end of pregnancy.

P. 1. Continue to discuss adjustment to pregnancy at visits.
2. Continue to discuss relationship with parents and father of child.
3. Schedule appointments so consistent personnel are present for support people.

Christine McFadden
15 years
Gestation length: 20 weeks

Problem: Psychological adjustment to pregnancy
    Milestone: Quickening

> S. States, "I like the feel of him moving. It's like he's touching me and saying everything's okay." Has bought one outfit for infant. Father of child (16-year-old high school junior) accompanied her for prenatal visit. Nervous, shy at being asked into examining room. Grew excited over listening to baby's heart sounds.
> Parents "still disappointed." "Won't talk about pregnancy."
> High school coach (once important to her) continues to ignore her.
> Has been told a cesarean section may be necessary for delivery. Asking questions about procedure.
> O. Appears to appreciate support of child's father.
> Appears distressed at discussing parents' attitude.
> A. Improved adjustment to unplanned pregnancy at quickening.
> Some improvement in support people.
> P. 1. Include father of child in prenatal care plans.
>   2. Discuss at visits concept of cesarean birth, working toward acceptance.
>   3. Continue to serve as support people as parents do not seem able to fill this role.

Problem-oriented Recording Progress Notes

Mary Kraft
22 years
First prenatal visit: LMP 9 weeks

Problem: Psychological adjustment to pregnancy

> S. Married 4 years; planned pregnancy after surgery for endometriosis 4 months ago. "Unbelievably happy" is reaction to pregnancy confirmation.
> Husband attends night school so "some nights are lonely."
> Family is out of town; she has few close friends, "One at work." Only black family in condominium and sometimes feels "out of place."
> Last pregnancy ended in spont. abortion at 2½ months. She asked, "How do I know that won't happen again?"
> O. Appears happy at discussing pregnancy, nervous at discussing lack of friends.
> A. Planned and desired pregnancy.
> Limited support people.
>
> Goals: a. Establish a satisfying relationship with at least one neighbor or new acquaintance outside work.
>   b. Able to use health personnel as her support people until outside sources are established.
>   c. Good beginning adaptation to pregnancy is continued (difficult to maintain due to prev. pregnancy loss)
>   d. Accept and view herself as mother by end of pregnancy.
>
> P. 1. Urge to communicate with family out of town by letter, telephone.
>   2. Urge to have husband accompany her for at least 1 prenatal visit.
>   3. Discuss way to fill in free time to counteract feelings of loneliness.
>   4. Discuss ways of meeting more people in order to establish her own network of friends outside husband's acquaintances.
>   5. Assure that pregnancy is going well (as appropriate) at visits because of prev. preg. loss to ensure mother-child bonding.
>   6. Schedule appointments so consistent health personnel are present for support people.

Mary Kraft
22 years
Gestation length: 20 weeks

Problem: Psychological adjustment to pregnancy
    Milestone: Quickening

> S. States, "I have never been so happy." "I'm past the point when I lost the last one, you know. I feel safe now."
> Has bought crib and wallpaper for baby's room.
> O. Appears happy discussing pregnancy.
> A. Good adaptation to pregnancy (nest building beginning).
> P. 1. Provide opportunities for discussion at visits so any problems that do arise can be aired.
> 2. Continue assurance that pregnancy is going well.

Problem-oriented Recording: Progress Notes

Angie Baco
42 years
First prenatal visit: LMP 12 weeks ago

Problem: Psychological adjustment to pregnancy

> S. Married, 6 previous pregnancies, 5 living children.
> Unplanned pregnancy. States, "I can't believe it; I can't get used to it. I can't see myself with a baby again."
> Husband is supportive (present with wife for visit). States, "We'll work things out." One daughter (20 years old and married) has baby 6 months old. Is supportive. Other children's reactions are mixed.
> No plans for abortion due to religious beliefs. A child who would be 8 died as newborn of congenital heart defect; 7-year-old has a learning disability. Patient states, "I think I'm too old to have well children; I must have been too old 8 years ago."
> O. Appears tense when discussing caring for new baby and outcome of last two pregnancies.
> A. Unplanned, unwanted pregnancy; no apparent acceptance of pregnancy yet.
> Concerned about health of coming child because of 7-year-old with learning disability and previous child with heart disease.

Goals: a. Accept pregnancy by quickening.
b. Establish better relationship with children.
c. Accept and view herself as mother of new baby by end of pregnancy.

> P. 1. Mark chart high-risk for maternal-child bonding.
> 2. Give assurance during pregnancy visits that pregnancy is going well (as appropriate) to develop concept of well child and improve maternal-child bonding.
> 3. Continue discussion of life changes and child rearing at further prenatal visits.
> 4. Urge husband to continue support (include in prenatal discussions about role changes).

Angie Baco
42 years
Gestation length: 20 weeks

Problem: Psychological adjustment to pregnancy
Milestone: Quickening

> S. States, "I don't go out as much now; I don't want people thinking I'm crazy, pregnant at my age. I suppose another girl wouldn't be bad; no more boys though."
> Husband accompanied her on visit; supportive. Is out of work (seasonal construction layoff). States, "Money is tight now, but we've been this way before." Wanted reassurance that baby "wouldn't be brain damaged like 7-year-old."
> O. —
> A. Adjustment to pregnancy still questionable at quickening.
> Financial situation compounding problem.
> P. 1. Refer for food stamps for financial help.
> 2. Continue to assure as appropriate that child is suffering no damage in utero.
> 3. Continue to discuss life adjustments to new child.
> 4. Mark definite high-risk for maternal-child bonding if no improvement by 1 month.

References

1. Bascom, L. Women who refuse to believe: Persistent denial of pregnancy. M.C.N. 2:174, 1977.
2. Brandwein, R. A. Women and children last: Divorced mothers and their families. Nurs. Digest 4:39, 1976.
3. Caplan, G. Concepts of Mental Health Consultations. Washington, D.C.: U.S. Children's Bureau, 1959.
4. Chao, Y. M. An habitual aborter's self-concept during the course of a successful pregnancy. Matern. Child Nurs. J. 6:165, 1977.
5. Cohen, D. S. Fears During Pregnancy. In K. A. Knafl and H. K. Grace (Eds.), Families Across the Life Cycle. Boston: Little, Brown, 1978.
6. Cohen, R. L. Maladaption to pregnancy. Semin. Perinatol. 3:15, 1979.
7. Degarmo, E. Fathers' and Mothers' Feelings About Sharing the Childbirth Experience. In L. K. McNall and J. T. Galeener (Eds.), Current Practice in Obstetric and Gynecologic Nursing. St. Louis: Mosby, 1976.
8. Duvall, E. Family Development. Philadelphia: Lippincott, 1971.
9. Erikson, E. H. Childhood and Society. New York: Norton, 1964.
10. Fawcett, J. Body image and the pregnant couple. M.C.N. 3:227, 1978.
11. Ferguson, I. A psychological approach to pregnancy and childbirth. Midwives Chron. 90:187, 1977.
12. Griffith, S. Pregnancy as an event with crisis potential for marital partners: A study of interpersonal needs. J.O.G.N. Nurs. 5:35, 1976.
13. Gruis, M. Beyond maternity: Post partum concerns of mothers. M.C.N. 2:182, 1977.
14. Hogan, L. R. Pregnant again—at 41. M.C.N. 4:174, 1979.
15. Horowitz, J. A., and Perdue, B. J. Single-parent families. Nurs. Clin. North Am. 12:503, 1977.
16. Kempe, C. H., and Helfer, R. (Eds.). Helping the Battered Child and His Family. Philadelphia: Lippincott, 1972.
17. Klepser, M. J. Grief: How long does grief go on? Am. J. Nurs. 78:420, 1978.
18. Lipkin, G. B. Parent-Child Rearing: Psychosocial Aspects. St. Louis: Mosby, 1978.
19. Macfarlane, A. The Psychology of Childbirth. Cambridge, Mass.: Harvard University Press, 1977.
20. Marquart, R. Expectant fathers: What are their needs? M.C.N. 1:32, 1976.
21. May, K. A. Psychologic involvement in pregnancy by expectant fathers. Nurs. Digest 4:8, 1976.
22. McNall, L. K. Concerns of Expectant Fathers. In L. K. McNall and J. T. Galeener (Eds.). Current Practice in Obstetric and Gynecologic Nursing. St. Louis: Mosby, 1976.
23. Newton, M. Meeting sexual and emotional needs during pregnancy. Fam. Health 9:15, 1977.
24. Rinquist, M. A. Psychologic Stress in the Last 3 Months of Pregnancy. In L. K. McNall and J. T. Galeener (Eds.). Current Practice in Obstetric and Gynecologic Nursing. St. Louis: Mosby, 1976.
25. Rose, J. The Prevention of Mothering Breakdown Associated With Physical Abnormalities of the Infant. In G. Caplan (Ed.). Prevention of Mental Disorders in Children. New York: Basic Books, 1961.
26. Rubin, R. Cognitive style in pregnancy. Am. J. Nurs. 65:97, 1965.
27. Rubin, R. Maternal tasks in pregnancy. J. Adv. Nurs. 1:367, 1976.
28. Snyder, C., et al. New findings about mothers' antenatal expectations and the relationship to infant development. M.C.N. 4:358, 1979.
29. Stichler, J. F., et al. Pregnancy: A shared emotional experience. M.C.N. 4:153, 1979.
30. Webster-Stratton, C., and Kogan, K. Helping parents parent. Am. J. Nurs. 80:240, 1980.

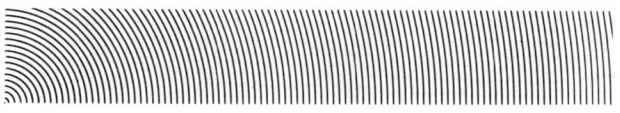

13. Growth and Development of the Fetus

Before the nineteenth century, people had a variety of concepts and superstitions concerning the fetus. Medieval artists depicted the child in utero as a miniature man. Leonardo da Vinci, in his notebooks of 1510 to 1512, made several sketches of unborn infants, indicating that he believed the fetus was immobile and essentially a part of the mother, sharing her blood and internal organs. During the seventeenth and eighteenth centuries, two separate theories were explored. According to one theory, the baby was contained fully formed in the mother's ovaries, and when male cells were introduced, the baby expanded to birth size. The second theory was that the child existed in the head of the sperm cell as a fully formed being, the uterus being used only as an incubator in which to grow. It was not until 1759 that Kaspar Wolff proposed that both parents contribute equally to the structure of the baby.

Fertilization: The Beginning of Pregnancy

As the ovum leaves the graafian follicle at ovulation, it is surrounded by a ring of mucopolysaccharide fluid (the zona pellucida) and a circle of cells (the corona radiata). These increase the bulk of the ovum, facilitating its migration to the uterus, and probably also serve as a protection from injury. The ovum and surrounding cells are propelled into a fallopian tube by currents initiated by the fimbriae, the fine hair-like structures that line the openings of the fallopian tubes. The ovum is propelled the length of the tube by peristaltic action of the tube and movement of the tube cilia. An ovum is capable of being fertilized for only 24 hours (48 hours at the most) after ovulation. After that time, it atrophies and becomes nonfunctional.

Ordinarily, only one ovum reaches maturity each month. A normal ejaculation of semen averages 2.5 ml of fluid. Each milliliter contains 60 to 100 million spermatozoa, or an average of 200 million per ejaculation. At ovulation there is a reduction in the viscosity of cervical mucus, making it easier for spermatozoa to penetrate it at this time. Spermatozoa deposited in the vagina during sexual intercourse generally reach the cervix of the uterus within 90 seconds after deposition and the end of the fallopian tubes in 5 minutes (this is the reason douching is an ineffective contraceptive measure unless it is done within 90 seconds of ejaculation). Spermatozoa move by means of their flagella (tails) through the cervix, the body of the uterus, and into the fallopian tubes, where one spermatozoon meets the waiting ovum.

The mechanism whereby spermatozoa are drawn

toward an ovum is unknown. It may be a species-specific reaction similar to an antibody-antigen reaction. Freshly ejaculated spermatozoa cannot fertilize ova; apparently some sort of change must occur in the head of the spermatozoon (capacitation) before it is capable of fertilization. This change takes place during passage through the uterus.

Fertilization (conception, impregnation, or fecundation), the union of ovum and spermatozoon, generally occurs in the outer third of a fallopian tube, the ampullar portion. All the spermatozoa that reach the ovum cluster around its protective layer of corona cells. Hyaluronidase (a proteolytic enzyme) is apparently released by the spermatozoa. This enzyme acts to dissolve the layer of cells protecting the ovum. Once a spermatozoon penetrates the zona pellucida, a reaction sweeps throughout the entire zona that makes it difficult for other spermatozoa to penetrate it. Similarly, only one spermatozoon is able to penetrate the cell membrane of the ovum. After it has done so, the cell membrane apparently becomes impervious to other spermatozoa.

The chromosomal material of the ovum and spermatozoon fuse, and the resulting structure is called a *zygote*. Since the spermatozoon and ovum each carry 23 chromosomes (22 autosomes and 1 sex chromosome) the fertilized ovum has 46 chromosomes.

If an X-carrying spermatozoon enters the ovum, the resulting child will have two X chromosomes and will be female (XX). If a Y-carrying spermatozoon fertilizes the ovum, the resulting child will have an X and a Y chromosome and will be male (XY).

Out of the fertilized ovum (the zygote) will form not only the future child but also the accessory structures he needs to support himself during intrauterine life: the placenta, the fetal membranes, the amniotic fluid, and the umbilical cord. These accessory structures plus the zygote are referred to as the *conceptus*.

Implantation

Once fertilization is complete, the zygote migrates toward the body of the uterus, aided by the currents initiated by the muscular contractions of the fallopian tubes. It takes three or four days for the zygote to reach the body of the uterus. During this time, mitotic cell division or cleavage begins at a rapid rate. The first cleavage occurs at about 24 hours; cleavage divisions continue to occur at a rate of one about every 22 hours. By the time the zygote reaches the body of the uterus, it consists of 16 to 50 cells. At this stage, because of its bumpy outward appearance, it is termed a *morula* (from the Latin word *morus*, meaning "mulberry").

The morula continues to multiply as it floats free in the uterine cavity for three or four more days. Large cells tend to mass at the periphery of the ball, leaving a fluid space surrounding an inner cell mass at one of the poles. At this stage, the structure is termed a *blastocyst*. The cells in the outer ring are known as *trophoblast cells*. They are the part of the structure that will later form the placenta and membranes. The inner cell mass is the portion of the structure that will later form the embryo.

After the 3rd or 4th day of free floating (about eight days from ovulation), the last residues of the corona and zona pellucida are shed by the growing structure. The blastocyst brushes against the rich uterine endometrium (in the second [secretory] phase of the menstrual cycle) and settles down into its soft folds (implantation, or nidation).

These stages are depicted in Fig. 13-1.

As the trophoblast cells on the outside of the blastocyst touch the endometrium, they produce proteolytic enzymes that dissolve the endometrial tissue they touch. This action allows the structure to burrow deeply into the endometrium and establish an effective communications network with the blood system of the endometrium. The touching or implantation point is usually high in the uterus and on the posterior surface. If the point of implantation is low in the uterus, the growing placenta may occlude the cervix and make delivery of the child at term difficult.

Implantation is an important step in pregnancy; as many as 50 percent of zygotes never achieve it. In these instances, a pregnancy ends as early as eight to ten days after conception, often before the woman is even aware it had begun. Occasionally, a small amount of vaginal spotting appears with implantation, since capillaries are ruptured by the implanting trophoblast cells. A woman who has particularly scant menstrual flows may mistake implantation bleeding for her menstrual period, and the predicted date of delivery of her baby (based on the time of her last menstrual period) will then be calculated one month late.

The Decidua

When conception has occurred, the corpus luteum in the ovary continues to function rather than to atrophy. Thus the endometrium of the uterus, instead of sloughing off as in a normal menstrual cycle, continues to grow in thickness and vascularity. The en-

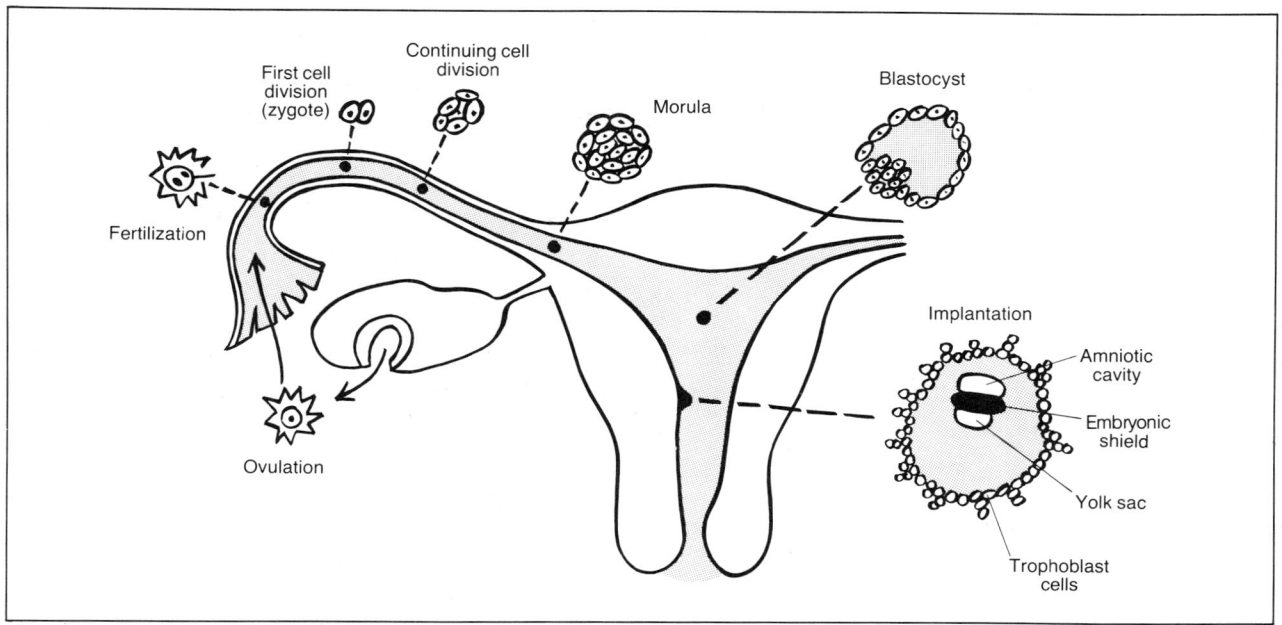

Fig. 13-1. Schema of ovulation, fertilization, and implantation. At the time of implantation, the blastocyst is already differentiated into germ layers (ectoderm, mesoderm, and entoderm). Cells at the periphery of the structure are trophoblast cells that mature into the placenta.

dometrium is now termed *decidua* (the Latin word for "falling off"), since it will be discarded following the birth of the child. The decidua has three separate areas: the *decidua basalis,* or the part of the endometrium lying directly under the embryo (or the portion where the trophoblast cells are invading maternal blood vessels); the *decidua capsularis,* or the portion of the endometrium that stretches or encapsulates the surface of the trophoblast; and the *decidua vera,* or the remaining portion of the uterine lining (Fig. 13-2).

As the zygote grows during pregnancy, it pushes the decidua capsularis before it like a blanket. Eventually, enlargement brings the structure into contact with the opposite uterine wall. Here, the decidua capsularis fuses with the endometrium of the opposite wall. This is why, at delivery, the entire inner surface of the uterus is stripped away and the organ becomes highly susceptible to hemorrhage.

Chorionic Villi

Once implantation is achieved, the trophoblastic layer of cells of the blastocyst begins to mature rapidly. As

Fig. 13-2. Division of uterine decidua into three areas.

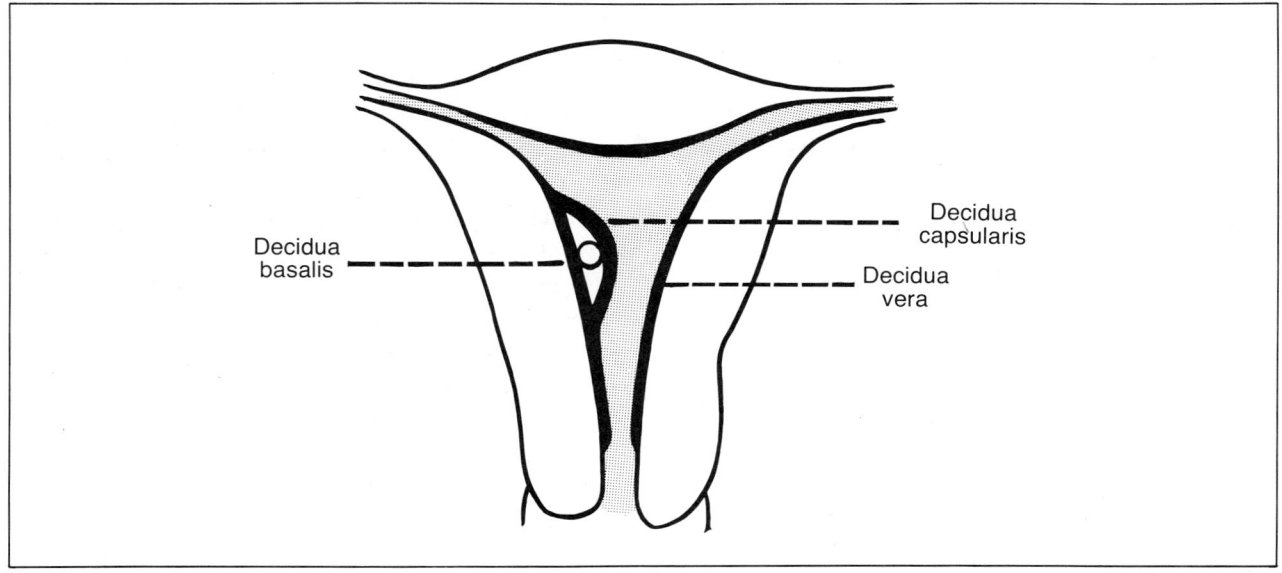

Growth and Development of the Fetus

early as the 11th or 12th day, miniature villi, or probing "fingers," reach out from the single layer of cells into the uterine endometrium; these are termed *chorionic villi*. At term, nearly 200 such villi will have formed.

Chorionic villi have a central core of loose connective tissue surrounded by a double layer of trophoblast cells. The central core contains fetal capillaries. The outer of the two covering layers is termed the *syncytiotrophoblast*, or the *syncytial layer*. The inner layer, known as the *cytotrophoblast*, or *Langhans' layer*, is present as early as 12 weeks of gestation, appears to be functional early in pregnancy, and disappears at about the 4th or 5th month. Apparently, its cells protect the growing embryo and fetus from certain infectious organisms, such as the spirochetes of syphilis. This is why syphilis is considered to have high potential for fetal damage late in pregnancy, when Langhans' cells are not functioning. Langhans' cells appear to offer little protection against viral invasion.

The syncytial layer of cells seems to be instrumental in the production of various placental hormones, such as human chorionic gonadotropin, human placental lactogen, estrogen, and progesterone.

The Placenta
CIRCULATION

The placenta arises out of trophoblast tissue and thus is fetal in origin. It serves as the fetal lungs, kidneys, and gastrointestinal tract and as a separate endocrine organ throughout pregnancy. It offers some protection to the fetus against invading microorganisms or chemical substances.

As early as the 12th day of pregnancy, maternal blood begins to collect in spaces (intervillous spaces) surrounding the chorionic villi. By the 3rd week, oxygen and other nutrients, such as glucose, amino acids, fatty acids, minerals, and vitamins, diffuse from the maternal blood through the cell layers of the chorionic villi to the villi capillaries. From there, the nutrients are transported back to the developing embryo.

There is no direct exchange of blood between the embryo and the mother during pregnancy; the exchange is carried out by selective osmosis. This osmosis is so effective that all but a few substances cross the placenta into fetal circulation. It is important that a woman take no drugs other than those prescribed for her during pregnancy because almost all drugs cross into the fetal circulation.

Substances cross the placenta by four separate processes: diffusion, facilitated diffusion, active transport, and pinocytosis. These are much the same processes that allow substances to pass from the gastrointestinal tract into the bloodstream in adults.

Diffusion
When there is a greater concentration of a substance on one side of a semipermeable membrane than on the other, substances of correct molecular weight cross the membrane from the area of higher concentration to the area of lower concentration. Oxygen and carbon dioxide cross the placenta by simple diffusion.

Facilitated Diffusion
In order that the fetus receive enough concentrations of necessary growth substances, some substances cross the placenta more rapidly or more easily than would occur if only simple diffusion were operating. Glucose is an example of a substance that crosses by this process. Fetal plasma maintains a glucose level about 60 to 70 percent that of the maternal concentration.

Active Transport
Essential amino acids and water-soluble vitamins cross the placenta against the pressure gradient. Amino acid concentrations in the fetal plasma are twice what they are in the mother, a situation that must occur to provide building substances for active fetal growth.

Pinocytosis
Pinocytosis is absorption by the cellular membrane of intact microdroplets of plasma and dissolved substances. Globulins, lipoproteins, phospholipids, and other molecular structures that are too large for diffusion and that cannot participate in active transport cross in this manner. Unfortunately, viruses that then infect the fetus may also cross in this manner.

As the number of chorionic villi increases, the villi form a network of communication with the maternal blood that becomes more and more complex. The intervillous spaces grow larger and larger and become separated by a series of partitions, or septa. On a mature placenta there are as many as 30 separate segments, called *cotyledons*. These compartments are what make the maternal side of the placenta at term look rough and uneven.

The placental circulation is depicted in Fig. 13-3. Maternal blood reaches the intervillous spaces through coiled or spiral endometrial uterine arteries, which open at the bases of the septa or directly onto the floor of the intervillous spaces. About 100 mater-

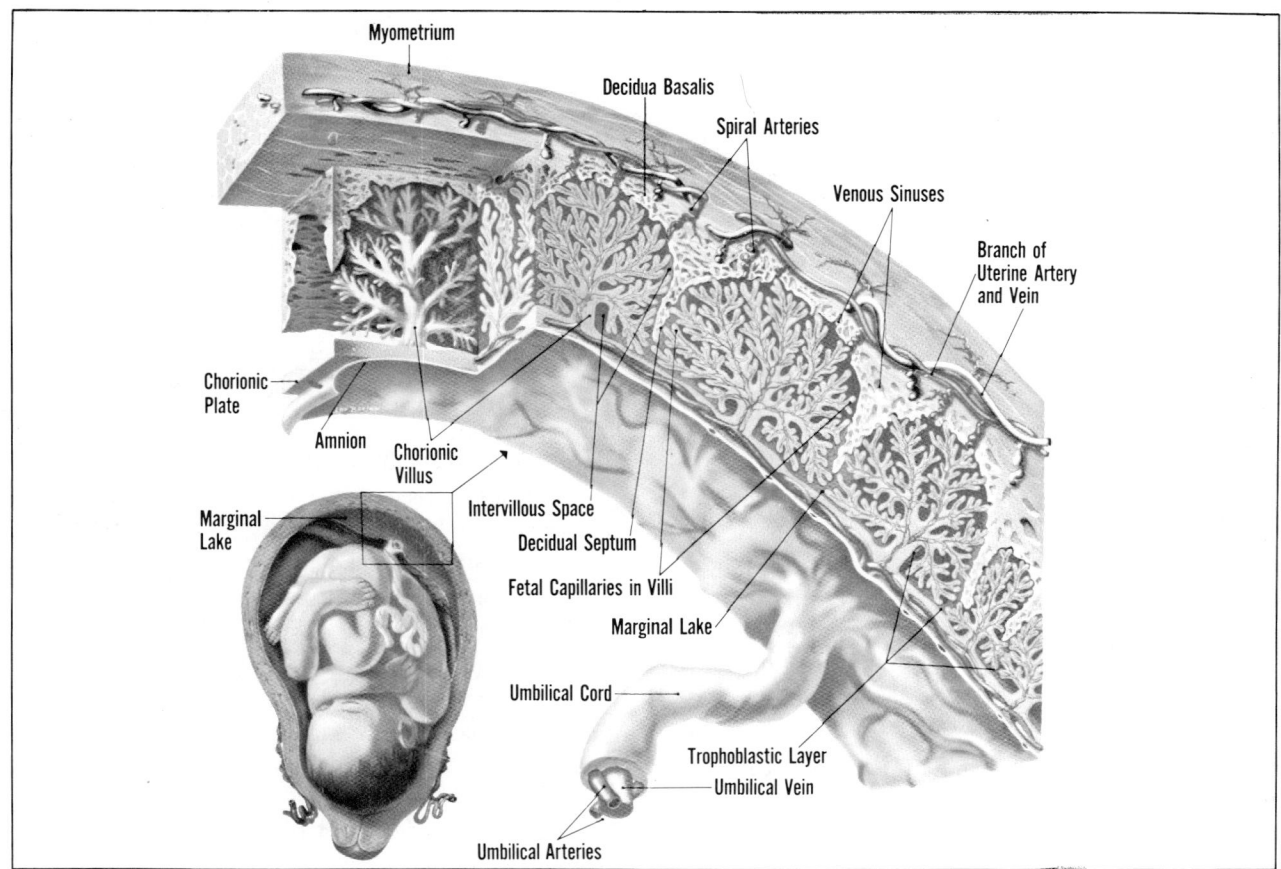

Fig. 13-3. Schema of placental circulation. (From Clinical Education Aid, *No. 2, Ross Laboratories, Columbus, Ohio, 1960).*

nal arteries supply the mature placenta. In order to provide enough blood for exchange, the rate of uteroplacental blood flow in pregnancy increases from about 50 ml per minute at 10 weeks to 500 to 600 ml per minute at term. No additional maternal arteries appear to be added after the first three months of pregnancy, but to accommodate the increased blood flow, the arteries increase in size. Systemically, the mother's heart rate, total cardiac output, and blood volume all increase to supply the placenta.

Uterine perfusion is most efficient when the mother lies on her left side. This position lifts the uterus away from the vena cava and prevents blood from being trapped in the vena cava and unable to circulate.

In the intervillous spaces, maternal blood jets from the arteries in streams or spurts. It is propelled from compartment to compartment by the currents initiated and not through definite anatomical channels that conduct it from artery to spaces around the villi to maternal vein. Thus, its movement appears to be controlled physiologically rather than anatomically. As the blood circulates around the villi, it gradually loses its momentum and is crowded toward the placental floor. From there, it enters the orifices of maternal veins and is returned to the maternal circulation.

At term, a placenta measures about 15 by 20 cm. It is 2 to 3 cm thick. It weighs 400 to 600 gm, or one-sixth of the weight of the baby.

ENDOCRINE FUNCTION OF THE PLACENTA
Human Chorionic Gonadotropin

The syncytial layer of the chorionic villi secretes a number of hormones or enzymes during pregnancy. The first hormone to be produced is human chorionic gonadotropin (HCG). It was previously assumed that this hormone was produced by the inner layer of cells, Langhans' layer, because its course closely approximates the course of that layer of cells. Chorionic gonadotropin can be demonstrated in maternal blood serum as early as before the first missed menstrual period (on the 6th or 7th day after implantation). It reaches a peak level at about the 60th day of pregnancy. Production of the hormone appears to diminish between the 2nd and 5th months.

The purpose of HCG is to act as a fail-safe measure to ensure that the corpus luteum of the ovary continues to function. Falling levels of progesterone therefore do not cause endometrial sloughing and pituitary gonadotropins do not increase to induce a new menstrual cycle.

Kangaroos and opossums are examples of a species (marsupials) that apparently do not have a pregnancy-prolonging factor such as chorionic gonadotropin. Pregnancy in a kangaroo or an opossum ends while the fetus is still grossly immature. The offspring matures by being sheltered in the mother's abdominal pouch at greater risk to the fetus than if it had remained in utero.

At about the 2nd month of pregnancy in the human, the syncytial cells of the developing placenta begin to produce progesterone, becoming an independent source of this hormone. The production of progesterone probably accounts for the fall in the production of HCG at that time.

Chorionic gonadotropin is an important hormone in pregnancy, not only because its action guarantees the production of progesterone by the corpus luteum but also because its presence in the mother's blood and urine serves as the basis for pregnancy testing. The hormone is present in blood almost immediately. It is present in urine in significant titer for these purposes from about a week after the first missed menstrual period (the 35th day) through the 100th day of pregnancy. Before or after those times, a false-negative result from a pregnancy test may be reported. The mother's urine will be completely negative for HCG within one to two weeks after delivery, proving that all the placental tissue has been delivered.

Estrogen

Estrogen is a second product of the syncytial cells of the placenta. Estrogen contributes to the mother's mammary gland development in preparation for lactation and stimulates the uterus to grow to accommodate the developing fetus. It is excreted by the mother in urine as estriol. Assessing the amount of estriol excreted serves as a test of fetal welfare because the immediate precursor of estrogen synthesis by the placenta is a compound produced by the fetal adrenal gland. When a fetus is in difficulty, the production of this fetal adrenal compound is decreased, estrogen cannot be synthesized, and estriol excretion in maternal urine will then be decreased.

Progesterone

Estrogen is often referred to as the "hormone of women"; progesterone as the "hormone of mothers." Its presence is indisputably necessary to maintain the endometrial lining of the uterus during pregnancy. A second function of this hormone appears to be induction of quiescence of the uterine musculature during pregnancy, which prevents premature labor. Such quiescence is probably produced by a change in electrolytes (notably potassium), which decreases the contraction potential of the uterus. Progesterone is synthesized from cholesterol; it is excreted in the maternal urine as pregnanediol. Assay of this compound can be used as a measure of placental, and therefore indirectly of fetal, well-being.

Human Placental Lactogen

Human placental lactogen (also called *chorionic somatomammotropin*) is a hormone with both growth-promoting and lactogenic properties. It is produced by the placenta beginning as early as the 6th week of pregnancy. It then increases in amount to peak level at term. It can be assayed in both maternal blood and urine. It functions to promote mammary gland growth in preparation for lactation in the mother (accounting for its name). This hormone appears to have an important role in regulating maternal glucose, protein, and fat levels so that adequate amounts of these are always available to the fetus.

Human Chorionic Thyrotropin

Human chorionic thyrotropin is a glycoprotein similar to thyroid-stimulating hormone produced by the adult pituitary. It seems to have thyroid-stimulating activity in the mother to help her body increase metabolic rate and better adapt to the demands of pregnancy.

Corticosteroids

It was previously thought that the placenta produced corticosteroids, as cortisol levels in pregnant women are raised two or three times above their nonpregnant rates. This rise appears to be due to an increase in maternal sources, however, not placental sources.

The Umbilical Cord

As chorionic villi form and begin to function, they join together into larger and larger veins and arteries, until they become the umbilical cord. Also called the *funis* (Latin for "cord"), the umbilical cord is about 53 cm (21 inches) in length at term. It is about 2 cm (¾ inch) in thickness. It contains one vein (carrying blood from the placental villi to the fetus) and two arteries (carrying blood from the fetus back to the placental villi). The remnant of the yolk sac (see p. 152) may be found in the fetal end of the cord as a white fibrous streak at term. The bulk of the cord is a gelatinous mucopolysaccharide called *Wharton's jelly*, which gives the cord body and prevents pressure on the vein and arteries. The outer surface is covered with amniotic membrane.

About 1 percent of all infants are born with a cord that contains only a single artery. About 15 percent of these infants are found to have congenital anomalies, particularly kidney and heart anomalies.

Smooth muscle is abundant in the arteries of the cord; the constriction of these circular muscles after birth contributes to hemostasis and helps prevent hemorrhage of the newborn through the cord. The rate of blood flow through an umbilical cord is rapid (350 ml per minute at term). This rapid flow makes it unlikely that a cord will twist or knot enough to interfere with the fetal oxygen supply. In 20 percent of all deliveries, a loose loop of cord is found around the fetal neck. If this loop of cord is removed before the shoulders are extruded, so that there is no traction on it, it is not constricted, and nutrition supply to the fetus remains unimpaired.

Since the umbilical cord appears to contain no nerve supply, it can be cut at birth without discomfort to the child or mother.

The Membranes and Amniotic Fluid

The chorionic villi in the medial surface of the trophoblast (those that are not involved in implantation because they do not touch the endometrium) gradually thin and leave the medial surface of the structure smooth (the *chorion laeve,* or smooth chorion). The smooth chorion eventually becomes the *chorionic membrane*, the outermost fetal membrane. A second membrane lining the chorionic membrane, the *amniotic membrane*, or amnion, then begins to form (Fig. 13-4). Early in pregnancy, these membranes become so adherent they seem as one at term. Like the umbilical cord, they apparently have no nerve supply. Thus, when they rupture at term, neither mother nor child experiences any sensation. These membranes cover the fetal surface of the placenta and give it its typical shiny look.

Within the amnion and chorionic membrane is a clear albuminous fluid (liquor amnii, or amniotic fluid), in which the embryo (later the fetus) floats. This fluid is constantly being newly formed and reabsorbed, so it is never stagnant. It is produced, evidently from the cells of the amniotic membrane, at a rate of about 500 ml per 24 hours. At term, the average amount of fluid present is 1,000 ml. The fetus swallows the fluid rapidly, and it is absorbed across the fetal intestine into the fetal bloodstream and by the umbilical arteries exchanged across the placenta. Some fluid is probably absorbed in direct contact with the fetal surface of the placenta. If for any reason the fetus is unable to swallow (esophageal atresia or anencephaly are the two most common reasons), hydramnios, or excessive amniotic fluid (over 2,000 ml), will result. Early in fetal life, as soon as the fetal kidneys become active, fetal urine adds to the quantity of the amniotic fluid. A disturbance of kidney function may cause oligohydramnios, or a reduction in the amount of amniotic fluid (under 300 ml).

Amniotic fluid is an important protective mechanism. It shields the fetus against pressure or a blow to the mother's abdomen. It also protects the fetus from

Fig. 13-4. Membranes, with embryo lying within amniotic sac.

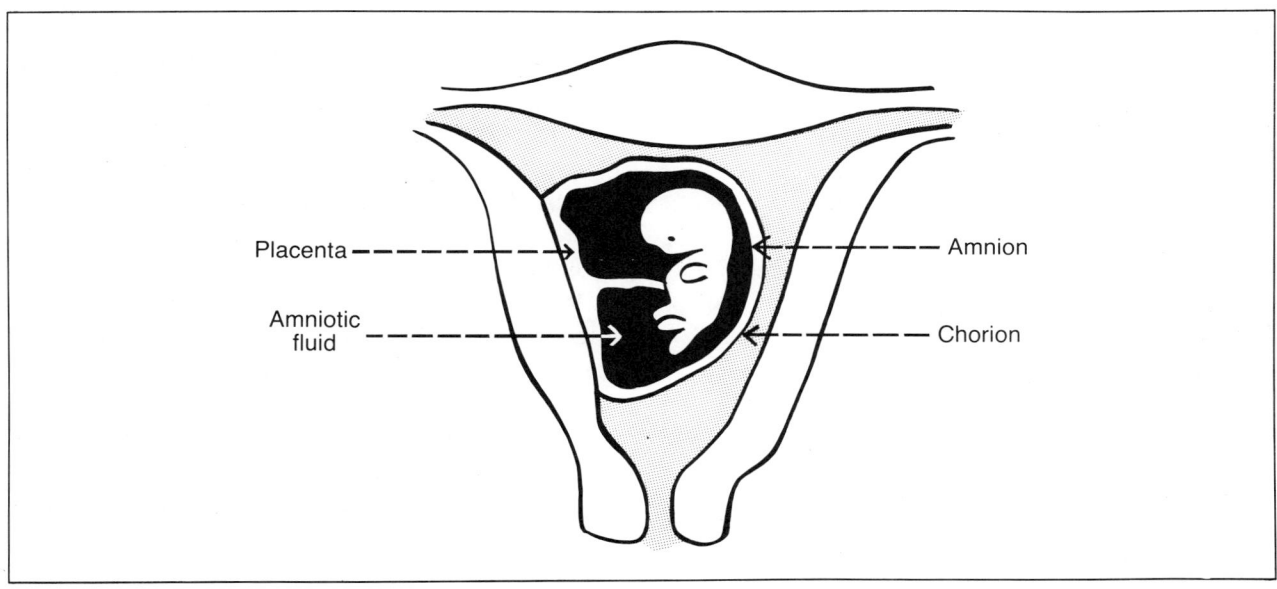

changes in temperature, since liquid changes temperature more slowly than air. Because it allows the fetus freedom to move, it probably aids muscular development.

Even if the membranes rupture prior to birth and the bulk of the amniotic fluid is lost, some will always surround the fetus in utero because of the constant formation of amniotic fluid. Amniotic fluid is slightly alkaline, with a pH of about 7.2. This might be important at the time of rupture, in differentiating it from urine, which is acidic (pH 5.0 to 5.5). The specific gravity of amniotic fluid is only slightly heavier than that of water—1.005 to 1.025.

Origin and Development of Organ Systems

The fertilized ovum is a *zygote* until implantation. From implantation to the end of the 5th to 8th week, it is an *embryo*. From the 5th to 8th week until the end of pregnancy, it is a *fetus*. These terms used to describe fetal growth are summarized in Table 13-1.

From the beginning, development of the fetus proceeds in a cephalocaudal (head to tail) direction; head development occurs first, then development of middle and lower body parts. That a baby is born with cephalocaudal development still incomplete is apparent by a newborn's ability to lift up his head but not to walk, to be able to control sucking and swallowing functions but not urinary or bowel function.

Fetal development follows the principle of *induction*; one tissue transmits a stimulus to an adjoining tissue to begin development. If at any point the stimulus is inadequate or for some reason the adjoining tissue cannot respond, growth or development of body parts will not proceed beyond that point. Thalidomide, a drug that caused infants to be born without arms or legs if taken by the mother during early pregnancy, is an example of a substance that interferes with induction. In some instances, interference with induction leads to the double formation of structures, such as double ureters.

PRIMARY GERM LAYERS

At the time of implantation, the blastocyst has already differentiated to a point at which two separate cavities appear in the inner structure: a large one, the *amniotic cavity*, and a smaller one, the *yolk sac*. These are illustrated in Fig. 13-1.

The walls of the amniotic cavity are lined with the cells of the primary germ layer, the *ectoderm*; the cavity is filled with amniotic fluid. The yolk sac is lined by another distinctive layer of cells, the *entoderm*. In chicks the yolk sac serves as a supply of nourishment for the embryo throughout its development. In human reproduction, the yolk sac appears to supply nourishment only until implantation. It then provides a source of red blood cells until the embryo's hematopoietic system is mature enough to perform this function (at about the 3rd month of intrauterine life).

Between the amniotic cavity and the yolk sac is a third layer of primary cells, the *mesoderm*. The embryo will begin to develop at the point where these three cell layers meet: the *embryonic shield*. The growing structure is called an embryo from implantation to the 5th to 8th week of pregnancy and a fetus thereafter.

Each germ layer of primary tissue develops into distinctive body systems. The mesoderm is responsible for formation of the supporting structures of the body (connective tissue, bones, cartilage, muscle, and tendons), the upper portion of the urinary system (the kidneys and ureters), the reproductive system, the heart, the circulatory system, and the blood cells.

The entoderm germ layer develops into the lining of the gastrointestinal tract, the respiratory tract, the tonsils, the parathyroid, thyroid, and thymus glands, and the lower urinary system (bladder and urethra). The ectoderm germ layer develops into the nervous system, the skin, hair, and nails, the sense organs, and the mucous membranes of the anus and the mouth.

It is helpful to know which structures arise from each germ layer because coexisting congenital defects found in newborns usually arise from the same layer. For example, a tracheoesophageal fistula (both organs arising from the entoderm) is a common birth anomaly. Heart and kidney defects (both organs arising from the mesoderm) are often found together. It is rare, however, to see a newborn with a heart malformation (arises from the mesoderm) and a lower uri-

Table 13-1. Terms Used to Denote Fetal Growth

Time Period	Common Name
From ovulation to fertilization	Ovum
From fertilization to implantation	Zygote
From implantation to 5 to 8 weeks	Embryo
From 5 to 8 weeks until term	Fetus
Low-birth-weight infant (previously termed a premature infant)	Infant born before the 37th week of intrauterine growth

nary malformation (bladder and urethra arise from the entoderm). Some infections, such as rubella, affect all three germ layers and cause congenital anomalies in a myriad of body systems, irrespective of their origin.

Knowing the origins of body structures helps you to understand why certain screening procedures are ordered for newborns with congenital malformations. A kidney x-ray examination, for example, may be ordered for a child born with a heart defect. A child with a malformation of the urinary tract is often investigated for reproductive abnormalities as well.

CIRCULATORY SYSTEM

All organ systems are complete, at least in a rudimentary form, at 8 weeks' gestation (the end of the embryonic period). The cardiovascular system is one of the first systems to become functional in intrauterine life.

Formation of the Heart

The heart begins to form as early as the 16th day of life. The circulatory system progresses from simple blood cells joined to the walls of the yolk sac, to a network of blood vessels, to a single heart tube, which begins to beat as early as the 24th day of life. The septum that divides the heart into chambers develops during the 6th or 7th week, and the heart valves begin to develop in the 7th week. An electrocardiogram may be recorded on a fetus as early as the 11th week, although the accuracy of such ECGs is in doubt until about the 5th month of pregnancy.

Fetal Circulation

As early as the 3rd week of intrauterine life, fetal blood has begun to exchange nutrients across the chorionic villi with the maternal circulation. Fetal circulation (Fig. 13-5) differs from extrauterine circulation in several respects. During intrauterine life the fetus derives its oxygen not from oxygen exchange in the lungs but from oxygen exchange at the placenta. The excretion of CO_2 also occurs at the placenta. Blood does enter lung vessels while the child is in utero, but this blood flow is to supply the cells of the lungs themselves, not for oxygenation. The major difference, then, between circulation in utero and after birth is that in the fetus the blood largely bypasses the lungs and primarily serves to carry nutrients to and from the placenta.

Blood arriving from the placenta (blood with a high oxygen content) enters the fetus through the umbilical vein (called a vein even though it carries oxygenated blood, because the direction of the blood is toward the fetal heart) and into an accessory vein, the *ductus venosus*. The ductus venosus supplies blood to the fetal liver and empties into the inferior vena cava, through which blood flows to the right side of the heart. As the blood enters the right atrium, the bulk of it is shunted into the left atrium through an opening in the atrial septum, the *foramen ovale*. From the left atrium it follows the course of normal circulation into the left ventricle and into the aorta.

Some of the blood that enters the right atrium leaves it by the normal circulatory route, that is, through the tricuspid valve into the right ventricle. Blood leaves the right ventricle through the pulmonary artery in the normal manner. A small portion of this blood flow services the lung tissue; the larger portion is shunted away from the lungs, through the *ductus arteriosus*, directly into the aorta.

Two umbilical arteries (called arteries because they carry blood away from the fetal heart, even though they are now transporting unoxygenated blood) transport most of the blood flow from the descending aorta back through the umbilical cord to the placental villi, where new oxygen exchange takes place.

The shunts of fetal circulation are necessary to supply the most important organs of the fetus: the brain, liver, heart, and kidneys. The ductus venosus supplies the liver, and the foramen ovale allows oxygenated blood to move directly to the left side of the heart and the aorta, the vessel from which the arteries arise that supply the brain, heart, and kidneys.

The fetus exists at a blood oxygen saturation level about 80 percent that of a newborn. The rapid rate of the fetal heartbeat during pregnancy (120 to 160 beats per minute) is necessary to supply oxygen to cells when blood cells are never fully saturated. Fortunately, fetal hemoglobin has a higher dissociation level than adult hemoglobin so that, again, the movement and release of oxygen are facilitated. Despite this low blood oxygen level, carbon dioxide does not accumulate in the fetal system because of rapid diffusion into maternal blood.

Fetal Hemoglobin

Fetal hemoglobin differs from adult hemoglobin in several ways. It has a different composition (two alpha and two gamma chains as compared with two alpha and two beta chains of adult hemoglobin). It has a greater oxygen affinity, which makes it more efficient. It is more concentrated (at birth, hemoglobin is about 17.1 gm per 100 ml and hematocrit is about 53 percent). These same changes occur in people who live at high altitudes, where the atmosphere has a reduced oxygen content. The change from fetal hemoglobin to adult hemoglobin begins before birth and accelerates following birth.

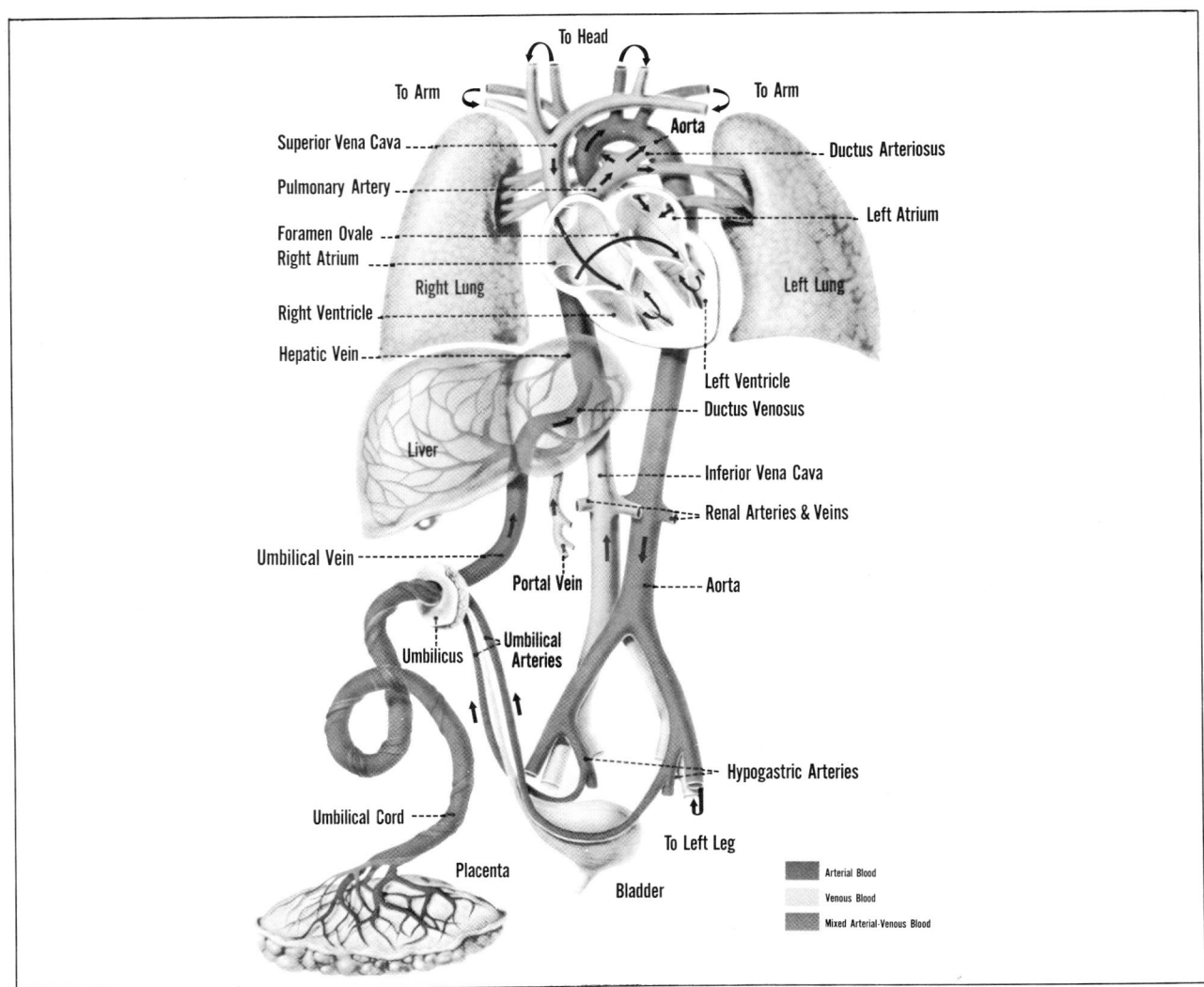

Fig. 13-5. Fetal circulation. (From Clinical Education Aid, No. 1, Ross Laboratories, Columbus, Ohio, 1963.*)*

RESPIRATORY SYSTEM

At the 3rd week of life, the respiratory and digestive tracts exist as a single tube. This is the reason that tracheoesophageal fistulas are a common newborn anomaly. By the end of the 4th week, a septum begins to divide the two systems. At the same time, lung buds appear on the trachea.

Until the 7th week of life the diaphragm does not completely divide the thoracic cavity from the abdomen. During the 6th week of life, lung buds may extend down into the abdomen, reentering the chest only as the chest's longitudinal dimension increases and the diaphragm becomes complete (the end of the 7th week). If the diaphragm fails to close completely, the stomach, spleen, liver, or intestines may enter the thoracic cavity. The child will then be born with a diaphragmatic hernia, compromising the lung and perhaps displacing the heart.

Alveoli begin to form between the 24th and 28th weeks. The alveoli are supplied by capillaries as they develop. Both capillaries and alveoli must be developed before gas exchange can occur in the fetal lungs. This is why 28 weeks is a practical lower limit of prematurity or the earliest gestation age at which a fetus can survive in an extrauterine environment.

At about the 6th month of pregnancy, some of the alveolar cells begin to secrete *surfactant,* a phospholipid substance. Surfactant decreases alveolar surface tension on expiration. This prevents lungs from collapsing on expiration and greatly adds to the infant's ability to maintain respirations in the outside environment. Surfactant has two components: lecithin and sphingomyelin. Early in the formation of surfactant, sphingomyelin is the chief component; at about 35 weeks there is a surge in the production of lecithin, and lecithin becomes the chief component.

Lack of surfactant is a factor in the development of respiratory distress syndrome (RDS), formerly called hyaline membrane disease. The maturity of lung tissue in a fetus can be estimated by the proportion of lecithin to sphingomyelin found in the amniotic fluid on amniocentesis.

As early as during the first three months of pregnancy the fetus begins to make spontaneous respiratory movements. These movements continue throughout pregnancy. Although babies are born with fluid in their lungs, it is not amniotic fluid but a specific lung fluid that has a low surface tension and low viscosity and is capable of being rapidly absorbed after birth. The presence of this fluid aids in the expansion of the alveoli at birth.

NERVOUS SYSTEM

Like the circulatory system, the nervous system begins to develop extremely early in pregnancy. During the 3rd and 4th weeks of life, at a time when the woman may not even realize that she is pregnant, active formation of the nervous system has already begun, and the sense organs are developing along with it.

By the 3rd week of gestation, a *neural plate* (a thickened portion of the ectoderm) is apparent in the developing embryo. The top portion of the neural plate differentiates into the neural tube, which will form the central nervous system (brain and spinal cord), and the neural crest, which will develop into the peripheral nervous system.

Although all parts of the brain (the cerebrum, the cerebellum, the pons, and the medulla oblongata) form in utero, the brain is not mature at birth. It continues rapid growth during the first year; growth continues at high levels until 5 or 6 years of age. Thus the newborn infant still has many findings of neurological immaturity such as a positive Babinski sign (toes flare on stroking of the bottom of the foot).

The neurological system seems particularly prone to insult during the early weeks of the embryonic period. All during pregnancy and at birth it is vulnerable to damage from anoxia.

ENDOCRINE SYSTEM

The fetal adrenal glands play a direct role in placental estrogen production, as they supply a precursor of estrogen synthesis. One of the theories of why labor begins is that the uterus receives a message from the fetal adrenals that the fetus is mature and ready to be born.

DIGESTIVE SYSTEM

Once the digestive tract is separated from the respiratory tract (at about the 4th week), the intestinal tract grows very rapidly. During the 6th week of intrauterine life the abdomen becomes too small to contain the intestine, and a portion of the intestine enters the base of the umbilical cord. Intestine remains in the base of the cord until about the 10th week, until the fetal trunk has extended and enlarged the abdominal cavity so it can accommodate all the intestinal mass. If intestinal coils remain outside the abdomen, in the base of the cord, a congenital anomaly, *omphalocele*, develops.

Meconium forms in the intestines as early as the 16th week. It is the end product of fetal metabolism, consisting of cellular wastes, bile, fats, mucoproteins, mucopolysaccharides, and portions of the vernix caseosa, the lubricating substance that forms on the infant's skin at the 5th month of intrauterine life. Meconium is black or dark green and it is sticky in texture. It derives its dark color from bile pigments. White meconium is a sign of biliary obstruction. Children with cystic fibrosis have such thick, tenacious meconium that they may have bowel obstruction and intestinal perforation and die in utero.

The gastrointestinal tract is sterile before birth. Because vitamin K is synthesized by the action of bacteria in the intestines, vitamin K levels may be low in the newborn infant.

Sucking and swallowing reflexes are not mature until the fetus is about 32 weeks or weighs 1,500 gm. That this function, so necessary for survival outside the uterus, develops so late in pregnancy has implications for nursing care of the fetus born before this time.

Ability of the gastrointestinal tract to secrete enzymes essential to the digestion of carbohydrate and protein is mature at 36 weeks. Amylase, an enzyme found in saliva and necessary for digestion of complex starches, is not mature until 3 months after birth. Lipase, an enzyme needed for fat digestion, is not available in many newborns. This fact has implications for newborn nutrition.

The liver is active throughout gestation, functioning as a screen between the incoming blood and the fetal circulation. It is still immature at birth, however. Two of the biggest problems of infants in the first 24 hours of life are hypoglycemia and hyperbilirubinemia, both related to immature liver function.

SKELETAL SYSTEM

In the first two weeks of fetal life, cartilage prototypes provide position and support. Ossification of bone tissue begins in the 3rd month. The ossification process continues all through fetal life and until adulthood. Carpal, tarsal, and sternal bones do not generally ossify until birth is imminent. A fetus cannot be detected by x-ray until a degree of ossification has taken place. A fetal x-ray film has been demonstrated as early as the 14th week of gestation, but on the average it is not accurate until the 5th lunar month.

REPRODUCTIVE SYSTEM

Whether the child will be male or female is determined at the moment of conception by a spermatozoon carrying an X or a Y chromosome. At about the 6th week of life, the gonads (ovaries or testes) form. When testes form, the secretion of androgen apparently influences the sexually neuter genital duct to form other male organs (maturity of the wolffian, or mesonephric, duct). In the absence of androgen secretion, female organs form (maturation of the müllerian, or paramesonephric, duct). This is an important phenomenon, because if the mother ingests androgen or androgen-like substances during this stage of pregnancy the child, although chromosomally female, may be more male than female in appearance at birth. This has sometimes been the result in children whose mothers were given synthetic progesterone to prevent spontaneous abortion, since a certain form of synthetic progesterone, no longer used during pregnancy, had an androgen-like action.

Masculinization may also occur in female infants with andrenogenital syndrome, a genetic disease in which there is deficient production of cortisol and excess production of androgen by the adrenal gland. These female infants are born with a clitoris that resembles a penis, and if close inspection is not carried out at birth, they may be assumed to be males with cryptorchidism (undescended testes). Males with this syndrome are born with abnormally enlarged genitalia.

Testes in a normal male tend to descend from the pelvic cavity where they first form into the scrotal sac late in intrauterine life, in the 7th to 9th month. Thus many male low-birth-weight infants are born with undescended testes. These children should be followed closely to see that the testes descend when the child reaches the 7th to 9th month of gestation age, since testicular descent does not always occur as readily in extrauterine life as it does during intrauterine existence.

URINARY SYSTEM

Although kidneys form early in intrauterine life, they do not appear to be essential for life before birth. Rudimentary kidneys are present as early as the end of the 4th week. Urine is formed by the 12th week and is excreted into the amniotic fluid by the 4th month of gestation. At term, fetal urine is excreted at the rate of 500 ml per day. The complex structure of the kidneys is gradually developed during pregnancy and for months afterward. The loop of Henle, for example, is not fully differentiated until the child is born. Glomerular filtration and concentration of urine in the newborn are not efficient, since the kidney is not fully mature at birth.

Early in the embryonic stage of urinary system development, the bladder extends to the umbilical region. On rare occasions, an open lumen between the urinary bladder and the umbilicus fails to close. This is a patent urachus and is discovered at birth by the persistent drainage of a clear, acid-pH fluid from the umbilicus.

IMMUNOLOGICAL SYSTEM

Maternal antibodies cross the placenta during the third trimester of pregnancy to give a fetus passive immunity against diseases for which the mother has antibodies. These usually include poliomyelitis, rubella (German measles), rubeola (regular measles), diphtheria and tetanus, infectious parotitis (mumps), and pertussis (whooping cough). The antibodies are of the IgG class of immunoglobulins.

Little or no immunity to varicella (chickenpox) or to herpes simplex virus (the virus of cold sores) is transferred to the fetus, and thus the newborn is always potentially susceptible to these diseases. Herpes simplex virus causes a systemic disease in the newborn that may be fatal. It is important, therefore, to screen a woman in labor for herpes simplex infections so that the newborn can be isolated from contact with this potentially hazardous virus.

Since the passive immunization passed placentally lasts about two months for diphtheria, tetanus, and pertussis; "baby shots" against these illnesses are typically begun at 2 months' extrauterine age. Passive antibodies to measles have been demonstrated to last over a year; consequently, the immunization for measles is not given until 15 months' extrauterine age.

A fetus is capable of antibody production late in a pregnancy. The average fetus is not called upon to use this function, however, because he will make antibodies only when stimulated by an invading antigen and no antigen invades his intrauterine space. Babies whose mothers have a rubella infection during pregnancy typically have IgA or IgM antibodies in their blood serum at birth. Because these antibodies do not cross the placenta, their presence in a newborn is proof that the fetus has been challenged by disease invasion and has actively produced antibodies.

Monthly Estimates of Fetal Growth and Development

During pregnancy, women often ask, "What is my baby like now?" "Does it have arms or legs yet?" "When can you tell if it is a girl or a boy?" "What day will it be born?" It is helpful to be able to describe to mothers the developmental milestones of intrauterine life.

Discussing intrauterine life is confusing because the life of the fetus is generally measured from the time of ovulation, while the length of the pregnancy is generally measured from the first day of the last menstrual period. Because ovulation takes place about two weeks after the last menstrual period, the ovulation age of the fetus is always two weeks less than the length of the pregnancy or the gestation age of the fetus.

Both the length of the pregnancy and the life of a fetus are measured in lunar months (four-week periods) rather than in calendar months. In lunar months a pregnancy is 10 months long; a fetus grows in utero 9½ lunar months. The relationship of ovulation age to gestation age is shown in Fig. 13-6.

METHODS OF ESTIMATION
Haase's Rule
Using Haase's rule, the expected size of a fetus can be approximated. This rule states that the length of the embryo in centimeters can be calculated during the first 5 months of gestation by squaring the number of the month of the pregnancy; in the 6th to 10th month, by multiplying the number of the month by 5. For example, a 4-month-old fetus is approximately 16 cm long; an 8-month-old fetus is 40 cm long.

Expected Date of Confinement
It is impossible to predict the date of confinement (the day of birth of a child) with a high degree of accuracy. As mentioned, the average length of a pregnancy from ovulation is 9½ lunar months, or 38 weeks, or 266 days; from the last menstrual period, a pregnancy is 10 lunar months, or 40 weeks, or 280 days. In actuality, fewer than 5 percent of pregnancies end exactly 280 days from the last menstrual period; fewer than half end within one week of the 280th day.

Nägele's Rule
Nägele's rule is the standard method used to predict the length of a pregnancy. To calculate the expected

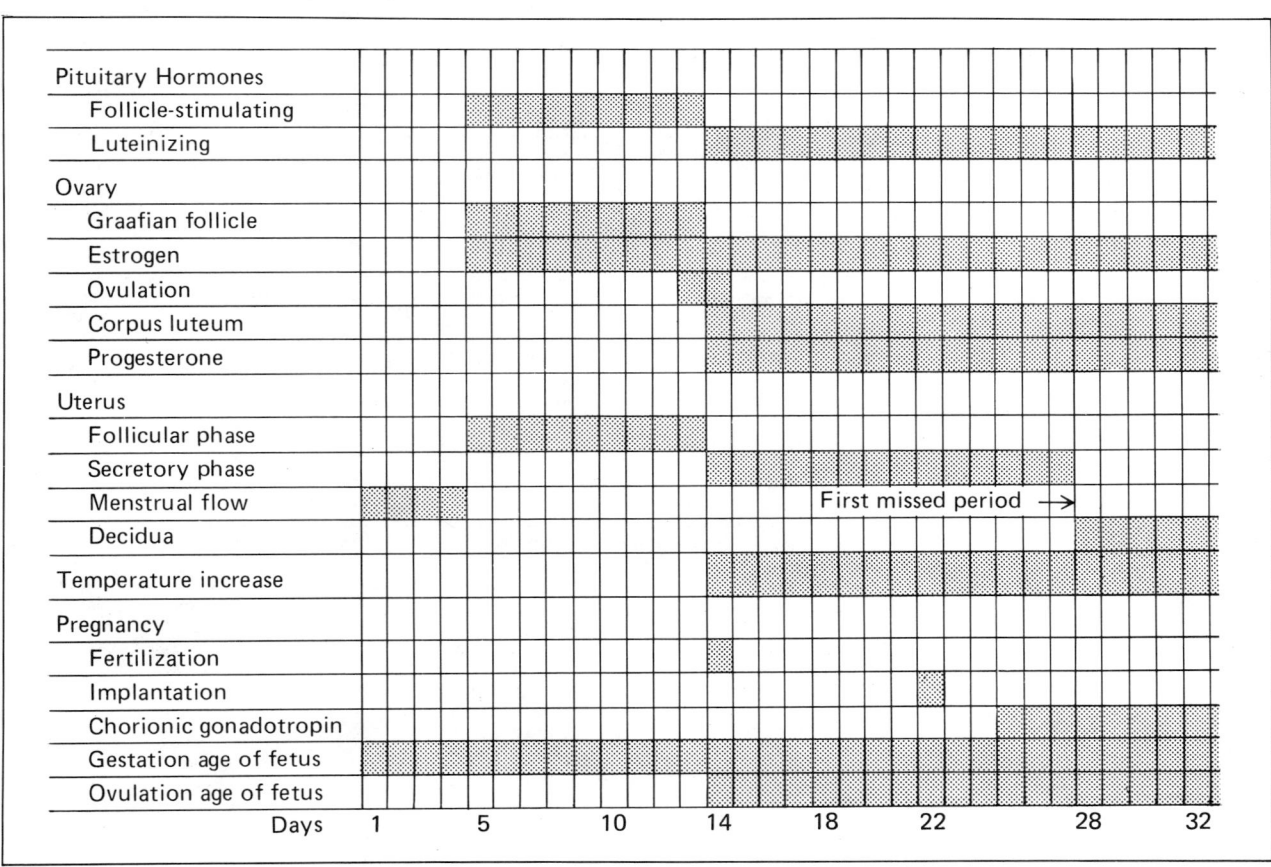

Fig. 13-6. Relationship of ovulation age to gestation age.

Growth and Development of the Fetus 157

date of confinement (EDC) by this rule, count backward 3 calendar months from the first day of the last menstrual period and add 7 days. For example, if the last menstrual period began May 15, you would count back 3 months (April 15, March 15, February 15), add 7 days, and the EDC would be February 22.

If fertilization occurred early in the menstrual cycle, the pregnancy will probably end "early"; if ovulation and fertilization occurred later in the cycle, the pregnancy will end "late." Because of these normal variations, a pregnancy ending two weeks before or two weeks after the calculated EDC is considered well within the normal limit.

FETAL DEVELOPMENTAL MILESTONES

Fetal developmental milestones are shown in Table 13-2. The following discussion of fetal development milestones is based on gestation weeks because it is helpful when talking to expectant parents to be able to correlate fetal development to the way they measure

Table 13-2. Timetable of Normal Fetal Development

Age (weeks)	Gross Appearance	Cardiovascular	Digestive	Respiratory	Urogenital	Nervous System	Sense Organs	Musculo-skeletal
1st	Fertilization. Cleavage of zygote. Blastocyst enters uterine cavity.							
2nd	Blastocyst enlarges. Implantation.							
3rd	Head and tail folds.	Primitive vascular system established. Heart tube.	Buccopharyngeal membrane breaks down. Foregut. Midgut. Hindgut.			Neural plate. Neural folds. Partial fusion of neural folds.		Somites appear.
4th	Body narrow and tubular; C-shaped. Limb buds appear. Placenta begins to form.	Heart is enlarged and beating. Partitioning of atrium begins. Hemopoiesis in yolk sac.	Esophagus, stomach, liver, and pancreatic buds.	Laryngo-tracheal tube, trachea, lung buds.	Mesonephros rapidly forming.	Neural tube. Three primary vesicles of brain.	Optic placode and auditory vesicle present.	Most somites formed. Myotome, sclerotome, and dermatome.
5th	Head increases greatly in size. Face is forming. Limb buds show limb, forelimb, hand or foot.	Cardiac septa developing. Atrioventricular cushions fusing.	Stomach starts to rotate. Midgut forms loop. Urorectal septum.	Lobes of lung formed.	Genital ridges. External genitalia.	Cerebral hemisphere.	Lens vesicle. Auditory vesicle.	Condensation of mesenchyme to form cartilage and muscle.
6th	Head dominant. Oral and nasal cavities confluent. Curvature of embryo diminished. Fingers and toes recognizable.	Heart now has definitive form. Foramen primum closes. Aortico-pulmonary septation. Hematopoiesis in liver.	Upper lip forming. Dental laminae. Palatal processes. Pleuroperitoneal canals close. Midgut loop herniates. Cecum and appendix. Vitello-intestinal duct atrophies.	Bronchi dividing.	Paramesonephric ducts. Sex cords start to develop in testis. Cloaca divided.	Flexures of brain obvious.	Nasolacrimal duct.	Chondrification. Intramembranous ossification.
8th	Head nearly as large as rest of body. Facial features more distinct. Eyes directed more anteriorly. Neck established. Limbs more developed. Digits of hands and feet separated. Fetus covered with epitrichium. Retrogression of tail.	Ventricular septum completed in week 7.	Enamel organs. Small intestine rotating in umbilical cord. Cloacal membrane has broken down.	Bronchioles dividing.	Genital tubercle and genital swellings further developed. Still sexless. Mesonephros fully developed. Metanephric duct branching to form collecting tubules. Testes and ovaries recognizable.	Rapid growth of CNS. Expansion of forebrain vesicle.	Eyes converging. Eyelids developing. External nares plugged. Auricle of external ear forming.	Fetal muscular movement commences. Endochondral ossification. Smooth muscle.

Table 13-2 (Continued)

Age (weeks)	Gross Appearance	Cardiovascular	Digestive	Respiratory	Urogenital	Nervous System	Sense Organs	Musculo-skeletal
12th	Rapid growth in fetal length. Head still relatively large. Eyes look anteriorly. External ears on side of head. Eyelids fused. Nails. Sex recognition possible.	Hematopoiesis in liver and spleen.	Nasal septum and palate fusion complete. Midgut loop returns to abdominal cavity.	Lungs are of definitive shape.	Kidneys have started to secrete urine. External genitalia sufficiently developed to identify sex. Testes close to future deep inguinal ring.	Brain and spinal cord well developed. Cauda equina.	Eyelids fuse. Nasal septum fuses with palate.	Ossification centers forming. Tooth buds present.
16th	Further rapid growth in fetal length. Head still relatively large. Eyes widely separated but eyelids fused. Lanugo present. Auricles of ear high up on side of head. Fetus looks human.	Hematopoiesis in bone marrow commences.	Ascending and descending colon retroperitoneal. Meconium starts to accumulate. Fetus swallowing amniotic fluid.		Mesonephros involuted. Definitive lobulated kidney present. External genitalia well developed.	Cerebellum prominent. Myelination begins in spinal cord.	Eyes, ears, and nose in final positions.	Joint cavities.
20th	Lanugo covers entire body. Hair present on head. Mother detects quickening.	Fetal heartbeat heard with stethoscope.	Meconium reaches rectum.					Distinct movements of limbs felt by mother (quickening).
24th	Skin wrinkled and red. Vernix caseosa present. Head still relatively large. Face childlike. Eyebrows and eyelashes present. Eyelids open.			Pulmonary alveoli appear.		Myelination begins in brain.	Eyelids reopen.	Movements stronger.
28th	Skin wrinkled. Fetal contours more rounded. Hair on head longer.				Testes in inguinal canal.			
32d	Fetus looks wrinkled and scraggy. Subcutaneous fat appearing. Lanugo hair has disappeared from face. Vernix caseosa thick. Nails reach end of fingers.							
36th	Fetus looks plumper and rounder.				Left testis in scrotum.	Cerebral fissures and convolutions rapidly developing.		Movements much stronger.
40th	Fetus fully developed. More subcutaneous fat present. Lanugo hairs disappear. Nails project beyond ends of fingers and toes.	Fetal hemoglobin begins conversion to adult hemoglobin.		Bronchioles and alveoli still developing.	Both testes in scrotum. Kidneys lie opposite L2.	Lower end of spinal cord at L3.	Paranasal sinuses are rudimentary.	Bones of skull are firm. Circumference of skull larger than rest of body.

Source. Adapted from R. S. Snell, *Clinical Embryology for Medical Students* (2nd ed.). Boston: Little, Brown, 1975.

pregnancy, or in gestation weeks (dated from the first day of the last menstrual period).

End of First Lunar Month (4 Gestation Weeks)
At the end of the first month the human embryo is a rapidly growing formation of cells, not resembling a human being yet. Very shortly, the head will become prominent, comprising about a third of the entire structure. The back is bent so that the head almost touches the tip of the tail (yes, a human embryo does have a tail at this point). The heart (still rudimentary) appears as a prominent bulge on the anterior surface. The arms and legs are bud-like structures. Rudimentary eyes, ears, and nose are discernible.

End of Second Lunar Month (8 Gestation Weeks)
Length, crown to rump, 1.3 cm (0.5 inch); weight, 1 gm (1/30 ounce). Organogenesis is complete at the end of eight weeks. With organogenesis, the structure is termed a *fetus* for the remainder of the pregnancy (*fetus* is from a Latin word meaning "offspring"). The heart has a septum and valves and is beating rhythmically. The facial features are definitely discernible. Legs, arms, fingers, toes, elbows, and knees have developed. Although the external genitalia are present, male and female are not distinguishable. The primitive tail is undergoing retrogression. The abdomen appears large as fetal intestine is growing rapidly. A sonogram taken at this time demonstrates a gestational sac and is diagnostic of pregnancy (Fig. 13-7).

End of Third Lunar Month (End of First Trimester) (12 Gestation Weeks)
Length, crown to rump, 6.5 cm (2.6 inches); weight, 20 gm (1¾ ounces). For ease of discussion, pregnancy is generally divided into three segments (trimesters), each of three months' duration. At the end of the 3rd month the fetus is at the end of the first trimester of pregnancy. Nail beds are forming on fingers and toes. The fetus is capable of spontaneous movements, although they are usually too faint to be felt by the mother. Some reflexes are present, notably the Babinski reflex. Ossification centers are forming in bones, and tooth buds are present. (The latter point is important to know, because if tetracycline is taken by the mother after this point in pregnancy the child may have tetracycline-stained, or brown, teeth.) Male and female fetuses are distinguishable by outward appearance. Kidney secretion has begun, although urine may not yet be evident in amniotic fluid. The heartbeat may be audible by a Doppler instrument, allowing the mother to hear the beat.

End of Fourth Lunar Month (16 Gestation Weeks)
Length, crown to rump, 11 cm (4.4 inches); weight, 124 gm (4 ounces). It may be possible to hear fetal heart sounds through an ordinary stethoscope at the end of the 4th lunar month. (The fetal heart rate is between 120 and 160 beats per minute throughout pregnancy.) The formation of lanugo (the fine, downy hair on the back and arms of newborns, apparently serving as a source of insulation for body heat) is well formed by this month. At this time the fetus actively swallows amniotic fluid, demonstrating an intact swallowing reflex. Ossification of bones is com-

Fig. 13-7. A sonogram showing implantation, or the characteristic circular ring present at 6 weeks' gestation.

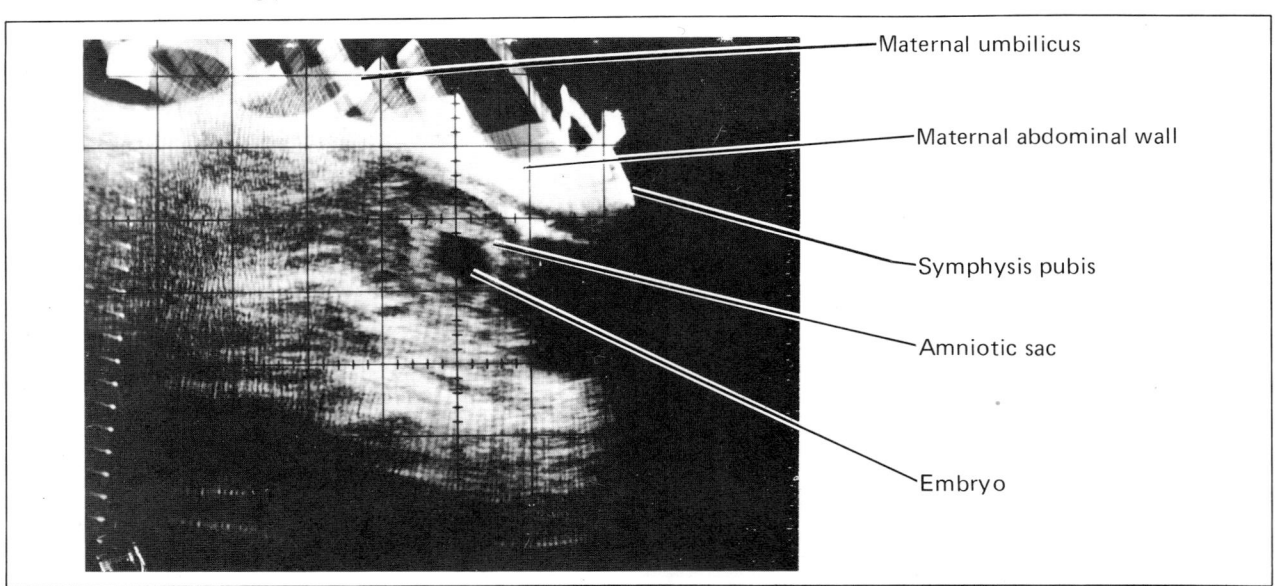

plete enough to allow the fetal skeleton to show on x-ray films.

End of Fifth Lunar Month (20 Gestation Weeks)
Length, crown to rump, 15 cm (6 inches); weight, 248 gm (8 ounces). During the 5th month of intrauterine life the spontaneous movements of the fetus become strong enough for the mother to feel. The sensation is like the fluttering of wings or fluid moving rapidly through the bowels. This event is termed *quickening*. It is a major milestone in pregnancy. For many women it is the first time the pregnancy, that they are actually going to have a child, seems real to them. It is such an exciting event in a first pregnancy that most mothers can remember for the rest of their lives not only at what month in pregnancy quickening occurred but exactly where they were when it happened.

A 20-week-old fetus is capable of antibody production but apparently produces few antibodies until challenged by antigens at the time of birth.

Twenty weeks is sometimes spoken of as the age of "viability," since a few infants born at this age have survived. The designation is mainly academic, however, because the average fetus born at this time does not have enough lung surfactant (necessary to keep the lungs from collapsing on exhalation) for respiration.

End of Sixth Lunar Month (End of Second Trimester) (24 Gestation Weeks)
Length, crown to rump, 20 cm (8 inches); weight, 600 gm (1⅓ pounds). Passive antibody transfer from mother to fetus probably begins as early as the 5th lunar month, certainly by the 6th lunar month.

Infants born before antibody transfer has taken place have no natural immunity and need more than the usual protection against infectious disease in the newborn period.

Vernix caseosa, a cream-cheese-like substance that apparently serves as a protective skin covering, begins to form during the 6th lunar month. Active production of lung surfactant begins, and features as detailed as eyebrows and eyelashes are being defined.

When a fetus reaches 24 weeks, or 601 gm, he has reached a practical lower age of viability if he is cared for after birth in a modern intensive care facility.

End of Seventh Lunar Month (28 Gestation Weeks)
Length, crown to heel, 37 cm (14.4 inches); weight, 1.1 kg (2½ pounds). The lung alveoli begin to mature, and surfactant can be demonstrated in amniotic fluid. The eyelids of the fetus have been fused since the 3rd lunar month. Now the membrane that had fused them dissolves, the eyes can open, and the pupils are capable of reacting to light.

Many women believe that a fetus born in this month has a better chance of surviving than one born in the 8th month. This belief is probably associated in part with the notion that seven is a lucky number and in part with a superstition handed down from ancient Greek times, when physicians thought that a fetus always attempts to escape the uterus during the 7th month. The fetus who is strong succeeds. If he fails, he again attempts escape at the 8th month. However, the fetus that succeeds on this try is so weak from the two attempts that he dies. The theory is doubly fallacious. The fetus appears to be a passive, not an active, passenger during delivery, and the more months he has to mature in utero, the more capable he is of surviving.

The vessels of the retina are susceptible to damage from high oxygen concentrations at seven months (an important point to be aware of when caring for low-birth-weight infants who need oxygen).

End of Eighth Lunar Month (32 Gestation Weeks)
Length, crown to heel, 43 cm (17 inches); weight, 1.6 to 1.8 kg (3½ to 4 pounds). Subcutaneous fat begins to be deposited in the fetus during this month, and he loses his former stringy, "little-old-man" appearance. The fetus is aware of sounds outside his mother's body, he has an active Moro reflex, and some have assumed delivery position (vertex or breech).

End of the Ninth Lunar Month (36 Gestation Weeks)
Length, crown to heel, 46 cm (18 inches); weight, 2.2 to 2.7 kg (5 to 6 pounds). In the last 2 months of intrauterine life, body stores of glycogen, iron, carbohydrate, and calcium are augmented; additional amounts of subcutaneous fat are deposited. The testes in the male begin to descend into the scrotal sac.

At this time the sole of the foot has only one or two crisscross creases. A full crisscross pattern will be evident at term. The amount of lanugo present begins to diminish.

Many babies turn in utero during this month into a vertex or head-first presentation.

End of Tenth Lunar Month (40 Gestation Weeks)
Length, crown to heel, 50 cm (20 inches); weight, 3.1 to 3.4 kg (7 to 7½ pounds). Because the length of menstrual periods varies, a pregnancy is considered normal if it ends between 38 and 42 weeks (36 to 40 ovulation weeks).

The fetus kicks actively during this month, hard enough to cause the mother considerable discomfort. Fetal hemoglobin begins its conversion to adult hemoglobin. The conversion is so rapid that at birth about 20 percent of hemoglobin will be adult in character.

Vernix caseosa, the creamy protective film that covers the skin at birth, is fully formed. Fingernails extend over the tips of fingers. Creases on the soles of the feet cover at least two-thirds of their surface.

In primiparas (women having their first babies) the fetus often sinks into the birth canal during these last two weeks, giving the mother a feeling that her load is being lightened. This event is termed *lightening*. It is a fetal announcement that the third trimester of pregnancy has ended and birth is at hand.

Figures 13-8 and 13-9 illustrate the comparative size and appearance of human embryos and fetuses at different stages.

Teratogens

A fetus can reach maturity in optimal health only if he receives sound genes (see Chap. 34) from his parents and he develops in an optimal intrauterine environment, protected from the influence of teratogens. A *teratogen* is any factor, chemical or physical, that affects the fertilized ovum, the embryo, or the fetus adversely. Today, many teratogenic factors can be isolated, yet the causes of many anomalies occurring in utero are still unknown.

Several factors influence the amount of damage a teratogen can cause. Strength is obviously one. Radiation is a known teratogen, but in small amounts (everyone is exposed to some radiation every day) it causes no damage. In large doses, however, such as a pregnant woman being treated for cancer of the cervix would receive, it can cause serious defects or death.

The timing of the teratogenic insult makes a significant difference. If a teratogen is introduced at the time when the main body systems are being formed (in the 2nd to 8th week of embryonic life), more harm can be expected than if the teratogen is introduced at the 8th or 9th month of pregnancy,

Fig. 13-8. Comparative sizes of the human embryo at nine different ages. (From L. Arey, Developmental Anatomy [7th ed.]. Philadelphia: Saunders, 1965.)

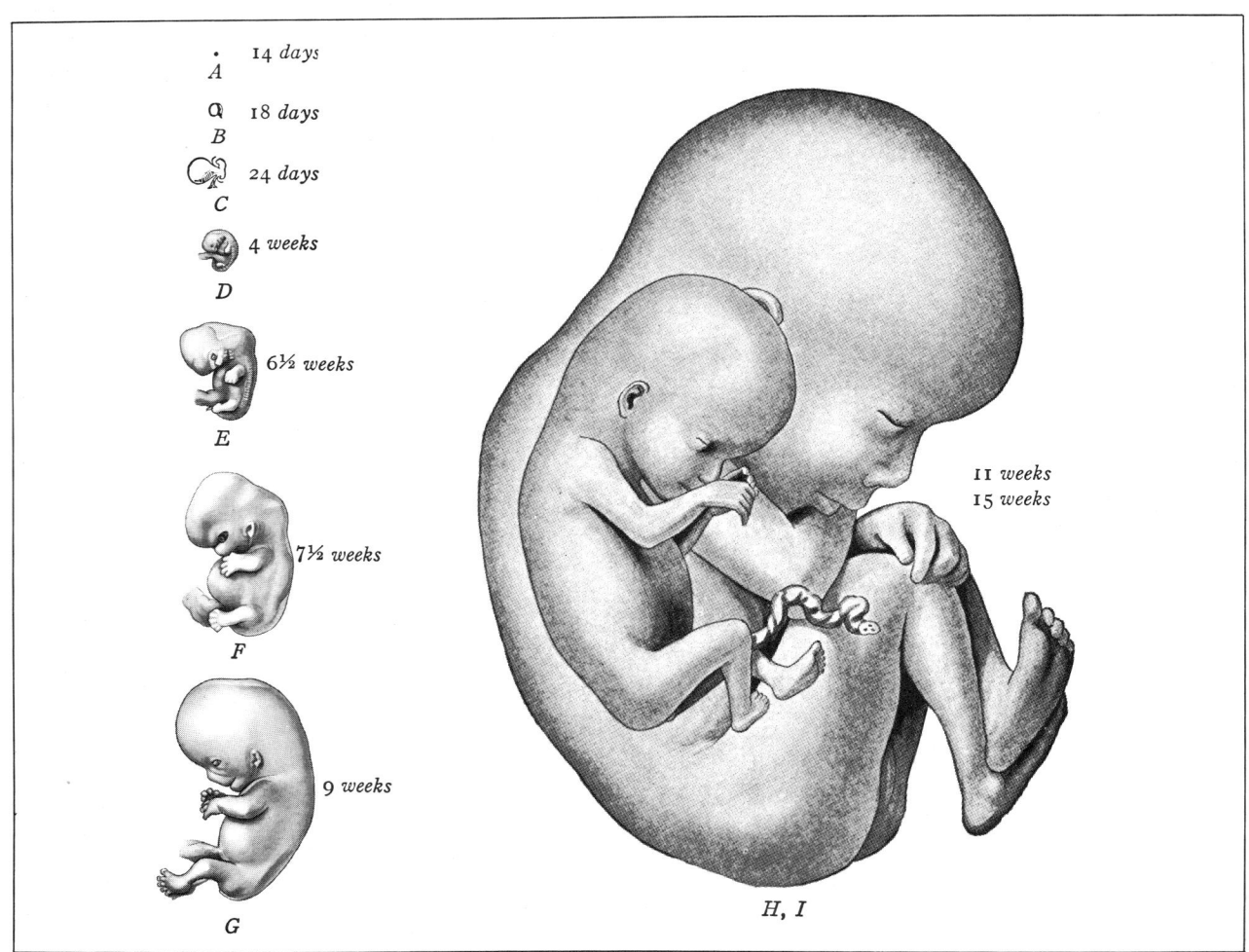

Table 13-3. Embryological Abnormalities by Time in Ovulation Weeks

Anatomical Tissue	Time (Approximate Range in Weeks)
Brain	2–11
Eyes	3–7
Cardiovascular	3–7
Renal	4–11
Genital	4–14
Lips and palate	7–10

Source. Adapted from D. Cavanagh and M. R. Talisman, *Prematurity and the Obstetrician*. New York: Appleton-Century-Crofts (Division of Prentice-Hall, Inc.), 1969.

when all the organs of the fetus are formed and are merely maturing. The times when different anatomical areas of the fetus are most likely to be affected by teratogens are given in Table 13-3.

Two known exceptions to the rule that deformities usually occur in early embryonic life are the effects caused by the organisms of syphilis and toxoplasmosis. These two infections can cause abnormalities in organs that were originally formed normally. This possibility has implications for a nurse working with pregnant women. The woman who contracts syphilis late in pregnancy needs treatment just as surely as the one who enters pregnancy with the infection. She should feel free to tell the health care personnel who care for her that she has been exposed to syphilis. If a nurse has moralized or made moral judgments about a woman early in pregnancy, the woman will be unlikely to mention this new contact. Thus, the nurse, by lack of understanding and compassion, will have indirectly prevented the mother from receiving treatment and, in a way, acted as a human teratogen.

A third factor determining the effects of a teratogen is that each teratogen generally has an affinity for specific tissue, so that its effect can sometimes be predicted. Lead, for instance, attacks and disables nervous tissue. Thalidomide causes limb defects. Tetracycline causes tooth enamel deformities and possibly long bone deformities. The rubella virus, on the other hand, can affect many organs, the eyes, ears, heart, and brain being the four most commonly attacked.

Nurses who are involved in prenatal care should be familiar with the various categories of teratogens described in the sections that follow. Many of the questions asked at prenatal visits are directly related to determining whether any teratogen interferences could have occurred since the last visit. A great deal of prenatal health teaching is based on helping the mother-to-be understand how to avoid teratogens.

MATERNAL INFECTION

Both bacterial and viral infections can cause damage to a fetus. Preventing and predicting fetal injury from infection is complicated, because a disease may be subclinical (without symptoms in the mother) and yet injure the fetus.

Rubella

The best example of a viral infection that causes extensive fetal damage is the rubella (German measles) virus. Its teratogenic effects were first discovered following a rubella epidemic in Australia in 1939–1940. Because there had been no major rubella outbreaks in the preceding 17 years, the majority of women of childbearing age had no immunity to the disease, and many contracted it during pregnancy. Of the infants born to these women, a large fraction had the classic sequelae: deafness, mental and motor retardation, cataracts, cardiac defects (patent ductus arteriosus and pulmonary stenosis being the most common), retarded intrauterine growth (small for gestation age), thrombocytopenic purpura, and dental and facial clefts, such as cleft lip and palate.

The greatest risk to the embryo from rubella virus is during the organogenesis period in early pregnancy. The frequency of defects is about 50 percent if infection occurs in the first eight weeks of pregnancy, 20 percent in the 9th through the 16th weeks. The risk is minimal later in the second trimester and apparently nil thereafter. In addition, there is about a 30 percent chance of spontaneous abortion or stillbirth if the infection occurs in the first trimester.

All women of childbearing age should be vaccinated against rubella so that this teratogen can be eradicated. A woman who is not vaccinated before pregnancy cannot be vaccinated during pregnancy because the vaccine utilizes a live virus that has effects similar to those occurring with a subclinical case of rubella. Immediately following a pregnancy, all women who have low rubella titers should be vaccinated, so that they will have the needed protection against rubella during their next pregnancy. Screening postpartum mothers to discover those with low or unknown titers should be a responsibility of the nurse in a postpartum unit.

Infants who are born of mothers who had rubella during pregnancy may be capable of transmitting the disease for up to 12 months after birth. The infant should be isolated in the newborn period from other newborns, and the mother should be made aware of the possibility that her infant might infect pregnant women. (Think of all the pregnant women who enjoy visiting a new baby, for a glimpse of what is to come!)

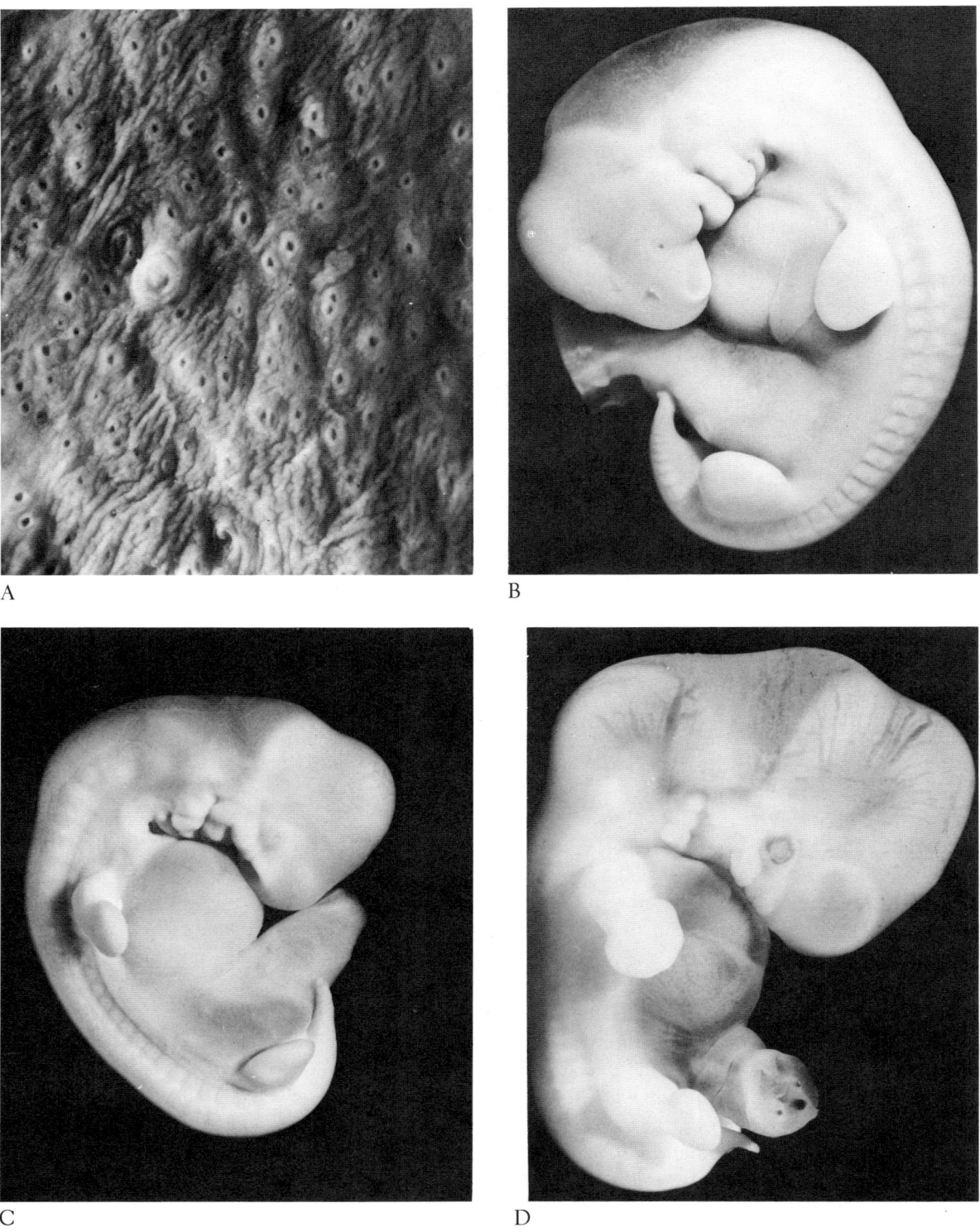

Fig. 13-9. Human embryo at different stages of development. A. Surface view of a human implantation on the uterus 7 to 8 days after conception. The openings of uterine glands of the epithelium appear as dark spots surrounded by light circles. B. Embryo at 32 days. Notice the primitive tail. The heart fills a large portion of the upper torso. C. Embryo at 37 days. The abdominal contents are beginning rapid growth. D. Embryo at 41 days. Arms and legs are becoming clearly defined. The tail is retrogressing. E. Embryo at 48 days. Fingers and toes are formed. The bulk of the fetal intestine is protruded into the umbilical cord. F. Embryo at 48 days, surrounded by amniotic membrane and fluid, the opened chorion, and the projecting chorionic villi. G. Embryo at 57 days (8 weeks). Organogenesis is complete. (Courtesy of Carnegie Institution of Washington, Department of Embryology, Davis Division.)

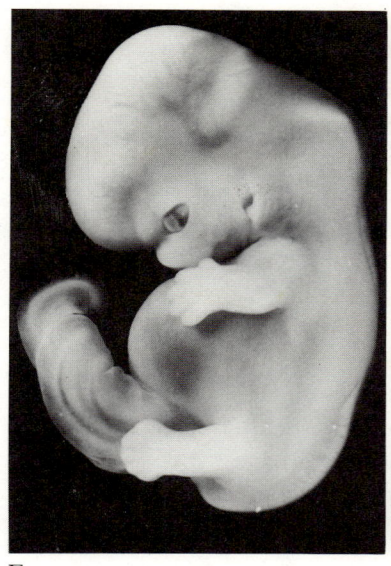 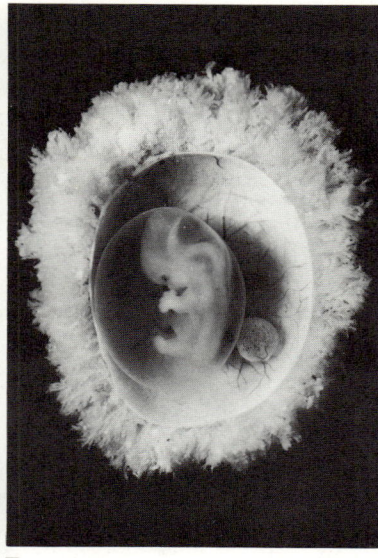 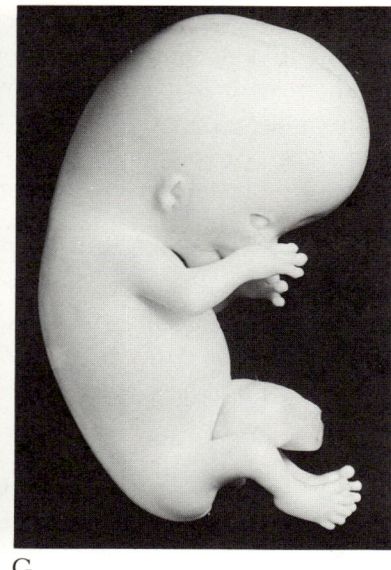

E F G

Nurses with low rubella titers should avoid caring for these infants.

Cytomegalic Inclusion Disease

Cytomegalic inclusion disease (salivary gland disease) is another viral disease that can cause extensive damage to a fetus. It is transmitted by droplet infection from person to person. The mother has almost no symptoms and so is not aware that she has contracted an infection, yet the infant may be born with severe brain damage (hydrocephalus, microcephaly, spasticity), eye damage (optic atrophy, chorioretinitis), or chronic liver disease. The child's skin may be covered with large petechiae (blueberry-muffin lesions).

Herpes Simplex II Virus Disease

Herpes simplex I virus is the causative agent of the common cold sore. When herpes simplex lesions occur on genitals, they are generally caused by a second virus, or herpes simplex II.

The fetus is usually exposed to the herpes II virus not through placental transmission but at birth as he passes through the birth canal and contacts infected genital secretions.

The infant appears well at birth but begins to develop fever, lethargy, and meningitis-encephalitis symptoms in a matter of hours. Although the prognosis for newborns who contract the infection is better than ever before, as many as 75 to 80 percent of infants will die or be left with extensive central nervous system damage. Women in labor should be observed closely to see whether herpes lesions (grouped painful pinpoint vesicles) are present on the vulva or vagina. If they are, the baby should be delivered by cesarean section to avoid virus contact. Because there is a close association between herpes simplex I and II virus, personnel with herpes infections should not work with newborn infants.

Other Virus Diseases

It is difficult to demonstrate other viral teratogens because of the phenomenon of subclinical infection, but the rubeola virus and the coxsackievirus are probably associated with defects; mumps, smallpox virus, and viral hepatitis may be related. Influenza virus is suspected of being a cause of malformation, probably of heart defects, and poliomyelitis will cause poliomyelitis in the fetus.

A baby born with central nervous system damage or anomalies may have a TORCH (*T*oxoplasmosis, *R*ubella, *C*ytomegalic inclusion disease, and *H*erpes II) screen ordered. This is a test to detect if antibodies against the common infectious teratogens are present in the newborn's serum.

Additional Infections

SYPHILIS. Syphilis, a spirochete infection, may cause damage to a fetus. This occurs after the 18th week of intrauterine life, when the cytotropic layer of the placental villi has atrophied and no longer protects against it. Deafness, mental retardation, osteochondritis, and fetal death are possible effects. The placenta of infants with congenital syphilis is generally large in size, constituting about 25 to 30 percent of fetal body weight, as compared with the normal 16 to 20 percent. Women should have a serology determination for syphilis at a first prenatal visit. If treated at that point, syphilis can be eradicated before it affects the fetus. If the infection is not detected or treated during pregnancy, the baby will be born with signs such as extreme rhinitis (snuffles) and a characteristic syphilitic rash, signs that help to identify him as a high-risk baby at birth.

TOXOPLASMOSIS. Toxoplasmosis, a protozoan infection, may be contracted by the mother by eating undercooked meat, although the organism is found most commonly in cat stool or in soil or cat litter. The mother has almost no symptoms of disease. Following placental transfer of the infection, however, the infant may be born with central nervous system damage, hydrocephalus, microcephaly, intracerebral calcification, and retinal deformities.

It is not necessary to remove a cat from a home during pregnancy as long as the cat is healthy; on the other hand, taking in a new cat is probably not wise. Pregnant women should be careful not to change a cat litter box or work in soil in an area where they notice cats defecate. They should be cautioned to avoid undercooked meat.

DRUGS

It is difficult to establish a drug as a teratogen because proof that a drug causes malformations or death in a fetus requires administration of the drug to a woman during pregnancy and observation of the effects on the fetus. Such experimentation is neither ethical nor legal.

Many women do not realize the danger of exposing their unborn children to drugs because they picture a placental "barrier" that acts as a shield against drugs. Not all drugs cross the placenta (heparin, for example, because of its large molecular size, does not), but most do. Women take some drugs because they do not think of over-the-counter medications as drugs.

The average number of drugs (over and above nutritional supplements and simple home remedies) that a woman takes during a pregnancy is about four. The most frequently consumed drugs are acetylsalicylic acid (aspirin), antihistamines, tranquilizers, antiemetics, laxatives, and nasal decongestants. In addition, a half ounce of pesticide per citizen per day is manufactured in the United States, and every day millions of cars and buses spew forth huge amounts of carbon monoxide. It seems highly likely that some of these substances affect women during pregnancy.

Over a dozen drugs and other substances are documented as being harmful to the fetus. More and more are identified every year. It is important, therefore, to understand two principles relating to drug intake during pregnancy. The first is that *any* drug under certain circumstances may be detrimental to fetal welfare; therefore, during pregnancy, no woman should take any drug not prescribed by her physician or without consulting her physician. The second is that no woman of childbearing age (14 through 40) should take any drug other than those prescribed by a physician who is aware of her age, since a fetus is as endangered when a woman taking drugs becomes pregnant as when a pregnant woman takes drugs.

The most dramatic example of a drug that is known to affect fetal development is thalidomide, which causes amelia or phocomelia (total or partial absence of extremities) in 100 percent of instances if taken between the 34th and 45th days of pregnancy. Interestingly, thalidomide caused no deformities in rats on which it was tested, only in humans.

Other drugs capable of being teratogenic are the following.

Chemotherapeutic Agents

The antimetabolites aminopterin, amethopterin (methotrexate), chlorambucil, and 6-mercaptopurine are known to cause malformation and abortion. All the antimetabolite and cytotoxic drugs are suspected of causing fetal injury.

Thyroid Agents

Propylthiouracil, a thyroid inhibitor, can cause congenital goiter. Ingesting iodides, such as potassium iodide, may also enlarge the fetal thyroid gland. Excessive enlargement causes tracheal compression and difficulty with respiration at birth. Iodides are contained in many over-the-counter cough suppressants, often taken by women who are unaware that they are harmful. Radioactive iodine (^{131}I) is contraindicated in pregnancy because there will be uptake by the fetal thyroid as well as by the maternal thyroid.

Analgesics

Narcotics all cross the placenta readily. When given during labor, meperidine (Demerol) has been associated with decreased responsiveness in newborns, which may interfere with mother-child interaction. When women take narcotics continually during pregnancy, small-for-date infants and congenital anomalies may be the result. Infants from such pregnancies may be born as addicted as their mothers and they may suffer extreme withdrawal reactions. This group includes infants born to mothers who have been placed on methadone for narcotic withdrawal.

Acetylsalicylic acid (aspirin), taken by many mothers for simple headaches (and not thought of by many as a drug, because it is so common), has been implicated in prolonged bleeding time in the newborn (which could lead to intracranial hemorrhage from birth pressure), a decreased albumin-binding capacity (which may lead to hyperbilirubinemia in the newborn), and perhaps prolonged gestation (which can lead to impaired central nervous system function due to lack of fetal nutrition).

Hormones
Synthetic progestins (ethisterone, norethisterone) or androgenic steroids given to women during pregnancy tend to masculinize the female fetus. Diethylstilbestrol given during pregnancy has been associated with the development of vaginal cancer in females when they reach the age of puberty. Corticosteroids cause cleft palate deformities in animal models, although apparently not in humans.

Diuretics
The excessive use of diuretics such as the thiazides may lead to electrolyte imbalance in the infant. This is an important point to remember, since diuretics, although not usually recommended, may be prescribed for women with symptoms of hypertension of pregnancy. Make certain that such women do not act on the principle that if a little of the medication is good for them, a lot will be even better.

Sedatives
Infants of mothers who receive a barbiturate during labor may be born depressed. The infant of the mother who has taken barbiturates continually during pregnancy may be born addicted and have withdrawal symptoms. These withdrawal symptoms may occur two to four weeks after birth, when the infant is at home, away from medical care, and so tend to be extremely serious.

Antacids
Antacids are not considered by many women to be drugs because they are largely over-the-counter medications. The sodium in them may lead to electrolyte disturbances in the mother and fetus. Products that contain bromides may cause bromide intoxication (lethargy, a bromide rash, mental retardation).

Psychotropic Drugs
Diazepam (Valium), one of the drugs prescribed to the general population to relieve anxiety, may cause infants to have poor sucking reflexes and hypotonia. Lithium, used by women with severe anxiety, has been implicated in congenital anomalies and in lethargy and cyanosis in the newborn.

Hypotensive Agents
Reserpine, given to women for treatment of high blood pressure during pregnancy, tends to cause nasal congestion, respiratory distress, cyanosis, and muscle flaccidity in the infant.

Antibiotics
Streptomycin may be associated with 8th cranial nerve deafness. The sulfonamides, given near term, interfere with bilirubin binding and may lead to kernicterus (high, destructive levels of bilirubin in brain tissue). Tetracycline may lead to brown-stained teeth and long bone deformities. Chloramphenicol, given near term, may cause shock and collapse in the newborn (the "gray baby" syndrome). Fortunately, ampicillin is a broad-spectrum antibiotic that can be given during pregnancy. It should be noted if mothers who are having urine collected for estriol levels are taking ampicillin, as it may reduce estriol excretion.

Anticoagulants
Coumarin may cause hemorrhage in the fetus or newborn. This can be severe enough to lead to fetal or newborn death.

Vitamins
Vitamins are another category of drugs that women may not consider medicine. Vitamins A and D have been implicated in congenital deformities; excessive vitamin K can lead to hyperbilirubinemia in the newborn. Pyridoxine (vitamin B_6) may cause withdrawal seizures. Women with tuberculosis may take pyridoxine to complement the action of isoniazid. It is good to ask a pregnant woman not only whether she is taking the vitamin prescribed, but how many she is taking. The woman who is taking three or four tablets a day instead of the one prescribed for her (hoping that her infant will be the brightest, strongest baby ever) may actually be harming her infant.

Anticonvulsant Agents
Diphenylhydantoin (Dilantin) has been associated with congenital anomalies (cleft lip and palate, congenital heart disease). Trimethadione (Tridione) and paramethadione (Paradione) may lead to similar defects. It is difficult to evaluate the effects of anticonvulsants on fetuses because, if a woman has a seizure during pregnancy, the accompanying anoxia and acidosis may be the factors that lead to the fetal insult. Even though Dilantin, especially, may be responsible for a syndrome in infants very similar to the fetal alcohol syndrome, women who have seizures uncon-

trolled except by such an agent may have no choice but to continue to take it during pregnancy.

Hypoglycemic Agents
Most diabetic women of childbearing age are juvenile diabetics and therefore take injectable insulin rather than hypoglycemic agents. Insulin is one of the rare substances that does not cross the placenta because of its large molecular size. Oral hypoglycemic agents do cross the placenta, however, and may lead to hypoglycemia in newborns.

Hallucinogenic Agents
Lysergic acid diethylamide (LSD) may cause breakage of chromosomes in the mother or father that will result in congenital deformities in children. Marijuana, on the other hand, a drug frequently attacked as being dangerous, has not been implicated in fetal deformities.

Alcohol
It has been known for years that babies of mothers who consume a large quantity of alcohol during pregnancy have a high incidence of congenital deformities and mental retardation. It was assumed that the defects were the result of the mother's poor nutritional state (drinking alcohol rather than eating food), not the direct result of the alcohol.

Alcohol by itself has now been isolated as a teratogen. Mothers who consume over 3 ounces a day may have babies born with a *fetal alcohol syndrome*, which includes being small for gestation age, mental retardation, and a particular craniofacial deformity. Mothers should be advised to limit alcohol consumption during pregnancy to under an ounce a day (remembering that they cannot save a week's limit for Saturday night and ingest it all then, because on that one day they could cause damage). This limitation of alcohol will be difficult for the woman whose life-style includes the ingestion of more alcohol than that daily or who is addicted to alcohol and feels a need for more than that quantity daily.

Immunological Agents
Live virus vaccines, such as measles, mumps, rubella, and poliomyelitis vaccines, are contraindicated during pregnancy because pregnancy can cause the actual virus infection in the fetus. Care must be given to ascertain that adolescents are not pregnant before they are included in routine immunization programs.

ENVIRONMENTAL TERATOGENS
Lead poisoning is generally considered a problem of early childhood. It is also a fetal hazard, since lead is teratogenic if consumed by a woman during pregnancy. Preschool children ingest lead by eating paint chips or wall plaster; women ingest it by drinking moonshine liquor distilled in an apparatus using lead pipes or by "sniffing" gasoline (a form of drug abuse). Making moonshine is still a common practice in some rural areas of the southeastern United States. If you are working with pregnant women in such areas you should be aware of the possibility that some women may be ingesting lead from this source. Lead ingestion during pregnancy leads to mental retardation and central nervous system damage to the fetus.

Mercury can cause mental retardation and central nervous system motor damage in a fetus. Mercury is an ingredient of pesticides. Naphthalene, the ingredient of mothballs, if ingested, can cause hemolysis. Mothballs are sometimes ingested by girls attempting suicide or trying to cause an abortion. Carbon monoxide, if inhaled in sufficient quantities, can bring about severe fetal central nervous system damage because it replaces oxygen at the placental exchange site. Pregnant women should be cautious about driving cars that have defective mufflers or waiting for cars to be repaired in unventilated repair shops.

The amount of DDT that can be utilized as a pesticide today is severely limited because DDT can cause fetal deformities. Fluoride, in appropriate amounts, helps to strengthen teeth against cavities. In large amounts, fluoride stains teeth. Many city water supplies are fluoridated. A pregnant woman needs to use common sense and not take a fluoride supplement if fluoride is present in her drinking water.

LABOR AND DELIVERY MEDICATIONS
The use of oxytocin as a medicine to induce labor is now seriously limited because infants born after its use tend to develop electrolyte disturbances and hyperbilirubinemia due to competitive albumin binding. Depressive responses at birth have been associated with the use of analgesics in labor, particularly meperidine (Demerol) and morphine. The use of general anesthetics leads to anesthetized infants, as anesthetic agents cross the placenta readily and reach levels in the fetus equal to those in the mother. Local anesthesia injected as a paracervical block may lead to fetal bradycardia; injected as a spinal or caudal anesthetic, it may produce hypotension in the mother, resulting in reduced placental blood flow. The precautions necessary to observe when using analgesics or anesthetics in labor are discussed in detail in Chap. 23.

RADIATION

Radiation has been proved to be a teratogen to unborn children. It produces a range of malformations, depending on the stage of development of the embryo or fetus and on the length of exposure. It does the most damage during the first two to six weeks after conception (during a time when many women are not aware that they are pregnant). As a rule, therefore, all women of childbearing age should be exposed to x-rays only in the first 10 days following a menstrual period (a time when pregnancy is unlikely because ovulation has not yet occurred), except, of course, in emergency situations.

Radiation of the pelvis should be avoided during pregnancy; it should be undertaken at term in pregnancy only if the data the x-ray will reveal cannot be obtained by any other means and will be important for delivery. Thus, x-ray examination is used to determine, for example, whether the fetal head can be delivered through the vaginal route or whether it is too large (x-ray pelvimetry); as a safeguard before using oxytocin for assistance in or induction of labor; and to verify suspected fetal malposition. Sonography is replacing x-ray examination for confirmation of situations such as multiple pregnancy as sonography does not appear to be teratogenic.

If the woman needs nonpelvic radiation during pregnancy (dental x-rays, a limb x-ray after a fall), her pelvis should be shielded by a lead apron during the procedure. Even fluoroscopy, which uses lower radiation doses than does regular x-ray photography, can cause deformation of the fetus and should be avoided during pregnancy—again, except in an emergency.

There is evidence that x-rays have long-lasting effects on the health of the child. There appears to be an increased risk of cancer before age 10 in children exposed to x-rays while in utero [30]. There is a possibility that the exposure of the fetal gonads could lead to a genetic mutation that would not be evident until the next generation.

These restrictions in the use of x-rays have special meaning for female nurses. If you are asked to assist with a patient in an x-ray room and you are in the postovulatory phase of a menstrual cycle, you have a right to demand lead shielding as pelvic protection. Do not be swayed when x-ray technicians say, "It's just one time," or "It's the buildup of radiation that counts." Protection that is suggested for women in general should be demanded by nurses.

SMOKING

Cigarette smoking by a pregnant woman has been shown to have teratogenic effects on the fetus. Although the teratogenic factor in cigarettes may be the nicotine, cigarettes are discussed separately from other drugs because it is difficult for the woman who smokes to equate smoking with drug ingestion.

There is firm evidence that children born of cigarette smokers are smaller for gestation age than children born to nonsmoking mothers. There is further evidence that these children continue to be underweight for some time in early life. The effect is apparent when the mother smokes more than 10 cigarettes a day and thus is related to the quantity of cigarettes smoked [13]. If a woman cannot stop smoking during pregnancy (and it is realistic to accept the fact that many women cannot), reducing the number of cigarettes smoked per day will help diminish the adverse effects on the fetus.

Although not proved, it is believed that the decrease in weight in the infants of smoking mothers probably results from vasoconstriction of the uterine vessels, limiting the blood supply to the fetus.

A second sound reason women should at least limit the number of cigarettes smoked per day is to protect their own health. A child needs a well mother during his years of growing up. Losing a mother from lung cancer is as deleterious to his psychological health as the original smoking may be to his physical health.

EMOTIONAL STRESS

There are many old wives' tales about the "marking" of infants in utero: If a woman sees a mouse during pregnancy, her child will be born with a furry or mole-like birthmark; eating strawberries causes strawberry birthmarks; looking at a handicapped child while pregnant will cause a child in utero to be handicapped the same way. Common sense and awareness of fetal-maternal physiology have dispelled these superstitions. There is growing evidence, however, that an emotionally disturbed pregnancy, one filled with anxiety and worry beyond the usual amount associated with pregnancy, may have some effect on the unborn child. Anxiety produces physiological changes through its effect on the sympathetic division of the autonomic nervous system. The main changes are an increase in heart rate, constriction of the blood vessels, a decrease in gastrointestinal motility, and dilatation of coronary vessels. This effect is sometimes called the *fight or flight syndrome*. If the anxiety is prolonged, there is a possibility that the constriction of uterine vessels will interfere with the blood supply to the fetus.

These phenomena are characteristic only of long-term, extreme stress, not of the normal anxiety of pregnancy. Illness or death of the husband, difficulty with relatives, marital discord, and illness or death of another child are examples of stress situations that might provoke excessive anxiety.

Helping a woman resolve these problems during pregnancy is not easy, because they are usually complex. If maternal stress is a teratogen, however, securing counseling for the woman under emotional stress during pregnancy is as important as ensuring her good physical care.

POOR NUTRITION

Although *excessive* intake of some nutrients, namely, vitamin A, riboflavin, zinc, and manganese, has been shown to cause malformation in animals, the usual problem in human mothers is *under*nutrition. Cretinism (hypothyroidism), for example, can occur in a fetus if his mother's iodine intake is inadequate during pregnancy. Lack of folic acid (necessary for cell formation and tissue growth) may result in malformations such as cleft lip or anencephaly. Lack of vitamin D may cause bone deformity (prenatal rickets).

General malnutrition results in babies that are small for their gestation ages and in an increase in low-birth-weight and fetal deaths. These effects may be related to deficiency of a number of nutrients in the fetus. There appears to be a strong correlation between the occurrence of iron deficiency anemia in the mother and low birth weight of the baby.

Protein intake in the mother is a major factor in maintaining the health of the unborn. The low-birth-weight rate of newborns increases when the maternal diet contains less than 50 gm of protein per day. The greatest damage from poor protein intake tends to occur in early pregnancy. This fact puts women of childbearing age on notice that it is essential to maintain themselves on an adequate protein diet. By the time they realize they are pregnant, and begin to eat a proper diet, teratogenic effects may already be present.

Interestingly, more mentally retarded children are born in the late winter and early spring months (that is, were conceived the previous spring and summer) than at other times of the year. Perhaps in early pregnancy during hot weather the mother lowers her total intake, including her intake of protein.

Pica, or the ingestion of substances other than foodstuffs, is not uncommon in the southern United States and is sometimes found in women who have migrated to the north. Clay, starch, and raw flour are the three substances most often eaten by pregnant women with pica. Few women can explain why they enjoy eating these substances. Some may use them to try to obtain relief from morning sickness; others simply feel a craving for the substance.

Clay eating may lead to iron deficiency anemia, since the presence of clay in the stomach interferes with the absorption of iron. Starch eating adds "empty calories" to the woman's diet and may prevent her from eating the nutritious diet she should have during pregnancy. Pica in children is associated with iron deficiency, and children who are iron deficient tend to crave non-food substances. Which occurs, then, is hard to determine: Is the woman iron deficient and so craves starch, or does she crave starch and then become iron deficient?

Pregnant women need guidance in selecting a healthy diet, in taking the vitamins, iron, and folic acid preparations prescribed for them by their physician (iodized salt may or may not be advised, depending on the geographical section of the country), and in taking *only* those prescribed.

Suggestions for diet counseling during pregnancy are given in Chap. 18.

MATERNAL ILLNESS

Certain disease states and other conditions in the mother can have teratogenic effects. Among them are maternal diabetes, maternal heart disease, maternal age, and maternal blood incompatibility. Because these situations involve nursing care applicable to the mother as well as to the fetus, they are discussed in Chap. 33. Maternal fever early in pregnancy (4 to 6 weeks) may cause in the fetus abnormal brain development and possibly seizure disorders, hypotonia, and skeletal deformities due to hyperthermia.

Assessing Fetal Well-Being and Maturity

Toward the end of pregnancy most women wish they could have a glimpse of their unborn child to see whether it is a boy or girl and to assure themselves that the child is doing well and is ready for extrauterine life. Often, those caring for the woman during pregnancy would also find this information helpful. Although knowledge of the fetus has not yet advanced to the point where information about a fetus is available to a mother or to health care personnel who are merely curious, a great deal about the health of the unborn child can be learned through various techniques when this information is essential.

MATERNAL HISTORY

The history of the current pregnancy, the woman's general health, the outcome of previous pregnancies, and her health during those pregnancies are good indexes to predict the outcome of a current pregnancy.

It is time-consuming to take a good initial history, but the potential dangers of, for example, a prediabetic condition or a blood incompatibility make it important to discover such conditions early in pregnancy.

Obtaining thorough initial and interval histories is a task a nurse with extended skills in interviewing can perform. The benefits of extensive interviewing are always surprising, both in terms of the amount of information that can be gained and in terms of the rapport that being listened to (*really* listened to) establishes with mothers.

ESTIMATION OF FUNDAL HEIGHT

Fundal height should be measured at each prenatal visit as a means of assessing fetal growth and well-being. It is a helpful determination, since the increase in the size of the uterus directly reflects the increase in the size of the fetus.

A rule of thumb for establishing correct fundal height is as follows: The measurement in centimeters from the top of the pubic bone to the top of the fundus equals the age in weeks of the fetus. In other words, if fundal height is 16 cm, the size of the fetus is comparable to that of a fetus of 16 weeks. If fundal height is 20 cm, the size of the fetus is comparable to that of a fetus of 20 weeks. A fundal height much greater than this suggests multiple pregnancy, miscalculated due date, hydramnios (increased amniotic fluid volume), or hydatid mole (see Chap. 33). A fundal measurement much less than this suggests that the fetus is failing to thrive or that an anomaly such as anencephaly is developing.

Another rule of thumb stresses that the rump to shoulder measurement is more meaningful than fundal height. Weight of the fetus may be calculated during the last half of pregnancy by multiplying the rump to shoulder measurement by 100. When this measurement is 25 cm, the fetus is, in terms of weight, ready to be born ($25 \times 100 = 2,500$ gm, or 5½ pounds).

ABDOMINAL SOUNDS AND MOVEMENTS

Fetal heart sounds are a good indication of fetal well-being. Typically, these are first heard with a stethoscope between the 16th and 20th weeks, so that auscultating them at this time is an assessment of well-being as well as a means of establishing or confirming the expected date of confinement (due date) of the pregnancy. Fetal heart rates can be heard as early as the 11th or 12th week by the use of an ultrasonic Doppler technique.

Quickening, or the feeling of life by the mother, is much less reliable as a sign of well-being. A woman who wants to have a baby very badly can be deceived by her own desire into "feeling" quickening when in reality there is no child inside her. A woman who has previously felt movement and reports that she no longer feels it needs to be seen immediately; she may be reporting fetal death.

ELECTROCARDIOGRAPHY

Fetal electrocardiograms (ECGs) may be recorded as early as the 11th week of pregnancy. The ECG is inaccurate before the 5th month, however, because until this time the fetal cardiac electrical signal is so weak that it may be masked by the mother's. It may be a helpful tool in differentiating between an intrauterine tumor and a viable pregnancy, however.

All fetal hearts should be monitored by an ECG technique or Doppler technique during labor, when the fetus is under a high degree of stress. Techniques of fetal heart monitoring and the associated nursing care required are discussed in Chap. 22.

X-RAY FILMS

Aside from being contraindicated during pregnancy unless they can supply information that cannot be established in any other way, fetal x-ray films are grossly unreliable for estimating fetal age or assessing fetal health. Fetal x-ray examination at term may be helpful in determining maturity. If the distal femoral and proximal tibial epiphyses are both present, the fetus is undoubtedly mature.

Fetal death may also be established by x-ray picture. Between 48 and 72 hours after death, fetal skull bones override, and the spine becomes extremely curved. If a radiopaque substance is introduced into the amniotic fluid and none of it appears in the fetal intestinal tract within 12 to 24 hours, the fetus either has an obstructing esophageal atresia that prevents him from swallowing or may be presumed to be dead.

SONOGRAPHY

Sonography may be used early in pregnancy to diagnose pregnancy (as early as 6 weeks' gestation age). Later in pregnancy it can be used to confirm the presence, size, and location of the placenta and to establish that the fetus is increasing in size. It may be used at term to predict maturity (Fig. 13-10).

In the sonogram technique, intermittent sound waves of high frequency (above the audible range) are projected toward the mother's uterus. The sound frequencies that bounce back are displayed on a screen, and those from tissues of various thicknesses and properties will have a different appearance. A permanent record can be made by timed Polaroid photography.

Growth and Development of the Fetus

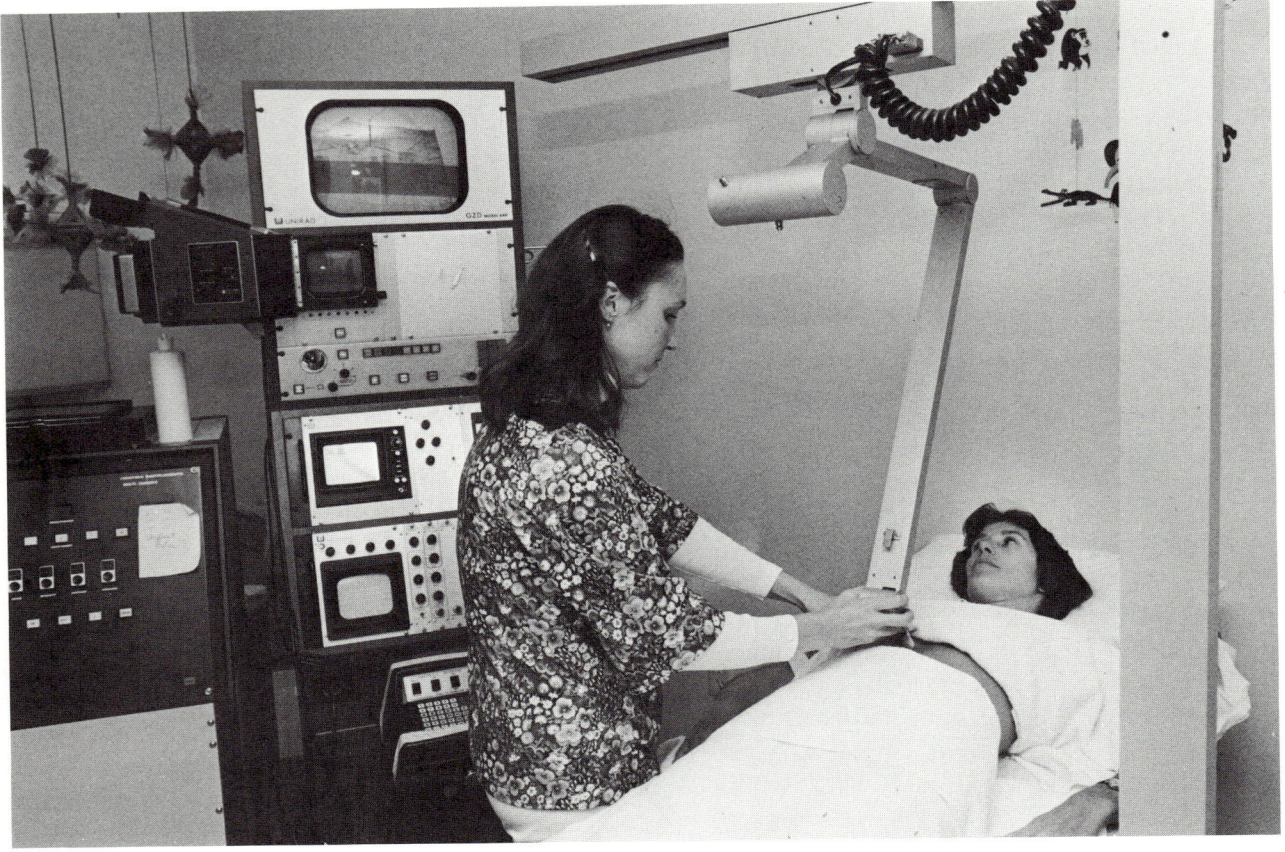

Fig. 13-10. A sonogram being recorded. (Courtesy of the Department of Medical Photography, Children's Hospital, Buffalo, N.Y.)

Sonography diagnoses the pregnancy by demonstrating the presence of a gestational sac. At almost the same time (six to eight weeks of pregnancy), movement of the fetal heart can be demonstrated. As sonography appears to have no effect on the fetus, it can be used to assess fetal well-being by identifying the fetal heartbeat at any point in pregnancy. Various growth anomalies, such as hydrocephalus, anencephaly, and spinal cord defects, can be detected on sonograms.

Sonography may be used to predict the maturity of the fetus by measuring the biparietal diameter (side-to-side measurement) of the fetal head on the permanent record. Thompson et al. [32] have determined that when the biparietal diameter of the fetal head is 8.5 cm or more, in 90 percent of pregnancies the infant will weigh more than 2,500 gm (5½ pounds).

Sonography appears to be safe for both mother and fetus. It involves no discomfort for the fetus, and the only discomfort for the mother is that a contact lubricant must be applied to her abdomen at the beginning of the scan. Figure 13-11 is a sonogram of a fetus at near term.

ASSAY OF MATERNAL URINE

There are a number of constituents of maternal urine that can be assayed to help determine fetal well-being and maturity.

Estriol

Estrogen is supplied by the placenta from precursors produced largely from the fetal adrenal glands. Measuring estriol, the breakdown product of estrogen, in urine, therefore, is a measure of both placental function and fetal well-being.

Estriol secretion rises about a thousand-fold during pregnancy. At the 7th week of gestation, the excretion rate is about 0.4 mg per day; by the 20th week it is between 1 and 3 mg per day. From the 20th week to the termination of pregnancy the rate increases even more rapidly, reaching 12 to 50 mg per day at term. Estriol levels fall rapidly when the fetus is in jeopardy or dies. Late in pregnancy (after the 34th week), a level under 1 mg is usually evidence of a dead fetus; levels between 1 and 4 mg suggest that the fetus is in serious danger. Levels between 4 and 12 mg suggest retarded fetal development.

Since estriol levels in urine are influenced by the efficiency of maternal kidney function, they vary widely from woman to woman. For this reason it is

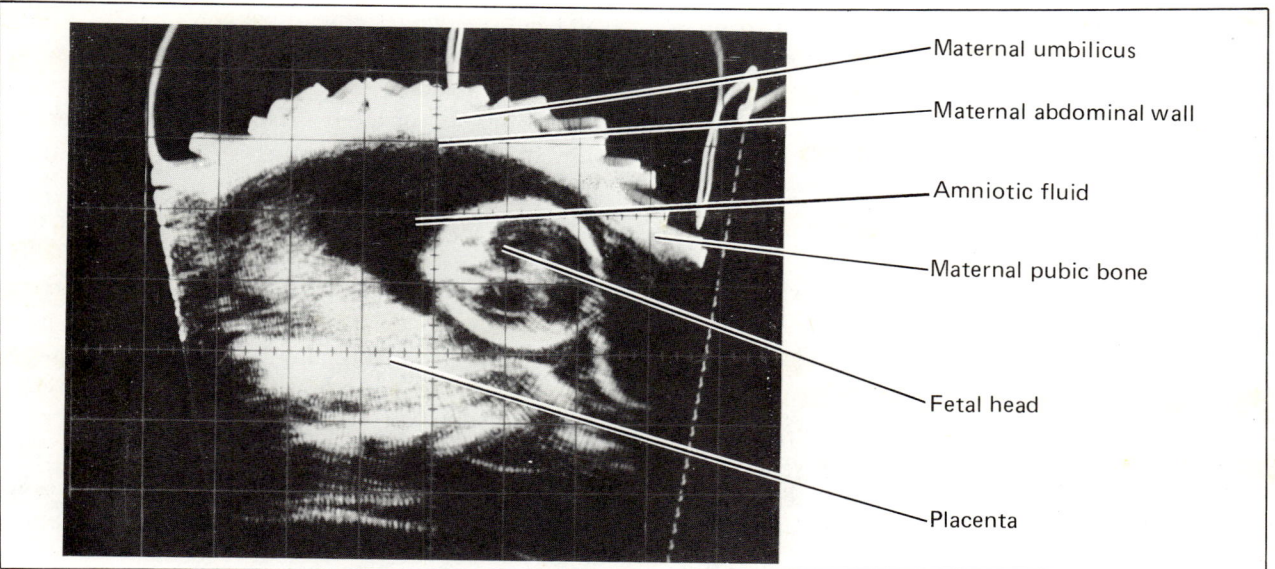

Fig. 13-11. A sonogram at 39 weeks' gestation. The biparietal diameter of the fetus measures only 7.7 cm. There is more amniotic fluid present than there normally would be (hydramnios). The abdominal wall appears shaggy, because of the scanning technique. (Courtesy of Richard W. Munschauer, M.D., Children's Hospital, Buffalo, N.Y.)

important that a woman who will be depending on assay of estriol levels late in pregnancy have a number of 24-hour urines collected at about the 30th week of pregnancy to serve as her individual baseline level. Urines being assayed for estriol are often analyzed for creatinine too. If the level of creatinine in the urine specimen is low, either the woman's kidney function is impaired (the fetus and placenta are both fine; the fault is with her kidneys) or part of the 24-hour specimen has been lost. This double check on the intactness of the specimen prevents overreading of the seriousness of low estriol levels.

Estriol levels in maternal urine are typically low in pregnancies in which the fetus is anencephalic (little head and brain development) because the fetus does not produce ACTH by his pituitary to stimulate adrenal function to produce the precursor of estrogen. Estriol levels may be low in women with pregnancy-induced hypertension or diabetes, demonstrating the poor placenta-blood interchange that is occurring. Estriol levels are not a helpful determination in a fetus who has damage due to Rh incompatibility, because with this complication, although the fetus's blood is threatened, his adrenal gland is not impaired, and estrogen production remains high (until, of course, the fetus is so severely compromised that he cannot maintain any body function).

Ampicillin causes low excretion of estriol. Women being treated with ampicillin must have estriol levels analyzed with this in mind; the fact that they are currently being treated with ampicillin must be marked clearly on the laboratory slip.

Estriol determinations are helpful in assessing placental health in the fetus who is overdue—that is, has remained in utero more than two weeks beyond the calculated due date. As long as estriol secretions remain at a high level, 12 to 50 mg per day, the likelihood is great that the birth date was calculated incorrectly and the pregnancy is not truly overdue.

Pregnanediol

The chemical determination of urinary pregnanediol is sometimes of use in determining the efficiency of placental function. Pregnanediol is the breakdown product of progesterone; indirectly, it measures the ability of the placenta to produce progesterone. A woman with a history of repeated spontaneous premature labor might have this determination made weekly or every two weeks during pregnancy. If serial determinations of urinary pregnanediol are consistently lower than normal, progesterone therapy may be indicated. It is inadvisable to give progesterone in large doses in early pregnancy until urinary human chorionic gonadotropin levels are also assayed. If these levels are low, placental growth may be faulty; hence, progesterone therapy to keep the decidua from sloughing off and ending a faulty pregnancy might be ill advised.

Bacteriuria

The urine of women should be screened for asymptomatic bacteriuria during pregnancy as a further test of fetal well-being, since there is a higher-than-usual incidence of low-birth-weight infants (27 percent versus 7 to 10 percent) in women with bacteriuria.

Collection of 24-Hour Urine Specimens

Whether or not maternal urine can be assayed depends on the reliability with which it is collected. Many women are instructed how to make the collection correctly and then collect their own 24-hour urine specimen at home. Others are hospitalized for 24 hours for the collection. Either way, the responsibility for giving accurate instructions falls to the nurse.

A 24-hour urine collection begins with a "discard" urine. If a urine is not discarded to begin a collection, you are actually measuring not only all urine the woman produced from 8:00 one morning to 8:00 the next, but also the urine that was in her bladder when you started. If the urine collection begins in the morning, it would include urine that has been in her bladder from the time she went to bed the night before, 8 hours earlier or longer. At the end, therefore, you have not a 24-hour urine but a 32-hour urine. Estriol levels might be low in the urine but because the urine is actually 32 hours, not 24, they might seem normal. A fetus in distress would go unrecognized.

Women are often reluctant to discard this first urine and need to be given the explanation of why they must discard it. Otherwise, they may think that every little bit will help in the analysis and not realize that they are interfering with the analysis by saving this.

The beginning of the 24-hour period is timed from the time of the *discard urine*. If the woman does not remember this step, but times from the first urine she is to save, she will again be compromising the analysis of the specimen. Suppose, for instance, she does not void again for 6 hours following the discard urine. If she times the 24-hour specimen from the first voiding, she is again adding too many hours (24 plus the 6 extra hours since the discard). Following the discard urine, the woman saves all urine for the next 24 hours. She should void as closely as possible to the time of the end of the collection (24 hours after the time of the discard specimen). The procedure is summarized in Table 13-4.

Urine should be saved in a clean container furnished by the hospital laboratory or clean quart jars the woman can supply herself. Refrigerating it keeps the bacteria count down. When women move their bowels, they invariably also void. Caution them to void *before* moving their bowels to avoid loss of urine.

ASSAY OF MATERNAL SERUM

Determinations of the levels of various hormones in maternal blood are being made more and more frequently as assessments of fetal well-being.

Diamine Oxidase

Diamine oxidase (DAO) is an enzyme that is typically found in high levels in maternal blood during pregnancy. The origin of diamine oxidase is the maternal decidua beneath the placenta. Large amounts of histamine are present in fetal tissue (the same quantity as is present in any rapidly growing tissue such as tumor or a healing wound). Diamine oxidase is formed from histamine. The level of diamine oxidase is two or three times above nonpregnancy levels by the 6th week of gestation. It reaches 100 units by 11 weeks, 500 units at 21 weeks. If levels of DAO are within the normal range during the first and second trimester, the fetus is probably actively growing (why high levels of histamine are present) and a normal outcome of the pregnancy can be predicted. A level that does not rise suggests improper or retarded fetal growth. Unfortunately, levels of DAO do not fall rapidly enough after fetal distress occurs in a healthy fetus to be used as a prediction of fetal distress in a previously healthy fetus.

Oxytocinase

Oxytocinase is an aminopeptide enzyme apparently produced by the syncytiotrophoblast layer of the placenta. It seems to inactivate maternal oxytocin so that the uterus remains quiet during pregnancy. Assay of maternal levels of oxytocinase is an indirect assay of placental function. Levels increase steadily from about the 11th week of pregnancy until term. They are typically low after a pregnancy becomes post-term.

Alkaline Phosphatase

Alkaline phosphatase is an enzyme originating in the placenta. It is released from placental tissue following

---

Table 13-4. Twenty-four-Hour Urine Collection

Day 1, 8:00 A.M.
  Void and *discard* urine, but *time* the beginning of collection from this point. Save all urine passed until
Day 2, 8:00 A.M.
  Void at this time (24 hours after beginning) to end collection. Add this specimen as final specimen to collection.
If a second 24-hour urine collection is to begin, consider the last specimen from the first collection period the discard specimen for the second collection.

injury to the placenta the way heart enzymes are released after heart damage. Assay of maternal plasma for alkaline phosphatase might be helpful if placental infarcts or trauma are suspected.

Human Placental Lactogen

Human placental lactogen (HPL) is an enzyme formed by the syncytiotrophoblast layer of the placenta. Levels of HPL can be detected in maternal plasma as early as the 6th week of gestation. They increase throughout pregnancy until the 36th week, after which they stay the same until term.

Since the half-life of HPL is short (about 20 minutes), the level decreases rapidly following delivery. It may be used to monitor placental function during pregnancy. A level of under 4 µg per milliliter after 30 weeks' gestation suggests that the placenta is not functioning adequately to support a growing fetus.

Plasma Estriol

Plasma estriol levels rather than urinary estriol levels may be monitored to determine the adequacy of the fetal-placental unit. If kidney function in the woman is impaired, plasma estriol level (because it is not being excreted) will be falsely high.

Electrophoretic Bands

A characteristic electrophoretic protein band appears to be present in over 80 percent of pregnant women during the third trimester of pregnancy. Its function is not well understood, but its absence in some women who deliver congenitally deformed infants is suggestive of its importance to a healthy pregnancy.

AMNIOCENTESIS

Amniocentesis is aspiration of amniotic fluid from the pregnant uterus for examination. It can be done in a physician's office or an ambulatory clinic as early as the 14th to 16th week of pregnancy.

It is an easy procedure, with a failure rate of only about 5 percent. However, it may be frightening to a woman and not totally without risk to the fetus because it involves penetrating the integrity of the amniotic sac. The following complications occur in rare instances: hemorrhage from penetration of the placenta; infection of the amniotic fluid; puncture of the fetus; and irritation of the uterus, which can initiate labor prematurely.

In preparation for amniocentesis, the woman is asked to void (to reduce the size of the bladder, so that it is out of the field). She lies in a supine position on the examining table and is draped for privacy, but with her abdomen exposed. The position of the fetus

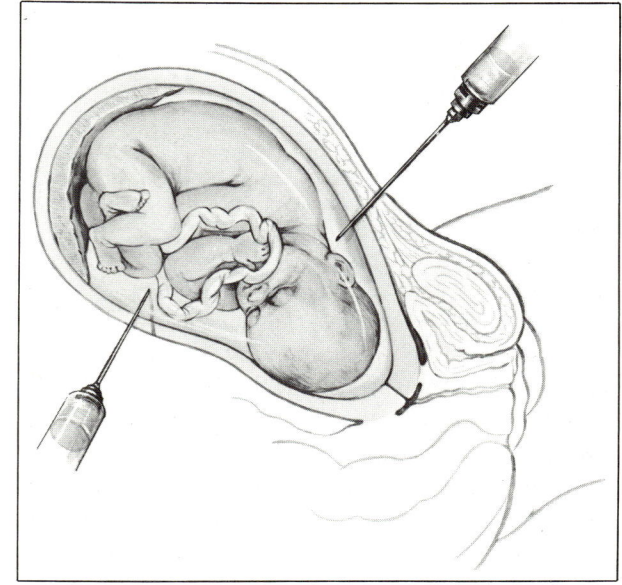

Fig. 13-12. Technique of amniocentesis. The needle is inserted by the back of the neck or by the small body parts to avoid the placenta. (Courtesy of Walter M. Wolfe, M.D., Department of Obstetrics and Gynecology, University of Louisville School of Medicine.)

is determined by palpation and by location of the fetal heart sound. Both the position of the fetus and the placenta may be located by sonogram. The woman's abdomen is washed with an antiseptic solution, and the skin is infiltrated with a local anesthetic, causing momentary pain, since abdominal skin is tender. This is the extent of the pain the woman will experience; she may feel a sensation of pressure as the needle for the actual aspiration is introduced.

As soon as the local anesthetic has taken effect, a 3½-inch 20- or 22-gauge spinal needle is inserted into the abdomen and into the amniotic cavity over the small parts of the fetus or at the back of the fetal neck (Fig. 13-12). This avoids penetrating the fetal trunk, with possible danger to internal organs or penetration of the placenta. A syringe is attached to the needle, and 10 to 20 ml of fluid is withdrawn. The needle is then removed, and the woman rests quietly for a short period. The fetal heart sounds are rechecked, and the woman is assured that they are still of good quality. The amniotic fluid is immediately placed in an opaque container so that if bilirubin pigment is present it will not change composition with light. The fluid is then centrifuged to remove blood particles. The time during pregnancy at which amniocentesis is done depends on the reason it is being done. These times are shown in Table 13-5.

Amniocentesis can reveal information in a number of areas.

Table 13-5. Timing of Amniocentesis Procedures

Chromosome determination	16 weeks
Rh isoimmunization	20–28 weeks
Maturity determination	34–42 weeks
Assessment of fetal well-being	34–42 weeks
Amniography	20–42 weeks

Significance of Color

Normal amniotic fluid is the color of water. A yellow tinge suggests a blood incompatibility (the yellow resulting from the presence of bilirubin released with the hemolysis of red blood cells). A green color suggests meconium staining, traditionally associated with fetal distress, but more precise studies than naked-eye observation are necessary to establish its significance. Meconium staining in amniotic fluid does not always signal fetal distress but is certainly ominous if the fetal heart rate is below 100 or over 170 beats per minute.

Estriol

The amount of amniotic estriol progresses steadily from early pregnancy to term. Late in pregnancy an amniotic fluid level under 100 µg per liter suggests fetal distress.

PCO_2

Acid-base measurements of amniotic fluid provide reliable indications of fetal welfare. Fetal distress from hypoxia results in fetal acidosis due to accumulating PCO_2. The pH of amniotic fluid is greatly reduced (acidotic) following a fetal death.

Creatinine

Creatinine in amniotic fluid is probably contributed by fetal urine. The amount of creatinine increases progressively as pregnancy advances. A value of 2 mg per 100 ml of fluid is a significant indicator of fetal maturity.

Lecithin-Sphingomyelin Ratio

Lecithin is one of the protein components of the lung enzyme surfactant that the alveoli begin to form about the 22nd to 24th weeks of pregnancy. Following amniocentesis, the ratio of lecithin to sphingomyelin may be determined quickly by a shake or bubble test, or sent for laboratory analysis. To do a shake test, amniotic fluid is placed in a test tube, ethanol alcohol is added to it, and the mixture is shaken. If stable bubbles appear, the lecithin-sphingomyelin (L-S) ratio is greater than 2:1 and the pulmonary system is sufficiently mature for birth. If the bubbles are unstable, the L-S ratio is below 2:1—that is, not enough lecithin is present to ensure lung function if the fetus should be delivered at this point.

More accurate information on lecithin production may be accomplished by laboratory analysis. Lecithin is produced by two pathways. In the early weeks of pregnancy, the route of production (the methyl-transferase reaction) is easily interfered with by anoxia or acidosis. The second pathway for lecithin production (the phosphocholine transferase reaction) begins to operate only at about 35 weeks. Usually when the second pathway is fully operative, the fetus is truly ready to be born in terms of lung maturity, as this second pathway is much more stable. Infants of severely involved diabetic mothers may have false mature readings of lecithin because the stress to the infant in utero tends to mature lecithin pathways early. Fetal values must be considered in light of the presence of maternal diabetes, or the infants may be delivered with mature lung function but be immature overall (fragile giants) and so not do well in postnatal life.

Bilirubin Determination

Determining the presence of bilirubin is important when a blood incompatibility is suspected. If the fetal red blood cells are being destroyed by maternal antibodies (as happens with an Rh incompatibility), the massive breakdown of red blood cells will release a great deal of indirect bilirubin into the fetal bloodstream. Indirect bilirubin crosses the placenta and is converted by the maternal liver into direct bilirubin, which is then converted into bile and excreted in maternal stool and urine (see Chap. 38 for a full description of Rh incompatibility physiology). If the fetus has a high level of indirect bilirubin due to abnormal cell breakdown, the fetus itself begins to convert some indirect bilirubin to direct bilirubin and excretes a portion of it as urobilinogen in urine. As urobilinogen-tainted urine is added to the amniotic fluid, the amniotic fluid becomes yellow in color.

The amount of bilirubin present in the amniotic fluid can be analyzed by spectrophotometric analysis. When a monochromatic light is shone on amniotic fluid, the amount of light absorbed depends on the differing amounts of products (bilirubin, protein, uric acid, meconium, etc.) in the fluid. The presence of bilirubin shows a great deal of absorption at 450 mμ wavelength. If the amounts of light absorbed at wavelengths between 350 and 650 mμ are graphed, this dramatic increase in absorption by bilirubin at 450 mμ is called a bulge or lump on the graph. Specimens of amniotic fluid for bilirubin analysis must be blood-free or the oxyhemoglobin of the blood will show a deceptive 450 mμ bulge (a false positive).

Chromosomes

Study of amniotic fluid for chromosome analysis is done early in pregnancy so that if a significant chromosomal abnormality is detected the woman may choose to abort the fetus. The earliest that there is enough amniotic fluid present to ensure a successful tap is 14 weeks. A few fetal skin cells are always present in amniotic fluid. These are the cells to be cultured and stained for chromosomal analysis. It is important that a specimen for chromosome analysis be blood-free, as cells will not grow in bloody fluid. When the cells have grown and are in a mitotic division stage, the stage at which chromosomal contents are best visualized, the cells are stained and examined microscopically. They can be photographed through the microscope, the various chromosome pictures cut out, and the individual chromosomes aligned into a karyotype or chromosome analysis format. The chromosomal diseases that can be detected by prenatal amniocentesis and their significance to health are discussed in Chap. 34.

Inborn Errors of Metabolism

Some inherited diseases that are caused by inborn errors of metabolism can be detected by amniocentesis. In order for a condition to be identified this way, the enzyme defect must be known and must be present in the amniotic fluid as early as 14 to 16 weeks' gestation. Phenylketonuria, for example, a defect that causes serious mental retardation unless the child's diet is carefully controlled, cannot be detected this early in pregnancy because phenylalanine hydroxylase, the defective enzyme, is not present in amniotic fluid this early in pregnancy. Enzyme defects that can be detected in amniotic fluid and their significance to health are also discussed in Chap. 34.

Alpha Fetoprotein

Alpha fetoprotein is produced by the fetal liver. If the fetus has an open spinal cord defect, such as anencephaly or myelomeningocele, alpha fetoprotein will be present in the amniotic fluid because of leakage of cerebrospinal fluid containing the protein into the amniotic fluid. If the defect in the spinal column is fully covered by skin, no alpha fetoprotein will be present in amniotic fluid. Another common method of assessing spinal cord development is by sonogram. Amniography or fetoscopy may also be helpful.

Other Measurements

Amniotic fluid may also be tested for the following: kinds of cells present (the presence of 20 percent heavily fat-laden cells suggests maturity of sebaceous glands); protein levels (there apparently is a decrease in protein values as pregnancy advances); and osmolality (osmolar concentration decreases as pregnancy progresses).

In spite of the slight risk associated with amniocentesis, it appears to be the most accurate method available for predicting the maturity of the fetus and certain aspects of its well-being, such as the presence or absence of a chromosome abnormality.

Women need support during the procedure, since it is intrusive and there are slight risks involved.

FETOSCOPY

Actually visualizing the fetus by inspecting it through a fetoscope (an extremely narrow, hollow tube inserted by amniocentesis technique) is helpful in assessing fetal well-being in some instances. Intactness of the spinal column can be confirmed by this method. Biopsies of fetal tissue and fetal blood samples can be removed through a fetoscope for analysis.

AMNIOGRAPHY

Injection of a contrast medium into the amniotic fluid, followed by x-ray examination, may be done to localize the placenta. A medium such as Ethiodan coats the fetal skin and so will show soft tissue abnormalities such as meningocele on the film. X-rays must always be used with caution during pregnancy because of their known teratogenic effects, so amniography is generally considered a second method of choice to other nonteratogenic approaches.

OXYTOCIN CHALLENGE TEST OR CONTRACTION STRESS TEST

Any woman who is at risk of having uteroplacental insufficiency, as can occur with diabetes mellitus, pregnancy-induced hypertension, or cyanotic heart disease, or who has a history of previous stillbirth, intrauterine growth retardation, or prolonged pregnancy may have an oxytocin challenge test (OCT) to determine whether the fetus is receiving adequate oxygen in utero and to assess whether the fetus will be able to do well during labor.

Women are asked to eat a full meal before they come for an OCT because with a full stomach a fetus is often quieter than otherwise and bowel sounds are quieter. The woman is placed in a semi-Fowler's position (not flat, so hypotension is avoided). A baseline blood pressure and pulse rate are obtained.

OCT tests may be done in pregnancy as early as the 28th week of gestation. External fetal and uterine monitors are placed on the woman's abdomen, and a baseline recording is made for about 10 minutes of uterine activity and fetal baseline heart rate. If there is enough uterine activity (Braxton Hicks contractions) so that a contraction is occurring at a rate of 3 per 10 minutes, a simple rhythm strip test can be done. If contractions are less than this, a dilute intravenous solution of oxytocin will be started until uterine contractions are 3 per 10 minutes.

Normally, a fetal heart rate slows with the beginning of a uterine contraction as the oxygen supply to the fetus is compromised and slight fetal myocardial hypoxia occurs. If the placenta is functioning well, however, as the uterine contraction ends, the fetal heart rate rises immediately to its precontraction level.

A fetal heart rate that dips with the contraction and stays down past the end of the contraction (termed *late deceleration*) is a sign that the placenta is not functioning adequately. An oxytocin challenge test is *positive* if three late decelerations occur in a 10-minute period. The fetus would be compromised to a point of injury during labor, when contractions are much longer and much more frequent than those created here.

A *negative* test denotes that the placenta is adequate and probably will be adequate for at least one more week. Tests may also be interpreted as suspicious (there was some late deceleration, but the pattern was not persistent), hyperstimulation (contractions were so close together than even a fetus with a well-functioning placenta would have late decelerations), or unsatisfactory (for some reason, the monitor recording was not adequate for interpretation).

The woman's blood pressure and pulse rate must be taken every 10 minutes during an OCT to be certain that hypotension is not occurring. The woman can be assured that, although she will have uterine contractions, they will be light enough not to be painful (more of a feeling of pressure). If tetanic contractions occur (contractions coming so close together that there is no room for placenta filling between them), the oxytocin infusion should be turned off immediately, the woman turned on her left side (to free the vena cava and cause a large return of blood to the placenta for better oxygenation), oxygen administered by mask, and a physician notified.

OCTs are contraindicated for women who have a placenta previa (a placenta covering the cervical os), multiple pregnancy, premature rupture of the membranes, incompetent cervix, or a previous classical cesarean section. In these women, the possibility of

Fig. 13-13. A rhythm strip for fetal condition being recorded. A simple rhythm strip can give the same information as an oxytocin challenge test without the risk of infusing oxytocin. (Courtesy of the Department of Medical Photography, Children's Hospital, Buffalo, N.Y.)

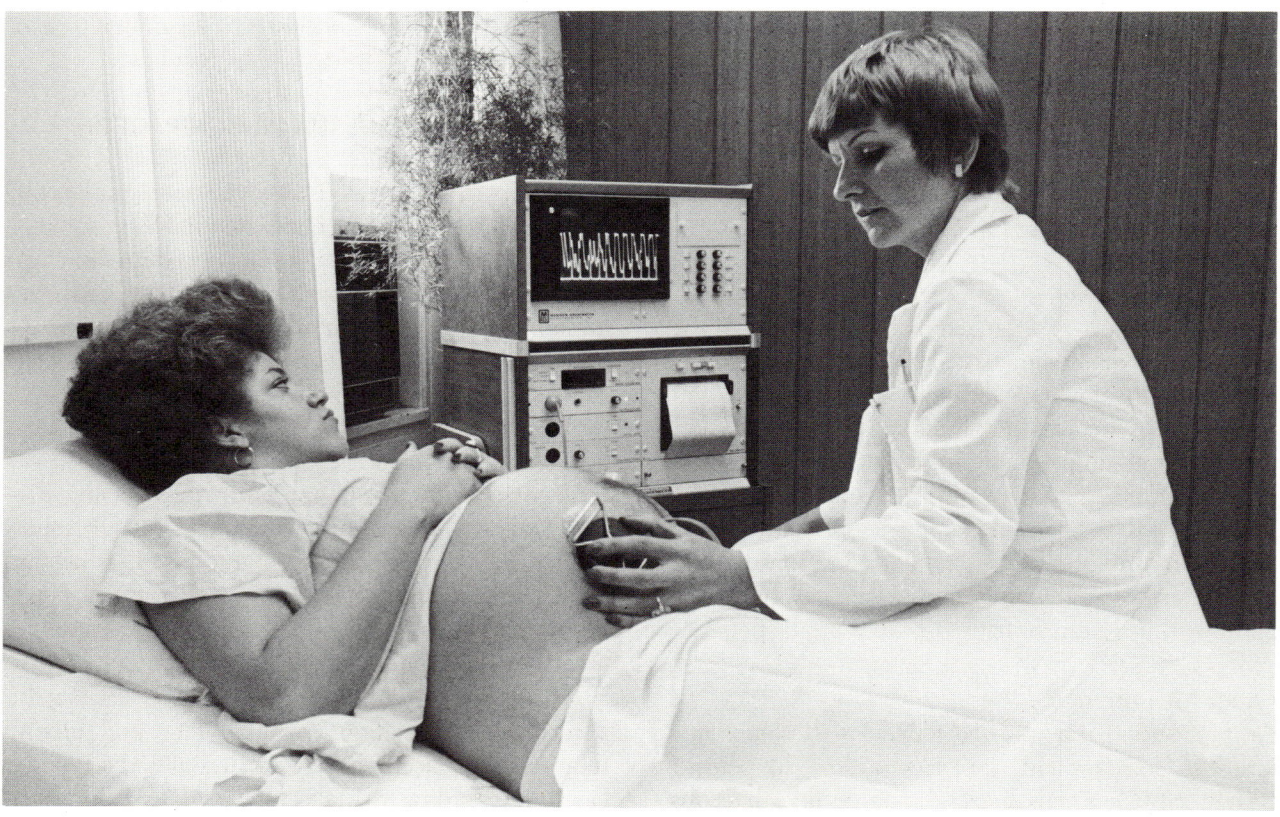

initiating labor by beginning even a dilute solution of oxytocin is too great a risk. The test takes about 2 hours. The uterus and fetal monitors are left in place until uterine contractions have quieted again to 3 or fewer contractions per 10 minutes and there is no danger that the initiation of contractions will lead to labor and delivery with the woman at home.

Oxytocin challenge tests offer a great deal of information about fetal well-being. If the fetus is stressed by this simple exercise, he will not be able to remain in utero safely much longer; plans for delivery will be undertaken. Some infants will be delivered by cesarean section so as not to be stressed by labor; in other cases women may be able to deliver vaginally but must lie in a lateral position during labor (the position that increases blood flow to the placenta) and have oxygen administered by mask during labor.

RHYTHM STRIPS OR NONSTRESS TEST

Because there is some risk in administering oxytocin to cause uterine contractions in that the contractions may not stop again, but go on to become active labor, assessment of the fetus is being done more and more by a simple rhythm strip (Fig. 13-13). Uterine and fetal monitors are attached externally. In many women late in pregnancy there are enough Braxton Hicks contractions present so that the fetal heart rate in connection with these contractions can be analyzed. In pregnant women who do not have natural uterine contractions, the response of the fetal heart rate to fetal movement can be used (a nonstress test). When the fetus is felt to move (place your hand on the woman's abdomen to feel movement), the fetal heart rate should increase, just as anyone's heart rate increases on exercise. It should decrease again at the point you feel the fetus quiet (about 15 seconds). If there is no variability in heart rate to fetal movement, it suggests poor oxygen perfusion, and the fetus is at risk in utero.

A nonstress test is scored as follows:

Reactive: There is fetal heart rate acceleration of 15 beats per minute associated with fetal movement and normal baseline fetal heart rate variability of 6 beats per minute or greater.
Nonreactive: There are no fetal heart rate accelerations or inadequate acceleration (under 15 beats per minute) or there is low fetal heart rate variability (under 6 beats per minute) throughout the testing period.
Sinusoidal: There is a smooth undulating fetal heart rate pattern with a frequency of oscillations of 2 to 5 per minute and an amplitude of 5 to 10 beats per minute. The meaning of a sinusoidal pattern is unclear.
Unsatisfactory: The tracing is not satisfactory for interpretation.

In order for a tracing to be interpreted it is generally accepted that there must be at least four fetal movements present.

Fetal assessment, once limited to listening to fetal heartbeats by an ordinary stethoscope, has progressed greatly in recent years. Waiting for test results on fetal well-being is a very stressful time for a woman. She needs support from health care personnel during the time she has to wait for results and at a time she must be given less than favorable news about her unborn child.

Problem-oriented Recording: Progress Notes

Christine McFadden
15 years
Gestation length: 16 weeks approx. (LMP unknown)

Problem: Fetal assessment

> S. No radiation, medications, spotting since LMP. Unsure of date of LMP (about 16 weeks). Has been diving on school team from high board with 2 "wrong dives" hitting abdomen hard against water. Now no longer diving.
> Nonsmoker, no alcohol consumption. Evasive about usual use of marijuana. None since she thought she might be pregnant.
> O. Uterine height 4 cm above symphysis.
> Fetal heart tones by Doppler at 150.
> A. Uterine height consistent with 16-week pregnancy.
> Fetal heart tones within normal limits.
>
> Goals: a. Take no nonprescribed medication during pregnancy.
> b. Keep sports activities to sensible levels.
> c. Carry pregnancy to term.
>
> P. 1. Schedule for sonogram for estimation of pregnancy length (LMP not known).
> 2. Caution about medication, drug and alcohol use during pregnancy.

3. Abdominal trauma no problem now; has stopped school diving. Caution to phone clinic for advice if in doubt about what is appropriate sports activity.

Problem-oriented Recording: Progress Notes

Mary Kraft
22 years
Gestation length: 9 weeks

Problem: Fetal assessment

S. No radiation, spotting since LMP. Heavy smoker—2 packs/day. Alcohol—1–2 martinis/day.
Takes Sudafed, 60 mg daily for "sinus headache."
Had one prev. pregnancy, ending in spont. abortion (no known cause) 2 years ago.

O. Uterine height, not palpable above symphysis.
No fetal heart sounds by Doppler.

A. Fetal threat present due to level of alcohol and smoking abuse.

Goals: a. Decrease smoking to below 10 cigarettes daily.
b. Limit alcohol consumption to 1 oz daily.
c. Carry pregnancy to term.

P. 1. Refer to M.D. for evaluation of safety of sinus medication during pregnancy.
2. Urge to quit smoking or decrease number of cigarettes smoked per day to under 10.
3. Urge to decrease alcohol consumption to 1 oz daily.
4. Sonogram scheduled for fetal growth evaluation because of heavy smoking.

Problem-oriented Recording: Progress Notes

Angie Baco
42 years
Gestation length: 12 weeks

Problem: Fetal assessment

S. No medication except aspirin gr. 10, 2 days ago, for headache.
No spotting, falls, radiation since LMP. Nonsmoker. Alcohol consumption, 2 beers/month.
States she doesn't want amniocentesis done for genetic studies (aware that she is high-risk for Down's syndrome) as she would not abort in any event.
Had gestational diabetes with last pregnancy; no symptoms present here yet. Last child weighed 9 lb 3 oz at birth.

O. Uterine height, barely palpable above symphysis.
Heart tones by Doppler 130.

A. Uterine growth comparable with 12-week pregnancy.
No symptoms of gestational diabetes yet.

Goals: a. Take no nonprescribed drugs during pregnancy.
b. If gestational diabetes occurs, observe diet, insulin, urine testing program to bring pregnancy to term.

P. 1. Schedule for glucose tolerance test next week to assess possibility of gestational diabetes with this pregnancy.
2. No amniocentesis scheduled as per patient preference.
3. Mark chart as high-risk for genetic interference (mother 42 years of age).
Possible large size (last pregnancy 9 lb 3 oz).
History of gestational diabetes and congenital heart disease in past pregnancies.
4. Caution about medication, alcohol consumption during pregnancy.

References

1. Bahr, J. E. Rising perinatal infections: Herpes virus hominis type 2 in women and newborns. *M.C.N.* 3:16, 1978.
2. Berger, G. S., et al. Fetal crown-rump length and biparietal diameter in the 2nd trimester of pregnancy. *Am. J. Obstet. Gynecol.* 122:9, 1975.
3. Bolognese, R., and Schwartz, R. H. *Perinatal Medicine*. Baltimore: Williams & Wilkins, 1977.
4. Bross, I. D., and Netarajan, N. Genetic damage from diagnostic radiation. *J.A.M.A.* 237:2399, 1977.
5. Broussard, P. M. The Oxytocin Challenge Test. In L. K. McNall and J. T. Galeener (Eds.). *Current Practice in Obstetric and Gynecologic Nursing*. St. Louis: Mosby, 1976.
6. Brown, S. G. The devastating effects of congenital rubella. *M.C.N.* 4:171, 1979.
7. Butnarescu, G. F. *Perinatal Nursing*. New York: Wiley, 1978.
8. Campbell, J. A. (Ed.). *Obstetric Diagnosis by Radiographic, Ultrasonic, and Nuclear Methods*. Baltimore: Williams & Wilkins, 1977.
9. de Vlieger, M. (Ed.). *Handbook of Clinical Ultrasound*. New York: Wiley, 1978.
10. Feldman, G. L. The fetal trimethadione syndrome. *Am. J. Dis. Child.* 131:1389, 1977.
11. Giacoia, G., and Yaffe, S. Drugs and the Perinatal Patient. In G. Avery (Ed.). *Neonatology*. Philadelphia: Lippincott, 1975.
12. Gordis, E., and Kreek, M. J. Alcoholism and drug addiction in pregnancy. *Curr. Pract. Obstet. Gynecol.* 1:5, 1977.
13. Gravida's smoking seen handicap to offspring. Editorial. *Obstet. Gynecol. News* 5:12, 1970.
14. Gullekson, D. J., et al. Maternal drug use during the perinatal period. *Fam. Community Health* 1:31, 1978.
15. Hanson, J. W., et al. Fetal alcohol syndrome experience with 41 patients. *J.A.M.A.* 235:1458, 1976.
16. Hill, R. M. Drugs that an unborn baby can't tolerate. *R.N.* 40:35, 1977.
17. Hill, R. M., et al. Utilization of over-the-counter drugs during pregnancy. *Clin. Obstet. Gynecol.* 20:381, 1977.
18. Kantor, G. K. Addicted mother, addicted baby—a challenge to health care providers. *M.C.N.* 3:281, 1978.
19. Ledger, W. J. Antibiotics in pregnancy. *Clin. Obstet. Gynecol.* 20:411, 1977.
20. Luke, B. Maternal alcoholism and the fetal alcohol syndrome. *Am. J. Nurs.* 77:1924, 1977.
21. Meyer, M. B. How does maternal smoking affect birth weight and maternal weight gain? *Am. J. Obstet. Gynecol.* 131:888, 1978.
22. Miskin, M., et al. Ultrasound in Prenatal Genetic Diagnosis. In D. White (Ed.). *Ultrasound in Medicine*. New York: Plenum Press, 1975.
23. Miyamoto, A. T. Diagnostic Ultrasound in Obstetrics. In J. A. Campbell (Ed.). *Obstetrical Diagnosis by Radiographic, Ultrasonic and Nuclear Methods*. Baltimore: Williams & Wilkins, 1977.
24. Moore, K. L. *The Developing Human: Clinically Oriented Embryology* (2nd ed.). Philadelphia: Saunders, 1977.
25. Neeson, J. D. Herpes virus genitalis: A nursing perspective. *Nurs. Clin. North Am.* 10:599, 1975.
26. Noller, K. L., et al. Identification, examination and management of diethylstilbestrol-exposed offspring. *Clin. Obstet. Gynecol.* 19:699, 1976.
27. Pitkin, R. M. Risks Related to Nutritional Problems in Pregnancy. In S. Aladjem (Ed.). *Risks in the Practice of Modern Obstetrics*. St. Louis: Mosby, 1975.
28. Smith, D. W. Teratogenicity of anticonvulsive medications. *Am. J. Dis. Child.* 131:1337, 1977.
29. Sokol, R. J., et al. Maternal-fetal risk assessment: A clinical guide to monitoring. *Clin. Obstet. Gynecol.* 22:547, 1980.
30. Stewart, A., and Kneale, G. W. Radiation dose effects in relation to obstetric x-rays and childhood cancers. *Lancet* 1:1185, 1970.
31. Taft, L. T. Child development: Prenatal to early childhood. *J. Sch. Health* 48:281, 1978.
32. Thompson, H. W., et al. Fetal development as determined by ultrasonic pulse echo techniques. *Am. J. Obstet. Gynecol.* 92:44, 1965.
33. Wallis, S., et al. Intrauterine infection of the fetus. *Nurs. Times* 74:912, 1978.
34. Weiss, R. N., et al. Origin of amniotic fluid alpha-feto-protein in normal and defective pregnancies. *Obstet. Gynecol.* 47:697, 1976.

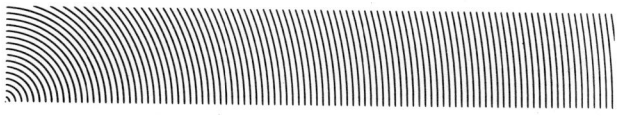

14. Physiological Changes in Pregnancy

The physiological changes of pregnancy affect all organ systems of the woman's body. They are temporary, for the duration of the pregnancy, and at the end of pregnancy the woman returns virtually to her prepregnant state. These changes enable her to provide oxygen and nutrients for the growing fetus and extra nutrients for her own increased metabolism. They ready her body for labor and delivery, and for lactation if she chooses to breast-feed her baby.

Local Changes
UTERUS

The most obvious alteration in the woman's body during pregnancy is the increase in the size of her uterus that is necessary to accommodate the growing fetus. Over the 10 lunar months of pregnancy, the uterus increases in length from approximately 6.5 cm to 32 cm; in depth, from 2.5 cm to 22 cm; and in width, from 4 cm to 24 cm. Its weight increases from 50 to 1,000 gm. At the beginning of pregnancy the uterine wall is about 1 cm thick, and its cavity is barely large enough to hold 2 ml. The wall first hypertrophies and thickens to about 2 cm. Then it begins to thin, so that by the end of pregnancy it is about 0.5 cm thick and very supple. At term the uterus can hold a 7-pound fetus plus 1,000 ml of amniotic fluid, a total of about 4,000 gm.

This great uterine growth is due to development of the decidua and formation of a few new muscle fibers, but the increase in capacity is principally due to the stretching of existing muscle fibers. By the end of pregnancy, muscle fibers in the uterus are two to seven times longer than they were pregestationally. The uterus is able to withstand this stretching of its muscle fibers because of the formation of extra fibroelastic tissue between fibers, which bind them close together.

At the end of the 12th week of pregnancy the growing uterus is large enough to be palpated as a firm spheroid on the abdominal wall above the symphysis pubis. An important factor in uterine growth is its constant, steady, predictable increase in size. By the 20th or 22nd week of pregnancy it reaches the level of the umbilicus. By the 36th week it touches the xyphoid process and makes breathing difficult for the woman. About two weeks before term in a primigravida (a woman in her first pregnancy), the fetal head settles into the pelvis preparatory to delivery, and the uterus returns to its height at 32 weeks. This is called *lightening*, because the easier breathing pattern seems to lighten the woman's load. When lightening will occur is not predictable in women who

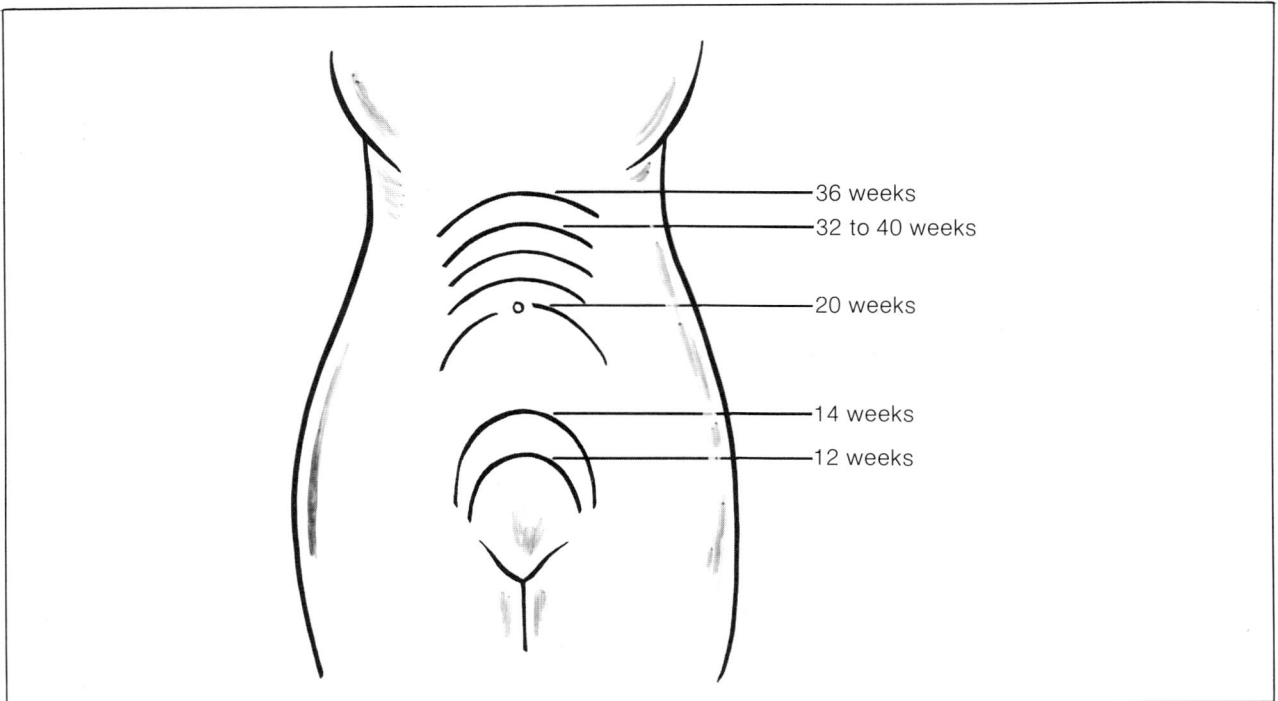

Fig. 14-1. Fundus height at various lunar months of pregnancy.

have had one or more children. In these women it may not be felt until the morning of delivery.

The fundus of the uterus usually remains in the midline during pregnancy, although it may be pushed slightly to the right side because of the larger bulk of the sigmoid colon on the left. The changes in fundus height during pregnancy are shown in Fig. 14-1.

As the uterus increases in size, it pushes intestine to the sides of the abdomen and elevates the diaphragm at term. The slender woman may worry that there is not room inside her abdomen for the uterus to increase in size as it should and her baby will feel crowded. She can be assured that abdominal contents can be shifted readily to accommodate the size of the uterus (Fig. 14-2).

CERVIX

During pregnancy, the cervix of the uterus becomes more vascular and edematous. The cervical glands undergo hyperplasia as they distend with mucus, and mucus plugs or obliterates the cervical canal. This mucous plug, the *operculum*, seals out bacteria during pregnancy and helps prevent infection in the fetus and membranes.

The consistency of a nonpregnant cervix may be compared to that of the nose. The changes of pregnancy cause a softening, so that the consistency of a pregnant cervix more closely resembles that of an earlobe. This softening is one of the diagnostic signs of pregnancy. Just prior to beginning labor the cervix might be described as having the consistency of butter; it is "ripe" for delivery.

VAGINA

An increase in the vascularity of the vagina, beginning early in pregnancy, parallels the vascular changes in the uterus. The resulting increase in circulation changes the color of the vagina from its normal light pink to a deep violet. The vaginal epithelium and underlying tissue become hypertrophic in preparation for great distention at birth. This increase in the activity of the epithelial cells results in a white vaginal discharge throughout pregnancy.

The secretions of the vagina during pregnancy have a pH of 4 or 5 (due to an increased lactic acid content) and therefore are resistant to bacterial invasion. The change in pH unfortunately favors the growth of *Candida albicans*, a species of yeast-like fungi. A candidal infection is manifested by an itching, burning sensation in addition to the discharge. A nonpregnant woman needs medication for such an infection to relieve discomfort. A pregnant woman needs medication not only to relieve discomfort but to prevent transmission of the infection to the infant as he passes through the birth canal at term. Candidal infection is manifested as *thrush* in the infant.

Many women are reluctant to tell a physician that they have an infection in this part of their body.

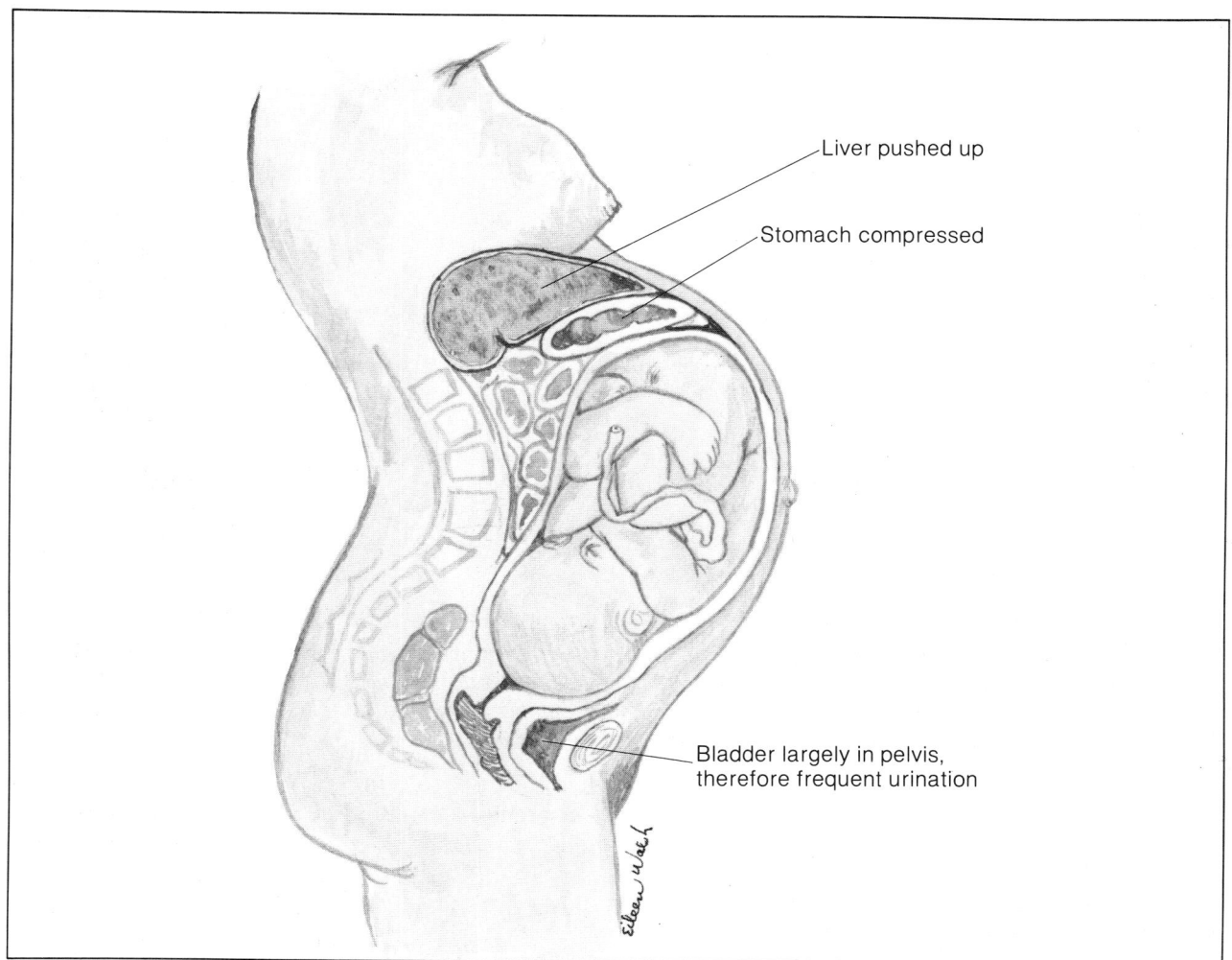

Fig. 14-2. Crowding of abdominal contents late in pregnancy.

Therefore, it should be a nursing responsibility to inquire whether any symptoms of this nature exist.

OVARIES

Ovulation stops with pregnancy, as does menstruation, because of lack of activity of follicle-stimulating hormone. The corpus luteum increases in size on the surface of the ovary until about the 24th week of pregnancy, when the placenta takes over the chief function of providing progesterone and estrogen and the corpus luteum is no longer essential for the continuation of the pregnancy.

ABDOMINAL WALL

As the uterus increases in size, the abdominal wall must stretch to accommodate it. This stretching (and possibly increased adrenal cortex activity) causes rupture and atrophy of the connective layer of the skin, and pink or reddish streaks (striae gravidarum) usually appear on the sides of the abdominal wall and sometimes on the thighs (Fig. 14-3). In the weeks following delivery, the striae gravidarum lighten to a silvery-white color (striae albicantes or atrophicae) and are barely noticeable.

Occasionally, the abdominal wall cannot stretch enough, and the rectus muscles are actually separated, a condition known as *diastasis*, which will be manifested after pregnancy as a bluish groove at the site of separation.

The umbilicus is stretched by pregnancy to the extent that by the 28th week it is usually pushed so far outward that its depression becomes obliterated and smooth. In some women it tends to appear as if it has turned inside out and protrudes as a round bump at the center of the abdominal wall.

INTEGUMENTARY CHANGES

In addition to the striae gravidarum that appear on the abdominal wall, there are other skin changes with pregnancy.

Extra pigmentation generally appears on the ab-

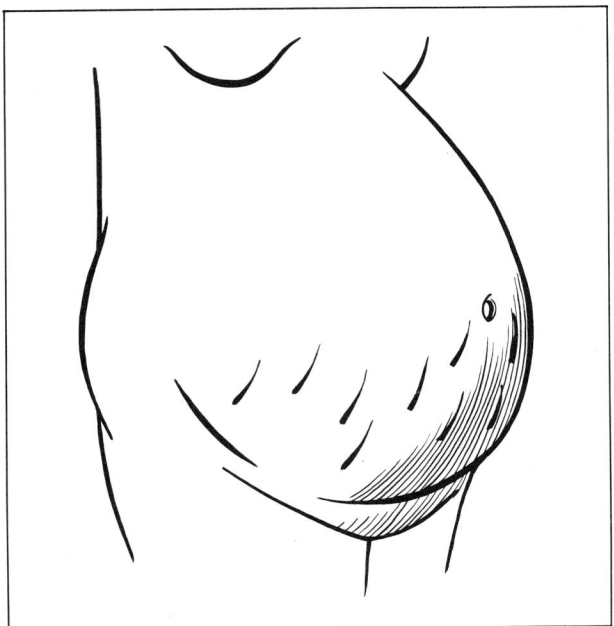

Fig. 14-3. Striae gravidarum. In the later months of pregnancy, reddish, slightly depressed streaks often develop in the skin of the abdomen and sometimes of the breasts and thighs. Following pregnancy, these fade to glistening silvery lines.

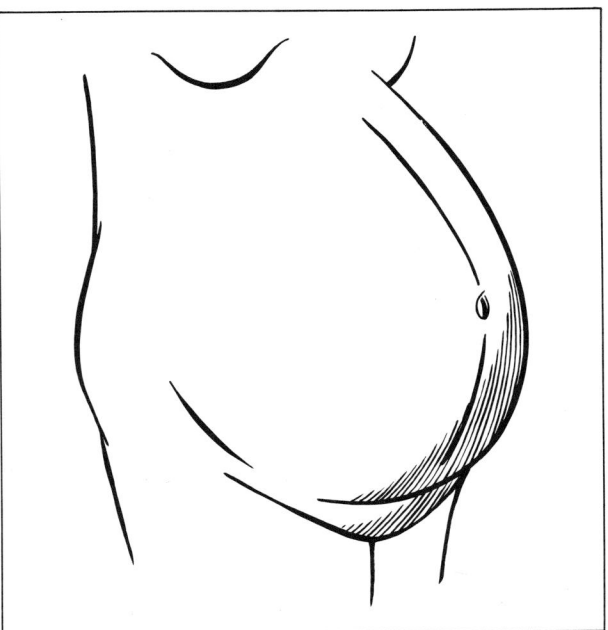

Fig. 14-4. Linea nigra. In many pregnancies, the abdominal skin at the midline becomes markedly pigmented, assuming a brownish-black color.

dominal wall. A brown line (linea nigra) may be present, running from the umbilicus to the symphysis pubis and separating the abdomen into a right and left hemisphere (Fig. 14-4). Darkened brown areas may appear on the face, particularly on the cheeks and across the nose. This is known as *melasma* (chloasma) or the "mask of pregnancy." The increases in pigmentation are due to melanocyte-stimulating hormone (MSH), secreted by the hypophysis (pituitary). With the fall in the level of the hormone after pregnancy, the areas lighten and disappear.

Vascular spiders (small, fiery-red branching spots) are sometimes seen on the skin of pregnant women, particularly on the thighs. These probably result from the increased level of estrogen in the body.

There is an increase in the activity of sweat glands throughout the body. This may be manifested as an increase in perspiration that can become annoying in its extent by the end of pregnancy.

BREAST CHANGES

Subtle changes in the breasts may be one of the first physiological changes of pregnancy the woman notices. She may experience a feeling of fullness or tingling, due to the increased stimulation of estrogen in the body. As pregnancy progresses, the breast size increases because of hyperplasia of the mammary alveoli and fat deposits. The areola of the nipple darkens in color and its diameter increases from about 3.5 to 5 or 7.5 cm (1½ to 2 or 3 inches). There is darkening of the skin surrounding the areola in some women, forming a secondary areola. As vascularity of the breasts increases, blue veins may become prominent over the surface. The sebaceous glands of the areola (Montgomery's glands) enlarge and become protuberant.

Early in pregnancy the breasts begin readying themselves for the secretion of milk. By the 16th week, *colostrum*, a thin, watery, high-protein fluid and the precursor of breast milk, may be expelled from the nipples.

Systemic Changes

Although the physiological changes the woman notices first and finds most interesting are those of the reproductive system and breasts, changes occur in almost all body systems.

RESPIRATORY SYSTEM

The increased level of progesterone during pregnancy appears to set a new level in the hypothalamus for acceptable blood carbon dioxide levels (PCO_2), as during pregnancy a woman's body tends to maintain a partial pressure of CO_2 at closer to 32 mm Hg than the normal 40 mm Hg.

This low PCO_2 level in the mother causes a favorable CO_2 gradient at the placenta (the fetal CO_2 level is higher than that in the mother), so CO_2 crosses readily from the fetus to the mother.

To keep the mother's pH level from becoming acidotic from the load of CO_2 shifted to her by the fetus, increased ventilation (mild hyperventilation) to blow off carbon dioxide begins early in pregnancy. Ventilation capacity rises by as much as 40 percent by term. The increased ventilation may be so extreme that the woman develops a respiratory alkalosis. To compensate for this, plasma bicarbonate is excreted by the kidneys in larger than normal amounts. With greater urine output, additional sodium is lost and therefore additional water. The effect is *polyuria*, an early sign of pregnancy.

The change in CO_2 level and the compensating mechanisms can be described as a chronic respiratory alkalosis fully compensated by a chronic metabolic acidosis.

As the uterus enlarges during pregnancy, a great deal of pressure is put on the diaphragm and ultimately on the lungs. The diaphragm may be displaced by as much as 1 inch upward. This crowding of the chest cavity causes an acute sensation of shortness of breath late in pregnancy, until lightening relieves the pressure.

Even with all the other respiratory changes happening, vital capacity (the maximum volume exhaled following a maximal inspiration) of the woman does not change during pregnancy. Although lungs are crowded in the vertical dimension, they can expand horizontally, and the woman expands her rib cage further with each inspiration. Residual volume (the amount of air remaining in the lungs following expiration) is decreased by the pressure of the diaphragm. Tidal volume (the volume of air inspired) is increased as the woman draws in extra volume to increase the effectiveness of air exchange.

The net effect of these respiratory changes is often felt by the woman as a chronic shortness of breath. She needs to take a deep breath periodically or sit down to "catch her breath." She waits for her breathing rate to slow in a sitting position. It does not. Women need a clear explanation that a breathing rate more rapid than normal (18 to 20 breaths per minute) is physiological for pregnancy and the way things should be. When you are taking vital signs on pregnant women you also should remember that the respiratory rate is normally elevated.

The slight increase in pH due to the increased expiratory effort slightly increases the binding capacity of maternal hemoglobin and so the oxygen content of

Table 14-1. Respiratory Changes During Pregnancy

Vital capacity	No change
Tidal volume	Increased
Respiratory rate	Increased
Residual volume	Decreased
Plasma PCO_2	Decreased
Plasma pH	Increased
Plasma PO_2	Increased

maternal blood (the level of PO_2) rises from a normal level of about 92 mm Hg to a level of 106 mm Hg early in pregnancy.

Changes in respiratory function during pregnancy are summarized in Table 14-1.

Another change that often occurs in the respiratory system is marked congestion or "stuffiness" of the nasopharynx, a response to increased estrogen levels. Women may worry that this stuffiness indicates an allergy or a cold. Some women take over-the-counter cold medications or antihistamines to try to relieve the congestion before they realize that they are pregnant. Some continue to take the medication, not mentioning it to their physician because they think it is a separate problem and not pregnancy-related. Asking a woman at prenatal visits if she is taking any kind of medicine or if she has noticed or been bothered by nasal stuffiness is a nursing responsibility.

TEMPERATURE

Early in pregnancy there is a slight increase in temperature, because of the activity of the corpus luteum (the temperature elevation that marked ovulation is sustained). As placental function is substituted for that of the corpus luteum at about 16 weeks, the temperature generally decreases to normal.

Some women associate this slight rise in temperature (99.6°F orally) together with the nasal congestion of pregnancy as a sure sign that they have a cold and need medication for it.

CIRCULATORY SYSTEM
Blood Volume

To provide for an adequate exchange of nutrients in the placenta and for blood to compensate for blood loss at delivery, the circulatory blood volume of the woman's body increases at least 30 percent (possibly as much as 50 percent) in pregnancy. The increase is gradual, beginning by the end of the first trimester. It reaches its peak at about the 20th to the 24th week and continues at this high level through the last trimester.

As the plasma volume first increases, the concentration of hemoglobin and erythrocytes may decline, giving the woman a pseudoanemia. The woman's body compensates for this change by producing more red blood cells, so that the concentration of red blood cells reaches normal levels again.

Almost all women need some iron supplementation during pregnancy; they usually have comparatively low iron stores (less than 500 mg) because of their monthly menstrual loss. The fetus requires about 350 to 400 mg of iron in order to grow. The increases in the circulatory maternal red cell mass require an additional 400 mg of iron. This is a total increased need of about 800 mg. As the average woman's store of iron is less than this, she should take in additional iron during pregnancy or she will develop a true anemia.

A hemoglobin concentration less than 10.5 gm per 100 ml, or a hematocrit value below 30 percent, is generally considered a true anemia for which iron therapy above normal supplementation is advocated.

The increase in blood volume helps not only to better the performance of the placenta but to compensate for blood loss at delivery. Blood loss for a normal vaginal delivery is about 300 to 400 ml. Blood loss from a cesarean section is higher, about 800 to 1,000 ml.

In order to handle the increase in blood volume in the circulating system, a woman's cardiac output increases significantly, by 25 to 50 percent, heart rate by 10 beats per minute. Like the circulating volume increase, the bulk of the cardiac work increase occurs during the first trimester, a small amount occurring in the last trimester. This rise in circulating load has implications for the woman with cardiac disease. A woman whose heart has difficulty moving her normal circulating load may be overwhelmed by the requirements placed on it by pregnancy. The average woman's heart has great ability to adjust to these changes, however. Although significant changes are occurring inside her related to her circulatory system, she is not even aware that they are happening.

Because the diaphragm is elevated by the growing uterus late in pregnancy, the heart is shifted to a more transverse position in the chest cavity. The heart may then appear enlarged on x-ray examination. Some women have audible functional (innocent) heart murmurs during pregnancy, probably on account of the altered heart position.

During the last trimester of pregnancy, blood flow to the lower extremities is impaired by the pressure of the expanding uterus on veins and arteries, which slows circulation. This decrease in blood flow in the venous system leads to edema and varicosities of the vulva, rectum, and legs.

Palpitations

Palpitations of the heart are not uncommon, particularly on quick motion, during pregnancy. A woman should be warned that palpitations may occur, so that she will not be frightened when they do. Palpitations in the early months of pregnancy are probably due to sympathetic nervous system stimulation; in later months, they may result from increased thoracic pressure caused by pressure of the uterus against the diaphragm.

Blood Pressure

Despite the hypervolemia of pregnancy, the blood pressure does not normally rise, as the increased heart action takes care of the greater amount of circulating blood.

In many women blood pressure decreases slightly during the second trimester because of the lowered peripheral resistance in the woman's circulation, which is due to the rapidly expanding placenta. During the third trimester, blood pressure rises again to first-trimester levels.

Determining normal blood pressure in pregnant women is as difficult as it is in the population at large. Average blood pressures for adult women are shown in Table 14-2. During pregnancy, a mean arterial pressure of 90 mm Hg or more in the midtrimester is an ominous sign. A mean arterial pressure above 105

Table 14-2. *Average Blood Pressures in American Females*

		White Women		Black Women	
	Age	Average (mm Hg)	S.D.	Average (mm Hg)	S.D.
Systolic	Under 20	111.0	13.7	112.7	13.2
	20–29	116.9	13.8	119.1	14.7
	30–39	121.4	16.3	128.1	20.2
	40–49	129.3	19.6	138.3	22.8
Diastolic	Under 20	69.3	9.8	70.0	10.1
	20–29	73.7	7.2	75.4	9.7
	30–39	76.9	10.7	82.0	13.0
	40–49	80.6	11.6	86.9	13.9

S.D. = standard deviation.
Source. Adapted from J. Stamler et al., Hypertension screening of one million Americans. J.A.M.A. 235:2299, 1976. Copyright 1976, American Medical Association.

mm Hg in the third trimester is generally regarded as hypertension.

To determine a mean arterial pressure, subtract the woman's diastolic reading from the systolic reading. This difference is the *pulse pressure*. Divide the pulse pressure by one-third and add that number to the diastolic pressure. If a woman's blood pressure is 120 over 70, for example, her pulse pressure is 50 (120 − 70). One-third of 50 is 16.6. Adding 16.6 to the diastolic reading (70) gives a mean arterial pressure of 86.6, which is a normal mean arterial pressure for a pregnant woman.

If a woman's blood pressure is 140 over 80, her pulse pressure is 60 (140 − 80). One-third of 60 is 20. Adding 20 to the diastolic reading (80) gives a mean arterial pressure of 100, which is ominously high for a pregnant woman.

The Roll-over Test

When one turns from a prone position to a supine position, the blood pressure usually falls. Interestingly, if a woman is about to develop hypertension of pregnancy, her blood pressure will show an increase when she turns from a side-lying position to a supine position. Many physicians include roll-over tests as part of routine health surveillance during pregnancy. This is a simple test that can be done by a nurse (directions are given in Chap. 17). It can be helpful in isolating women who will develop hypertension of pregnancy (one of the three commonest causes of maternal mortality in pregnancy) before clinical symptoms become apparent. Preventive measures to stop the blood pressure from rising can then be instituted.

Blood Constitution

The level of circulating fibrinogen, a constituent of the blood necessary for clotting, increases during pregnancy, probably because of the increased level of estrogen. This is a safeguard against major bleeding should the placenta be dislodged and the uterine arteries or veins open. Total white cell count rises slightly, probably as both a protective mechanism and a reflection of the woman's total blood volume. The total protein level of blood decreases, perhaps reflecting the amount of protein needed by the fetus. Because the circulating system has a lowered total protein load, fluid will readily leave the intravascular spaces to equalize osmotic pressure. Hence the very common ankle and foot edema of pregnancy (not to be confused with nondependent edema, which is a symptom of pregnancy-induced hypertension).

Table 14-3. Changes in the Cardiovascular System During Pregnancy

	Prepregnancy	Pregnancy
Cardiac output		25–50% increase
Heart rate		10 beats/min increase
Plasma volume (ml)	2,600	3,600
Blood volume (ml)	4,000	5,250
Red cell mass (cu mm)	4,200,000	4,650,000
Leukocytes (cu mm)	7,000	10,500
Total protein (gm %)	7.0	5.5–6.0
Fibrinogen (mg %)	300	450
Blood pressure		Decreases in second trimester; at prepregnancy level in third trimester

Changes in the cardiovascular system during pregnancy are summarized in Table 14-3.

GASTROINTESTINAL SYSTEM

As the uterus increases in size, it tends to displace the stomach and intestines toward the back and sides of the abdomen. At about the midpoint of pregnancy, the pressure may be sufficient to slow intestinal peristalsis and the emptying time of the stomach, leading to heartburn, constipation, and flatulence. Relaxin, a hormone produced by the ovary, may contribute to decreased gastric motility; so may the decrease in blood supply to the gastrointestinal tract (blood is drawn to the uterus). Progesterone, also, has an effect on smooth muscle, making it less active.

Nausea is one of the first sensations the woman may experience with pregnancy (sometimes before the first missed menstrual period). This is most apparent early in the morning, on rising, or when she becomes fatigued during the day. Known as *morning sickness*, it is probably a systemic reaction to decreased glucose levels, glucose being utilized in great quantities by the growing fetus, and to increased estrogen levels.

The nausea subsides after the first three months, and the woman may acquire a voracious appetite. Although the acidity of the stomach secretion decreases during pregnancy, heartburn may result from the reflux of stomach contents into the esophagus, because of the displaced position of the stomach and the relaxed cardioesophageal sphincter.

Decreased emptying of bile from the gallbladder may result in reabsorption of bilirubin into the maternal bloodstream, giving rise to symptoms of generalized itching (subclinical jaundice). A woman with previous gall stone formation may have an increased tendency to stone formation during pregnancy. Women with peptic ulcer generally find their condition improved during pregnancy because the acidity of the stomach is decreased.

Some women notice hypertrophy at their gumlines and bleeding of gingival tissue when they brush their teeth. This is probably a local response to increased levels of estrogen. It is annoying but not a serious problem.

Our grandmothers expected to lose a tooth a pregnancy, as a growing fetus requires so much calcium to make bones. If a woman ingests a good diet during pregnancy, including a quart of milk a day or a calcium supplement if she cannot drink milk, this becomes an old wives' tale. Some women do not go to the dentist during pregnancy because they are afraid that he will want to take an x-ray film and this will harm their growing baby. Lack of dental care can be very damaging to teeth. Women can have dental x-ray examinations during pregnancy, provided their abdomen is protected with a lead apron. Dental care should be continued during pregnancy the same as any other time in life. Before extensive dental work involving a local anesthetic or nitrous oxide inhalation is done, however, the woman should consult her obstetrician.

URINARY SYSTEM

During pregnancy, the kidneys must excrete not only the waste products of the woman's body but those of the growing fetus as well. Thus, urinary output gradually increases and specific gravity decreases during pregnancy.

Occasionally, a trace of albumin will be present in urine, due to congestion in renal capillaries. Glomerular filtration rate (GFR) and renal plasma flow are both most effective when a person lies in a lateral recumbent position (on the side). Women should be advised to rest and sleep in this position during pregnancy in order to assist the kidneys to function most efficiently.

Both the glomerular filtration rate and the renal plasma flow increase 30 to 50 percent. The rise is consistent with that of the circulatory system increase, peaking at about 24 weeks. This efficient GFR level leads to a lowered blood urea nitrogen (BUN) and low creatinine levels in maternal plasma. A BUN of 15 mg per 100 ml or higher and a creatinine over 1 mg per 100 ml are considered abnormal and reflect kidney difficulty in handling the increased blood load. The higher GFR leads to increased filtration of glucose into the renal tubules. Because reabsorption of glucose by the tubal cells occurs at a fixed rate, there will be some accidental spilling of glucose into urine during pregnancy. Lactose, the sugar of breast milk, which is being produced by the mammary glands but is not utilized during pregnancy, will also be spilled into the urine.

Although some spilling of glucose may occur, the finding of glucose in a routine sample of urine from a pregnant woman is considered abnormal until proved otherwise, as it can be a sign of gestational diabetes (see Chap. 33).

To differentiate what sugar is spilling into urine, a test material for urine analysis specific for glucose (Tes-Tape) must be used. A urine test method which is positive for all sugars (Benedict's solution) will give false positives as it will report the presence of the harmless lactose as well.

The ureters increase in diameter in order to accommodate the greater urine flow. Bladder capacity increases to about 1,500 ml. The uterus tends to rise in the right side of the abdomen, since it is pushed slightly in that direction by the greater bulk of the sigmoid colon. The consequent pressure on the right ureter may result in urine stasis and pyelonephritis if it is not relieved.

The woman may notice urinary frequency the first three months of pregnancy until the uterus rises out of the pelvis and relieves pressure on the bladder. Frequency of urination may return at the end of pregnancy as lightening occurs and the fetal head exerts pressure on the bladder once more.

Changes in the urinary tract during pregnancy are summarized in Table 14-4.

SKELETAL SYSTEM

As pregnancy advances, there is a gradual softening of the pelvic ligaments and joints to allow for pliability

Table 14-4. Urinary Tract Changes During Pregnancy

Glomerular filtration rate	Increased
Renal plasma flow	Increased
Blood urea nitrogen	Decreased
Plasma creatinine level	Decreased
Renal threshold for sugar	Decreased
Bladder capacity	Increased
Diameter of ureters	Increased
Frequency of urination	Present first trimester, last two weeks of pregnancy

and to facilitate passage of the baby through the pelvis at the time of delivery. This is probably due to the influence of the ovarian hormone *relaxin*. Excessive mobility of the joints may cause discomfort, and a wide separation of the symphysis pubis may occur.

In order to change her center of gravity and make ambulation easier, a woman tends to stand straighter and taller than usual during pregnancy. This stance is frequently referred to as "pride of pregnancy."

ENDOCRINE SYSTEM

The most striking change in the endocrine system during pregnancy is the addition of the placenta as an endocrine organ, producing large amounts of both estrogen and progesterone. Many women experience palmar erythema during early pregnancy as a response to high estrogen levels.

The pituitary gland is affected by pregnancy in that, under the influence of high estrogen and progesterone levels, the production of follicle-stimulating hormone and luteinizing hormone is halted.

There is increased production of growth hormone and melanocyte-stimulating hormone (the reason skin pigment changes occur in pregnancy). Late in pregnancy, the posterior pituitary begins to produce oxytocin that will be needed to aid in initiation of labor. Prolactin production is also begun late in pregnancy to aid in lactation at birth.

The thyroid gland is significantly altered. The gland enlarges in early pregnancy. Levels of protein-bound iodine (PBI), butanol extractable iodine (BEI), and thyroxine iodine (T_4) are all elevated. The result is an elevation of basal metabolic rate by about 20 percent.

These thyroid changes, along with emotional lability, tachycardia, heart palpitations, and increased perspiration, may lead to a mistaken diagnosis of hyperthyroidism if it has not been determined that the woman is pregnant.

The parathyroid glands, which are necessary for the metabolism of calcium, also increase in size during pregnancy. Since calcium is an important ingredient of fetal growth, the hypertrophy is probably necessary to satisfy the increased need for calcium.

Glucocorticoid levels increase in pregnancy, perhaps because of increased plasma binding rather than increased production by the adrenals. The pancreas increases production of insulin in response to the higher glucocorticoid levels, estrogen, progesterone, and human placenta lactogen, all of which tend to make insulin not as effective as normally. Thus a woman who is diabetic and taking insulin before pregnancy will need more insulin during pregnancy. A woman who is prediabetic may develop overt diabetes for the first time during pregnancy.

Table 14-5. Average Weight Gain in Pregnancy

System	Pounds	Kilograms
Fetus	7.0	3.1
Placenta	1.5	0.6
Amniotic fluid	2.0	0.9
Uterus	2.5	1.1
Blood volume	3.5	1.5
Breasts	1.5–3.0	0.6–1.3
Body fluid	8.0	3.6
Total	26.0–27.5	11.4–12.1

Weight Gain

All the physiological changes of pregnancy and the growth of the fetus tend to result in a weight increase of about 25 to 30 pounds (11.3 to 13.1 kg). A portion of the weight gain can be easily accounted for and is shown in Table 14-5. The remainder of the weight gain comes from the greater-than-normal accumulation of fat and fluid that is characteristic of pregnancy.

During the first three months of pregnancy, weight gain is usually slight (2 to 4 pounds). If the woman has a great deal of nausea, she may actually lose a small amount of weight. During the second and third trimesters she generally gains about a pound a week. A typical graph of weight gain is shown in Fig. 14-5. Whether a woman is taking in a diet sufficiently high in protein and whether her vital signs, particularly blood pressure, remain normal for her are equally as important as the fact she is gaining weight at this rate.

Women who are underweight coming into pregnancy may easily gain (and should gain) more weight than the average woman during pregnancy. An obese woman may gain less. As a rule, women should not diet to lose weight during pregnancy lest nourishment to the fetus be decreased.

Weight gain should be higher for a multiple pregnancy than for a single pregnancy. There is a high correlation between adequate weight gain in pregnancy and adequate birth weight and well-being of newborns. Nurses in the past have been overly conscientious about trying to force women to limit the amount of weight gained during pregnancy. It is true that a rapid increase in weight is a danger sign, since it may herald the onset of pregnancy-induced hypertension. However, weight gain during pregnancy can be kept in a better perspective if you remember that it is the

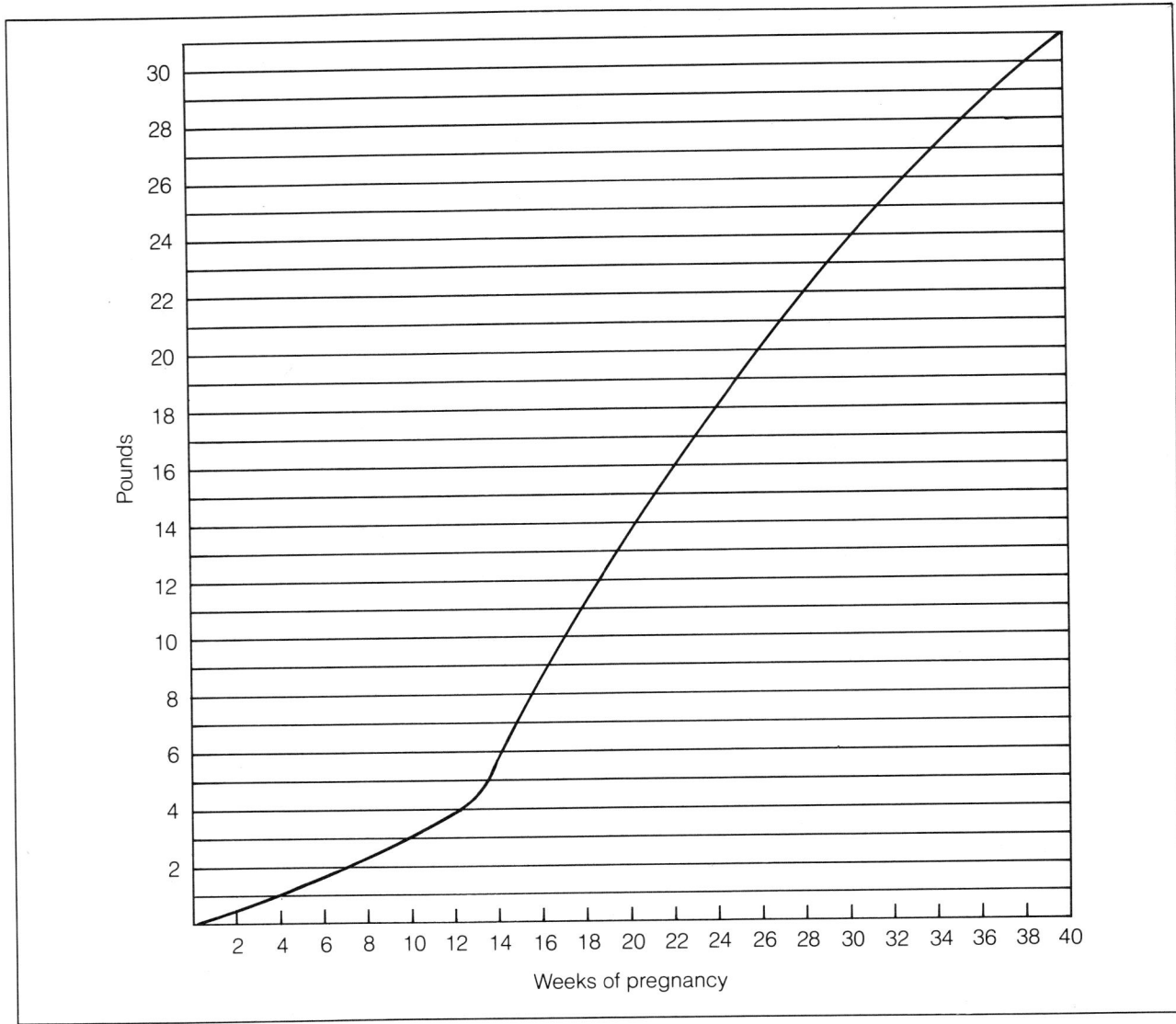

Fig. 14-5. Normal weight gain during pregnancy.

pregnancy-induced hypertension that causes the increase in weight, not the increase in weight that causes the hypertension.

Effects of Physiological Changes

The physiological changes of pregnancy may appear insignificant if taken one by one, but together they add up to a major change.

Every woman of childbearing age has a mental picture of herself. She has a good idea how she will look in a dress before she tries it on in a store. She chooses a certain style of furniture for her house or takes a vacation in a certain place because it says "this is me."

Then, in nine months, she gains 25 to 30 pounds, and her figure changes so drastically that none of her prepregnancy clothes fit. Toward the end, the extra weight and the strain of waiting make her feel tired and short of breath. Endocrine changes make her moody and perhaps quick to cry. She may never have been concerned with her health before, and now, every month (toward the end of pregnancy, every week), she must think about it as she reports for a prenatal checkup. She may worry that she will never lose all the weight she has gained, that the ugly stretch marks on her abdomen will remain forever, and that she will always be as tired or as nauseated as she is now.

At prenatal visits, women need help in voicing their concerns over the physiological changes of pregnancy. The worry these changes may cause, if the woman is not forewarned that they are a normal and necessary but transitory part of pregnancy, compounds an already stressful situation.

References

1. Danforth, D. (Ed.). *Obstetrics and Gynecology* (3rd ed.). New York: Harper & Row, 1977.
2. Grollman, S. *The Human Body: Its Structure and Physiology* (4th ed). New York: Macmillan, 1978.
3. Gusdon, J. P., et al. A clinical evaluation of the roll-over test for pregnancy-induced hypertension. *Am. J. Obstet. Gynecol.* 127:1, 1977.
4. Hytten, F. E. Physiological Adjustments in Pregnancy. In R. R. MacDonald (Ed.). *Scientific Basis of Obstetrics and Gynecology*. Edinburgh: Churchill Livingstone, 1978.
5. Jacobson, H. N. Weight and weight gain in pregnancy. *Clin. Perinatol.* 2:243, 1975.
6. Marchant, D. J. Alterations in anatomy and function of the urinary tract during pregnancy. *Clin. Obstet. Gynecol.* 21:855, 1978.
7. Peach, E. H. Counseling sexually active very young adolescent girls. *M.C.N.* 5:191, 1980.
8. Pitkin, R. M. Risks Related to Nutritional Problems in Pregnancy. In S. Aladjem (Ed.). *Risks in the Practice of Modern Obstetrics*. St. Louis: Mosby, 1975.
9. Sciarra, J. J., and Gerbie, A. B. *Gynecology and Obstetrics*. New York: Harper & Row, 1978.

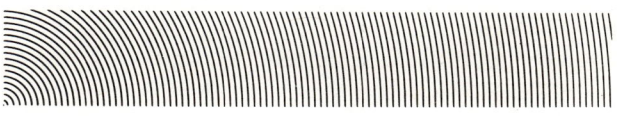

15. The Diagnosis of Pregnancy

The diagnosis of pregnancy is an important event because for many women medical confirmation that they are pregnant makes the pregnancy real for the first time. Further, it is an important step toward acceptance of the pregnancy and of the eventual outcome of the pregnancy, the newborn child.

A woman may be only one hour "more pregnant" when she leaves the physician's office or prenatal clinic than she was when she entered it, but if pregnancy has been confirmed, she invariably feels "more pregnant." From that day on, she is determined to eat a proper diet, give up or cut down on her cigarette smoking, and stop taking over-the-counter medications. A woman may not take these measures before confirmation of her pregnancy, which is one good reason early diagnosis is important. Further, if the woman does not wish to continue the pregnancy, early diagnosis is imperative so that abortion can be carried out at the earliest stage possible.

Pregnancy is diagnosed on the basis of the symptoms the woman reports and the signs the physician or nurse can elicit. These signs and symptoms are traditionally divided into three classifications: presumptive, probable, and positive.

Presumptive Signs
AMENORRHEA
In a healthy woman who has menstruated previously, the absence of menstruation strongly suggests that impregnation has occurred. However, amenorrhea may announce the initiation of menopause rather than pregnancy, or menstruation may be delayed because of a change in climate, worry (perhaps over becoming pregnant), chronic illness, such as severe anemia, or stress. Occasionally, the spotting that may occur with implantation is mistaken for a menstrual flow. For all these reasons, amenorrhea is only a presumptive sign of pregnancy.

FATIGUE
Early in pregnancy, perhaps before the first missed menstrual period, most pregnant women have episodes of fatigue and drowsiness. They probably occur because the rapid growth of the fetus at this stage utilizes the woman's glucose stores and leaves her with a low blood glucose at certain times during the day. However, fatigue has many causes, among them illness, overexertion, and depression. Thus, fatigue is no more than a presumptive sign of pregnancy.

NAUSEA AND VOMITING
At least 50 percent of women experience some nausea early in pregnancy; about 33 percent have some vom-

iting. These often occur on arising (morning sickness) but may occur any time during the day and in many women are most acute when they are fatigued or are preparing meals. Morning sickness may precede the missed menstrual period but generally occurs at about the same time. It normally disappears by the end of the 12th week of pregnancy. Because nausea and vomiting have many other causes, such as a gastrointestinal disorder, emotional stress, and infection, they are not reliable indications of pregnancy.

FREQUENT MICTURITION

The expanding uterus puts pressure on the base of the bladder, causing the woman to feel as though she needs to urinate frequently. This is a presumptive sign of pregnancy when coupled with a missed menstrual period. It could also be caused by a mild urinary tract infection, however, and so has limited value in diagnosing pregnancy.

BREAST CHANGES

Breast changes, namely, a feeling of fullness coupled with an increase in the diameter and darkening of the areola, the enlargement of Montgomery's glands, and the secretion of colostrum, are presumptive signs of pregnancy. They are most significant in women having their first pregnancy. In a woman who has nursed a child in the past year, they are sometimes almost unnoticeable. Breast changes occur early, at about the 6th week of pregnancy.

VAGINAL CHANGES

As vascular activity increases in the vagina, the walls of the vagina deepen in color, becoming violet, in contrast to the normal nonpregnant pink. This is known as *Chadwick's sign*. Since it may occur in any condition in which vaginal vascularity is increased (for example, in the presence of a rapidly growing uterine tumor), it is only a presumptive sign of pregnancy. Increased color is present at the 6th week of pregnancy.

SKIN CHANGES

Striae gravidarum, linea nigra, and melasma are skin changes that generally appear only with pregnancy. However, striae may occur with any rapidly expanding abdominal mass. The linea nigra may remain on the abdomen for a while following a pregnancy and so may be misleading in the diagnosis of a new pregnancy. These changes take place during the second trimester; in any event they would rarely be the first thing noticed.

QUICKENING

Quickening is the woman's first perception of movement by the fetus. It was once believed that the child lay lifeless in the woman's body until a point in pregnancy when "soul" or life was instilled into it. *Quick*, as used in biblical references ("the quick and the dead"), means "alive"; *quickening* is the old term for the "instillation of life into the fetus."

The first time the woman feels the child move is not a true measure of movement because the fetus has been making faint, undetectable movements since early in pregnancy. Once quickening has occurred (usually at 18 to 20 weeks), the woman should continue to feel movements of the fetus. The strength of the movement will vary with the thickness of the uterus and abdominal wall and the position and strength of the fetus. Any time that 24 hours pass without any discernible movement, the woman should ask to have the fetal heart sounds auscultated. If they are present, despite the decrease in movement observed, it can be assumed that the fetus is well. Movements are generally best felt when the woman lies on her back.

Although a woman's statement that she "feels life" should be a reliable sign of pregnancy, it cannot be accepted as any more than a presumptive sign. Occasionally, the movement of gas in the intestine may simulate such a sensation.

Probable Signs

UTERINE CHANGES

The changes in the size, shape, and consistency of the uterus beginning early in pregnancy are more reliable indications that pregnancy has occurred than are the presumptive signs.

Bimanual examination (one finger of the examiner in the vagina, the other hand on the abdomen) demonstrates that the uterus is more anteflexed, larger, and softer to the touch than normal. About the 6th week of pregnancy (at the time of the second missed menstrual period) the lower uterine segment just above the cervix becomes so soft that when it is compressed between the examining fingers by bimanual examination the wall cannot be felt or feels as thin as tissue paper. This extreme softening of the lower uterine segment is known as *Hegar's sign* (Fig. 15-1).

During the 16th to 20th weeks of pregnancy, when the fetus is still small in relation to the amount of amniotic fluid present, ballottement (from the French word *balloter*, meaning "to toss about") may be demonstrated. On bimanual examination, if the lower

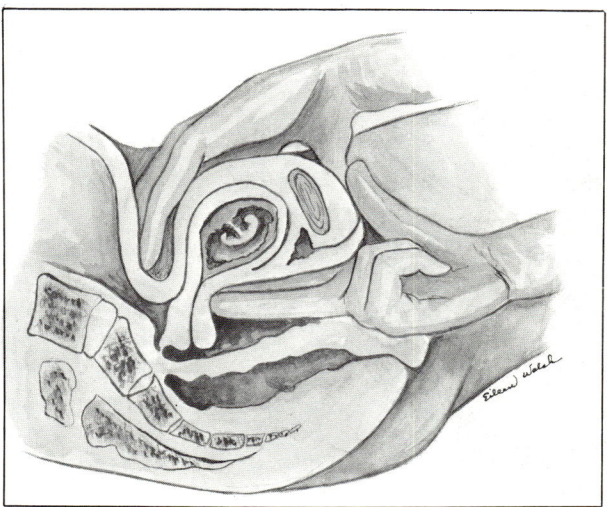

Fig. 15-1. Hegar's sign. When the lower uterine segment is compressed between the examining fingers, it feels as thin as tissue paper.

uterine segment is tapped sharply by the lower hand, the fetus will bounce or rise in the amniotic fluid up against the top examining hand. This phenomenon is interesting but can be simulated by a pedunculated uterine tumor and so is only a probable sign of pregnancy.

As the blood supply to the cervix increases in amount, the consistency of the cervix changes from that of the tip of the nose to one resembling an earlobe. This marked softening (*Goodell's sign*) occurs at about the time of the second missed menstrual period. It is only a probable sign, since it is not a reliable phenomenon. (One method of remembering which name applies to which sign of pregnancy is to remember that Chadwick's, Goodell's, and Hegar's signs occur in alphabetical order from the lower reproductive tract upward; i.e., Chadwick's sign is a vaginal change, Goodell's sign a cervical change, and Hegar's sign a uterine change.)

Enlargement of the uterus at a slow, steady rate is also an important sign of pregnancy. The uterus should rise above the symphysis pubis by the 12th week, reach the umbilicus at about the 20th or 24th week, and reach the xyphoid process at the 36th week. Although enlargement at this predictable rate rarely occurs with other phenomena, it can occur with a uterine tumor. Thus, increase in size, like the other uterine changes, is only a probable sign of pregnancy.

FETAL OUTLINE

About the 24th week of pregnancy, the uterine wall has become thinned to such a degree that a fetal outline within the uterus may be palpated and identified by a skilled examiner. However, since a tumor with calcium deposits occasionally simulates fetal outline, even this sign does not constitute a positive confirmation of pregnancy.

BRAXTON HICKS CONTRACTIONS

Uterine contractions begin early in pregnancy, at least by the 12th week, and are present throughout the rest of pregnancy, becoming stronger and harder as the pregnancy advances. They may be felt by the woman as periods in which hardness or tightening is felt across her abdomen. An examining hand may be able to feel the contraction as well. These "practice contractions" are termed *Braxton Hicks contractions*, or *Hicks' sign*. They serve as warm-up exercises for labor and become so strong and noticeable in the last month of pregnancy that they may be mistaken for labor contractions (false labor). They can be differentiated from true labor contractions on internal examination by the absence of cervical dilatation. These contractions always accompany pregnancy to some degree, but because they could be caused by any growing mass in the uterus, they are not positively diagnostic of pregnancy.

SONOGRAPHY

As indicated in Chap. 13, high-frequency sound waves projected toward a woman's abdomen are useful in demonstrating fetal maturity. This technique may also be used to diagnose pregnancy (Fig. 15-2). In the event of pregnancy, a characteristic ring, indicating the gestational sac, will be revealed on the oscilloscope as early as the 6th week of amenorrhea. This method of determination also gives information about the site of implantation. It is helpful if the woman having a sonogram for early pregnancy diagnosis has a urine-filled bladder, as a full bladder pushes the uterus up out of the pelvis and also helps with transmission of the ultrasound.

PROGESTERONE WITHDRAWAL TEST

In the progesterone withdrawal test, progesterone is given orally or intramuscularly to the woman. If she is not pregnant, a menstrual flow will occur within three to five days because of the withdrawal effect of the decreased level of synthetic progesterone. If the woman is pregnant, the corpus luteum or the placenta produces enough hormone to neutralize the effect of the declining synthetic hormone level, and no bleeding occurs. Women sometimes call this test an "abortion shot." When they fear they are pregnant, they see a physician, who gives them an injection, and within a

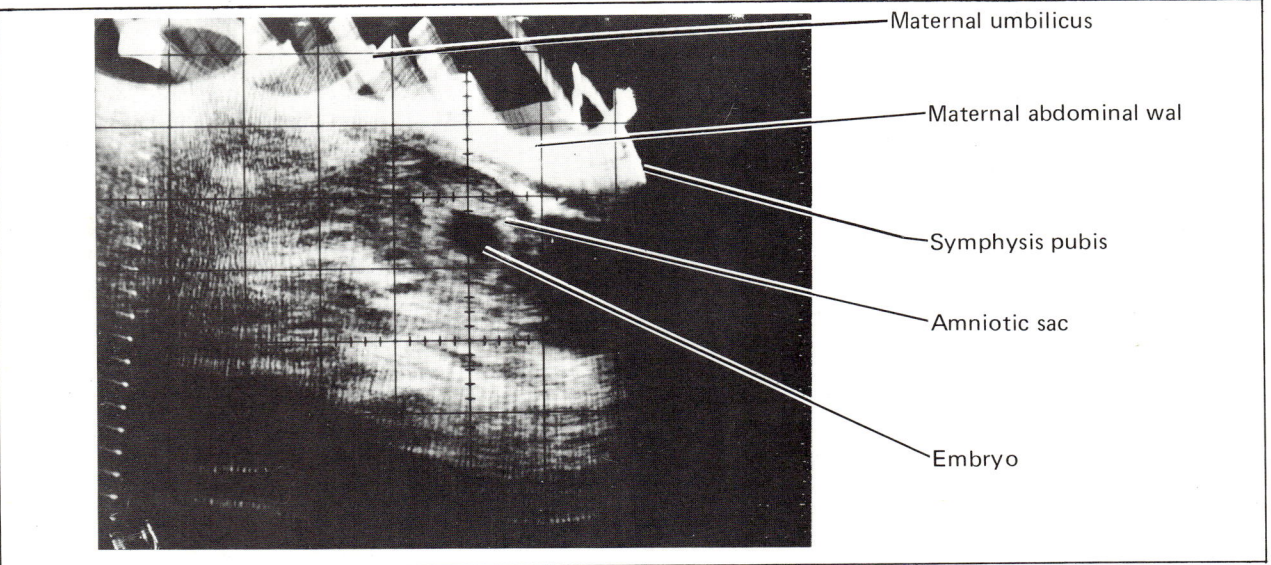

Fig. 15-2. Sonogram showing the characteristic circle diagnostic of pregnancy.

few days they have a normal menstrual period. In reality, the physician has merely demonstrated that they are not pregnant. Today, when immunological tests can offer quick diagnostic results, progesterone withdrawal tests are rarely used.

LABORATORY TESTS

The commonly used laboratory tests for pregnancy are based on the presence of human chorionic gonadotropin (HCG), a hormone produced by the chorionic villi, in the urine or serum of pregnant women. HCG is present in the bloodstream by the 8th to 10th day of pregnancy; it may not be present in urine in quantities great enough to use for testing until the 40th day of gestation. In the past, biological tests were the type of test used. These were based on the principle that when urine containing HCG is injected into various animals, the hormone present produces characteristic effects in the animal, indicating pregnancy.

Aschheim-Zondek Test

The Aschheim-Zondek test, devised in 1927, was the first laboratory test for pregnancy. Although it is rarely used today, the name is often applied erroneously to any pregnancy test. For an Aschheim-Zondek test, five immature female mice are injected with quantities of urine over a two-day period, and 100 hours from the first injection the mice are killed and their ovaries are examined. If HCG was present in the injected urine, hemorrhagic graafian follicles or corpora lutea will be present. Although an Aschheim-Zondek test is 97 percent accurate, its usefulness is limited by the number of animals required, the long waiting period for test results, and the time required by laboratory personnel to perform the test.

Friedman's Test

In Friedman's test, devised in 1929, urine is injected into an isolated virgin rabbit over a two-day period. The animal is killed on the third day and the ovaries are inspected. If HCG was present in the urine injected, there will be formation of corpora lutea, as in an Aschheim-Zondek test. The Friedman test also is 97 percent accurate, but its disadvantage is the cost involved in isolating the rabbit for 30 days prior to the test and sacrificing the animal.

Rat Ovarian Hyperemia Test

In the rat ovarian hyperemia test, urine is injected into immature rats, and their ovaries are inspected 16 to 24 hours later. Gross hyperemia (an excess of blood) indicates pregnancy.

Hogben Test

For the Hogben, or *Xenopus*, test, a female African clawed toad (*Xenopus laevis*) is used. Within 8 to 16 hours after injection of urine the animal will extrude large numbers of eggs if the urine is positive for HCG.

Male Frog Test

In the male frog test, urine is injected into male frogs. If HCG is present in the injected urine, spermatozoa can be detected microscopically in the frog's cloacal fluid 2 hours after the injection. This test has the advantage of having only a 2-hour waiting period; false-positive readings may result if the test frog spontaneously ejaculates, which is particularly likely to happen during the mating season. This test may also be performed on toads.

Immunological Tests

A number of tests involving hemagglutination inhibition, complement fixation, or precipitation reactions are now available (immunological tests), and these are most used today. These are office, clinic, or home procedures. Test-tube tests take about 2 hours; slide tests take only a few minutes. In the most common slide test today, latex particles coated with HCG and an anti-HCG rabbit serum are used. The anti-HCG serum is first mixed with the urine, then the HCG particles are added. Failure of the mixture to agglutinate (form clumps) is a positive test; it means the urine contained HCG and the HCG in the urine neutralized (reacted with) the antiserum before the latex-coated HCG particles were added.

Home Pregnancy Tests

Several brand name kits for pregnancy testing based on immunological reactions are available as over-the-counter purchases. These have a high degree of accuracy if the instructions are followed. It is convenient for women that such kits are available, as waiting for a physician's appointment to have a pregnancy diagnosed is an anxious, stressful time for many women. In most tests, a positive test is indicated by the formation of a dark ring in the test tube.

One of the chief reasons women go for early prenatal care is not that they are so certain they need a health checkup but that they wish to have the pregnancy officially diagnosed. There may be a tendency for women to diagnose their pregnancies at home by means of a test kit, then not to go for prenatal care until something seems to be wrong or late in pregnancy. Women need to be cautioned that prenatal care is important to safe pregnancy outcome and not to use a home test kit to replace it.

Women who are taking psychotropic drugs may have false-positive results on immunological tests. Women on oral contraceptives may also have false-positive results; for such a test to be accurate, oral contraceptives should be discontinued five days before the test. A woman who has proteinuria, is postmenopausal, or has hyperthyroid disease may also show a false-positive result.

A woman in early pregnancy, with an incomplete or a missed abortion, or with an ectopic pregnancy, may have a false-negative result.

Radioimmunoassay Tests

Radioimmunoassay techniques on blood serum make it possible to demonstrate the presence of HCG earlier than ever before, and pregnancy can be diagnosed as early as eight days after implantation.

URINE COLLECTION. Urine for pregnancy tests must meet certain criteria if false-negative test results are to be avoided. When women are asked to bring in a specimen from home, they must be given correct instructions on the method of collection. Since the urine should be concentrated, ideally the woman should have nothing to drink after about 8:00 P.M. the evening before the test. The first morning voiding should be collected in a dry, clean jar. If more than an hour will pass before the sample will be used, it should be refrigerated, since HCG is unstable at room temperature.

Because all the laboratory tests for pregnancy are inaccurate to some degree, positive results from these tests are considered probable rather than positive signs of pregnancy.

Positive Signs

There are only four positive signs of pregnancy: fetal heart sounds, fetal movements felt by the examiner, fetal heart movement on sonogram, and x-ray film outline of the fetal skeleton.

FETAL HEART SOUNDS

Although the fetal heart has been beating since the 24th day after conception, it is audible by auscultation of the abdomen with an ordinary stethoscope only at about 18 to 20 weeks of pregnancy. Fetal heart sounds are difficult to hear when abdomens have a great deal of subcutaneous fat or in uteri with a greater-than-normal amount of amniotic fluid. They are heard best when the position of the fetus is determined by palpation and the stethoscope is placed over the area of the fetus's back.

Fetal heart rate usually ranges between 120 and 160 beats per minute. An ordinary bell stethoscope may be used to auscultate heart sounds, but special fetal heart stethoscopes are available. One such stethoscope rests on the examiner's head and allows for bone conduction of the sound as well as air conduction to the eardrum. Others have a diaphragm that is larger than normal.

Ultrasonic monitoring systems that convert ultrasonic frequencies to audible frequencies (Doppler technique) are extremely helpful in detecting fetal heart sounds. Because they broadcast the sound, they have the added advantage of allowing the woman as well as the examiner to hear the heart sounds. Fetal heart sounds may be heard as early as the 11th week of gestation by this method. Hearing fetal heart sounds may be another important step in helping the woman accept the reality of the pregnancy.

In addition to the fetal heartbeat, two other sounds are often heard on auscultation, namely, the funic and uterine souffle. *Souffle* means "blowing." The funic souffle is the murmur of the blood rushing through the umbilical cord. Because this is part of the fetal circulation, the rate of the sound parallels the fetal heart rate. Blood moving through the distended maternal arteries creates the uterine souffle, which, because it represents maternal blood movement, has the same rate as the maternal pulse (about 70 to 80 beats per minute).

FETAL MOVEMENTS FELT BY THE EXAMINER

Movements of the fetus perceived by the woman may be misleading. Those felt by an objective examiner are much more reliable and constitute a positive sign of pregnancy. Such movements may be felt by the 24th week of pregnancy unless the woman is extremely obese.

HEART MOVEMENT BY SONOGRAM

By using a "real-time" technique of ultrasound, after a gestational sac has been identified, movement of the fetal heart may be demonstrated as early as 7 weeks gestational age.

X-RAY OUTLINE OF SKELETON

A roentgenogram showing the outline of a fetal skeleton is proof that pregnancy exists. Such an outline can be apparent as early as the 14th week of gestation; it is readily apparent after the 20th week. Although this is a positive sign of pregnancy, there are few instances that warrant its use as a diagnostic method, since x-rays may be teratogenic to the growing fetus.

Problem-oriented Recording: Progress Notes

Christine McFadden
15 years

Problem: Diagnosis of pregnancy

S. Unsure of last menstrual period (about 4 months ago). Has nausea every morning; has vomited last two mornings. Breast tenderness, feels tired. Definite increase in abdominal size. Thinks she has felt "something twisting inside me." Has been sexually active; no contraceptive used.
O. Uterus palpated 4 cm above symphysis pubis. Secondary alveoli present on breasts; colostrum expressed from nipples. Fetal heart tones present by Doppler at 150.
A. Pregnancy of about 16 weeks' length by positive sign criteria (M.D. to confirm).

Goals: a. Make firm decision on whether to continue or end pregnancy by one week.
b. Arrange appointments for prenatal care around school schedule so she can remain in school and prenatal care can be optimal if pregnancy will continue.
c. If decision is to end pregnancy, to return here for contraceptive counseling to prevent a second unwanted pregnancy.

P. 1. Mark for M.D. evaluation and physical exam.
2. Schedule for routine blood work and urinalysis.
3. Discuss plans for continuing pregnancy or abortion to end pregnancy.
4. If decision in one week is to end pregnancy, schedule appointment.
5. Evaluate in terms of physical, developmental, and psychological readiness for childbearing due to age.
6. Refer to M.D. for future prenatal visit schedule due to age if pregnancy is to be continued.

Problem-oriented Recording: Progress Notes

Mary Kraft
22 years

Problem: Diagnosis of pregnancy

S. Last menstrual period 37 days ago. Did home pregnancy test: result positive. Some nausea in morning; some breast tenderness.
O. Has been trying to conceive since surgery for endometriosis 4 months ago.

Uterus not palpable above symphysis.
No fetal heart sounds heard by Doppler.
Slight linea nigra present on abdomen.
A. Presumptive possibility of pregnancy (M.D. to confirm).

Goals: a. Continue the pregnancy.
b. Arrange appointments for prenatal care around work schedule so prenatal care can be optimal.
c. Husband wants to be included in pregnancy care and active participant at delivery.

P. 1. Mark for M.D. evaluation and physical exam.
2. Schedule routine blood work and urinalysis (include serum HCG for pregnancy confirmation).
3. Schedule for further visits based on M.D. confirmation of pregnancy and recommendations.

Problem-oriented Recording: Progress Notes

Angie Baco
42 years

Problem: Diagnosis of pregnancy

S. Last menstrual period 12 weeks ago. Was using vaginal foam for contraception. Has mild nausea in A.M.; frequency of urination, some breast tenderness.
O. Uterus palpable slightly above symphysis pubis.
Fetal heart tones by Doppler at 120.
A. Pregnancy of 12 weeks' duration by positive sign criteria (M.D. to confirm).

Goals: a. Continue the pregnancy.
b. Discuss the meaning of pregnancy for self and family to clarify meaning of pregnancy in own mind.
c. Schedule appointments for prenatal care around family commitments so close family support is maintained and prenatal care is optimal.

P. 1. Mark for M.D. evaluation and physical exam.
2. Schedule routine blood work and urinalysis.
3. Refer to M.D. for any additional assessment interventions such as sonogram or amniocentesis (age 42 years).

References

1. Anderson, S. G. Real-time sonography in obstetrics. *Obstet. Gynecol.* 51:284, 1978.
2. Corson, S. L. Ultrasound in obstetrics and gynecology. *J. Reprod. Med.* 20:1, 1978.
3. Donald, I. Further developments in diagnostic sonar in obstetrics and gynecology. *Obstet. Gynecol. Annu.* 6:23, 1977.
4. Ger, R., et al. Using sonography to help solve ob/gyn problems. *Patient Care* 13:54, 1979.
5. Kremkau, F. W., et al. Diagnostic ultrasound and its obstetrical applications. *Am. Fam. Physician* 17:148, 1978.
6. Landesman, R. What is the new advance in clinical laboratory testing for pregnancy? *Am. J. Obstet. Gynecol.* 130:242, 1978.
7. Mukheyie, T. K., et al. Evaluation of a new direct latex agglutination tube test for pregnancy. *Am. J. Obstet. Gynecol.* 131:701, 1978.
8. Plano, V. F. The newer pregnancy tests. *J.A.O.A.* 77:100, 1977.
9. Roy, S., et al. Diagnosis of pregnancy with a radioreceptor assay for HCG. *Obstet. Gynecol.* 50:401, 1977.
10. Sokol, R. J., et al. Maternal-fetal risk assessment: A clinical guide to monitoring. *Clin. Obstet. Gynecol.* 22:547, 1980.
11. Thompson, H. E. Ultrasound: The method. *Perinatal Care* 2:6, 1978.
12. Vengadasalam, D., et al. An evaluation of intramuscular progesterone for the diagnosis of early pregnancy. *J. Reprod. Med.* 20:260, 1978.
13. Wesley, G. D. Laboratory pregnancy testing. *Nurs. Times* 74:25, 1978.

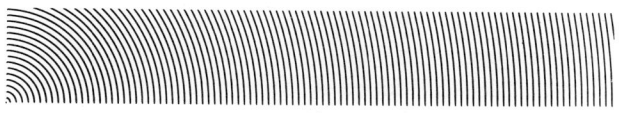

16. The First Prenatal Visit

Ideally, prenatal care begins in the mother's childhood. It includes a good calcium and vitamin D intake during infancy and childhood, so that the woman's pelvis is wide and not contracted by rickets or other malformations. It includes a good overall diet, so that both the woman and her husband enter pregnancy in the best state of health possible. It includes adequate immunization against contagious diseases during childhood, so that the woman will be protected against diseases such as rubella during pregnancy.

It includes the instillation of positive attitudes and concepts about sexuality, womanhood, and childbearing, so that the woman can enter pregnancy in good psychological health, unburdened by old wives' tales. It involves prompt and effective treatment of venereal diseases and other pelvic inflammatory diseases, so that the woman will be fertile and as free as possible from such complications of childbearing as ectopic pregnancy. It involves the utilization of family planning information, so that each pregnancy can be planned and the child desired.

A woman is wise to consult a physician for a premarital examination for reassurance about her fertility, for detection of gross problems that need correction, and for authoritative birth control information. If she did not have a premarital examination, a prepregnancy examination is her next wisest choice. Her hemoglobin level and blood type (including Rh factor) can be determined at this time; minor vaginal infections such as those arising from *Candida* can be corrected to ensure fertility; and the woman can be counseled on the importance of a good protein diet and early prenatal care in the event she does become pregnant. X-ray pelvimetry may be done at this time to ensure pelvic adequacy for delivery. X-ray photography for this purpose is not recommended during pregnancy; having the information already on file is helpful.

Prenatal care is an important aspect of childbearing from a nursing standpoint because a great deal of the care involves listening, counseling, and supporting, which are three areas of nursing expertise.

For prenatal care, a woman may choose to go to a clinic, a physician in general practice, or an obstetrician. Most important is that the woman initiates prenatal care early in pregnancy; the risk of infant mortality can be greatly lessened by doing so.

In the first prenatal visit, an extensive history is taken, and the woman has a physical examination, including a pelvic examination. Blood work and a urinalysis are done, and pelvic measurements may be taken to determine pelvic adequacy. The woman is also given appropriate guidance and instruction. The entire history necessary for a first visit (and succeeding ones also) can be obtained by a nurse skilled in the technique of patient history taking.

Conducting an Initial Interview

In interviewing expectant mothers, one encounters a welter of contradictions. On the one hand, a woman is likely to want to talk about her past health and present pregnancy. Thus, an interview should go smoothly and should easily be productive. On the other hand, the woman may never have been interviewed by a health care person in depth before, and so she may want very much to talk but may not feel free to do so. She may not regard the information that she has to supply as important, perhaps unaware that she is the only person who knows the answers to certain vital questions ("How do you feel about being pregnant?" or "What have you been taking for your morning nausea?"), and so she answers questions vaguely. She may be afraid of criticism, of herself or of her views, and so resists expressing herself. Also, she has outside pressures on her mind: the children coming home from school, dinner to prepare, a bus to catch. Later in pregnancy she may feel discomfort from having to sit still so long.

If an interview is going to be productive, all these factors must be considered, and some way must be found to modify their effects on the results obtained.

SETTING

Interviewing is best accomplished in a private, quiet setting. Trying to talk to the woman in a crowded hallway, or a waiting room full of other patients, is never effective. It will yield no more than superficial facts (name, address, birth date, social security number, and so on).

The woman should be invited to sit down. Your provision of a chair in privacy suggests that you have reserved this time just to talk to her. This helps her to feel that she is not imposing on you if she describes her feelings or concerns in depth.

You must be seated also. Perching on the edge of a desk or cart or leaning against a wall suggests you have only a few minutes to spare, and she had better limit her answers to a simple yes or no to avoid trespassing on your time.

It is helpful if the receptionist in the clinic or office—or you yourself, if you are the one making the appointments—cautions patients that the first visit will of necessity be a long one. This will prevent the woman from trying to sandwich the visit in between other errands and from having to terminate the interview because of another appointment. If a woman who has been cautioned that the visit will be lengthy tries to hurry matters, it might mean nothing, but it would be an interesting finding to note. Along with other observations it might indicate that she is trying to ignore her pregnancy or is so worried that you or the physician will discover her pregnancy is not going well that she prefers to keep the visit short.

ESTABLISHING RAPPORT

Women need to feel that they are important, that what they have to say is important, before they can begin to answer questions in any depth. The private, personal setting conveys this; being certain to call the woman by her correct name conveys it. Knowing what name to call patients is always a problem in nursing. If you are a student or a new graduate, and the woman is older than you are, you have to remember what your mother taught you: not to call persons older than you by their first names. On the other hand, if the woman is close to your age (and women of childbearing years fall into a relatively young age group), ask if she would like you to call her by her first name. You will notice that obstetricians invariably call their patients by their first names. This is a personal, concerned touch that most women appreciate. (As long as the woman's age or her personal preference does not interfere, this is an effective technique for you, too.)

Calling a woman by her first name may solve the problem of what to call an unmarried pregnant woman. Addressing her as Ms. Smith may be an answer. A more straightforward one is to call her Miss Smith, because, contrary to what you may think, an unmarried pregnant woman usually wants you to know she is unmarried. She does not want you to think she lives in a little cottage, complete with roses at the doorstep, a brick walk, and a white picket fence. She lives at home; her parents are angry with her because she is pregnant; her boyfriend has disappeared; girls she thought were her friends are shying away from her. Calling an unmarried pregnant woman *Mrs.* Smith may make you feel better. It does not take away any of her guilty feelings or make the pregnancy any easier to accept, and it may convince her that you are either hard of hearing or so grossly unconcerned that you cannot remember that she is not married.

Make certain the woman knows *your* name and understands your *role* correctly. If she views you as a secretary, she will be willing to discuss superficial facts (name, address, phone number, and the like) but will resist discussing more intimate things (her feelings toward this pregnancy, the difficulty she has reworking old fears, how scared she is about delivery).

Do not be a "form filler-inner." If you do nothing during the interview but read questions from a form and fill in spaces, you might as well hand the woman the form and let her fill it in herself. She can establish no more rapport with you on this basis than she could achieve with a computer.

TYPES OF QUESTIONS

History taking is basic data gathering. It seems simple: You want an answer, and so you ask a question. *How* you ask a question, however, will yield different kinds of answers. Using fact-finding and open-ended questions and supportive statements produces in-depth results. Vague, compound, critical, or overly sophisticated questions limit your effectiveness as an interviewer.

The *fact-finding question* is straightforward: "How much do you normally weigh?" "What was the date of your last menstrual period?" These are questions that generally evoke a simple answer: "I weigh 110 pounds." "My last period was March 21st."

The *open-ended question* is one that gives the woman freedom to answer in a number of ways. It is good to begin and end all sections of an interview with an open-ended question to see whether the woman will spontaneously come up with information you might not have elicited. An example of an open-ended question is, "Why did you come to the office today?" The woman may answer in a variety of ways: "I'm pregnant." "I think I'm pregnant." "I hope I'm pregnant." "I'm afraid I'm pregnant." "I'm pregnant. *Do* something about it." The depth of information gained in the words *think*, *hope*, and *afraid* is much more than you would secure by asking a fact-finding question such as, "Are you here because you think you are pregnant?"

The *vague question* is an open-ended question gone wrong. It is so open-ended that the woman does not know how to answer it. It baffles her and makes the interview a trying rather than a comfortable experience. "What about your general health?" is an example of such a question. The only answer a woman might give to that is, "*What* about it?" Instead, ask exactly what you want to know about her health. "Have you ever had any serious illness?" "Have you ever been hospitalized?" "Are you currently being treated for any disease?"

In a *multiple*, or *compound, question*, two fact-finding questions are intertwined. "Do you have nausea and vomiting?" is such a question. If the woman has nausea but no vomiting, she is likely just to say yes or no (she does not want to delay matters by going into detail). Neither answer elicits the facts, however. It is better to ask single questions: "Do you have nausea?" "Do you have vomiting?"

A *leading question* is one that by its structure suggests the answer. Because she wants to please you (you are in authority), she will answer in the manner you suggest. "You don't have any spotting, do you?" is such a question. Perhaps she actually does have spotting, but you imply she should not, so she will try to accommodate you by saying, "No, I don't." "Are you happy to be pregnant?" is another example. Because you have implied that she ought to be happy, she may feel trapped into answering affirmatively, despite her true feelings.

SUPPORTING STATEMENTS

Many women "toss" comments to see if they will catch your attention. These are generally indicative of strong feelings, so strong that some urging is needed to elicit them. At the same time, women are so worried with these concerns that they cannot keep them totally repressed. A woman in this conflict will be helped by your reassurance that she is free to discuss whatever is on her mind, that this clinic or this office is interested in more than her physical symptoms, her blood pressure, or the amount of her weight gain.

Her statement might be, "This better be a boy." Then silence. A supportive response from you might be, "Tell me why you say that." Such a request lends weight to her statement and makes it important enough for her to discuss. Suppose a woman says, "My first baby was stillborn." The woman looks as if she would like to say more, to tell you about that pregnancy, that baby. But, after all, she is here because of a new pregnancy. Can you afford to spend time discussing that earlier pregnancy? Do you want to discuss it? Is there a place for that information on the form in front of you? You do have time, because how she accepts this pregnancy is going to be largely dependent on how well she handled the outcome of the earlier one. A supportive statement such as "That must have been hard on you" will help her to talk about it.

TRANSITION STATEMENTS

Transition in interviewing is bridging the parts of the interview, or allowing you to move smoothly from one portion of an interview to another. It is basically an explanation of what is coming next. "I'm going to ask you some questions now about illnesses in your family" sets the stage and guides the woman's thoughts to that channel. It is disconcerting to jump to a new topic without such a statement. For example, if you ask, "Are you managing all right with your diet?" and immediately afterward ask, "Is there any diabetes in your family?" the woman may put the two statements together and conclude that you know something about her the physician did not discuss with her, namely, that she is becoming diabetic. It will be difficult for her to concentrate on any other subject when she is needlessly preoccupied with anxiety about diabetes.

CRITICAL REMARKS

If you think of history taking as simple data gathering, you can avoid making critical remarks ("You shouldn't do that." "Why on earth do you think that?"). Such remarks made in response to the woman's comments will limit the information you can obtain at an interview. The woman did not come to the clinic (or office) to be criticized. She came to be told she is or is not pregnant. She may not come back. Or she may come back, but she will be very careful in the future to slant her answers to obtain your approval. Remember that your eyebrows or your facial expression can reveal your disapproval just as readily as what you actually say. During the interview, the woman will observe your facial expressions and your tone of voice for clues to your attitudes.

Parts of an Interview

An initial interview has several purposes: to gain information about the woman's physical and psychosocial health, to establish rapport, and to obtain a basis for anticipatory guidance at the conclusion of the visit. Thus, it consists of several parts.

INTRODUCTION

It is surprising how many professionals neglect to extend the simple courtesy of introducing themselves to patients. "Hello, Mrs. Smith, I'm Cynthia Harper, a registered nurse" takes less than a minute, yet identifies you and your role. It is so much simpler for patients if they have to call a clinic or office to be able to identify someone by name rather than saying, "I spoke to the little blonde girl. I don't know if she was a nurse or not."

PURPOSE OF THE INTERVIEW

Women need an explanation of why they are being asked so many questions. It is helpful if they know what areas you are going to be discussing. Thus, explaining the purpose of the interview is the second step. "I'm going to be talking to you today in order that Dr. Weber and I can get to know you better. I'm going to begin by asking you about any concerns you have. Then I'll ask you questions about your family, your past health, and any previous pregnancies you have had. We'll talk in detail about the reason you've come into the office today."

CHIEF CONCERN

A woman makes an appointment at a physician's office or at a clinic because she has a special problem or need that is uppermost in her mind. Perhaps she has rehearsed various ways of wording the problem on her way to the appointment, so that her pain, or her fear, or her hope can be precisely conveyed. Until she has voiced this chief concern, it is hard for her to concentrate on other matters and give an accurate report of her history. An obstetrical history therefore begins with an attempt to elicit this chief concern: "Why did you come to the clinic today?" or "Why did you make your appointment?"

After she has stated her chief concern, explore the concern in greater detail. You need to know the duration, intensity, frequency, and description of a symptom, her actions with respect to it, and any associated symptoms she has. Suppose, for example, that her chief concern is nausea and vomiting. You need to know how long she has noticed these symptoms (duration); whether she has actually vomited or is just nauseated, and how late into the day she experiences the nausea (intensity); whether she notices it every day or only occasionally (frequency); exactly what she is describing (vomiting of undigested food or bile-stained fluid) (description); what she has tried to do to relieve the nausea and vomiting (eating dry crackers, taking an over-the-counter medication) (her actions); whether or not she has a fever or diarrhea (associated symptoms). You may discover by gathering all this information that the woman has gastroenteritis, not morning sickness, that her problem is a virus, not a pregnancy.

Following an in-depth look at the chief concern, ask, "Is there anything else that concerns you?" Because the woman's first response was respected and treated by you as important, she is likely to feel free to mention any further concerns she has.

FAMILY SETTING

Many physicians leave the social history or family setting until the end of the interview. However, using this technique is similar to interviewing in the dark and switching on the light only for the last few sentences. In order to interview a woman intelligently you need to know whether she lives alone or with a husband or family. If she lives alone, whom does she approach for emotional support or advice or help with problems? What is the source and level of her income? One of the hardest questions for nurses to ask is, "Are you married?" One method of avoiding this question is to ask, "Who else lives at home with you?" The married woman answers, "My husband and my 4-year-old son." The single woman answers, "No one" or "My parents and my brothers and sisters." If this method of discovering marital status makes you more comfortable than would asking for the status directly, use it. Remember, however, that most unmarried women *want* you to know they are unmarried and will just as readily answer a direct question, "Are you married?"

It is good to know the size of the apartment or house in which the woman lives. If she is expecting a baby, you are going to be talking to her in the coming months about a bedroom or space for the baby's bed. It is important to know whether the essential rooms are on the ground floor or upstairs, since she may be restricted from climbing stairs more than once or twice a day following delivery or during the last part of pregnancy.

Before you can begin to offer the woman any more than stereotyped health instruction, it is important to know her husband's age, educational level, and occupation, the shift he works on, her age and educational level, whether or not she is employed, and what kind of work she does (does it involve heavy lifting, long hours of standing in one position, handling of a toxic substance?).

As mentioned in Chap. 12, situations such as changing status from independence to dependence because of stopping work, chronic illness at home, the death of a significant person during pregnancy, the infidelity of a husband, geographical moves, financial hardship, or lack of support people may be injurious to the woman's ability to accept her pregnancy and child. No one in the clinic or office will be aware of these potentially harmful situations if you do not ask the questions about family setting that expose them.

PAST MEDICAL HISTORY

A number of diseases pose potential difficulty during pregnancy. These include kidney disease, heart disease (coarctation of the aorta and rheumatic fever are the two that cause problems most often), hypertension, venereal disease, diabetes, thyroid disease, recurrent convulsions, gallbladder disease, urinary tract infections, varicosities, and tuberculosis. These conditions are important to ask about when taking the past history, since they may become active during or immediately following pregnancy. It is important to know whether the woman had such childhood diseases as mumps (infectious parotitis), measles (rubeola), German measles (rubella), or poliomyelitis. From this information an estimate can be made as to the antibody protection she has against these diseases in case she is exposed to them during her pregnancy. If pregnant, she can be immunized against poliomyelitis by the Salk (killed virus) vaccine. She *cannot* be immunized against the others, since the vaccines used against them contain live viruses, as does the oral (Sabin) poliomyelitis vaccine.

It is important to learn of any drug sensitivities, so that prescription of drugs that might harm her will be avoided during pregnancy. A complete allergy history is vital, since women with allergies of any magnitude should probably breast-feed rather than bottle-feed their infants in order to avoid the possibility of milk allergy in the infant. This choice will be the woman's, not yours or the physician's to make. However, you need the information for appropriate counseling.

Any past surgical procedures are important. Adhesions resulting from past abdominal surgery may cause difficulty with the growth of the uterus. Because of the known deleterious effect of smoking on the growth of a fetus, the woman's smoking history should be obtained. Ask about alcohol consumption, since excessive alcohol intake may lead to poor nutrition or be responsible for a fetal alcohol syndrome in the baby. Ask whether any medication, prescribed or over-the-counter, is being taken so the effect of these on a growing fetus can be evaluated.

HISTORY OF FAMILIAL ILLNESS

Because some diseases are familial or inherited, the woman should be asked what diseases tend to occur in her and her husband's families. The most common ones to ask about are heart defects, hypertension, tuberculosis, diabetes, recurrent convulsions, allergies, congenital anomalies, and multiple births (document whether these are fraternal or identical births). Also important might be a history of large or small babies, frequent miscarriages, or cesarean sections in family members.

GYNECOLOGICAL HISTORY

A woman's past experience with her reproductive system has some influence on how well she accepts a pregnancy. You need to know the age of menarche and whether or not she was prepared for it. A woman who was told in advance that menstruation would occur as a normal part of being a mature woman and having babies is bound to feel more comfortable about womanhood and childbearing than the woman who was not prepared.

You also need to know the interval, the duration, and the amount of menstrual flow. Does she have discomfort? If she describes menstrual cramps as "horrible" and wonders how she "lives through them some months," imagine what her concept of labor must be like! To face an experience such as labor, she will need more counseling as pregnancy progresses than does the average woman.

It is also essential to secure information about any gynecological surgery or problem the woman has had. If she has had a tubal operation, such as surgery for an ectopic pregnancy, the risk of a tubal pregnancy this time is theoretically higher for her than for the woman who has not had such an operation. If she has had uterine surgery, her child may have to be delivered by cesarean section rather than vaginally. Ask what birth control methods, if any, she has been using. Occasionally, a woman becomes pregnant with an intrauterine device in place. Ask whether she has one. She will need to have it removed or infection during pregnancy may result.

PREVIOUS PREGNANCIES

Do not assume that the current pregnancy is the first simply because a woman is very young or says she has been married only a short time. Ask. You need to obtain the facts about past pregnancies as well as eliciting the woman's subjective feelings about these pregnancies. You need to know the child's sex and place and date of each previous birth. It is good to review the pregnancy briefly. Was it planned? Did she have any complications such as spotting, swelling of her hands or feet, falls, surgery? Did she take any medication? Did she receive prenatal care? What was the duration of gestation? What was the duration of labor? Was labor what she expected? Worse? Better? What was the type of delivery? What was the type of anesthetic? What was the infant's birth weight? What was the condition of the infant at birth? Did he cry right away? Did he have any blueness? Did he become yellow during his hospital stay? (Avoid the terms *cyanosis* and *jaundice* since many women do not know what they mean.) Did he require any special equipment? Was he discharged from the hospital with her? What is his present state of health?

What was the outcome of the pregnancy for *her*? Did she have stitches following delivery? Did she have any complications?

Ask about any previous miscarriages or abortions. Did she have any complications during or following them? *Abortion* is the medical term for any pregnancy terminated before the age of viability. The *age of viability* is the earliest age at which a fetus could survive if he were born at that time, generally accepted as 20 weeks, or a fetus above 400 gm. Although you chart both induced and spontaneous pregnancy terminations in the same way, women appreciate your separating the terms into *miscarriage* (a spontaneous abortion) and *abortion* (used in its more limited meaning of induced or therapeutic or planned termination of pregnancy) when you are talking to them. If her blood type is Rh negative, ask if she received RhoGAM immunoglobulin after miscarriages or abortions so you will know whether Rh sensitization could have occurred.

After a history of previous pregnancies is obtained, the woman's status with respect to the number of children above the age of viability she has previously delivered (para) and the number of times she has been pregnant including this pregnancy (gravida) is determined. A woman who has had two previous pregnancies, has delivered two children, and is pregnant now is para 2, gravida III. A woman who has had two abortions at three months (under the age of viability) and is now pregnant is a para 0, gravida III. A woman pregnant for the first time is a *primigravida*. A woman who has been pregnant before is a *multigravida*. A woman who has delivered one child is a *primipara*; two or more children, a *multipara*.

A pregnant woman who had the following past history—in 1968, a boy born weighing 7 pounds, now alive and well; in 1969, a girl born weighing 7½ pounds, now alive and well; in 1972, a girl born weighing 4 pounds, now alive and well—would have her pregnancy information summarized as follows: para 3; gravida IV; premature births, 1; abortions, 0; living children, 3.

PRESENT PREGNANCY HISTORY

It is a good idea to establish a baseline health picture at the initial visit, so that if on subsequent visits a symptom is mentioned you can check your records to see whether it is truly a new symptom. It may be that the woman is just becoming more aware of it.

You need to know whether or not the pregnancy was planned. "All pregnancies are a bit of a surprise. Is that how you reacted to this one?" is the kind of statement that will give you this information if you feel uncomfortable asking it directly. Other ways to word such a question are, "Some unmarried girls want to have babies and some don't. How was it with you?" or "Some married couples plan on having children right away, some plan on waiting. How was it with you?"

Ask the date of the last menstrual period and whether the woman has had signs of early pregnancy, such as nausea, vomiting, breast changes, fatigue, and heartburn. Is she having any minor discomforts of pregnancy, such as constipation, backache, frequent urination? Has she felt quickening yet? At this point in pregnancy, how does she feel about the pregnancy? Has she reached a point where she can say she wants this child growing inside her? Is she taking any medication, prescribed or over-the-counter? Has she experienced any of the danger signals of pregnancy, such as bleeding, continuous headache, visual disturbances, edema of the hands and face?

REVIEW OF SYSTEMS

A review of systems takes about 10 minutes. You will be amazed at the results obtained by telling a woman you are going to start at the top of her head and go through to her toes asking about body parts or systems and diseases she has had in these body systems. She recalls diseases she forgot to mention earlier, diseases that are important to your history.

The following body systems and conditions should constitute the minimum covered in a review of systems:

1. *Head*. Headache? Head injury? Seizures? Dizziness? Syncope?
2. *Eyes*. Vision? Glasses needed? Diplopia? Infection? Glaucoma? Cataract? Pain? Recent changes?
3. *Ears*. Infection? Discharge? Earache? Hearing? Tinnitus? Vertigo?
4. *Nose*. Epistaxis? Discharge? How many colds a year? Allergy? Postnasal drainage? Sinus pain?
5. *Mouth and pharynx*. Dentures? Condition of teeth? Toothache? Any bleeding of gums? Hoarseness? Difficulty in swallowing? Tonsillectomy?
6. *Neck*. Stiffness? Masses?
7. *Breasts*. Lumps? Secretion? Pain? Tenderness? Does she know how to do a breast self-examination?
8. *Respiratory system*. Cough? Wheezing? Asthma? Shortness of breath? Pain? Serious chest illness such as tuberculosis or pneumonia?
9. *Cardiovascular system*. History of heart murmur? Rheumatic fever? Hypertension? Any pain? Palpitations? Any heart disease? Anemia?
10. *Gastrointestinal system*. Vomiting? Diarrhea? Constipation? Change in bowel habits? Rectal pruritus? Hemorrhoids? Pain? Ulcer? Gallbladder disease? Hepatitis? Appendicitis?
11. *Genitourinary system*. Infection? Hematuria? Frequent urination? Venereal disease?
12. *Extremities*. Varicose veins? Pain or stiffness of joints?

CONCLUSION OF THE INTERVIEW

End an interview by asking if there is something you have not covered that the woman wants to discuss. Resist explaining your clinic appointment system or giving prenatal health information until the woman has had a physical examination and a confirmation of pregnancy. If she is hoping she is not pregnant or is not ready to accept her pregnancy, she is not ready to listen to health instruction.

Because initial history taking is time-consuming, the use of forms the patient fills in herself is often advocated. Pregnancy is such a personal experience that it seems callous to depersonalize it in this way. A better solution to the time problem is for nurses to learn good interviewing technique so they can secure thorough and meaningful health histories. The rapport that is established by face-to-face interviewing gives a woman the feeling that she is more than just a file card. It may be as important in bringing her back to a clinic or a physician's office as her desire to be assured that physically her pregnancy is progressing normally.

The Husband's Role in an Initial Interview

Because most appointments in clinics or physicians' offices are made for daytime hours, few husbands or prospective fathers accompany women for prenatal visits. Further, they may regard prenatal visits as women's business and suspect they would not be welcome if they came. Perhaps nurses, who set the tone in clinics and offices, do not always make them feel welcome.

If a man accompanies his wife, or a woman who is not his wife but is bearing his child, should he be included in an initial interview? As a whole, interviewing is most effective if it is a one-to-one interaction. A woman may be unwilling to mention certain of her concerns with her husband present for fear of worrying him. The husband may not be the father of her child, and she may be unable to voice her concern over this fact or alert you to the possibility she is worried about blood incompatibility because another man is the father.

However, if childbearing is a family affair, it is just as important to determine the father's degree of acceptance of the pregnancy and of being a father as it is to establish how far the woman has come in the process of acceptance. The main areas you should investigate with the father are his present health, his feelings and concerns about the pregnancy, and his knowledge of pregnancy and childbirth. Following the confirmation of pregnancy, he should be present when health care information is given.

The Physical Examination

At the initial visit, following the history taking, the woman will have a physical assessment. She should undress, put on a gown, and empty her bladder. The latter is necessary for the pelvic, or internal, examination. Save the urine for albumin and sugar tests and for microscopic examination to detect the presence of bacteria.

The woman should be weighed to obtain a base weight for comparison with all future weights. Ask her her usual weight to determine how much weight she has already gained. Blood pressure, respirations, and pulse should also be measured to obtain baseline data. A sudden increase in blood pressure or in weight is a danger sign in pregnancy; a sudden increase in pulse or respirations may be equally serious.

Some women may need reassurance that a full physical examination is necessary for the physician to be certain that she is entering pregnancy in as good a physical condition as possible. The examination will be a general physical (conducted by a physician or by a nurse in an extended role) and will include the following:

1. Examination of the eyes by inspection (a funduscopic examination is helpful to establish whether or not papilledema is present).
2. Examination of the ears, nose, and throat, noting the condition of the teeth and gums and palpating the neck for lymph nodes and thyroid.
3. Palpation and auscultation of heart sounds; percussion and auscultation of breath sounds.
4. Examination of the breasts for cysts or lumps. Every woman of childbearing age should be aware of how to examine her own breasts monthly. If a woman has not been doing this routinely, teaching her how during prenatal visits is good health education. As this is also good information to review with women in the postpartal period, it is discussed in Chap. 26.
5. Examination of the abdomen to discover masses other than the growing uterus; auscultation of fetal heart sounds if pregnancy is sufficiently advanced; measurement of the height of the fundus (Fig. 16-1).
6. Inspection of the back for spinal disorders and of the rectum for hemorrhoid development.
7. Inspection of the lower extremities for varicosities.

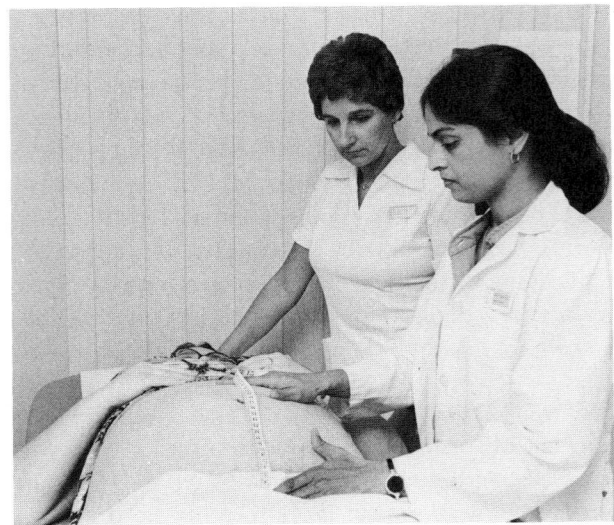

Fig. 16-1. Measuring fundal height. Height is measured from the superior aspect of the pubis to the fundal crest. (Courtesy of the Department of Medical Photography, Children's Hospital, Buffalo, N.Y.)

MEASUREMENT OF FUNDAL AND UTERINE HEIGHTS

Fundal height is measured from the notch above the symphysis pubis to the superior aspect of the uterine fundus. Uterine height should be plotted on a graph such as the one shown in Fig. 16-2. If this is not currently done by the prenatal care physician, the plotting of uterine growth can be an independent nursing function.

Plotting uterine growth at each visit in this way allows variations in fetal growth to become apparent. Further investigation, such as a sonogram, can then be made to determine the cause of the growth increase or retardation.

PELVIC EXAMINATION

A pelvic examination is included in a first visit and requires the following equipment: speculum, spatula for cervical scraping, clean examining glove, lubricant, glass slide for plating the Papanicolaou smear, and culture tube and sterile cotton-tipped applicator for obtaining a culture. A good examining light and a stool of correct sitting height are also necessary.

For a pelvic examination, the woman lies in a lithotomy position (on her back with her thighs flexed and her feet resting in the table stirrups). Her buttocks should extend slightly beyond the end of the examining table. Her abdominal muscles will be more relaxed if she has a pillow under her head.

She should be properly draped (a draw sheet over her abdomen and extending over her legs). It is helpful if the foot of the examining table does not face the examining room door so that if someone should walk

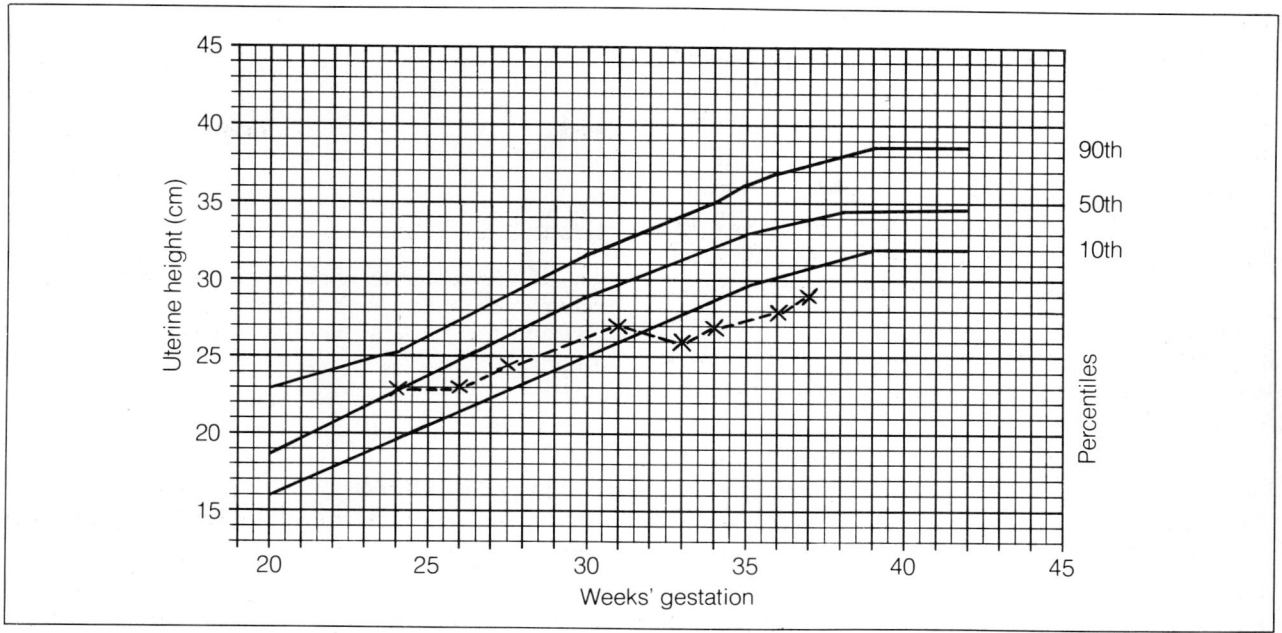

Fig. 16-2. Uterine height percentiles. Subject was a fetus with intrauterine growth retardation. (From J. M. Belizan, et al. Diagnosis of intrauterine growth retardation by a simple clinical method: Measurement of uterine height. Am. J. Obstet. Gynecol. 131:643, 1978.)

in unexpectedly the woman will not feel exposed. She should have an opportunity to talk with her physician in a sitting position before being placed in a lithotomy position, for the sake of her self-esteem.

It is a courtesy to a woman, especially on an initial pregnancy visit, for a nurse to be in the room with her for the pelvic examination. If this is a first pregnancy, it may well be the first time the woman has been in a physician's office since she finished receiving her childhood immunizations, and she may never have had a pelvic examination before. There are so many stories about how painful these examinations are that the woman tenses just thinking about it. When pelvic muscles are tight and tense, not only is the examination painful, but the physician has difficulty assessing the status of the pelvic organs.

You can help a woman to relax during the examination in a number of ways. One is by remaining in the room. Having someone with her whom she knows (and following an extensive interview the woman surely will feel that she knows you) is supportive. Being with her means being at the head of the table, near to her, not at the foot of the table, "where the action is." Being near to her enables you to touch her hand or cheek if she needs the support of physical contact. An explanation of what is happening or what is going to be done by the nurse or physician is an aid to relaxation. Remember that while this may be the thousandth pelvic examination for you, it could be the first for her. Meaningful conversation with the woman may be helpful, but conversation with the physician over her head is *not*. Suggesting that the woman breathe in and out (not hold her breath as she is prone to do) may help her relax.

A pelvic examination begins with inspection of external genitalia. Things that are noted are signs of inflammation, irritation, or infection, such as redness, ulcerations, or discharge.

Herpes simplex II virus infections appear as clustered pinpoint vesicles on an erythematous (reddened) base. They are painful when touched or irritated by underclothing. The presence of herpes lesions on the vulva or vagina at the time of delivery will necessitate cesarean section, in order to prevent exposing the fetus to the virus during passage through the birth canal. Management of the newborn with herpes is discussed in Chap. 38. As there may be an association between cervical cancer and herpes simplex II virus infections, the presence of a herpes infection should be noted clearly in the woman's record so she can be followed in the future by cytological smears (Pap smears) for cervical cancer.

To check whether Skene's glands are infected, the physician inserts a gloved finger into the woman's vagina and presses it against the anterior vaginal wall to see if any pus can be extruded from the openings to the glands at the urethral opening. To check for possible infection of Bartholin's glands, the sites of Bartholin's glands (5 and 7 o'clock) are palpated between the vaginal finger and the thumb of the same hand. If a discharge is produced from any of these gland ducts (Skene's or Bartholin's), it is cultured. Infection here could be caused by something as simple as streptococci; it often is gonorrhea.

To assess whether either a rectocele (a forward pouching of the rectum and posterior vaginal wall due to loss of posterior muscular support) or a cystocele (an inward pouching of the bladder and anterior vaginal wall due to loss of muscular support) is present, the physician asks the woman to bear down as if she were moving her bowels while he gently separates the labia to view the vaginal walls.

To view the uterine cervix, the vagina must be opened with a speculum (Fig. 16-3). Knowing how to insert a vaginal speculum is useful for nurses. No lubricant other than warm water should be used over the speculum blades; a lubricant might interfere with the interpretation of the Papanicolaou smear that will be taken. Warm water rather than cold water should be used, so that the woman does not contract her vaginal muscles on feeling the cold instrument.

A speculum is introduced with the blades in a closed position and directed toward the posterior rather than the anterior vaginal wall because the posterior wall is less sensitive. A speculum enters most readily if it is inserted at an oblique angle (the crease of the blades directed to 4 or 8 o'clock), then rotated to a horizontal position when fully inserted (the crease of the blades pointing to a 3 or 9 o'clock position). When fully inserted and rotated to a horizontal position, the blades are opened so the cervix is visible and secured in the open position by tightening the thumb screw at the side.

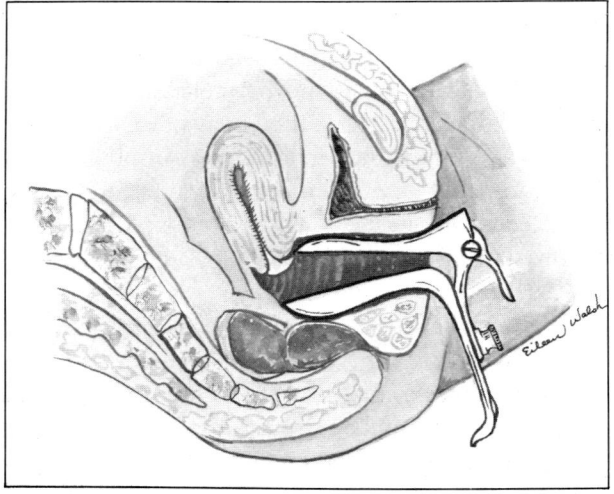

Fig. 16-3. A vaginal speculum in place.

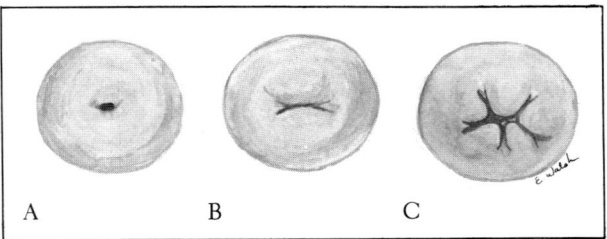

Fig. 16-4. Appearances of the cervix in nulliparous and multiparous women. A. Nulliparous cervix. B. Cervix after childbirth. C. "Stellate" cervix, seen after mild cervical tearing.

The cervix is inspected for its position (a retroverted uterus has a cervix tipped forward; an anteverted uterus has its cervix tipped posteriorly), its color (a nonpregnant cervix is light pink; in pregnancy it changes to almost purple); and any lesions, ulcerations, discharge, or otherwise abnormal appearance.

In a nulligravida (a woman who has never before been pregnant), the cervical os is round and small. In a woman who has had a previous pregnancy, the cervical os has much more of a slit-like appearance (Fig. 16-4). If the woman had a cervical tear during a previous delivery, the cervical os may appear as a transverse crease the width of the cervix or as a typical star-like (stellate) formation. If a cervical infection is present, the epithelium of the cervical canal enlarges and spreads onto the area surrounding the os, giving the cervix a reddened appearance (termed *erosion*). This area bleeds readily if it is touched.

Carcinoma of the cervix appears as an irregular granular growth at the os. Cervical polyps (red, soft pedunculated protrusions) may also be seen at the os.

Papanicolaou Smear

Three separate specimens are usually obtained for a Papanicolaou smear: one from the endocervix, one from the cervical os, and one from the vaginal pool. For the first specimen, take a sterile cotton applicator, wet it with saline, and insert it through the speculum into the os of the cervix. Gently rotate it clockwise, then counterclockwise. Remove it without touching the sides of the vagina and paint a glass slide using a gentle touch so as not to destroy cells. Spray the slide with a fixative to preserve the cells.

To take a cervical specimen, press the longer end of the scraper supplied for the test on the os of the cervix; rotate it to scrape cells in a circle around the os. Smear the scraper onto a slide and spray with fixative.

For the third specimen, place a cotton applicator at the posterior fornix just below the cervix (the vaginal pool); roll it gently to pick up secretions collecting there. Remove it carefully and prepare a third slide.

Pap smear reports are classified according to the findings, as follows:

Class I	Normal; no atypical cells are present.
Class II	Normal, although there are atypical benign cells present.
Class III	Suspicious cells, possibly malignant, are present.
Class IV	Signs of malignancy are present.
Class V	Cells definitely malignant are present.

Vaginal Inspection

Before the speculum is removed, a culture for gonorrhea is generally taken. This is done by a gentle swab of the cervix by a cotton-tipped applicator.

A speculum must be unlocked to be removed. The excessive stretching that will occur if it is removed in an open position is very painful. If the speculum is kept partially open as it is removed, however, the sides of the vagina can be inspected as it is withdrawn. Any areas of inflammation, ulceration, lesions, or discharge are noted. In a nonpregnant woman, vaginal walls are light pink; pregnancy turns them dark blue to purple. Such a vaginal inspection is critically important in a woman whose mother took diethylstilbestrol during pregnancy, who is prone to develop vaginal cancer.

Trichomoniasis, a protozoal infection, generally gives signs of redness, a profuse whitish bubbly discharge, and petechial spots on the vagina. Candidal (*Monilia*) infection typically presents with thick white vaginal patches that may bleed if scraped away. Gonorrhea infection typically presents with a thick greenish-yellow discharge and extreme inflammation. A urethral infection may be present as well with gonorrhea. Vaginal cancer (a condition always to be considered in a woman whose mother took diethylstilbestrol) presents as an abnormal ulceration or growth on the vaginal wall.

Bimanual Examination

Following the speculum examination, the physician performs a bimanual (two-handed) examination to assess the position, contour, consistency, and tenderness of pelvic organs. The index and middle finger of the right hand are lubricated and inserted into the vagina and the walls of the vagina palpated for abnormalities. The left hand is then placed on the woman's abdomen and pressed downward toward the hand still in the vagina until the uterus can be felt between the two hands. Some physicians like a low stool supplied at this point so they can rest their right elbow against their raised knee in order to maintain enough pressure to palpate adequately.

The physician continues to move his hands and identifies the right and left ovaries by the same method. Ovaries are normally slightly tender. The pressure caused by palpation may cause the woman some discomfort at this point.

Abnormalities that can be noted by bimanual examination are ovarian cysts, enlarged fallopian tubes (perhaps from pelvic inflammatory disease), and an enlarged uterus. An early sign of pregnancy (Hegar's sign) is elicited on bimanual examination. If a uterus is extremely retroverted it may not be palpable abdominally.

Rectovaginal Examination

Following a bimanual pelvic examination, the physician withdraws his hand from the vagina and reinserts only his index finger in the vagina, his middle finger in the rectum. By palpating the tissue between the examining fingers, he can assess the strength and irregularity of the posterior vaginal wall and the posterior cervix. This maneuver may be slightly uncomfortable for the woman because of the rectal pressure involved. Some physicians prefer to use a clean pair of gloves before they perform a vaginal-rectal examination so that they will not spread an infection from the vagina to the rectum. Following the rectal examination, if the examiner has to reexamine the vagina for any reason, he must use clean gloves in order to avoid contaminating the vagina with fecal material.

After completing the examination, the physician needs a tissue to wipe away excess lubricant from the vaginal and rectal openings. If the physician omits this step, it should be done by you before you help the woman sit up again. Remember to wipe front to back so that you do not carry rectal contamination forward to the vaginal introitus.

ESTIMATING PELVIC SIZE

If, on this initial visit, the physician establishes that the woman is pregnant, and if she has never given vaginal birth before, pelvic measurements (see p. 215) will usually be taken to assure the physician that the size and shape of her pelvis is within normal limits and will allow a child to pass safely through its bony canal at delivery. Some physicians prefer to delay taking these measurements until later in pregnancy, when the woman's perineal muscles are more relaxed and the measurements can be accomplished with a little more ease. However, there is danger in waiting too long, because if the pelvis is too small, the fetal head will not deliver and a cesarean section will be necessary in order to effect a delivery that is safe for both mother and infant. Pelvic measurements must be taken at least by the 24th week of pregnancy because by this time there is danger that the fetal head will reach a size that will interfere with safe passage if the measurements are small.

Once a woman has given vaginal birth, her pelvis has been proved adequate, and it is not necessary to take her pelvic measurements again unless she has an intervening history of pelvic accident.

Structure of the Pelvis

The pelvis is a bony ring formed by four united bones: the two innominate (hip bones), which form the anterior and lateral portion, and the coccyx and sacrum, which compose the posterior aspect (Fig. 16-5).

The *innominate bones* are divided into three parts: ilium, ischium, and pubis. The *ilium* is the upper and back portion. The flaring superior border forms the prominence of the hip, or the crest of the ilium. The *ischium* is the inferior portion. At the lowest portion of the ischium are the ischial tuberosities, the part on which you sit. The *pubis* is the anterior portion of the innominate bone. The symphysis pubis is the junction of the innominate bones in front of the pelvis.

The *sacrum* is actually composed of five bones so tightly fused together that they seem one. There is a marked anterior projection of the sacrum at the point where it joins the lumbar vertebrae. This is the *sacral prominence*, a landmark to be identified in securing pelvic measurements.

The *coccyx* is also composed of five very small bones fused together. There is a degree of movement possible in the joint between the sacrum and the coccyx (the *sacrococcygeal joint*). This is important because the movement permits the coccyx to be pressed backward, allowing more room for the fetal head as it passes through the bony pelvic ring at delivery.

For obstetrical purposes, the pelvis is further divided into the false pelvis (the superior half) and the true pelvis (the inferior half) (Fig. 16-6). The *false pelvis* supports the uterus during the late months of pregnancy and aids in directing the fetus into the *true pelvis* for delivery. The false pelvis is divided from the true pelvis by an imaginary line, the *linea terminalis*. This line is drawn from the sacral prominence along the ilium on both sides to the superior aspect of the symphysis pubis. Above the line is the false pelvis; below it is the true pelvis.

The linea terminalis not only separates the false from the true pelvis but also marks the *inlet*, the entranceway to the true pelvis. A view down at the inlet shows that the passageway tends to appear heartshaped because of the jutting sacral prominence. It is wider transversely than in the anteroposterior dimension.

The *pelvic cavity* is the space between the inlet and the outlet (the most inferior portion of the true pelvis). This space is not a straight passage but is curved like a stovepipe. In order to travel through this portion of the pelvis, the fetus has to accommodate himself to this curved structure.

The *outlet* is the inferior portion of the pelvis, or that portion bounded in the back by the coccyx, on the sides by the ischial tuberosities, and in the front by the inferior aspect of the symphysis pubis and the

Fig. 16-5. Structure of the pelvis.

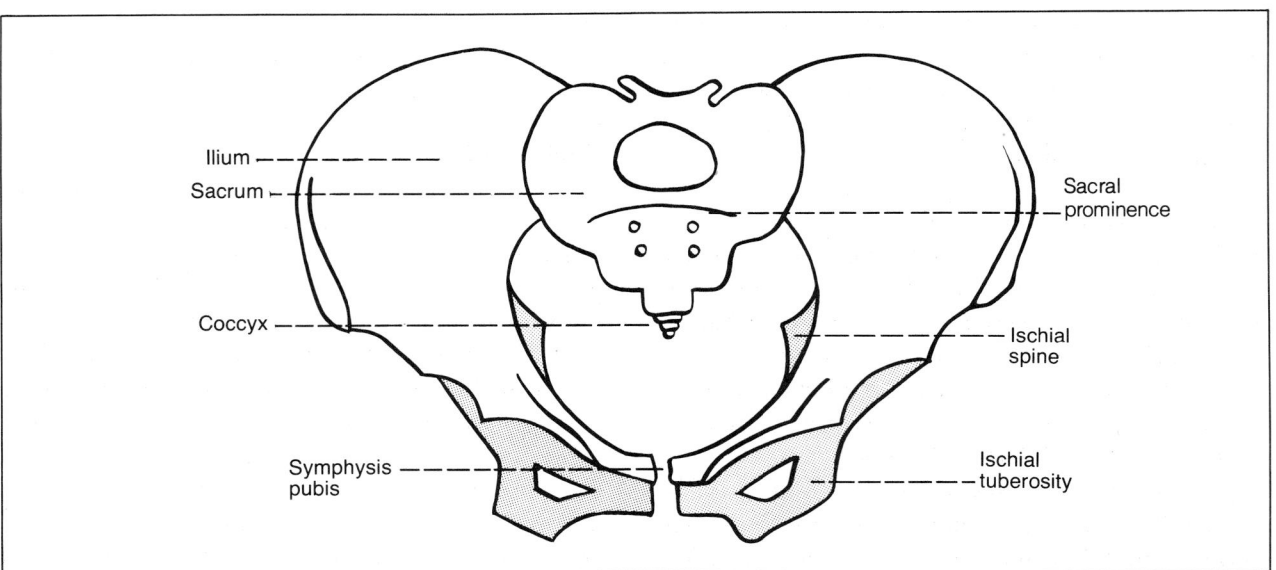

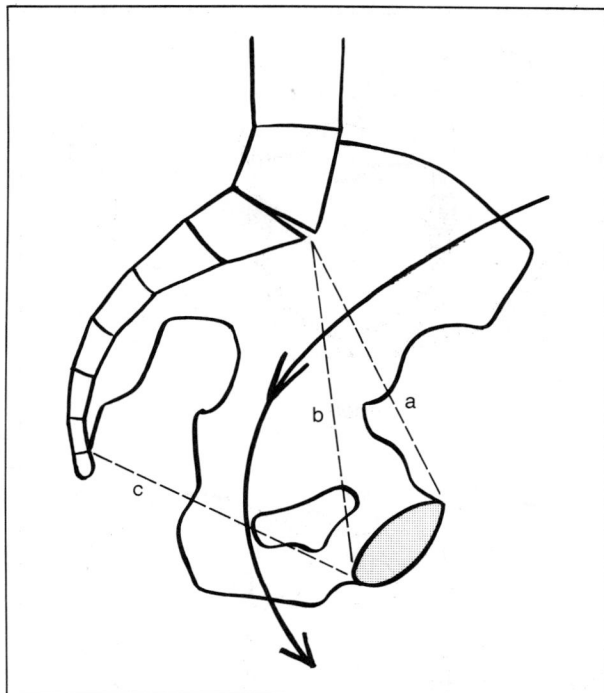

Fig. 16-6. True and false pelvis. A. Linea terminalis (pelvic inlet). B. True conjugate diameter. C. Pelvic outlet. Portion above linea terminalis is false pelvis; portion below is true pelvis. Arrows show "stovepipe" curve that the fetus must follow to delivery.

pubic arch. In contrast to the inlet of the pelvis, the greatest diameter of the outlet is its anteroposterior diameter.

It is important to be able to picture the route a fetus must take to traverse the pelvis for a vaginal delivery. To enter the inlet, the fetus must present the widest diameter of the head to the transverse diameter of the pelvis. The fetus must then move through the curved pelvic cavity. At the outlet, he must turn to present the widest diameter of his head to the anteroposterior diameter of the pelvis, since that is now the widest diameter of the pelvis.

There are physiological reasons for the design of the pelvis. The curved structure prevents rapid propulsion of a fetus; the snugness of the cavity compresses the chest of the fetus as he passes through, helping to expel lung fluid and mucus and preparing the lungs for good aeration at birth. The actual mechanics of the birth process are discussed in Chap. 21.

Pelvic Variations

It is impossible to predict from the outward appearance of a woman whether or not her pelvis is adequate for the passage of a fetus through its center. Some women look as if they have wide pelves but in reality have only wide iliac crests and a normal or smaller-than-normal internal ring. Other women appear small because the ilial crests are nonflaring, but the internal pelvis, the part that must be sufficiently large for childbirth, is of average size, and they give birth vaginally without difficulty. Differences in pelvic contour and development occur because of hereditary factors, disease (e.g., rickets, which may cause contraction of the pelvis), or injury (inadequate repair following accidents).

Types of Pelves

Four main types of pelves are found in women (Fig. 16-7):

1. *Gynecoid pelvis*, the "normal" female pelvis. The inlet is well rounded forward and back. It is ideal for childbirth.
2. *Anthropoid pelvis*. In this pelvis the transverse diameter is narrow and anteroposterior diameter of the inlet is larger than normal. This does not accommodate a fetal head as well as the gynecoid pelvis.
3. *Platypelloid pelvis*. In this pelvis, the inlet is an oval, smoothly curved, but the anteroposterior diameter is shallow.
4. *Android pelvis*, or "male" pelvis. The inlet has a shallow posterior portion and a pointed anterior portion.

Although any of these types of pelves may be adequate for childbearing, the gynecoid pelvis is the one designed for this function. A fetal head might have difficulty fitting into or passing through the other three types, particularly the android pelvis, because of its pointed, rather than rounded, aspects.

Pelvic Measurements

Pelvic measurements are made to determine whether or not the normal vaginal route of delivery will be safe for both the infant and mother. Because an x-ray is not an acceptable technique to use early in pregnancy (it is a potential teratogen to the fetus), this information must be obtained manually.

Traditionally, pelvic measurements have been made by the physician. However, there is no reason they cannot be made, recorded, and interpreted by a nurse who has learned the necessary techniques and appreciates the need for accurate measurements and correct interpretation of her findings.

EXTERNAL MEASUREMENTS. External measurements of the pelvis, once made routinely, offer so little information that they are no longer done.

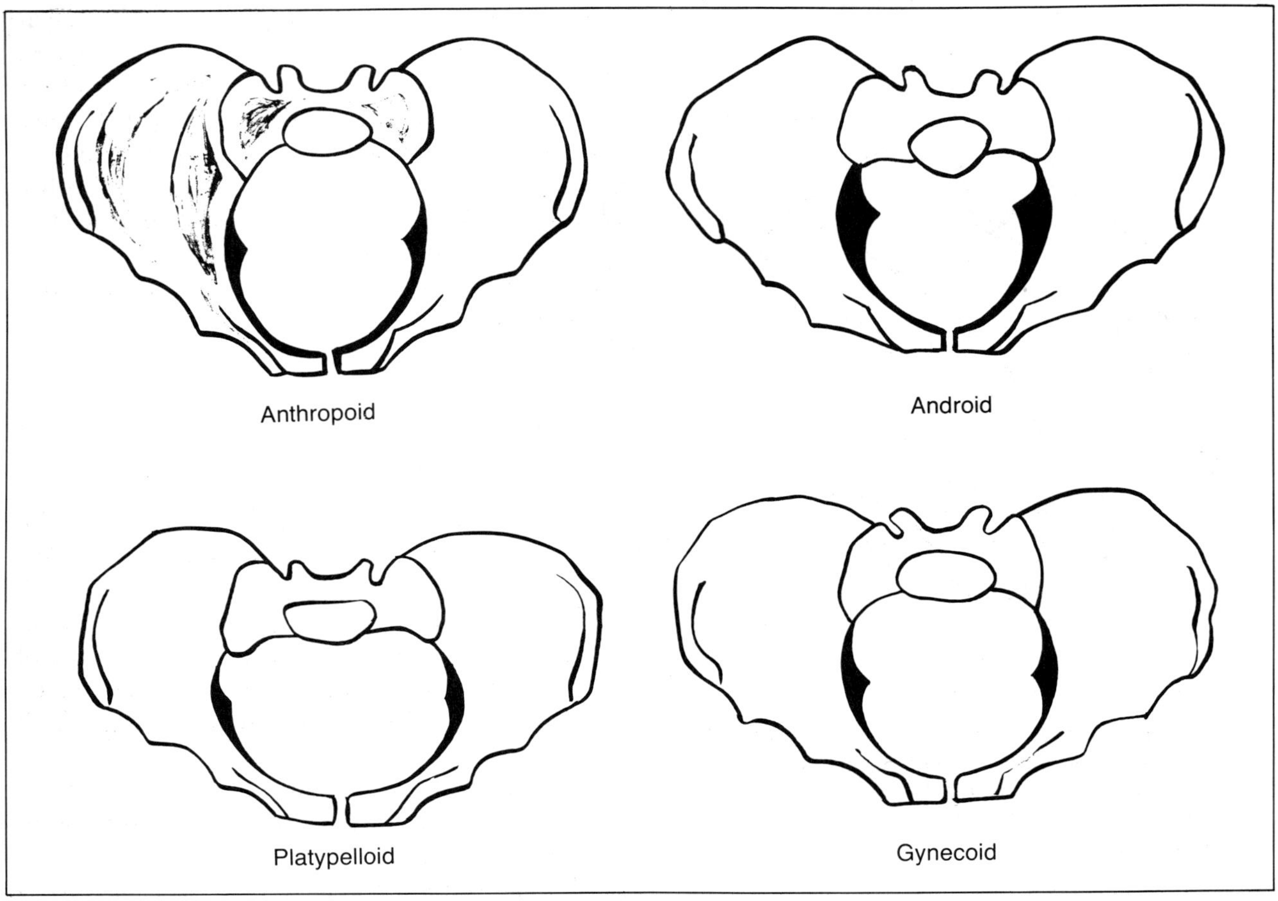

Fig. 16-7. Types of pelves.

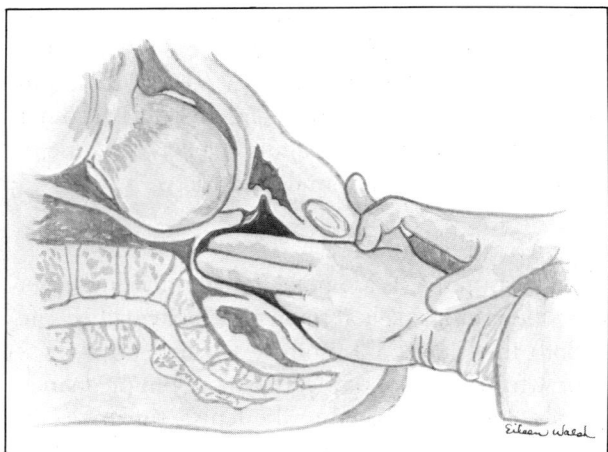

Fig. 16-8. Measurement of diagonal conjugate diameter.

INTERNAL MEASUREMENTS. Internal measurements give the actual diameters of the inlet and outlet. The following are the ones taken most often:

1. The *diagonal conjugate*, the distance between the sacral prominence and the inferior margin of the symphysis pubis (Fig. 16-8), is the most useful measurement for estimation of pelvic size. It is measured by having the woman lie in a lithotomy position. The examiner introduces two fingers vaginally and presses inward and upward until the middle finger touches the sacral prominence. The part of the hand that touches the symphysis pubis is marked by touching it with the examiner's opposite hand. The examining hand is then withdrawn, and the distance between the tip of the middle finger and the marked point of the glove is measured by a ruler or, for greater accuracy, by a pelvimeter. If this measurement is more than 12.5 cm, the pelvic inlet is rated as adequate for childbirth. It is less time-consuming for both the woman and the health care personnel if the physician or nurse who initially performed the pelvic examination takes this measurement at the same time.

2. The *true conjugate*, or *conjugate vera*, is the measurement between the posterior surface of the symphysis pubis and the anterior surface of the sacral prominence. This measurement cannot be made directly, but it can be estimated from the measurement of the diagonal conjugate, as follows: The usual depth of the symphysis pubis is

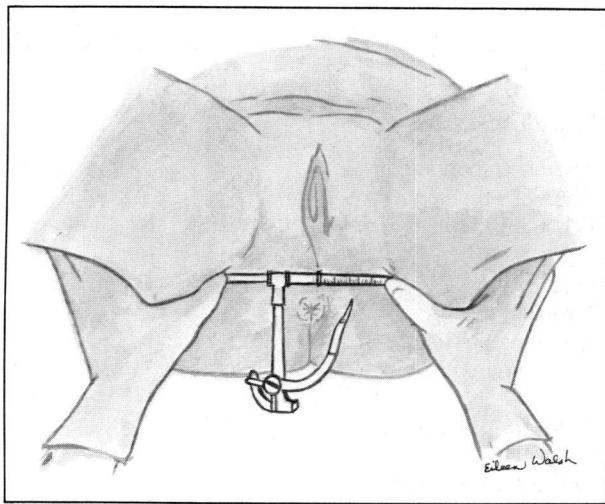

Fig. 16-9. Measurement of intertuberous diameter.

1.5 to 2 cm. If this distance is subtracted from the diagonal conjugate measurement, the distance remaining will be the true conjugate, or the actual diameter of the pelvic inlet through which the fetal head must pass. The average true conjugate diameter is therefore 12.5 cm minus 1.5 or 2 cm, or 10.5 to 11.0 cm.

3. The *ischial tuberosity diameter*, the measurement between the ischial tuberosities, or the transverse diameter of the outlet, is made at the medial and lowermost aspect of the ischial tuberosity at the level of the anus (Fig. 16-9). A Williams or Thomas pelvimeter is generally used. The diameter is usually 11 cm.

The pelvic measurements ordinarily taken and their average diameters are as follows:

Measurement	*Diameter*
Diagonal conjugate	12.5 cm
True conjugate	10.5 to 11 cm
Ischial tuberosity	11 cm

LABORATORY STUDIES
Blood Studies

The following blood studies are usually done at the first prenatal visit:

1. Complete blood count, hemoglobin, or hematocrit, to determine the presence of anemia. A hematocrit is a simple test that may be done in a matter of minutes in the office by a technician or nurse skilled in the technique. Black women may have a blood sample taken to be tested for sickle cell trait or disease if they have not had this done before.
2. A Venereal Disease Research Laboratories (VDRL) test or rapid plasma reagin (RPR) test to determine the presence of syphilis. Syphilis should be treated early in pregnancy before fetal damage occurs. A serological test for gonorrhea is now available and may be drawn on women suspected of having the disease.
3. Blood typing (including Rh factor), so that blood can be made available if the woman has bleeding early in her pregnancy and to provide for additional care when a blood incompatibility with the fetus is suspected.
4. An antibody titer for rubella, to determine whether or not the woman is protected against the disease in case of exposure during pregnancy.

If the woman has a history of previous unexplained fetal loss, has a family history of diabetes, has had babies that were large for gestation age (9 or more pounds at term), is obese, or has glycosuria, she should be given a glucose loading or tolerance test toward the end of the first trimester of pregnancy to rule out gestational diabetes. Since fasting is required before a glucose tolerance test, arrangements for the test are usually made at the first prenatal visit.

Urinalysis

A urinalysis is performed to assay for albuminuria, glycosuria, and pyuria. All three of these tests are office procedures, done by means of test strips and microscopic examination of the urine.

Chest X-ray Examination

If the woman has a history of tuberculosis or is from an area where tuberculosis is a major health problem, the physician may order a chest x-ray. A woman is sometimes reluctant to have this done because she has read that radiation is harmful to a growing fetus. Her fear is well founded. She needs to be assured that she will be provided a lead apron to cover her abdomen to protect the fetus and that only her chest will be exposed.

A tuberculin skin test is another screening method, and it is safe to use during pregnancy. Only those who have a positive reaction will require subsequent x-ray studies.

It is important to screen for tuberculosis early in pregnancy because it is a chronic and debilitating disease and thus increases the risk of abortion. Further, the change in the shape of the lung tissue as the

Table 16-1. Antepartum Fetal Risk Score

CATEGORY I

Baseline Data (Prepregnancy)

Age 15 or under	1
Age 35+	1
Age 40+	2
Para 0	1
Para 5+	2
Interval <2 years	1
Isolation: 50+ miles from medical care	2
Weight <100 lb (45 kg)	1
Weight 200 lb or more (90 kg)	2
Diabetes	
Class A	1
Class B, C, D	2
Class F, R	3
Chronic renal disease	1
Chronic renal disease with diminished renal function	3
Preexisting hypertension	
140+/90+	1
160+/110+	2
Interpregnancy cardiac failure	2
Rh-isoimmunized mother (1:8 AHG+)	
With homozygous husband	2
With previously affected infant (regardless of outcome)	3

Reproductive History

Abortion, spontaneous
Abortion, therapeutic
Pelvic infection, postabortal or postpartum

Fetal death
Neonatal death
Surviving premature infant
Surviving infant, low birth weight for date

Antepartum hemorrhage
Toxemia
Difficult midforceps
Cesarean section
Hysterotomy
Myomectomy
Major congenital anomaly
Cervical incompetence
Large infant: 10 lb or more (4.5 kg)
Malpresentation

One instance of above	1
Two or more instances of the above (in one or more pregnancies)	2

Score (circle one)   0   1   2   3

CATEGORY II

Present Pregnancy

Bleeding early (<20 wk)	
Alone	1
With pain	2
Bleeding late (>20 wk)	
Ceased	1
Continues	2
With pain	3
With hypotension	3
Spontaneous premature rupture of membranes	1
With latent period 24 hours	2
Asymptomatic bacteriuria	1
Toxemia grade I	1
Toxemia grade II	3
Eclampsia	3
Hydramnios (single fetus)	3
Multiple pregnancy	2
Gestational diabetes	
Diagnosis before 36 wk	1
Diagnosis after 36 wk	2
Decreasing insulin requirement (50% + reduction in 48 hr)	3
Maternal acidosis	3
Maternal pyrexia (39°C or over)	1
Maternal pyrexia + FHR > 160	2
Rising Rh antibody titer (2 tube+)	2

No antepartum care	2
Less than 3 visits	1
Heart disease: AHA functional Class III or IV	2
Anemia	
10 gm or less	1
10 gm after 36 wk	2
8 gm or less	2
Megaloblastic anemia	2
Specific Infections	
Untreated syphilis	2
Toxoplasmosis	2
Hepatitis	1
Vaccination during pregnancy	1
Rubella titer rising significantly	
6 wk	3
12 wk	2
12 wk	1
Inhalation anesthesia (emergency)	1
Abdominal operation	2
Cervical suture (cerclage)	3
Pelvic irradiation diagnostic 12 wk	1

Score (circle one)   0   1   2   3

Table 16-1. (Continued)

CATEGORY III

Gestation Age Achieved

28 weeks or under	4	37 weeks or under	1
32 weeks or under	3	42 weeks or over	1
35 weeks or under	2	43 weeks or over	2

Score (circle one)   0 1 2 3 4

Total Score (0–10) =

Source. J. W. Goodwin and P. T. Hewlett. The strategy of fetal risk management. *Can. Family Physician* 19(4):54, 1973. (Modification of score devised by J. W. Goodwin, J. T. Dunne, and B. W. Thomas, *Can. Med. Assoc. J.* 101:458–464, 1969.) Reprinted by permission of author and publisher.

---

growing uterus presses on the lungs may reactivate old lesions.

Dental X-ray Studies

If many dental caries are present at the time of the first prenatal examination, the woman may be referred to her dentist or a dental clinic. Carious teeth are a source of infection and should be treated before abscesses develop and cause more serious problems. Dental x-rays may be taken during pregnancy, but the woman should remind her dentist that she is pregnant and needs a lead apron to protect her abdomen.

Expected Date of Confinement

Once a woman is told that her pelvic examination and history suggest pregnancy, she will ask when the baby is due. Her due date, or expected date of confinement (so called because a long period of bed rest following childbirth used to be the norm), is calculated by Nägele's rule: count back three months from the first day of the last menstrual period and add seven days. This date is not hard and fast, since the actual date of delivery is influenced by the date of ovulation and impregnation. For the woman with a typical 28-day menstrual cycle, the date will be relatively accurate. The woman with a 40-day cycle does not ovulate until about the 26th day of her cycle, not the 14th, so her child will not be ready to be born until almost two weeks after this date. Be certain the mother understands that delivery two weeks before or two weeks after the expected date will be within normal limits.

If the woman does not know the date of her last menstrual period, the length of the pregnancy will be estimated from measurement of fundal size or by sonogram.

Risk Assessment

At a first prenatal visit, the total findings—psychosocial, financial, physical, and cultural—are assessed to determine whether this pregnancy will continue with a good outcome or whether it will probably end before term or with an unfavorable fetal outcome (a high-risk pregnancy).

Many factors enter into the categorization of high risk. A commonly used scale for risk assessment is shown in Table 16-1.

A score of more than 3 by Goodwin's scale identifies a fetus as being at high risk for damage. For example, the baby of a woman more than 35 years of age (score 1) in her first pregnancy (score 1) who had anemia of 10 gm or less (score 1) would by this scale be at high risk. The infant born of this woman would need close observation in the neonatal period until it was confirmed that he had no anomalies and was doing well. Category III is scored only after the baby is born.

The failure to identify risk potential in pregnancy leads to increased perinatal mortality. In prenatal offices where women are scheduled at the rate of one every 15 minutes for care, the physician cannot begin to deal with fetal risk assessment. Identifying fetuses at risk by using a standard scoring system such as Goodwin's can be an independent nursing function that can do much to increase the health of newborns and prevent unwanted fetal loss.

Risk assessment should be done at the first prenatal visit. It should be updated at each pregnancy visit or it will lose its effectiveness later in pregnancy.

Open Communication—Key to Nursing Care

Following the interview, the physical assessment, and the diagnosis of pregnancy based on the probable signs observed, the woman—and her husband, if he is present—should be given counseling on health maintenance during pregnancy. This is discussed in Chap. 17.

Be certain that a woman leaving the initial prenatal visit has a firm appointment to return to the clinic or physician's office. This may not seem important to her when her mind is full of all the new things that are happening to her, but it will be important the following month, when it is time for follow-up care.

During a normal pregnancy, return appointments are scheduled every month through the 32nd week of pregnancy, then every two weeks through the 36th week, and then every week until delivery. Women who are categorized as high risk will be followed more closely during pregnancy than this usual pattern.

It is helpful to give women pamphlets or booklets about prenatal care to read later; after their initial surprise wears off, they may be in a better frame of mind to grasp the material and enjoy reading it. Be sure you have read all the printed matter you give them, to be certain the advice it contains is consistent with that you have given orally and with the views of the physician with whom you work. A beautiful picture on the cover of a pamphlet does not ensure the quality of the advice inside.

Assure the woman she may call the office or clinic if she has any problems or questions during the coming month. Some women are raised with such awe of authority (and you and the physician represent authority) that they will worry about a problem for an entire month, but will not call unless you indicate beforehand that they are free to do so.

References

1. Ascher, B. H. Maternal anxiety in pregnancy and fetal homeostasis. *J.O.G.N. Nurs.* 7:18, 1978.
2. Aubrey, R. Identification of the High Risk Perinatal Patient. In S. Aladjem (Ed.). *Perinatal Intensive Care*. St. Louis: Mosby, 1977.
3. Belizan, J. M., et al. Diagnosis of intrauterine growth retardation by a simple clinical method: Measurement of uterine height. *Am. J. Obstet. Gynecol.* 131:643, 1978.
4. Chiota, B. J., et al. Effects of separation from spouse on pregnancy, labor and delivery, and the post partum period. *J.O.G.N. Nurs.* 5:21, 1976.
5. D'Angelo, L., and Sokol, R. J. Prematurity: Recognizing patients at risk. *Perinatal Care* 2:16, 1978.
6. Foster, R. S. How to encourage breast self examination. *Female Patient* 5:36, 1980.
7. Gohari, P., et al. Early diagnosis key to reduction of grave intrauterine growth retardation risk. *Contemp. Obstet. Gynecol.* 4:79, 1976.
8. Hill, R. M., et al. Utilization of over-the-counter drugs during pregnancy. *Clin. Obstet. Gynecol.* 20:381, 1977.
9. Hobel, C. J. Identification of the Patient at Risk. In R. H. Schwarz and R. J. Bolognese (Eds.). *Perinatal Medicine*. Baltimore: Williams & Wilkins, 1977.
10. Hogan, L. R. Pregnant again—at 41. *M.C.N.* 4:174, 1979.
11. Jones, M. B. Antepartum assessment in high-risk pregnancy. *J.O.G.N. Nurs.* 4:23, 1975.
12. Marshall, G. W., and Newman, R. L. The roll-over test. *Am. J. Obstet. Gynecol.* 127:623, 1977.
13. Rotterdam, H. Vaginal and cervical abnormalities in DES daughters. *Female Patient* 4:22, 1979.
14. Sciarra, J. J., and Gerbie, A. B. *Gynecology and Obstetrics*. New York: Harper & Row, 1978.
15. Skalnik, B. Radiation protection for pregnant personnel. *Appl. Radiol.* 7:84, 1978.
16. Snow, L. F., et al. The behavioral implications of some old wives' tales. *Obstet. Gynecol.* 51:727, 1978.
17. Sonstegard, L. Pregnancy-induced hypertension: Prenatal nursing concerns. *M.C.N.* 4:90, 1979.
18. Wells, G. M. Reducing the threat of a first pelvic exam. *M.C.N.* 2:304, 1977.
19. Wolkind, S., et al. Psycho-social correlates of nausea and vomiting in pregnancy. *J. Psychosom. Res.* 22:1, 1978.
20. Yeh, S., et al. A study of the relationship between Goodwin's high risk score and fetal outcome. *Am. J. Obstet. Gynecol.* 127:50, 1977.

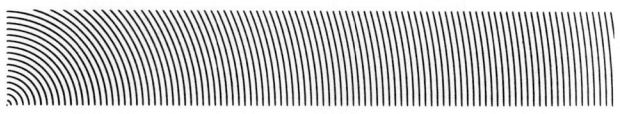

17. Health Maintenance During Pregnancy

After women learn that they are pregnant, some immediately want to know everything they should do to keep themselves well during pregnancy. Others are so surprised, so delighted, so disappointed, or so upset at the news that their only desire is to get away from the clinic or office as soon as possible to discuss it with someone close to them. You have to discover in each instance how receptive to instruction the woman will be. From the initial interview you have some indication of whether she is pleased or displeased with the pregnancy, whether she intends to continue it or to take active steps to discontinue it.

No matter how excited and pleased a woman is to be pregnant, she can assimilate only so much information at any one time. You will need to select from all the health information available those points that seem most relevant to the individual woman. The priority for discussing varicosity prevention, for example, would seem higher for a woman who has had varicosities in a former pregnancy than for one who is pregnant for the first time and is an avid sportswoman. Do not nag in health teaching. Rather, choose priorities and give meaningful, individualized health advice that will allow the woman to arrive at a plan of prenatal care that will suit her life-style and yet be consistent with good prenatal care. This kind of advice is much more likely to be followed than that given in a standardized "lecture" that the woman will instantly recognize is given to everyone.

Certain information is essential to provide at a first visit if the woman indicates that she intends to continue the pregnancy. These are the minor symptoms of pregnancy, personal care during pregnancy, and the danger signs of pregnancy.

Assessment of Minor Symptoms of Early Pregnancy

The topics included among the minor symptoms of pregnancy should be the normal accompaniments of pregnancy. *Minor* does not mean that they seem minor to the woman. A woman who is attempting to continue working, manage a household, attend to her children's needs, and participate in at least a few religious or community activities might be able to fit a pregnancy into that life with little difficulty if she did not have nausea and vomiting and so did not feel like her old self before 2:00 P.M. each day. It is reassuring to her to know that her nausea and vomiting are normal. However, they are by no means minor to her; they may be factors keeping her from enjoying and accepting this pregnancy.

The statement "Toothache is a normal consequence of carious teeth" is a true statement, but because it does not remove the pain it is not helpful. Comments such as "Backache is common," "Nausea and vomiting are to be expected," "Fatigue always occurs in early pregnancy" are reassuring but also not helpful. A comment such as "You want to be pregnant, don't you? You have to accept these things" is not helpful. The woman wants to be pregnant, true, but she does not want to be nauseated every morning. Why should she accept it?

It is as important, then, to be told how to relieve the minor discomforts or symptoms of pregnancy as it is to know what symptoms can be expected.

NAUSEA AND VOMITING

No definite reason has been established for the almost universal nausea and vomiting of early pregnancy. It may be due to sensitivity to the high gonadotropin levels produced by the trophoblast; to high estrogen levels; to lowered maternal blood sugar caused by the needs of the developing embryo; to lack of pyridoxine (vitamin B_6); to diminished gastric motility. It is aggravated by fatigue and may be aggravated by emotional disturbance.

Most women have some nausea during the first three months of pregnancy, and vomiting once a day is not uncommon. The sensation is usually most intense on arising but may occur while the woman is preparing meals and smelling food. Women who work nights and sleep days often experience "evening sickness," because that is the time of day they are arising.

Increasing glucose intake seems to relieve morning sickness better than any other remedy. The traditional solution is for women to keep dry crackers by the bedside and eat a few before rising; sourballs may serve the same purpose. The woman should eat a light breakfast or delay breakfast until 10:00 or 11:00 A.M., past the time her nausea seems to persist. It is essential for her to maintain a good food intake during pregnancy, so she has to compensate for missed breakfasts later in the day. They should not be skipped altogether.

If the woman is still having difficulty with nausea after trying to limit her morning intake, an antiemetic drug may be ordered for relief. Ask her at a first prenatal visit and at each succeeding visit for the first months of pregnancy how she is coping with the constant nausea. Ask her if she needs help. Many women are reluctant to say they need help unless you suggest it. Some may not know that there is help available. Others may feel that women are expected to endure morning sickness stoically and that asking for help will harm their image.

The drug most frequently prescribed for the normal nausea of early pregnancy is Bendectin, which is similar to the drugs prescribed for motion sickness. It is usually effective and completely eliminates morning sickness if taken daily. Like all drugs, Bendectin is now being investigated for possible teratogenic effects.

Women should be cautioned against taking home remedies, including antacids. Preparations containing sodium bicarbonate may cause fluid retention because of the sodium content. It is a sound rule that a woman should take *no* medication during pregnancy unless her physician specifically prescribes it or agrees to its use.

Morning sickness disappears spontaneously as the woman enters her 4th month of pregnancy. If it persists beyond the 4th month, its cause should be investigated. It may indicate the development of hyperemesis gravidarum, a complication of pregnancy (see Chap. 33).

PYROSIS

Pyrosis (heartburn) is a burning sensation along the esophagus caused by regurgitation of the gastric contents into the esophagus. In pregnancy, it may accompany nausea, but it may persist beyond the resolution of nausea and even increase in severity as pregnancy advances.

Pyrosis is probably caused by decreased gastric motility. It may be helped by eating small meals frequently and by not lying down immediately after eating. Aluminum hydroxide gel and magnesium hydroxide (Maalox) or aluminum hydroxide, magnesium hydroxide, and magnesium trisilicate (Gelusil) serve to reduce gastric acidity and may be prescribed for relief. Be certain the woman understands that this "chest" pain is from her gastrointestinal tract and that although it is called heartburn it has nothing to do with her heart.

GINGIVITIS

Turgescence of the gums in association with changes in salivary pH may cause bleeding and tenderness of the gingivae. It is generally slight. However, if a woman notices bleeding when she brushes her teeth, she may fear she is bleeding inside as well, endangering her baby. She needs assurance that this is a local problem, not a systemic one.

Gingivitis is sometimes caused by dietary deficiencies, particularly a lack of vitamin C. Ask the woman to list all the foods she has eaten the last two days and note whether or not she includes some citrus fruit or citrus fruit juice.

CONSTIPATION

Constipation tends to occur in pregnancy as the pressure of the growing uterus presses against the bowel and slows peristalsis. If you discuss preventive measures with the woman early in pregnancy, she may be able to avoid this problem. Encourage her to evacuate her bowels regularly (many women neglect this first simple rule), to increase the amount of roughage in her diet by eating raw fruits and vegetables, and to drink extra amounts of water daily.

The woman should not use home remedies to prevent constipation; she should avoid mineral oil especially. Mineral oil interferes with the absorption of fat-soluble vitamins (A, D, K, and E), which are needed for good fetal growth and maternal health.

Enemas should be avoided. Over-the-counter laxatives are contraindicated, as are *all* drugs during pregnancy unless specifically prescribed or sanctioned by the physician.

FATIGUE

Fatigue is extremely common in early pregnancy. It is probably due to increased metabolic requirements. Much of it can be relieved by increasing the amount of rest and sleep. Some women are reluctant to sleep or rest during the day because they fear being called lazy by their neighbors or husband. If they are working outside the home, they worry about being accused of not holding their own at their job.

Explain that their changing metabolism increases their need for rest during the early months. A good resting position is a modified Sims's position, with the top leg forward (Fig. 17-1). This puts the weight of the fetus on the bed, not on the woman, and allows good circulation in the lower extremities, which relieves the aching of poorly nourished leg muscles.

Women who continue employment during pregnancy should be reminded that they need rest as much as the woman who stays at home. The majority of women who are working at the time their pregnancy is confirmed continue working until the 7th or 8th month of pregnancy. A working woman might use a part of her lunch hour to sit in the ladies' room with her feet up on a chair, or at her desk with her feet elevated on an adjoining chair. After she returns home from work in the evening she may need to modify a customary routine from cooking dinner, doing the dishes, straightening up the house, and so on, to *resting*, then cooking dinner, doing the dishes,

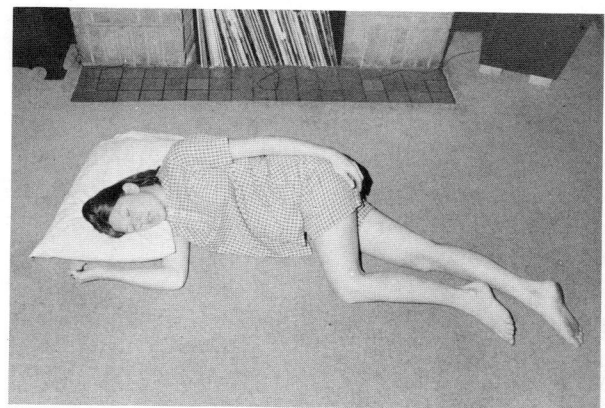

Fig. 17-1. Modified Sims's position as a rest position during pregnancy. The knees and elbows should be slightly bent, the muscles limp, and the breathing slow and regular. Notice that the weight of the fetus is resting on the floor.

and so on; or cooking dinner and then *resting while her husband does the dishes* (part of "*we* are having a baby at our house" for a husband who does not usually share in household chores).

Some women are reluctant to take the time out of their day for rest because they know that pregnancy is not an illness (and of course it is not), and so they proceed as if nothing is happening to them. Rarely is there justification during a normal pregnancy for women to take extra days off from work because of their condition, but it is unrealistic to proceed as if nothing is happening. Morning sickness increases with fatigue, and if a woman becomes too tired, she does not eat properly. If she is fatigued, preparing meals becomes too great an effort, and she does not eat properly. If she remains on her feet without at least one break during the day, the tendency for varicosities to develop increases, and so does the danger of thromboembolic complications.

Ask the woman at prenatal visits whether or not she plans to have and manages to have at least *one* short rest period every day.

POSTURAL HYPOTENSION

When advising women to rest during pregnancy, warn them that in late pregnancy lying down may cause postural hypotension. A pregnant woman who lies on her back for a long period may show signs and symptoms of shock. These include faintness and breathlessness, apprehension, low blood pressure, and sometimes a rapid and thready pulse. The phenomenon occurs because her posture (position) allows the heavy uterus to press back on the inferior vena cava and interfere with the return of blood from her lower extremities. The resultant pooling of blood produces the same symptoms as a sudden hemorrhage in which the same amount of blood was lost.

The treatment is simple: If the woman turns or is turned on her side, pressure is removed from the vena cava, blood flow is again adequate, and the symptoms quickly fade. When advising women to rest or sleep during pregnancy, recommend a left side-lying position, such as a modified Sims's position, to avoid this problem.

VARICOSITIES

Varicosities are common in pregnancy because the weight of the distended uterus puts pressure on the vessels returning blood from the lower extremities. This causes a pooling of blood in the vessels. The veins become engorged, inflamed, and painful. Varicosities are usually found in the lower extremities; they may extend to the vulva.

Women need to take precautions early in pregnancy to prevent the development of varicosities. Resting in a Sims's position or on the back with the legs raised against the wall for 15 to 20 minutes twice a day is a good precaution (Fig. 17-2).

Some women may need the support of elastic stockings or an Ace bandage for relief of varicosities. The stocking or bandage should be applied to the leg so that it reaches an area above the point of distention. The woman should apply the support before she arises in the morning; once she is on her feet, the pooling of blood has already begun, and the stockings or bandages will not be so effective. If a woman is going to buy stockings, be certain she understands they are to be medical support hose. Many panty hose manufacturers say their stockings give "firm support," and the woman may erroneously assume that this is sufficient for her.

Exercise is as effective as rest periods in alleviating varicosities, since it stimulates venous return. Most women state that they do not need set exercise periods during pregnancy because they work hard cleaning the house, or they have a job and get exercise there. If the woman analyzes the type of work she does, however, she will realize that a great deal of housework and office or factory work leads to stasis of lower-extremity circulation. The woman stands in one position to wash dishes, to iron, to make beds, to cook dinner; to file, to run a duplicating machine; to process a part on an assembly line. She needs to break up these long periods of standing still by a "walk break" at least twice a day, and her family would benefit by accompanying her. If her husband analyzes his workday, he will probably discover that he, too, walks very little during the day.

Vitamin C may be helpful in reducing the size of varicosities. It is apparently involved in the formation of blood vessel collagen and endothelium. Ask at prenatal visits whether or not vitamin C is included in the woman's diet. Ask her if she takes a walk every day, weather permitting.

MUSCLE CRAMPS

Decreased levels of serum calcium, increased levels of serum phosphorus, and, possibly, interference with circulation commonly cause muscle cramps of the lower extremities during pregnancy. They are best relieved by lying on the back and extending the involved leg. The woman should keep her knee straight and dorsiflex her foot (Fig. 17-3). With the leg in this position, it may help to knead the muscle until the hard "knot" is gone.

If the woman is having frequent leg cramps, the physician may prescribe aluminum hydroxide gel (Amphojel) in order to remove phosphorus from the intestinal tract and thereby lower its circulating level. Lowering milk intake may also help to reduce the phosphorus level. Elevating the lower extremities to improve circulation may be of benefit.

Muscle cramps are a minor symptom of pregnancy, but the pain may be extreme, and the intensity of the contraction is frightening. The woman needs reassurance that muscle cramps are normal in pregnancy.

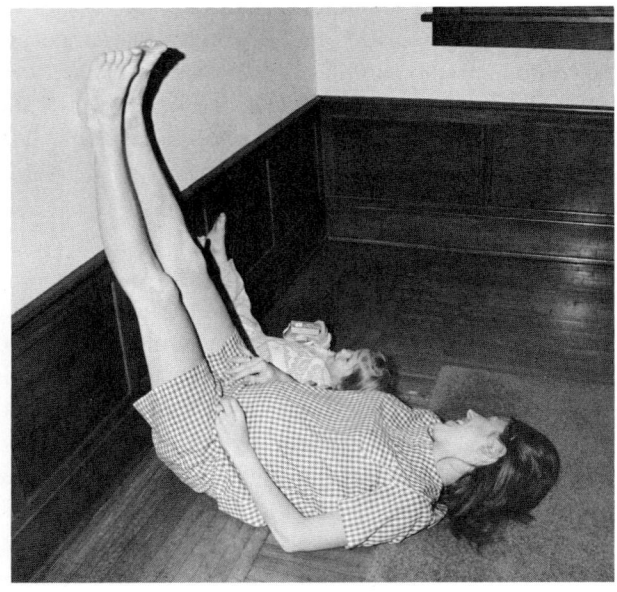

Fig. 17-2. Position to relieve varicosities. A 2-year-old daughter joins her mother in the exercise.

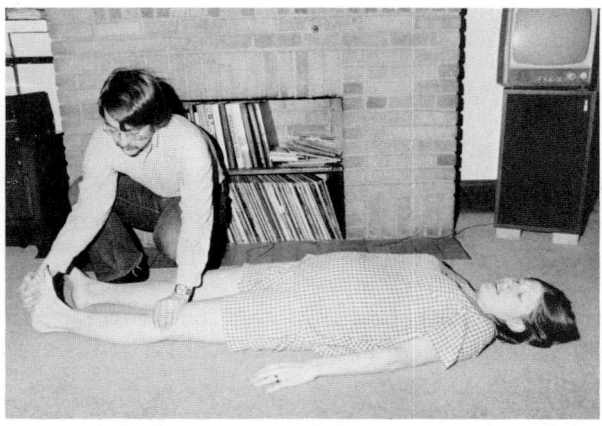

Fig. 17-3. Relieving a leg cramp in pregnancy. Pressing down on the knee and forcing the toes upward relieves most cramps. The husband assists here.

HEMORRHOIDS

Hemorrhoids, which are varicosities of the rectal veins, are common in pregnancy because of pressure on these veins from the bulk of the growing uterus. Preventive measures early in pregnancy may be effective in reducing their severity. Daily bowel evacuation not only helps to relieve constipation but also helps to prevent the formation of hemorrhoids. Resting in a modified Sims's position daily is helpful. At day's end, assuming a knee-chest position (Fig. 17-4) is an excellent way to reduce the pressure on rectal veins. A knee-chest position tends to make a woman feel light-headed; thus, at first, she should remain in this position for a few minutes only, gradually increasing the time until she can comfortably maintain the position for about 15 minutes. Stool softeners may be recommended for the woman who already has hemorrhoids.

PALPITATIONS

On sudden movement, such as turning over in bed, a pregnant woman may experience a bounding palpitation of the heart. It is probably due to the circulatory adjustments necessary to accommodate the increased blood supply during pregnancy. The sensation is frightening because the heart seems to skip a beat. Slower movements will prevent its happening so frequently. It is reassuring to know that palpitations are normal and to be expected on occasion.

VAGINAL PROBLEMS

Leukorrhea

Leukorrhea is a whitish, viscous vaginal discharge or an increase in the amount of normal vaginal secretions. It probably occurs because of the high estrogen levels and the increased blood supply to the vaginal epithelium and cervix in pregnancy. A daily bath is usually enough to control this problem. Some women feel they must wear sanitary pads. Women should be cautioned not to use tampons, since they may lead to stasis of secretions and possible subsequent infection.

Pruritus

Any woman who has vulvar pruritus needs to be seen by a physician, since this usually indicates infection. Be certain that when she is describing pruritus-like symptoms she is not really describing burning on urination, a sign of a beginning bladder infection.

Infections

The most frequent vaginal infections are trichomoniasis and candidiasis. Nystatin (Mycostatin) and aqueous gentian violet in either douche or suppository form are the two most commonly prescribed drugs for candidiasis. Flagyl (metronidazole), a drug used to treat trichomoniasis, is not recommended during pregnancy because it crosses the placenta and may be teratogenic.

It is dangerous for a woman to use a bulb-type douche apparatus while she is pregnant. It puts solution into the vagina under pressure, which can cause a circulatory embolism if the solution is pushed into the cervix and under the edge of the placenta and into maternal vessels. This is an important point to remember when talking to pregnant women about douching, because women are likely to regard the

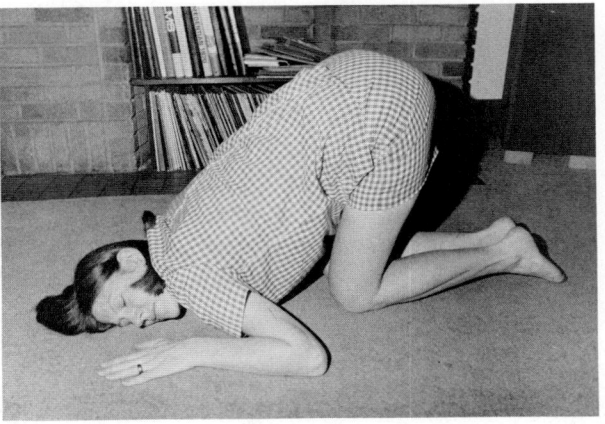

Fig. 17-4. Knee-chest position. This position allows for freer flow of urine from the kidneys (preventing urinary tract stasis and infection) and better circulation in the rectal area (preventing hemorrhoids), since the weight of the uterus is shifted forward.

bulb-type apparatus as more convenient and will buy this type if not cautioned against doing so.

A woman who is uncomfortable about discussing this part of her body or who associates vaginal infections with poor hygiene or venereal disease may be reluctant to mention an irritating vaginal discharge. Specifically ask each woman whether she has this problem. Specific management of vaginal infections is discussed in Chap. 33.

FREQUENCY OF URINATION

Frequency of urination is due to the pressure of the growing uterus on the anterior bladder. It begins in early pregnancy, lasts for about the first three months, then disappears until late in pregnancy, when it again becomes a problem. It disappears in midpregnancy because the uterus rises above the bladder; it returns in later pregnancy as the fetal head presses against the bladder.

When a woman is describing frequency of urination to you, be certain it is the only urinary symptom she has. Ask her whether she has burning as well, or whether she has noticed any blood in her urine (signs of urinary tract infection).

PALMAR ERYTHEMA

Palmar erythema or palmar pruritus occurs in early pregnancy and is probably caused by the increase in the level of estrogen. Constant redness or itching of the palms may make the woman think she is allergic to something. She spends much time and effort trying different soaps or detergents or attempting to implicate certain foods she has eaten recently. Calamine lotion may be soothing for this condition. As soon as the woman's body adjusts to the increased level of estrogen, the erythema and pruritus disappear.

ABDOMINAL DISCOMFORT

Some women experience uncomfortable feelings of abdominal pressure early in pregnancy. Women with a multiple pregnancy may notice this all through pregnancy. Women learn to relieve the feeling by putting gentle pressure on the uterine fundus. Pregnant women typically stand with their arms crossed in front as the weight of their arms resting on their abdomens relieves the discomfort.

When women stand up quickly, they often experience a pulling pain in the right or left lower abdomen from tension on the round ligaments. The pain is sharp and frightening. They can prevent this type of pain by always rising slowly from a lying to a sitting, or from a sitting to a standing, position. Since round ligament pain may simulate the abrupt pain that occurs with ruptured ectopic pregnancy (tubal pregnancy), a woman's description of sharp lower abdominal pain must be listened to carefully.

BREAST TENDERNESS

Breast tenderness is often one of the first symptoms noticed in early pregnancy. Exposure to cold air may make the tenderness more noticeable. For most women the tenderness is minimal. If it is enough to cause real discomfort, encourage the woman to wear a bra with a wide shoulder strap for support. Nipple fissure or other reason for the pain should be investigated.

Personal Care During Pregnancy

Because pregnancy is not an illness, the woman has to take few special care measures other than to use common sense. Women are likely to have heard many old wives' tales about what a woman can and cannot do during pregnancy. Thus, the bulk of teaching time in the personal care area is spent separating fact from fiction, enabling the woman to enjoy her pregnancy unhampered by unnecessary restrictions.

BATHING

At one time, bathing was restricted during pregnancy because it was feared that bath water would enter the vagina and cervix and contaminate the uterine contents. Further, it was believed that hot water touching the abdomen might bring on labor. Because the vagina is normally in a closed position, or the sides approximate each other, the danger that water will enter the uterus is minimal. The temperature of the water has no documented effect. Sweating tends to increase with pregnancy because the woman excretes waste products not only for herself but for the child within her, so daily bathing has now moved from a high place on the *don't* list to a high place on the *do* list.

As pregnancy advances, it may be hard for a woman to get in and out of a bathtub because of her problem in maintaining balance. If so, she should shower instead or take sponge baths, whichever her common sense tells her is better. If membranes rupture, bathing is contraindicated because then there *is* a danger of contamination of uterine contents. During the last month of pregnancy, when cervical dilatation may be beginning, some physicians restrict tub bathing for the same reason.

DOUCHING

Although women have increased vaginal discharges during pregnancy, douching is not advocated. If a woman feels this is necessary, her physician should specify the amount and kind of solution she may use. As indicated in the discussion of vaginal infections, she should never use a bulb-type syringe.

EXERCISE

Women need exercise during pregnancy to prevent circulatory stasis. For many women, teaching is centered on helping them realize the need for exercise and urging them to get enough. Others may have to be taught to restrict exercise or participation in sports. If a woman is a competent horsewoman, for example, there is little reason for her to discontinue riding until it becomes uncomfortable (as long as she does not have a history of abortion). However, pregnancy is no time to learn to ride because a beginning rider is in more danger of being thrown than is an experienced one. The same principles apply to skiing and bicycling. An accomplished skier or bicycler may continue her activity in moderation until balance becomes a problem, but pregnancy is no time to learn to ski or ride a bicycle because the lack of skill may result in many falls. Swimming is a good activity for pregnant women and, like bathing, is not contraindicated as long as the membranes are intact. Long-distance swimming to a point of fatigue is difficult to justify.

ALCOHOL CONSUMPTION

Alcohol consumption should be limited in pregnancy lest a fetal alcohol syndrome develop. This syndrome includes growth retardation, mental deficiency, and craniofacial or structural musculoskeletal anomalies in the infant. The exact amount of alcohol that will lead to damage to the fetus is not well documented, but as little as 1 to 3 ounces of alcohol a day during the early months of pregnancy may be dangerous; six alcoholic drinks a day, especially before the 5th month of pregnancy, is documented to be beyond safe limits.

Pregnancy may be the motivation a woman needs to seek help for excessive drinking. Be certain to ask about drinking habits on an initial interview; you may discover a woman in a vulnerable, ready-to-ask-for-help moment.

SMOKING

It is well documented that *smoking in excess* (more than 10 cigarettes per day) is harmful to fetal growth. However, it is often impossible for a smoker to stop if she has been smoking any length of time. She may be able to cut down on the number of cigarettes smoked per day. This possibility should be explored early in pregnancy.

It is difficult for a nurse who does not smoke to appreciate what a cigarette means to a smoker. If you are a nonsmoker, be aware that you are advising or asking the woman to give up something that you do not fully appreciate the need for.

EMPLOYMENT

Unless the woman's job involves handling toxic substances, lifting heavy objects, other kinds of excessive physical strain, or long periods of standing or having to maintain body balance, there are few reasons she cannot continue to be employed until at least the 7th month of pregnancy.

New rights for pregnant women were passed by Congress in 1978 (Public Law 95-555). As a result of these, an employer *cannot*

Deprive a woman of seniority rights, in pay or promotion, because she takes a maternity leave.
Treat a woman back from maternity leave as a new hire, starting over on the eligibility period for pension and other benefits.
Force a pregnant woman to leave if she is able to and wants to continue to work.
Refuse to hire a woman just because she is pregnant or fire her for the same reason.
Refuse to cover an employee's normal pregnancy and delivery expenses in the company health plan, or pay less for pregnancy than for other medical conditions.
Refuse to pay sick leave or disability benefits to women whose difficult pregnancies keep them off the job.

The only women not covered by this new law are those who work for companies with fewer than 15 employees.

In *Standards for Maternity Care and Employment of Mothers in Industry*, the Maternal Child Health Service of the United States reports that pregnant women should not work with any of the following substances: aniline, benzene and toluene, carbon disulfide, carbon monoxide, chlorinated hydrocarbons, lead and its compounds, mercury and its compounds, nitrobenzene and other nitro compounds of benzene and its homologues, phosphorus, radioactive substances, x-rays, and turpentine.

Remember that few women work for the sheer joy of working; the majority work to augment the family income. However, some prefer to work, and others begin working as a means of filling in empty hours or to exercise a skill they have worked hard to acquire, such as nursing. After they have worked for a while, they adapt their style of living to the added income. Giving it up then becomes as difficult for this woman as for the woman who began to work solely for additional income. More effective than counseling women to resign from their jobs during pregnancy, then, so they do have more rest, may be counseling them to reserve periods during the day for rest and urging them to eat a proper diet.

TRAVEL

Most women have questions about travel during pregnancy, especially as the summer months approach and they are planning vacations. Early in a normal pregnancy, there are literally no restrictions. Late in pregnancy, however, travel plans should take account of the possibility of early labor, requiring delivery at a strange hospital where the woman's obstetrical history is unknown.

If the woman plans to spend her vacation at a remote camp site, be certain that no matter what the month of her pregnancy she knows of a physician near the campsite who can provide medical attention if an unexpected complication should occur. If she is going to be away from home for an extended vacation, she will need to make arrangements to visit a physician in her vacation area at the times her regular prenatal visits would be scheduled. Ask her to make these plans far enough ahead of time for her records from your clinic or office to be copied and forwarded to the physician she will see (you need her written permission to send records). She should be sure to take enough of her prescribed medication and prescriptions for refills if necessary.

Advise a woman who is taking a long trip by automobile to plan frequent rest or stretch periods. Every 100 miles, or at least every 200 miles, she should get out of the car and walk a short distance. This practice will relieve stiffness and muscle ache and will improve lower-extremity circulation, preventing varicosities and hemorrhoids.

Pregnant women should use seat belts in automobiles, as should everyone else. Occasionally, uterine rupture has been reported from seat belt use, but, overall, the evidence suggests that seat belts reduce maternal mortality in car accidents. The use of shoulder harnesses should be encouraged as well.

Women may drive as long as they fit comfortably behind the steering wheel. Those who are susceptible to motion sickness should take no medication that is not specifically prescribed by their physician or discussed with their physician.

Traveling by plane shortens traveling time and is not contraindicated as long as the plane has a well-pressurized cabin (true of commercial airlines, but not of all small private planes). A well-pressurized cabin is important because low oxygen concentrations may occur at high altitudes if the cabin pressure is not stabilized. Low oxygen intake may lead to hypoxia, with possible brain damage to the fetus. Some airlines do not permit women who are more than seven months pregnant on board; others require written permission from the woman's physician. The woman will have to investigate the restrictions herself. Most travel agencies have this information.

Women who are traveling abroad may need extra vaccination protection for entry into certain countries or to safeguard their own health. Vaccinations are a form of medication in that they are intrusive and should not be taken without the physician's knowledge and approval. Live virus vaccination is contraindicated during pregnancy because the virus may cross the placenta and infect the fetus. Vaccines against smallpox, mumps (infectious parotitis), rubeola, rubella, yellow fever, or poliomyelitis (Sabin's vaccine) should *not* be administered to a pregnant woman. However, if the woman is in an area where smallpox or yellow fever is endemic, vaccination might be essential. Such immunization should be undertaken, however, with the understanding that fetal risk is involved.

The vaccine against cholera contains killed bacteria and thus may be given if the woman is exposed to the infection. It does not appear to be abortifacient. Tetanus and diphtheria toxoids are apparently safe.

The field of immunization is a constantly changing one, since new discoveries are continually being made. Before you give advice on immunizations to a pregnant woman, check with the public health authorities in your community.

Following delivery of the child, the woman should be urged to have the standard immunizations (especially rubella vaccine), so that during the next pregnancy the problem of whether or not vaccinations should be given will not arise.

CLOTHING

The day when a woman had to purchase a completely new maternity wardrobe is fast disappearing. This has an economic advantage, but it may be disappointing to a woman who wants to announce her pregnancy early by putting on maternity clothes.

A young woman today usually needs little guidance in selecting proper clothing for her expanding abdomen. She may wear an abdominal support in early pregnancy if she wishes (for *support*, not to compress and constrict her abdomen). She should avoid garters and panty girdles, since they impede lower-extremity circulation. She may need to purchase larger-size bras as her breasts enlarge. Otherwise, the rule is common sense and comfort.

INTERCOURSE

Some women do not ask questions about sexual relations during pregnancy because they have inhibitions about broaching the subject. Most women have questions, however, about restriction of intercourse during pregnancy.

Old wives' tales about intercourse in pregnancy abound: Intercourse on the date her period would have been expected (if the woman had not become pregnant) will initiate labor; orgasm will initiate labor, but relations without orgasm will not; intercourse during the fertile days of a cycle will cause a second pregnancy or twins; intercourse might cause rupture of the membranes. If a woman has such concerns, she needs to voice them. Then they can be dispelled as the old wives' tales they are, and she will not refrain from intercourse when she desires it or worry needlessly that intercourse is harming her child.

Women who have a history of repeated abortion may be advised to avoid intercourse during the time of the pregnancy when the previous abortions occurred. Women whose membranes have ruptured or who have vaginal spotting should be advised against intercourse in order to prevent infection. Otherwise, there are no sexual restrictions during pregnancy.

As pregnancy advances and the woman's abdomen increases in size, she and her husband may need to use new positions for intercourse. A side-by-side position, or the woman in a superior position, may be more comfortable. As vaginal secretions change, the woman may find a lubricant helpful. If she begins to experience discomfort, mutual masturbation or oral-genital relations might be satisfying to both partners. However, advise caution about male oral–female genital contact, since accidental air embolism has been reported from this act during pregnancy.

Many nurses are not accustomed to discussing sexual relations and therefore ignore the subject as if it were not a concern during pregnancy. Couples who are having problems in this area are thus left feeling as though there were something basically wrong with them or their relationship, rather than being assured that such difficulties are normal in pregnancy. You should be as familiar with this aspect of pregnancy and as ready to offer helpful suggestions about it as you are about the problems of constipation, nausea, or bathing.

NUTRITION

Good nutrition is extremely important during pregnancy. The essentials of a proper diet need review. These are discussed in Chap. 18.

Danger Signs of Pregnancy

An important part of health teaching at a first prenatal visit involves instructing the woman about the danger signals to which she should be alert during pregnancy. Assure her you have no reason to think she is going to experience any of these things; that you have every reason to believe she is going to have a normal, uncomplicated pregnancy (if that is true); but that if any of these things occur, she should inform the physician or the clinic by telephoning immediately. Be certain you give her an alternate number to call in the event the physician's office or clinic is closed. Emphasize that these danger signals do not mean something bad has happened to her or her baby; they will merely alert her to the possibility that something *may* happen. It is important for her to report them immediately, so that they can be dealt with *before* something harmful occurs.

VAGINAL BLEEDING

A woman should report vaginal bleeding no matter how slight; some of the serious bleeding complications of pregnancy begin with *slight* spotting. If you are talking to the woman on the telephone, ask her how she discovered the spotting. If she discovered it on toilet paper after voiding, she is probably reporting actual vaginal bleeding. If she reports spotting on her underpants, she may be reporting spotting from hemorrhoids. When a woman has spotting, the physician will either see her or offer her advice on the telephone, depending on the length of her pregnancy and the individual circumstances.

PERSISTENT VOMITING

It is not uncommon during the first trimester of pregnancy for a woman to vomit once or twice a day. Persistent vomiting is never normal; vomiting that continues past the 4th month of pregnancy may be considered persistent.

CHILLS AND FEVER

Pregnancy is not an illness, and thus chills and fever, symptoms of infection, are never normal. They may be evidence of an intrauterine infection, which is a serious complication for both the woman and baby. They may also be symptoms of a relatively benign gastroenteritis. However, the woman herself is incapable of making an informed decision as to the cause.

SUDDEN ESCAPE OF FLUID FROM THE VAGINA

When fluid is suddenly discharged from the vagina, it is evident that the membranes have ruptured; the fluid is amniotic fluid. This may be one of the first signs of labor. Mother and fetus are now both threatened, because the uterine cavity is no longer sealed against infection. If the fetus is small and his head does not fit snugly into the cervix, the umbilical cord may prolapse with the membrane rupture, the head may be compressed against the cord, and the fetus may be in immediate and grave danger.

PAIN IN THE ABDOMEN

Abdominal pain at any time is a signal that something abnormal is occurring. However, some women may think that it is normal in pregnancy because of the growing uterus and the deflection of their other organs from their usual alignment. They are wrong—an expanding uterus expands painlessly. Abdominal pain is announcing something else: a tubal (ectopic) pregnancy; a separation of the placenta; or something unrelated to the pregnancy but perhaps serious, such as appendicitis, ulcer, or pancreatitis.

When a pregnant woman stands up suddenly, particularly if she was sitting on the floor, she may experience sharp, fleeting pain in her groin from extension of the round ligament. Most women can distinguish this sensation of pulling from other abdominal pain, but some may report it as a danger signal of pregnancy.

DANGER SIGNALS OF PREGNANCY-INDUCED HYPERTENSION

Four symptoms signal developing pregnancy-induced hypertension:

1. Swelling of the face or fingers
2. Flashes of light or dots before the eyes
3. Dimness or blurring of vision
4. Severe, continuous headache

It is normal for a woman to have some edema of the ankles during pregnancy, particularly if she has been on her feet for a long period of time. Swelling of the hands (ask if she has noticed that her rings are tight) or face indicates edema too extensive to be normal. Visual disturbance or continuous headache may be a sign that cerebral edema is also present or that hypertension is becoming acute. Be certain the wom-

Table 17-1. Danger Signs of Pregnancy

Sign	Possible Importance
Vaginal bleeding	Placenta previa, premature separation of the placenta, premature birth
Persistent vomiting	Systemic infection; will lead to electrolyte and fluid disturbances
Chills and fever	Intrauterine infection
Sudden escape of fluid from the vagina	Premature ruptured membranes
Abdominal pain	Ectopic pregnancy, premature separation of the placenta, uterine rupture
Swelling of the face or fingers	Pregnancy-induced hypertension
Flashes of light or dots before the eyes	Pregnancy-induced hypertension
Dimness or blurring of vision	Pregnancy-induced hypertension
Severe, continuous headache	Pregnancy-induced hypertension

an is using her common sense and is not reporting symptoms she had before she became pregnant. If she had the same visual difficulties and headaches before pregnancy as she is having now, she may need to see an ophthalmologist rather than her obstetrician for help with the problem.

Danger signs of pregnancy are summarized in Table 17-1.

Nursing Interventions at Prenatal Visits

If the woman appears to have no health problem or other problem that would require additional supervision, she is usually advised to visit her physician once a month until the 32nd week of pregnancy and every two weeks thereafter until the 36th week, when the visits are increased to once a week until she delivers.

INTERVAL HISTORY

An interval history should be taken at each visit, updating occurrences from the last visit. The interval history begins with an introduction, an explanation of the purpose of the contact (which should be the rule in all patient contacts), and elicitation of the chief concern. Only a week may have passed since the woman's last visit, yet many things may have occurred that are causing her concern. For example, the *little* heart palpitation that she noticed in preceding months never bothered her, but the many palpitations she has been experiencing over the past week may be bothering her a great deal. Being two days past her due date may not have bothered her a week ago, but today the fact that she is nine days late may be extremely anxiety-provoking.

Remember that the woman's psychological adjustment to her pregnancy is just as important as her physical adjustment. If she voices a physical concern, be certain to ask about her psychosocial well-being. Many women take nine months to adjust to the fact that health care personnel are as interested in their psychosocial problems as in their physical problems; it may be as difficult for the woman to accept this concept as to accept her pregnancy.

After the woman has expressed her concerns, review the present pregnancy history, asking specifically about the danger signals. Be sure to allow time for her to bring up any problem she wishes to discuss with you or the physician on this visit.

Initial interviews are often more interesting than interval histories. Be sure you do not convey this feeling to the woman. A warm reception on the first visit and a less enthusiastic reception on subsequent visits will be disheartening and may result in missed appointments. For the woman, this pregnancy remains unique and special all during its course. The first visit was exciting because she was told she was pregnant. Today is the first day, or the first day in this pregnancy, that she has been three, or four, or five months pregnant, which is equally exciting. Share her enthusiasm and thereby help her to enjoy her pregnancy to the fullest.

URINALYSIS

At each prenatal visit, a woman is asked to bring a first-voided morning specimen of urine. As mentioned, glucose spills into urine easily during pregnancy. The first voiding in the morning is most likely to be free of glucose. Finding glucose in this urine is thus probably significant. If for any reason the woman does not bring a urine sample—and sometimes it is inconvenient for her to carry such a specimen on a bus or to have it in her purse if she has to pay a cab driver—she should be given a clean specimen cup and asked to void at the office or clinic.

At each visit, this urine is tested for glucose and albumin by you or by a technician. If the woman has any symptoms suggestive of urinary tract infection—pus or blood in her urine, frequency of urination (more than occurs normally with pregnancy), lower abdominal pain, slight fever, burning on urination—she should be instructed to void a clean-catch urine specimen, as follows:

She first washes her perineum from front to back with sterile cotton balls saturated with a soap or antiseptic solution. She then rinses it with cotton balls saturated with sterile water. After drying the urethral opening and vulva (always working front to back to avoid bacterial contamination from the rectum), the woman should begin to void. After a moment, she should place a sterile cup or container under the stream of urine to collect a midstream specimen for examination.

If the physician wishes to examine the specimen microscopically, the urine is transferred to a test tube and spun in a centrifuge for about 5 minutes. A few drops of the sediment are smeared on a slide, and the slide is examined under a microscope for a preliminary reading. The presence of bacteriuria can be suggested by this method. For assessment of the types of organisms present, the urine is plated on agar media, sent to a laboratory for a culture and sensitivity study, or placed in a culture container supplied for that purpose.

PHYSICAL EXAMINATION AND BLOOD STUDIES

The woman's blood pressure and weight are measured at each office or clinic visit. The woman's abdomen is palpated, the fundal height is measured, and the fetal heart rate is recorded on each visit.

After the initial visit a woman is sometimes reluctant to return for further visits because she is concerned that each visit will entail a vaginal examination and drawing of blood. She can be assured that under normal circumstances blood will not be drawn again until the last trimester of pregnancy, when her finger will be pricked for a repeat hematocrit. She will not need another pelvic examination until about midway in pregnancy (to make certain that everything is proceeding well) and at term (to check on cervical dilatation). Vaginal examinations are always kept to a minimum to reduce the risk of introducing infection.

A woman with Rh-negative blood can expect to have blood drawn approximately three times during pregnancy, beginning at the 4th month, to determine antibody titer. A woman with anemia will have her blood assayed more frequently.

Assessment of Minor Symptoms of Mid or Late Pregnancy

At the midpoint of pregnancy (the 20th to 24th weeks) the woman is usually ready for further health teaching that relates to the new developments in the latter half of pregnancy. She should be informed of the signs and symptoms of beginning labor. As she starts to view the child within her as a separate person, she becomes interested in discussing and making plans for labor, delivery, and the infant's care. At the midpoint of a pregnancy it is good to review the precautions she should take to prevent constipation, varicosities, and hemorrhoids and to describe the new minor symptoms that may now be expected.

BACKACHE

As pregnancy advances, postural changes will be necessary to maintain balance, and the muscle strain involved will cause backaches. Shoes with a moderate height heel reduce the amount of spinal curvature necessary to maintain an upright posture. Encouraging the woman to walk with her pelvis tilted forward (putting pelvic support under the weight of the fetus) is also helpful. Too often, women are observed at a prenatal visit only lying in a lithotomy position on an examining table. Make it a nursing responsibility to assess the manner in which the woman walks and what type of shoes she is wearing as she moves from the waiting room to the examining room. This assessment can reveal a lot about the cause of her backache. Advising the woman to squat and not to bend over to pick up objects may also help. She may need a firmer mattress during pregnancy than she did before; sliding a board under the mattress serves the same purpose and is cheaper than buying a new mattress. Pelvic rocking, an exercise described in Chap. 19, also helps to relieve backache.

Backache can be an initial sign of bladder or kidney infection. Thus, you need a detailed account of the woman's symptoms to make sure she is describing only backache. The woman should not take muscle relaxants or analgesia for back pain without first consulting her physician (as she should take no medication without first consulting her physician during pregnancy).

DYSPNEA

Shortness of breath occurs in pregnancy as the expanding uterus puts pressure on the diaphragm and causes some lung compression. A woman may notice this mostly at night, when she lies flat, and she will definitely notice it on exertion. As pregnancy progresses, she may require two or more pillows in order to sleep at night. She needs to limit her activities to a point before she becomes short of breath. Remember that anxiety adds to the sensation of breathlessness. Worry over dyspnea may make her more dyspneic, which is one reason this is an important minor symptom to review.

ANKLE EDEMA

Most women experience some swelling of the ankles and feet during late pregnancy. It is most noticeable at the end of the day. Women are often conscious of it first because they kick off their shoes at a restaurant or party and then are unable to put them on again comfortably.

Ankle edema of this nature, as long as proteinuria and hypertension do not accompany it, is a normal occurrence of pregnancy. It is probably caused by reduced blood circulation in the lower extremities due to uterine pressure, and general fluid retention. This simple edema can be relieved by resting in a side-lying position. Elevating the legs is also helpful. Women should avoid constricting panty girdles or knee-high stockings, as these impede circulation.

Women need reassurance that ankle edema is normal during pregnancy. Otherwise, they worry that it is a beginning sign of pregnancy-induced hypertension. On the other hand, do not dismiss a report of lower-extremity edema until you are certain that the woman does not evidence any signs (proteinuria, hypertension, edema of other, nondependent parts, sudden increase in weight) that might indicate pregnancy-induced hypertension.

ROLL-OVER TEST

That pregnancy-induced hypertension may occur in later pregnancy may be predicted by the roll-over test. This assessment can be done as an independent nursing assessment if it is not routinely incorporated in physician care. At a prenatal visit between the 28th and 32nd week of pregnancy, the woman lies in a left lateral recumbent position on the examining table for 15 minutes. At the end of 15 minutes her blood pressure is taken for a baseline reading. The woman is then helped to turn onto her back and her blood pressure is again recorded. If her diastolic pressure is 20 mm Hg or more in a supine position than in a left lateral position, the woman is likely to develop pregnancy-induced hypertension as pregnancy progresses. This assessment is deceptively simple for a tool that has such a high predictive reliability.

FREQUENCY OF URINATION

Frequency of urination usually ceases after the first trimester of pregnancy. Unless a woman is cautioned that the sensation returns after lightening (the settling of the fetal head into the inlet of the pelvis), she may think she has a urinary tract infection.

WEIGHT GAIN

By the midpoint of pregnancy, the woman begins to gain weight faster than she did in early pregnancy. For some women this is an encouraging sign, since they interpret it to mean that the fetus is growing and thriving. Others, unaware that it would happen, become afraid that they will be criticized for gaining too much weight and so may miss appointments or go on diets that lack essential nutrients.

The average weight gain in mid and late pregnancy is about a pound a week. A sharp, sudden weight gain may indicate fluid retention or developing hypertension of pregnancy. Be careful when talking to women about weight gain that you do not put the "cart before the horse." The hypertension does not develop because of the gain in weight; the gain in weight is evidence that hypertension and edema are developing.

CONTRACTIONS

Beginning as early as the 3rd month of pregnancy, the uterus "practices" contractions in preparation for labor (Braxton Hicks contractions). Early in pregnancy, these contractions are not noticeable. In mid and late pregnancy, the contractions become stronger, and the woman who tenses at the sensation may even experience some minimal pain. She needs reassurance that the contractions are normal and that they are not a sign of beginning labor. However, they are a positive sign that her pregnancy will end. Late in pregnancy, some women feel as if they have been pregnant forever and are much in need of this type of reassurance.

BREAST CHANGES

At about the 16th week of pregnancy, colostrum secretion begins in the breasts. The sensation of a fluid discharge from the breasts will be frightening unless the woman is forewarned that it is likely to happen at about this time. Instruct her to wash her breasts with clear water daily in order to wash the colostrum away and minimize the risk of infection from organisms growing in this medium.

Personal Care Update

An updating of personal hygiene information is helpful to women at the midpoint of pregnancy. If the physician with whom you work restricts sexual relations or bathing during the last month of pregnancy, the woman will need to be reminded of these restrictions and have the available alternatives discussed with her. She should be cautioned once more against douching, since it becomes more and more hazardous the closer she comes to delivery and cervical dilatation.

Many physicians advise no special breast care other than gentle cleansing once a day with clear water for all their patients. Others advocate that women who plan to breast-feed take certain measures beginning at about the midpoint of pregnancy. These are discussed in Chap. 30.

Preparation-for-Childbirth Classes

All women should be encouraged to attend preparation-for-childbirth classes or classes for expectant parents. The curriculum of these classes is discussed in Chap. 19.

Signals of Beginning Labor

By the 28th week of pregnancy, review with the woman the events that signal the beginning of labor. These include

Lightening (settling of the fetal head into the pelvis)
"Show" (slight blood-streaked vaginal discharge)
Rupture of the membranes (sudden gush of clear fluid from vagina)
Excess energy
Uterine contractions

LIGHTENING

Lightening is the settling of the fetal head into the inlet of the true pelvis. It occurs approximately two weeks before labor in primiparas but at unpredictable times in multiparas. The woman notices that she is not so short of breath as she was; her abdominal contour is definitely changed; and on standing she may experience sciatic pain from the lower fetal position.

SHOW

Show is the common term for the release of the cervical plug (operculum) that formed during pregnancy. It consists of a mucous, often blood-streaked vaginal discharge and indicates that cervical dilatation is beginning.

RUPTURE OF THE MEMBRANES

A sudden gush of clear fluid (amniotic fluid) from the vagina indicates rupture of the membranes. The woman should telephone the clinic or office at once if labor begins this way. If the physician is concerned about possible cord prolapse, he may want to see her immediately.

EXCESS ENERGY

Feeling extremely energetic is a sign of labor that is important for women to recognize. It occurs as part of the body's physiological preparation for labor. If they do not recognize the sensation for what it is, they will use this burst of energy to clean, iron, and cook, depleting it and entering labor exhausted. Recognizing this symptom as an initial sign of labor, they will conserve the energy for labor, the purpose for which nature provides it.

UTERINE CONTRACTIONS

For most women, labor begins with contractions. True labor contractions usually start in the back and sweep forward across the abdomen like a band tightening. They gradually increase in both frequency and intensity. Advise the woman to telephone the clinic or office when contractions begin, to alert the health care personnel that she is in labor. Inform her at what point in labor her physician wants her to come to the hospital, but be sure she knows this is not a hard-and-fast rule. If she should become exceptionally anxious, be home alone, or have a long drive to the hospital, she should have the option to arrive at the hospital ahead of time.

Preparation for the Baby's Care

Once a woman feels the fetus stir, she is usually ready to start making plans to care for the coming baby. She does not need a great deal of equipment to care for an infant at home, and if she buys only the essentials, she will minimize the financial burden of the new baby on the family. On the other hand, every woman needs to buy some new clothes and equipment as part of "nest building" to make the pregnancy and therefore the baby seem more real.

SLEEPING ARRANGEMENTS

A newborn should have a bed of his own. It can be a crib, bassinet, cradle, or baby buggy; if the family cannot afford anything else, it can be a padded dresser drawer.

Newborns generally enjoy being swaddled or tightly wrapped and so sleep more soundly in a bassinet or cradle than in a large crib. However, when they begin to turn over, at about 2 months of age, they will need a larger bed. Thus, if finances are a major problem, the woman would be well advised to buy only a crib. If she swaddles the infant and places a blanket roll behind his back, he will feel snug and content in his crib.

If parents are going to repaint a crib, they should be sure the paint is lead-free, since the infant is likely to chew on the crib rail as he grows older. Lead poisoning may result if a lead-base paint is used. Paint or wallpaper peeling anywhere in the house should be removed or covered by paneling, especially in the child's room. As a temporary measure until the walls are repaired, the crib will have to be placed in the center of the room. Children like to chew on peeling paint chips, since paint tastes sweet, and they will taste and eat them again and again. Crib rails should be sturdy so they will not break, and the space between them should be narrow enough to keep the infant from putting his head in between the rails and possibly being suffocated. A crib bumper provides the same insurance.

The crib mattress should be firm and should be covered by a waterproof material. It is not necessary to purchase special crib sheets, which are expensive for their size; regular bed sheets folded over or cut down can be used. Regular pillowcases make satisfactory bassinet mattress covers.

Wool blankets are not the best choice. They may cause allergies and are not easy to wash and dry. Rings or clamps should not be used to anchor the blanket to the side rails of the crib, since the baby may become strangled in such clips. Another good safety rule to emphasize concerns pillows: *never use a pillow in a crib*. When the infant is old enough to graduate to a bed, he is also old enough to sleep on a pillow without danger of suffocation.

A newborn sleeps best in a room by himself where he will not be awakened by people moving around and talking. If he is awake and needs something, the healthy newborn will cry vigorously and loudly enough to be heard all over the house. However, the mother who feels she will be too anxious if the infant is separated from her might place the infant's crib next to her own bed. Encourage her never to plan to sleep with the baby. An infant can be injured by an adult who rolls over on him during the night, and he can be suffocated by the pillows.

If a woman is planning on sleeping with her infant, explore the reason with her. Perhaps she cannot afford to buy a crib and needs financial assistance to do so. Perhaps someone in her family lost a child from sudden infant death syndrome (gently sleeping one hour, found dead the next); a woman who has this kind of fear needs to have the crib in the room with her, to hear the baby breathing and be sure this is not happening to him. Perhaps there are rats in the home, and she fears they may attack her baby; she feels he would be safer with her than in a separate crib. This is a legitimate fear and involves yet another solution:

The woman needs to be told how to free her home from rodents and make it a safe place for an infant.

If you come from a middle-income home, you may tend to think of homes as places with several bedrooms, green lawns, and adequate plumbing, heating, and refrigeration. A large proportion of babies are born to such homes. Smaller proportions are born to affluent homes or to homes that lack the necessities for adequate infant care and safety.

It is good to explore the woman's preparations for the baby with her, to reveal inadequacies that may exist. Ask whether the baby will have his own bed. Ask about refrigerator space. Is there adequate heat? Newborns need a temperature of 70° to 75°F during the day and at least 60° to 65°F at night. Are heating facilities adequate to maintain this temperature?

SELECTING A LAYETTE

In selecting clothes for a newborn several principles should be kept in mind:

1. Clothes should be easy to launder. Since newborns spit up and wet through several layers of clothing, all their clothes have to be changed after a feeding. Everyday clothes should be simple, with no trimming to irritate sensitive skin or complicate laundering. The woman will probably want to choose one dress-up outfit, but even this should be easy to launder.
2. Clothes should be easy to put on the baby. Shirts that open in the front and are fastened by ties or snaps are easier to put on newborns than those that slip over the head. Plastic pants that snap at the sides go on more easily than those with elastic tops.
3. Clothes should be large enough to allow for growth. A baby will outgrow a 3-month or even a 6-month size before he wears it out. Size 12 months, although large for a newborn, allows for growth.

Diapers

The selection of diapers involves a major decision; the child will wear diapers long after he has outgrown his baby clothes. The choices available are cloth diapers, disposable diapers, or a diaper service. The woman's choice will be based on the experiences of her friends and neighbors and the washing facilities she has available. If she has no washing machine, she will find a diaper service or disposable diapers more convenient than a daily trip to the laundromat.

At first thought it seems as if a diaper service or buying disposable diapers is expensive. This makes purchasing cloth diapers seem a preferable choice. However, when the costs of water, bleach, softener, soap, wear and tear on a washing machine, and replacing worn-out diapers are added in, the expense is probably comparable. Mothers often use a cloth diaper to cover their shoulder while burping the baby, so they may want to buy some even if they are not going to be using them as diapers.

Basic Layette

A basic layette for a newborn should consist of

6 shirts
6 nightgowns or kimonos
6 receiving blankets
1 bunting or heavy blanket
6 diaper pads or plastic pants
1 sweater, cap, and bootie set
1 outfit for dress-up
1 rubber sheet to protect the mattress
3 or 4 dozen diapers (or about 10 disposable diapers per day)
4 rustproof diaper pins

As mentioned, special sheets are not necessary; nor are special towels and washcloths as long as freshly laundered ones are used for the baby. Additional purchases might include a baby bathtub, additional basic clothing, baby lotion, oil, or powder, as preferred, and a diaper pail if cloth diapers are to be used.

Most women make the decision whether to breast-feed or bottle-feed the baby during pregnancy. If the decision is to bottle-feed, the woman will need to purchase equipment for this as well. Both breast-feeding and bottle-feeding are discussed in Chap. 30. Home care of the newborn is discussed in Chap. 31.

Arrangements for Labor and Delivery

Be sure to review the arrangements the woman needs to make for labor and delivery. No matter how calm a woman seems when discussing these arrangements, all women have some fear that at the last minute they will forget what is expected of them and, for example, will go to the wrong hospital or fill in the wrong form.

Some clinics and physicians ask women to preregister for delivery, so that on the day of labor they need spend no time filling out forms. The woman needs to be certain that she knows the way to the hospital, knows who is going to drive her there, and has alternate transportation if that person is not available. If she has children, she must arrange for their care and perhaps for someone to do the cooking while she is hospitalized.

True, these are arrangements the woman has to make for herself, but asking about whether or not she has made them may be the incentive she needs to get her plans under way. Pregnancy is a stress situation, and people under stress do not think as clearly or objectively as they normally do. For her safety and her child's, if the woman seems to require assistance, help her to make some of these decisions.

Open Communication — Key to Nursing Care

Women do not always express their dissatisfaction with a clinic or physician's office. They make their feelings known by missed appointments or failure to return at all.

It is a good practice to take a minute at visits to ask whether the woman has any difficulty getting to the clinic or the office. If her income is marginal, the cab or bus fare involved may be a major obstacle. She may have trouble arranging for a babysitter for a particular time of day. Her husband may be using their car every day. Her appointments might need to be scheduled for times more convenient for her. She may need a referral to a social worker to arrange financial assistance.

Many obstetricians and general practitioners do not charge for individual prenatal visits. Rather, they charge for prenatal care, labor, and delivery all in one fee. In this system, the fee is the same no matter how many visits prenatal care entails. This encourages a woman to keep appointments in order to get the most for her money. Clinic fees can generally be adjusted to the income of patients, so that the cost of prenatal care will not present an obstacle to obtaining it.

A major reason for dissatisfaction and missed appointments is a woman's feeling that she was treated as a number, not as a person, while in the clinic or office. It is a nursing responsibility to set the tone in clinics and offices and to make patients feel a pervading concern for them as individuals. Whenever the frequency of missed appointments is high, the amount of personal interest that is being shown or not shown to patients is one of the first items to be investigated.

Problem-oriented Recording: Progress Notes

November 6
Mary Kraft
22 years
Gestational length: 13 weeks

Problem: Constipation

> S. Problem for last 2 weeks. Regularly has BM daily; now q 3rd day. Stool hard, black in color (taking iron supplement). Includes 2 glasses of water, fruits and vegetables daily.
> O. Appears distressed when discussing problem.
> A. Constipation due to normal changes in pregnancy.
>
> Goals: a. Alleviation of constipation by 1 week.
> b. Able to explain reason for problem.
> c. Able to voice concept that she knows this will not affect health of child or be a permanent problem.
>
> P. 1. Assure that constipation is often a normal consequence of pregnancy.
> 2. Encourage to include high-fiber foods in diet (given list).
> 3. Encourage to rest in lateral Sims's or legs-elevated position 2 × per day to prevent constipation leading to formation of hemorrhoids.
> 4. Refer to M.D. for stool softener or additional interventions.

November 13
Mary Kraft
22 years
Gestational length: 14 weeks

Problem: Constipation

> S. (Telephone call.) Constipation only slightly improved. Stool still hard and bowel movements have become painful. Drinking 4 glasses of water daily; taking a source of bran daily (bran cereal or bran muffins). Has not been taking stool softener prescribed as she is

concerned about taking medication during pregnancy.

O. —

A. Constipation continuing due to inadequate patient compliance.

P. 1. Urge to take stool softener and counseled regarding safety of prescribed medication during pregnancy.
2. Reassure again that constipation is a normal occurrence in pregnancy.
3. Urge to continue program of resting in lateral Sims's or legs-elevated position daily to prevent hemorrhoid formation.
4. To call again if after taking stool softener for 1 week constipation is not relieved.

December 8
Mary Kraft
22 years
Gestational length: 17 weeks

Problem: Constipation

S. Constipation no longer a problem. BM now q day; taking stool softener daily. Stool soft, no pain.

O. Appears relaxed on discussing problem.

A. Constipation relieved by use of stool softener and diet modification.

P. 1. Assure again that medication will not be harmful to fetus or her during pregnancy.
2. Urge to continue to take medication and maintain high-fiber diet.
3. Refer to M.D. to check if medication should be reduced to every other day or any other change necessary.

References

1. Berg, M., et al. Prenatal care for pregnant adolescents in a public high school. *J. Sch. Health* 49:32, 1979.
2. Bonebrake, C. R., et al. Routine chest roentgenography in pregnancy. *J.A.M.A.* 240:2747, 1978.
3. Brant, H. A. Improving the quality of antenatal care. *Nurs. Mirror* 147:7, 1978.
4. Brant, H. A. Prevention of handicap: The quality of prenatal care. *Midwives Chron.* 91:315, 1978.
5. Brown, M. S. A cross cultural look at pregnancy, labor and delivery. *J.O.G.N. Nurs.* 5:35, 1976.
6. Christianson, R. E. Studies on blood pressure during pregnancy. *Am. J. Obstet. Gynecol.* 125:509, 1976.
7. David, M. L., et al. First trimester pregnancy. *Am. J. Nurs.* 76:1945, 1976.
8. Doering, S. C., and Entwisle, D. R. Preparation during pregnancy and ability to cope with labor and delivery. *Am. J. Orthopsychiatry* 45:825, 1975.
9. Graven, S. N. Perinatal health promotion—an overview. *Fam. Community Health* 1:1, 1978.
10. Jacobson, H. N. Weight and weight gain in pregnancy. *Clin. Perinatol.* 2:233, 1975.
11. Kimbrough, C. A. The search for labor information during pregnancy. *Matern. Child Nurs. J.* 6:107, 1977.
12. Kuntz, W. D. Pregnant working women: What advice should you give them? *Contemp. Obstet. Gynecol.* 15:69, 1980.
13. May, K. A. Active involvement of expectant fathers in pregnancy, some further considerations. *J.O.G.N. Nurs.* 7:7, 1978.
14. McKay, S. R. Smoking during the childbearing years. *M.C.N.* 5:46, 1980.
15. Meeks, L., et al. Patient education through pregnancy counseling: A preventive approach. *Health Educ. Monogr.* 9:42, 1978.
16. Rich, O. J. The sociogram: A tool for depicting support in pregnancy. *Matern. Child. Nurs. J.* 7:1, 1978.
17. Sciarra, J. J., and Gerbie, A. B. *Gynecology and Obstetrics.* New York: Harper & Row, 1978.
18. Steinman, M. E. Reaching and helping the adolescent who becomes pregnant. *M.C.N.* 4:35, 1979.
19. Sumner, G. Giving expectant parents the help they need: The ABC's of prenatal education. *M.C.N.* 1:220, 1976.
20. Warshaw, L. J. Pregnancy and work. *Occup. Health Nurs.* 26:7, 1978.
21. Westbrook, M. T. Analyzing effective responses to past events: Women's reactions to a childbearing year. *J. Clin. Psychol.* 34:967, 1978.

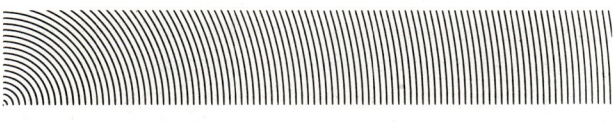

18. Nutrition and Pregnancy

A good diet cannot guarantee a good pregnancy outcome, but it makes an important contribution to it. The nutritional state that a woman brings into pregnancy and her nutrition during pregnancy both have a direct bearing on her well-being and on that of her child.

The classic study of Burke and her co-workers [4] in 1943 established the high correlation between maternal diet and infant health. Among 284 women whose prenatal diet was evaluated, only 42 had a good or excellent diet; their infants (96 percent) were in good or excellent health at birth. Of 40 women rated as having a poor or very poor diet, only 8 percent had babies rated as in good or excellent health; 27 percent of their infants were in fair health and 65 percent in poor health. Babies included in the "poor" category were either stillborn, premature, or functionally immature, died within three days of birth, or had congenital defects.

Poor nutritional intake may play a part in poor neurological and bone growth, in premature birth, and in premature separation of the placenta. There is also a correlation between inadequate protein intake during pregnancy and small-for-gestation-age newborns.

Nutritional Requirements

That the pregnant woman must "eat for two," then, is not just an old wives' tale but a scientific fact. Although the pregnant woman may not have to increase the *quantity* of her intake to provide for the child forming inside her, an increase in the *quality* of her intake is usually necessary. Good nutritional counseling during pregnancy should help a woman gain an appropriate amount of weight during pregnancy, decrease pregnancy-induced hypertension, provide an environment in which a fetus can gain appropriate weight, prepare her body for lactation and feeding of her baby, and acquire nutritional knowledge that she can use with her child all the years of his growing up.

In past years, when weight gain in pregnancy was severely limited, to under 20 pounds, women were reluctant to talk about their dietary intake at prenatal visits. Some of them were forced to lie about what they were really eating in order to gain approval from health personnel. They were so worried about being weighed in at visits that they did not eat at all the day before coming for a visit. Now that a more lenient weight gain is recommended, women are more relaxed about discussing what they eat and are receptive to nutritional counseling and advice.

The recommended dietary allowances for girls and

women and the requirements that pregnancy adds are given in Table 18-1.

CALORIES

As can be seen in the table, an additional 300 calories, or a total caloric intake of 2300 to 2700 calories, is recommended to meet the increased needs of pregnancy. In addition to supplying the fetus and placenta, a good pregnancy diet must provide for the mother's increased metabolic rate and her increased work load from the extra weight she must carry.

The physiological changes of pregnancy, such as the 30 to 50 percent increase in blood volume and blood constituents, require an increase in the amount of protein and iron ingested. If a woman does not take in enough calories, her body will utilize protein for energy, depriving the fetus of the protein he needs. In addition, the breakdown of protein leads to ketoacidosis.

Even in obese women, a pregnancy diet should never contain fewer than 1500 calories. A diet low in calories is almost automatically low in protein, a lack that will be detrimental to fetal growth. The use of saccharin as a sugar substitute in not recommended, as the woman needs the sugar (and the safety of saccharin for the population as a whole is still seriously questioned from a carcinogenic standpoint).

In planning for increased caloric intake, be sure that the woman will add calories by eating foods rich in protein, iron, and other essential nutrients, rather than just eating empty-calorie foods such as pretzels and doughnuts. Some women worry about total caloric intake during pregnancy because they fear gaining so much weight that they will be overweight permanently. If a woman increases her total caloric intake by adding nutritious foods, thereby building mainly protein and iron stores, this will not be a problem, and she can be assured of that.

A method of determining nonpregnant ideal caloric intake is to compute 40 calories per kilogram of ideal body weight. Ideal female weight for height is shown in Table 18-2.

PROTEIN

If protein needs are met, overall needs are likely to be met (with the exceptions of ascorbic acid, vitamin A, and vitamin D) because of the association of other nutrients with protein foods. If protein is inadequate in the diet, iron, B vitamins, calcium, and phosphorus will undoubtedly be inadequate also. Vitamin

Table 18-1. Maternal Daily Dietary Allowances

	Recommended Daily Allowances for Nonpregnant Women				Recommended Daily Allowances to Be Added for Pregnancy
	Age 11–14	Age 15–18	Age 19–22	Age 23–50	
Calories (kcal)	2400	2100	2100	2000	+300
Protein (gm)	46	46	44	44	+30
Vitamin A (μg)	800	800	800	800	+200
Vitamin D (μg)	10	10	7.5	5	+5
Vitamin E (mg)	8	8	8	8	+2
Ascorbic acid (mg)	50	60	60	60	+20
Folic acid (μg)	400	400	400	400	+400
Niacin (mg)	15	14	14	13	+2
Riboflavin (mg)	1.3	1.3	1.3	1.2	+0.3
Thiamine (mg)	1.1	1.1	1.1	1.0	+0.4
Vitamin B_{12} (μg)	3.0	3.0	3.0	3.0	+1.0
Vitamin B_6 (mg)	1.8	2.0	2.0	2.0	+0.6
Calcium (mg)	1200	1200	800	800	+400
Phosphorus (mg)	1200	1200	800	800	+400
Iodine (μg)	150	150	150	150	+25
Iron (mg)	18	18	18	18	+30–60
Magnesium (mg)	300	300	300	300	+150
Zinc (mg)	15	15	15	15	+5

Source. Food and Nutrition Board, *Recommended Daily Dietary Allowances*. Washington: National Academy of Sciences, National Research Council, 1979.

Table 18-2. Ideal Female Weight for Height in Pounds

Height (with 2-Inch-Heel Shoes)		Small Frame	Medium Frame	Large Frame
Feet	Inches			
4	10	92–98	96–107	104–119
4	11	94–101	98–110	106–122
5	0	96–104	101–113	109–125
5	1	99–107	104–116	112–128
5	2	102–110	107–119	115–131
5	3	105–113	110–122	118–134
5	4	108–116	113–126	121–138
5	5	111–119	116–130	125–142
5	6	114–123	120–135	129–146
5	7	118–127	124–139	133–150
5	8	122–131	128–143	137–154
5	9	126–135	132–147	141–158
5	10	130–140	136–151	145–163
5	11	134–144	140–155	149–168
6	0	138–148	144–159	153–173

Source. Metropolitan Life Insurance Company, Health and Safety Education Division, Actuarial Tables, 1959.

B_{12} is found exclusively in animal protein and so will be insufficient if animal protein is totally excluded from the diet.

The intake of protein should be increased 30 gm per day above normal during pregnancy. Extra protein is best supplied by meat, poultry, fish, yogurt, eggs, and milk because the protein in these forms contains all eight essential amino acids or is *complete*. The protein in nonanimal sources does not contain all eight essential amino acids and so is termed *incomplete*. It is possible, however, by choosing non-animal proteins carefully, to provide all amino acids in the diet. Proteins that when cooked together provide all eight essential amino acids are termed *complementary proteins*. Examples are beans and rice, legumes and rice, or beans and wheat.

Meat, the richest source of protein, is expensive. Poultry, cheese, eggs, and peanut butter are usually less expensive. A woman who comes from a family with a tendency to high cholesterol levels probably should not eat more than one egg per day. Because liver is such a rich source of protein, it is good for a woman to include it in her diet at least once a week. Women who do not like the taste of liver can eat it as liverwurst or liver spread or include it in meatloafs. Lunch meats (bologna, salami) should not be included as staples in the diet because their salt content is exceptionally high.

Milk is a rich source of protein, but some women resist drinking it because it is also a high-calorie food. However, skim milk, either liquid or dry, supplies the same protein as regular milk but half the calories. Thus, there is no need to eliminate this essential food to prevent too much weight gain.

Some women find it difficult to drink a quart of milk a day because they simply do not like its taste. Buttermilk can be substituted, or chocolate or another flavoring can be added to make milk palatable. Yogurt or cheese may also be substituted for milk, or milk may be incorporated into custards, eggnogs, or cream soups.

Common foods from each basic food group are contrasted as to protein content in Table 18-3.

FAT

There is only one fatty oil, linoleic acid, that cannot be manufactured in the body from other sources and is therefore essential. The oils that people use in salads or for cooking—corn, safflower, peanut, and cottonseed oil—contain linoleic acid.

FAT-SOLUBLE VITAMINS

Fat-soluble vitamins are absorbed across the villi of the intestine with fat. A pregnant woman should not use mineral oil as a laxative if these important vitamins are to be absorbed and not eliminated from the body with stool. Fat-soluble vitamins are vitamins A, D, K, and E. Table 18-4 contrasts common foods from each food group as to vitamin A content.

Vitamin A

Vitamin A promotes growth and reproduction of body cells, maintains healthy skin and mucous membrane, and is beneficial to vision. It is found in yellow and dark-green vegetables, butter, and margarine. Vegetables not only provide a good source of this vitamin but are also a good source of protein and add bulk to the diet to aid bowel movements.

Oral contraceptives may deplete vitamin A stores, so the woman who has been using oral contraceptives prior to pregnancy needs to include good sources of vitamin A in her early pregnancy diet.

Vitamin D

Because metabolism of calcium and phosphorus depends on vitamin D, this vitamin must be present in the diet to ensure good bone growth and proper mineralization of bones and teeth in the fetus. Some vitamin D is formed by exposure of skin to sunlight.

Table 18-3. Protein Content of Common Foods

Food	Amount	Protein Content (gm)
Meat		
Beef, rib roast	3 oz	17
Bologna	2 slices	3
Chicken	1 drumstick	12
Clams (raw)	3 oz	11
Haddock	3 oz	17
Ham	3 oz	18
Hamburger	3 oz	21
Liver, beef	3 oz	22.5
Vegetables and fruits		
Carrots	1	1
Collards	1 cup	5
Corn	1 ear	3
Lima beans	1 cup	16
Peanut butter	1 tbsp	4
Peas, dried, split	1 cup	20
Spinach	1 cup	5
Apple	1	Trace
Banana	1	1
Orange	1	1
Watermelon	1 wedge	2
Breads and grains		
Bagel	1	6
Bread, rye	1 slice	2
Bread, white	1 slice	2
Bread, whole wheat	1 slice	3
Cornmeal	1 cup	11
Oatmeal	1 cup	5
Rice, white	1 cup	4
Spaghetti	1 cup	5
Dairy products		
Butter	1 pat	Trace
Cheese (American)	1 oz	7
Egg	1 whole	6
Ice cream	1 cup	6
Margarine	1 pat	Trace
Milk	1 cup	9
Yogurt	1 cup	8

Source. *Nutritive Value of Foods*, U.S. Dept. of Agriculture, Home and Garden Bulletin No. 72, 1970.

Fortunately, most commercial milk today is fortified with 400 I.U. (10 μg) of vitamin D per quart, so a quart of milk taken daily will supply most of the vitamin D the woman requires.

Vitamin K

Vitamin K promotes the formation of prothrombin and fibrin to ensure efficient blood clotting. In case a bleeding complication should occur in pregnancy, adequate levels of this vitamin will help safeguard both mother and fetus. Vitamin K is found in green, leafy vegetables, soybeans, fish meal, and vegetable oils. Since it is also formed by bacterial action in the intestines, some of the vitamin is available to the body even if it is not supplied in the diet.

Vitamin E

The relationship of vitamin E to good nutrition has not been clearly determined. Wheat germ, nuts, eggs, and legumes are rich sources.

WATER-SOLUBLE VITAMINS

Vitamin C

Vitamin C, or ascorbic acid, is necessary for protein utilization and absorption of iron and for the formation of bone and connective tissue. It also appears to augment resistance to infection. It is not stored in body tissues and so must be taken in daily. It is found largely in citrus fruits and in tomatoes, broccoli, brussel sprouts, and cabbage. The daily amount recommended for the pregnant woman is 70 to 80 mg. The safety of taking excessive amounts of vitamin C to prevent colds is not established; this should not be tried during pregnancy. Common foods from the four basic food groups are contrasted as to their content of vitamin C in Table 18-4.

Vitamin B Complex

The principal B vitamins are thiamine, riboflavin, niacin, pyridoxine (B_6), folic acid, and B_{12}. They are essential for proper nerve growth, for the maintenance of good vision, and for conversion of carbohydrate to energy, and they aid in the digestion and assimilation of food. They are found in protein foods, namely, meat, eggs, enriched breads, enriched cereals, and dairy products.

Women who have been using oral contraceptives prior to pregnancy may have B_6 (pyridoxine) deficiencies and may need additional supplements during pregnancy. Common foods from the four basic food groups are contrasted as to vitamin B_1 (thiamine) and B_2 (riboflavin) content in Table 18-5.

Folic Acid

Although folic acid (folacin) belongs to the B vitamin group, it warrants separate discussion.

It was thought previously that a diet high in iron would be sufficient for adequate hemoglobin formation in the fetus. It is now recognized that folic acid is also necessary. In a pregnant woman with low levels of folic acid, a megaloblastic anemia or a low red cell count and low hemoglobin may develop. If the woman manifests such symptoms at the time she delivers, the infant may be anemic as well. Both the

Table 18-4. Vitamin A and Vitamin C Content of Common Foods

Food	Amount	Vitamin A (I.U.)	Vitamin C (mg)
Meat			
Beef, rib roast	3 oz	70	0
Bologna	2 slices	0	0
Chicken	1 drumstick	50	0
Clams (raw)	3 oz	90	8
Haddock	3 oz	0	2
Ham	3 oz	0	0
Hamburger	3 oz	30	0
Liver, beef	3 oz	45420	22.7
Vegetables and fruits			
Carrots	1	5500	4
Collards	1 cup	10260	87
Corn	1 ear	310	7
Lima beans	1 cup	0	0
Peanut butter	1 tbsp	0	0
Peas, dried, split	1 cup	100	0
Spinach	1 cup	14580	50
Apple	1	50	3
Banana	1	230	12
Orange	1	260	66
Watermelon	1 wedge	2510	30
Breads and grains			
Bagel	1	30	0
Bread, rye	1 slice	0	0
Bread, white	1 slice	Trace	Trace
Bread, whole wheat	1 slice	Trace	Trace
Cornmeal	1 cup	620	0
Oatmeal	1 cup	0	0
Rice, white	1 cup	0	0
Spaghetti	1 cup	0	0
Dairy products			
Butter	1 pat	170	0
Cheese (American)	1 oz	350	0
Egg	1 whole	590	0
Ice cream	1 cup	590	1
Margarine	1 pat	170	0
Milk	1 cup	350	2
Yogurt	1 cup	170	2

Source. *Nutritive Value of Foods*, U.S. Dept. of Agriculture, Home and Garden Bulletin No. 72, 1970.

woman and the infant respond well to the administration of folic acid during pregnancy. In addition, low levels of folic acid in the woman may be associated with premature separation of the placenta or spontaneous abortion. For these reasons most pregnant women are given a folic acid supplement of 400 to 800 µg per day. Oral contraceptives may deplete serum folic acid levels. Women who were taking oral contraceptives prior to pregnancy are probably most in need of supplementation.

CALCIUM AND PHOSPHORUS

Because the skeleton and teeth of the fetus constitute a major portion of its structure, extra calcium and phosphorus are needed during pregnancy. Calcium is provided by milk (a quart a day supplies three-fourths of a day's requirement), cheddar cheese, and green, leafy vegetables. Phosphorus is found in organ meats, whole grain products, milk, nuts, and eggs. In order for the woman to absorb and utilize calcium and phosphorus, she must also have adequate amounts of vitamin D.

Before nutrition counseling in pregnancy became as common as it is today, a woman expected to lose "a tooth a child"; or believed that the fetus drew calcium from her teeth as he grew. The calcium in teeth is not as readily absorbable as that of bone, so this may have always been an old wives' tale. With a good calcium

Table 18-5. Thiamine and Riboflavin Content of Common Foods

Food	Amount	Thiamine (mg)	Riboflavin (mg)
Meat			
Beef, rib roast	3 oz	1.05	0.13
Bologna	2 slices	0.04	0.06
Chicken	1 drumstick	0.03	0.15
Clams (raw)	3 oz	0.08	0.15
Haddock	3 oz	0.03	0.06
Ham	3 oz	0.40	0.16
Hamburger	3 oz	0.07	0.18
Liver, beef	3 oz		
Vegetables and fruits			
Carrots	1	0.03	0.03
Collards	1 cup	0.27	0.37
Corn	1 ear	0.09	0.08
Lima beans	1 cup	0.25	0.11
Peanut butter	1 tbsp	0.02	0.02
Peas, dried, split	1 cup	0.37	0.22
Spinach	1 cup	0.13	0.25
Apple	1	0.04	0.02
Banana	1	0.06	0.07
Orange	1	0.13	0.05
Watermelon	1 wedge	0.13	0.13
Breads and grains			
Bagel	1	0.14	0.10
Bread, rye	1 slice	0.05	0.02
Bread, white	1 slice	0.06	0.05
Bread, whole wheat	1 slice	0.09	0.03
Cornmeal	1 cup	0.46	0.13
Oatmeal	1 cup	0.19	0.05
Rice, white	1 cup	0.23	0.02
Spaghetti	1 cup	0.20	0.11
Dairy products			
Butter	1 pat	—	—
Cheese (American)	1 oz	0.01	0.12
Egg	1 whole	0.05	0.15
Ice cream	1 cup	0.43	2.23
Margarine	1 pat	—	—
Milk	1 cup	0.07	0.41
Yogurt	1 cup	0.10	0.44

Source. *Nutritive Value of Foods*, U.S. Dept. of Agriculture, Home and Garden Bulletin No. 72, 1970.

intake during pregnancy, this prediction certainly does become just another old wives' tale today. Common foods from the four basic food groups are contrasted as to calcium content in Table 18-6.

IODINE

Iodine is essential for the formation of thyroxine and therefore for the proper functioning of the thyroid gland. Iodine deficiency may cause goiter in the woman or fetus; in extreme instances, it may cause cretinism in the fetus. In areas where water and soil are known to be deficient in iodine, it is suggested that the woman use iodized salt and include a serving of seafood in her diet at least once a week.

IRON

A fetus at term has a hemoglobin of about 17 gm per 100 ml of blood. This high hemoglobin level is necessary to oxygenate his blood, since in the fetal circulation venous and arterial blood are so mixed that 100 percent oxygenation of red blood cells is not attained. In addition to needing iron to build this high level of hemoglobin late in pregnancy, the fetus needs iron for storage in the liver, to last through the first three months of life, when intake will consist mainly of milk, which is low in iron.

The woman needs additional iron to build the increased red cell volume of pregnancy and to replace iron lost in blood at delivery.

Table 18-6. Calcium Content of Common Foods

Food	Amount	Calcium Content (mg)
Meat		
Beef, rib roast	3 oz	8
Bologna	1 slice	2
Chicken	1 drumstick	6
Clams (raw)	3 oz	59
Haddock	3 oz	34
Ham	3 oz	8
Hamburger	3 oz	10
Liver, beef	3 oz	9
Vegetables and fruits		
Carrots	1	18
Collards	1 cup	289
Corn	1 ear	2
Lima beans	1 cup	55
Peanut butter	1 tbsp	9
Peas, dried, split	1 cup	28
Spinach	1 cup	167
Apple	1	8
Banana	1	10
Orange	1	54
Watermelon	1 wedge	30
Breads and grains		
Bagel	1	9
Bread, rye	1 slice	19
Bread, white	1 slice	21
Bread, whole wheat	1 slice	24
Cornmeal	1 cup	24
Oatmeal	1 cup	22
Rice, white	1 cup	21
Spaghetti	1 cup	11
Dairy products		
Butter	1 pat	1
Cheese (American)	1 oz	198
Egg	1 whole	27
Ice cream	1 cup	194
Margarine	1 pat	1
Milk	1 cup	288
Yogurt	1 cup	294

Source. *Nutritive Value of Foods*, U.S. Dept. of Agriculture, Home and Garden Bulletin No. 72, 1970.

Women in low-income groups find it hard to include enough iron in their diets, since the foods richest in iron (organ meats; eggs; green, leafy vegetables; whole grain or enriched breads; dried fruits) are also the most expensive foods. The recommended daily allowance of iron is 18 mg. An average diet takes in 6 mg of iron per 1000 calories. If the woman eats a 2400-calorie diet daily, she takes in 12 to 15 mg of iron. Since only 10 to 20 percent of dietary iron is absorbed, however, she is actually taking in less than this amount. Therefore, a prenatal diet should be supplemented with 30 to 60 mg of iron per day. The woman should not regard this medication as a substitute for eating iron-rich foods; it is intended as a supplement to an iron-rich diet. Oral iron compounds turn stools black and tend to cause constipation in some women. Common foods compared as to iron content are shown in Table 18-7.

FLUIDS

Extra amounts of water are needed during pregnancy for good kidney function, since the woman must excrete waste products for two. Two glasses of fluid daily

Table 18-7. Iron Content of Common Foods

Food	Amount	Iron Content (mg)
Meat		
Beef, rib roast	3 oz	2.2
Bologna	1 slice	0.7
Chicken	1 drumstick	0.9
Clams (raw)	3 oz	5.2
Haddock	3 oz	1.0
Ham	3 oz	2.2
Hamburger	3 oz	3.0
Liver, beef	3 oz	7.5
Vegetables and fruits		
Carrots	1	0.4
Collards	1 cup	1.1
Corn	1 ear	0.5
Lima beans	1 cup	5.9
Peanut butter	1 tbsp	0.3
Peas, dried, split	1 cup	4.2
Spinach	1 cup	4.0
Apple	1	0.4
Banana	1	0.8
Orange	1	0.5
Watermelon	1 wedge	2.1
Breads and grains		
Bagel	1	1.2
Bread, rye	1 slice	0.4
Bread, white	1 slice	0.6
Bread, whole wheat	1 slice	0.6
Cornmeal	1 cup	2.9
Oatmeal	1 cup	1.4
Rice, white	1 cup	1.8
Spaghetti	1 cup	1.3
Dairy products		
Butter	1 pat	0.0
Cheese (American)	1 oz	0.3
Egg	1 whole	1.1
Ice cream	1 cup	0.1
Margarine	1 pat	0.0
Milk	1 cup	0.1
Yogurt	1 cup	0.1

Source. *Nutritive Value of Foods*, U.S. Dept. of Agriculture, Home and Garden Bulletin No. 72, 1970.

over and above the daily quart of milk is a recommended fluid intake.

FLUORIDE

Since fluoride aids in the formation of sound teeth, a pregnant woman should drink fluoridated water. In an area where water is not fluoridated, supplemental fluoride may be recommended. Fluoride in large amounts causes brown-stained teeth, so the woman must not take the supplement more often than prescribed.

SODIUM

It was formerly recommended that salt be restricted during pregnancy in order to minimize fluid retention. Thus, a woman had to try to eat tasteless, unappetizing food in the early months of pregnancy, when nausea and vomiting makes food unappetizing at best. As a result, many women did not eat at all, and the protein contents of their diets fell below the recommended levels.

Although substantial sodium is retained during pregnancy, it is a normal adjustment to the increased intravascular and interstitial fluid volume, not excessive retention. In many women, the increase in glomerular filtration rate actually promotes sodium loss. While the total blood volume increases during pregnancy, the functional blood volume may be less than normal because the placenta is utilizing so much for exchange. Depleting sodium by diuretics or decreased intake may reduce the blood volume to a point where the placental exchange will be compromised.

Unless the woman is hypertensive or has heart disease when she enters pregnancy, she should continue to put salt into food as she normally does. Many women find the idea that they do not need to restrict salt during pregnancy contrary to what they were told during their last pregnancy. They welcome the change in philosophy but question it. Be certain you have the reason salt is allowed straight in your own mind so you can explain it correctly: Salt does not cause hypertension of pregnancy. It is necessary for regulating fluid balance in the body and the fetus and so should not be restricted during pregnancy.

FIBER

Eating fiber-rich foods daily is a natural way of preventing constipation, as the bulk of the fiber in the intestine aids evacuation. A food has high fiber content when it consists of parts of the plant cell wall that are resistant to normal digestive enzymes of the small intestine. Crude fiber content refers to how much fiber is left after intestinal breakdown. Table 18-8

Table 18-8. Crude Fiber Content of Various Foods

Food	Crude Fiber (%)
Bran	10.0–13.5
Whole grain	1.0– 2.0
Nuts	2.0– 5.0
Legumes (cooked)	1.5– 1.7
Vegetables	0.5– 1.5
Fruits (fresh)	0.5– 1.5
Fruits (dried)	1.0– 3.0

Table 18-9. Quantities of Food Necessary During Pregnancy

Food Group	Active Nonpregnant Woman	Pregnant Woman
Meat	2 servings of meat, fowl, or fish daily; 3–5 eggs per week	4 servings of meat, fowl, or fish daily; or 1 egg and 3 servings of meat, fowl, or fish daily
Vegetables:		
Dark green or deep yellow	1 serving (at least 3 times per week)	2 servings daily
Other vegetables	1 or more servings daily	1 serving daily
Fruits:		
Citrus, melon, strawberries, tomato	1 serving daily	1 or more servings daily
Other fruits	1 serving daily	1 serving daily
Breads and cereals	4 or more servings daily	4 servings daily
Milk	1 pint (two 8-oz glasses) daily	1 quart (four 8-oz glasses) daily
Additional fluid	Ad lib	At least 2 glasses daily

contrasts various foods as to crude fiber content. Bran is the seed coat of grain kernels. Refined grains have had the bran and germ removed and have much less fiber content.

Daily Needs

Table 18-9 lists the quantities of each food that will supply the calories and nutrients recommended in Table 18-1. In discussing diet with a woman, remember that she will more readily grasp what amounts are required if you talk in terms of servings of food rather than about milligrams or percentages.

The following foods can be substituted for those in Table 18-9.

1 8-oz glass whole milk:	1 glass skim milk
	1 glass buttermilk
	½ cup cottage cheese
	¼ cup nonfat or whole dry milk
	½ cup ice cream
	1¼ oz cheddar cheese
1 serving vegetable or fruit:	1 medium potato, tomato, or piece of fruit (used whole)
	½ grapefruit
	1 cup tomato juice (has vitamin C content of ½ cup orange juice)
2–3 oz lean meat:	2 oz poultry or fish
	2 eggs
	1 oz cheddar cheese
	4 tablespoons peanut butter
	1 cup cooked dried beans, peas, or nuts
	½ cup cottage cheese
Bread or cereal:	½–¾ cup cooked or ¾ cup ready-to-serve cereal
	½–¾ cup cooked macaroni, spaghetti, or rice

A typical day's menu based on these requirements might be the following:

Breakfast:	1 glass orange juice (8 oz)
	1 slice toast with butter or fortified margarine
	1 egg
	1 serving sausage
	Supplemental vitamin, folic acid, and iron capsule
Snack:	1 glass milk (8 oz)
	1 piece fruit
Lunch:	1 peanut butter and jelly sandwich
	1 cup tomato soup
	1 glass milk (8 oz)
Afternoon snack:	1 glass milk (8 oz)
	Celery sticks and canned chick peas
Dinner:	1 serving roast beef
	1 medium potato
	1 serving corn
	1 dinner roll or 1 slice bread
	Green salad with French dressing
	Fruit Jell-O
	1 glass water (8 oz)
Bedtime snack:	1 glass milk or 1 cup cocoa (8 oz)

A less typical menu, but one that is adequate during pregnancy, is the following:

Breakfast:	1 orange
	Pieces of tuna fish
Morning snack:	1 glass milk (8 oz)
	1 apple
	1 serving grits
Lunch:	1 hamburger on a bun
	1 serving cole slaw
	1 serving french fries
	1 serving ice cream
	1 glass soft drink (noncaffeine)
Dinner:	1 serving pigs' knuckles
	1 serving collard greens
	1 serving rice
	1 glass milk (8 oz)
Bedtime snack:	1 eggnog (8 oz milk)
	Supplemental vitamin, folic acid, and iron capsule

Be careful when you are assessing a woman's diet that you assess it according to whether it contains sufficient amounts of the basic food groups, not in terms of your own preference or eating habits.

Nutritional Problems in Pregnancy

Nutritional problems may occur in pregnancy as a result of a number of factors.

CRAVINGS

Cravings for food during pregnancy are so common that they can be considered a normal part of pregnancy. These strange desires for food may reflect a need to gain attention or may be a reaction to the woman's imposed dependent state. A woman may feel helpless because she has just left her job, or she may feel unattractive in her pregnant state. She can demonstrate that she is neither helpless to manipulate her environment nor unattractive in her husband's eyes if she can send him to the store for fresh strawberries she "absolutely must have."

Nutrition and Pregnancy

Because these cravings are usually for high-carbohydrate foods, such as chocolate, doughnuts, and sponge cake, they may reflect a physiological need for more carbohydrate in the diet. Women who crave citrus fruit during pregnancy are not said to have cravings but "an awareness of good nutrition." Is there really a difference?

Cravings may be the same kind of phenomenon as the thirst of patients who have been told they can have no fluids by mouth. When drinking was permitted, they were not thirsty; as soon as they are told they cannot drink, their thirst becomes overpowering.

Now that women are allowed more calories in their daily diets, cravings are seen less often than they used to be. Allowing a few of the extra calories to include the food the woman craves prevents her from cheating on her diet just to include this item and reduces her guilt feelings about eating during pregnancy.

PICA

Some women report an abnormal craving for nonfood substances (termed *pica*) during pregnancy. The commonest form of pica is a craving for clay or laundry starch. It is seen most often in the southeast, but occurs everywhere. If a woman is eating large quantities of starch or clay, her diet becomes deficient in protein, iron, and calcium.

Encouraging the woman to stop eating clay may be ineffective. By the time she reaches childbearing age, she may have had this habit for a long time. For a nurse, who is unlikely to eat clay, discouraging the habit presents the same problem as discouraging smoking when she is a nonsmoker: How can you understand the urge the woman feels for this substance? Do not scold or nag. Stress instead that despite her habit of eating clay or starch, her diet must be high in protein, vitamins, and iron.

Many people with pica have iron deficiency anemia, and correcting the anemia reduces pica. It is as if the body knew that it needed something and devised this abnormal craving for an inedible substance. During pregnancy, the possibility of iron deficiency anemia must always be considered.

UNDERWEIGHT

Fashion's concentration on slim female figures makes it easy to overlook the health problem of the woman who is underweight. A woman who enters a pregnancy underweight needs dietary counseling just as much as the overweight woman.

Underweight is defined as a state in which a person's weight is 10 to 15 percent less than ideal weight (see Table 18-2). Because underweight may signify underlying disease, it is important that it be recognized during pregnancy. Most people who are underweight have reduced resistance to disease, tire easily, and have an accompanying iron deficiency anemia.

Underweight can occur because of poverty and inability to buy adequate food, although many poor women are obese because starch foods are cheaper than meat, eggs, or cheese. It may be due to excessive worry or stress, which has led to loss of appetite. It may be due to depression, which causes a chronic loss of appetite. A great deal of underweight is caused by an insufficient intake of food due to chronic poor nutritional habits.

Nutritional counseling with underweight women, therefore, may not be easy, as you may be asking the woman to change lifelong habits of eating, at a time when she is worried and under stress and change is difficult for her. Diet counseling during the first trimester of pregnancy, when the woman has even mild nausea and vomiting, will be extremely difficult (she wants to eat nothing; you want her to eat more than ever before).

Asking a woman to list what she has eaten in the last twenty-four hours is often an effective means of pointing out to her how inadequate her intake is. If you just ask her if she eats well, she will say that she does. When she looks at a list of what she has eaten, however, and all she sees is a cup of coffee for breakfast, a container of yogurt and a glass of diet soft drink for lunch, a pork chop, salad, and a second cup of coffee for dinner, she can better appreciate how little this actually is.

Caloric intake for the underweight woman may need to be 500 to 1000 calories above that ordinarily specified during pregnancy (2300 to 2700 calories). Working out well-planned meals rather than depending on quick takeout foods is generally helpful to increase the total intake of calories. Additional calories might be added in the form of a concentrated formula.

A 500-calorie increase over normal calorie requirements should result in a weight gain of a pound per week. Be certain when the total weight gain during pregnancy is calculated at each office visit that this pound per week is subtracted, or the total weight gain of the woman may seem excessive when it is actually healthy.

If underweight is making the woman tired, she needs to be urged to take adequate rest periods daily in order to feel sufficiently energetic to prepare nutritious meals and gain adequate weight.

OBESITY

Obesity is a serious problem among women in the United States. Approximately 20 percent of American women are overweight. Women from poverty areas tend to be more overweight than others because they may not be so aware of the comparative levels of carbohydrates in foods and because many starchy foods (macaroni, spaghetti) are cheaper than less caloric but more nutritious foods such as meat and cheese. Native American women have an exceptionally high ratio of obesity.

By definition, a person is *overweight* if she is 10 percent above the desirable weight for her height and age group; *obese* if she is more than 10 percent above her desirable weight. Obesity is generally accepted to be the result of excessive caloric intake and decreased energy expenditure.

Diet counseling with obese women during pregnancy may be difficult because overeating has many causes. For some women, overeating is a coping mechanism for stress. As pregnancy is a stress, for such women to change food intake patterns at this time may be very hard. Other women overeat because their parents did and they were raised to consume a diet over-rich in calories. Changing this pattern means changing a lifelong habit. If their husband or children also enjoy an excessive intake of calories, in order to effect change in the woman's diet you have to change her whole family's eating patterns.

Obesity is a problem during pregnancy because the woman's circulatory volume increases 30 to 50 percent and her metabolism must increase to meet the demands of the pregnancy, putting additional stress on a possibly already overworked body. It is often difficult to hear fetal heart tones on an obese woman; palpating for position and size of the fetus is difficult. If a cesarean section is needed at delivery, it is difficult to do because of the excessive adipose tissue that must be cut in order to reach the uterus. Ambulating during pregnancy and immediately afterward is more difficult for an obese woman and so thrombophlebitic disease may occur more frequently.

Pregnancy is not a good time for a woman to undertake a reducing diet, however, because if carbohydrates are reduced too much, the body will utilize protein and fat for energy. This situation will deprive the fetus of protein and can lead to ketoacidosis in the woman and an environment detrimental to fetal growth. A pregnancy diet, therefore, in even the most obese woman, should never be below 1500 to 1800 calories.

Overweight women tend to exercise less than those of normal weight (exercising is more awkward and more tiring, and they may feel self-conscious dressed in certain sports clothing). They need to be urged to undertake at least a minimum activity program such as a walk around the block daily in addition to adjusting caloric intake.

Table 18-10 contrasts the nutritional worth of some common snack foods with their caloric totals. Helping a woman look at her diet in terms of empty-calorie foods in contrast to nutritional-calorie foods may help her to eat more sensibly during pregnancy. Early in pregnancy when she is eager to appear pregnant, she may be very resistant to any limitation of intake. She needs to understand that a fetus grows best on nutritional foods, not necessarily those with the most calories.

FOOD ALLERGIES

Women who are allergic to specific foods should not eat them during pregnancy (nor at any other time, for that matter). Many women do not have food allergies, but certain foods make them uncomfortable when they eat them. It is good to ask what these foods are before beginning any nutritional counseling because women do not eat these foods even if you recommend them. If you are aware of them, you can suggest alternative foods that can be eaten.

Table 18-10. Food Values of Common Snack Foods

Food	Protein	Calcium	Iron	Vitamin A	Vitamin C	Calories
Carbonated cola, 8 oz	0	0	0	0	0	145
Doughnut, plain	1	13	0.4	30	Trace	125
Brownie	1	9	0.4	20	Trace	85
Apple pie, 1 slice	3	11	0.4	40	1	350
Fudge, 1 piece	Trace	22	0.3	Trace	Trace	115
Cheese pizza, 1 slice	7	107	0.7	290	4	185

Source. *Nutritive Value of Foods*, U.S. Dept. of Agriculture, Home and Garden Bulletin No. 72, 1970.

CONSTIPATION

Because of the reduced activity of the gastrointestinal tract during pregnancy (from pressure of the growing uterus and the placental hormone relaxin) many women experience constipation during pregnancy. This leads to a feeling of bloating or fullness and lack of appetite. Women need to include an adequate intake of fiber-rich foods so they have enough bulk in the intestines to promote peristalsis. Preventing constipation by nutritional intervention is preferable to treating constipation with laxatives or enemas.

LACTOSE INTOLERANCE

The sugar in milk is lactose. In the intestine, lactose is broken down into glucose and galactose by the enzyme lactase. In most of the world's population lactase is present in infants but disappears by school age. This is the same phenomenon that occurs in dogs. Puppies can drink milk, but dogs drink water. Blacks, Native Americans, and Oriental persons tend to have the highest percentage of lactose intolerance (about 70 percent of mature American blacks cannot drink milk). Persons most likely to be able to tolerate milk are North Europeans and their descendants.

When persons who are lactose-intolerant drink milk, they report symptoms of nausea, diarrhea, cramps, gas, and a general feeling of bloatedness. Some express these symptoms as simply, "I don't like milk."

Women who cannot drink milk may be able to eat cheese because the processing of cheese changes the lactose content. They will need a calcium supplement (1,200 mg daily) and a vitamin D (400 I.U.) supplement. Because milk is a good source of protein, you need to take a thorough diet history to see whether, without milk, the woman is taking in enough protein.

Many baby magazines, television ads, and government pamphlets on pregnancy mention over and over that it is important to drink milk during pregnancy, but you need to spend time reassuring women who cannot drink milk that it really is *not* necessary. It is never the milk per se that is good for them; it is the nutrients of milk, which can be provided in other ways.

A number of newborns are born lactose intolerant and have trouble digesting breast milk or formula. These infants have the same symptoms (watery diarrhea, cramps, irritability). They need to be placed on lactose-free formulas so they obtain sufficient nutrition. There is no need for a woman to worry during pregnancy that her child will be born with this problem, however. Most lactose intolerance comes with maturity, not in the infant period.

TEENAGE PREGNANCIES

Good nutrition is often a problem with pregnant teenagers because of the dual demands of pregnancy and adolescence. The girl must take in enough food to provide not only for fetal growth but for her own growth as well. A part of adolescents' search for identity involves a turning away from foods that their mothers saw as important for them (milk, warm cereal, vegetables, fruit). Teenagers indulge themselves instead in foods that their mothers usually disapprove of, such as pizza, Coca-Cola, potato chips, or organic foods that their mothers do not understand the need for (if, indeed, the teenagers themselves understand). In helping the teenager plan a diet for pregnancy, you should respect her right to reject traditional foods as long as her diet includes sufficient nutrients. Pizza and a glass of milk is a lunch that provides all basic food groups (meat: pepperoni; bread: pizza crust; fruit and vegetable: tomato sauce; milk: the glass of milk). A hotdog "with everything" and milk provides the same nutrition.

Counseling with adolescents may be very difficult because they often are not responsible for cooking the food they eat. You may need to speak to the mother about foods to prepare before you can alter a teenager's diet pattern.

The pregnant teenager needs a high caloric intake (2400 to 2700 calories) to supply energy for her high level of activity. The nutrients most poorly supplied by a teenage diet tend to be calcium, iron, vitamin A, and total calories. Look for sources of these when analyzing a teenage pregnancy diet.

DECREASED NUTRITIONAL STORES

A woman with high parity or a short interval between pregnancies may have depleted nutritional stores. Women who have been dieting rigorously to lose weight prior to pregnancy may have depleted their nutritional reserves to such an extent that they have little to draw on during the first part of pregnancy, when they may not be able to eat well because of the normal nausea and vomiting of pregnancy. They need to be identified so that nutritional counseling can be begun early and symptoms of nausea and vomiting limited; then they can eat adequately.

MULTIPLE PREGNANCY

In a multiple pregnancy, the growing demands of multiple fetuses may overtax a woman's nutritional reserves. It is important that multiple pregnancy be recognized early and dietary supplements added as needed.

SMOKING, ALCOHOLISM, AND DRUG DEPENDENCY

Women who smoke excessively may eat less than nonsmokers because they finish their meals with a cigarette rather than with dessert. They smoke a cigarette rather than eat a snack. Smoking may dull their taste sense, and foods do not seem as appetizing to them as to others. Women who stop smoking, in contrast (and many women choose to decrease or stop smoking during pregnancy—and *should* do so), snack excessively. In nutritional counseling, it is important to analyze a day's intake for both groups and see that a woman's intake is adequate or to urge her, as long as you cannot control her snacking, to make her snacks nutritious ones.

Aside from having definite teratogenic effects of its own, alcohol may further compromise a successful pregnancy. Women who drink alcohol excessively may do so at the expense of eating. In order to metabolize large quantities of alcohol, the body utilizes large quantities of thiamine. Alcoholic women often suffer thiamine shortages and need to take a thiamine supplement and eat foods high in this vitamin during pregnancy.

Women who are drug-dependent may have difficulty supporting their drug habit and buying nutritious food also. If they are drug-dependent on a hallucinogen or euphoric drug, they may not feel hungry and may skip meals for days. Enrolling these women in drug withdrawal programs such as a methadone program, where a drug is supplied for them daily, helps them to be able to afford food. It also keeps them in contact with health care personnel who can urge them to continue prenatal care.

CONCURRENT MEDICAL PROBLEMS

Women who have medical problems such as kidney disease, diabetes, or tuberculosis need special dietary considerations because of the specific metabolic disorders that can occur with these diseases. Nursing interventions with women with these medical problems are discussed in Chap. 33.

Cultural Influences

Adults tend to eat the foods they ate as children. Women during pregnancy do not want to change from these cultural patterns. For many women, because they prepare foods for their husbands and families as well as for themselves, this would involve changing the food patterns of others besides themselves.

In nutritional counseling, therefore, you need to be aware of the cultural patterns of the population with which you work. Then you can suggest foods that fit within personal preferences.

CHINESE DIET PATTERNS

There are four main areas in China, and the diet pattern in each area varies. People from the *Mandarin*, or northern, area eat a diet rich in sweet and sour dishes with noodles as a staple. *Shanghai* is the coastal region, and fish and seafood are popular dishes there. In the southern, or *Cantonese* area, pork, chicken, and dumplings filled with meat (Dim Sum) are popular. Inland China, or the *Szechwan* area, is known for hot foods, highly seasoned with pepper.

Most people in the United States with a Chinese heritage eat a diet rich in vegetables (bean sprouts, broccoli, mushrooms, bamboo shoots)—stirfried (cooked quickly) so they retain their nutrients well. Since meat is served mixed with vegetables, the proportion of meat eaten daily may be small. Rice, rather than potatoes or bread, is a staple. Encourage pregnant women to eat enriched rice if possible for its added vitamin content. Milk is not a popular beverage because of lactose intolerance in Oriental people. Bean curd is a good source of protein and calcium, eaten often to take the place of milk. Soybeans, mustard greens, collard greens, and kale are vegetables with high calcium. Ice cream is an enjoyable source of calcium. The problem that may arise for women eating a Chinese diet during pregnancy is lack of protein due to small meat servings.

JAPANESE DIET PATTERNS

In a Japanese diet, little milk or cheese is used. Eggs, bean curd (tofu), spinach, broccoli, mustard greens, tomatoes, and eggplant are sources of protein and calcium. As with Chinese diet patterns, meat is generally served with vegetables; the small amount of protein taken in may be a problem in pregnancy.

PUERTO RICAN DIET PATTERNS

In many Puerto Rican homes, the midday meal is the large meal of the day. Although many types of meat are used, they are often cooked as stews, so individual portions of meat or protein may be small. Beans and rice are often cooked together, a good source of complementary proteins. Many Puerto Rican women do not drink milk (lactose intolerance) but do add some to coffee. Black malt beer (malta) is a nonalcoholic beverage thought to be nutritious and hence popular during pregnancy. Folic acid deficiency may be a problem for Puerto Rican women. Foods rich in folic acid are green, leafy vegetables, liver, fish, meat,

Nutrition and Pregnancy

poultry, legumes, and whole grains. These should be encouraged. Obesity is a common nutritional problem.

MEXICAN-AMERICAN DIET PATTERNS

The Mexican-American diet is a blend of Spanish, Native American, and Anglo-Saxon diet patterns. Corn is the basic grain used. *Tortillas* (flat cakes made from ground corn) are a staple of the diet. *Enchiladas* and *tacos* are filled tortillas. Since meat is generally used with beans (pinto and garbanzo) or tomato sauce, individual portions of meat may be small. Milk is limited although it is used in custards and rice puddings. During pregnancy, vitamin A and folic acid deficiency may be problems. Obesity is a common Mexican-American health problem.

BLACK DIET PATTERNS

Meat in a "soul food" diet is often pork (pigs' feet, ham hocks, chitterlings, or spareribs). Vegetables are often cooked with salt pork for long periods, so water-soluble vitamins are lost in cooking. Mustard greens, collards, black-eyed peas, corn, and sweet potatoes are popular vegetables. Grits, cornbread, and rice are staples. Little milk is consumed (lactose intolerance), but large quantities of cheese may be eaten as macaroni and cheese. Problems that a pregnant woman may encounter are low hemoglobin levels from the sparsity of meat, obesity, and chronic hypertension from the increased sodium intake from salt pork.

JEWISH DIET PATTERNS

The Jewish dietary laws (*kashruth*) are followed to varying degrees in Jewish homes. Orthodox Jewish families follow them strictly; Reformed Jewish families give them no great emphasis; Conservative families practice at individual levels. The word *kosher* means "fit or clean." Grains, fruits, and vegetables are kosher. Meat and poultry are not kosher and must be made kosher by being soaked in salted water to remove all blood. Only animals that are "four-footed, cloven-hoofed, and chew a cud" are used (beef and lamb). Pork and fish without scales and fins, such as shellfish, are prohibited. Milk and meat cannot be eaten together (creamed meat soups). No cooking is allowed on the Sabbath (sundown Friday through Saturday evening) in strict homes. Yom Kippur (Day of Atonement) is a 24-hour period of fasting.

Nutritional problems of following a Jewish diet may be increased cholesterol levels due to high levels of saturated fat.

EUROPEAN DIET PATTERNS

Diet patterns vary widely in persons from European cultures. Diet faults tend to cluster around overcooked vegetables, which then have less than desirable levels of water-soluble vitamins, lack of fresh fruits, and excessive bread or pasta intake. In pregnant women, lack of vitamin C and obesity may be common nutritional problems.

Fad Diets

Every year new diets to help people lose weight painlessly are introduced. As a rule of thumb, pregnant women should not be on reducing diets, so there is no place for these in a pregnancy diet. It is helpful to be familiar with some of the basic principles of these diets, however, as many women enter pregnancy on them or have recently been on them.

NATURAL FOOD DIETS

Foods that remain in their natural state with a minimum of processing and contain no artificial ingredients are "natural foods." There can be no harm from eating only natural foods unless it restricts the woman's diet in some important nutrient area.

ORGANICALLY GROWN FOOD DIETS

Foods grown without the use of pesticides, fumigants, or synthetic fertilizers and containing no preservatives or synthetic coloring agents are "organically grown foods." These must be purchased in specialty shops and are 30 to 100 percent more expensive than other foods because of low crop yields. Women who eat only organically grown food may be reluctant to take vitamin supplements during pregnancy. Chemically, natural and synthetic vitamins are the same; buying them at a health food store does not improve the quality.

ZEN MACROBIOTIC DIET

Macrobiotic means "large or long life." The combination of a macrobiotic diet and a pseudo-Oriental philosophy seems to appeal to younger women and teenagers. Foods are chosen on the basis of Yang (hot, masculine) or Yin (cold, feminine) properties. There are 10 levels of diets. The simplest level includes cereal, vegetables, fruits, seafoods, and desserts, and very limited fluid. The strictest level is composed only of brown rice and, again, very limited fluid. Women ingesting a macrobiotic diet for long periods run the risk of scurvy, anemia, hypoproteinemia, hypercalcemia, and emaciation due to starvation. It is certainly not an adequate pregnancy diet.

STILLMAN DIET

The Stillman diet allows the person to eat unlimited amounts of meat, fish, and eggs; eight glasses of water and a vitamin supplement are taken daily. It is an unbalanced diet, high in saturated fat, and not recommended in pregnancy.

MAYO DIET

The Mayo diet includes high protein intake along with a generous supply of grapefruit, which supposedly has a fat-dissolving capability. There is no scientific basis for the diet, and it is not adequate during pregnancy.

ATKINS DIET

The Atkins diet includes no carbohydrate sources the first week, to promote ketosis. It is high in saturated fat. Ketosis is a state to be avoided during pregnancy as it is teratogenic to a growing fetus.

VEGETARIAN DIETS

There are many different types of vegetarian diets. Some people on vegetarian diets eat no animal or dairy products (vegans); some allow milk and eggs (lacto-ovo vegetarians); some eat fish and chicken but no red meat. A vegetarian diet can be a complete diet if the person is knowledgeable about complementary proteins and includes these in the diet. Concerns for a pregnant woman on this diet may be lack of vitamin B_{12} (meat is the chief source of this), perhaps calcium (encourage dark-green vegetables as sources), and vitamin D (fortified milk is the main source of this). Most women who are vegetarians are very knowledgeable about their diets and are able to point out to you what foods are high in various nutrients and how they incorporate these in their diets. They can be a helpful source of nutritional information for you.

Nutritional Counseling

Two subjects that are not always taught well in schools of nursing are nutrition and pharmacology. On in-service units, nutrition has become largely the province of the dietitian. You order the diet, and it comes from the kitchen fully prepared and labeled. All you do is set the meal tray in front of the patient. Long gone are the days when you had to determine what foods should be included in a specific diet, and then ladle them out of a central serving cart onto a patient's plate.

In an ambulatory setting, such as a prenatal clinic or physician's office, you often do not have the luxury of a dietitian nearby. Even if you do, you can still handle the diet counseling necessary for a normal pregnant woman, provided you see this aspect of care as important and so spend the extra time and preparation required to be informed about nutrition. Doing all other counseling—talking about bathing, exercise, clothing, travel, rest—then passing nutrition counseling on to another person gives nutrition a different value from the other health topics. It makes it seem complicated (if you cannot handle it, how can a woman alone in her kitchen handle it?), impersonal (you see the woman month after month; she sees a dietitian once or twice), and unimportant (it was not important enough for you to handle). Are these things you want to imply?

In nutritional counseling, there are a number of concerns to keep in mind.

Food has a psychological as well as a nutritional meaning to people. Under stress, some people nibble and eat constantly; some have anorexia. Pregnancy is a type of stress, so at a time when the woman's eating patterns should be optimal, they may be at their worst. Nibblers should be encouraged to choose raw vegetables and fruit (canned chick-peas and raisins are very high in iron) or hard-boiled eggs as snack foods. Women with poor appetites may need nutritional boosts such as commercial milk additives; they may find that six small meals a day suit them better than three large ones.

Most people think they eat a good diet, or at least an adequate diet. Before you can begin to talk to a woman about improving her diet, you have to demonstrate to her first that her diet *needs* some revamping. One method of doing this is to ask her for a "typical day" history. What did she eat for breakfast yesterday? For a snack? For lunch? For dinner? After dinner? This method yields much more accurate information about actual intake than if you ask how often during the week she eats citrus fruit, or how much milk she drinks a day. A woman who does not know what citrus fruit is cannot answer the first question, but she *can* tell you she had an orange for breakfast. A woman who knows how much milk she ought to drink a day will probably say she drinks a quart. However, if asked to list the foods she ate the day before, she may report that she drank only one glass of milk all day.

After you have a day's list of food, compare the amounts on the list with a chart showing nutrient values (all nutrition books and local health departments have them). Establish priorities where the diet seems to be most deficient. Do not ruin your gain at that point by saying, "You must drink more milk. Add a glass at breakfast and another for dinner." The woman may hate milk, and she may feel that you are forcing health care values on her without considering her preference. State instead, "You need more calcium in your diet. Could you drink more milk? Could you eat more cheese? Have you ever tried yogurt?"

Diets have to be tolerable or people will not follow them more than a few days. Since pregnancy lasts nine months, the woman herself must make the choices of specific foods in the various food groups you indicate are important in pregnancy. Otherwise, your clinic or office will be full of women who give lip service to good nutrition ("I'm eating everything you say") but who are not eating well at all.

Meal planning involves the entire family. The woman may be receptive to changing her eating habits but may have difficulty carrying out recommendations if her family resists change. With a teenage girl, it is often important to speak to her mother or whoever prepares the meals at home in order to effect a change.

Food is costly. In order to provide the extra servings required during pregnancy, you are asking a woman to spend more on food for herself per week than she is used to spending. Women generally view this increased expense as an investment in their child's health and so do not regard it as a burden. The family on a marginal income, however, may be willing to shoulder the additional cost but will have trouble finding the money. The woman with this problem needs a review of her diet to make certain she is not buying only starchy foods because they are more filling and cheaper than protein foods. She needs help in securing any financial assistance that is available, such as food stamps or nutrition aid programs.

Most women who receive public assistance or whose household has a limited income are eligible for a food stamp program. Any food except alcohol or pet food may be purchased with food stamps. This can mean considerable savings and can mean the difference between a poor and an adequate diet during pregnancy.

Food supplements for pregnant and lactating women may also be provided by the Special Supplementary Food Program for Women, Infants and Children (WIC). To be eligible for this program, a woman must live in a low-income area serviced by an approved health care center that administers the program. She must be considered by health officials to be at nutritional risk because of inadequate nutrition or income. Any woman with anemia, inappropriate growth patterns (underweight, overweight), high-risk pregnancy (increased parity, short interconceptual interval, or previous low-birth-weight child) is generally eligible for this aid.

In a WIC program, every month the woman receives 31 quarts of milk, 2½ dozen eggs, 4 packages of iron-fortified cereal, and 6 cans of fruit or vegetable juice. Equal amounts of Swiss, American, or cheddar cheese may be substituted for milk for those women who cannot drink milk.

A number of adolescent girls who come for prenatal care derive a portion of their daily food intake from school lunches, which are provided free to students with limited incomes. A class A school lunch consists of 8 ounces milk, 2 ounces protein, one serving whole or enriched grain product, ¾ cup vegetables, and ¾ cup fruit. How these dietary specifications are actually provided depends on the individual school dietitian.

Be familiar with the usual dietary patterns in the part of the country or the ethnic group of the woman with whom you are working. Collard or dandelion greens, for example, may not appeal to you as vegetables, but nutritionally they compare favorably to spinach or broccoli, two vegetables you may customarily recommend. There is no reason to try to convert women to your eating habits if their way is only "different," not "inadequate."

Statements such as "Eat high-protein foods" are meaningless for many women. Food, after all, does not come from the supermarket labeled "high-protein food." Women need advice given in more specific terms—for example, "Eat three servings of some kind of meat every day."

The word *diet* has come to mean a form of unpleasant food denial. It is better to talk about the "foods that are best for you during pregnancy" rather than a "pregnancy diet." The former has a positive sound and is closer to what you will be encouraging the woman to eat. A list of prenatal instructions listing proper foods is good to distribute to women as long as it is short and clear, like Table 18-9. Complicated lists of foods or a list of *don'ts* will land in the wastepaper basket rather than being used and followed.

Socioeconomic level is not a criterion for judging good nutritional intake. Some women with ample money to spend actually feed their families less nutritionally well than those who have to live on a lower budget. Each family and woman must be evaluated individually.

Because a little supplementation is good during pregnancy, a woman may think that a lot will be even better for her. She should be cautioned against taking vitamins indiscriminately. Overconsumption of vitamin A has been shown to be associated with congenital defects in animals. The woman should take the supplement her physician recommends and no others, just as she avoids any medication during pregnancy that is not specifically prescribed or approved by her physician.

Be certain to comment on the things the woman is doing *correctly*. This is an elemental rule of teaching that almost every teacher forgets in his or her zeal to create a perfect student.

Problem-oriented Recording: Progress Notes

Christine McFadden
15 years

Problem: Nutrition in pregnancy

> S. Patient is student in high school; no previous pregnancies.
> Food at home prepared by mother.
> Eats breakfast at home, lunch at high school cafeteria, dinner often at fast-food takeout on way to part-time job.
> 24-hour diet history:
> > Breakfast: 2 slices toast, 1 glass orange juice
> > Lunch: grilled cheese sandwich, 1 glass milk
> > Dinner: 1 hamburger, 1 serv. french fries, 1 cup coffee
> > Snacks: 6–8 cookies, 1 bag pretzels, 1 glass cola
>
> Doesn't dislike milk or vegetables; just doesn't eat them.
> Admits to being poor medicine taker.
> O. Prepregnancy weight: 115; appropriate for height.
> Weight today (last menstrual period about 16 weeks ago): 122. Appears pale, although hemoglobin is 11 gm.
> A. Weight gain appropriate for this point in pregnancy.
> Food intake inadequate for pregnancy (little protein, no vegetables except french fries, little milk, high caffeine).
>
> Goals: a. Pregnancy weight gain to total 25–30 pounds.
> > b. Hemoglobin to remain above 11 gm.
> > c. Able to describe adequate pregnancy diet at next visit.

> > d. To take vitamin and iron supplement daily.
>
> P. 1. Diet to be 2700 calories (to allow for teenage growth).
> 2. Counsel *re* pregnancy diet and difficulty with cafeteria and fast-food sources.
> 3. Help to design a compliance chart to record vitamin and iron supplement daily for better compliance.
> 4. Review diet next visit (to bring up any problems she encounters).
> 5. Strong support for following improved diet (few support people around her to reinforce actions).

Problem-oriented Recording: Progress Notes

Mary Kraft
22 years

Problem: Nutrition in pregnancy

> S. Patient is housewife; part-time job in public library.
> Cooks for self and husband; "not a good cook." Often cooks just for herself as husband attends night school. Culture: black.
> One previous pregnancy ending in spont. abortion 2 years ago.
> Has "always had a weight problem" she keeps under control by "eating almost nothing."
> 24-hour diet history:
> > Breakfast: 1 cup black coffee
> > Lunch: None
> > Dinner: 1 serv. macaroni and cheese; 1 serv. greens, 1 cup coffee
> > Snacks: 2 glasses milk, 1 candy bar
>
> Finances adequate.
> O. Prepregnancy weight: 110 (10 pounds under desirable weight).
> Weight today (last menstrual period 9 weeks ago): 111.
> Appears thin; hemoglobin 11 gm.
> A. Food intake inadequate for pregnancy (low total calories, low protein, no fruit, high caffeine).
>
> Goals: a. Pregnancy weight gain to total 35–40

pounds (10 pounds underweight prepregnancy).
b. Hemoglobin to remain above 11 gm.
c. Able to describe adequate pregnancy diet at next visit.
d. To take vitamin and iron supplement daily.

P. 1. Diet to be 2900 calories daily (500 additional calories to increase weight).
2. Counsel *re* pregnancy diet and need to increase intake.
3. Return in 1 week for nurse appointment for further nutrition review and suggestions.
4. To bring suggestions that might make cooking for herself in evening or at noon easier or more fun.
5. Respect cultural influences on diet; wants to raise children with knowledge and appreciation of black culture.

Problem-oriented Recording: Progress Notes

Angie Baco
42 years

Problem: Nutrition in pregnancy

S. Patient is housewife; cooks for 5 children (ages 20, 19, 18, 15, and 7) and husband. Enjoys cooking; has won prizes at county fair for cakes and pies.
Culture: Italian. Is reluctant to take an iron supplement because it might cause constipation; no objection to vitamins.
Finances adequate. Had weight gain of 50 pounds last pregnancy, mild gestational diabetes.
24-hour diet history:
Breakfast: 1 serv. oatmeal with milk and honey, 1 glass orange juice, 2 slices cinnamon bread with butter
Lunch: 1 serv. tomato soup, bacon and cheese sandwich, 2 pieces cherry pie, 1 glass lemonade
Dinner: 1 serv. spaghetti and meatballs, 1 serv. green salad, 2 slices bread and butter, 2 pieces carrot cake, 1 glass milk, 1 cup coffee
Snacks: 2 slices cinnamon toast, 2 oranges

O. Prepregnancy weight: 144 (30 pounds above ideal weight). Weight today (12 weeks since LMP): 150. Hemoglobin 11.5 gm.

A. Prepregnancy obesity—already 7-pound weight gain. Inadequate pregnancy diet (little milk, high total calories but questionable protein intake).

Goals: a. Weight gain to be 30–40 pounds.
b. To increase exercise daily.
c. Hemoglobin to remain above 11 gm.
d. Able to describe adequate pregnancy diet at next visit.
e. To take vitamin and iron supplement daily.

P. 1. Pregnancy diet to be limited to 2400 calories.
2. Counsel pregnancy diet and need to limit high-calorie but not high-protein foods.
3. To try vitamin and iron supplement for 1 week and see if constipation occurs.
4. Husband to accompany her at next visit to talk about family's cooperation in limiting high-calorie foods.
5. Give generous support for attempts at compliance; difficult for her to change diet pattern.
6. Encourage to attempt walk daily to increase exercise.

References

1. Adams, S. O., et al. Effect of nutritional supplementation in pregnancy. *J. Am. Diet. Assoc.* 72:144, 1978.
2. Ancri, G., et al. Comparison of the nutritional status of pregnant adolescents with adult pregnant women. *Am. J. Clin. Nutr.* 30:568, 1977.
3. Brown, P. T., and Bergan, J. G. The dietary status of "new" vegetarians. *J. Am. Diet. Assoc.* 67:455, 1975.
4. Burke, B. S. Nutritional studies during pregnancy. *Am. J. Obstet. Gynecol.* 46:38, 1943.
5. Cohen, A. W., and Gabbe, S. G. When obesity complicates pregnancy. *Contemp. Obstet. Gynecol.* 15:45, 1980.

6. Feigenberg, M., et al. Nutritional counseling for middle class gravidas. *J.O.G.N. Nurs.* 6:19, 1977.
7. Food and Nutrition Board. *Recommended Daily Dietary Allowances*. Washington: National Academy of Sciences, National Research Council, 1979.
8. Holey, E. S. Promoting adequate weight gain in pregnant women. *M.C.N.* 2:86, 1977.
9. Jacobson, H. N. Current concepts in nutrition: Diet in pregnancy. *N. Engl. J. Med.* 297:1051, 1977.
10. Johnson, E. M., et al. Physicians' opinions and counseling practices in maternal and infant nutrition. *J. Am. Diet. Assoc.* 73:246, 1978.
11. Kaminetsky, H., and Baker, H. Micronutrients in pregnancy. *Clin. Obstet. Gynecol.* 20:363, 1977.
12. Lappe, F. M. *Diet for a Small Planet*. New York: Ballantine Books, 1975.
13. Lindenbaum, J., et al. Oral contraceptive hormones, folate metabolism and the cervical epithelium. *Am. J. Clin. Nutr.* 28:346, 1975.
14. Luke, B. Lactose intolerance during pregnancy: Significance and solutions. *M.C.N.* 2:92, 1977.
15. Martinez, O. Effect of oral contraceptives on blood folate levels in pregnancy. *Am. J. Obstet. Gynecol.* 128:255, 1977.
16. Natow, A., et al. Integrating the Jewish dietary laws into a dietetic program. *J. Am. Diet. Assoc.* 67:14, 1975.
17. Osancova, K., et al. Diet and weight gain in pregnancy in relation to the birth weight and height of the infant. *Nutr. Metab.* 1:216, 1977.
18. Parker, S., and Bowery, J. Folacin in diets of Puerto Rican and black women in relation to food practices. *J. Nutr. Educ.* 8:73, 1976.
19. Pirani, B. B., et al. Smoking during pregnancy. Its effect on maternal metabolism and fetoplacental function. *Obstet. Gynecol.* 52:257, 1978.
20. Pitkin, R. M. Nutrition during pregnancy: The clinical approach. *Curr. Concepts Nutr.* 5:27, 1977.
21. Pitkin, R. M. Nutritional influences during pregnancy. *Med. Clin. North Am.* 61:3, 1977.
22. Rosso, P. Maternal nutrition, nutrient exchange and fetal growth. *Curr. Concepts Nutr.* 5:3, 1977.
23. Worthington, B. S. Nutritional considerations during pregnancy and lactation. *Fam. Community Health* 1:13, 1978.

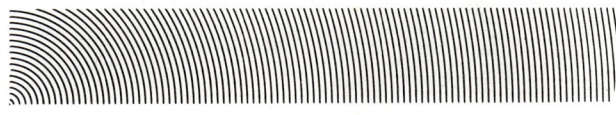

19. Preparation for Parenthood

Although parenthood is the occupation most closely involved in protecting the physical and mental health of the next generation, it is one of the few occupations that require no formal course of instruction, no examinations to test the person's competency to fulfill this role, and no refresher course to ensure that the parent is following up-to-date concepts of child rearing.

In most communities today, courses are available for prospective parents. Every pregnant woman, whether primipara or grand multipara, should be asked during the prenatal period whether or not she would be interested in participating in a course that will help to prepare her for giving birth or raising her child. You should be familiar with the material offered by these courses so that you can be certain the ones you are advocating present adequate and accurate information. Nurses are the people in the community most often asked to conduct educational programs for prospective parents, and thus you may be asked to present such a program. If there are no preparation-for-parenthood classes in your community, you *should* organize and teach such classes.

Prospective parents usually are not ready for participation in such programs early in pregnancy. They need time to accept the pregnancy, to work through what it feels like to be having a child, to think about being a mother or father. At the time of quickening, when they can feel the child stir and move, attending classes may become part of nest building. Mention early in pregnancy that such courses are given; at quickening (18 to 20 weeks) suggest the concrete opportunities available.

The programs offered are of two principal types: In one the course of normal pregnancy and beginning child care are discussed, and in the other active preparation for childbirth is taught.

Expectant Parents' Classes

Parents, like all students, learn best when material is presented in a variety of ways. Some topics, such as childbearing anatomy, are best taught by lecture. A topic such as the psychological aspects of pregnancy is best taught by group interaction. Imagine how you, if you were pregnant, would respond to a nonpregnant nurse standing in front of a classroom telling you how it feels to be pregnant. You would want to tell *her* how it feels. You would want to talk to the other pregnant women in the group and see if they feel as you do, to assure yourself that you are responding normally to this pregnancy. Some topics are best taught if both men and women are present; others, such as the man's feelings toward pregnancy, might be best handled in a group attended only by prospective fathers.

COURSE PLANNING

Most preparation-for-parenthood programs are planned to cover 4 to 8 hours of time spaced over a four- to eight-week period. The curriculum should be individualized for the group and that group's particular needs. If all the women in the group already have children, for example, they may not feel a need for a tour of a maternity unit as part of the program; instead, they may want a review of what is new in baby food or child care. If all the women are teenagers, they may be most interested in what is going to happen to their bodies during pregnancy, or what sports activities are safe to continue during pregnancy. They probably will want a tour of the maternity unit included.

It is good to begin a first class by passing out cards to the members of the group and asking them to write down the topics they most want to hear discussed at sessions. Asking members to put their interests in writing is often more productive than asking the group for oral suggestions. Some people, particularly fathers-to-be, are not willing to admit before a group of strangers that they do not know very much about childbirth or children. However, they will express their needs in writing: "Tell us how to space babies better." "Does the baby feel anything when it's being born?" "Do I *have* to eat liver?"

Some people have not thought through what they expect or want from the course. They have come because they want to learn, assuming the course would consist of a series of preplanned lectures. They need help in selecting topics that will be of interest to them. Review with them topics that other groups have asked to have discussed or the time-honored concerns in pregnancy. This introduction will stimulate individual ideas.

A typical course plan for eight weeks might be as follows:

Lesson 1: Introduction of group members
Anatomy and physiology of childbearing
Fetal growth
Lesson 2: Personal care of the woman during pregnancy
Lesson 3: Feelings toward pregnancy
Lesson 4: What you always wanted to know about labor and delivery (but were afraid to ask)
Lesson 5: The postpartum period
What it feels like to be a new parent
Lesson 6: Infant care
Lesson 7: Tour of a maternity unit
Plans for hospitalization
Lesson 8: Family planning

Some group leaders like to proceed without any set plan, just asking at every meeting what the group would like to discuss that evening. Use this technique judiciously unless you are skilled in group dynamics. Otherwise, every week the topic will be decided on by the most talkative members of the group, and less voluble members will sit through eight sessions with few of their questions answered.

Collecting the topics that people would like to hear discussed, then organizing the material for presentation, is a good compromise between an entirely open group and formal, stiff lectures. It assures everyone in the group that his or her topic will be discussed. It assures you that the essential information of pregnancy and childbirth will be covered and allows you time to prepare for classes—and preparation is necessary if you are to cover a topic thoroughly.

Specific suggestions as to the material that might be included in each of the lessons follow.

LESSON 1: GROUP INTRODUCTION

Because members of the group learn as much (perhaps more) from interaction with each other than from an instructor, they first need to become acquainted with one another. Arrange your classroom so the chairs are in a circle, not in rows. Provide cocoa or cold drinks if at all possible within your setting and budget.

Begin by suggesting that couples introduce themselves, giving their names, indicating whether or not this is their first baby, and mentioning anything else interesting about themselves that they want to share with the group. Fathers will usually identify themselves at the first meeting by their occupations: "I'm Bob Jones, an accountant. This is our first baby." Women, too, generally introduce themselves in terms of occupations (listen for "I'm *only* a housewife"; such a woman may need assurance that she is a worthwhile person who is capable of carrying a pregnancy to completion) and sometimes in terms of interests: "Hi, I'm Betty Jones. I'm not working now. I volunteer at the hospital."

Introductions are helpful in breaking the ice, and they provide you and the other group members a background against which to evaluate each other's opinions. Bob Jones, for example, throughout the course, asks questions like "What costs more, a diaper service or disposable diapers?" "Does anyone here think it's worthwhile to buy an expensive crib?" "How much is the hospital bill likely to be?" As an accountant, he is oriented toward money; his thoughts gravitate to that value first. Betty, on the other hand, is more concerned with feelings. She says, "I don't think I could watch my baby being born. I'd be too scared." "Do you think dogs get jealous of new babies?" "Sometimes I wish I weren't pregnant."

Listening to introductions and being aware of what values people are placing on things help you to answer questions more pertinently during the course. When Bob Jones asks the group or you, "Which is better, a spinal or a general anesthetic?" he may actually mean, "Is there a difference in cost?" His wife, asking the same question, might mean, "Which is better for the baby?"

If a group member has raised a question that is obviously of interest to the group, the topic should be explored following introductions. If not, a review of female anatomy and the growth of the fetus in utero is a good place to begin. It is always surprising how little many women know about their own bodies (how much did you know before you took anatomy and physiology?), and men know even less.

Many old wives' tales will surface during the discussion: Is it true a baby carried in the upper part of the uterus is a boy, and one carried in the lower part is a girl? How do I know the baby is growing where it's supposed to and isn't lost in the abdomen somewhere? Don't women produce an egg for a girl one month, an egg for a boy the next? How does a baby breathe when it's in all that fluid? These are concerns that mothers-to-be and fathers-to-be carry with them throughout the pregnancy if they do not have an opportunity to voice them and have them clarified.

LESSON 2: PERSONAL CARE

In discussing personal care during pregnancy, you will present material that will be essentially what you give to women at prenatal visits. The difference in parents' classes is that the husband is present. He hears of the need for rest periods, better nutrition, and planned exercise. For women who go to physicians who do not include teaching as part of prenatal visits, this may be new and extremely welcome information.

LESSON 3: FEELINGS TOWARD PREGNANCY

Feelings toward pregnancy may be best handled if the fathers are allowed a session from 7:00 to 8:00 P.M., followed by the women at 8:00 to 9:00 P.M. If you have two instructors, two separate meetings can be planned for 7:00, with the men talking among themselves, the women among themselves, and then everyone meeting together for the last hour. It is as important for a husband to appreciate how his wife feels as it is for him to talk about how *he* feels about being a father. It is equally important for a wife to learn that pregnancy is a stress for her husband as well as for her.

After it has been brought out by you or the group that pregnancy is a stress period, that wives become irritable and perhaps cry easily, it is not unusual for a man to slump back in his chair, tremendously relaxed, and say, "I thought it was something *I* did. You mean it's normal for her to act that way?"

Nurses usually find it easier to talk about the physical aspects of pregnancy, so there is a tendency for them to omit a class on feelings about pregnancy when planning a program for prospective parents. Remember that parents protect the mental health of the next generation. They cannot do this well unless they themselves are in good mental health. Marital discord (with so many quarrels that their causes are quickly forgotten) is not conducive to sound child rearing and mental health. Initiating a discussion about the psychological changes in women and men during a pregnancy should help to lay a foundation for better parent-child relations and is a good mental health measure.

LESSON 4: LABOR AND DELIVERY
Signs of Beginning Labor

Primiparas are always anxious to have the signs of beginning labor reviewed one more time. They are often worried that they will sleep through labor and deliver the infant at home. Some primiparas arrive at the labor wing of a hospital on the day of delivery completely exhausted because they have been afraid to sleep soundly for the past month. It helps to be reassured that *no one sleeps* through active labor.

Medication in Labor

Most women today are aware that they will have some say about the amount of medication they will be given for discomfort in labor and about the type of anesthesia that will be used for delivery. In order for a woman to be able to make a responsible choice as to whether she wants pain relief in labor or not, she needs to have the options for anesthesia explained to her in this class.

Be sure she understands two general rules of thumb concerning analgesia and labor: Usually, no analgesia is given in labor until the cervix is dilated 3 to 4 cm. It is also not given if delivery is anticipated within an hour. With this knowledge, a woman will understand why she cannot always have pain relief at the exact time she wants it. Be certain that women realize that

Preparation for Parenthood

relaxation is one of their greatest assets in the first stage of labor, that pushing is reserved for the second stage.

Dilatation and Effacement
It is good to discuss the terms that apply to the progress of labor. Let the woman know that cervical dilatation is measured by (1) effacement and (2) dilatation. If on examining her the physician reports that she is making little progress in dilatation, tell her to ask him how she is doing in effacement. This prevents her from becoming discouraged because nothing appears to be happening.

Hospital Regulations
Familiarize yourself with the policies of the various hospitals where the women will deliver. Will the father of the child be allowed to stay with the woman in labor? Will he be allowed in the delivery room? Will he be able to see the baby with her or only through the nursery room glass? Will she be allowed to breast-feed her baby in the delivery room? Is a birthing room available?

Exercises and Breathing Techniques
Every woman should learn muscle-strengthening exercises as well as breathing techniques to limit the amount of discomfort she will have in labor. As indicated, analgesia is not given in labor until the cervix is dilated 3 to 4 cm. Meanwhile, contractions have been bitingly painful for an hour or more. Even when medication is given, it will only take the edge off the pain. Thus, common sense dictates that if a woman can take away the rest of her discomfort by correct breathing patterns she will be foolish to enter labor without learning these patterns.

Women who show an interest in this kind of preparation for labor should be enrolled in a series of classes specifically designed for labor preparation following the completion of expectant parents' classes. A woman should be cautioned that this training is basic preparation for minimizing her discomfort and helping to shorten the length of labor. It will not make her knowledgeable enough to supervise her own labor and delivery. In the event a deviation from the normal occurs, she must be ready and willing to place herself entirely in her physician's hands.

LESSON 5: THE POSTPARTUM PERIOD
The postpartum period does not seem very important when a woman in pregnant. It seems too far away to be real, and her imagination carries her only as far as the day of delivery. It will be helpful to discuss what she can expect in the hospital in the hours after delivery, however. Knowing that she will stay in a birthing room or go to a recovery room for a period of time and that she will be under close observation there saves both her and her husband unnecessary worry. Knowing that the baby will be taken to a special observation or careful-watch nursery for the first 8 to 12 hours, if that is hospital policy, relieves anxiety about his welfare.

The members of the group will probably be timid at first in discussing what it feels like to be a new parent. All they can do is project how they think they will feel. In most groups, however, there is at least one person who is sure what it will be like. Remembering that this person said, "I think I'll be *scared*. I think I'll feel so *responsible*" will be very reassuring to every couple the day they bring their baby home from the hospital. They will know that they are experiencing a common apprehension.

LESSON 6: INFANT CARE
As a woman passes the point of quickening, she becomes interested in child care. She wants to know the kinds of things she needs to buy and how many of each item should be purchased. She appreciates a baby bath demonstration, and it makes a pregnancy and a coming child seem very real. Thoughts such as "I wouldn't be sitting here watching a woman demonstrate how to bathe a baby unless I'm going to have one, right?" and "I'm really going to have a baby" are going through her mind.

About the fifth month of pregnancy, women begin to make a choice as to whether they will breast-feed or bottle-feed their infants. In order to make an informed decision, they should know all the ramifications of both methods. There is a feeling currently that a woman must be either for breast-feeding or against it, as though there were a fence between the two methods and a woman must get firmly on one side or the other of it. Be certain that you are not giving off signals as to which side of the fence you are on. You can help women make this decision, but the woman and her infant are the ones who have to live with it, and it has to be the right one *for them*.

LESSON 7: PLANS FOR HOSPITALIZATION
Allow time for open discussion on whatever topic the group chooses. Conclude the evening with a discussion of what the woman will need to take to the hospital with her and a tour of the maternity unit. In some courses the parents might be asked to complete their hospital admission forms at this time.

LESSON 8: FAMILY PLANNING

A review of the various methods of family planning available is helpful as the last class.

Many couples have difficulty terminating the last class. They put on their coats, yet stand by the doorway, reluctant to say good-bye. They are saying, without words, that the series of meetings was worthwhile, that they were scared, confused, and concerned and now are grateful because you took the time to listen to them and to respect their fears. They may leave the meeting room without saying thank you. They are, after all, young and not fully aware themselves why they are standing there so long. They are just aware that it seems the thing to do. As the women's abdomens have expanded over the past eight weeks, their self-esteem and their ability to cope with this new experience have grown as well.

Preparation-for-Childbirth Classes

Some unfortunate connotations have come to be associated with the term *natural childbirth*. Women who chose this method of delivering their child were at one time labeled "fanatics" or "martyrs." Women who entered labor saying they wanted to deliver naturally, then asked for analgesia or an anesthetic, were "failures." These connotations prevented many women from attending classes in preparation for childbirth. They would have liked to be as prepared for childbirth as possible, to have their child as naturally as possible, to limit discomfort, if possible; on the other hand, they did not want to be trapped into having to "tough it out." It seemed easier just to give up the idea altogether. Today it is generally accepted that being prepared for childbirth is not just a nicety reserved for a few; it is every woman's right.

A great deal of the confusion regarding preparation for childbirth classes would be cleared away if the terminology used to describe the process were always consistent. The term *natural childbirth* should be reserved for instances in which the woman wants no analgesic, no anesthetic, no instruments used, no health care personnel in attendance, and no hospital environment. The woman who chooses to prepare herself for childbirth but still wants to deliver in the secure environment of a hospital or alternate birth center, with health care personnel and safety equipment surrounding her, who agrees that if deviations from the normal occur during labor and delivery she will follow her physician's judgment as to analgesia or anesthesia, is choosing *prepared childbirth*. This term puts matters in the proper perspective. In prepared-childbirth classes, the woman learns exercises to strengthen her pelvic and abdominal muscles and make them more supple and exercises to help her manage her discomfort in labor. She is under no commitment to go a step farther than she wishes. She is not putting her wishes above those of the physician or other health care personnel but is actually aiding them in the safe delivery of her child.

Being prepared for childbirth does not necessarily make childbirth less hazardous, nor does it prevent such complications as hemorrhage, infection, and pregnancy-induced hypertension. (Does that trigger a flash of recognition? Those are the three main causes of maternal mortality.) Prepared childbirth may actually call for more labor room personnel in attendance, because women who want to assist in their labor but are unsure of themselves need the presence of a competent support person.

Prepared childbirth requires a change in the attitude of the labor room nurse from "Bite the bullet" to "Let me show you how you can minimize the bite of that contraction"; or from "You're having a baby, what can you expect?" to "Let me teach you what you can expect."

EXERCISES FOR CHILDBEARING

The purposes of doing exercises during pregnancy are to promote comfort, facilitate labor and delivery, and strengthen muscles so that they will revert to their normal condition and functioning quickly and efficiently following childbirth.

A woman may begin exercise periods as early in pregnancy as she likes. Many women are not interested in these activities until the time of quickening. For some women it is good to begin at this midpoint of pregnancy. They are then less inclined to lose interest before delivery and thus defeat the purpose of the exercises they have done.

A woman has to use common sense in exercising. First of all she should set aside a specific time each day for the task; otherwise her participation will be sporadic. Initially, she should do each exercise only a few times, gradually increasing the number she does at each session. She should not participate in an exercise program without her physician's approval. She should not attempt exercise if any of the danger signals of pregnancy appears, and she should never exercise to a point of fatigue.

The following exercises are designed to stretch the perineal muscles and to make them more supple. A supple perineum offers less resistance to the fetal head at delivery and is more likely to stretch rather than to tear.

Tailor Sitting

All kindergarten children know how to tailor sit. Women have to be retaught. To do this correctly, the woman should not put one ankle on top of the other but should place one leg in front of the other (Fig. 19-1). As she sits in this position, she should gently push on her knees (pushing them toward the floor) until she feels her perineum "stretch." This is a good position to use to watch television, to read, to talk to friends. It is good to plan on sitting in this position for at least 15 minutes every day. By the end of pregnancy, the woman should be so supple that when she tailor sits her knees will almost touch the floor if pushed to that position.

Squatting

Squatting (Fig. 19-2) also stretches the perineal muscles. A woman should practice this position for about 15 minutes a day. Women in nonindustrial cultures squat many times a day—to tend a fire, to pick up a child, to wash vegetables—but women in the United States rarely squat. Most women need a demonstration of squatting. Otherwise, they have a tendency to squat on tiptoes, a more ladylike position. In order for the pelvic muscles to stretch, the woman must keep her feet flat on the floor. This is a position a woman can assume while watching television, talking on the telephone, reading, or perhaps peeling potatoes. Incorporating squatting into her daily activities reduces the amount of time she has to devote to her daily exercises.

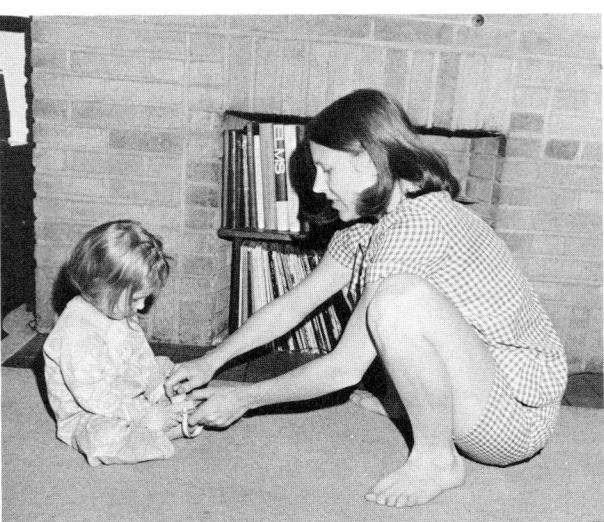

Fig. 19-2. Squatting helps to stretch the muscles of the pelvic floor. Notice that the feet are flat on the floor for optimum stretching. The woman assumes the position here instead of stooping to help her child with a toy.

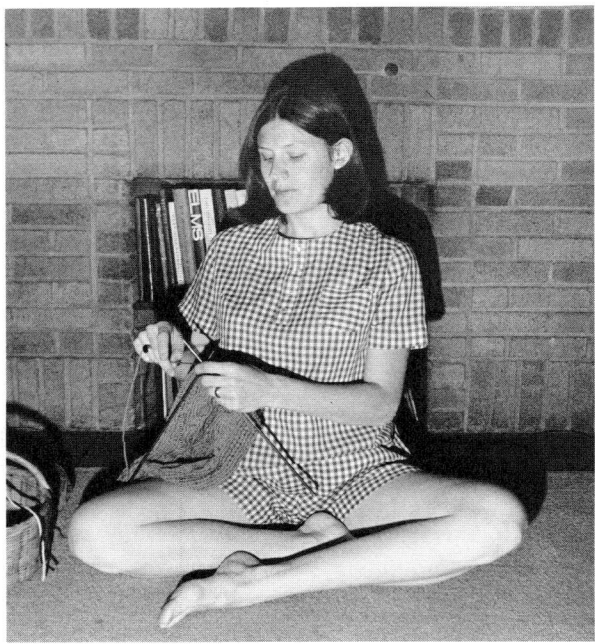

Fig. 19-1. Tailor sitting strengthens the thighs and stretches perineal muscles. Notice that the legs are parallel so that one does not compress the other. A woman should use this position for television watching, telephone conversations, or sitting jobs such as knitting.

Pelvic Floor Contractions

Pelvic floor contractions can be done during the course of daily activity as well. While working around the house or sitting at her desk, the woman can tighten the muscles surrounding her urethra, relax, tighten the muscles surrounding her rectum, relax, tighten her entire perineum, relax. She can repeat this sequence 50 to 100 times daily. Another method is to start to void, then tighten the perineum until the urine stream stops, begin again, stop again. Perineal muscle–strengthening exercises are often called Kegal exercises and are helpful in the postpartum period as well to promote perineal healing.

Abdominal Muscle Contractions

Abdominal muscle contractions help strengthen abdominal muscles during pregnancy and therefore help retain abdominal shape following pregnancy. Strong abdominal muscles contribute to effective second-stage pushing during labor. These contractions can be done in a standing or lying position along with pelvic floor contractions. The woman merely tightens her abdominal muscles, then relaxes, and she can repeat the exercise as often as she wishes during the day.

Another way to do the same thing is to practice

"blowing out a candle." The woman takes a fairly deep inspiration, then exhales normally; then holding her finger about 12 inches in front of herself as if it were a candle, exhales forcibly, pushing out residual air from her lungs. Try it. You can feel your abdominal muscles contract as you reach the end of your forcible exhalation.

Pelvic Rocking

Pelvic rocking (Fig. 19-3) helps relieve backache during pregnancy and early labor. It can be done in a variety of positions: on "all fours," lying down, sitting, or standing. No matter what position is used, the exercise is the same. The back is hollowed and then arched upward like a startled cat's. The woman should do this at the end of the day about five times, to relieve back pain and make her more comfortable for the night.

Because many of these exercises can be incorporated into daily activities, they take little time from a woman's day. If practiced during pregnancy, because they strengthen abdominal and perineal muscles they can make a real difference in the length and the comfort of her labor.

METHODS OF MINIMIZING THE DISCOMFORT OF CHILDBIRTH

Remember the senior prom in high school that you planned and planned and made paper flowers for by the thousands? Remember staying up all night to help decorate the gym? Were you ever so exhausted and yet so satisfied before or since? Your active participation in the event made it meaningful to you. Active participation in childbirth can have the same effect. Prepared childbirth gives the woman the means to participate in the event.

There are two major approaches to prepared childbirth: the Dick-Read method and the Lamaze, or psychoprophylactic, method. Both methods are based on two premises. The first is that discomfort during labor can be minimized if the woman comes into labor informed about what is happening and prepared with breathing exercises to use during contractions. In both methods, therefore, the woman learns about her body's response in labor and the mechanisms involved in childbirth and practices breathing exercises during the months of pregnancy prior to delivery. The second premise is that discomfort during labor can be minimized if the woman's abdomen is relaxed and the uterus is allowed to rise freely against the abdominal wall with contractions. The methods differ only in the means by which they achieve this relaxation.

A woman may use a prepared-childbirth method with or without medicine for pain, with or without additional anesthesia for delivery. Breathing exercises are not necessarily an end in themselves; they are merely another adjunct or means of pain relief in labor.

The Lamaze (Psychoprophylactic) Method

The Lamaze method of prepared childbirth is the method most often taught in the United States today. It is based on the theory that through stimulus-response conditioning women can learn to use controlled breathing automatically and therefore to relax automatically during labor. The method was developed in Russia but was popularized by a French physician, Ferdinand Lamaze.

When it was first introduced in the United States in the 1950s, the method met with a great deal of resis-

Fig. 19-3. Pelvic rocking is helpful in relieving backache during pregnancy and labor. A. In the first movement, the back is hollowed and the head raised. B. In the second movement, the back is arched and the head lowered.

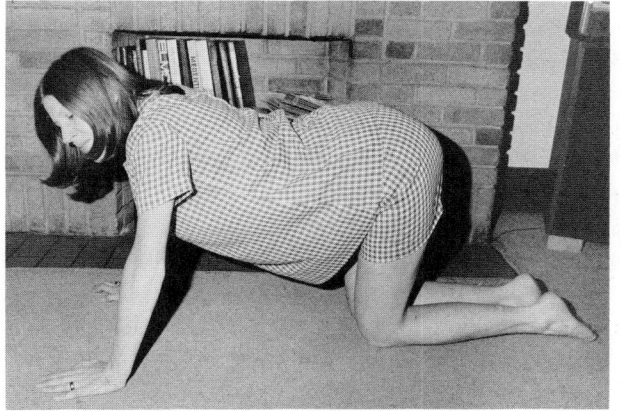
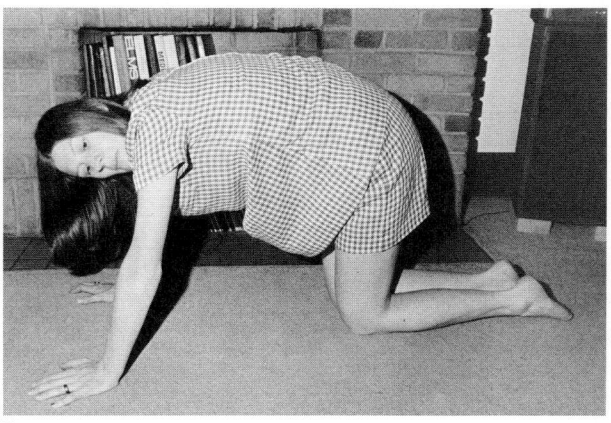

A B

tance from health care personnel. A woman skilled in this method was perceived as a zealot who would be ready to jeopardize her child's health if necessary to prove the worth of the system. In some cases that assessment was justified. She tended to view health care personnel who were telling her that she needed an anesthetic for delivery as people bent on undermining her beliefs rather than as conscientious people trying to explain, for example, that her particular complication required that forceps and therefore a spinal anesthetic were necessary for delivery to ensure her child's safety.

Women themselves sometimes objected to what they considered being placed in the same category as dogs, since the experiments of the Russian physiologist Ivan Pavlov with dogs are the basis for psychoprophylactic childbirth. Recent studies document that the Lamaze method of prepared childbirth not only reduces pain in labor but appears to have fetal benefits as well. In a study of 500 patients [11], Lamaze-prepared women had one-fourth the number of cesarean sections, one-fifth the amount of fetal distress, and one-third the number of postpartal infections as control women without Lamaze preparation.

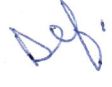

The word *psychoprophylaxis* is a combination of what is attempted by the method: preventing pain in labor (prophylaxis) by use of the mind (psyche).

Three main premises are taught the woman in the prenatal period: (1) Pain does not have to occur with contractions, (2) conditioned reflexes can replace pain sensations in labor, and (3) sensations can be inhibited from reaching the brain cortex and registering as pain.

A great deal of time in Lamaze classes is spent reviewing or teaching reproductive anatomy and physiology and the process of labor and delivery. Thus the couple is familiar with what will happen to the woman in labor and the nature of contractions. The implications for nurses working with a Lamaze-prepared woman in labor are that the woman is usually very aware of the normal course of labor, she is likewise very aware, when a complication begins to develop, that something out of the ordinary is happening.

Time in preparation classes is also spent on learning conditioned reflexes. While conducting studies of salivation in dogs, Pavlov noticed that every time he put out food for his dogs, the dogs salivated at the mere sight of it. To learn more about this phenomenon, he tried ringing a bell each time he presented food and found that after a time the dogs salivated at the sound of the bell even when meat was not offered. This is called a *conditioned response*. The same training technique is applied to the birth process in the Lamaze method. The woman is conditioned to relax automatically on hearing a command ("Contraction beginning") or on the feel of a contraction beginning. Learning by conditioning is especially applicable to basic, simple responses, such as those in childbirth, in which it works wonderfully well.

In order to use the third premise in labor, that sensations coming into the brain can be inhibited from registering, the woman is taught to focus on her breathing patterns or a specified object, blocking out other phenomena. The effectiveness of focusing can be observed in athletes who hurt themselves in basketball or football games but do not feel the pain until after the game, their concentration on winning being so great during the game. A mother, running to scoop her child away from danger, will manifest the same inhibition phenomenon, not even aware that she has wrenched her ankle in the process of rescuing her child until the child is safe.

Women who use a Lamaze method of preparation for childbirth arrive at the hospital in good control of contractions and, because they are so knowledgeable about what is to happen during labor, extremely cooperative and helpful. Women using this method deliver children in a way that is close to the long-hoped-for "painless childbirth."

In order to use the Lamaze method, the responses to contractions must be recently conditioned to be effective (since conditioned responses die out if not reinforced). It is generally recommended, therefore, that women do not begin classes in this method before the 26th week of pregnancy. They then continue the classes to the end of pregnancy. Such timing corresponds nicely to that of the psychological nest building that occurs at about the same time.

All instructors teach muscle-strengthening exercises such as Kegal exercises and abdominal strengthening as part of muscle preparation. Breathing exercises taught vary from teacher to teacher but have common features. Typical exercises taught are the following.

THE CLEANSING BREATH. To begin all breathing exercises, the woman breathes in deeply and then exhales deeply, a "cleansing breath." To end each exercise she repeats this step. It is an important one to take as it limits the possibility of hyperventilation with rapid breathing patterns; it ensures a full fetal oxygen supply.

CONSCIOUSLY CONTROLLED BREATHING. In consciously controlled breathing, the woman lies on her back on the floor with a pillow under her head and a small one under her knees, if she needs it for comfort. She inhales comfortably but fully, then exhales, with her exhalation a little stronger than her inhalation.

She practices breathing in this manner at a controlled pace, about six to nine breaths per minute.

LEVELS OF BREATHING. When the woman has mastered the preceding exercise, she is ready to learn different levels or rates of consciously controlled breathing.

1. Level A consists of comfortable but full respirations at a rate of about six to nine breaths per minute. This level is used for early contractions.
2. Level B is lighter breathing than level A. The rib cage should expand, but the diaphragm barely moves. The rate of respirations is 22 to 30 per minute. This is a good level of breathing for contractions when cervical dilatation is between 4 and 6 cm.
3. Level C breathing is shallow, mostly at the breast bone. The rate is 50 to 70 breaths per minute. As the respirations become faster, the exhalations should be a little stronger than the inhalations for good air exchange and to prevent hyperventilation. If the woman practices saying "out" with each exhalation, she almost inevitably will make exhalation stronger than inhalation. The woman uses this level for transition contractions.
4. At level D the woman breathes naturally, at no particular rate. She runs through a tune inside her head and taps the rhythm on the floor or her abdomen, concentrating on nothing but the rhythm and the tune.

An alternative method of breathing is a "pant-blow" pattern, such as taking four to eight quick breaths (in and out), then a forceful exhalation. Because this type of breathing sounds like an imitation of a train (breath-breath-breath-huff), it is sometimes referred to as "choo-choo" breathing.

Once a woman has mastered the levels of breathing, her next step is to learn to shift from one level to the other on command, so at the sound of "Contraction beginning" she breathes at 12 breaths a minute; at the sound of "Contraction getting harder," 22 breaths a minute; "Harder still," 70 breaths a minute, and so on. These are basic shifts she will use in labor.

NEUROMUSCULAR DISSOCIATION. After a week of practice on the breathing levels, the woman is taught a role-playing drill for labor. She maintains all her muscles in a state of relaxation except for one specific muscle group, which she contracts. This is similar to what she must do in labor; when her uterus is contracted, all her other muscles must be relaxed. The drill is carried out as follows:

The woman contracts her left arm and, with someone telling her when to change, takes 3 breaths at level A, then 4 to 6 breaths at level B, then 8 to 10 breaths at level C, then 15 to 20 breaths at level D. She then comes down through levels C, B, and A. She practices the same shifting of breath levels using different muscle groups to represent the uterus: the right arm and right leg, the left arm and right leg, the right arm and left leg. A woman who can successfully perform the various levels of breathing and change from one to the other on command is prepared to handle labor contractions.

Figure 19-4 illustrates the use of levels of breathing. An early labor contraction is mild. When the contraction begins, the person with the woman (the monitor) says, "Contraction beginning." The woman breathes at level A; she feels no bite from the contraction and so does not need to shift. Later in labor, the contraction is stronger and longer. Now, at the sound of "Contraction beginning," the woman begins level A breathing (3 breaths), shifts to level B (4 or 6 breaths), and then to level C (10 breaths). The contraction is lessening. She shifts down to level B (4 or 6 breaths), then to level A (3 or 4 breaths). The contraction is gone. Her monitor tells her when to shift breathing levels: "Contraction beginning, getting stronger, stronger, getting weaker, weaker, almost gone, gone." These words indicate to her when to shift up or down. In the space of time before transition, when contractions are longest and strongest, the woman will need to utilize her level D breathing as well.

A woman needs practice during pregnancy to perfect different levels of breathing. Because of the practice required, this method cannot be taught readily to unprepared women in early labor.

EFFLEURAGE. One further exercise in the Lamaze technique is effleurage, which is light abdominal massage, done with just enough pressure to avoid tickling. It is used in connection with breathing levels. To ensure that she is maintaining a steady rhythm of massage, the woman should trace a pattern on her abdomen with her fingertips such as the one shown in Fig. 19-5. The rate of effleurage should remain constant, even though breathing rates change. Effleurage decreases sensory stimuli to the abdominal wall and prevents local discomfort.

FOCUSING. Focusing intently on an object is another method of keeping sensory input from reaching the cortex of the brain. The woman brings with her into the hospital a photograph of her husband or other children or a graphic design or just something that appeals to her. She concentrates on it during contractions. Be careful that you do not step in

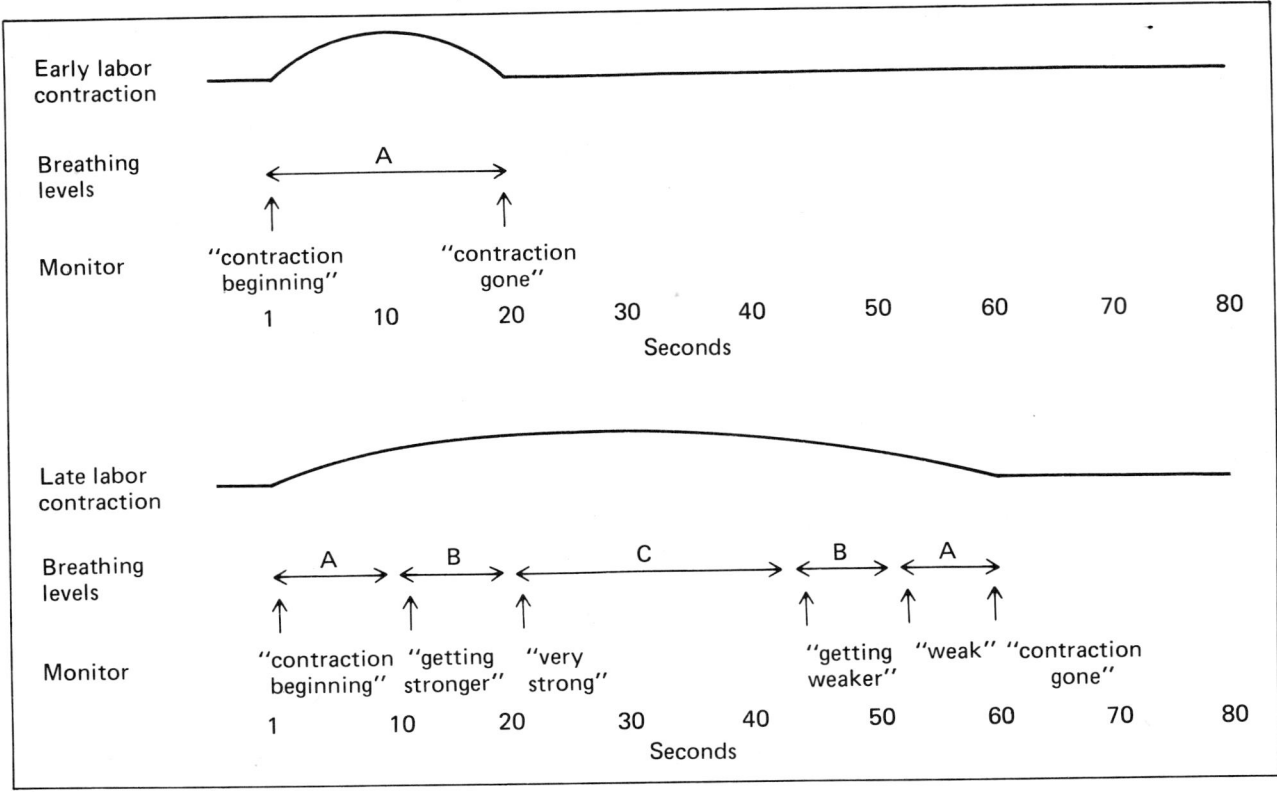

Fig. 19-4. Examples of Lamaze breathing patterns. A, B, and C are levels of breathing.

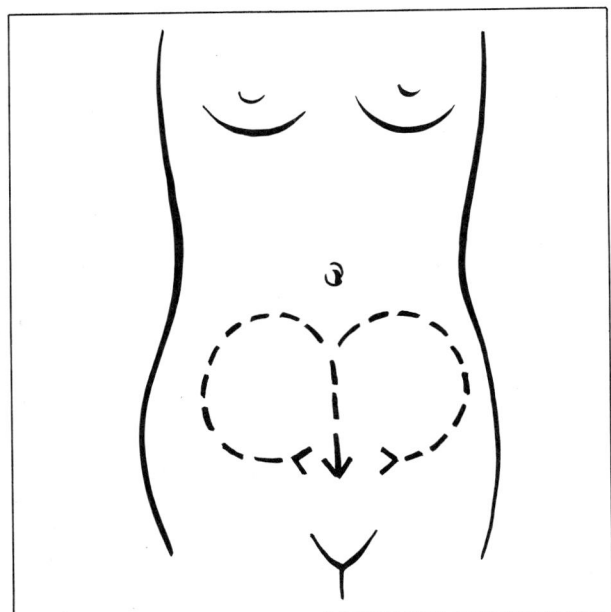

Fig. 19-5. Effleurage patterns. Effleurage is light massage, performed with only enough pressure to avoid tickling. It desensitizes the abdominal skin, in turn relaxing the underlying muscles. During uterine contractions, the woman traces the pattern on her bare abdomen with her fingers.

her line of vision during a contraction and break her concentration.

EATING. Women are usually cautioned not to eat once they begin labor, to prevent vomiting and aspiration in the event a general anesthetic is used. Women using the Lamaze technique are sometimes instructed to eat a full meal when labor first begins and to continue to eat, or at least to drink, during labor in order to maintain their energy level; orange juice, oranges, and lollipops are suggested for maintaining a good energy level.

As long as it can be assumed that hospital rules are made primarily to ensure a healthy outcome to both child and mother, a compromise of the rules with respect to eating in labor may perhaps be reached. Probably all women need calories during labor. Why not provide them with lollipops instead of the traditional ice chips? Because digestion slows during labor and no woman can be certain that a general anesthetic will not be necessary, however, eating a complete meal early in labor appears to be an unnecessary handicap to her physician.

NURSING SUPPORT. Remember that a woman prepared by the Lamaze method is taught not to rest between contractions; she is taught to be alert and ready to respond to her next contraction. She will want the lights on, possibly a radio on. Do not urge her to lie down and rest or sleep. She may not even want to lie down, since she may incorporate a pant-blow type of breathing for contractions just before transition that involves her sitting upright. Most women appreciate the use of a fetal heart monitor, as it alerts them to when a contraction is beginning long before a hand on the abdomen can do that.

Many Lamaze-prepared women need to have a person beside them to give them their breathing pattern cues. Women who write articles on Lamaze childbirth in women's magazines invariably begin their articles with "Labor began when my husband, who was to serve as my coach, was out of town." The article then recites page after page of unkind, unsympathetic, or ill-mannered statements made to them during labor by nurses. When one is depending on a support person to be with her, not only because this is a new experience (lying on the living-room rug practicing contractions is *not* the same as having the real labor contractions), but also because she believes his presence is necessary for enabling her to reduce labor pain, and that person is not available, surely everything that comes after that moment could easily be viewed as unkind, unsympathetic, and ill-mannered.

A Lamaze monitor, however, can be *anyone* who knows the methods and the correct words to say (Fig. 19-6). Every nurse who works on a labor unit should be as skilled in the technique as she is at listening to fetal heart sounds. Often, if a woman has to be admitted without her monitor, a course instructor will come if she requests it. If not, offer your services. Ask her what specific words her husband or monitor uses. Stay with her and say them: "Contraction beginning, contraction getting stronger, stronger, on the top, getting weaker now, still weaker. That's it. Contraction gone." The words are not magic or complicated. Being able to assist a woman in labor is not magical or complicated. It is merely demonstrating the essence of nursing: caring and concern.

The Dick-Read Method

The Dick-Read method is based on the approach proposed by Grantly Dick-Read, an English physician. The premise of the method is that fear leads to tension, which leads to pain. If you can prevent this chain of events from occurring, or break the chain between fear-tension or tension-pain, you can reduce the pain of childbirth contractions.

When women know what is going to happen in labor, their fears diminish. This is the reason a class on labor and delivery should be included in preparation-for-parenthood courses. Women can prevent themselves from becoming tense if they learn how to

Fig. 19-6. Practicing breathing exercises in a class for expectant parents. (Courtesy of the Department of Medical Photography, Children's Hospital, Buffalo, N.Y.)

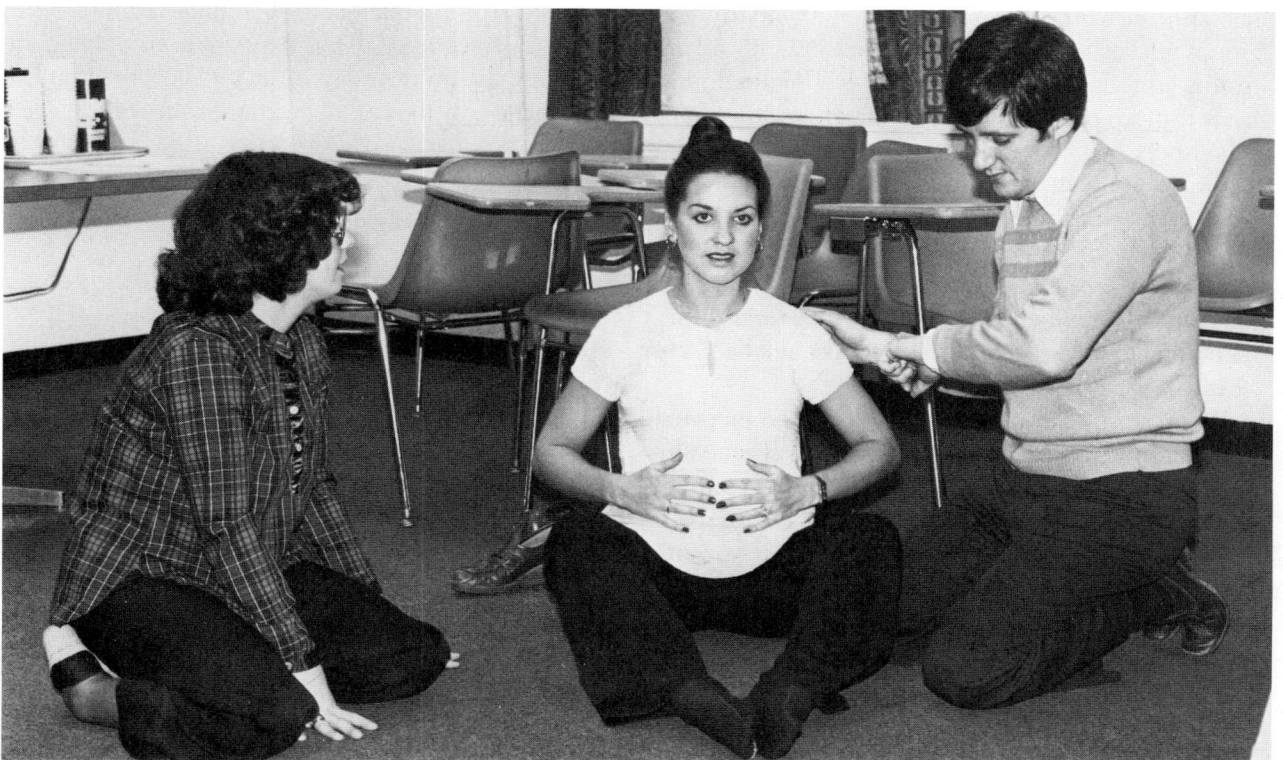

relax and have a definite pattern of breathing they can initiate and concentrate on during contractions.

Relaxation during labor, therefore, is an important part of the Dick-Read method. Most labor rooms are structured for this approach to childbirth. The rooms are nonstimulating (few accessories, plain walls), and the woman is either by herself or with only one other woman. Although this is not as popular a method of instruction for prepared childbirth as the Lamaze method in the United States today, it is helpful for the nurse to be familiar with the Dick-Read method because it is often easier to teach its breathing techniques to women who appear at the door of a labor room totally unprepared as a way of giving them some quick help in labor.

WHOLE-BODY RELAXATION EXERCISE. Being told to relax and being able to relax are not the same thing; a woman has to learn *how* to relax. A relaxation position that is generally taught during pregnancy is a modified Sims's position. The woman lies on her side, with a pillow under her head. She allows the weight of her abdomen to rest against the mattress or floor. No body part should rest on another, but each should be supported by the mattress or floor. In order to become thoroughly relaxed, the woman should contract and relax all her muscles from her head down to her toes as follows: wrinkling her forehead, then relaxing the forehead muscles; tensing all the facial muscles, relaxing them; tensing her neck, relaxing it; tensing her right arm, relaxing it; tensing her left arm, relaxing it; and so on. With all muscle groups relaxed, many women can fall instantly asleep in this position. They can use the technique during labor to sleep or nap between contractions to prevent exhaustion.

After resting in this position the woman should never rise quickly or she will become extremely light-headed and dizzy. To rise from the floor, she should first push herself up onto her hip with her hand and elbow, then over onto her hands and knees, then finally up on her feet. This should be done slowly, as in a slow-motion film.

When caring for a woman who has been prepared for labor by the Dick-Read method, you will generally find that she assumes this position between contractions. It is sometimes awkward for you because you cannot hear the fetal heart sounds then. If you are going to auscultate for the sounds with a stethoscope, you may have to ask the woman to turn on her back.

Some women dislodge an external fetal heart monitor as they turn to this position. If a woman has been trained to use the position, however, it is important to encourage her to maintain it. It reduces pressure from the uterus against the vena cava and actually is the preferred position for all women in labor.

ABDOMINAL BREATHING. Abdominal breathing is the second relaxation technique that women are taught by this method. Abdominal breathing not only prevents the woman from tensing her whole body (because she is busy concentrating on what she is doing) but also forces the abdominal muscles to rise, giving the uterus room to rise freely and easily with a contraction and maintaining a good blood supply to the uterus. (One theory proposed to account for the pain of contractions is that contractions cause ischemia in the uterus and thus pain, in the same way as poor lower-extremity circulation causes ischemia of a leg and thus leg cramps.) Removing the pressure of the abdominal wall also prevents the uterus from "bumping" against it with each contraction, presumably reducing local tenderness and so pain.

To do abdominal breathing, the woman lies on her back and inhales slowly, using her abdominal muscles. If she is truly using them, her abdominal wall will rise with the inhalation. She then exhales slowly, allowing the abdominal wall to return gradually to its normal position (Fig. 19-7). When a woman first begins to learn abdominal breathing, she finds she can breathe this way for only about 20 seconds (a 10-second inhalation and a 10-second exhalation). (Try it. Unless you are an accomplished swimmer, you will find it hard work to maintain abdominal control longer than 20 seconds.) If the woman begins doing this exercise 10 times a day at about the 5th month of pregnancy, by the end of pregnancy she will be able to

Fig. 19-7. Abdominal breathing. When the woman inhales using her abdominal muscles, she can feel her abdominal wall rise.

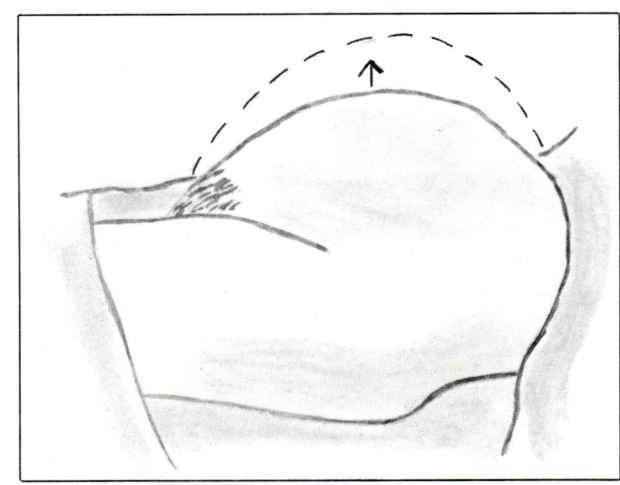

270 *The Prepartal Period: Preparing for Parenthood*

maintain a well-paced 30-second inhalation and a well-paced 30-second exhalation. The inhalation-exhalation time should be built up gradually during pregnancy: 20 seconds total time (inhalation and exhalation) the 1st week; 25 seconds the following week; 30 the 3rd week; and so on until the total time is 60 seconds. She should count as she breathes, so that she knows it is taking 60 seconds. The woman has to concentrate on exhaling steadily; this is hard to do, and there is a tendency to hurry it.

In early labor, the total length of uterine contractions is about 20 seconds. As labor increases in intensity, the contractions grow longer, ultimately 50 to 60 seconds. Thus, the woman who can handle a 60-second controlled breath can reduce discomfort in labor up through transition, until she experiences the welcome and wonderful compulsion to push with contractions. Abdominal breathing up to 70 seconds' duration gives a woman extra assurance that she will be able to handle her longest contractions. However, few women can achieve this much control. While the woman is learning this technique, it is important that she put her hand on her abdomen and actually feel the abdominal wall rise. Otherwise, she cannot be sure that she is breathing correctly.

Abdominal breathing can be taught to a woman who comes into labor totally unprepared as an emergency method of reducing labor discomfort. However, a woman so taught is not able, without practice, to maintain more than a 20-second total breath. By the time she arrives at the hospital, she is already tense and frightened and so dreads the next contraction that she has difficulty relaxing enough to give the method a fair try. She can do no more than 20-second breaths, but she can lengthen their period of effectiveness by attempting one abdominal breathing pattern immediately following the first. This is difficult to do, because as she finishes her first breath, the contraction is still strong. Thus, she may be unable to keep her mind on concentrated breathing and inhale regularly again. Such a woman needs a support person with her.

Abdominal breathing patterns are charted in Fig. 19-8.

GENERAL RULES

Once the woman has learned to do breathing exercises in a reclining position, she needs to practice them standing—while she is doing dishes, ironing, or

Fig. 19-8. Abdominal breathing patterns. The woman who trained before childbirth and uses practiced abdominal breathing can effectively breathe through contractions. A woman who learns the technique in labor (unpracticed abdominal breathing) will still be able to reduce the discomfort of contractions.

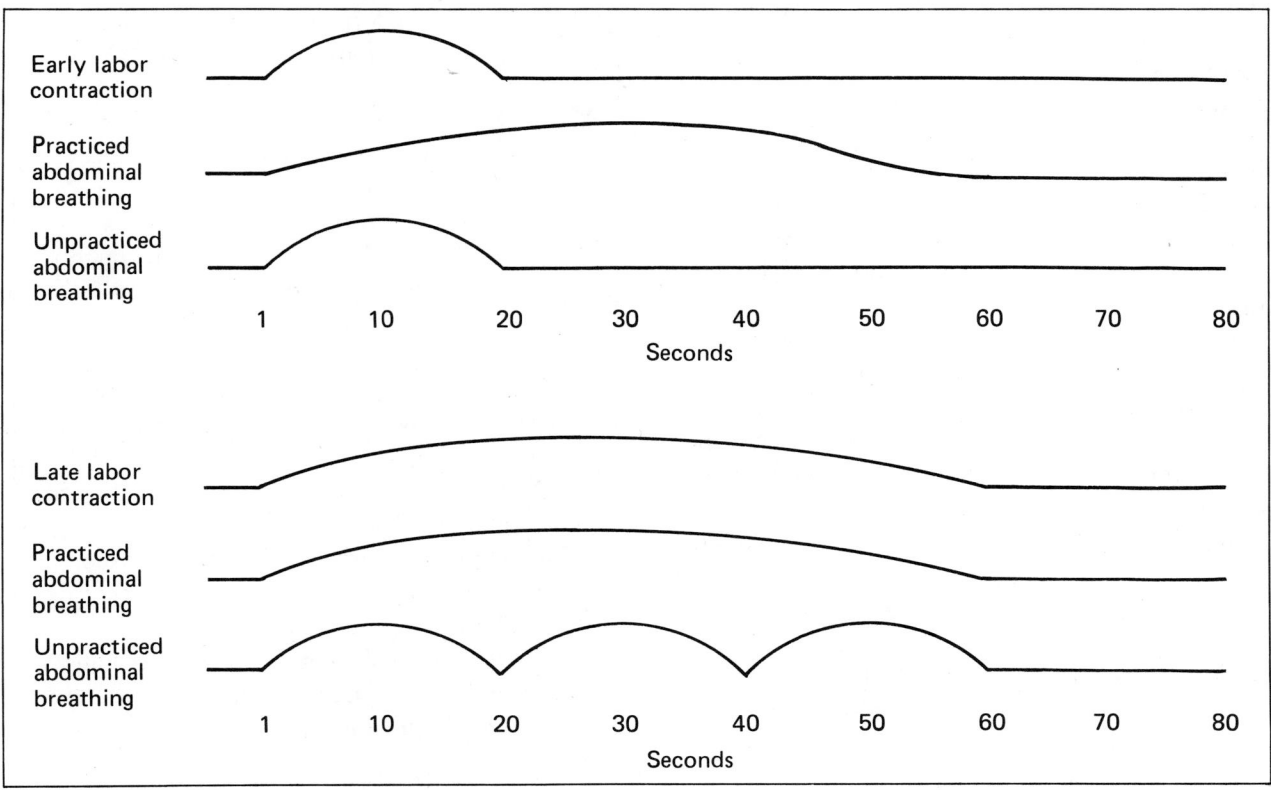

Preparation for Parenthood 271

running a duplicating machine. Once labor starts, she should begin to use the technique with the first contraction. The advantage of being able to use it effectively in a standing position is that she can handle her contractions and yet continue with the normal activities that women are engaged in when labor begins (picking up around the house, packing a suitcase, ironing, cooking, and so on). She should not save the technique for use later in labor, when contractions become more intense, since at that time the local tenderness of the uterus and the awareness that contractions are starting to hurt may make it difficult for her to relax.

Using breathing with the first contraction is rewarding. It puts a woman in control of a new, potentially frightening situation.

It is important not to interrupt women doing exercises in labor. Once their concentration is disrupted, they feel the bite of the contraction; and when they have been using breathing exercises and so reducing pain sensations, suddenly feeling the real force of a contraction is frightening. The woman tenses, the pain becomes worse, she becomes more frightened, and she may doubt her ability to breathe constructively in the face of such sharp pain. Allow the woman to finish breathing with her contraction, then ask your question or announce what procedure you need to do next. Or ask your question, but wait patiently for 60 seconds for the answer.

Once the transition stage of labor is over and the woman feels she has to push, she needs no further breathing exercises. Pushing feels good by itself. Pushing does not need to be practiced during pregnancy; effective pushing can be taught during labor when the woman is at the second stage or pelvic division of labor. During the pelvic division of labor, when the fetus is at the pelvic floor, it is better for the woman not to push if the baby's head is to be born easily, between contractions. In order to stop pushing, the woman may need to pant (small, short breaths that prevent her from using her abdominal muscles to push). The sensation of pushing can be compared to the sensation you feel when you have a strong urge to move your bowels; it feels good, and so it is almost impossible not to push. Panting must be shallow, or the woman will hyperventilate, become dizzy, and may even faint. Panting, like pushing, is an activity that can be taught when it is needed.

The time will come when *all* women will participate in some kind of prepared childbirth. This does not mean that all women will lie in labor rooms and breathe with their contractions in special ways. All women should not be expected to react this way during childbirth any more than all women should be expected to react the same way to any stress situation. All women should be offered the option of prepared childbirth, however, so that those who want to use these techniques and participate actively in the birth of their children can do so. Women who come to a hospital ready to use these techniques in labor should have the support of labor room personnel. Nurses who are serving as community instructors and nurses in the hospital need to work in better harmony, so that each knows what the other is doing. Such cooperation would benefit both the parents and the child about to be born.

Problem-oriented Recording: Progress Notes

Christine McFadden
15 years

Problem: Preparation for childbirth

S. "I'm really scared thinking about labor but I don't want to take a course if I'm going to end up having a c-section."

O. —

A. No interest in formal preparation for labor as cesarean section may be necessary.

Goals: a. Be familiar with process of labor and delivery by 36th week of pregnancy.
b. Maintain muscle-strengthening exercises for postpartal healing.
c. Be familiar with anesthetic options and cesarean section process by 36th week of pregnancy.

P. 1. Encourage Kegal exercises and abdominal strengthening exercises at prenatal visits.
2. Include labor and delivery information in prenatal discussion at 30th week of pregnancy as no formal class will be taken.
3. Include newborn expectations and care at 36th week of pregnancy.
4. Mention possibility of more preparation later in pregnancy in hopes she changes her attitude toward preparation.

Problem-oriented Recording: Progress Notes

Mary Kraft
22 years

Problem: Preparation for childbirth

> S. "Both my husband and I want to know everything we can learn about labor. He wants to be there for the whole thing."
>
> O. —
>
> A. Need to enroll in preparation-for-childbirth class.
>
> Goals: a. Able to discuss normal patterns of labor and delivery and means to control pain of labor.
> b. Be active participant in labor and delivery.
> c. To take formal preparation course.
>
> P. 1. Explain differing preparation-for-childbirth courses available to couple.
> 2. Patient to call if any difficulty enrolling in chosen course.
> 3. Provide discussion room at prenatal visits for questions that may arise from course information.
> 4. Mark chart for M.D. discussion of analgesic and anesthetic as couple wants to be well informed, but probably won't use in labor.

Problem-oriented Recording: Progress Notes

Angie Baco
42 years

Problem: Preparation for childbirth

> S. "I want as much medicine as possible in labor, so I'm as sleepy as possible."
> Husband expresses no interest in seeing child born. States, "I didn't see any of the others."
>
> O. —
>
> A. No interest in formal preparation-for-childbirth course, possibly because pregnancy is not fully desired as yet.
>
> Goals: a. Be prepared within the limits acceptable to her by 36th week of pregnancy.
> b. Be able to discuss possibility of cesarean section or induced delivery on account of gestational diabetes.
>
> P. 1. Include labor and delivery information in prenatal visits at 30th week of pregnancy as no formal class will be taken.
> 2. Encourage Kegal exercises and abdominal strengthening exercises at prenatal visits.
> 3. Mark chart for M.D. discussion of analgesic and anesthetic for labor as patient desires to use medication in labor.

References

1. Anderson, J. A clarification of the Lamaze method. *J.O.G.N. Nurs.* 6:53, 1977.
2. Beck, N. C., et al. Natural childbirth. A review and analysis. *Obstet. Gynecol.* 52:371, 1978.
3. Cave, C. Social characteristics of natural childbirth users and nonusers. *Am. J. Public Health* 68:898, 1978.
4. Charles, A. G., et al. Effects of psycho-prophylactic preparation for childbirth. *Am. J. Obstet. Gynecol.* 131:44, 1978.
5. Cogan, R. Practice time in prepared childbirth. *J.O.G.N. Nurs.* 7:33, 1978.
6. Dick-Read, G. *Childbirth Without Fear: The Original Approach to Natural Childbirth* (4th ed.). H. Wessel and H. F. Ellis (Eds.). New York: Harper & Row, 1972.
7. Doering, S. C., and Entwisle, D. R. Preparation during pregnancy and ability to cope with labor and delivery. *Am. J. Orthopsychiatry* 45:825, 1975.
8. Greene, J. W. Maternal and fetal outcome of Lamaze prepared patients. *Obstet. Gynecol.* 51:723, 1978.
9. Halstead, J., et al. Evaluation of a prepared childbirth program. *J.O.G.N. Nurs.* 7:39, 1978.
10. Hawkins, M. Fitting a prenatal education program into the crowded inner city clinic. *M.C.N.* 1:226, 1976.
11. Hughey, M. J. Maternal and fetal outcome of Lamaze prepared patients. *Obstet. Gynecol.* 51:653, 1978.

12. Huprich, P. A. Assisting the couple through a Lamaze labor and delivery. *M.C.N.* 2:245, 1977.
13. Maternity Center Association. *Psychophysical Preparation for Childbearing: Guidelines for Teaching* (2nd ed.). New York: Maternity Center Association, 1965.
14. Roberts, J. Priorities in prenatal education. *J.O.G.N. Nurs.* 5:17, 1975.
15. Scott, J. R., et al. Effect of psychoprophylaxis on labor and delivery in primiparas. *Obstet. Gynecol. Surv.* 31:714, 1976.
16. Summer, G. Giving expectant parents the help they need: The ABC's of prenatal education. *M.C.N.* 1:220, 1976.
17. Tricker, I. Painless childbirth. *Nurs. Times* 74:225, 1978.
18. Wapner, J. The attitudes, feelings and behaviors of expectant fathers attending Lamaze classes. *Birth Fam. J.* 3:5, 1976.
19. Webster-Stratton, C., and Kogan, K. Helping parents parent. *Am. J. Nurs.* 80:240, 1980.

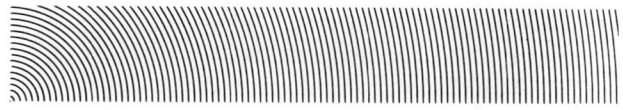

UNIT III. Utilizing Nursing Process: Questions for Review

1. Teratogens may affect fetal growth at any stage of fetal development. The neurological system is most at threat during what weeks of development?
   a. 2nd through 11th
   b. 4th through 18th
   c. 12th through 32nd
   d. 16th through 18th

2. Which of the following is not known to have teratogenic properties?
   a. Tetracycline
   b. Radiation
   c. Toxoplasmosis
   d. Ampicillin

3. During pregnancy, the blood pressure in the woman normally
   a. Increases with each month of pregnancy
   b. Decreases in the second trimester
   c. Decreases with each month of pregnancy
   d. Increases about 30 percent the last trimester

4. Kidney changes which can be expected with pregnancy are
   a. Decreased glomerular filtration rate
   b. Increased creatinine excretion
   c. Decreased glucose secretion
   d. Increased glomerular filtration rate

5. Which of the following situations is recognized as a situation that might lead to poor adaptation to pregnancy?
   a. A move away from home
   b. Loss of financial support
   c. Illness in an older child
   d. All of the above

6. If a pregnancy is unwanted at conception, the milestone at which most women change their attitudes toward the pregnancy is
   a. The 1st week
   b. Quickening
   c. The 7th month
   d. Lightening

7. A *probable* sign of pregnancy is
   a. Chadwick's sign
   b. Nausea and vomiting
   c. A positive urine pregnancy test
   d. Amenorrhea

8. A *positive* sign of pregnancy is
   a. A positive urine pregnancy test
   b. Fetal movement felt by examiner
   c. Hegar's sign
   d. Uterine contractions

9. During pregnancy, the best position for a woman to nap in is
   a. On her stomach with a pillow under her breasts
   b. On her side with the weight of the uterus resting on the bed
   c. On her back with a pillow under her knees
   d. None of the above

10. To prevent hemorrhoids, a woman should
    a. Eat a low-fiber diet
    b. Wear knee socks for support
    c. Do no walking
    d. Rest in a knee-chest position twice a day

11. The B vitamins are important in a pregnancy diet. Which of the following foods is the best source of vitamin B_{12}?
    a. Carrots
    b. Hamburger
    c. Milk
    d. Cottage cheese

12. An iron supplement during pregnancy is needed
    a. Over and above a high iron intake
    b. Only in women who are anemic
    c. Only in multiple pregnancies
    d. Only if the woman does not like meat

13. Nausea in normal pregnancy does not last beyond
    a. 4 weeks
    b. 12 weeks
    c. 16 weeks
    d. 20 weeks

14. When a pregnant woman lies on her back she may develop
    a. Postural hypotension
    b. Varicosities
    c. Uterine cramping
    d. A postural vaginal discharge

15. A general safe rule regarding douching during pregnancy is
    a. It is never safe.
    b. A bulb-type syringe should never be used.
    c. The solution used should never be acid.
    d. The height of the douche container should never be over 6 inches.

16. A danger sign of pregnancy is
    a. Uterine enlargement to the umbilicus by 20 weeks
    b. Severe, continuous headache
    c. No fetal heart sounds by auscultation by 12 weeks
    d. None of the above

17. Tailor sitting during pregnancy
    a. Improves the blood supply to the uterus
    b. Strengthens abdominal muscles
    c. Decreases respiratory effort
    d. Stretches perineal muscles

18. Pelvic rocking during pregnancy
    a. Should hurt or will not be effective
    b. Stretches perineal muscles
    c. Relieves backache
    d. May cause mild abdominal cramping

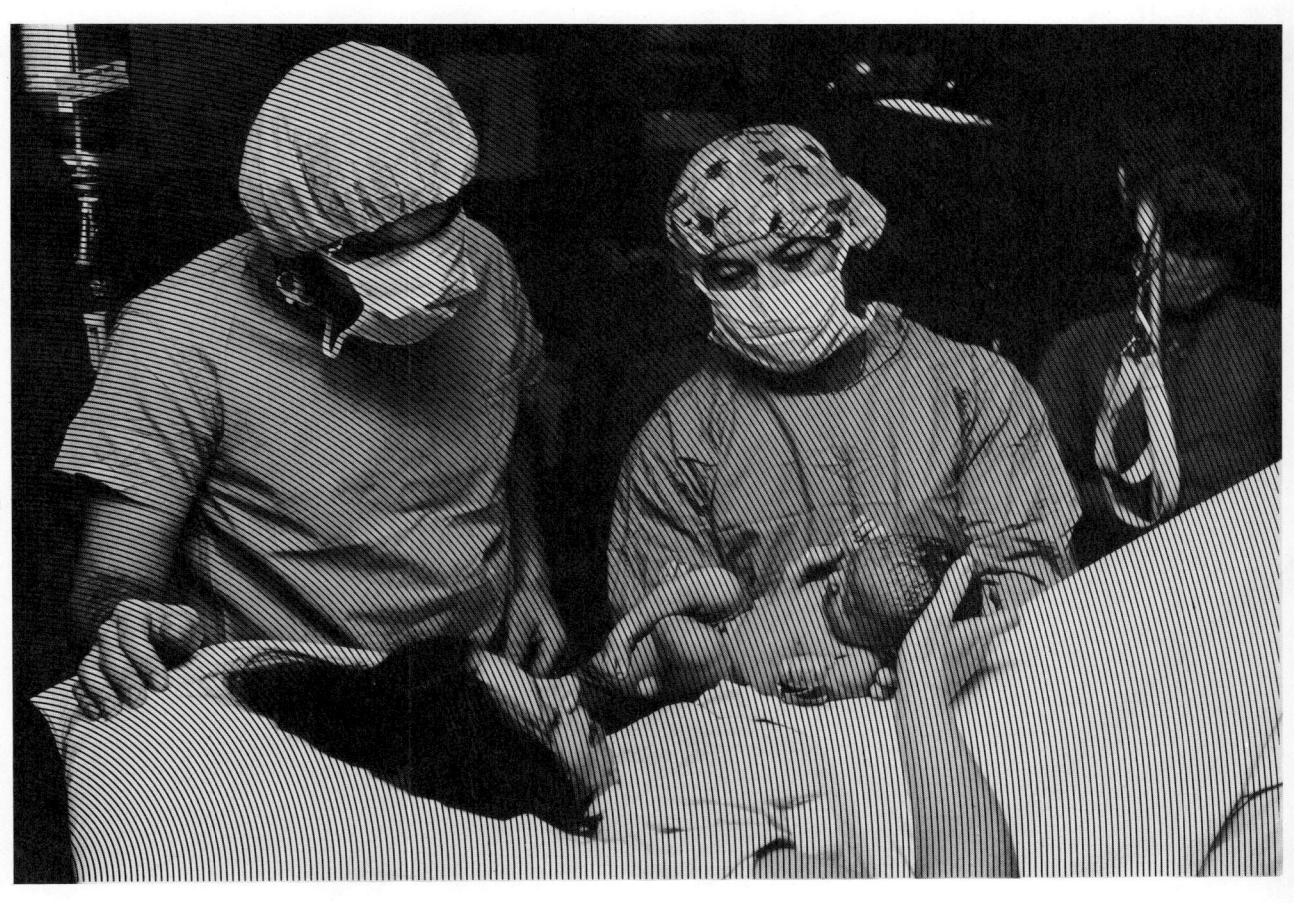

IV. Period of Parturition: Becoming a Parent

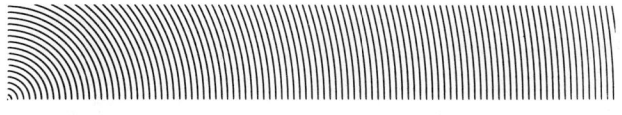

20. Psychosocial Aspects of Labor

Fear of the unknown is a universal fear, and labor is an unknown. Whether this is the first, second, or fifth pregnancy for a woman, it is the first time she has been in labor with this child. Even though it is not her first labor, then, it is still an unknown.

There are countless old wives' tales about how awful labor is. A woman who discovered that labor was not all bad with a first birth may begin to worry, therefore, that she experienced the exception, not the rule, her first time, and that this labor will surely be a horrible one.

Not only is labor an unknown, but for most healthy women a hospital admission to have a baby is their 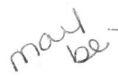 first hospital admission. Things that are routine to other types of hospital patients, such as Gatch controls for beds, call-light buttons, or the rattle of a food tray in the hallway, are strange. She needs comprehensive care so she can be assured that, although she is in a strange place and what is happening to her internally feels strange, she is not among strangers.

Readiness for Labor

Her readiness for labor has a great deal to do with how a woman perceives labor. At the time of quickening, women begin to view being pregnant in a positive light. They begin the psychological work of thinking of themselves as pregnant, of adjusting to their changing body image. They begin to like the sensation of seeing themselves in this new way.

At about the 28th week of pregnancy, women move into a new phase—that of not thinking of themselves so much as being pregnant, but of thinking of themselves as having a child. They change from thinking about clothing for themselves to thinking about clothing for a baby. Again, this is an enjoyable step in pregnancy.

Late in pregnancy, as their due date approaches, thoughts change once more. The woman moves from anticipation and planning for a baby to anxiety to get the pregnancy over. She is like a person who has stayed at the prom too long and recognizes that the lavender and gold boughs she first walked under are not as grand as she thought, but actually purple and yellow crepe paper hanging from basketball hoops. The baby is a weekend guest who has stayed well past Monday morning.

These feelings bring odd sensations and questions. What kind of mother will she be if she is tired of the child and the child is not even born yet? What kind of woman is she no longer to enjoy being pregnant?

Having such thoughts lowers her self-esteem at a time when she needs high self-esteem because she is shortly going to be exposed to sensations she has never felt before (and so difficult to describe that no matter how many books she reads about childbirth she will never truly be prepared for it until she experiences it). Reassurance that the feeling of entertaining an unwelcome guest are normal is helpful in maintaining self-esteem.

The Stress of Labor

Ability to tolerate stress (to cope adequately) depends on one's perception of the event, support people available, and past experiences with coping (see Chap. 1). Women who have attended preparation-for-labor classes and are knowledgeable about the physiological process of labor are better prepared to have a factual perception of the birth process than are those who know little about what will happen to them in the next few hours. By teaching such classes, nurses contribute greatly to helping women tolerate the stress of labor.

FATIGUE

By the time her due date approaches, a woman is generally tired from the burden of carrying an extra 20 to 30 pounds of weight with her every second of her day. Most women do not sleep well during the last month of pregnancy because they have backache in a side-lying position; they turn on their back and the fetus kicks and wakens them; they turn to their side and their back aches—and so on. Some women do not sleep well the last two weeks of pregnancy because they are afraid they will sleep through labor contractions and the baby will be born at home, away from professional supervision.

Sleep hunger makes it difficult for them to perceive situations clearly or to adjust rapidly to new situations. It makes the process of labor loom as an overwhelming experience they surely will not be able to endure. It makes a little deficiency—a wrinkled draw sheet —appear as a threatening discrepancy in their care.

PAIN

Women who arrive at a labor wing of a hospital are in pain. It is an extremely organized woman who can finish locating shirts so her husband has something to wear the three or four days that she will be hospitalized, ride in the car while she and her husband drop off a crying 2-year-old at her mother's home, ride farther to the hospital, then walk from the parking lot into the hospital and still remember to breathe at a prepared rate through contractions. Once she is in a labor bed in a controlled environment free from outside interferences, she can quickly begin to control breathing patterns and reduce the pain of labor contractions to a feeling closer to irritation than pain. But at the door to a labor unit, she is in pain. Pain reduces the ability to cope with everything and may make her quick-tempered and quick to criticize anything around her.

FEAR

Women enjoy a review of physiological happenings in labor because they like to be reminded that this is not a strange bewildering experience but a well-known and documented process. This puts a fence around it, controlling the enormity of it. A good explanation of what will happen in labor and a review for those who have had classes in preparation for labor are always welcome, therefore. Explaining that contractions are a certain length and a certain firmness and are following the expected course is always gratefully received.

Being taken by surprise—labor moving faster than they thought it would or slower than they thought—is frightening. It brings to a woman's mind the horror stories of labor that she has heard from her mother or friends. A television drama or novel in which a woman died in childbirth is suddenly recalled. This might be the day, the time, the hour, *she* is to die.

Fear increases when women are left alone. You cannot realistically be at the bedside of all the women on a labor unit all the time if you are the only nurse assigned to the unit. You can convey the feeling to patients, however, that your concern is with them even when you are physically absent. Saying that you are going to be gone for a few minutes and then being gone for only a few minutes, returning promptly, making it obvious that you are checking often, is reassuring intervention.

Reducing Stress in Labor

Ways to reduce stress in labor center around helping the woman to perceive labor clearly despite her fear, pain, and fatigue that make this difficult and around providing support people for her, either from her family or friends or from health personnel.

SUPPORT PEOPLE

The husband or the father of the child or someone else that the woman chooses should be admitted to the labor or birthing room with the woman. He or she should be able to follow the woman into the delivery room or remain with her in a birthing room through delivery. Having someone with her is important to a woman in early labor; later, as contractions become intense and hard, her interest turns inward to the functioning of her body and she may actually be unaware that anyone else is in the room. This is an important point to remember. As contractions grow harder and more intense (the transition stage of labor) being in the room becomes more and more important for the husband or father. He may not view being with his wife in early labor as that important. To the woman, the beginning of labor, when everything is still so new and she is still so unused to the sensation of contractions, may be the time she needs a support person the most.

TEACHING

Familiarity is always comforting. Nothing feels like coming home. It is helpful if a woman has had a tour of the hospital labor unit where she will deliver. She then has some idea in advance about the physical aspects of the unit and knows some of the personnel. If this is not the case, you need to make her feel at home promptly on admission.

Introduce yourself. Be certain that all who care for her introduce themselves and explain what they will be doing. Women under stress are very aware of social amenities, of friendliness or the lack of it. They are *afraid* of being alone with strangers when their child is born. If all personnel on a labor unit wear scrub dresses or suits with only small badges for identification, introductions become extremely important. If a woman needs help in labor, she wants to be certain that the person she calls is a nurse, not a technician or a nurse's aide.

Ask whether the woman has attended classes on labor; how much she knows about labor. Fill in what is needed well in advance of when it is needed. It is good practice to ask whether there is anything about labor that concerns her particularly. Women often respond with a question such as "Is it really as bad as everyone says?" Despite attendance at preparation-for-labor classes, most prominent in her mind at this point is what her mother told her 10 years ago. Knowing in early labor what her misbeliefs are leaves time to try and correct them before labor gets so intense that listening to explanations becomes difficult.

In one study [10] investigators reported that if a mother communicated all positive aspects of labor to her daughter, the daughter was unprepared for the intensity of labor and therefore had a difficult labor. If the mother's description of labor was very bad, the daughter was unable to relax enough to appreciate what was happening to her and viewed labor as very difficult.

A middle ground seems to be the appropriate answer to how bad labor contractions are. They do hurt, but with a few simple breathing exercises, a positive approach, and people around her who care, labor becomes an event to be cherished rather than dreaded.

Labor rooms are traditionally kept free of articles that collect dust so that they can be easily cleaned. Consequently they seem bare and unwelcoming compared to other hospital rooms. The woman needs to be told why labor rooms are structured to be functional rather than beautiful. Women protect their unborn children against threat. That is one of the psychological reactions to pregnancy. They may react badly, therefore, to having their child born in dreary, tasteless surroundings. Fortunately, more hospitals are providing birthing or perinatal rooms for women in labor, and these are decorated in a home-like and comfortable atmosphere.

Women in labor need to have their call bell answered promptly. They are very aware of how many minutes elapse between their ring and a response. An intercom system saves steps for nursing personnel, but it is a poor excuse for communication on a labor service. A voice from a wall offers little comfort. It conveys instead a feeling that walking the 20 steps to the room is an effort. This time the woman only wants her supply of ice chips replenished. But what, she wonders, if she begins hemorrhaging acutely (the imagination can work overtime when one is in labor), how will the voice from the wall appreciate the seriousness of her condition? Suppose she dies while the voice from the wall asks, "Can I help you?"

There is no substitute for personal touch and contact during labor. Patting a woman's arm while you tell her that she is progressing in labor, brushing a wisp of hair off her forehead, wiping her forehead with a cool cloth—these are indispensable methods for conveying concern. A woman who is touched, who experiences the warmth and friendliness of human contact during labor, a time when she is physically dependent, will handle her newborn (who is also physically dependent and undergoing an adjustment not unlike the one she has just gone through) more warmly and affectionately.

Be wary of making careless remarks just outside the door. Because the woman and her husband are so concerned with what is happening to them, they interpret anything they hear as relating to them. "We've got a problem" said outside the door is interpreted as meaning *they* are having a problem. Laughter outside a door is interpreted as laughter *at them.* A whisper about the terrible food in the hospital cafeteria is interpreted as a whisper *about them.* Avoid this kind of situation by remaining alert to the sensitivities of the woman in labor.

When coping levels are low, it is easy to be frustrated with things such as hospital forms. Being asked to wait while forms are filled out or a nursing shift changes is an intolerable delay that no professional nurse should ever be a part of. If forms are necessary, the husband or whoever accompanies the woman can be asked to fill them in. He can be invited to join his wife in her room as soon as they are completed. If the woman has no one with her, there will be time for her to fill out the forms after the physical admission procedures have been carried out. If she is in active labor, there will be time to fill in the forms after the baby is delivered.

Stages of Labor

Labor has three separate time periods—the time from beginning cervical dilatation through full dilatation (the preparatory, dilatational, and deceleration sequence); the time from full dilatation until the fetus is pushed through the birth canal and born (the pelvic division or traditional second stage); and the time during which the placenta is delivered (the placental stage)—and each stage feels so different that it evokes a different reaction. Care must be individualized for the woman, depending on the stage of labor she is in.

THE TIME DURING CERVICAL DILATATION

The time span during which cervical dilatation occurs is the longest time interval in labor (about 12 to 14 hours in a nullipara, 8 hours in a multipara). At first it is exciting to feel labor contractions. They are little more than menstrual cramps; they project a this-is-really-happening quality. Soon, however, if the woman is not concentrating on controlled breathing exercises, they become biting in their intensity; they last longer and longer. Despite the fact that she is becoming more and more uncomfortable, nothing seems to be happening. She cannot see cervical dilatation. She begins to worry that something is going wrong. Nine months are over; victory is so near, yet it is escaping her.

Women need to be given reports in labor on what is happening so that they do not grow discouraged or fearful at the seeming lack of progress.

Control

A woman wants to remain in control of herself during labor. She is most comfortable, after all, if she is in control of her emotions at the supermarket or in her own kitchen or at the office and would like to be now as well. Women respond to stressful and painful situations differently, however. Some women handle the stress of labor by being extremely quiet. Others feel most comfortable when they can show their emotions. There is no reason that women all have to react the same in labor. Your role is to help each woman express her feelings in the way she chooses, without concern that she must be pushed into a mold or will be reminded later that she screamed instead of breathed with labor contractions.

Do not be fooled into thinking that all women who appear calm during labor are in control of their emotions. Fear also calms people into immobility. But quietness from fear will not foster a good mother-child interaction later on. It is an outward projection of good behavior at the expense of mental health.

Feelings of Responsibility

The feeling of what having a child means may become real for a woman for the first time during the first stage of labor (Fig. 20-1). Some women want to talk about what it will be like to have a child beginning today. Often during their pregnancy they have talked about what it will be like to have a child, but

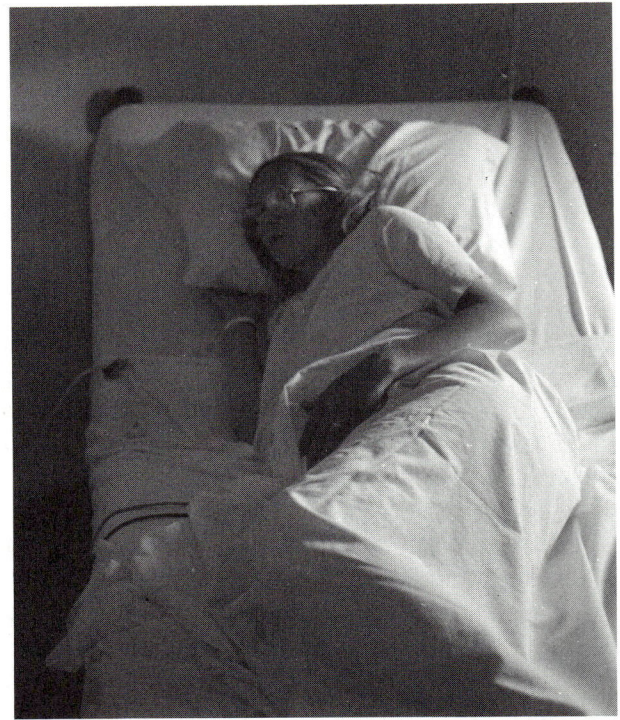

Fig. 20-1. Labor is a time for introspection, for asking, "What kind of mother will I be?" Note side-lying position, the best physiological position for labor.

never before about having a child *today*. Thoughts arise such as, "Never again for 18 years will I sleep soundly through a night. Never again will I be able to just run out to the library to return a book, soak for hours in a tub, take off for a weekend trip at a moment's notice. After *today*, a child will always be there, needing to be dressed and fed and cared for. Am I really ready for this?"

The mother who already has a child at home may worry that she will not have time to care for this new child. She seems to be busy every moment with her one child! How can she be sure she has a big enough heart to love two children? How can she love them equally? These thoughts were present in pregnancy also, but never before did she have to consider them important until *today*.

During early labor a woman may begin to worry about the sex of the child she is having. All during pregnancy she relied on the tried and true cliché "As long as it's healthy, I don't care" as her answer to which sex she preferred. And it did not matter because having the child was too far down the road to be real. Today, in a matter of hours, it will matter. She will make herself and her husband either very happy or at least moderately disappointed; perhaps very disappointed. In pregnancy she could control many things: what medication she took, how carefully she ate, how much rest and exercise she managed, the quality of her prenatal care. Now she may feel frustrated that she had no control over the sex of her child, a difference that can be important to her. *Today*.

These feelings of increased responsibility coupled with fatigue and pain increase her anxiety. They may make her view her husband sitting in a chair by her bed—smiling and seemingly enjoying himself, stretching lazily, chatting and joking with nurses—as taking this process too lightly, irresponsibly. She may worry that the task of child rearing will fall to her alone, the responsible person here.

Remembering that the first stage of labor is a time for introspection helps you to plan nursing care. A woman needs time just for working through a final rounding out of pregnancy tasks (throwing aside the daughter role; after today she is a mother, not a daughter); she also needs time to talk about those things that can be worked through best by talking (magically, mothers are no more busy with two children than they were with one; even if she feels not ready to be a mother yet, in the next day or two she will be with her baby under the supervision of knowledgeable people to help her be ready). She needs time alone with her support person to discuss with him or her how she feels about having this child. She may need time without her support person to voice worries she does not want to burden that person with.

Each labor is different. Each woman in labor reacts differently to the process depending on her background and her personality. For most women, the dilatational time of labor has two common entities: It is long, and it is frustrating when nothing seems to be happening. Any intervention aimed toward helping the woman understand what is happening and reducing stress is therapeutic in the first stage.

THE PELVIC DIVISION OR SECOND STAGE OF LABOR

With full dilatation, the second stage of labor begins. During this stage the fetus is pushed through the birth canal. Now the nature of contractions changes, from a crescendo-decrescendo pattern that caused dilatation to an overwhelming desire to push or bear down as if to move the bowels. The feeling is so intense there is nothing she can do to stop it.

Even women who take preparation-for-labor classes are surprised at the intensity of this form of contraction. An instructor spent some time in class telling them they would have to push to expel the fetus. They were still not prepared for the sensation that they are not doing or controlling the pushing; their uterus is controlling it, whether they are ready or not. The worry about having this baby today can reach a point of panic with the second stage of labor.

Because the feeling of pushing is so strong, most women react by tensing their abdominal muscles, trying to resist the sensation, and it becomes painful and even more frightening. They expect this new form of contraction to be even more painful than the type they have had before. It takes a few minutes for them to appreciate that if they relax or push with the contraction all pain disappears. The process can be compared to that of a swimmer's, whose muscles ache so with fatigue that he feels he cannot take another stroke, suddenly realizing he has his second wind and stroking is pain-free. It is the same as sliding down the other side of the mountain after the arduous climb to the top.

Women need to have someone with them as they enter this stage of labor to reassure them that what they are going through is normal; that in another minute, as soon as they get used to this sensation of pushing, having the baby can be fun.

Some women react to this change of contractions by growing increasingly argumentative or angry, by crying or screaming. Family support people may not be adequate at this point. The woman momentarily wants someone with her to give more knowledgeable support that everything is all right than a family member may be qualified to give.

In the first moments of the pelvic division of labor (often called *transition*) a woman is so acutely attuned to what is happening to her body that she does not "hear" instructions well. If she is going to be moved from a labor room to a delivery room at this time, it is difficult for her to understand your "Move over to the cart." She may ignore her husband's questions as if he had said nothing. It is good for her to know that these are typical reactions; it is important for family support people to know that this inward turning is a normal part of labor. Being aware of these things reduces the impact of the strange abdominal sensation to an acceptable, conquerable level.

THE PLACENTAL STAGE OF LABOR

The third stage of labor is delivery of the placenta. Expulsion of the placenta may be effected by the mother's bearing down as she did during the second stage of labor, or the physician may exert gentle pressure on the uterine fundus to aid in delivery.

Following the delivery of the placenta, any perineal stitches needed are put in place. The suturing of the perineum is a long, tedious procedure from the mother's viewpoint. There is a tendency for everyone in a delivery room to be involved in something else at this point. The physician and his or her assistant are occupied with the stitching, which is an important repair, requiring careful inspection to avoid overlooking a cervical or vaginal laceration that could lead quickly to postpartum hemorrhage. You are busy with care of the newborn. The father is looking at the bassinet off to the side rather than at his wife. The job is over, tension is gone, the staff members begin to talk among themselves, ignoring the mother.

The mother may feel rejected, perhaps like the discarded packing crate in which a new appliance arrived. The health care personnel seem to be much more interested in trying out the new "appliance," commenting on its lusty cry, its weight, or its sex, than in seeing to the "carton" that allowed the appliance to be shipped safely.

A woman is as vulnerable to hurt in the immediate postpartum period as she was during pregnancy and early labor. Be certain that she is included in explanations, that you appreciate how anticlimactic she feels (an "after-the-prom" feeling). Otherwise, the "postpartum blues" can begin minutes after birth.

The Father and Labor

It is well documented that husbands (or fathers of children) offer a high degree of support during labor, and it should not be hospital policy to exclude them. In most hospitals that do exclude them it is the nurses who have structured the policy, believing that husbands interfere with procedures. Changing these rules is the nursing staff's responsibility. A professional nurse should not associate herself with a labor unit in which such an obsolete policy is still followed.

A husband is awkward in the hospital. Remember, this may be the first time he has been in a hospital. He will push a chair into a corner and sit there out of the way unless he is urged to pull it up to his wife's bedside. He will say too little or too much, as people do when they are nervous. He may attempt to act unconcerned by reading a newspaper or book.

A husband is as vulnerable as his wife during labor—perhaps more so because he is helpless to do anything to aid in the progress of labor. He may be used to being the doer, the decision maker, and for the next 12 hours he will be forced into the role of a passive observer. This may make him quick-tempered and irritable. He is also probably as fatigued as his wife. She has not slept soundly for the past month, but neither has he. There may be things at work this day that need his supervision. Part of his attention may be on them. For the next three days other children are his responsibility. Part of his attention may be on wondering how they are. He is drawn in many directions, trying to give support in a process he does not fully understand. No wonder husbands and fathers have such bad reputations in labor rooms. It is their nervousness and their fatigue, not their unwillingness or inability to help, that are at fault.

The husband needs as much reassurance as the wife that everything is going well in labor. A frequent "Your wife is fine, she's doing great" is very reassuring to a man who knows more old wives' tales than you do and all of them are about the terrible things that happen to women in childbirth. He needs to be included in explanations of progress: "Mary is in early labor. Her contractions are about 40 seconds long and 10 minutes apart. The bottom of the uterus, the part called the cervix, is just beginning to open, to dilate." Like every husband, he wants to know how long it will be before the baby is born. Give him an approximation of time based on the averages but stress that each labor is unique (otherwise, he may hold you accountable if it takes longer; he may be used to working within honored time limits).

He can be given some tasks to do while his wife is in labor. He can time the duration and frequency of contractions. He can rub his wife's sacral area if that part of her back is causing a great deal of discomfort. He will recognize these chores as being little more than the modern hospital's way of assigning him "Water to boil," but nonetheless, he generally welcomes having something to do.

Do not feel compelled to keep him busy, however. His most important contribution is just to be there, to be a supportive, comforting, loving presence. If he does nothing more than hold his wife's hand for the 12 hours she is in labor, he has contributed in a unique way to the birth of his child. He has provided a caring atmosphere for his child to be born into. In a world of plastic plants and pervading uninvolvement such contributions cannot be discounted.

The husband whose wife is going to deliver by a Lamaze prepared method of childbirth has an active role to play as he serves as her coach throughout labor. Be certain to reassure him that, although he will take an active part, you will also be readily available as a support person. It is frightening for him to think that the good or bad outcome of this labor rests solely on him.

It may be difficult for a husband to appreciate how important it is for his wife to have him with her in labor. If she is using breathing exercises and has reduced the pain of labor to controllable stinging sensations, he may view this as an easy time free from stress. He may need a reminder that although the pain is gone from labor contractions the banding or tightening feeling remains; the unknown aspect of labor is still present. And these feelings are just as stressful as pain.

He may fail to realize that his wife's personality changes during the second stage of labor are normal and reprimand her for not cooperating or for growing agitated. A warning ahead of time is helpful.

The feeling of responsibility that engulfs the woman in labor may be experienced by the husband at this time also. He may not like his job very much. If there were just he and his wife, he would quit work that day and try something new. But after today there will be a baby to support too. He is not as free to take chances as he was yesterday. Life is closing in on him *today*, making him grow up whether he is ready or not.

He needs time alone with his wife during labor for the opportunity to share with her his feelings about his child—his feelings of being a father. On the other hand, he may need talk time with health personnel and generally appreciates having someone present in the room with him who knows more about labor than he does. It is difficult for him to be supportive when he is concerned about his wife's safety.

One interesting study [2] showed that when fathers were present during labor the first stage of labor for primiparas was 3½ hours shorter and the first stage for multiparas was 1½ hours shorter than in control labors where fathers were not present. The first stage progresses most rapidly if the mother is relaxed, and this decrease in labor time probably reflects the degree of relaxation which an effective support person can help supply.

The Unmarried Woman in Labor

If women have no support person with them in labor, they need to be able to use you as their support person. Often young girls are not aware that they could have asked the father of their child to accompany them. They may want to phone him to tell him they are in labor.

Young girls may need a review of anatomy so they are certain they understand what happens in labor. They may be worried that the baby will tear them because they are not yet fully grown. They require frequent reassurance that everything is going well and not only the baby but they too are safe from harm.

Unmarried women should have time during labor to complete their pregnancy work just as married women do: to think about what it will be like to be a mother, to care for a child. If they have made a decision to place the baby for adoption, they need time to think about whether this is still what they want now that the day of birth has arrived. It is much easier to decide to place a baby for adoption during pregnancy when the event seems far away than during labor when the decision involves something that is happening *today*.

Because the acceptance of the pregnancy may have come late in pregnancy for unmarried women who did not plan on having a child, they may not have completed the psychological tasks of pregnancy by the time they are in labor. Not being ready for this baby may make labor more difficult. In a study of 48 women [5] it was shown that women who were not ready for child rearing had longer labors (16.8 hours) than women who were ready (7.3 hours).

The Unmarried Man and Labor

Only in the last few years have unmarried partners been welcome in labor rooms. An unmarried father-to-be, although he has been told that he is welcome, may have grave doubts that this is indeed the case. He needs to be included in explanations of labor progress and aspects of care, as appropriate. The fact that he has chosen to include himself in the labor experience shows his commitment as a support person and probably his value to the woman as an important person in her life.

Home Births

Because labor units of hospitals were for many years managed with operating room–like efficiency, warmth and humaneness were sometimes overlooked in favor of routines or rules. This circumstance has made delivering a baby at home, where warmth and familiarity are the chief ingredients, an attractive alternative. When a woman delivers at home, however, she sacrifices the safety of having backup equipment and care available should something be wrong with her infant at birth or happen to herself during labor or delivery.

Nurses can be instrumental in making the milieu of labor units so accepting and humane that women do not have to choose an unsafe alternative in order to have their baby surrounded by the people important to them. Understanding the psychological reactions to labor and delivery in order to give helpful support in labor is vital to creating an atmosphere where women do feel comfortable and want to come for care.

Problem-oriented Recording: Progress Notes

Christine McFadden
15 years
Para 0, gravida 1, premature 0, abortion 0, stillborn 0, living children 0

Problem: Psychological adjustment to labor

> S. States, "I hate this. I didn't want this baby. I don't want to go through with this. I just want a c-section to get this over." Has no support person with her. Has been told that her pelvic measurements are borderline and a cesarean section may be necessary. Grandmother purchased baby items to be ready for birth; Chris did not participate in preparation. Attended no preparation-for-labor classes.
> O. Appears tense, frightened.
> A. Extremely frightened by labor; no effective support person present.
> Goals: a. Learn ways to participate in labor rather than be passive observer.
>   b. Able to accept labor by vaginal delivery if possible.
>   c. Able to accept c-section decision if this decision is made.
> P. 1. Ask if family support person should be called.
>   2. Provide continuous nursing support.
>   3. Review physiology of labor so she fully understands it.
>   4. Give good explanations of all equipment used, procedures done.
>   5. In postpartal period assess adequacy of maternal-child relationship because of poor preparation for labor.

10:00 A.M. Interim assessment

> S. States, "I hate Mark [father of child] for putting me through this. I hate my parents." Mother is coming to be support person for her but has not arrived yet. Asked that father of child not be notified of labor.
> O. Extremely tense; appears frightened and lonely.
> A. Primipara with inadequate support from family members.
> Feelings of resentment against child and child's father.
> P. 1. Continue nursing support.
>   2. Support grandmother as needed when she arrives.
>   3. Offer opportunity to discuss feelings about labor and coming child.

11:00 A.M. Interim assessment

> S. Has been told that cesarean section will be necessary for safe delivery of baby because of borderline pelvic measurements and lack of progress in labor. Seems relieved at decision and now she will have no more uterine contractions. Asking to be put to sleep immediately for surgery. Mother is with her; appears concerned about surgery. Asking questions about what this will mean in future years for daughter regarding other pregnancies. Relationship with daughter appears strained,

but the daughter asked for her to come so some meaningful relationship must be present.
- O. Appears more relaxed on hearing surgery decision.
- A. Primipara with poor adjustment to pregnancy and labor not unhappy with cesarean decision.
- P. 1. Educate regarding anatomy of cesarean section operation.
  2. Continue support until anesthetized; follow-up in recovery room.
  3. In postpartal period assess for maternal-child attachment because of delivery under general anesthetic.
  4. Assess daughter-mother relationship more thoroughly (patient will be living at home following delivery).

Problem-oriented Recording: Progress Notes

Mary Kraft
22 years
Para 0, gravida 2, premature 0, abortion 1, stillborn 0, living children 0

Problem: Psychological adjustment to labor

- S. States, "I thought labor would be worse than this; so far this is all downhill." Using breathing exercises learned in prenatal class; has husband with her for support person. Baby planned; has clothing, etc., ready for baby. States she doesn't care about sex of child. Asked for birthing room; husband wants to be with her for delivery as well as labor.
- O. Appears relaxed, but tired.
- A. Primipara psychologically prepared for labor and new child.

Goals: a. Participate in labor rather than be passive observer.
b. Complete labor as a family unit.

- P. 1. Offer support as necessary.
  2. Offer education of labor happenings as necessary.

Interim assessment: Birth of Child

- S. States, "I wanted a boy, I really did." (Had 6 lb 5 oz boy.) Husband states he also wanted boy. Mother anxious to hold baby and breast-feed.
- O. Appears happy. Appears to enjoy breast-feeding.
- A. Couple with filled expectations at birth.
- P. 1. Encourage rest to prevent exhaustion from excitement.
  2. Support rooming-in unit for postpartal care.
  3. Assess mothering ability in postpartal time as routine (no problem anticipated).

Problem-oriented Recording: Progress Notes

Angie Baco
42 years
Para 6, gravida 7, abortion 0, premature 0, stillborn 0, living children 5

Problem: Psychological adjustment to labor

- S. States, "Well, here I am, all the way to 37 weeks." Seems sad that pregnancy will be induced this morning because of gestational diabetes but happy that pregnancy came this far. States that she knows more about labor than everyone here (6 previous labors) but seemed grateful for explanation of admission procedures. Baby not planned initially, but has baby items ready, name for baby chosen. Says she wants a girl, but boy would be "okay." She wants to deliver in a delivery, not a birthing, room, *"in case the baby isn't all right."* Husband not sure he wants to see delivery; says "we'll see" when time comes. Did not see any previous births. Couple's last child had congenital heart disease, died 4 days after birth.
- O. Appears relaxed although bites lip when not actively engaged in conversation.
- A. Multipara anxious in labor due to previous poor outcome of pregnancy; adaptation may be difficult if baby is a boy.

Goals: a. Complete labor as a family unit.
b. Be able to face and accept a possible poor outcome.

P. 1. Provide adequate support because of anxiety.
2. Support husband as necessary (he is not certain he is ready for poor outcome to pregnancy).
3. Reassure frequently that labor is going well and fetus is doing well (as appropriate).
4. Assess mother-child relationship in postpartal period on account of mother's perception that infant may be ill.
5. Assess mother-child relationship in postpartal period if child is a boy (having boy only "okay," not desired).

References

1. Anderson, C. Operational definition of "support." *J.O.G.N. Nurs.* 5:17, 1976.
2. Bradley, R. A. Fathers' presence in delivery rooms. *Psychosomatics* 3:474, 1962.
3. Card, J. J., et al. Teenage mothers and teenage fathers: The impact of early childrearing on the parents' personal and professional lives. *Fam. Plann. Perspect.* 10:199, 1978.
4. Chiota, B. J., et al. Effects of separation from spouse on pregnancy, labor and delivery and the post partal period. *J.O.G.N. Nurs.* 5:21, 1976.
5. Davids, A., et al. Psychological study of emotional factors in pregnancy: A preliminary report. *Psychosom. Med.* 23:93, 1961.
6. Degarmo, E. Fathers' and Mothers' Feelings About Sharing the Childbirth Experience. In L. K. McNall and J. T. Galeener (Eds.), *Current Practice in Obstetric and Gynecologic Nursing.* St. Louis: Mosby, 1976.
7. Freeman, M. H. Giving family life a good start in the hospital. *M.C.N.* 4:51, 1979.
8. Hrobsky, D. M. Symposium on parenting: Transition to parenthood, a balancing of needs. *Nurs. Clin. North Am.* 12:457, 1977.
9. Kimbrough, C. A. The search for labor information during pregnancy. *Matern. Child. Nurs. J.* 6:107, 1977.
10. Levy, J., and McGee, M. Childbirth as crisis. *J. Pers. Soc. Psychol.* 31:171, 1975.
11. Shannon-Babitz, M. Addressing the needs of fathers during labor and delivery. *M.C.N.* 4:378, 1979.

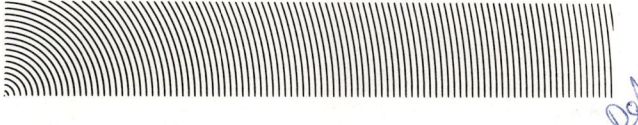

21. The Labor Process

Labor is the series of events by which the products of conception are expelled from the woman's body. The terms *childbirth, accouchement, confinement, parturition,* and *travail* are all synonyms for labor. *Labor* is an apt term because a great deal of work is involved in the process of birth. For the woman and the fetus alike, it is a time of change, both a time of ending and a time of beginning.

Fetal Cranial Determinations
STRUCTURE AND DIAMETERS OF FETAL SKULL

The position the fetus assumes just prior to delivery determines to a great degree whether or not his entrance into the world will be free of complications. Two main conditions in terms of size and presentation must coexist before labor and delivery can proceed without mishap: The fetal head must not be too large to fit through the birth canal, and the birth canal must not be too small to accommodate the fetal head. Thus, there are two separate causes to consider should a difficulty arise: It may be due to either a fetal or a maternal problem.

The maternal pelvic measurements that are taken to predict the adequacy of the maternal pelvis were discussed in Chap. 16. In most instances of disproportion, the pelvis is the organ at fault. This is an important point to understand when discussing with parents why an infant cannot be delivered vaginally. It is one thing to learn that a child cannot be born vaginally because the mother's pelvis is too small and another to learn that the infant's head is too large. The first fact is merely unfortunate; the second implies that something is wrong with the baby. A thought of that kind can interfere with the establishment of the good maternal-child relationship that is necessary for the child's sound mental health.

When the fetus is causing the problem, it is often because the fetal head is presented to the birth canal at less than its narrowest diameter, not because the head is actually too large. In order to understand how such a presentation occurs, you must have some acquaintance with the bones, fontanelles, and suture lines of the fetal skull (Figs. 21-1 and 21-2).

The cranium is composed of eight bones. The four superior ones—the frontal bone, the two parietal bones, and the occipital bone—are the important bones in terms of obstetrics. The other four (sphenoid bone, ethmoid bone, and two temporal bones) do not play a large part in obstetrics, since they lie at the base of the cranium and therefore are never presenting parts.

The two parietal bones of the skull are joined by a

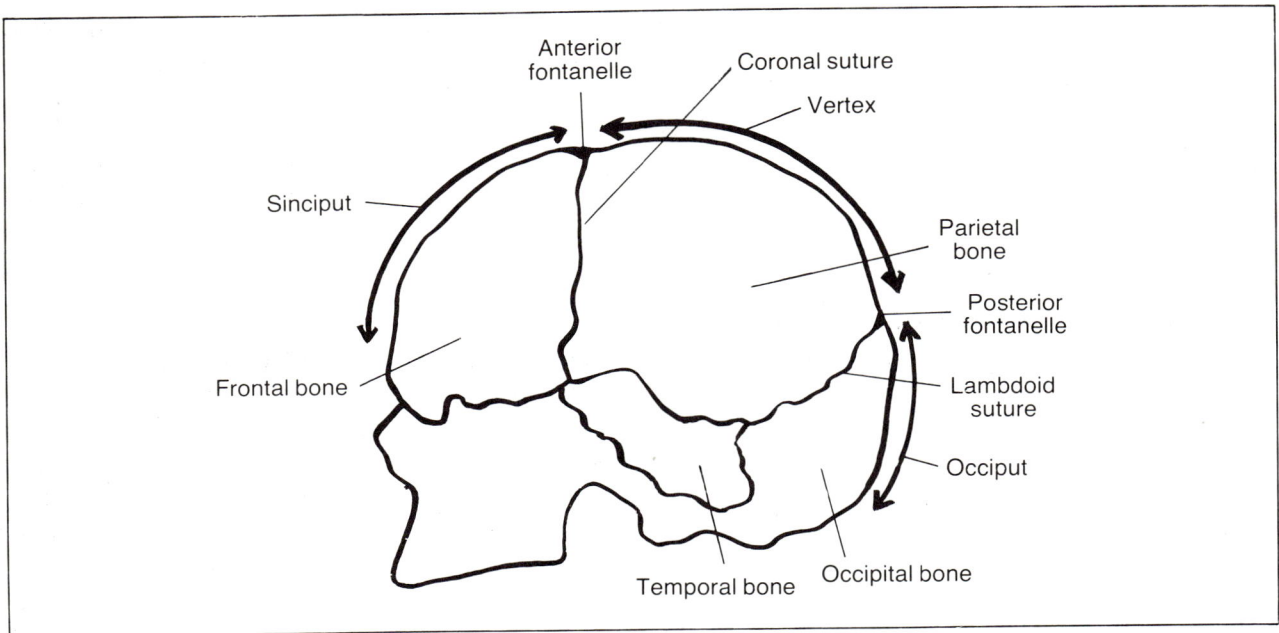

Fig. 21-1. The fetal skull (lateral view).

membranous interspace, the sagittal suture line. The coronal suture line is the line of junction of the frontal bone and the two parietal bones. The lambdoid suture line is the line of junction of the occipital bone and the two parietal bones. The suture lines are important in delivery because they allow the cranial bones to move and overlap, thus molding or diminishing the size of the skull so that it can more readily pass through the birth canal.

At the junction of the main suture lines are significant membrane-covered spaces, the fontanelles. The *anterior fontanelle* lies at the junction of the coronal and sagittal lines. Because the frontal bone consists of two fused bones, four bones (counting the two parietal bones) are actually involved at this junction, making the anterior fontanelle diamond-shaped. It measures approximately 3 to 4 cm in its anteroposterior diameter and 2 to 3 cm in its transverse diameter.

Three bones (the two parietal bones and the occipital bone) are involved at the junction of the lambdoid and sagittal suture lines; thus the *posterior fontanelle* is triangular. It is smaller than the anterior fontanelle, measuring about 2 cm across its widest part. Fontanelle spaces compress during delivery to aid in molding of the fetal head.

The shape of a fetal skull causes it to be wider in its anteroposterior diameter than in its transverse diameter. To fit through the birth canal, the fetus must present the smaller diameter (the transverse diameter) to the smaller diameter of the maternal pelvis; otherwise progress will halt and birth cannot be accomplished.

At the pelvic inlet, for example, the fetus must present the narrowest diameter, the biparietal diameter (about 9.25 cm) (Fig. 21-3) to the anteroposterior diameter of the pelvis (a space about 11 cm wide). At the outlet, this narrow diameter must be presented to the transverse diameter, a space about 11 cm wide. If the anteroposterior diameter of the skull (a measurement wider than the biparietal diameter) is presented to the anteroposterior diameter of the inlet, engagement, or the settling of the fetal head into the pelvis, may not occur. If the anteroposterior diameter of the skull is presented to the transverse diameter of the outlet, arrest of progress may occur at that point.

The diameter of the anteroposterior fetal skull depends on where the measurement is taken. The nar-

Fig. 21-2. The fetal skull (from above).

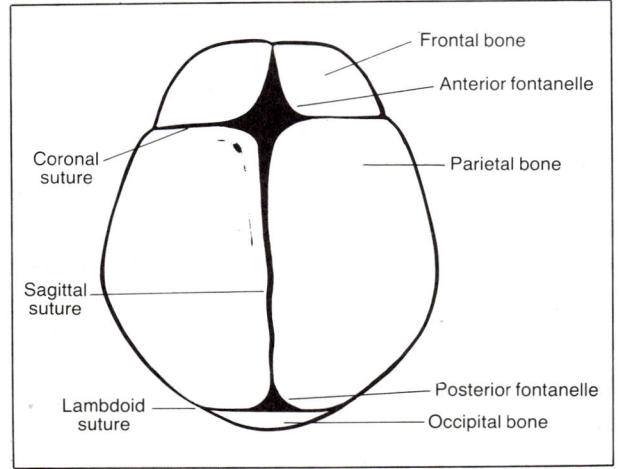

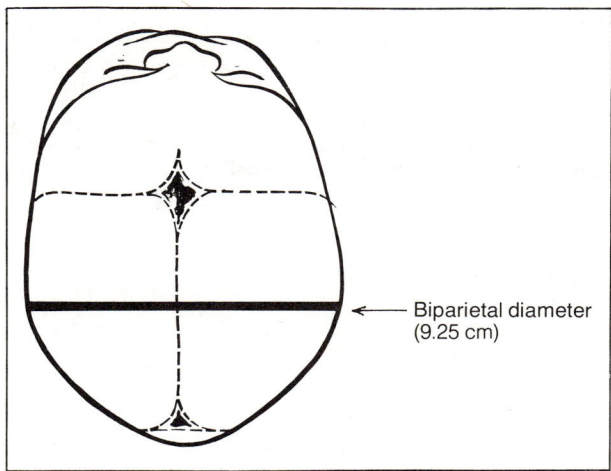

Fig. 21-3. Biparietal diameter.

rowest diameter (about 9.5 cm) is from the inferior aspect of the occiput to the center of the anterior fontanelle (the suboccipitobregmatic diameter). The occipitofrontal diameter, measured from the bridge of the nose to the occipital prominence, is about 12 cm. The occipitomental diameter, which is the widest anteroposterior diameter (about 13.5 cm), is measured from the chin to the posterior fontanelle. These diameters are shown in Fig. 21-4.

Which one of these anteroposterior diameters is presented to the birth canal depends on the degree of flexion of the fetus's head. In full flexion the head flexes so sharply that the chin rests on the thorax, and the smallest anteroposterior diameter, the suboccipitobregmatic, will be presented to the birth canal. If the head is held in moderate flexion, the occipitofrontal diameter will be presented. In poor flexion (the

Fig. 21-4. Anteroposterior diameters of the skull. A. Suboccipitobregmatic diameter (9.5 cm). B. Occipitofrontal diameter (12 cm). C. Occipitomental diameter (13.5 cm).

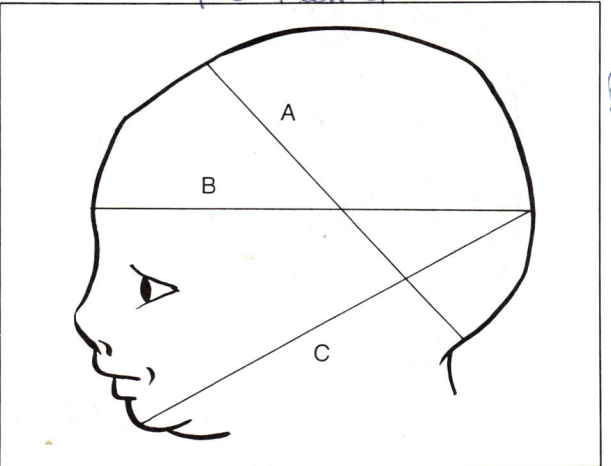

head hyperextended) the largest diameter, the occipitomental, will be presented.

This anteroposterior diameter must fit through the transverse diameter of the pelvic inlet, a space of about 12.5 to 13.5 cm; and at the outlet, through the anteroposterior diameter of the pelvis, a space of 9.5 to 11.5 cm. It follows that a fetal head presenting a diameter of 9.5 cm will fit through a pelvis much more readily than if the diameter is 12.0 or 13.5 cm. This relationship is shown in Fig. 21-5. Diameters of the fetal skull are summarized in comparison with pelvic diameters in Table 21-1.

MOLDING

Molding is the change in the shape of the fetal skull that occurs during labor to reduce the engaging diameters and make passage of the fetal head easier.

Molding is produced by the force of uterine contractions. The change in shape is possible because the bones of the fetal skull are not yet completely ossified and therefore do not form a rigid structure. Skull bones overlap so that the head becomes narrower but longer.

At birth, the overlapping of the sagittal suture line and generally the coronal suture line can be easily palpated in the newborn skull.

In a brow presentation, there is little molding because frontal bones are fused. Because molding does not occur readily in brow presentations, the labor will undoubtedly be arrested and the fetus be unable to pass through the pelvis. In a breech presentation, no skull molding occurs, and the fetal head presents a delivery problem.

Fetal Presentation and Position

In addition to being familiar with the component parts and diameters of the fetal head, you should be able to use with understanding the terms describing fetal presentation and position.

ATTITUDE

Attitude is a term to describe the degree of flexion the fetus assumes (Fig. 21-5). A fetus in good attitude is in complete flexion: The spinal column is bowed forward; the head is flexed forward so much that the chin touches the sternum; the arms are flexed and folded on the chest; the thighs are flexed onto the abdomen; and the calves of the legs are pressed against the posterior aspect of the thighs. A good attitude is advantageous for delivery not only because it helps the fetus present the smallest anteroposterior diameter of the skull to the pelvis but also because it puts the whole

The Labor Process 291

Table 21-1. Diameters of Fetal Skull Compared to Female Pelvic Diameters

Diameter	Measurement	Average Diameter (cm)
Anteroposterior Fetal Skull Diameter		
Suboccipitobregmatic	Inferior aspect of occiput to center of anterior fontanelle	9.5
Occipitofrontal	Bridge of nose to occipital prominence	12.0
Occipitomental	Chin to posterior fontanelle	13.5
Transverse fetal skull diameter, biparietal	Distance between parietal prominences	9.25
Anteroposterior pelvic diameters		
Diagonal conjugate	Inferior margin of symphysis pubis to sacral promontory	12.5
True conjugate	Internal aspect of symphysis pubis to sacral promontory	11.0
Transverse pelvic diameter, ischial tuberosities	Between ischial tuberosities at the level of the anus	11.0

Fig. 21-5. Fetal attitude. A. Fetus in full flexion presents smallest (suboccipitobregmatic) anteroposterior diameter of skull to inlet in this good attitude. B. Fetus is not as well flexed (military attitude) as in A and presents occipitofrontal diameter to inlet. C. Fetus in complete extension presents wide (occipitomental) diameter. D. Fetus in partial extension (brow presentation).

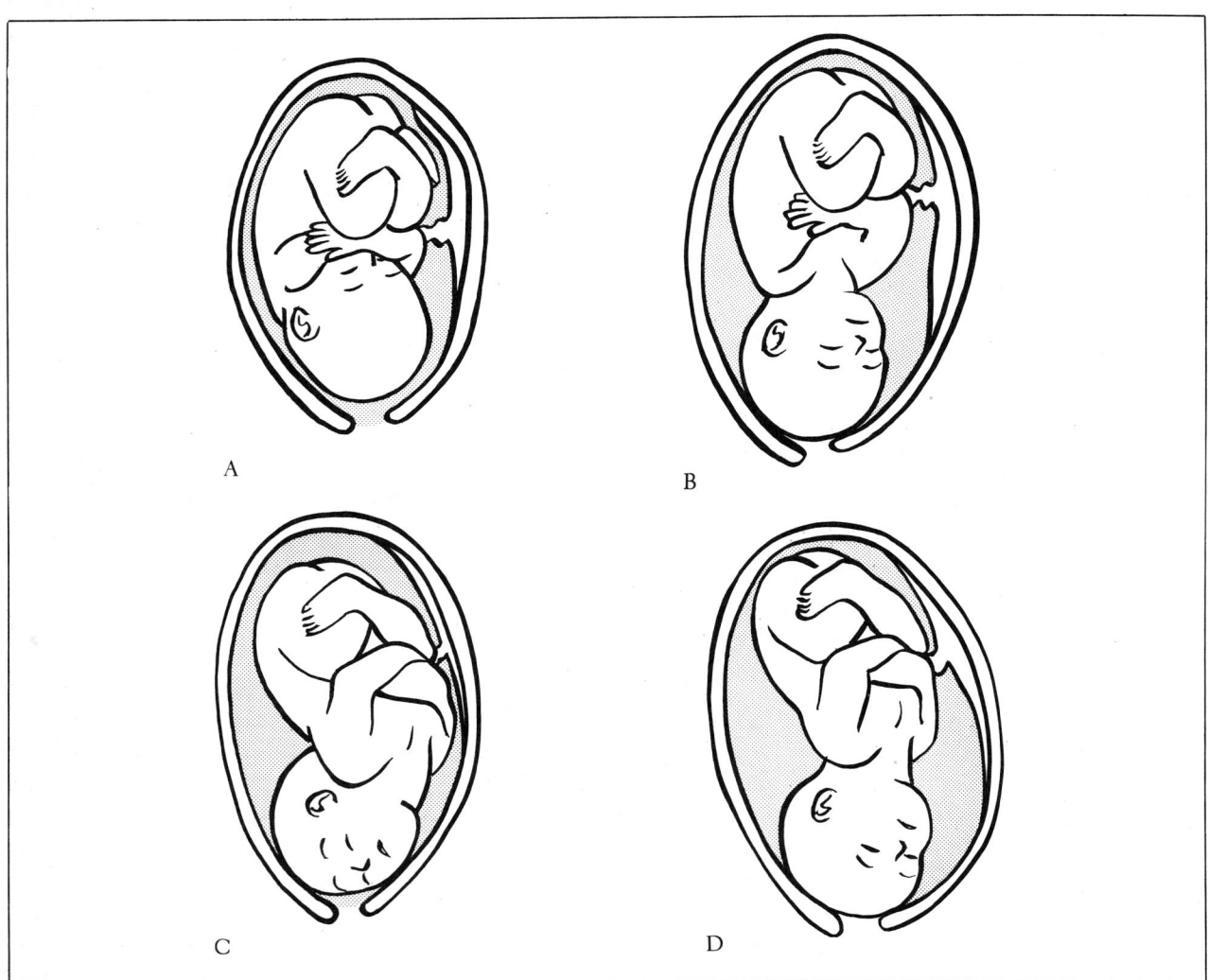

292   Period of Parturition: Becoming a Parent

body into an ovoid shape, occupying the smallest space possible.

ENGAGEMENT

The presenting part of the fetus is said to be *engaged* when it has settled far enough into the pelvis to be at the level of the ischial spines. Engagement means that lightening has occurred. Nonengagement of the head at the beginning of labor in a primipara indicates a possible complication; an abnormal presentation or position, abnormality of the fetal head, or a cephalopelvic disproportion may be preventing the head from engaging. In multiparas, engagement may or may not be present at the beginning of labor. A presenting part that is not engaged is said to be "floating."

STATION

Station refers to the relationship of the presenting part of the fetus to the level of the ischial spines (Fig. 21-6). When the presenting part is at the level of the ischial spines, it is at a 0 station (synonymous with *engagement*). If the presenting part is above the spines, the distance is measured and described as −1 cm (minus 1 station), −2 cm (minus 2 station), and so on. If the presenting part is below the ischial spines, the distance is determined (+1 cm, +2 cm, and so on) and designated as a plus 1 station, a plus 2 station, and so on. At a plus 3 or 4 station the presenting part is at the perineum and can be seen if you separate the vulva (synonymous with *crowning*).

PRESENTATION OR LIE

Presentation is the relationship between the long axis of the fetal body and that of the woman's body, that is, whether the fetus is lying in a horizontal or a vertical position. About 99 percent of fetuses lie in a vertical presentation (with their long axis parallel with the long axis of the woman). Vertical presentations are further classified as cephalic presentations (the head is the presenting part, i.e., first contacts the cervix) or breech presentations (the breech, or buttocks, is the portion to contact the cervix first).

Cephalic presentations (see Fig. 21-7) may be vertex presentations, in which the head is sharply flexed (good attitude), making the vertex (the parietal bones) the presenting part; or with poor flexion they may be brow presentations, face presentations, or chin (mental) presentations.

Three types of breech presentation are possible (Fig. 21-8): complete breech (the thighs are flexed on the abdomen and the legs on the thighs); frank breech (the thighs are flexed and the legs extended, so that they rest on the anterior surface of the body); footling breech (one or both legs are extended, becoming the presenting parts).

A very few fetuses (under 1 percent) lie horizontal to the long axis of the woman's body, or in a *transverse lie*. Since this position causes the shoulder to be the presenting part of the body, it is also called a *shoulder presentation* (Fig. 21-9). Transverse lies are rare and are usually due to relaxed abdominal walls from grand multiparity or to pelvic contraction or placenta previa. Most infants in a transverse lie must be delivered by cesarean section.

POSITION

Position is the relationship of the presenting part to a specific quadrant of the woman's pelvis. For convenience in defining position, the maternal pelvis is divided into four quadrants: right anterior, left anterior, right posterior, and left posterior. Four parts of the fetus have been chosen as points of direction in order to describe the relationship of the presenting part to one of the pelvic quadrants. In a vertex presentation, the occiput is the chosen point; in face presentations, it is the chin (mentum); in breech presentations, it is the sacrum; in shoulder presentations, it is the scapula or the acromial process of the scapula.

The fetal position is left occipitoanterior (LOA), for example, in a vertex presentation (the fetus is in good attitude in a vertical cephalic lie) when the occiput of the fetus points to the left anterior quadrant of the mother. When the occiput points to the right posterior quadrant, the position is right occipitoposterior (ROP). LOA is the most common fetal position and right occipitoanterior (ROA) the second most frequent position. Table 21-2 presents a summary of possible

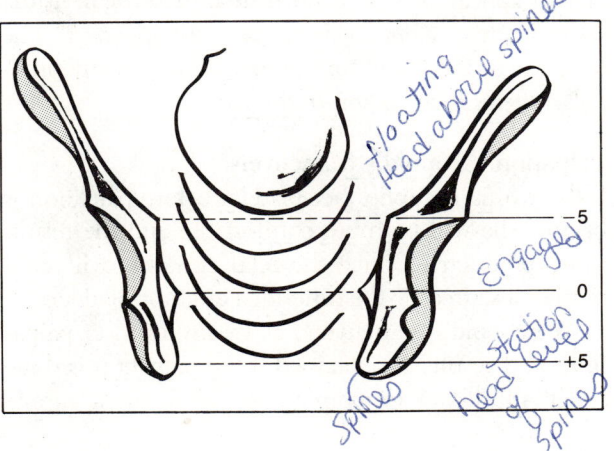

Fig. 21-6. Station (anteroposterior view). Station, or degree of engagement, of the fetal head is designated by centimeters above or below the ischial spines. At −5 station, head is "floating." At 0 station, head is "engaged." At +5 station, head is at outlet.

The Labor Process 293

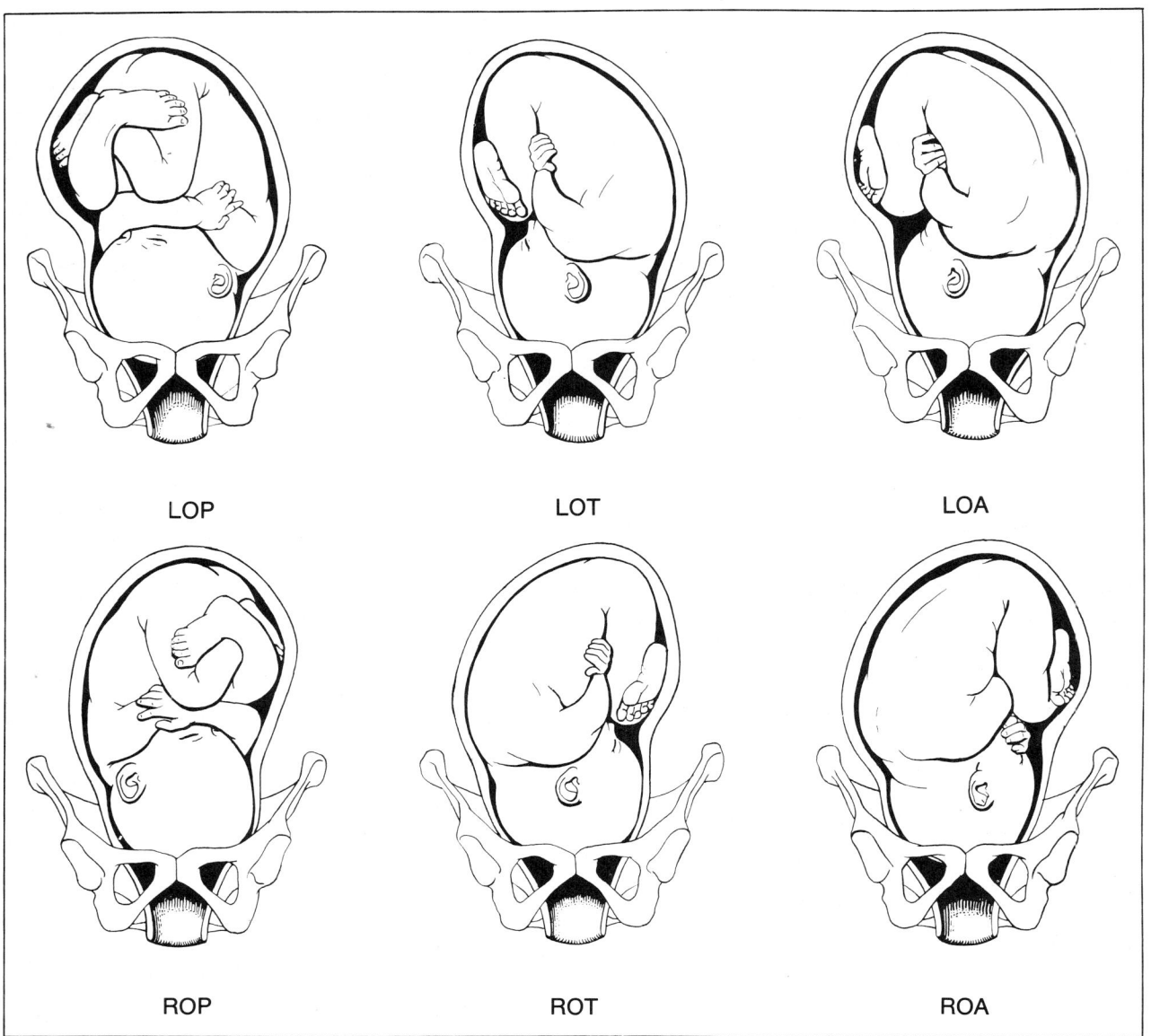

Fig. 21-7. Cephalic presentations. All are vertex presentations. A = anterior, L = left, O = occiput, P = posterior, R = right, T = transverse. (From Clinical Education Aid, No. 18, Ross Laboratories, Columbus, Ohio, 1958.)

positions, and two common positions in cephalic presentations are depicted in Fig. 21-10.

DETERMINING FETAL PRESENTATION AND POSITION

It is important to recognize the fetal position in order to predict the course of labor. There are four methods: (1) combined abdominal inspection and palpation, (2) vaginal or rectal examination, (3) auscultation, and (4) sonography or x-ray examination. X-ray examination is rarely used routinely because of its potential teratogenic effect.

Inspection

In trying to determine fetal position, it is worthwhile to spend some time observing the woman's abdomen. Ask yourself the following: What is the longest diameter in appearance? Is it horizontal or vertical? If the fetus is active, where is the movement apparent? The long axis is the length of the fetus. The activity probably reflects the position of the feet.

Palpation: Leopold's Maneuvers

If the woman empties her bladder before palpation is begun, she will be more comfortable and the results more productive, since the fetal contours will then not be obscured by the distended anterior bladder.

In Leopold's maneuvers, as in any form of palpation, best results are obtained if the palpation is done systematically. The woman should lie in a supine

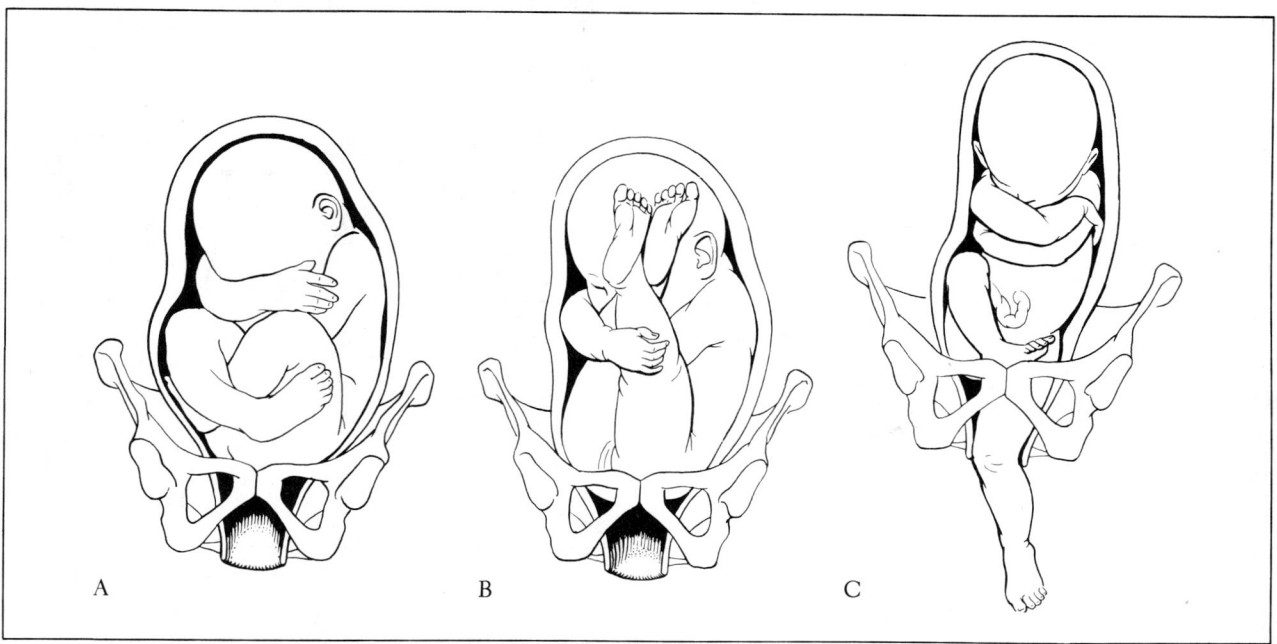

Fig. 21-8. Breech presentation. A. Complete breech. B. Frank breech. C. Footling breech. (From Clinical Education Aid, No. 18, Ross Laboratories, Columbus, Ohio, 1958.)

position with her knees flexed slightly so that her abdominal muscles are relaxed. Be certain your hands are warm (by washing them in warm water first if necessary); cold hands cause abdominal muscles to contract and tighten. Use gentle but firm motions.

FIRST MANEUVER. Palpate the superior surface of the fundus (Fig. 21-11A). What is the consistency? A head feels more firm than does a breech. What is the shape? A head is round and hard; the breech is less well defined. What is the mobility of the palpated part? A head moves independently of the body; the

Fig. 21-9. Transverse or shoulder presentation. (From Clinical Education Aid, No. 18, Ross Laboratories, Columbus, Ohio, 1958.)

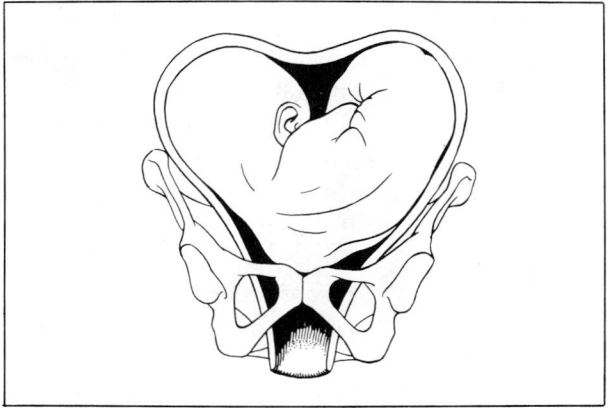

breech moves only in conjunction with the body. Form an opinion of what portion of the fetus lies in this fundal area.

SECOND MANEUVER. Palpate the sides of the uterus to determine which direction the fetal back is facing (Fig. 21-11B). This maneuver is accomplished most

Table 21-2. Possible Fetal Positions

Vertex presentation
   LOA = Left occipitoanterior
   LOP = Left occipitoposterior
   LOT = Left occipitotransverse
   ROA = Right occipitoanterior
   ROP = Right occipitoposterior
   ROT = Right occipitotransverse

Breech presentation
   LSA = Left sacroanterior
   LSP = Left sacroposterior
   LST = Left sacrotransverse
   RSA = Right sacroanterior
   RSP = Right sacroposterior
   RST = Right sacrotransverse

Face presentation
   LMA = Left mentoanterior
   LMP = Left mentoposterior
   LMT = Left mentotransverse
   RMA = Right mentoanterior
   RMP = Right mentoposterior
   RMT = Right mentotransverse

Shoulder presentation
   LSCA = Left scapuloanterior
   LSCP = Left scapuloposterior
   RSCA = Right scapuloanterior
   RSCP = Right scapuloposterior

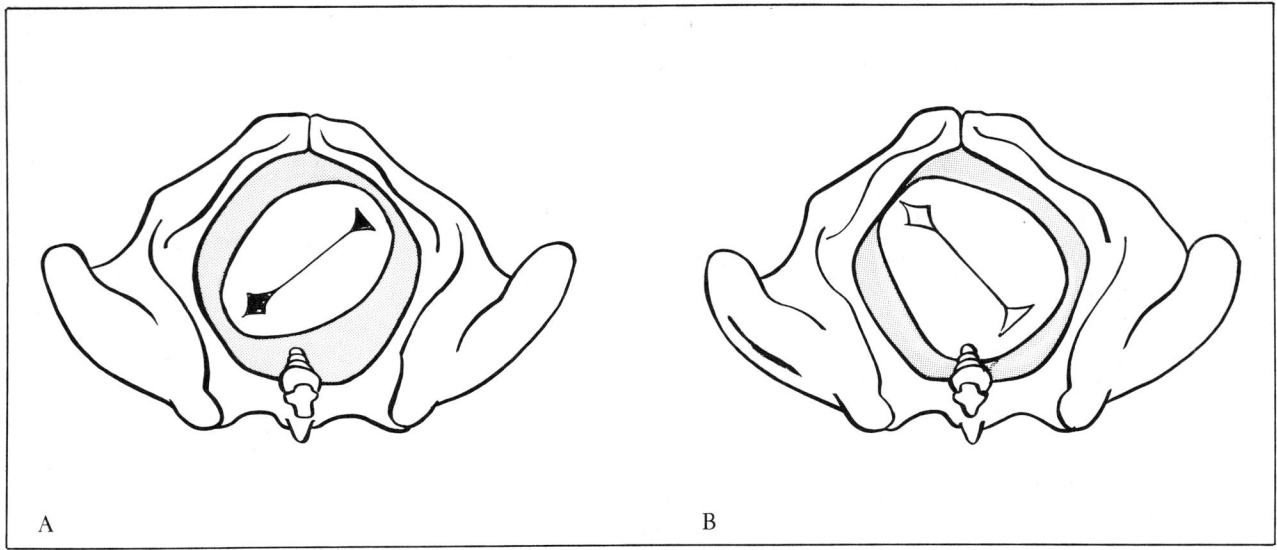

Fig. 21-10. Fetal presentation views from the outlet. A. Right occipitoanterior (ROA). B. Right occipitoposterior (ROP).

successfully if the left hand is held stationary on the left side of the uterus while with the right hand you palpate the opposite side of the uterus from top to bottom. Next, hold the right hand stationary to immobilize the uterus, and palpate top to bottom on the left side. You will find one side a smooth, hard, resistant surface (the back), while on the opposite side you will feel a number of angular nodulations (the knees and elbows of the fetus).

THIRD MANEUVER. Next, palpate to discover what is at the inlet of the pelvis (Fig. 21-11C). Gently grasp the lower portion of the abdomen just above the symphysis pubis between your thumb and index finger and try to press your thumb and finger together. If the presenting part moves upward to allow you to press your hand together, the presenting part is not engaged (not firmly settled into the pelvis). Is it firm (the head)? Or is it soft (the breech)?

FOURTH MANEUVER. Assuming you have found the fetus to be in a cephalic presentation, you will now want to determine the fetal attitude (degree of flexion). Place your fingers on both sides of the uterus about 2 inches above the inguinal ligaments (Fig. 21-11D). Press downward and inward. The fingers of one hand will slide along the uterine contour and meet no obstruction; this is the back of the fetal neck. Your other hand will meet an obstruction an inch or so above the ligament; you are touching the fetal brow. The position of the fetal brow should correspond to the side of the uterus you have designated as containing the elbows and knees of the fetus. If the fetus is in a poor attitude, you will meet an obstruction on the same side as the fetal back; that is, your fingers will touch the hyperextended head.

Some information as to the infant's anteroposterior position may also be gained from this final maneuver. If the brow is very easily palpated (as if it lies just under the skin), the fetus is probably in a posterior position (the occiput is pointing away from you).

Leopold's maneuvers therefore tell you about the presentation, presenting part, position, and attitude of the fetus, which are all important facts to know to help predict the course of labor. It is difficult to palpate fetal contours in an obese woman or one with hydramnios (excessive amniotic fluid).

Auscultation

Fetal heart sounds are transmitted through the convex portion of the fetus, since that is the part lying in close contact with the uterine wall (Fig. 21-12). In a vertex or breech presentation, fetal heart sounds are best heard through the fetal back; in a face presentation the back becomes concave, and they are best heard through the more convex thorax.

In breech presentations the sounds are heard most clearly high in the uterus at the woman's umbilicus or above. In cephalic presentations, they are heard loudest low in the abdomen. In ROA position the sounds are heard best in the right lower quadrant; in LOA position, in the left lower quadrant. In posterior positions (left or right occipitoposterior—LOP or ROP) the heart sounds are loudest in the maternal side. Figure 21-13 shows typical sites where heart sounds can be heard.

Hearing the fetal heart sounds in these positions

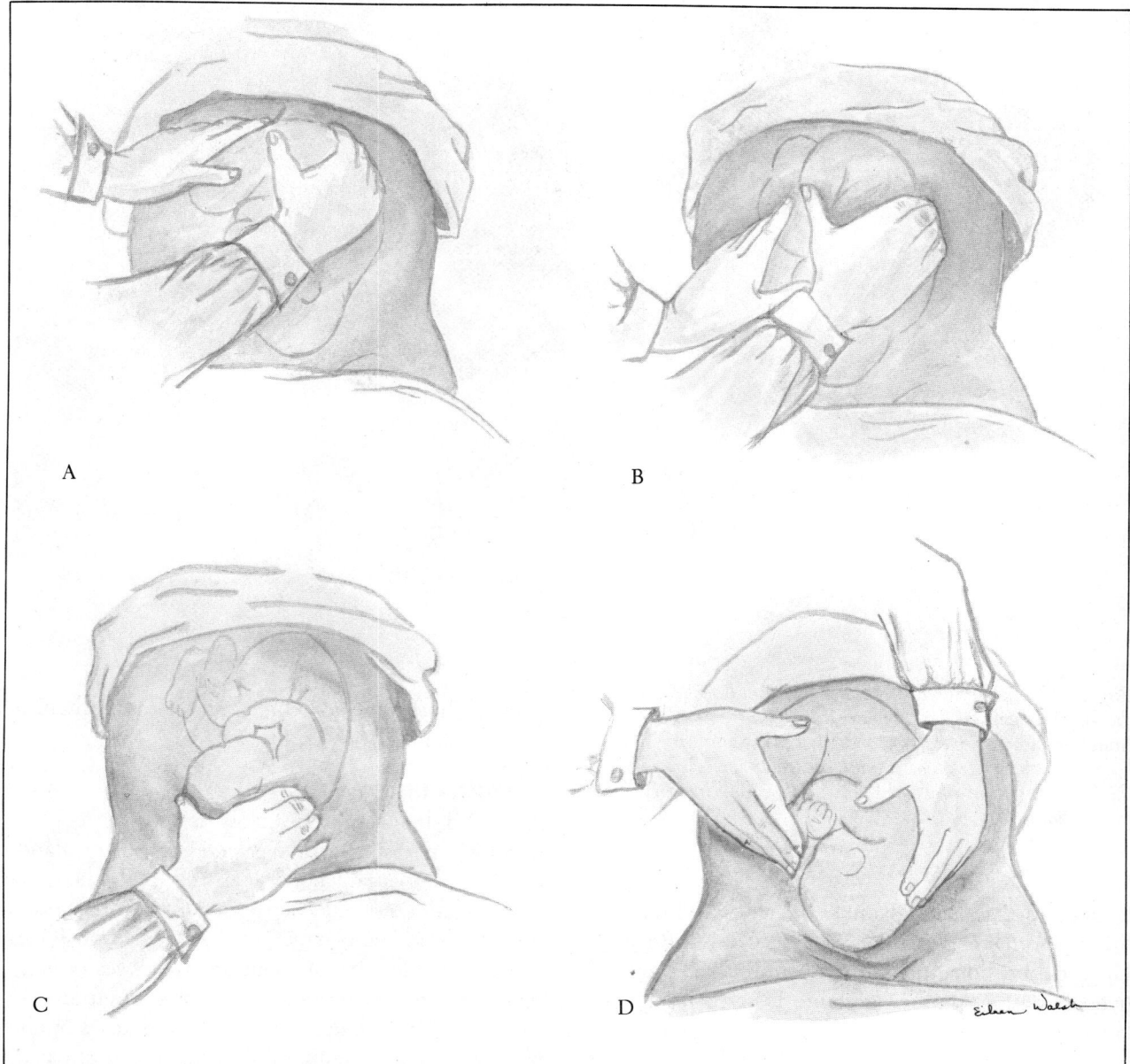

Fig. 21-11. Leopold's maneuvers. A. First maneuver. B. Second maneuver. C. Third maneuver. D. Fourth maneuver.

provides confirmatory information about fetal position. Conversely, recognizing the fetal position aids you in locating fetal heart sounds.

Vaginal Examination

After cervical dilatation has begun, the presenting part can be identified on vaginal examination. If it is a cephalic presentation, the positions of the fontanelles and the suture lines of the skull are palpated and identified, supplying information about the position and attitude of the fetus.

Sonography and X-ray Examination

In women who are obese or have such rigid abdominal walls that abdominal palpation is difficult, or in whom a poor fetal position is suspected, sonography or x-ray studies may be done to determine presentation, presenting part, position, flexion, and degree of descent of the fetus. Sonogram determination has the advantage of being assumed harmless to the fetus. X-ray films are ordered only when the information cannot be obtained in any other way.

Theories of Labor Onset

Labor normally begins when a fetus is sufficiently mature to cope with extrauterine life, yet not too large

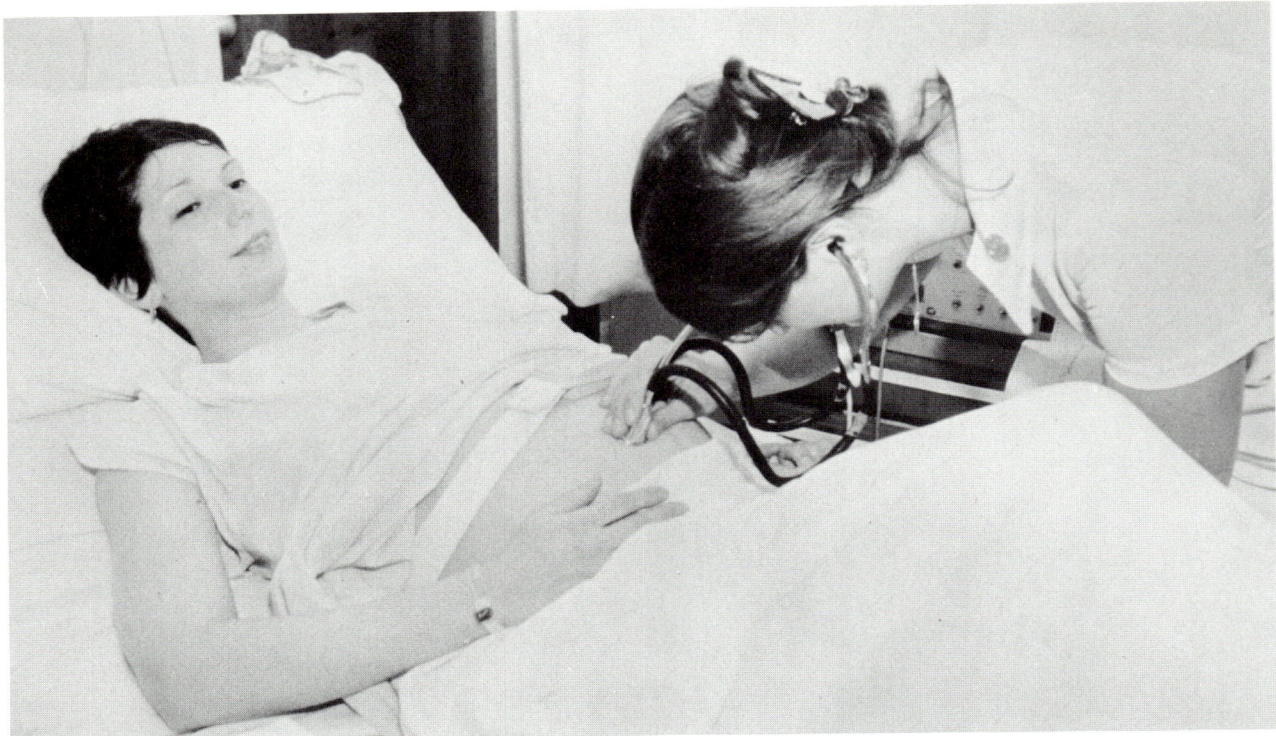

Fig. 21-12. *Taking fetal heart rate by auscultation. Nurse checks fetal heart rate before beginning continuous electronic monitoring. Strap on abdomen is external tokodynamometer to record uterine contractions. (Courtesy of the Department of Medical Photography, Children's Hospital, Buffalo, N.Y.)*

to cause mechanical difficulties in delivery. However, the trigger that converts the random, painless Braxton Hicks contractions into strong, coordinated, productive labor contractions is obscure. In some instances, labor begins before the fetus is mature (premature birth); in others, labor is delayed until the fetus and the placenta have both passed beyond the optimum point for birth (postmature birth).

A number of theories of why labor occurs have been suggested.

UTERINE STRETCH THEORY

Any hollow body organ stretched to capacity will contract and empty. A distended bladder empties by incontinence. A distended stomach empties by vomiting. By analogy, a uterus stretched to capacity by a mature fetus may also be "ripe" for emptying. This is an old theory of the cause of labor onset. Stretch may play a role in the initiation of labor, but by itself it does not seem an adequate precipitating cause. It is true that labor generally begins earlier in multiple than in single gestations, but in a single premature birth the uterus empties before it is stretched to capacity. Thus, some additional or different mechanism must be involved.

OXYTOCIN THEORY

A second long-accepted theory is that oxytocin, a hormone released by the posterior pituitary gland, initiates labor contractions. It is well established that oxytocin administered to a woman during labor acts to strengthen uterine contractions, assisting labor. It can be demonstrated that at about the 37th week of pregnancy the uterus becomes increasingly sensitive to oxytocin. (*Oxytocinase*, an enzyme produced by the placenta that apparently inhibits the action of oxytocin on uterine tissue, decreases at this time.)

Oxytocin is present in maternal blood during labor. Interestingly, it is also present under other stress situations. Thus, it may be present in the bloodstream because labor is a stress, not because it *initiates* contractions.

Animal studies have shown that despite destruction of the posterior pituitary so extensive as to preclude the production of oxytocin labor still occurs at the end of the normal gestation period.

PROGESTERONE DEPRIVATION THEORY

It is well known that progesterone is essential for maintaining a pregnancy. When the corpus luteum of pregnancy is removed in rabbits, prompt delivery of the products of conception occurs. The suggestion is that progesterone levels fall just prior to the onset of

A

B

C

D

E

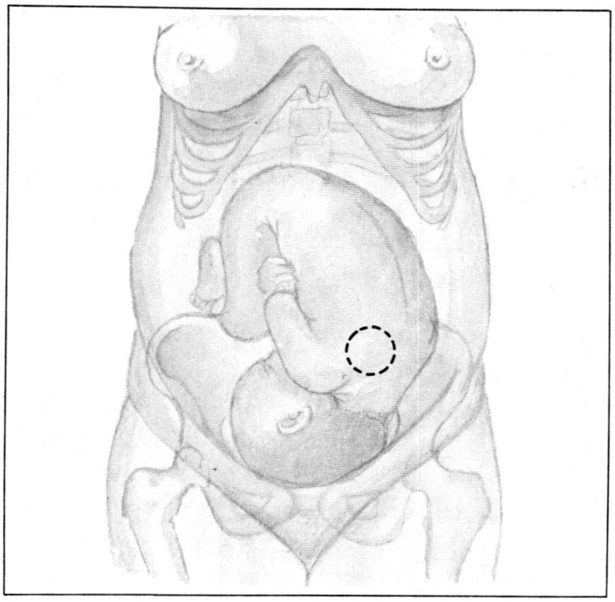

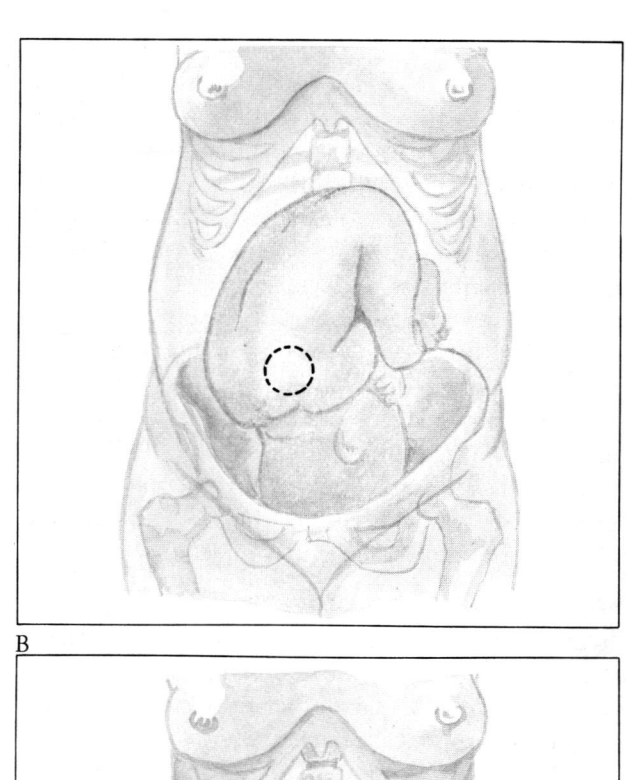

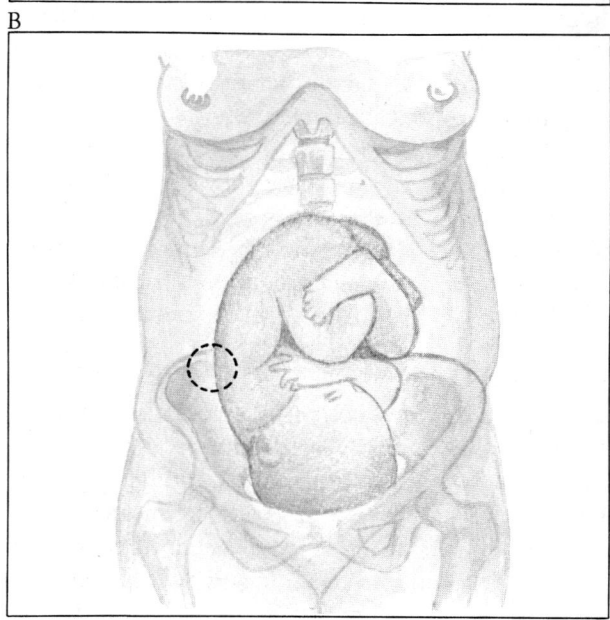

Fig. 21-13. Locating fetal heart sounds by fetal position.
A. LOA. B. ROA. C. LOP. D. ROP. E. LSA.

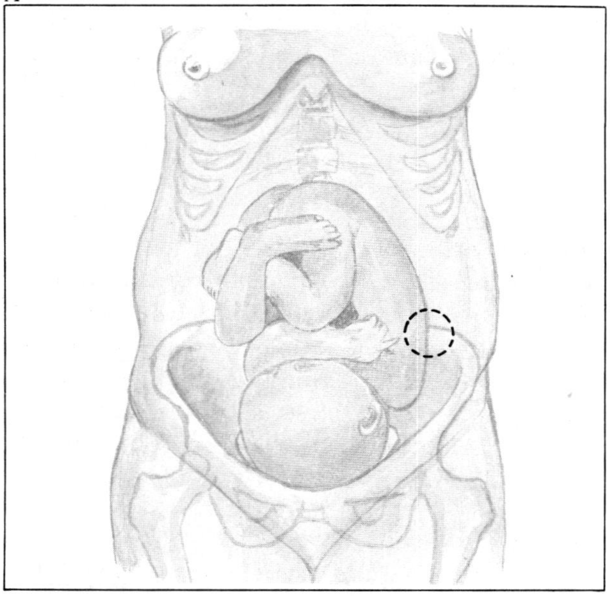

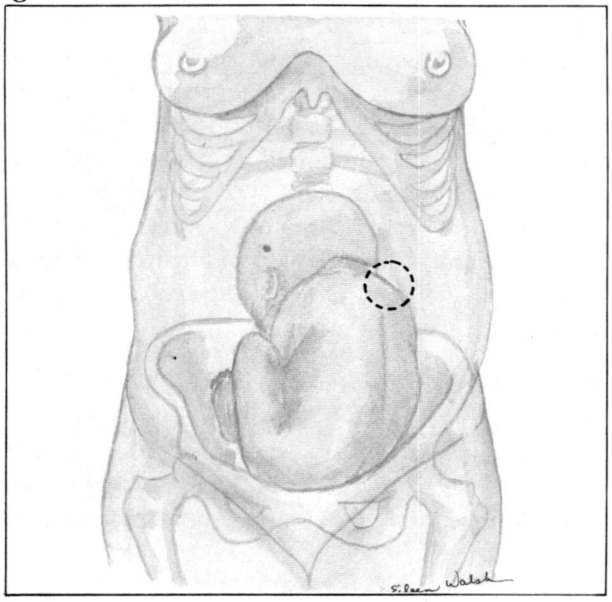

labor. This is not well documented, however, except by the observations of Haskins [9] that the placentas of women delivered by cesarean section in whom labor did not occur contain twice as much progesterone as the placentas of women who had been in labor, and by the findings of Kumar et al. [10] that in the majority of premature births the placentas contain less progesterone than those of infants delivered at term.

Exactly how progesterone can prevent contractions is puzzling. Daniel et al. [6] suggest that progesterone tends to maintain a high concentration of potassium and a low concentration of sodium chloride and water in the myometrium at the placental site. This high level of potassium may cause a myometrial block. As progesterone production falls, the block lessens, and efficient, coordinated uterine contractions occur.

FETAL ADRENAL RESPONSE THEORY

Interestingly, in 400 B.C. Hippocrates wrote that the fetus initiated labor. Two thousand years later, new research begins to suggest that his hunch was accurate. In experiments in lambs, when a fetal lamb had its pituitary gland removed in utero, labor did not begin. Labor could be initiated, however, by injecting the lamb fetus with ACTH. Removal of both adrenal glands in the fetal lamb produced the same results. Labor in these pregnancies could be initiated by the administration of cortisol. Fetal adrenal glands, therefore, appeared to be responsible for the "trigger" that initiated labor.

If the same phenomenon occurs in humans, these are the events that seem to take place: Estriol produced by the fetal adrenals is conjugated in the placenta into estrogen from early in pregnancy. As estrogen formed by fetus and placenta reaches a certain level, maternal decidua begins to synthesize and produce prostaglandin PGF2a. That prostaglandins can initiate uterine contractions has been established by the usefulness of prostaglandins in therapeutic abortion. Findings that support this theory are as follows: The adrenal glands in babies born by spontaneous labor are heavier than those of infants born by cesarean section or when labor is induced. Inhibitors of prostaglandin synthesis such as aspirin may delay labor in women. PGF2a and its immediate precursor are found in increased amounts in amniotic fluid during early spontaneous labor.

Signs of Labor

During the 40 weeks of gestation, subtle physiological and psychological changes have taken place in the gravid woman preparatory for labor. At the same time, fetal growth and development progress, finally bringing the fetus to the point where he can survive in an extrauterine environment.

By the end of pregnancy, women feel so short of breath, have so many minor discomforts (e.g., backache, frequency of urination), and have planned for so long that, however much they may dread the beginning of labor because of the stories they have heard, they rarely fail to feel relief on realizing that the time for labor is at hand.

PRELIMINARY SIGNS
Lightening
In primiparas, lightening occurs about 10 to 14 days before labor begins. It changes the shape of the woman's abdominal contour, since the fetus settles into the brim of the pelvis (engagement). Lightening gives the woman relief from the diaphragmatic pressure and shortness of breath she has been experiencing, or "lightens" her load (hence its name). The woman may have shooting pains in her legs from pressure on the sciatic nerve following lightening. She will certainly notice an increase in frequency of urination from the increased pressure on the bladder. In multiparas, lightening usually occurs on the day of labor or even after labor has begun.

Loss of Weight
A weight loss of 2 to 3 pounds may occur a day or two before the onset of labor. This is probably due to the decrease in progesterone and estrogen production, leading to a decrease in fluid retention. It is important to warn women about this weight loss, since they may associate it with fetal weight loss and worry that the fetus has died in utero.

Increase in Level of Activity
A woman may wake on the morning of labor full of energy, in contrast to her feelings during the previous month. The increase in activity is due to an increase in epinephrine, secreted to prepare her body for the work or labor that is ahead. Women need to be told that this energy is to assist them in labor. Otherwise, they will use it to clean house, iron, or shop, and will arrive at the hospital exhausted and unable to participate in labor. If the woman is extremely fatigued when she enters labor, uterine contractions cannot be maintained and she may need medication to help her achieve adequate contractions.

Braxton Hicks Contractions
In the last week or days before labor begins, the woman usually notices extremely strong Braxton Hicks contractions, which she may interpret as true labor contractions. They can be differentiated from

true labor contractions in a number of ways. True contractions may be slightly irregular at first, but become regular and predictable within a matter of hours; false contractions remain irregular. True contractions are generally felt first in the lower back and sweep around to the abdomen in a wave; false labor contractions are generally confined to the abdomen. True contractions increase in duration, frequency, and intensity; false contractions do not. True contractions continue no matter what the woman's level of activity; false contractions often disappear if the woman ambulates. The ultimate distinction is the presence or absence of cervical dilatation. Over a few hours' time, true contractions cause effacement and dilatation of the cervix; false contractions cause no cervical changes.

Women, particularly primiparas, have great difficulty in distinguishing between the two forms of contraction. A woman sometimes comes to the hospital and is admitted to the labor unit because the false contractions so closely simulate real labor. It is discouraging for a woman who is having discomfort (and false or not, strong Braxton Hicks contractions cause discomfort) to be told that she is not in true labor and should return home to wait for true contractions to begin. It is something like waking Christmas morning and being told that Christmas has been postponed for a week. Such women need sympathetic support. They do not find their situation amusing. They can be assured that misinterpreting labor signals is a natural mistake. They can be told that if false contractions have become so strong they can be mistaken for true labor, true labor is not far away.

Ripening of the Cervix

Ripening of the cervix is an internal sign, of which the woman is not aware; it is seen only on pelvic examination. The physician will look for this sign at the pregnancy's predicted term. All during pregnancy, the cervix feels softer than normal and has the consistency of an earlobe (Goodell's sign). At term, the cervix becomes still softer, until it can be described as "butter-soft," and tips forward. This is ripening, an internal announcement that labor is close at hand.

Rupture of the Membranes

Labor may begin with rupture of the membranes, which the woman experiences as either a sudden gush or scanty, slow seeping of clear fluid from the vagina. Women worry when labor begins with rupture of the membranes because of old wives' tales that such labors are "dry" and thus difficult and long. Actually, amniotic fluid continues to be formed until delivery of the membranes, after the child is born, and so no labor is ever dry. Early rupture of the membranes causes the fetal head to settle snugly into the pelvis and may actually shorten labor.

A woman who experiences rupture of the membranes as a sudden gush of fluid should lie down with her feet elevated. Someone should telephone her physician, who will probably instruct her to come into a hospital so that it can be determined whether the fetal head is firmly engaged and fitting snugly into the pelvic brim. If it is not, the umbilical cord may prolapse into the vagina after the membranes supporting it are ruptured. A prolapsed cord may be compressed by the fetal head, and the fetus's oxygen supply may be compromised.

If membranes rupture more than 24 hours prior to the delivery of the child, intrauterine infection is a possible consequence. Labor is generally induced at the end of 24 hours following membrane rupture if it has not begun spontaneously by that time, provided the woman is estimated to be at term. An antibiotic may be ordered for the woman to protect the fetus against infection, although there is no established proof that amnionitis will be prevented by such a measure.

Ask the woman whose membranes have ruptured (many women refer to "the bag of waters breaking") if she noticed the color of the fluid. Green staining means the fluid was contaminated with meconium, a possible sign of fetal distress. Yellow staining may mean blood incompatibility. Pink staining may indicate slight bleeding, such as occurs with a placenta at the edge of the cervix (placenta previa).

Show

The pressure of the descending presenting part of the fetus causes rupture of minute capillaries in the mucous membrane of the cervix. This small amount of blood mixes with mucus and is evident as a pink or brown (old blood) vaginal discharge when the mucous plug (operculum) that has filled the cervical canal during pregnancy is released. Show should be no more than a pinkish discharge. Fresh bleeding accompanying the operculum discharge is abnormal and is a danger sign of labor, usually signaling placental bleeding. Show is proof that cervical dilatation is beginning; with dilatation, the operculum can no longer be contained in the canal.

SIGNS OF TRUE LABOR
Uterine Contractions

The surest sign that labor has begun is the initiation of effective, productive uterine contractions.

Uterine contractions are involuntary. The woman has no more control over their duration, intensity, or progress than she does over her heartbeat. However, she can control the degree of discomfort contractions give her if she uses the exercises she has learned in preparation-for-labor classes.

Labor contractions begin at "pacemaker" points in the myometrium of the uterus near the uterotubal junctions. The contraction sweeps down over the uterus as a wave. After a short rest period, another contraction is initiated and the downward wave begins again.

In early labor, the uterotubal pacemakers may not be working in a synchronous manner; in this event contractions are sometimes strong, sometimes weak, and not very regular. This mild incoordination of early labor improves after a few hours, however, as the pacemakers begin to function smoothly.

In some women contractions appear to originate in the lower uterine segment rather than in the fundus. These are reverse, ineffective contractions, which actually cause contraction rather than dilatation of the cervix. That contractions are being initiated in a reverse pattern is difficult to tell from palpation. It can be suspected if a woman tells you that she feels pain in her lower abdomen before the contraction is readily palpated at the fundus. It is truly revealed only when cervical dilatation does not occur.

Other women seem to have additional pacemaker sites in other portions of the uterus, in which case severe incoordination of contractions will occur. Uncoordinated contractions slow labor and may lead to failure to progress in labor and fetal distress because they do not allow for adequate placental filling. Evaluating the rate and intensity and pattern of uterine contractions is an important nursing responsibility with a woman in labor.

Uterine contractions have three phases: a first phase during which the intensity of the contraction increases (the increment or crescendo phase), a second phase during which the contraction reaches its height (apex), and a third phase during which the intensity decreases (decrescendo). The first phase is longer than the other two phases combined. A uterine contraction is diagrammed in Fig. 21-14.

Uterine contractions can be palpated by placing your hand on the woman's fundus. They should be assessed in terms of three characteristics:

1. DURATION. The duration of a contraction is the length of the contraction from the time you can feel it on the uterus until it can be felt to relax again. The woman will not feel it as soon as you do, but deter-

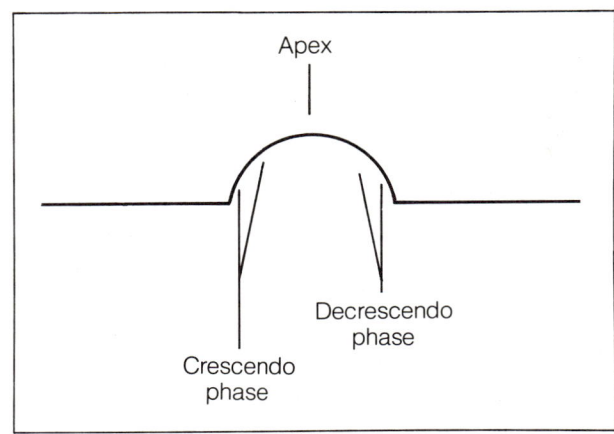

Fig. 21-14. Three phases of a uterine contraction.

mine time from your objective view, not hers, for consistency.

If labor is being electronically monitored, the duration of a contraction is measured from the point at which it reaches 20 mm Hg on the monitor screen or tape until, after increasing, it returns to 20 mm Hg again. The woman feels the contraction when the pressure reaches about 25 mm Hg.

2. INTENSITY. Intensity is the strength of a uterine contraction. Contractions are *mild* if the uterus can be easily indented with your fingers at the height of a contraction, *moderate* if indentation is becoming difficult, and *strong* if the uterus cannot be indented by examining fingers. Always feel for intensity gently; the fundus grows sensitive to manipulation as labor progresses, and the feel of probing fingers becomes painful.

If a uterine monitor is being used, a *mild* contraction is one in which pressure is about 30 mm Hg. A *strong* contraction has a pressure reading of 50 mm Hg. *Moderate* contractions, therefore, are those with pressures between 30 and 50 mm Hg.

3. FREQUENCY. Frequency is the rate at which contractions are occurring. Frequency is timed from the *beginning* of one contraction to the beginning of the next. The interval may be 40 to 50 minutes at the beginning of labor but gradually decreases until contractions are no more than 2 minutes apart in the second stage of labor. It is important that a relaxation interval always be present, even if it is only a minute in length, to allow time for uterine blood vessels to fill and continue to supply adequate nutrients and oxygen to the fetus during labor.

Effacement

Effacement is the shortening and thinning of the cervical canal from its normal length of 1 to 2 cm to a

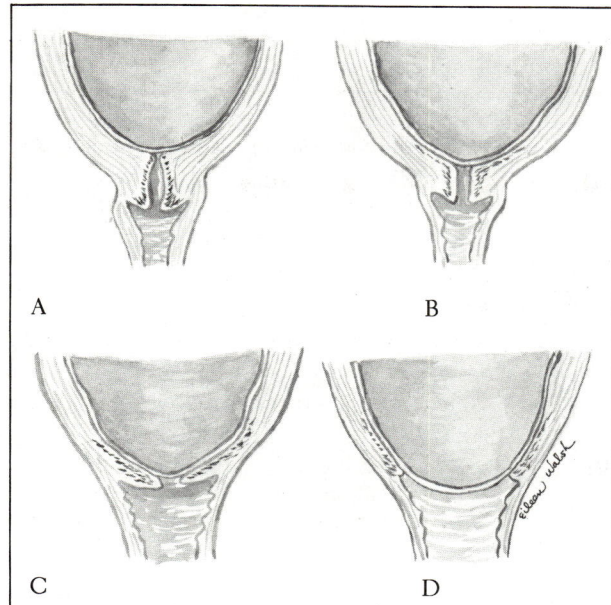

Fig. 21-15. Effacement and dilatation of cervix. A. Beginning labor. B. Effacement is beginning; dilatation is not apparent yet. C. Effacement is almost complete. D. After complete effacement, dilatation proceeds rapidly.

structure with paper-thin edges in which no canal distinct from the uterus appears to exist. It is illustrated in Fig. 21-15.

In primiparas, effacement is accomplished before dilatation begins. This is an important phenomenon to point out to a woman during her first labor. She will become discouraged if, for example, at 12:00 noon the physician reports to her that she is 2 cm dilated and reports again at 4:00 P.M. that she is still 2 cm dilated; it will seem to her that absolutely nothing has happened in four hours. However, effacement is happening, and when effacement is complete, dilatation will then progress rapidly.

In multiparas, dilatation may proceed before effacement is complete. Effacement must occur at the end of dilatation before the fetus can be safely pushed through the cervical canal or cervical tearing may result.

Dilatation

Dilatation (Fig. 21-15) denotes the enlargement of the cervical canal from an opening a few millimeters wide to one large enough to permit passage of the fetus (about 10 cm).

Dilatation occurs for two reasons: Uterine contractions gradually increase the diameter of the cervical canal lumen, and the presenting part of the fetus presses against the cervix. If the membranes are intact, they push ahead of the fetus and serve as an opening wedge; if they are ruptured, the presenting part will serve this same function. Excessive pressure against the cervix, such as would occur if the woman pushed during this stage, interferes with dilatation by causing edema of the cervix. The best action of the woman during the stage of dilatation is to relax, so that she does not push with contractions.

There is an increase in the amount of show as dilatation begins, since the last of the operculum is dislodged, and minute capillaries in the cervix rupture.

Uterine Changes

As labor contractions progress, the uterus is gradually differentiated into two distinct portions. The upper portion becomes thicker and active, preparing it to exert the strength necessary to expel the fetus when the expulsion phase of labor is reached. The lower segment becomes thin-walled, supple, and passive, so that the fetus can be pushed out of the uterus easily.

As the lower segment thins and the upper segment thickens, the boundary between the two portions becomes marked by a ridge on the inner uterine surface, the *physiological retraction ring*. This is normal in labor. In a difficult labor, particularly in obstructed labor, when the fetus is larger than the birth canal, the round ligaments of the uterus may become tense during dilatation and expulsion and may be palpable on the abdomen. The normal physiological retraction ring may become prominent and observable as an abdominal indentation. This is termed a *pathological retraction ring*, or *Bandl's ring*. It is a danger sign of labor that may signify impending rupture of the lower uterine segment if the obstruction to labor is not relieved.

A comparison of false labor and true labor signs is shown in Table 21-3.

Divisions of Labor

Labor has traditionally been divided into three stages: a first stage of dilatation (where the uterus dilates or opens), a second stage (during which the infant is actually born), and a third or placental stage (during which the placenta is delivered). Some authorities term the first hour following delivery of the placenta the "fourth stage" of labor, to emphasize the importance of the close observation needed at that time to ensure safety of the mother. This is a misleading term, however, particularly as regards planning nursing intervention. Active nursing intervention to en-

Table 21-3. Characteristics of True Labor Versus False Labor

Characteristic	False Labor	True Labor
Contractions		
Location	Often felt in abdomen	Often felt in back and sweep forward onto abdomen
Regularity	Irregular	Become regular
Intensity	Mild	Become increasingly stronger
Frequency	No change	Become gradually more frequent
Show	None	Present
Amniotic fluid	None present	Membranes may rupture with amniotic fluid present
Cervical dilatation	None	Gradual progression of effacement and dilatation
Effect of ambulation	Contractions often fade on ambulation	Contractions continue no matter what the position or activity

sure safety of the mother should be engaged in during the entire pregnancy, labor and delivery, and the postpartal period, not just in the first hour after birth. Newer terminology in reference to labor also makes use of this term obsolete.

Friedman [7] has classified the first and second stages of labor into divisions according to the objective being accomplished during each timed interval. These new divisions are a *preparatory* division, a *dilatational* division, and a *pelvic* division.

THE PREPARATORY DIVISION

The preparatory division consists of two phases: a latent phase and an acceleration (active) phase. It is that time in labor from the onset of regular perceived contractions to the end of the acceleration phase. During the latent phase (that period of labor beginning at the onset of regular perceived uterine contractions and ending at the point where rapid cervical dilatation begins), contractions are mild and short (20 to 30 seconds in length). In a woman who is psychologically prepared for labor and who does not tense at each tightening sensation in her abdomen, beginning contractions cause only minimal discomfort. The woman can continue to walk about and make preparations for her hospital stay, such as last-minute packing of her suitcase or preparing her children for her departure and giving instructions to the person who will take care of them while she is away.

Contractions gradually increase in duration and intensity. The cervix dilates from 0 to 2 cm during this phase. The phase lasts about 6 hours in a nullipara, 4.5 hours in a multipara. A woman who enters labor with a "nonripe" cervix or one that is not soft will have a longer than usual latent phase. Analgesia given too early in labor will prolong this phase. The latent phase can be prolonged when a cephalopelvic disproportion exists.

The acceleration phase is the remainder of the first division of labor. During this phase, cervical dilatation begins to be accomplished more rapidly; contractions are stronger (30 to 45 seconds long; 3 to 5 minutes apart). This phase lasts about 3 hours in a nullipara, 2 hours in a multipara. Although this is a difficult time for a woman in labor (contractions begin to "bite" or cause true discomfort), it is also an exciting time because she can realize that something is changing. It may be a frightening time as she realizes that this labor is truly progressing; she can never go backward.

THE DILATATIONAL DIVISION

The second division of labor, the dilatational division, is that time period during which cervical dilatation proceeds at its most rapid pace (also termed the *period of maximum slope*). Analgesic administration has little effect on progress at this point. Cervical dilatation proceeds at an average rate of 3.5 cm per hour in nulliparas, 5.9 cm per hour in multiparas.

Most women assume that dilatation occurs at a steady rate throughout labor. They may grow discouraged at realizing that in the 10 hours previous to this (the latent and acceleration phases) their cervix has only dilated 4 cm. They imagine that labor will last at least 15 hours more. In nulliparas, however, cervical dilatation from 4 to 8 cms will take only 1 to 2 hours more; in multiparas, it may be as short as half an hour. During this division, contractions grow strong, and hard and frequent (45 to 60 seconds in duration; 2 to 3 minute intervals).

THE PELVIC DIVISION

The pelvic division includes a deceleration phase and a fetal descent phase. Deceleration is a misnomer in that the process of labor does not actually slow at this point; the final degrees of cervical dilatation are achieved and the cervix retracts over the presenting part. Contractions are so hard that the uterus feels like wood at the peak of a contraction, and they are quite long (60 to 70 seconds in duration). If the membranes have not previously ruptured or been ruptured by amniotomy, they will rupture as a rule at full dilatation. Show will be present as the last of the operculum is released. This phase averages about 1 hour in a nullipara, one-half hour in a multipara.

With retraction of the cervix over the presenting part, fetal descent and negotiation of the pelvis occurs rapidly. The woman may experience momentary nausea or vomiting, since pressure is no longer exerted on the stomach because of the downward movement of the fetus. Contractions change from the characteristic crescendo-decrescendo pattern she has grown accustomed to, to an overwhelming, uncontrollable urge to push or bear down with contractions as if she were moving her bowels. She pushes with such force that she perspires and the blood vessels in her neck become distended.

As the woman undergoes these changes, she may experience a feeling of panic or acute anxiety and become argumentative or irritable. Up to this point, she may have felt in charge of her labor, aware that she could control the degree of pain or discomfort by breathing exercises. Now the sensation in her abdomen is so intense that it may seem as though labor has taken charge of her. A few minutes before, she enjoyed having her forehead wiped with a cool cloth; now she may knock your hand away. A minute before, she enjoyed having her husband rub her back; now she may resist his touch or thrust him away.

It takes a few contractions of this new kind for her to realize that everything is still all right, just different; to appreciate that it feels good, not frightening, to push with contractions. In actuality, the need to push becomes so intense that she cannot stop herself from pushing. She barely hears the conversation in the room around her. She does not hear your instructions. All of her energy, her thoughts, her being are directed toward delivering her child.

A woman may have sharp cramps in the calves of her legs as the fetus is pushed against pelvic nerves. These cramps are relieved in the same way as are the cramps that tend to occur during pregnancy, namely, by straightening the leg and dorsiflexing the foot. The cramp may recur with the next contraction, however.

As she pushes, using her abdominal muscles and the involuntary uterine contractions, the fetus is pushed out of the dilated uterus through the birth canal (Fig. 21-16).

Fetal Position Changes

Passage of the fetus through the birth canal involves a number of different position changes to keep the smallest diameter of the fetal head (in cephalic presentations) always presenting to the smallest diameter of the birth canal. The position changes are termed *descent, flexion, internal rotation, extension, external rotation,* and *expulsion* (Fig. 21-17).

DESCENT. Descent begins with engagement. In primiparas, descent occurs approximately two weeks before labor. In multiparas, it occurs with the beginning of labor or at the pelvic division. Descent is the downward movement of the biparietal diameter of the fetal head to within the pelvic inlet. Full descent occurs when the fetal head extrudes beyond the dilated cervix and touches the posterior vaginal floor. When the signs of the second stage of labor are apparent, the fetal heartbeat should be recorded, since this is a particularly dangerous point for the fetus; as he moves downward into the birth canal, the cord may be compressed.

FLEXION. As descent occurs, pressure from the pelvic floor causes the head to bend forward onto the chest. The smallest anteroposterior diameter (the suboccipitobregmatic diameter) is the one presented to the birth canal in this flexed position.

INTERNAL ROTATION. The head enters the pelvis with the fetal anteroposterior head diameter in a diagonal or transverse position. The head flexes as it touches the pelvic floor, and the occiput rotates until it is superior, or just below the symphysis pubis, bringing the head into the best diameter for the outlet of the pelvis (the anteroposterior diameter is now in an anteroposterior plane of the pelvis). The shoulders, coming next, are also brought into an optimum position to enter the inlet.

EXTENSION. As the occiput is born, the back of the neck stops beneath the pubic arch and acts as a pivot for the rest of the head. The head thus extends, and the foremost parts of the head, the face and chin, are born.

EXTERNAL ROTATION. In external rotation, almost immediately after the head of the infant is born, the head rotates from the anteroposterior position it assumed to enter the outlet back to the diagonal or transverse position of the early part of the second stage. The aftercoming shoulders are thus brought into an anteroposterior position, which is best for en-

The Labor Process

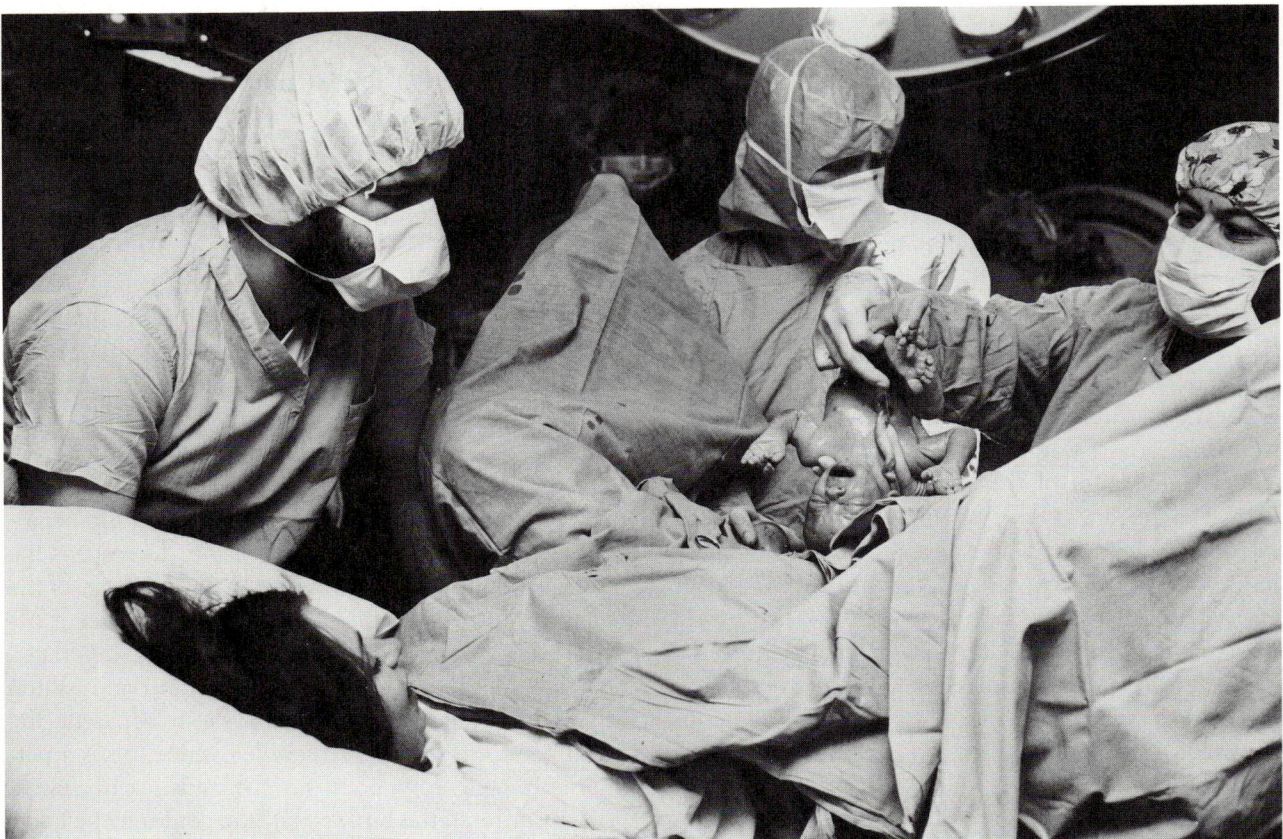

Fig. 21-16. New parents watch their baby being born. (Courtesy of the Department of Medical Photography, Children's Hospital, Buffalo, N.Y.)

tering the outlet. The anterior shoulder stops under the symphysis pubis, allowing the posterior shoulder to be delivered first, assisted perhaps by upward flexion of the infant's body.

EXPULSION. Once the shoulders are delivered, the rest of the baby is delivered easily and smoothly because of its smaller size. This is expulsion and the end of the pelvic division of labor (Fig. 21-18).

The principal clinical features of the divisions of labor are shown in Table 21-4. Newer divisions of labor and characteristics are contrasted to traditional stages of labor in Table 21-5. Divisions of labor are shown diagrammatically in Fig. 21-19.

GRAPHING LABOR PROGRESS

Graphing labor progress can be an independent nursing function. Using square-ruled graph paper, number the left side of the graph 1 to 10 (representing centimeters of cervical dilatation). Number the bottom line to represent hours of labor. Number the right side of the graph −3 to +4 to represent the station of the fetal presenting part.

After each cervical examination, plot the extent of cervical dilatation and the fetal descent on the graph. The pattern of cervical dilatation when graphed in this way is typically an S-shaped curve. The descent pattern of the fetus typically forms a downward curve. The sharp downward shape of fetal descent should cross the dilatation line at the same time as maximum cervical dilatation occurs (phase of maximum slope). A typical labor graph is shown in Fig. 21-20.

Prolonged Latent Phase

A latent phase that is more than 20 hours in a nullipara and 14 hours in a multipara is a prolonged latent phase.

Protracted Active-Phase Dilatation

If the phase of maximum slope occurs at a rate less than 1.2 cm per hour for multiparas and 1.5 cm per hour for nulliparas, it is a protracted or abnormally extended phase.

Prolonged Deceleration Phase

If a deceleration phase is longer than 3 hours in a nullipara, 1 hour in a multipara, the phase is abnormally long or protracted.

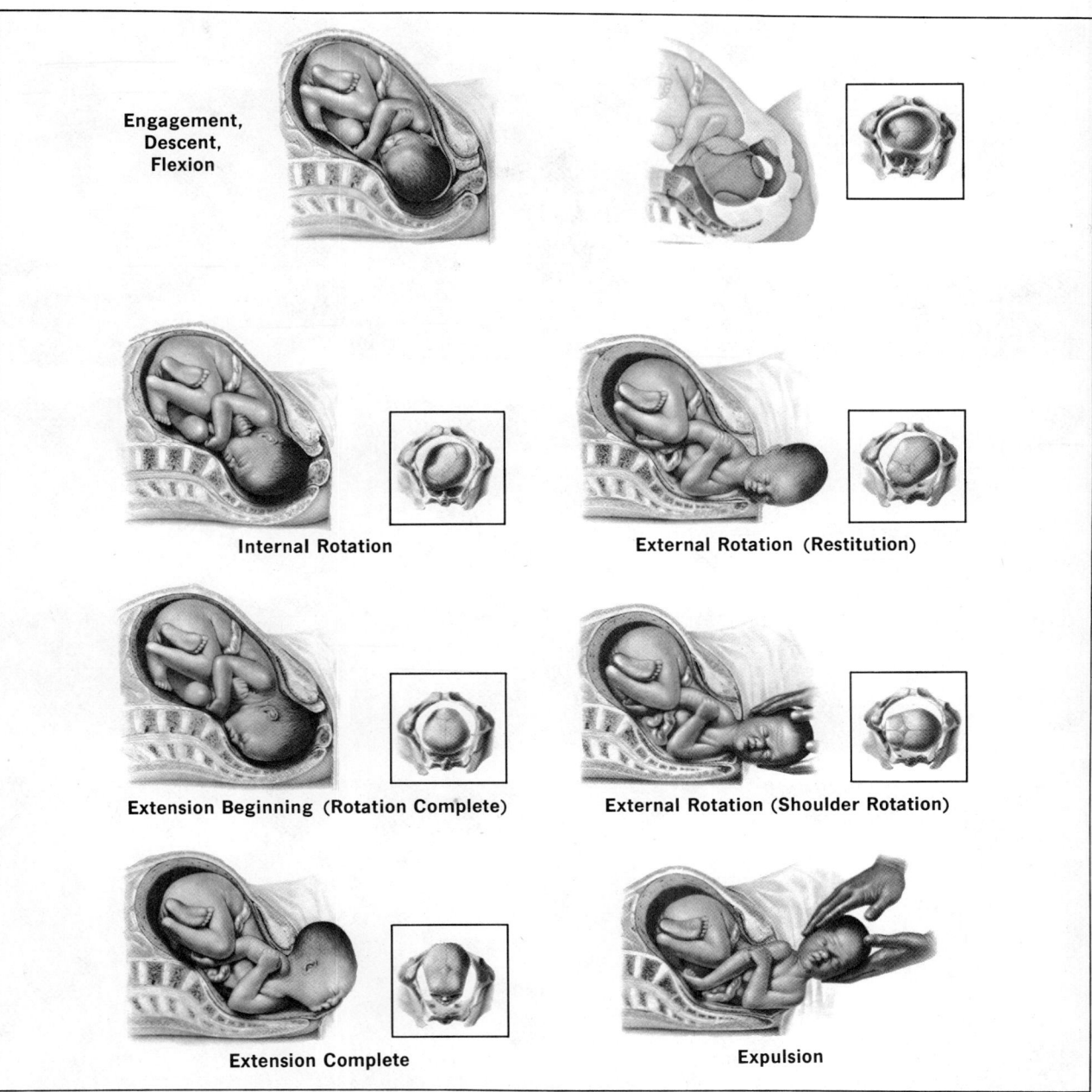

Fig. 21-17. Mechanism of normal labor in left occipitoanterior position. (From Clinical Education Aid, No. 13, Ross Laboratories, Columbus, Ohio, 1964.)

Protracted Descent
The slope of fetal descent is normally greater than 1 cm per hour in nulliparas, 2 cm per hour in multiparas. A descent under these limits is considered a protracted descent.

Secondary Arrest of Dilatation
This is cessation of progressive dilatation in the active phase before full dilatation.

Arrest of Descent
This is cessation of progressive linear descent occurring in the pelvic division.

These abnormal patterns are shown in Fig. 21-21.
Plotting the duration of labor phases offers a way to recognize any indication that something is wrong with the labor. The management of prolonged labor or arrest of labor is discussed in Chap. 35.

PLACENTAL STAGE OF LABOR
The *placental stage* begins with delivery of the infant and ends with the delivery of the placenta. Two sepa-

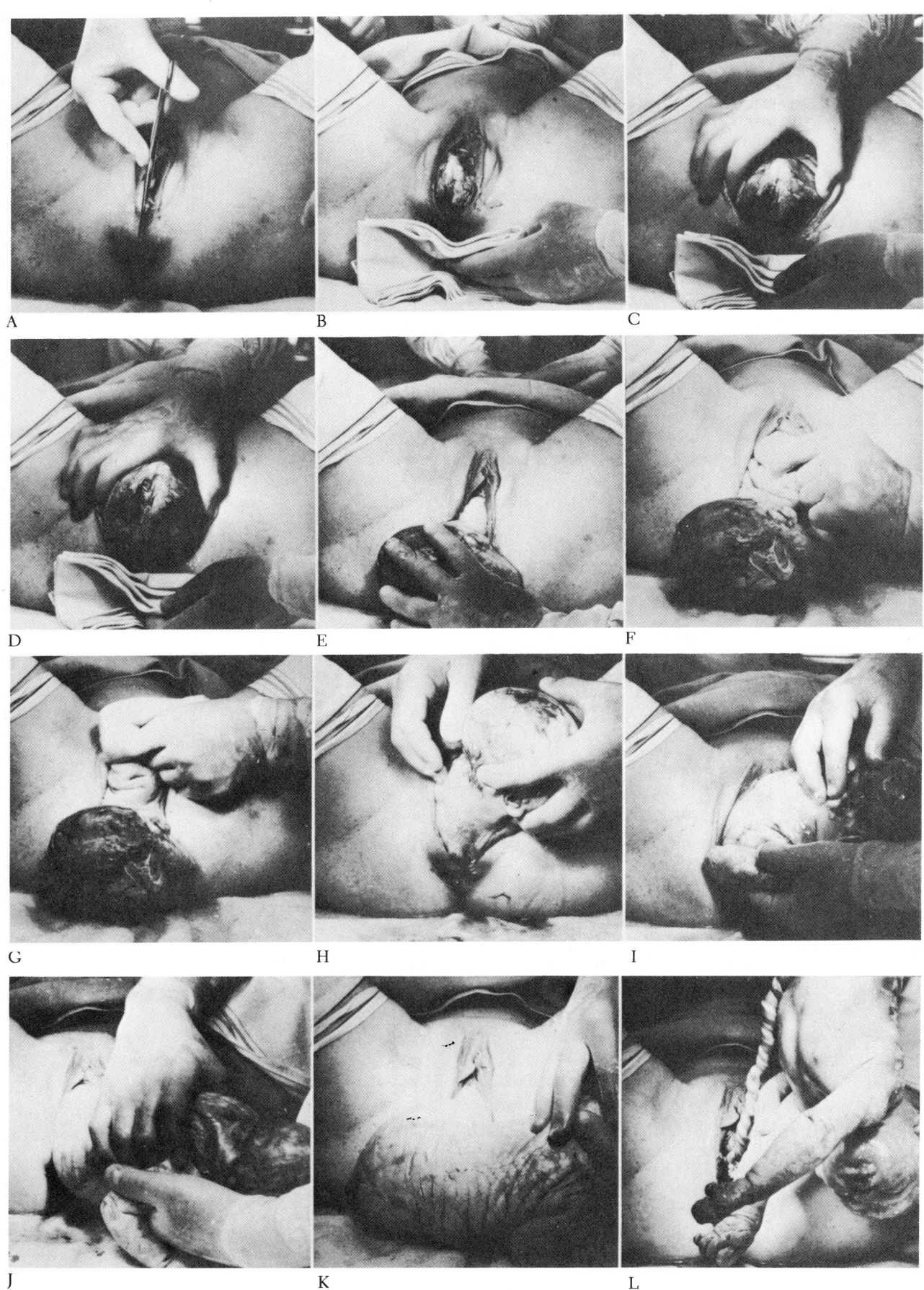

308 *Period of Parturition: Becoming a Parent*

Table 21-4. Principal Clinical Features of the Divisions of Labor

Characteristic	Preparatory Division	Dilatational Division	Pelvic Division
Functions	Contractions coordinated, polarized, oriented; cervix prepared	Cervix actively dilated	Pelvis negotiated; mechanisms of labor; fetal descent; delivery
Interval	Latent and acceleration phases	Phase of maximum slope	Deceleration phase and second stage
Measurement	Elapsed duration	Linear rate of dilatation	Linear rate of descent
Diagnosable disorders	Prolonged latent phase	Protracted dilatation; protracted descent	Prolonged deceleration; secondary arrest of dilatation; arrest of descent; failure of descent

Source. E. Friedman, *Labor, Clinical Evaluation and Management* (2nd ed.). New York: Appleton-Century-Crofts, 1978.

Table 21-5. Divisions of Labor

| Assessment | Preparatory Division | | Dilatational Division | Pelvic Division | |
	Latent Phase	Acceleration Phase	Phase of Maximum Slope	Deceleration Phase	Fetal Descent
Time interval	6.1 hours nullipara	3.4 hours nullipara	1–2 hours nullipara (3.5 cm/hr dilatation rate)	0.7 hour nullipara	0.7 hour nullipara (3.6 cm/hr rate)
	4.5 hours multipara	2.1 hours multipara	½–1 hour multipara (5.9 cm/hr dilatation rate)	0.3 hour multipara	0.3 hour multipara (7.0 cm/hr rate)
Contractions					
Duration	20–30 seconds		30–60 seconds	60–70 seconds	
Frequency	5–20 minutes		3–5 minutes	2 minutes	
Intensity	Mild (30 mm Hg)		Moderate–strong (30–50 mm Hg)	Strong (50–100 mm Hg)	
Fetal descent	Station 0 in nullipara		+1 to +2	+2 to +4	
	Station 0 to +2 in multipara		+1 to +2	+2 to +4	
Cervical dilatation	0–2 cm	2–4 cm	4–8 cm	8–10 cm	

|———————— Traditional first stage ————————| |———— Traditional transition period and second stage ————|

Source. Adapted from E. Friedman, *Labor, Clinical Evaluation and Management* (2nd ed.). New York: Appleton-Century-Crofts, 1978.

rate phases are involved: a placental separation phase and a placental expulsion phase.

Following the birth of the infant, the uterus can be palpated as a firm, round mass just inferior to the level of the umbilicus. After a few minutes of rest, uterine contractions begin again, and the organ assumes a discoid shape. It retains this new shape until the placenta has separated, about 5 minutes after delivery of the infant.

Placental Separation

Placental separation takes place automatically as the uterus resumes contractions. With a contraction, there is such a disproportion between the placenta itself and its attachment site as the uterus contracts down on an almost empty interior that folding and separation of the placenta occur. Active bleeding on the maternal surface of the placenta begins with sep-

Fig. 21-18. Birth of a baby. (From D. Danforth [Ed.], Textbook of Obstetrics and Gynecology [2nd ed.]. New York: Harper & Row, 1971. Reproduced with permission.)

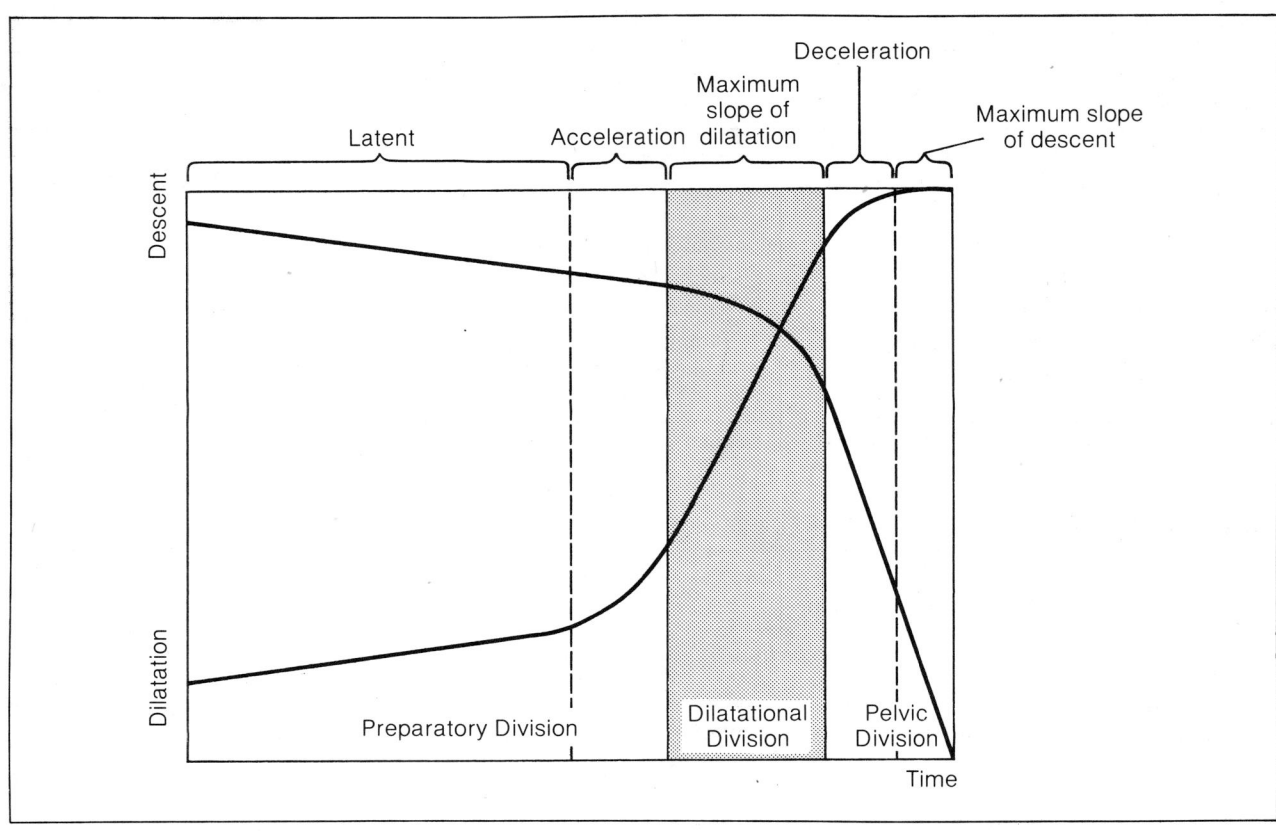

Fig. 21-19. Divisions of labor (From E. Friedman, Labor, Clinical Evaluation and Management [2nd ed.]. New York: Appleton-Century-Crofts, 1978.)

Fig. 21-20. Normal labor graph.

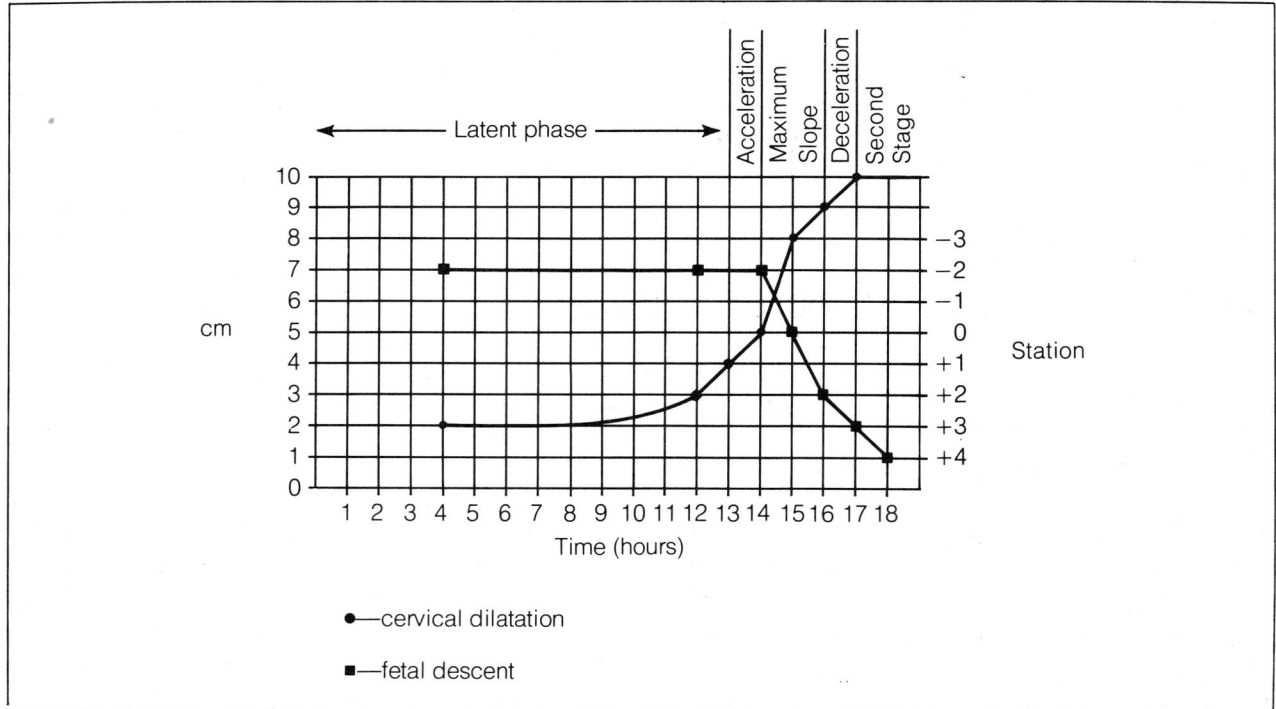

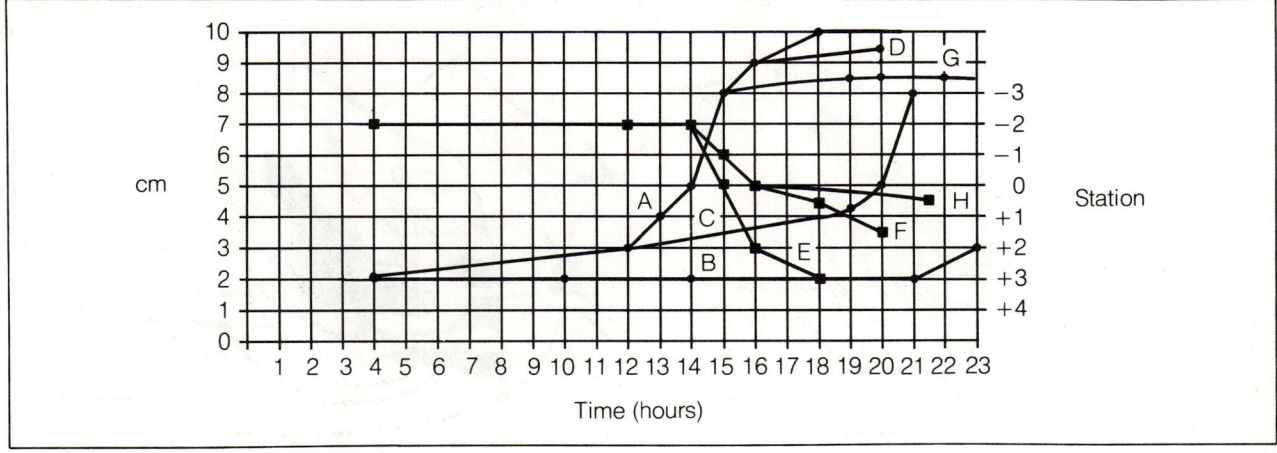

Fig. 21-21. Abnormal labor graph. A = normal labor curve, B = prolonged latent phase, C = protracted active-phase dilatation, D = prolonged deceleration phase, E = normal descent, F = protracted descent, G = secondary arrest of dilatation, H = arrest of descent.

aration; the bleeding helps to separate the placenta still further by pushing it away from its site. As separation is completed, the placenta sinks to the posterior aspect of the lower uterine segment or the upper vagina.

The occurrence of separation is suggested by a number of signs: a sudden gush of blood from the vagina; the extension of the umbilical cord 3 or more inches out of the vagina; a change in the uterus as it becomes firmer and round in shape again and rises high in the abdomen to the level of the umbilicus.

If the placenta separates first at its center and last at its edges, it tends to fold on itself like an umbrella and presents at the vaginal opening with the fetal surface evident (Fig. 21-22A). It appears shiny and glistening from the fetal membranes. This is called a *Schultze presentation*. About 80 percent of placentas separate and present this way. If the placenta separates first at its edges, it slides along the uterine surface and presents at the vagina with the maternal surface evident (Fig. 21-22B). It looks raw, red, and irregular because its cotyledons show. This is a *Duncan presentation*. The two presentations have long been remembered by nurses by their associating "shiny" (the fetal membrane surface) with Schultze and "dirty" (the irregular maternal surface) with Duncan (Fig. 21-23).

Bleeding occurs with placental separation as part of the normal consequence of the process, before the uterus can contract enough following placental delivery to seal maternal sinuses. The normal blood loss is 250 to 300 ml.

Placental Expulsion

Expulsion of the placenta may be effected by the mother's bearing down as she did during the second stage of labor; or, if she is anesthetized, by the physician's gentle pressure on the fundus of the uterus (after he has first established that the uterus is firm and contracted). If pressure is applied to a uterus in a noncontracted state, it may evert (turn inside out). This is a grave complication of delivery; in an everted uterus, the maternal blood sinuses are open, and gross hemorrhage occurs.

If the placenta does not deliver spontaneously, the physician will have to remove it manually. With delivery of the placenta, the third stage of labor is over.

Danger Signals of Labor

There is a wide variation in the pattern of labor contractions and maternal response to labor and delivery. Certain signals alert you that the course of events is deviating too far from normal.

FETAL DANGER SIGNALS
Fetal Heart Rate

Monitoring fetal heart rates and reporting deviations from the normal are primary responsibilities of the nurse during labor. As a rule of thumb, fetal heart rates over 160 beats per minute (marked fetal tachycardia) or below 100 beats per minute (marked fetal bradycardia) are signals that the fetus is experiencing distress. Stage II and variable dip patterns on fetal monitors are just as important signs of fetal distress as tachycardia or bradycardia. The fetal heart rate may return to within 101 to 159 beats per minute between these patterns and give you a false feeling of security if you are relying only on the first rule of thumb.

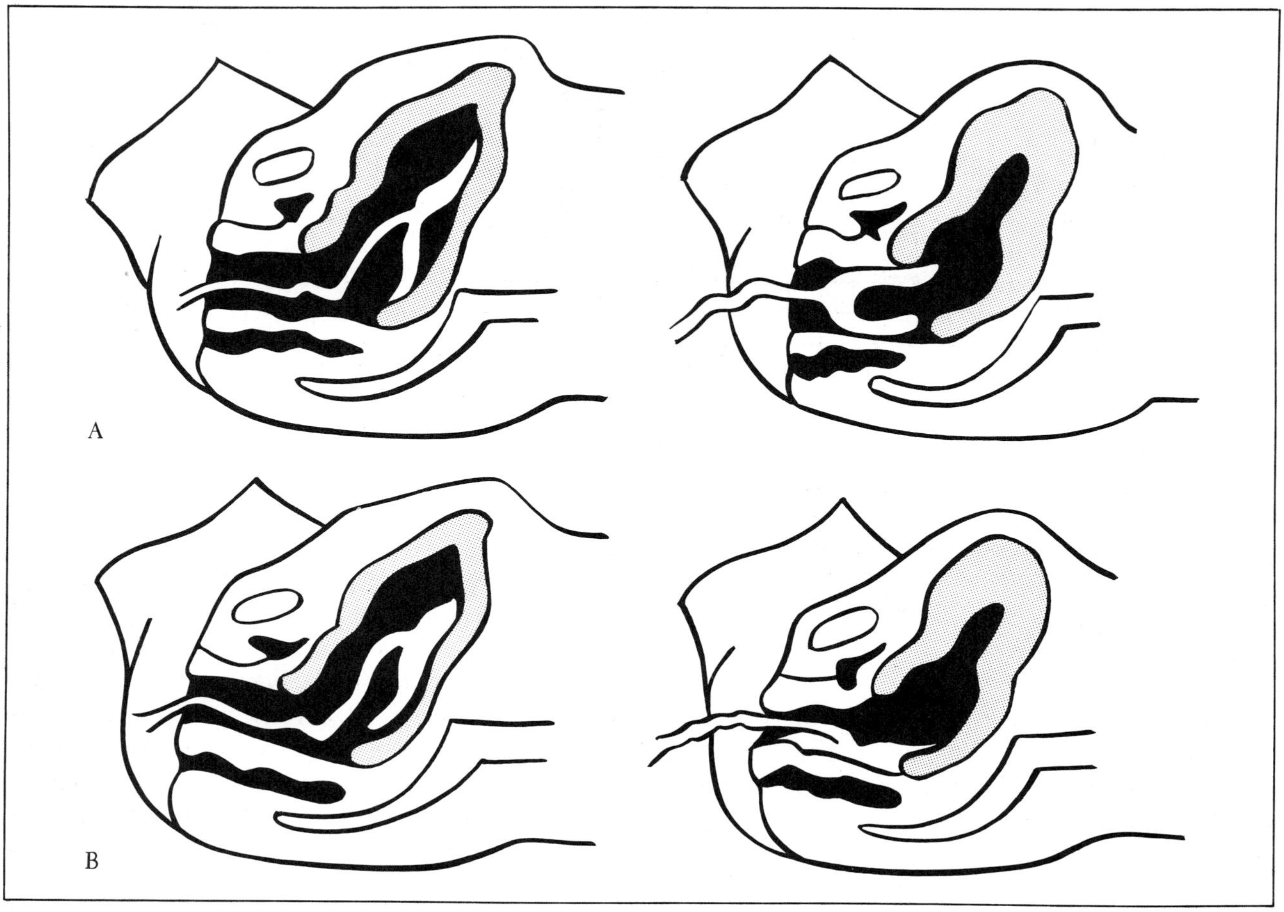

Fig. 21-22. Delivery of the placenta. Note the change in contour of the mother's abdomen after separation of placenta. A. Placenta separates first at center and delivers fetal surface in evidence (Schultze presentation). B. Placenta separates first at edge and delivers with maternal surface in evidence (Duncan presentation).

Fig. 21-23. Maternal (left) and fetal (right) surface of the placenta. (From Clinical Education Aid, No. 2, Ross Laboratories, Columbus, Ohio, 1960.)

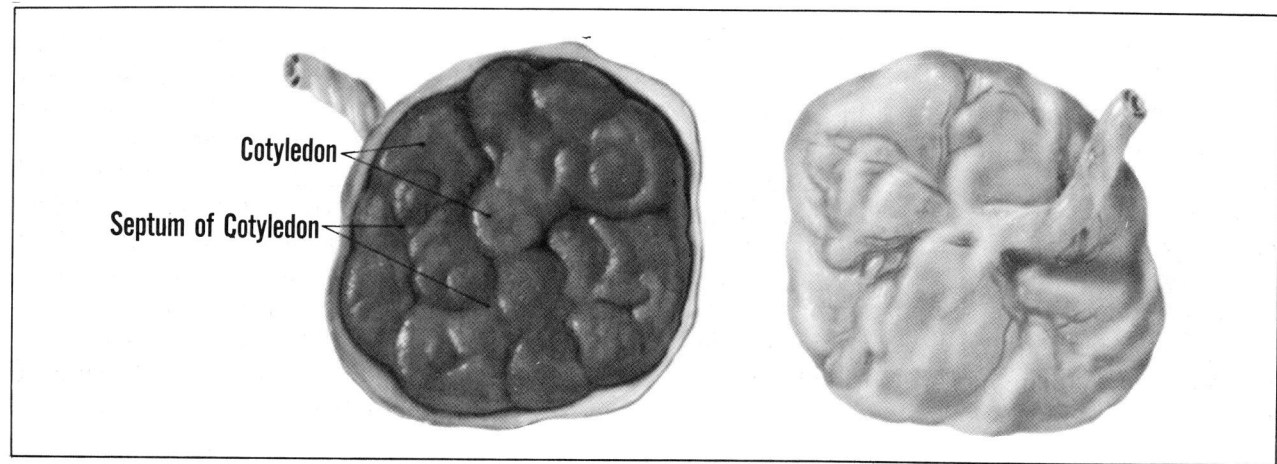

Meconium Staining

Although meconium staining of the amniotic fluid is not always a sign of fetal distress, its correlation with fetal distress is high. It may indicate that a vagal reflex of the fetus, due to hypoxia, has increased bowel motility and caused loss of rectal sphincter control, leading to the escape of meconium into amniotic fluid.

Meconium staining may be normal when the presentation is breech, since pressure on the buttocks can cause meconium loss. Meconium staining should always be reported, so that the physician can make a determination as to its meaning and seriousness.

Hyperactivity

Ordinarily, a fetus is quiet and barely moving during labor. Hyperactivity of the fetus may be a signal that he is suffering hypoxia.

Fetal Acidosis

When blood determinations are made on the fetus during labor by use of a scalp capillary technique, the finding of acidosis (blood pH below 7.2) is a certain sign that fetal well-being is becoming compromised.

MATERNAL DANGER SIGNALS

Blood Pressure

Blood pressure normally rises slightly in the second stage of labor. How high is high or how low is low depends on what blood pressure is normal for the woman in her nonpregnant state. A rule of thumb in labor is to report a systolic pressure over 140 mm Hg and a diastolic pressure over 90 mm Hg (the basic criteria for pregnancy-induced hypertension). A falling blood pressure is just as essential to report as an increasing one, since it may be the first sign of an occult intrauterine hemorrhage. A falling blood pressure is often associated with other clinical signs of shock, namely, apprehension, increased pulse rate, and pallor.

Pulse

Most women of childbearing age have an average pulse rate of 70 to 80 beats per minute. Pulse normally increases slightly during the second stage of labor because of the exertion involved in this stage. A maternal pulse more rapid than 100 beats per minute during the normal course of labor is unusual. In general, pulse rates over 100 should be reported as possible indications of hemorrhage.

Contractions

Uterine contractions become more frequent, more intense, and longer in duration as labor progresses. Contractions becoming less frequent or less intense or shorter in duration may indicate uterine exhaustion (inertia). This problem must be corrected or a cesarean section performed if delivery is to be achieved.

A period of relaxation must be provided between contractions if the intervillous spaces of the uterus are to fill and maintain an adequate supply of oxygen and nutrients for the fetus. As a rule of thumb, uterine contractions lasting longer than 70 seconds may begin to compromise fetal well-being and should be reported. The physician can then make a determination, based on the fetal heart sounds and the stage of labor, as to the effect, if any, of these long contractions on fetal or maternal well-being.

Pathological Retraction Ring

An indentation across the woman's abdomen where the upper and lower segments of the uterus join may be a sign of pending uterine rupture, or at least of uterine distress. For this reason, it is important to observe the contours of the woman's abdomen periodically during labor. If you are auscultating the fetal heartbeat by stethoscope, observation of the mother's abdomen is automatic. If an electronic monitor is in place, you have to remember to make these observations.

Abnormal Lower Abdomen Contour

A full bladder during labor may be manifested as a round, protruding bulge on the lower anterior abdomen. This is a danger signal for two reasons: the bladder may be injured by the pressure of the fetal head, or the pressure of the full bladder may not allow for descent of the fetal head.

Increasing Apprehension

Warnings of psychological danger during labor are as important to consider in assessing maternal well-being as are the traditional physical signs. A woman who is so frightened that she cannot cooperate in delivery needs more anesthetic than does the woman who is secure that everything that is happening to her is within normal expectations. The more anesthetic that is used, the greater the risk to mother and fetus. A woman who is becoming increasingly apprehensive despite clear explanations of unfolding events may be close to the pelvic division of labor. She may also be not "hearing" you because she has a concern that neither you nor her physician has met. Try an approach such as this: "You seem more and more concerned. Could you tell me what it is that is worrying you?" Seek consultants to investigate this apprehension as you would for a physical danger signal.

The Labor Process

References

1. Anderson, S. F. Childbirth as a pathological process: An American perspective. *M.C.N.* 2:240, 1977.
2. Angelini, D. Body boundaries: Concerns of a laboring woman. *Matern. Child. Nurs. J.* 7:41, 1978.
3. Beard, R. W. Controlling and quantifying uterine activity. *Contemp. Obstet. Gynecol.* 13:75, 1979.
4. Bell, M. L. The first stage of labour—how long? *Midwives Chron.* 91:84, 1978.
5. Blackwell, J. Labour pains. *Nurs. Mirror* 146:28, 1978.
6. Daniel, E. E., et al. Electrolytes in the human myometrium. *Am. J. Obstet. Gynecol.* 79:417, 1960.
7. Friedman, E. *Labor, Clinical Evaluation and Management* (2nd ed.). New York: Appleton-Century-Crofts, 1978.
8. Grace, J. T. Good grief: Coming to terms with the childbirth experience. *J.O.G.N. Nurs.* 7:18, 1978.
9. Haskins, A. L. The progesterone content of placentas before and after the onset of labor. *Am. J. Obstet. Gynecol.* 67:330, 1954.
10. Kumar, D., et al. Studies in human premature births. *Am. J. Obstet. Gynecol.* 81:126, 1963.
11. Liggins, G. C. What factors initiate human labor? *Contemp. Obstet. Gynecol.* 13:147, 1979.
12. Malinowski, J. S., et al. *Nursing Care of the Labor Patient.* Philadelphia: Davis, 1978.
13. Roberts, J. E. Maternal positions for childbirth: A historical review of nursing care practices. *J.O.G.N. Nurs.* 8:24, 1979.
14. Sciarra, J. J. *Gynecology and Obstetrics.* New York: Harper & Row, 1978.
15. Whitney, N. Uterine contractile physiology: Application in nursing care and patient teaching. *J.O.G.N. Nurs.* 4:54, 1975.

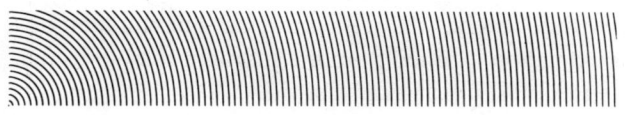

22. The Labor Experience: Nursing Interventions

Most physicians ask a woman to telephone them when she first believes she is in labor and to come to the hospital when her contractions are 5 to 10 minutes apart. Most women delay coming into the hospital as long as possible in order to shorten their hospital stay. Women who are anxious usually come in before the 10-minute limit has been reached. Watch for this woman. Waiting in the hospital for contractions to increase in intensity is much more tedious than staying at home. If she is there early, she is there for a reason you should explore with her.

Assessment on Admission to the Hospital

A woman plans well if she has a suitcase packed by two weeks before the expected delivery date, since two weeks before or after the expected date of confinement is a normal time for labor to begin. Despite all the situation comedy programs to the contrary, unless she is a grand multipara, once labor begins, she has ample time to finish packing and make a safe trip to the hospital.

It is reassuring to a woman to know what hospital entrance she should use. She is under stress, and people under stress are sensitive to annoyances that otherwise would not concern them at all. For the same reason, hospital forms should be simple; preferably, just a signature should be required. It is equally helpful if the woman has had a tour of the labor and delivery unit during her pregnancy in conjunction with a preparation-for-labor class. Check whether she has a support person with her and admit both the woman and her support person to a labor or birthing room.

INITIAL HOSPITAL INTERVIEW

Certain information must be obtained so that the physician can evaluate the extent of the woman's labor, her general physical condition, and her preparedness for labor and delivery and you can plan comprehensive nursing care. This procedure must take place quickly in order to recognize the woman who is admitted in very active labor or has a history of precipitous deliveries. Nevertheless, interviewing skill and tact must be used lest you leave the impression that you are more interested in the information than in the woman.

Ask her about her expected date of confinement; then you and the medical personnel can be alerted to the possibility of a premature birth. Ask questions to determine her stage of labor and whether any abnormality is readily apparent; you need to know the frequency, duration, and intensity of her contractions, the amount and character of show, and whether or not her membranes have ruptured. Ask when she last ate, to establish risk in case a general anesthetic must be planned. Ask whether she has any known allergies to drugs; then you will know if there will be an immediate problem with medication administration.

This information is scant but distinguishes for you the woman who is in very active labor and needs immediate care from the woman who has arrived at the hospital at the average time and will need paced interventions.

BIRTHING ROOMS, LABOR ROOMS

Traditionally, women completed their dilatational or first stage of labor in a labor room (a bare, easy-to-clean patient room), then at the pelvic or second stage of labor were transferred to a delivery room (designed as an operating room). In newer hospitals (or redesigned labor units) labor rooms have become birthing or perinatal rooms where the woman remains for all three stages of labor and the immediate period postpartum.

In the beginning of labor, the birthing room appears as a comfortable bedroom. At the second stage of labor, the bed converts to a delivery platform; cupboards at the sides are opened to reveal sterile packs of supplies; a screen or folding partition at the end of the room opens to disclose newborn care equipment.

The advantage of a birthing room is that the woman does not need to be transferred in the middle of labor. Also, the homelike atmosphere allows her to relax and fully participate in this rare life event.

INITIAL ASSESSMENT PROCEDURES

In order to establish the woman's physical well-being, her temperature, pulse, respiration, and blood pressure, as well as the fetal heartbeat, should be taken and evaluated. Though you have the woman's stated report of contractions, assess them yourself.

Length of Contractions

If you rest your fingers on the woman's abdomen at the fundus of the uterus *very gently*, you can determine the beginning of a contraction by the gradual tensing and upward rising of the fundus. You are usually able to feel this tensing about 5 seconds before the woman is able to feel the contraction. Therefore, do not rely on her to tell you when a contraction is beginning or you will underestimate the length of contractions. (You are able to feel a contraction when the intrauterine pressure reads about 20 mm Hg. The pain of a contraction is not felt until pressure reaches about 25 mm Hg.) The duration of a contraction is timed from the moment the uterus first tenses until it has relaxed again.

Intensity of Contractions

In addition to observing the duration of contractions, you need to make an estimation of intensity, or the strength of the contraction. Contractions are rated as mild (the uterus is contracting but does not become more than mildly tense), moderate (the uterus feels firm), or strong (the contraction is so intense the uterus feels as hard as wood at the peak of the contraction). The uterus cannot be indented by your fingertips in a strong contraction.

When estimating the intensity of contractions, check the fundus at the conclusion of the contraction to determine whether it relaxes or becomes soft to the touch. If it does, you know that the uterus is not in continuous contraction but is providing a relaxation time during which its blood vessels can fill to supply the fetus with adequate oxygen.

Frequency of Contractions

Next, time the frequency of contractions. The frequency is timed from the *beginning* of one contraction to the *beginning* of the next. Be certain you are not timing from the end of a contraction to the beginning of the next or you will report contractions as being closer together than they actually are. You need to time three or four contractions before you have any picture of the frequency at which they are occurring. The duration and frequency of contractions are depicted diagrammatically in Fig. 22-1.

Use as light a touch as possible on the woman's abdomen while you are timing contractions and estimating their strength (Fig. 22-2). The fundus of the uterus becomes sore if it has to push against extra weight with each contraction—unnecessary discomfort for a woman in labor.

RUPTURE OF MEMBRANES

In as many as 25 percent of labors, labor begins with spontaneous rupture of the fetal membranes. In most instances with rupture of membranes, there is a sud-

Fig. 22-1. Duration and frequency of contractions.

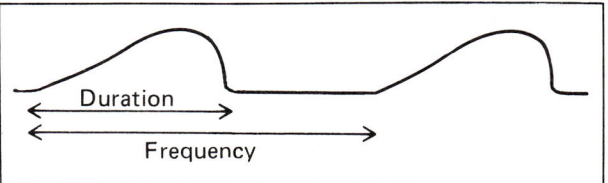

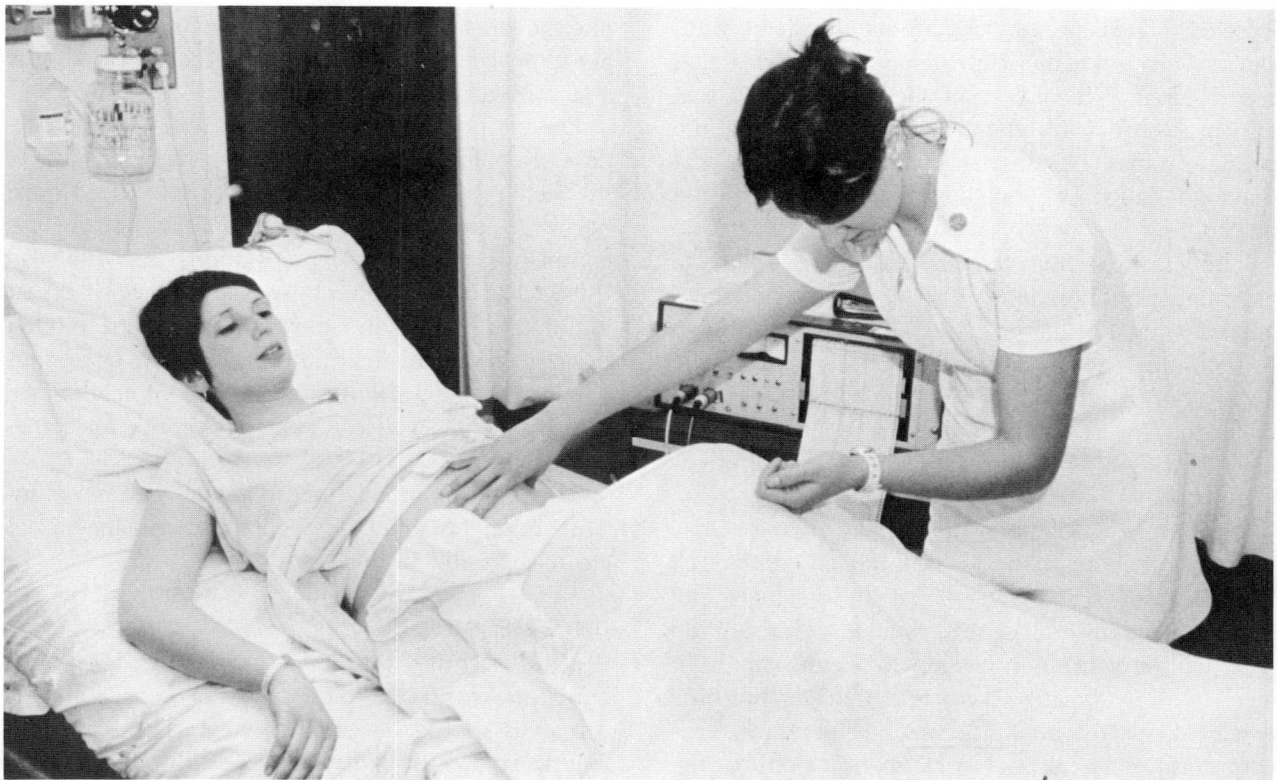

Fig. 22-2. Observing the frequency, duration, and strength of contractions. Note how the nurse's hand rests lightly on the mother's abdomen. She stands away from the bed so as not to obstruct the woman's line of vision as the woman studies a geometric wall picture to help her to concentrate on breathing patterns, a help to mothers prepared in the Lamaze method of childbirth. (Courtesy of the Department of Medical Photography, Children's Hospital, Buffalo, N.Y.)

den gush of amniotic fluid from the vagina. Women are startled by this sensation (it feels as if they have lost bladder control). It may happen while they are shopping or in a public place, and they may be embarrassed before they realize that the warm moist fluid on their perineum and legs is not urine but the announcement that labor is beginning. In other women, rupture of membranes is not a dramatic event but only a slow loss of fluid, and there is a question whether membranes have ruptured.

If there is a question as to whether or not the membranes have ruptured, a simple test with Nitrazine Paper may supply the answer. Vaginal secretions are acid; amniotic fluid is alkaline. If amniotic fluid has passed through the vagina, the pH of the vagina will probably be alkaline if tested by Nitrazine Paper.

Insert a sterile, cotton-tipped applicator deeply into the vagina and then touch it to a strip of Nitrazine Paper. Compare the paper with the chart accompanying it. If the paper indicates a pH below 6.5, the membranes are probably still intact. A pH over 6.5 indicates leakage of amniotic fluid. A false reading may occur in women with intact membranes who have a heavy, bloody show, since blood is also alkaline.

Ask the woman whose membranes ruptured at home what the color of the amniotic fluid was. It should be clear as water. Yellow-stained fluid may indicate a blood incompatibility between mother and fetus (the amniotic fluid is bilirubin-stained from the breakdown of red blood cells). Green-colored fluid indicates meconium staining. Meconium staining is often normal in breech deliveries because of buttock compression, which expels meconium into the fluid. In a vertex presentation, meconium staining generally indicates that the fetus has suffered anoxia in utero and the anoxia has led to spontaneous sphincter relaxation and meconium loss into amniotic fluid. This fetus needs immediate physician intervention. In either situation, the infant will be in danger following delivery as he will undoubtedly have aspirated some meconium into his trachea or lungs.

PREPARATION OF THE PERINEUM

At one time it was customary to shave the perineum of women preparatory to delivery. The area surrounding the vagina could then be cleaned and disinfected to help prevent contamination of the birth canal. Today, whether shaving is necessary or not is controversial. If the physician does not anticipate that an episiotomy will be needed, just cleansing the perineum may be all that is required. If perineal shaving is called for, you should be familiar with the procedure.

The cleaning and shaving procedure differs in technique from hospital to hospital, but the principles are the same. The hair over the pubis does not need to be removed, since the area will be covered with sterile towels during delivery. However, some physicians prefer to have this hair removed as well, so you will have to be familiar with the preference of the physician who is to perform the delivery.

You need a good light source in order to see exactly what you are doing. The perineal hair should be well lathered prior to shaving, so that the shaving is not painful and skin cuts can be avoided. The solution used will vary from institution to institution, from green soap to shaving cream to a mild dishwashing detergent mixed with warm water. The perineum is very sensitive to hot and cold, so be careful of the water temperature. Cold water will cause abdominal tension and discomfort if the woman should experience a contraction during the procedure. Despite the advantageous cumulative bactericidal and bacteriostatic properties of hexachlorophene, it should be avoided as a lathering agent until the long-range effects of absorption of this compound have been further documented.

After the perineal hair has been well lathered, begin at the mons veneris and stroke from above downward with a safety razor, around the vulva to the base of the perineal body. Be certain to stretch the skin from above as you work, so that the skin is taut and allows the razor to move easily. Use single strokes, front to back, rinsing the razor head after each stroke, so that pathogens from the anal area are not carried forward to the birth canal.

After the anterior portion of the perineum has been shaved, ask the woman to turn on her side to allow you to shave any hair surrounding the anal area. With the upper part of the woman's leg well flexed, you have a good view of the anal area in this side-lying position.

After all hair on the perineum has been shaved away, the perineum is then washed thoroughly. Some hospitals' policies specify cotton balls; others specify sterile sponges, disposable washcloths, or reusable washcloths. The solution varies also, but usually it is a mild antiseptic such as benzalkonium chloride (Zephiran Chloride) or green soap. Be certain to separate the labial folds so that any secretions in the folds are removed. Wash from front to back, cleaning the anal area last.

Provide privacy for the woman during the procedure. Remember, again, that she is very sensitive to the feeling tone of the persons caring for her. If she begins to experience a contraction while you are completing the perineal preparation, stop and wait until it has passed. On a busy labor service, it is easy to think, "I haven't time to wait. I have a dozen other things to do in this half hour." However, labor contractions at their strongest rarely last more than 60 seconds. Surely you can wait 60 seconds for someone's comfort.

After the woman's perineum has been cleansed, instruct her not to touch her genitals, to keep the area as clean as possible during labor.

URINE SPECIMEN

A urine specimen to be tested immediately for protein and glucose and sent to the laboratory for a complete urinalysis should be obtained next. The woman is able to void most easily if she is allowed to use the bathroom. A bedpan or receptacle placed on the toilet will allow for comfort and also will permit any material passed by the vagina to be preserved. If the woman describes any symptoms that suggest urinary tract infection (burning on urination, blood in her urine, extreme frequency, flank pain), you will need to obtain a clean-catch urine for culture. Women who report ruptured membranes should not be ambulated until it is confirmed that the fetal head is engaged so that the umbilical cord cannot slip past the loosely fitting head and prolapse, causing fetal distress.

ENEMA ADMINISTRATION

At one time every woman was given an enema in early labor. It was thought that cleansing the bowel at this point avoided the excretion of stool at the time of delivery and possible contamination of the birth canal. Moreover, it was hoped that the peristaltic action of the bowel would tend to increase uterine contractions and possibly speed labor. As some enema solution is retained in the lower bowel, however, because of pressure of the fetal head against the lower bowel, there is invariably some stool excretion at the time of delivery in any event. Whether enema administration speeds labor is debatable. An enema is therefore no longer a routine procedure but may be ordered depending on the individual physician's preference. An enema is not given to a woman who is near the pelvic division of labor for fear that as she bears down to expel the enema she will expel the fetus as well. Enemas are not given to women after membranes have ruptured because of the danger of contaminating the then unprotected birth canal and fetus from fecal contaminants.

Enemas are uncomfortable procedures to women not in labor. To a woman in labor they are doubly uncomfortable. A Fleet enema is not only the most convenient type to administer but the most comfortable for the woman because of the small amount of fluid that is injected and the speed with which it can be given. It may be difficult to insert an enema tip in the woman's rectum because of the pressure of the presenting part on the anal area and the presence of hemorrhoids that have developed during pregnancy. Be certain to provide privacy and explain that you are aware this is something the woman is not looking forward to. Assure her that you will be as gentle as possible and that if she tells you when she is beginning to have a contraction or any abdominal cramping you will stop the flow of fluid until her discomfort passes.

Following administration of the enema, allow the woman to get up and go to the bathroom. Tell her to wipe herself from front to back following expulsion of the enema, so that she does not carry fecal material forward to the birth canal. After she returns to bed, the perineal area should be rewashed to eliminate the possibility of fecal contamination.

OTHER PROCEDURES

Next, blood is drawn for hemoglobin or hematocrit reading, VDRL (serological test for syphilis), and blood typing. Thus everyone dealing with the woman can be assured that she is in good physical health, and the blood laboratory is alerted that a woman with a certain blood type is in labor.

Ideally, a fetal monitor to record fetal heart sounds and a monitor to record uterine contractions should be attached at this point to ensure accurate fetal assessment during the remainder of labor.

The nurse who is prepared to take an extended role may next take a more definitive history and perform a vaginal or rectal examination to determine the presence of effacement, degree of dilatation, and presentation, position, and station of the fetus.

HISTORY TAKING

The history taken at this point should include a review of the woman's pregnancy, with both physical and psychological events, and a review of past pregnancies, general health, and family medical information.

If the woman is in active labor, the history taken on arrival may be the only history obtained until after the baby is born. However, most women get to the hospital in time for thorough history taking.

Current Pregnancy History

To determine the state of the woman's health during this pregnancy, begin with an open-ended question such as "How did your pregnancy go?" or "How has your pregnancy been?" This type of question allows the woman to answer in any of a number of ways: "Too long," "Terrible," "Good, except that I worried so much," "All right, after I decided there wasn't much I could do about it," "Great." If you begin with a question such as "Any problems during this pregnancy?" you limit the woman to concrete problems (e.g., spotting, injuries) and thereby limit the amount of information you will obtain.

If the woman answers your opening inquiry with a noncommittal "Good" or "Fine," pursue some specific areas of the pregnancy: When was her last menstrual period? How many days does her average period last? How long is the interval between periods? (This helps to document the due date. If she has 40-day cycles, she will probably be in labor two weeks after her due date.) Did she have prenatal care? When did she first go for care? It is important to ask her the reasons for her actions. If she went exceptionally early, even before she missed a period, what was the reason? Was she frightened? Did she anticipate trouble with this pregnancy? If she went unusually late, why was that? Was she so secure in her own judgment that she did not feel a need for care? Was she hoping she was not pregnant and trying to delay the diagnosis to avoid facing the fact of the pregnancy? Was money such a problem that she could not afford care? The answers to these questions will be important in planning postpartal nursing interventions because she could be elaborating situations that will interfere with optimal mother-child bonding or future health care.

How often did her physician ask her to come to his office or clinic during pregnancy? This is a good question to validate her first response; that is, a woman who made weekly rather than monthly prenatal visits either has an extremely conservative obstetrician or has not had a "fine" pregnancy, despite what she says. Did she keep all her scheduled prenatal appointments? If not, why not? Financial or transportation problems? Was she afraid the physician would discover something wrong (no news is good news)? Was she fearful something would be wrong? Does she have a friend or a relative who has a child with a defect? Did she feel the office or clinic personnel were not interested in her, that she was only a number on a chart? Does that influence her feelings about this hospital staff? It is frightening to feel alone in labor even with people around you because a previous experience led you to believe that health care personnel are indifferent to you.

Ask about and explore any medical problems the woman had during pregnancy. Did she have any spotting? When? How long did it last? What did she do? If she called her physician, what did he say to do? Did she follow his instructions? What happened? How does she feel about the episode? Did it frighten her? Did her physician assure her that spotting in early pregnancy is usually benign? Is she still worried about it?

Did she notice any swelling of her hands or feet during pregnancy? If she had edema, what was its extent? Just in her ankles at bedtime? In her face when she awoke in the morning? How much weight did she gain during pregnancy? Was her physician happy with that weight gain?

Did she have any falls? When? How did she fall? How far did she fall? Did she have any aftereffects? Almost all women have a fall of some sort during pregnancy. If she delivers a healthy child, the incident will be as nothing. If she delivers a child with a congenital defect, she may blame herself for the problem. This kind of information prepares the health care personnel who will be dealing with the woman after delivery to help her work through her adjustment to a child who is not the perfect child she imagined she carried.

Did she have any infections? A rash that might suggest rubella (a pink macular rash lasting two or three days)? Herpes simplex lesions?

Did she take any medication during pregnancy? What kind? When? Did she drink alcohol? Does she smoke cigarettes? It is realistic to ask young women whether they took any hallucinogens or euphoric drugs during pregnancy or whether they smoke marijuana. If you convey the impression that you are interested in her welfare and that of her child (and such questions are important to the immediate welfare of the infant if the woman is addicted to drugs such as heroin or barbiturates), most women will answer truthfully.

Was the woman ill in any way during pregnancy? Did she have influenza? A bladder infection? Back pain? Varicosities? Hemorrhoids? When did she have the illness? What did she do about it? Did she take medication? Is she aware of a blood incompatibility? Does she know her blood type? Did she take vitamins or iron or folic acid during pregnancy? (If not, the hemoglobin of her child may need special attention to be certain it is adequate.)

Interviewing women in labor is difficult because you both are constantly interrupted by labor contractions. Impatience shows; remember that the longest contraction is rarely more than 60 seconds. The woman may concentrate so intently on a breathing exercise that a question asked just prior to a contraction is completely driven from her mind. As the contraction subsides, repeat the question as if you had not asked it before or as if you do not mind asking it again.

At the same time you are asking about the early part of pregnancy, ask whether or not the pregnancy was planned. You may find this an awkward question. It is not. It is a good question here because the manner in which the woman accepted her pregnancy has a great deal to do with how she will accept her child. You might word the question: Most pregnancies come as a surprise—is that how this was?

If she states that the child was unplanned, ask whether or not she was using a birth control measure. Many young girls have inaccurate birth control information and will need counseling in the postpartum period to provide themselves with better protection in the future.

As you pursue the history of the remainder of the pregnancy, attempt to identify a point at which the woman changed her mind about wanting a baby. Do not be naive. Not all children are wanted. It is normal not to want a baby if your circumstances make it difficult or impossible to supply all the love and care the child needs. Be careful that you do not sound judgmental. If you imply that the correct answer to the question "Did you plan this pregnancy?" is "I wanted this baby very much. I love him already," that is the answer you will get. This is not eliciting information; it is asking for compliance.

Does she remember at what month in pregnancy she felt the child inside her move (quickening)? The month quickening occurred helps you document the due date. The woman who is worried that her child may not be all right will probably remember exactly when she felt life. The woman who has four normal children at home and has every reason to think this child will also be normal may not have been sufficiently aware of quickening to time it accurately. Ask her to think in terms of holidays as a way of jogging her memory. She may recall that she felt the fetus move while she was at a Fourth of July picnic or on vacation.

Ask the woman who said she did not want the pregnancy whether feeling the child kick inside her made any difference. Many women will say that it did: "I guess that was the first time the pregnancy was real. I started to plan after that." If quickening did not change her attitude, can she name a point where it did change? Has she made everything ready for the baby? When did she begin to prepare for the baby? A woman who says she has done nothing either has been so worried that her child would be born imperfect or dead that she could not begin to look at tiny shirts or gowns, has divorced herself from emotional attachment to the baby, or has no money for baby clothing. She cares too much or too little or needs financial help.

It is good to ask her about the child's father's attitudes toward the pregnancy. How did he feel about her being pregnant? How has he acted since she started labor? Is he supportive when she is worried, or too "manly" to display emotions and consequently of little help to her?

Did she attend any classes in preparation for parenthood or labor? If she wants an anesthetic for delivery, does she prefer a particular type? Listen to her reply. Does she say a "general" because she is terrified of the pain her mother warned her of? Or because she is afraid the baby will be born dead and she wants to delay the inevitable? Has she heard scare stories about spinal anesthesia and is afraid of it even though she would like to be awake during her baby's birth? Does she want "nothing" because she really believes that is the way to have children, or is she determined to be a heroine, to prove something to her husband or herself?

Make certain she understands that her physician will have the ultimate say about whether an anesthetic is needed and the kind of anesthetic she receives, but that if there is a choice her wishes will be respected. If she indicates that she wants to be awake but wonders how she will react to the situation, assure her that seeing the birth of her child is an event that will happen only a few times in a lifetime. It is a moment to be treasured, and she will be among friends, who will not be critical of her reactions.

Ask next about her plans for the coming baby. Has she chosen a pediatrician? Does she plan to breast-feed or bottle-feed? It is important to know because if she is going to breast-feed she should not receive a lactation suppressant after delivery.

It is preferable to interview a woman in a private setting without her husband present. True, this is his child also, but the thoughts about the pregnancy are *her* thoughts. Whether or not she wants this child and what she is concerned about are things she can choose to share or not to share with her husband. If you interview her with her husband present, she may have to make a choice: either to give you wrong information or to admit a particular thought to her husband unwillingly. It is always poor judgment and poor health interviewing technique to force people to reveal confidences or to be untruthful.

Women who come into labor with concerns about the health of their unborn child may need extra help in the immediate postpartum period "binding in" or claiming their infant. Questions concerning psychological adaptation to pregnancy are therefore as important as those that deal with the woman's physical well-being throughout the pregnancy.

Past Pregnancy History

Ask, Has she ever been pregnant before? If so, what was the outcome? How were her other children born? Vertex? Breech? Cesarean section? What was the reason for cesarean section? What was the infant's birth weight? Were there any complications at birth? Was any special equipment used? Did the infant go to the regular nursery? Did the infant go home from the hospital with her? Did the infant have any jaundice or cyanosis? What is the present state of health of her child or children?

Were any of her children stillborn? Any prematurely born? Any miscarriages? Any abortions? (Women generally differentiate miscarriages from abortions and appreciate categorizing these separately.) Any complications for herself following any delivery? If there was infection or cervical tearing following previous childbirth, the cervical dilatation you are hoping for here may not occur with ease. It is best to be forewarned of this possibility. Ask the woman whether her blood type is Rh negative and whether she received Rh (D antigen) immune globulin (RhoGAM) following an abortion, a stillbirth, or a past delivery.

Past Health History

Ask, Has she ever had any surgery (surgical adhesions might interfere with free fetal passage); heart disease or diabetes (women with heart disease and diabetes need special precautions during labor and delivery); anemia (blood loss at delivery may be more important than normally); tuberculosis (tuberculosis lung lesions may be reactivated at delivery by changes in lung contour); kidney disease or hypertension (blood pressure will need to be watched even more carefully than normally); venereal disease (the infant may be exposed to the disease by vaginal contact if the disease is still active); herpes lesions (these can be transmitted to the fetus at birth if vaginal lesions are present)?

Family Medical History

Because some diseases are transmitted by genetic patterns and others tend to be familial, it is important to know whether any of these diseases are in either the mother's or the father's family. Adequate preparation for a child born with a disease can then be made. Does any family member have heart disease, a blood dyscrasia, diabetes, kidney disease, cancer, allergies, seizures, congenital defects, or mental retardation?

PHYSICAL EXAMINATION
General Examination
Following history taking, the woman needs a thorough physical examination, including a pelvic examination, to confirm the presentation and position of the fetus and determine the stage of dilatation. A nurse who is functioning in an extended role is able to perform such an assessment in consultation with a physician.

Physical assessment during labor begins, as does all physical assessment, with the woman's overall appearance. Does she appear tired? pale? ill? frightened? Is there obvious edema or dehydration? Are there open lesions anywhere?

Assess by palpation any enlargement of lymph nodes. Is there any suggestion of infection? Inspect the mucous membrane of the mouth and the conjunctiva of the eye for color. Does the color (paleness) suggest anemia? Does she wear contact lenses (they will have to be removed if a general anesthetic becomes necessary)? What is the condition of her teeth? Are they carious? Do any teeth appear abscessed (such as condition might account for a postpartum temperature)? Does she have a bridge or dentures or retainers (which might have to be removed if a general anesthetic becomes necessary)?

Is there evidence of erythema in the posterior pharynx? A streptococcal throat infection will require treatment to prevent transmission to the child. Does she have rhinitis? Any other cold symptoms? Examine the outer and inner surfaces of her lips carefully. Does she have herpes simplex? Type II (genital) virus is lethal to newborns. If herpetic lesions are present anywhere, the woman will probably be isolated from her child until the lesions crust.

Are her lungs clear? Does she have normal heart sounds and rhythm? Inspect and palpate her breasts. Are they free of cysts or lumps? Does she inspect her own breasts monthly? Do not try to teach breast self-examination while a woman is in labor; she will be unable to concentrate on what you are saying. If she needs instruction in this area, indicate it on her chart, so that the postpartum nursing staff can provide it before she leaves the hospital.

Estimate fetal size and presentation by Leopold's maneuvers if this judgment has not already been made. Palpate and percuss her bladder area (over the symphysis pubis) to detect a full bladder. Even though the woman has just voided, she might not have emptied her bladder sufficiently (retention) because of pressure of the fetal head. A full bladder is uncomfortable during labor and may impede the descent of the fetus. In addition, an overdistended bladder can be injured in labor under pressure of the fetus and will cause urinary retention in the postpartum period.

Inspect the lower extremities for edema and varicose veins. Women with large varicosities are prone to thrombophlebitis following delivery. Some physicians prefer not to use delivery room stirrups if varicosities are prominent during labor, since the stirrups may press against them. Severe edema suggests hypertension of pregnancy, so the extent and intensity of edema must be assessed.

Vaginal Examination
At one time the majority of examinations done during labor were done rectally because it was thought that the risk of spreading pathogenic bacteria from the distal vagina to the cervix was thereby reduced. If careful technique is used, however, and vaginal examinations are kept to the few required, they do not increase the incidence of infection. Further, they give more accurate and useful information than rectal examinations. The key words in pelvic examinations are *careful technique* and *few in number*.

For a vaginal examination, the woman should lie on her back with her knees flexed. Be certain to provide privacy by a curtain or by draping. Wash your hands well and pull on a sterile examining glove. Use a clean lubricating solution on your fingertips. Place your ungloved hand on the outer edges of the woman's vulva and spread her labia so you can inspect the external genitalia for lesions such as occur with infection, primary syphilis, or herpes infections (red, irritated mucous membrane, open ulcerated sores, clustered pinpoint papules). Look for escaping amniotic fluid or the presence of the umbilical cord or bleeding. If there is no bleeding or cord visible, introduce your index and middle fingers gently into the vagina, directing them toward the posterior vaginal wall, which is less sensitive than the anterior wall. Stabilize the uterus by placing your ungloved hand on the woman's abdomen and touch the cervix with your gloved examining fingers (Fig. 22-3). You should compare the width of your fingertips to a centimeter scale if you are going to do vaginal examinations so you know how wide your index and middle fingers are at the tip. An index finger averages about 1 cm; a middle finger about 1½ cm. If they can both enter the

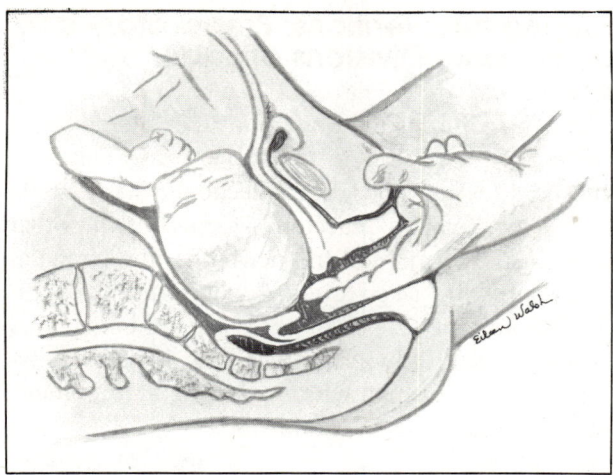

Fig. 22-3. Technique of vaginal examination.

cervix, the cervix is dilated 2½ to 3 cm. If there would be room for double the width of your examining fingers in the cervix, the dilatation is about 5 to 6 cm. When the space is four times the width of your fingertips, dilatation is complete—10 cm.

The last portion of the cervix to dilate is generally the anterior rim or lip. Feel for its presence.

Estimate the degree of effacement. A cervix before labor is 2 to 2½ cm thick. If it is only 1 cm thick now, it is 50 percent effaced. If it is tissue paper thin, it is 100 percent effaced. It is difficult to feel for dilatation with a 100 percent effaced cervix because the edges of the cervix are so thin; it is difficult to be certain whether you are touching fetal scalp or brushing against an edge of the paper-thin rim of cervix. Practice is necessary.

Estimate whether membranes are intact. The membranes (with a slight amount of amniotic fluid in front of the presenting head) are the shape of a watch crystal. With a contraction, they bulge forward and become prominent and can be felt much more readily.

Ask yourself, What is the level of the presenting part in relation to the level of the ischial spines? Is it above, below, or at the spines? How many centimeters above or below? What is the fetal presenting part? From Leopold's maneuvers you know what you think it is. Can you confirm that? Differentiating a vertex from a breech may be more difficult than would first appear. A vertex has a hard smooth surface; however, fetal hair massed together and wet may be difficult to appreciate through gloves. Palpating the two fontanelles, one diamond-shaped and one triangular, helps the identification. Buttocks feel softer and give under fingertip pressure. You can identify the anus because the sphincter action will "trap" your index finger.

What is the position? In a right occipitoanterior (ROA) position, the triangular fontanelle (the posterior one) will point toward the right anterior pelvic quadrant. In a left occipitoanterior (LOA) position, the posterior fontanelle will point toward the left anterior pelvis. In a breech presentation, the anus can serve as a marker for position. When the anus is pointing toward the left anterior quadrant of the woman's pelvis, the position is left sacroanterior.

Because nurses are traditionally women, they have an advantage over male physicians in their usually narrower fingers, which cause less pressure and less discomfort on vaginal examination. Be certain your fingernails do not extend beyond the edge of the fingertips of your examining fingers, so that there is no danger of piercing an examining glove.

Following a vaginal examination, withdraw your hand as gently as you introduced it. Wipe the perineum (front to back) to remove secretions or the examining solution, and replace the top sheet of the bedcovers.

Women are anxious to have frequent progress reports during labor, assuring them that their work is not in vain. Tell the woman immediately after the examination about the progress of dilatation. Most women are aware of dilatation but not the word *effacement*. Just "No further dilatation" is a depressing report. "You're not dilated a lot more, but a lot of thinning out is happening and that's just as important" is the same report given in a positive manner.

Vaginal examinations are never done in the presence of fresh bleeding, since this may indicate a placenta previa (implantation of the placenta so low in the uterus that it encroaches on the cervical os). Performing a vaginal examination might tear the placenta and cause hemorrhage, with resultant danger to both mother and fetus. If in doubt, err on the side of postponing a vaginal examination until a consultant arrives.

Rectal Examination

Because of the danger of introducing pathogenic bacteria into the birth canal during vaginal examination, some physicians prefer that rectal rather than vaginal examinations be done on patients in labor.

For a rectal examination you need a clean but not necessarily a sterile examining glove. Use only your index finger and tuck your thumb under your remaining fingertips as you examine, so that it does not touch the vaginal introitus and introduce infection (Fig. 22-4). Lubricate your finger well with water-soluble jelly, and introduce it into the rectum gently (remember that hemorrhoids develop in at least a

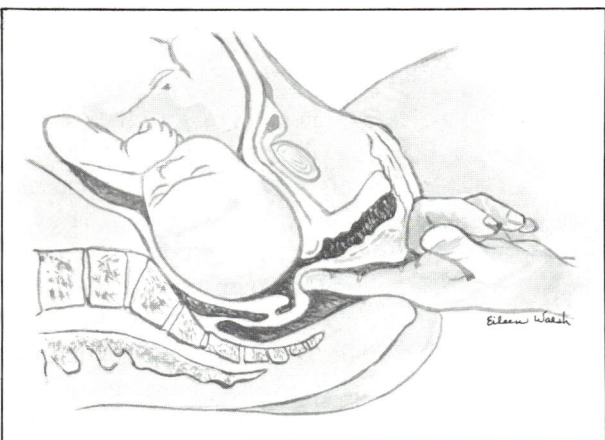

Fig. 22-4. Technique of rectal examination. Be certain that your thumb does not extend and contaminate the vaginal opening.

third of women during pregnancy). Slide your finger along the anterior wall of the rectum. The rectal and vaginal walls and the intervening tissue are all so thin at this point that you can feel the cervix through them; it will be felt as a circular ridge with a depression at the center. The extent of the depression is the dilatation. Estimate the degree of effacement (difficult to establish on rectal examination). Try to determine the presence of membranes (they perhaps can be felt only as they bulge into the cervix with a contraction). The position of the presenting part is much less accurately determined by this method, since it is hard to detect the fontanelles or determine their outlines through the rectal-vaginal septum.

Following the examination, the glove should be discarded if it is disposable or placed in a closed container to be sterilized if it is not. Even though the glove used for a rectal examination need not be sterile, it is good practice to place nothing but sterile gloves in labor rooms. This will prevent an erroneous exchange of gloves in which an examiner uses a clean but not sterile glove for a vaginal examination.

After finishing a vaginal or rectal examination plot the new degree of dilatation and descent of the presenting part on a labor progress graph.

The nurse who can assess a woman in labor this thoroughly is an indispensable asset to the physician who utilizes the labor unit where she works. Since physicians cannot realistically stay with all their patients throughout labor, they must rely on nurses to bear a major part of the responsibility for assessment and for safeguarding both mother and child.

Nursing Interventions: Preparatory and Dilatational Divisions of Labor

TEMPERATURE

The temperature of the woman in labor should be recorded on admission to the labor unit. This is a safeguard to rule out active infection, which would necessitate isolation procedures to protect the other women in the unit and the newborn. The temperature should be taken every 4 hours during labor. Temperatures over 37.2°C (99°F) should be reported to the attending physician; they may indicate dehydration in the woman who is awaiting an anesthetic and taking no fluids by mouth.

PULSE AND RESPIRATION

Pulse and respiration should be taken and recorded every hour during labor. A woman's pulse may be rapid on admission because she is nervous and anxious. After she has settled down and has been reassured that everything is going well, it should be in a range of 70 to 80 beats per minute. A persistent pulse rate over 100 suggests tachycardia from dehydration or hemorrhage.

BLOOD PRESSURE

Blood pressure also should be taken and recorded every hour during labor. It should be recorded between contractions, both for the woman's comfort and for best accuracy, since blood pressure tends to rise 5 to 10 mm Hg during a contraction. An increase in blood pressure may indicate the development of pregnancy-induced hypertension (a fourth of all instances of pregnancy-induced hypertension occur during labor and delivery). A decrease in blood pressure or a decrease in the pulse pressure (the difference between the systolic and diastolic pressures) may be indicative of hemorrhage.

FOOD AND FLUID INTAKE

How much fluid or solid food a woman is allowed to drink or eat during labor varies from physician to physician. When it may be necessary for delivery to take place under general anesthesia, she should have nothing to eat or drink during labor except ice chips or lollipops.

On many labor services, every woman in labor is treated as if she were awaiting a general anesthetic. One reason for continuing such a policy is that there is always a chance that any woman may ultimately require this type of delivery assistance; a policy of no food for anyone covers all eventualities. A second reason is that digestion in the stomach is slowed during labor, and thus no woman needs great amounts of food at this time. However, women in prolonged labor need to maintain an adequate fluid and caloric intake in order to prevent secondary uterine inertia (a cessation of labor contractions), as well as generalized dehydration and exhaustion. If oral fluids are contraindicated by the delivery plan, intravenous glucose solutions may be administered to maintain caloric reserve.

BLADDER CARE

A woman should be asked to void every 2 to 4 hours while in labor. She needs to be reminded to do so because she is concentrating on so many new sensations in her abdomen that she may misinterpret the discomfort of a full bladder as a part of her labor discomfort. If she cannot void and the bladder is distended, the woman may need to be catheterized. Catheterizing a woman in labor is uncomfortable for her and difficult for you because the vulva is edematous from the pressure of the fetal presenting part. The mother should be encouraged to void spontaneously if possible so that catheterization and the risk of introducing a urinary tract infection can be avoided. The relationship of a full bladder to ease of descent of the fetus is shown in Fig. 22-5.

ANALGESIA

Many women who plan to receive an analgesic for labor think that the minute they arrive at the hospital they will be given something for their discomfort. In order not to impede the progress of labor, analgesics are not routinely given to women until cervical dilatation has reached 3 to 4 cm in a primipara and 4 to 5 cm in a multipara. If analgesia cannot be given when a woman first enters the hospital because dilatation has not progressed sufficiently, she should be told why the medication is being withheld. Most women believe that an analgesic given in labor will take away all their discomfort. In most instances, this is not the case. The woman will still feel the tension of contractions along with some discomfort. The analgesic does take the biting edge off the contraction and makes it bearable, enabling her to work better with contractions.

The analgesics and anesthetics used in labor and delivery are discussed in Chap. 23.

POSITION OF THE WOMAN DURING LABOR

In early labor, a woman may be out of bed walking or sitting up in bed or in a chair, whatever position she prefers. Because the main piece of furniture in a labor

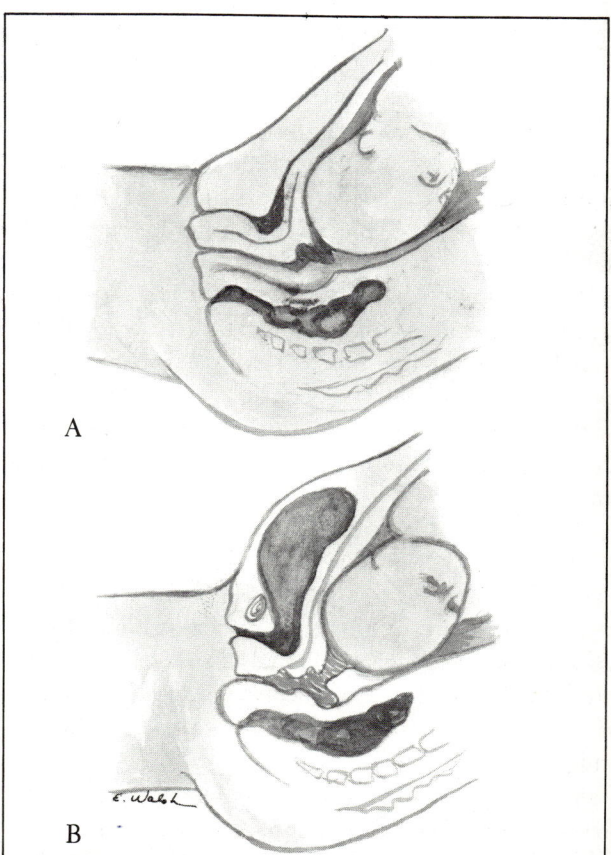

Fig. 22-5. Relationship of a full bladder to ease of descent of fetus. A. Empty bladder. B. Full bladder blocks descent.

or birthing room is a bed, most women assume that they are expected to lie in bed and must be assured otherwise. A woman whose membranes have ruptured should be kept flat until she has been checked by a physician because unless the head of the fetus is well engaged (firmly fitting into the pelvic inlet) an umbilical cord may prolapse into the vagina if she walks about.

Following the administration of medication such as a sedative or narcotic, the woman should lie down so that if she becomes dizzy she will not fall. As labor becomes advanced, lying down is her best position so that if delivery is precipitous (happens rapidly) the infant will not be born while she is ambulatory and suffer an injury.

Women with fetal heart monitors in place often assume that they must lie in bed so the monitor works properly. They may sit up in a chair by the side of the bed as long as the machine connections are long enough to reach that far.

Women should be encouraged to lie on their side during labor. This position causes the heavy uterus to

The Labor Experience: Nursing Interventions 325

tip forward away from the vena cava, allowing free blood return from the lower extremities and adequate placenta filling and circulation.

Most women are comfortable in this position and adjust to it readily. Check that the chair for the woman's support person is on the side of the bed she faces; otherwise, she will keep turning to her back to talk.

Some women have learned to do breathing exercises in a supine position and may need additional coaching to do them in a side-lying position. If a woman must turn to her back during a contraction in order to make her breathing exercises effective, help her to remember to return to her side between contractions.

FETAL HEART MONITORING

Although a fetus is passive in labor, he is subjected to extreme pressure by uterine contractions and during passage through the birth canal. Compression of the umbilical cord and the placenta by uterine contractions may compromise the fetal blood and oxygen supply.

Fetal distress occurs in about 10 percent of normal labors. Until irreparable damage has occurred, it is difficult to diagnose fetal distress with the standard methods of monitoring fetal heart rates, such as listening every 15 to 30 minutes to fetal heart sounds by means of a stethoscope. Errors in counting rates occur because the rate is so rapid. Periodic heart-rate sampling may miss a pattern of change for up to half an hour, during which irreversible damage or death may take place. It is difficult to hear fetal heart sounds by an auscultatory method during a contraction; thus, essential information on what is happening to the fetal heart rate during contractions is unavailable, further limiting the usefulness of the auscultatory method. Fetal heart rate should be counted every 30 minutes during beginning labor, every 15 minutes during active labor, and every 5 minutes during the second stage or pelvic division of labor.

If stethoscope monitoring is the only method available in a particular instance, Bonica and Hon [2] suggest that this procedure be followed: Count fetal heart rate for at least 20 consecutive periods. Start the count before the onset of a uterine contraction and continue for at least 2 minutes after the uterus is fully relaxed. Rest for 5 seconds and begin a count again. Record the average fetal heart rate for each period and the relationship of each period to a uterine contraction. Given these data, you can plot the relationship of the fetal heart sounds to the peak of uterine contractions. Fetal heart monitoring by electronic or ultrasonic techniques is always preferable to this method, however.

Fetal Heart Monitoring Devices

Several types of monitoring devices are now available for recording fetal heart rate and uterine contractions. In high-risk situations, techniques for analyzing fetal blood composition may also be utilized.

Fetal Heart Rate Patterns

Recording fetal heart rates during labor offers information on the fetal heart rate between contractions (the baseline rate) and during contractions.

BASELINE RATE. This is the rate of the fetal heart between contractions. It should be between 120 and 160 beats per minute. It fluctuates slightly (5 to 15 beats per minute) as the fetus moves or sleeps. This fluctuation is termed *baseline variability*. If no variability is present, the natural pacemaker activity of the heart (effect of the sympathetic and parasympathetic nervous systems) has probably been affected. This can be a response to narcotics or barbiturates administered to the mother in labor. Baseline variability increases when the fetus is stimulated; it slows when the fetus sleeps. Fetal hypoxia and acidosis as a cause must be investigated. Very immature fetuses will show diminished baseline variability because of immature overall nervous system stimulation and immature cardiac node function.

Beat-to-beat variability refers to the difference between successive heartbeats. A fetus who is withstanding the effects of successive labor contractions well has both beat-to-beat and baseline variability (sometimes referred to as *short-term* and *long-term variability*).

RATE DURING CONTRACTIONS. During a uterine contraction there is a brief deceleration in fetal heart rate, probably due to vagal compression. The rate rarely falls below 100 and returns quickly to between 120 and 160 beats per minute at the end of the contraction.

FETAL TACHYCARDIA. A fetal heart rate over the normal rate of 160 is fetal tachycardia. A rate of 161 to 180 is moderate tachycardia; higher than 180, marked tachycardia. A fetus in distress often has an increased heart rate of this nature before his heart rate begins to fall. Transient tachycardia occurs with fetal movements.

FETAL BRADYCARDIA. A fetal heart rate below the normal limit of 120 is fetal bradycardia. A rate of 100 to 119 is moderate bradycardia; under 100, marked bradycardia. Bradycardia almost always signifies fetal hypoxia.

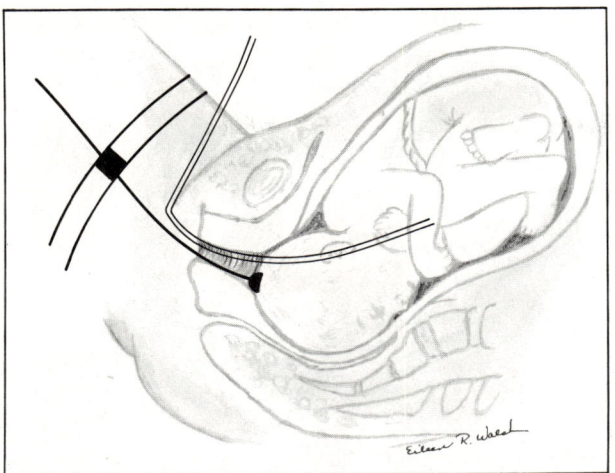

Fig. 22-6. An internal fetal heart rate monitor in place. Uterine contractions are monitored by the intrauterine catheter.

Internal Monitoring

The most reliable method of recording fetal heart sounds is by use of a fetal scalp electrode. When the fetal head is engaged, the woman's cervix is dilated 3 cm, and the membranes have ruptured, a fetal scalp electrode is inserted vaginally and attached to the fetal scalp. The fetal electrocardiograph signal obtained is amplified and fed into a cardiotachometer. The output from the cardiotachometer is then recorded on a permanent graph paper record. The quality and frequency of uterine contractions may be monitored at the same time by means of a Teflon catheter passed through the vagina into the uterine cavity (Fig. 22-6). The catheter is filled with saline and attached to a pressure recorder. As each contraction puts pressure on the uterine contents, the pressure exerted on the catheter is recorded. A correlation can then be made between the fetal heart rate (actually the fetal ECG) and uterine pressure from contractions.

External Monitoring

In a breech presentation or before the woman's cervix is sufficiently dilated, or because of a physician's preference, fetal heart rate can be monitored reliably by means of a Doppler ultrasonic system, by phonocardiography, or by abdominal electrocardiography. A Doppler ultrasonic monitoring sensor, one of the types most frequently used, is a small unit, about the size of a quarter. When taped to the woman's abdomen it converts fetal heart movements into audible beeping sounds. The sounds may be translated into electronic impulses and plotted on a permanent graph paper record, the same as with an internal monitor. An external tokodynamometer transducer used in connection with this gives a printout of the uterine contractions. Such a unit is held in place on the woman's abdomen by a cloth strap (Figs. 22-7 and 22-8).

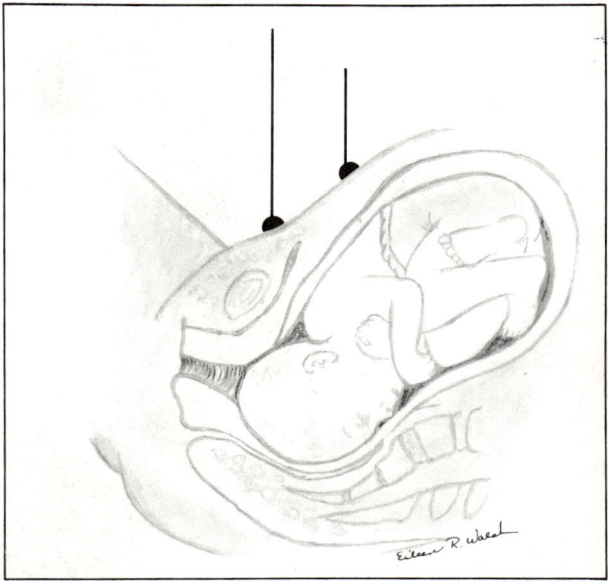

Fig. 22-7. Placement of external monitor leads for fetal heart rate and uterine contractions.

Fetal Distress Patterns

Either persistent bradycardia, persistent tachycardia or absence of beat-to-beat variability is an ominous sign in labor, indicating potential fetal distress. An initial baseline fetal tachycardia may develop into a deceleration response as labor progresses.

Hon and Paul [9] have further identified two fetal heart rate patterns that are indicative of fetal distress (Fig. 22-9).

EARLY DECELERATION (TYPE I). Early deceleration of fetal heart rate occurs at the beginning of a contraction, but the rate returns to the normal level by the end of the contraction. Compression of the head by pressure of uterine contractions initiates a vagal reflex in the fetus that causes the deceleration. This particular pattern appears to have no clinical significance.

LATE DECELERATION (TYPE II). Late deceleration is delayed until 30 to 40 seconds after the onset of the contraction and continues beyond the end of the contraction. This is an ominous pattern in labor because it suggests uteroplacental insufficiency or decreased blood flow through the intervillous spaces of the uterus during uterine contractions. Such a condition may occur with marked hypotonia or with abnormal uterine tonus caused by the administration of oxytocin. Immediate steps to correct the situation must be instituted: if oxytocin is being used, slowing

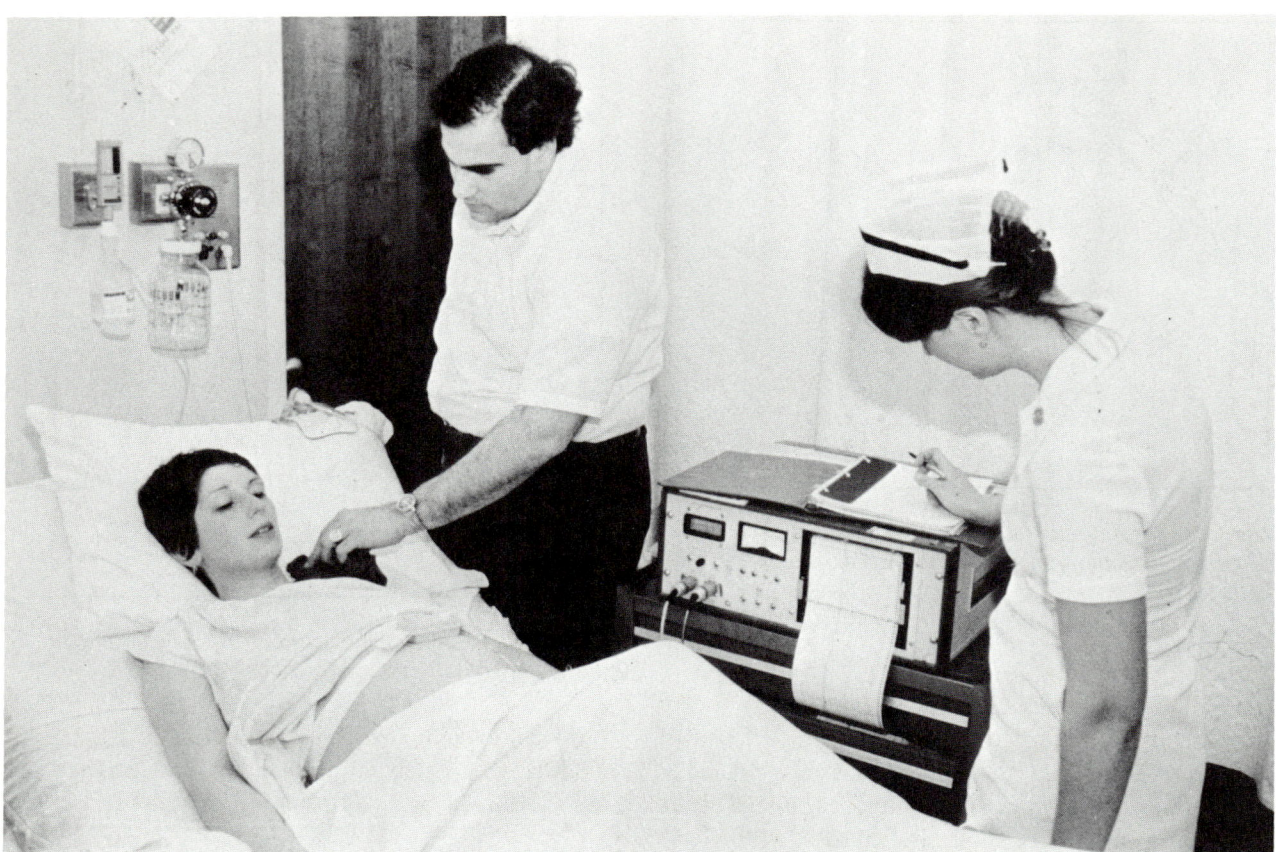

Fig. 22-8. *External electronic monitoring of fetal heart rate and uterine contractions. Husband wipes perspiration from wife's neck as she nears second stage of labor. Oxygen mask lies ready on pillow in case fetal heart rate pattern shows inconsistencies remediable by oxygen administration. The monitor for uterine contractions is evident; the external fetal heart monitor is obscured by the bed cover. (Courtesy of the Department of Medical Photography, Children's Hospital, Buffalo, N.Y.)*

the rate of administration or stopping it altogether; changing the woman's position from supine to lateral (to relieve pressure on the aorta and vena cava and supply more blood to the uterus); administering intravenous fluids or oxygen to the woman.

If the fetal heart rate alone is being recorded, the difference between type I and type II deceleration cannot be observed. Thus it is as important to record uterine contractions during labor as it is to record the fetal heartbeat.

VARIABLE PATTERN. The variable pattern of deceleration occurs at unpredictable times during contractions and indicates compression of the cord, which is an ominous development in terms of fetal well-being. However, because the pattern is variable, it can be completely missed if monitoring is not continuous. If this pattern is recognized on the monitor, changing the woman from a supine to a lateral position or to a Trendelenburg position is recommended. Administering oxygen to the woman may be helpful. If these measures do not right the fetal heart pattern, a cesarean section may have to be performed to save the fetus's life.

Figure 22-10 is a diagrammatic sampling of a labor room fetal heart rate record. At 10:00 A.M. the fetal heart rate averages 150 beats per minute. The dip is slight, occurs with contractions, and disappears at the end of the contraction (type I deceleration, a normal fetal heart rate pattern). As labor progresses, the deceleration pattern becomes type II at noon. Deceleration begins late in the contraction and lasts beyond it; tachycardia is also present. The woman is turned on her side, and oxygen is administered. At 12:10 P.M., 10 minutes later, no noticeable improvement is observed. At 12:15 the record shows a fetus in extreme distress. The late deceleration pattern continues. The baseline fetal heart rate is falling. This is the graph of a fetus dying. Ten minutes later, an infant, alive and well and with a 1-minute Apgar score of 9, was delivered by cesarean section. This is a common, everyday success story when monitoring equipment is correctly used.

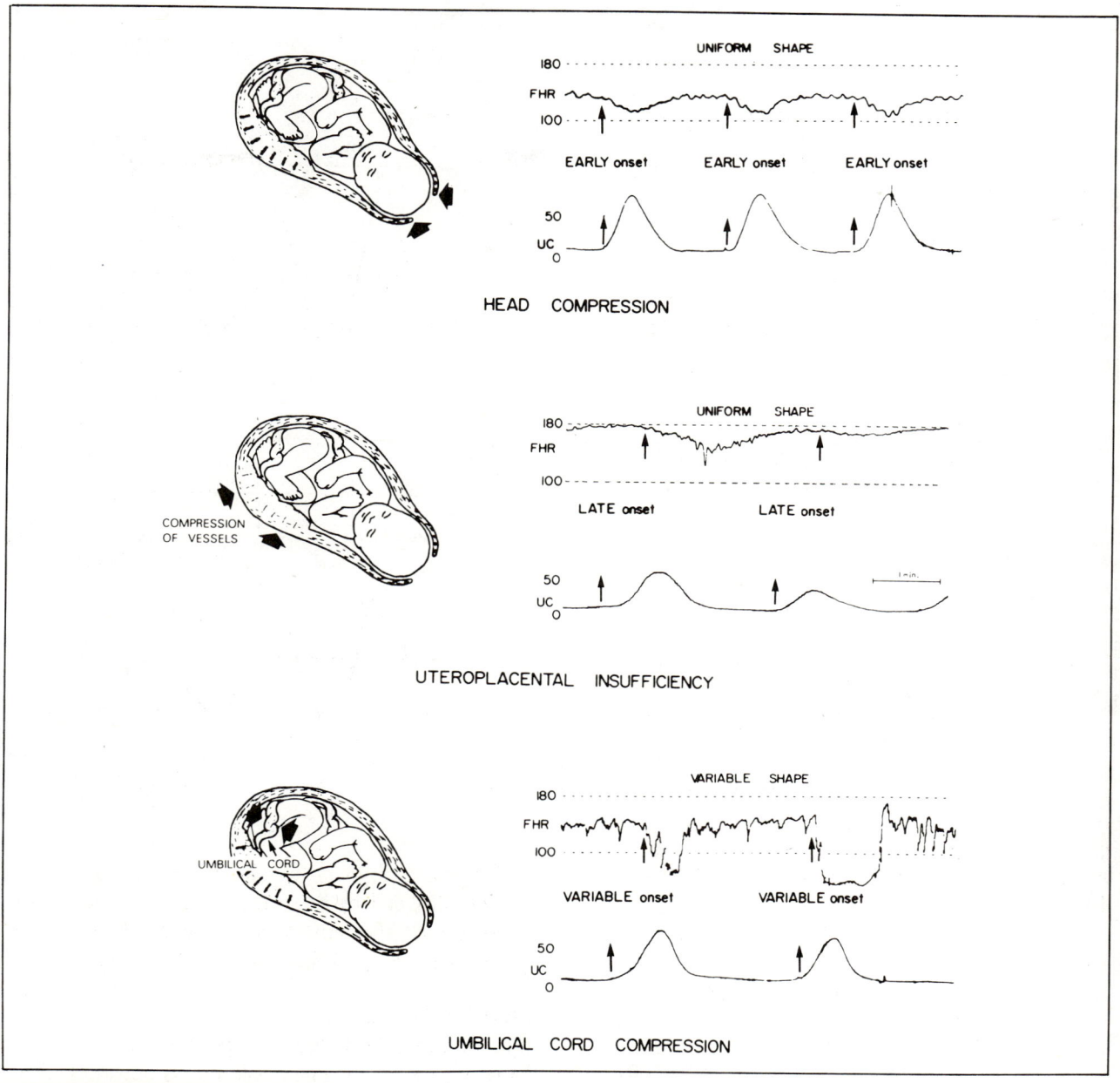

Fig. 22-9. *Fetal distress patterns.* (From E. H. Hon and R. H. Paul, A Primer of Fetal Heart Rate Patterns. New Haven, Conn.: Harty Press, 1970.)

SINUSOIDAL HEART RATE PATTERNS. In an infant who is severely anemic or hypoxic, central nervous system control of heart pacing may be so impaired that the fetal heart rate pattern resembles a frequently undulating wave. Although the cause of this pattern is poorly understood, it is being recognized as a pattern as equally ominous as a late deceleration or variable deceleration pattern.

UTERINE CONTRACTIONS BY MONITOR

When uterine contractions are being monitored by an internal pressure gauge, the frequency, duration, baseline strength, and peak strength of contractions all can be evaluated. Strength of the contraction is evaluated by the size of the peak of the contraction on the tracing. Equally important to evaluate is the return of the uterine tone to baseline strength between contractions. This ensures placental filling between contractions.

With latent contractions, the baseline level is under 5 mm Hg; with active contractions, it is about 12 mm Hg; during the second stage or pelvic division of labor, the baseline may be as high as 20 mm Hg. If baseline readings do not return to 20 mm Hg or below, uterine hypertonia and a compromise of fetal well-being are indicated. External monitors record only the frequency and duration of contractions.

The Labor Experience: Nursing Interventions

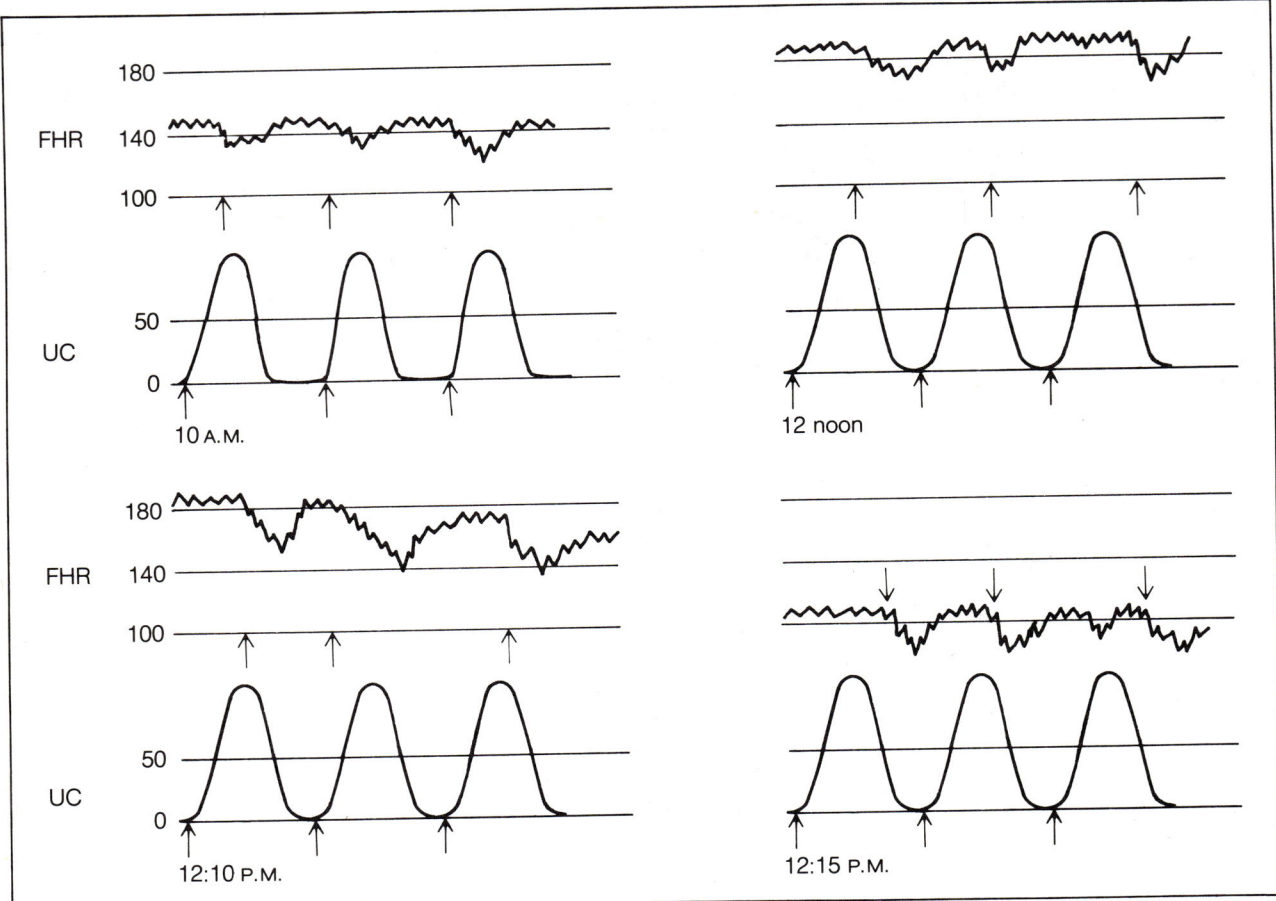

Fig. 22-10. Data recorded by fetal monitor. Note that by 12:15 P.M. the fetal heart rate (FHR) baseline is falling and the late deceleration pattern in uterine contraction (UC) continues.

INTERVENTIONS FOR FETAL HEART RATE OR UTERINE MONITORING ABNORMALITIES

In the event that variable deceleration, late deceleration, or increased uterine baseline levels occur, three quick interventions are helpful safeguards to prevent fetal anoxia.

1. Turn the woman to her side if she is not already in that position. The side-lying position reduces the pressure from the uterus on the vena cava and allows better placenta filling. It moves the weight of the fetus away from the cord if cord compression was occurring. If the woman is already on her side (she should be, in labor), turn her to the opposite side.
2. Administer oxygen to the mother by mask or nasal prongs at 5 to 7 liters per minute. Increasing the oxygen content in the maternal bloodstream will quickly increase that in the fetal bloodstream as well because of rapid oxygen diffusion.
3. Call for a physician's help. If a fetal heart rate is not corrected by these means, a cesarean section to remove the fetus from an environment that is no longer safe for him may be necessary.

FETAL BLOOD SAMPLING

By monitoring fetal blood composition, damage to the fetus may be determined before it is apparent in an ECG or an external monitoring system. Changes in blood composition are the cause of the alterations in fetal heart rate.

Fetal blood can be monitored by analysis of small samples of blood droplets collected from the fetal scalp as it presents to the cervix. It is not necessary or practical to monitor all fetuses by blood sampling during labor. The procedure is generally reserved for high-risk fetuses and is therefore discussed in Chap. 35.

NURSING CARE DURING A MONITORING PROCEDURE

A woman and her husband need a good explanation of why monitoring equipment is necessary. Most people associate monitors with intensive care units and thus with critical illness. A woman may interpret the presence of monitoring equipment at her labor bedside as a sign that something is going terribly wrong, that she or her baby is in grave danger.

Assure both parents that this is now a routine procedure. Tell them that the equipment provides more accurate information about the fetal heartbeat than a stethoscope does. If parents are informed that monitoring equipment is good for the welfare of their child, they will not only tolerate its presence but welcome it. The woman who is worried that something will happen to her child during labor is reassured by listening to the beeping sound of the fetal heart. Many women ask for a graph tracing to save for their child's baby book.

Occasionally, a woman finds the strap holding an external monitoring unit in place uncomfortable, or the snugness of the sensor head limits her ability to breathe deeply, as in abdominal breathing. Spreading talcum powder on the abdomen may make the strap more comfortable. Taking off the sensor periodically and allowing for a position change is helpful. If the woman changes her position herself (and she will change position during labor because she is human, not a machine), repositioning the sensor will be necessary. Remind her that this will happen—not so she will lie frozen in one position during labor, but so she will not think her baby's heart has stopped when her change of position shifts the beam of the sensor.

Occasionally, a woman will experience a supine hypotensive syndrome during labor. As she lies on her back, uterine pressure causes blood to pool in the inferior vena cava; she experiences sudden anxiety and shortness of breath. In this event she will need to be positioned on her side and the monitoring sensor shifted so that the heartbeat is again recordable.

Monitoring equipment is helpful to women who wish to use breathing exercises during labor. A contraction can be anticipated by observing the monitor printout rather than by a hand on the abdomen. A hand held constantly on an abdomen causes discomfort during labor.

Be careful that you do not fall into the habit of nursing the equipment and not the patient, communing with the monitor and not the woman and her husband. Monitoring equipment frees you from the task of listening to fetal heart rates every 15 or 30 minutes—not to spend more time at your desk or in the supply room or looking at the monitor, but to spend more time giving emotional support in labor.

Some nurses tend to be resentful of or resistant to using monitoring equipment for observation of the fetal heartbeat. Many perceive such equipment as unnecessary. Such a response can be compared to that of the nurse who resisted thermometers when they were first introduced because she was used to determining temperature by feeling brows; or to the response of the nurse who resisted blood pressure cuffs when they were first introduced because she found reading the dial and interpreting two figures too complicated. It has been documented that fetal heart monitoring is more accurate than intermittent stethoscope listening, and nurses have proved to be capable of interpreting the graphed patterns correctly. Therefore, opposition to the use of monitoring devices is difficult to justify.

It has also been proposed that the woman herself will object to a monitor. If she does, she is probably responding to the attitude of the nurse in the room, who is making it clear that she does not like the monitor. Surely no one doubts that a woman prefers to deliver a healthy, normal baby rather than a dead or mentally retarded one. If a monitor can make the difference—and monitors can—how can women object to them? In the near future, all women in labor may have fetal heart monitoring done by electronic devices as a primary prevention measure. Fetal heart monitoring by electronic devices will become a routine and primary nursing responsibility for the nurse in maternity nursing. This involves a dependent nursing function in that it is done under a physician's instructions; the attaching of the monitor, the reading and interpreting of the fetal heart pattern, the emergency measures to be taken if an abnormal fetal heart pattern is detected (such as turning the woman onto her side or administering oxygen), however, are independent nursing functions. Monitors and sensors do not interfere with the "naturalness" of labor; they strengthen the "naturalness" of having healthy children.

ROLE AS A SUPPORT PERSON

A great deal is written about the nurse's responsibility to help the woman maintain control during labor, as if labor and delivery are like an afternoon tea where a woman's manners are observed and her white gloves are inspected for spots. Labor is not like a tea party. It is a stress situation, and a woman has a right to react to the stress.

A better approach to helping a woman in labor is to reduce the stress as much as possible; with lessened stress, the woman can maintain her own self-control. Women are under stress in labor because it is an unknown, whether the labor is her first or her tenth; a tenth labor is the first time she has labored with this child. She is under stress because she is uncomfortable, because she is in an unfamiliar environment, among strangers.

There is no such thing as unacceptable behavior during labor. All the reading a woman does, all the questions she asks, cannot completely prepare her for the experience of labor and delivery. Despite how well she planned to cope with these strange sensations, she may be caught off guard by their strength when they really happen. If she chooses to scream with each contraction as a way of coping, and screaming works for her, it is acceptable behavior during labor. Doing breathing exercises to reduce the pain of contractions is more constructive for most women, but individuality in care should provide for those who choose to be more unorthodox.

The woman needs clear explanations of what is happening and what is going to happen. Include the husband in the plans. Help the woman with breathing patterns or relaxation techniques. Stay with her. Keep her from being frightened. If you do all these things, you will wonder what people are talking about when they say helping a woman to maintain control in labor is a problem. A timetable for nursing interventions during the first stage or preparatory and dilatational divisions of labor is shown in Table 22-1.

AMNIOTOMY

If membranes do not rupture spontaneously, the physician may choose to perform an amniotomy during the first stage of labor. After pulling on a sterile glove, he or she introduces a sterile, pointed instrument, such as a Kelly clamp, into the vagina and touches it against the pouching membranes. He snips the membranes to open them and allow amniotic fluid to drain.

It is more dangerous for a baby to be born with membranes intact than with them ruptured. If they are intact, he is born surrounded by amniotic fluid, and he may aspirate a quantity of the fluid with his first breath. There are many stories of babies born with the membranes intact (born "under the caul"). This was at one time considered good luck or an omen that the child was a special, protected child (Hamlet was born "under the caul"). In reality, the child born this way is more likely to have aspiration pneumonia than special powers.

Rupture of the membranes almost always makes labor proceed faster, since the head fits more snugly into the cervix and contractions seem to become more effective. The color of the amniotic fluid should be carefully noted for green or yellow staining, indicating possible fetal distress. Fetal heart rate should be taken following amniotomy. *After membranes ruptured.*

Since the membranes contain no nerve endings, amniotomy is not a painful procedure. The woman will experience some discomfort from the physician's gloved hand in the vagina, as she would in a pelvic examination during labor.

Nursing Interventions: Pelvic Division of Labor

If the membranes have not previously ruptured, the transition (deceleration phase) into the second stage or pelvic division of labor may be marked by a gush of amniotic fluid from the vagina resulting from the rupture of the membranes as the fetus is pushed into the birth canal. Show becomes prominent as the last of the operculum is released.

A woman needs someone with her as she enters the second stage of labor. The change in the nature of contractions from the crescendo-decrescendo pattern to the almost violent urge-to-push type is frightening.

Table 22-1. *Time Intervals for Nursing Interventions During First Stage of Labor (Preparatory and Dilatational Divisions)*

		Continued Frequency	
Intervention	Admission	Latent Phase	Active Phase
Assess and Record:			
Temperature	X	q4h (unless membranes are ruptured, then q2h)	q4h (unless membranes are ruptured, then q2h)
Pulse	X	q1h	q1h
Respirations	X	q1h	q1h
Blood pressure	X	q1h	q1h
Voiding	X	q2–4h	q2–4h
Fetal heart rate	X	Continuously by monitor or q30min	Continuously by monitor or q15min
Contractions	X	Continuously by monitor or q30min	Continuously by monitor or q15min
Provide:			
Ambulation	Until membranes rupture		
Support	X	Continuously	Continuously

Table 22-2. Time Intervals for Nursing Interventions During Second Stage of Labor (Pelvic Division)

Intervention	Beginning of Second Stage	Continued Frequency	After Birth of Infant	After Delivery of Placenta
Assess and Record:				
Temperature		q2h		X
Pulse	X	q1h	X	X
Respirations	X	q1h	X	X
Blood pressure	Following anesthetic administration	q1h	X	X
Fetal heart rate	X	Continuously by monitor or q5min		
Contractions	X	Continuously by monitor or q5min		
Provide:				
Support	X	Continuously	Continuously	Continuously

She may have cramps in the calves of her legs as the fetus compresses pelvic nerves and need help in relieving them by dorsiflexion of her feet.

Fetal heart sounds should be counted at the beginning of the second stage to be certain that the start of the baby's passage into the birth canal is not occluding the cord and interfering with fetal circulation. A timetable for interventions during the second stage of labor is shown in Table 22-2.

EFFECTIVE SECOND-STAGE PUSHING

For pushing during the second stage of labor to be most effective, the woman must push *with* contractions and rest between them. Pushing is best done from a semi-Fowler's position rather than flat. Place one or two pillows under the woman's head and let her flex her thighs on her abdomen. She will achieve the best effect if she grasps her legs just below the knees, takes a deep breath as a contraction begins, and pushes as if she were starting to move her bowels. Her effort should be as sustained as possible; short pushes do not move the fetus well forward. Pushing is exhausting but exhilarating. Best of all, when the woman is pushing, *really* pushing, the contractions become painless—a welcome relief after the long, hard, uncomfortable ones that preceded transition. At first she may be reluctant to push with contractions; she is afraid that pushing will hurt, and she has had enough pain. A few tentative pushes, however, will convince her that this stage holds for her the same exhilaration that a marathon runner feels with his "second wind." Pushing with contractions feels good.

As descent, flexion, internal rotation, and extension occur, the anus of the woman appears everted; stool may be expelled from the pressure exerted on it. As the fetal head touches the internal perineum, the perineum begins to bulge and appear tense. As the fetal head is pushed still tighter against the perineum, the fetal scalp becomes visible at the opening to the vagina. At first this is a slit-like opening, then oval, then circular. The circle enlarges from the size of a dime to that of a quarter to that of a half dollar. This is called *crowning*.

To keep the second stage from moving too fast in a multipara, it may be necessary to prevent her from pushing. The best way to accomplish this is to have her pant with contractions. Since it is difficult to push effectively when she is using her diaphragm for panting, she stops pushing. Remember that pushing is involuntary. No matter how much she wants to cooperate with you, stopping this overwhelming urge to push is almost beyond her power. Demonstrating "panting like a puppy" and panting with her may be most effective. Be sure that she is inhaling adequately or she will hyperventilate and become light-headed. Have her take deep breaths between contractions. Breathing into a paper bag also helps hyperventilation as it causes the woman to rebreathe carbon dioxide.

The multipara is generally taken to a delivery room, or the birthing room is converted into a delivery room, when the cervix reaches 7 to 8 cm dilatation. As a rule a primipara remains in a labor room and pushes with contractions until the baby's head has crowned the size of a quarter or half dollar.

DELIVERY

If the woman has been admitted to a birthing room, she completes delivery in the same room. The room is converted to a delivery room by the addition of sterile packs of supplies on waiting tables; the partition at the end of the room is opened to reveal the "baby island," or newborn care area.

If a labor room has been utilized, the woman must

be moved at the beginning of the second stage of labor to a central delivery room. Transfer to a delivery room at this point is awkward as her interest is on what is happening inside her. Also, she has grown used to the labor room surroundings, and being transferred to a sterile-appearing operating room is intimidating. Her support person may feel particularly threatened by the strange surroundings in a delivery room.

In either instance, what is going to happen in the next hour involves sensations that are difficult to appreciate until they are experienced. All the preparations thus far will not be enough to make a woman comfortable unless she has a support person with her. It will be important later that this person shared this moment with her; in years to come the couple will talk of it often. At present, however, delivery is such a new phenomenon for most people that much of a husband's effectiveness is lost during delivery. Health personnel who know what is happening and can give assurance that everything is going the way it should are indispensable in a birthing or delivery room at the second stage of labor.

A husband should be as welcome in a delivery room as he is in a labor room. Husbands do not faint any more often than do student nurses or medical students, and the woman needs her husband's support during this final phase of childbirth as much as she did during the previous phases. Do not feel compelled to keep a husband busy in the delivery room or birthing room so that he will stay out of trouble. Sitting on a high stool at the head of the table where his wife can see him and he can see the delivery in the table mirror is adequate. His role is support, not busywork.

If a woman is to be transported to a delivery room, it is easiest for her to be taken in her labor room bed. Then she will not have to slide onto a cart in the labor room and again to the delivery table in the delivery room.

A delivery room is intimidating because it looks like an operating room. Its dominant piece of furniture is the delivery table, a stainless steel obstetrics platform. An instrument table stands at its foot and holds the sterile instruments and supplies required during a delivery. A second table or stand with basins is also at the foot of the table; one basin will receive used sponges and the other will receive the placenta.

An "island" in the room is readied for the baby's care. The equipment should include a radiant-heat warmer, equipment for suction and resuscitation, and supplies for eye care and identification of the newborn. A transformed birthing room contains the same equipment; its appearance, however, is more homelike and friendly.

You need to scrub your hands for 3 minutes at the sink outside the delivery room and to pull on a clean gown over your labor room uniform, a cap over your hair, a mask over your nose and mouth, and cloth "boots" over your shoes to prevent static electricity. If the husband is going to join his wife in the delivery room, he must follow the same procedure.

In the delivery room, the woman is helped to slide over onto the delivery table. Delivery rooms are kept at about 68°F to reduce the danger that the gases used in some deliveries might explode. The woman may complain that the room or the sheets on the delivery table seem cold. More often, she is too involved in the final climactic moments to notice the change. Help her make the transfer from the bed or cart to the table between contractions, so that it is most comfortable for her; be sure the bed is held snugly against the delivery table so that she feels secure in the move. Since contractions will now be coming about every 1 or 2 minutes, this must be done quickly and efficiently, yet without seeming to rush.

Anesthesia

If a low spinal or a saddle block anesthetic is to be administered, the woman is asked to sit up on the side of the delivery table or bed or to turn on her side, depending on the anesthesiologist's preference. If she is going to do the former, she needs support; she is "front-heavy" and with a contraction becomes extremely uncomfortable. Her back should be held rounded and her head flexed forward on her chest to provide the anesthesiologist the widest possible exposure to the vertebral canal. She should lean her head against your shoulder for support. Plant your feet firmly; she is exhausted and may lean harder against you than you anticipate.

As soon as the anesthetic is injected, the anesthesiologist will wait a specified number of seconds (about 30) and then ask you to help the woman to lie down again. It is important that she lie down immediately. If she sits up too long, the anesthetic will not rise high enough in the spinal canal, and adequate anesthesia will not be achieved. On the other hand, if she lies down too soon, before the anesthesiologist says it is all right, the anesthetic may rise too high in the spinal canal, causing respiratory paralysis. This is the exception to the fundamental rule that you should always wait for contractions to pass before you reposition or talk to the woman. Ignore a beginning contraction if it is time to change position after the administration of a spinal anesthetic.

If the woman is to receive a general anesthetic, she remains supine on the table. Local or pundendal blocks are generally administered closer to delivery, after the woman's feet are placed in the stirrups.

Fetal Heart Monitoring

The fetal heartbeat should be continually monitored while the woman is on the delivery table. If the monitoring equipment is not portable and must be removed when the woman is taken to the delivery room, the fetal heart should be auscultated every 5 minutes.

Positioning on the Delivery Table

In most instances, when the physician has masked and scrubbed and donned a sterile gown and gloves, the woman's legs are covered by cloth boots to her knees. Her legs are raised to the table stirrups. It is important that both legs be raised at the same time to prevent muscle strain. It is also important that the strap holding the leg in the stirrup is secured snugly but not so tightly that it causes constriction. Remember that a woman who has received a spinal or general anesthetic will not be able to tell you that her leg has impaired circulation. Even with no anesthesia, she may be too involved in the delivery to feel the sensation of tingling, cramping, or pain in her leg until later. An alternative delivery position that may be used is a lateral Sims's position. This eliminates the need for stirrups and is perceived by some women as a more natural position for delivery. Stirrups, however, are not uncomfortable and provide the most advantageous position for viewing the perineum in order to detect lacerations or other problems at delivery. In a birthing room, a supine position without stirrups is often used (the position used for home delivery).

Delivery room tables have metal handles on their sides that the woman can grasp to continue her pushing effort. If a nurse is going to be in attendance at the head of the table (and one should be), there is no need to use wrist straps. It is frightening and demeaning to be strapped down to a table and may leave bitter memories of a delivery that otherwise would have been a fulfilling experience. The purpose of the straps is to prevent the woman from touching sterile drapes. This is not really a problem, and this practice should be allowed to become obsolete for the sake of human dignity.

Once the woman is placed in a lithotomy position by means of the stirrups, the table is "broken" (its lower half is folded downward) so that the physician can be in close proximity to the birth outlet. Never leave the foot of a broken delivery room table until you are replaced by the physician, so that if birth occurs precipitously, the infant will not be injured.

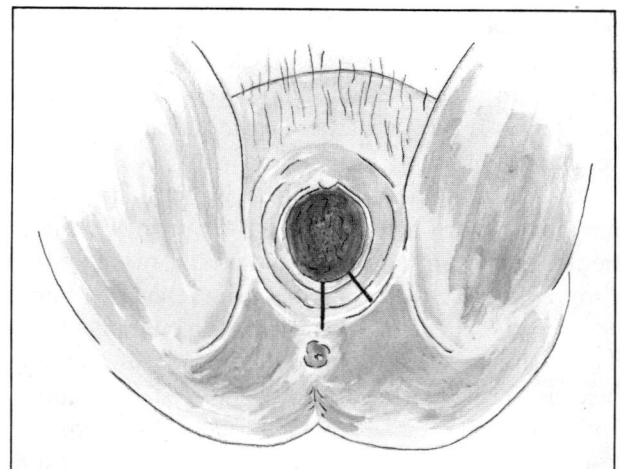

Fig. 22-11. Episiotomy incisions.

Episiotomy

Either the physician or the scrub nurse cleans the vulva and surrounding skin. Use a sterile glove and sterile compresses impregnated with whatever specific cleansing solution is designated by hospital procedure. Always scrub from the vaginal introitus outward, never from a distal area toward the birth canal. Use a clean compress for each stroke. Sterile drapes are placed around the perineum as the next step.

An episiotomy incision (Fig. 22-11) may be made. It is made with blunt scissors in the midline of the perineum (a midline episiotomy) or begun in the midline but directed laterally away from the rectum (a mediolateral episiotomy). Mediolateral episiotomies have the advantage over midline cuts in that, if tearing occurs beyond the incision it will be away from the rectum, with less danger of complication from rectal mucosal tears. However, midline episiotomies appear to heal more easily, cause less blood loss, and result in less discomfort to the mother in the postpartal period.

Episiotomies were once done only when tearing seemed imminent but are now considered a part of a normal delivery. They substitute a clean cut for a ragged tear, minimize pressure of the fetal head, and shorten the last portion of the second stage of labor.

The pressure of the fetal presenting part against the perineum is so intense that the nerve endings in the perineum are momentarily deadened. Thus, an episiotomy may be done in the woman who has received no anesthesia without her feeling the cut. There is a slight loss of blood at the time of the cut, but the pressure of the presenting part serves to constrict the cut edges and keep bleeding to a minimum.

The fetal head generally moves forward considerably with the tension of the perineum relieved. Fecal material may be expelled from the rectum as the rectum is compressed by the pressure of the fetal head. This is sponged away by the physician to prevent contamination of the birth canal.

As soon as the head of the fetus is prominently visible (about 8 cm across), the physician may place a sterile towel over the rectum and press forward on the chin of the fetal head while he presses the other hand downward on the fetal occiput (the Ritgen maneuver). This helps the fetus achieve extension, so that the head is born with the smallest diameter presenting, and it controls the rate at which the head is born.

Pressure should never be put on the fundus of the uterus to effect delivery. This may rupture or cause other damage to the uterus.

The woman who has not had anesthesia experiences the birth of the head as a flash of pain or a sensation of heat, as if someone had poured hot water on her perineum. It is a fleeting sensation and is not particularly uncomfortable.

Forceps

Forceps are metal instruments that may be used during normal labor to extract the fetus from the birth canal. The use of low or outlet forceps for this purpose is so common (especially when the woman has had anesthesia that is making second-stage contractions ineffectual) that it can be considered a routine procedure in delivery. The use of forceps shortens the second stage of labor, prevents excessive pounding of the fetal head against the perineum, prevents exhaustion from the woman's pushing effort, and can speed delivery in the event of fetal distress.

Forceps used to extract the head gently are applied when the fetal head is at the perineum (+3 or +4 station) and the sagittal suture line of the fetal head is in an anteroposterior diameter in relation to the outlet. Simpson's or Elliot forceps are the most common type of outlet forceps used. The blades of the forceps are slipped alongside the fetal head in the birth canal (they are designed to mold to the contour of a fetal head), and the handles of the instrument are joined and locked. Gentle traction is then exerted along the pelvic axis to deliver the head (Fig. 22-12).

In order for forceps to be used safely, it must be ascertained that the woman's pelvis is adequate, effacement is complete, the cervix is fully dilated, and the membranes are ruptured. Anesthesia must be used to attain sufficient perineal relaxation and prevent pain. Before the application of forceps, the physician must be certain of the position of the fetus to apply the forceps properly.

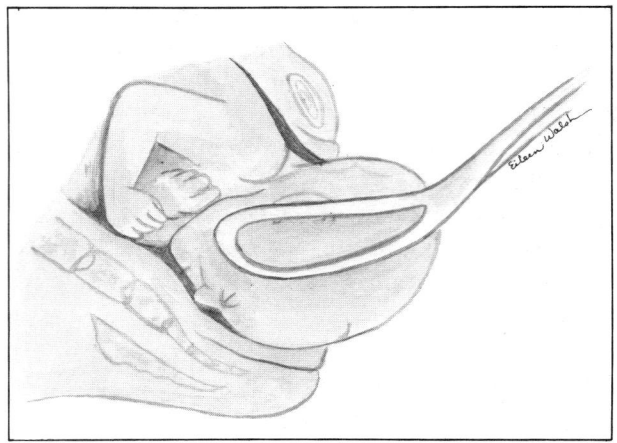

Fig. 22-12. Application of outlet forceps.

There are as many scare stories about the use of forceps as there are about the use of saddle block or spinal anesthetics. When forceps were first designed and used, some of these stories were undoubtedly true. With improvements in their design, and in the hands of a skilled obstetrician, forceps are now an adjunct rather than a deterrent to safe childbirth. Although forceps appear hard and cold and as if they would put pressure on a fetal head, they are so designed that pressure is put on the shank, not on the blade, and thus they actually *reduce* pressure to the fetal skull. Forceps marks from the pressure of a blade against the infant's cheek may be noticeable for 24 to 48 hours after delivery. These marks, which are usually no more than a linear ecchymosis, are normal and are not a complication of forceps use.

Checking the Position of the Umbilical Cord

Immediately following delivery of the head, the physician passes his fingers along the occiput to the newborn's neck to determine whether or not a loop of umbilical cord is encircling the neck. It is not uncommon for a single loop of cord to be positioned this way. If such a loop is felt, it is gently loosened and drawn down over the fetal head. If it is too tightly coiled to allow for this procedure, it must be clamped and cut before the shoulders of the infant are delivered. If it is not treated this way, interference with the fetal oxygen supply or tearing of the umbilical cord can result.

Birth

The shoulders and the remainder of the newborn must now be delivered to free the chest for the first breath. Gentle pressure is exerted on the side of the infant's head, and the anterior shoulder nestles against the symphysis to allow the posterior shoulder to be born. The remainder of the body is then delivered.

The child is born when his whole body is delivered. This is the time that should be noted and recorded as the time of birth—a nursing responsibility. (Most physicians regard it as their responsibility, or pleasure, to announce the sex of the infant.)

Cutting and Clamping the Cord

The infant is held with his head in a slightly dependent position to allow secretions to drain from his nose and mouth; his mouth is gently aspirated by a bulb syringe to remove more secretions. The cord continues to pulsate for a few minutes after birth, and then the pulsation ceases. As soon as pulsation has stopped, the cord is clamped 8 to 10 inches from the infant's umbilicus by two Kelly hemostats and cut between them. An umbilical cord clamp or tie is then applied.

There are a number of theories as to the optimum time for cutting the cord. Delaying the cutting until pulsation ceases allows 50 to 100 ml of blood to pass from the placenta into the fetus. This may help to prevent iron deficiency anemia in infants. On the other hand, late clamping of the cord may cause overinfusion with placental blood. The timing of cord clamping will therefore vary, depending on the individual physician and situation.

First Respirations

With birth, the infant cries and draws in his first breath. His most important transition to the outside world, the establishment of independent respirations, has been made. He will be handed to the nurse, who receives him in a sterile blanket. Wrap him snugly (he is slippery from being wet, and he must be kept warm). If his respirations are good, take him to the head of the table to show him to his mother and father. It is easy to omit this step in the excitement of the moment, the excitement of feeling that you and the physician have delivered the baby. Allow a few moments for adoration, then carry him to the heated crib provided for newborn care. The second stage of labor is now complete (Fig. 22-13).

Nursing Interventions: Placental Stage

The placenta is delivered either by the natural bearing-down effort of the mother or by gentle pressure on the contracted uterine fundus by the physician. Pressure is never applied to a uterus in a noncontracted state or it may evert and hemorrhage.

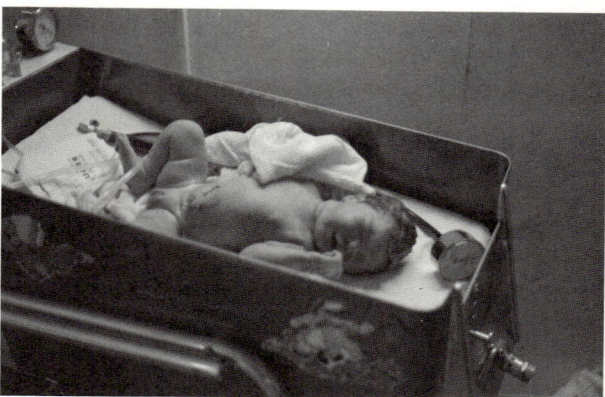

Fig. 22-13. A newborn baby minutes after birth.

Once the placenta is delivered, oxytocin, or ergonovine or one of its derivatives, or both, are generally administered on the physician's order. These medications increase uterine contractions and minimize bleeding.

One of the most widely used drugs is methylergonovine maleate (Methergine), a semisynthetic derivative of ergonovine. Methergine produces strong and effective contractions, and its effect lasts several hours. The usual dose is 0.2 mg (1 ml) given intramuscularly or intravenously. Another drug often used today is the synthetic oxytocin preparation Syntocinon. The usual dose is 10 units (1 ml) given intravenously or intramuscularly.

The administration of these drugs is the nurse's responsibility in most hospitals. She either administers the drug intramuscularly or adds it to an established intravenous line. Medication should not be given until the delivering physician indicates that it is the appropriate time. He may want it given as the fetal anterior shoulder is delivered or he may want to inspect the placenta first, to be certain that it is intact and without gross abnormalities and that none of its cotyledons remain in the uterus. Ergot derivatives cause hypertension by vasoconstriction and so must be used with caution in women with elevated blood pressure.

If the placenta does not deliver spontaneously, the physician will have to remove it manually. He needs fresh sterile gloves for this procedure in order not to introduce pathogens into the uterus.

PERINEAL REPAIR—ANESTHESIA

If suturing of the episiotomy is done immediately after the delivery of the placenta and inspection of the placenta by the physician, a woman who delivered without the aid of an anesthetic will theoretically still have so much natural pressure anesthesia of the perineum that she will not require an anesthetic. In actual practice, enough time has usually passed before the placenta is delivered (about 5 minutes) so that the woman needs injection of a local anesthetic in order to be comfortable during this procedure. Women who received a local block anesthetic such as a pudendal block before or those who have had spinal or general anesthesia do not need additional medication.

ASSESSMENT OF VITAL SIGNS

Take vital signs (pulse, respirations, and blood pressure) as the episiotomy is being sutured, to establish a postpartum baseline.

INTRODUCING THE INFANT

As soon as the immediate newborn care is complete (see Chap. 31), bring the infant to the table again, so that both mother and father can begin to get better acquainted.

A woman usually wants to touch her newborn (to prove to herself that he or she is *real*). She wants to have a complete look at the baby (to prove to herself that he has no defects). Remember the fall she had at the 5th month? Remember the day she did not feel the baby move for hours? She needs to be assured that nothing she did during pregnancy, or that happened to her during pregnancy, has hurt her baby. This is important reassurance for parents to be given if the parent-child relationship is to get off to a good start.

A mother may hold her baby if she wishes while she lies on the delivery table, but do not leave her alone with the infant because she is more tired than she realizes. If she wishes to breast-feed, this is an optimal time for her to begin. An infant sucking at the breast stimulates release of endogenous oxytocin, which aids in uterine contractions and involution or the returning of the uterus to its prepregnant state.

CHILLS

The mother usually becomes sensitive to the coolness of the delivery room at this time. She appreciates being covered with a warmed blanket. Mothers often experience a chill and shaking sensation 10 to 15 minutes after delivery. This is due in part to the low temperature of the delivery room but is primarily the result of exhilaration and exhaustion. It is a normal phenomenon, but it is frightening to the mother. She gets the same feeling as she did in labor, that her body is taking over and she is no longer in charge. She may associate the shaking chill with fever or infection and worry that she will be ill at a time when she most wants to be well to care for her new child. Reassure her that this is a normal happening. Fortunately, the sensation is transitory.

TRANSFER TO RECOVERY ROOM

When the episiotomy repair is complete (usually in about 10 minutes though it seems to the mother like half an hour), check the fundus height and consistency (see Chap. 26) for a baseline estimate. Check vital signs once more and help the mother slide to a recovery room bed or cart for transfer to the recovery room, or return the birthing room table to its original bed shape. Put a sterile perineal pad in place, held by a sanitary belt to absorb vaginal discharge (lochia).

If the father has not been in the delivery room, be certain the mother and he have an opportunity to talk together alone right after she leaves the delivery room. They have a great deal to discuss and fulfilled dreams to share (or crushed hopes if the child was the unanticipated sex).

Emergency Delivery of an Infant

Every nurse should have the knowledge and the ability to remain calm enough to deliver a baby in an emergency situation. Firemen, policemen, and taxicab drivers, who have much less knowledge of the birth process than a nurse, do this all the time.

Occasionally, a woman enters the hospital so far advanced in labor that delivery occurs before the resident or attending physician can arrive. Occasionally, despite the best-prepared labor unit, a multiparous woman, whose birth canal offers little resistance to birth, will deliver precipitously. The public health nurse may find herself summoned to assist at a home delivery. At any public event, a nurse may be called on to perform this service.

The first requirement in assisting at a precipitous delivery is calmness. Of all infants born, 95 percent are in a vertex presentation, and the majority are in an advantageous position (LOA or ROA). Thus, the probability is high that the delivery will be uncomplicated. Calmness on your part conveys to the woman (and to her husband if he is present) that there is reason for her to be calm as well. Relaxed, she can assist you—and the woman must assist; it is, after all, she, not you, who actually delivers the baby.

It is best if the woman does not push but pants with second-stage contractions as soon as the fetal head crowns, so that the fetal head will be born gently, without undue pressure. This limits tearing of the perineum and injury to the fetal head. Rest your hand on the fetal head to help control the fetus's egress. External rotation generally occurs spontaneously once the head is delivered. Have the mother pant once more during the final contraction to allow you time to check the neck of the infant for a loop of cord and to prevent the shoulders from being born too rapidly. If a loop of cord is present and slides free easily (and it usually does), pull it over the infant's head and free it; if it does not, it must be clamped or tied twice (with string ligatures, such as boiled shoelaces), then cut between the ties before the remainder of the child is delivered.

Take a clean piece of cloth and swab excess mucus from the infant's mouth. If it seems necessary, press down slightly on the side of the head until the superior shoulder impinges on the symphysis. A little upward pressure on the head delivers the inferior shoulder. With the inferior shoulder delivered, the superior shoulder slides out rapidly, and the remainder of the child's body is delivered smoothly. Be careful. The baby is very slippery.

Do not put traction on the cord as the body is delivered or you may cause a maternal hemorrhage by tearing or dislodging the placenta before it is ready to be delivered.

Hold the infant with his head slightly lowered, so that secretions drain from his mouth and throat. In a few moments he will draw in a quick breath and cry. The cry guarantees that he is breathing, because the sound is caused by the passage of air over the vocal cords. If he does not cry spontaneously (this is unlikely, since the mother has had no anesthesia to cause narcosis in the infant), do not attempt to spank him, tub him, jackknife him, or perform any of the actions you may have seen tried in the movies. Rub his back gently. If this is not effective in initiating respirations after 2 minutes, begin artificial respiration by mouth-to-mouth breathing (see Chap. 38).

If the infant is crying well and needs no special measures, do not attempt to cut the cord. Remember that the fetal vessels end in dead-end villi; the infant will not bleed from the placenta when the placenta is born. An infant can bleed from an insecurely tied cord, however, and cord ties are not as easy to tie as they look. The cord is wet, your hands are wet, you are nervous, and the string slips. The infant is perfectly safe with the umbilical cord left uncut.

Lay the infant on his mother's abdomen, face down, and wait for the signs that the placenta has separated: an extension of the umbilical cord, a spurt of new blood, a rising upward of the uterus. When these signs are evident, with gentle tension remove the placenta from the vagina. Do not attempt to push on the uterus to expel the placenta or you may cause inversion of the uterus. As soon as the placenta is delivered, the uterus will rise upward and contract against the abdominal wall. Since no oxytocin will be given, you will have to keep a hand on the fundus of the uterus, gently massaging it to help it to remain contracted (see Chap. 26).

Wrap the infant with the cord and placenta still attached in a warm blanket and arrange for transportation of infant and mother to a health care facility for follow-up care.

Problem-oriented Recording: Progress Notes

Christine McFadden
15 years

Problem: Progress in labor; admission assessment

> S. Screaming with each contraction; unable to utilize breathing exercises because of fright. Pelvic measurements are borderline; c-section possibly expected.
> O. Temperature 99; P 80, R 24, BP 110/80. Contractions average 20-sec duration, 10-min frequency, moderate intensity. Labor began 4 hours ago; effacement 50%; dilatation 3 cm. Station −2, vertex presentation, position ROA, FHR 130. Moderate amount pink-tinged show; membranes intact.
> A. Latent stage of labor; parameters within normal limits; known questionable pelvic adequacy.
>
> Goals: a. Labor completed within normal time limits.
> b. Learn to use breathing exercises to help with contractions.
> c. Fetal assessments remain within normal well limits.
> d. Able to establish a relationship with health personnel so she has support people meaningful to her during labor.
>
> P. 1. Admit to labor room.
> 2. Place external fetal and uterine monitors.
> 3. Notify private M.D. and house officer of admission.
> 4. Schedule sonogram or x-ray pelvimetry as ordered.
> 5. Partial perineal shave; no enema.
> 6. Vital sign and contraction assessment per routine.

Problem: Progress in labor; 10:00 A.M. interim assessment

> S. Asking to be told that progress is normal.
> O. Length of labor 8 hours. No further effacement or dilatation since admission. FHR 130; good variability. Station still −2.
> A. Doubtful progress in labor.
> P. 1. Pelvimetry scheduled, as ordered.
>   2. Establish cesarean-section nursing plan if decision is made.

Problem: Progress in labor; 11:00 A.M. interim assessment

> S. Has been told that a c-section is necessary. Mother has arrived as support person; seems concerned that c-section is necessary but relationship with daughter seems strained and cool.
> O. Vital signs stable as on admission. FHR 140 with good variability. Station—no progression.
> A. Primipara in need of cesarean section information.
> P. 1. Review anatomy so she is aware what will happen.
>   2. Discuss routine procedure of placing infant in Isolette for 24 hours post c-section.
>   3. Preparation of abdomen done.
>   4. No preoperative med. (Had Demerol 2 hours ago.)
>   5. Urge to void preop. Has not voided for 3 hours.
>   6. Continue support from nursing staff because of mother's questionable support.

Problem-oriented Recording: Progress Notes

Mary Kraft
22 years

Problem: Progress in labor; admission assessment

> S. Breathing regularly with contractions; lies supine to do breathing.
> O. Temperature 99.2, pulse 74, respirations 20, BP 110/78. Contractions 45-sec duration, 5-min frequency, moderate intensity. Labor began 7 hours ago. Effacement 70%; dilatation 2 cm. Station −1; vertex presentation, position LOA, FHR 120. Moderate amount pink-tinged show; membranes ruptured spontaneously just prior to coming to hospital. Fluid clear, no blood or meconium staining.
> A. Para 0, gravida 2 in latent stage of labor; assessments within normal limits. Caution: ruptured membranes.
> Goals: a. Labor and delivery completed within normal time limits.
>   b. Labor and delivery accomplished without medication or anesthetic interventions; to use breathing exercises.
>   c. Fetal assessments remain within normal limits.
>   d. Husband to be present for delivery.
> P. 1. Admit to birthing room.
>   2. Place external fetal and uterine monitors.
>   3. Encourage to lie on side, not back, for labor.
>   4. Notify private M.D. and house officer of admission.
>   5. Partial perineal shave. No enema given as membranes are ruptured.
>   6. Keep nonambulatory until checked by M.D.
>   7. Vital sign and contraction assessment per routine.

Problem: Progress in labor; interim assessment: beginning second stage of labor

> S. States, "I didn't know pushing would feel like this. How long does it take now?" Pushing effectively with contractions.
> O. Contractions 60-sec duration; frequency q2min; FHR 130, good variability. Crowning beginning; moderate amount of blood-tinged show evident.
> A. Para 0, gravida 2 in second stage of labor; parameters within normal limits.
> P. 1. Encourage pushing efforts.
>   2. Ready birthing room for delivery.

3. Ready baby care island for newborn care.
4. M.D. in attendance; no notification necessary.

Problem: Progress in labor; interim assessment: birth of child

S. States, "This has got to be the greatest moment in my life."
O. Delivered 6 lb 5 oz boy at 4:05. Breathed spontaneously. Apgar 8 at 1 min; 9 at 5 min. Delivered placenta at 4:20. Placenta intact, by gross inspection. Perineal sutures set by Dr. B. Blood loss estimated as 300 ml by M.D. Breast-fed on delivery table.
A. Second and third stage of labor complete.
P. 1. To remain in birthing room with infant and husband for first hour post partum.
2. Transfer to rooming-in unit following first hour of care.
3. Support breast-feeding decision especially in light of successful delivery room experience.

Problem-oriented Recording: Progress Notes

Angie Baco
42 years

Problem: Progress in labor; admission assessment

S. Has gestational diabetes. Knows she will use delivery room, not birthing room, because of possible high-risk fetus. Had past babies this way; accepting of it. Is aware that she is in very early labor but was instructed to come to hospital as soon as labor began. Husband with her as support person. Young child at home being cared for by married sibling. No worries about his care.
O. Temperature 98.8, P 86, R 24, BP 130/90. Contractions irregular, 20–30 sec duration; intensity mild; frequency q20min. Contractions began 1 hour ago. Effacement 50%; dilatation 2 cm; station −1; presentation vertex; position LOA, FHR 140.

A. Gestational diabetic in latent stage of labor; para 6, gravida 7.

Goals: a. Labor and delivery completed within normal time limits.
b. Fetal assessments remain within normal limits.
c. Be able to accept extra procedures or interventions necessary because of medical problem.

P. 1. Mark high-risk because of gestational diabetes and being grand multipara.
2. Admit to labor room.
3. Place external fetal and uterine monitor.
4. Routine vital sign and contraction assessment, except BP ½h (130/90 in early labor).
5. Notify house officer and private M.D. of admission.
6. Establish high-risk diabetic program of care as ordered.

References

1. Angelini, D. J. Nonverbal communication in labor. *Am. J. Nurs.* 78:1220, 1978.
2. Bonica, J. J., and Hon, E. H. Fetal Distress. In J. J. Bonica (Ed.), *Principles and Practice of Obstetric Analgesia and Anesthesia.* Philadelphia: Davis, 1969. Vol. 2.
3. Cahill, A. S. Dual-purpose tool for assessing maternal needs and nursing care. *J.O.G.N. Nurs.* 4:28, 1975.
4. Cirz, D. Nurses and the future in childbirth. *J.O.G.N. Nurs.* 7:25, 1978.
5. Cohen, W. R., and Rosen, R. Recognition and treatment of fetal distress during labor. *J.O.G.N. Nurs.* 5:565, 1976.
6. Freeman, R. Defining the role of antepartum monitoring. *Contemp. Obstet. Gynecol.* 13:65, 1979.
7. Hardy, C. T., et al. Hospital meets patient demand for "home style" childbirth. *Hospitals* 52:73, 1978.
8. Highley, B., et al. Safeguarding the laboring woman's sense of control. *M.C.N.* 3:39, 1978.
9. Hon, E. H., and Paul, R. H. *A Primer of Fetal Heart Rate Patterns.* New Haven, Conn.: Harty Press, 1970.
10. Hugo, M. A look at maternal position during labor. *J. Nurse Midwife.* 22:26, 1977.
11. Huprich, P. A. Assisting the couple through a Lamaze labor and delivery. *M.C.N.* 2:245, 1977.
12. Jennings, B. Emergency delivery: How to attend to one safely. *M.C.N.* 4:148, 1979.
13. Kerner, J., et al. An alternative birth center in a community teaching hospital. *Obstet. Gynecol.* 51: 371, 1978.
14. Lederman, R. P. Evaluating Uterine Contractions of

Women in Labor. In J. S. Malinowski, *Nursing Care of the Labor Patient*. Philadelphia: Davis, 1978.
15. Malinowski, J. S., et al. Interpreting Fetal Heart Rates. In J. S. Malinowski, *Nursing Care of the Labor Patient*. Philadelphia: Davis, 1978.
16. Mozingo, J. N. Pain in labor: A conceptual model for intervention. *J.O.G.N. Nurs.* 7:47, 1978.
17. Paul, R. H., and Miller, F. C. Antepartum fetal heart rate monitoring. *Clin. Obstet. Gynecol.* 21:375, 1978.
18. Phillips, C. R. The essence of birth without violence. *M.C.N.* 1:162, 1976.
19. Pillay, S. K., et al. Fetal monitoring: A guide to understanding the equipment. *Clin. Obstet. Gynecol.* 22:571, 1980.
20. Quilligan, E. J. Identifying true fetal distress. *Contemp. Obstet. Gynecol.* 13:89, 1979.
21. Sokal, R. J., et al. Slowing of active labor with internal fetal monitoring. *Am. J. Obstet. Gynecol.* 124:764, 1976.

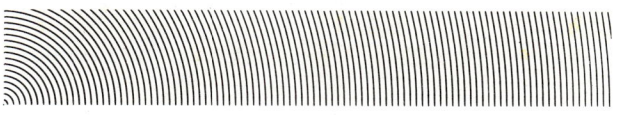

23. Analgesia and Anesthesia in Labor and Delivery

The contractions of the uterus are unique among involuntary muscle contractions in that they cause pain. (Contractions of the heart, stomach, and intestine involve involuntary muscles and do not cause pain.)

The pain that accompanies uterine contractions in labor occurs for several possible reasons. Uterine contractions cause anoxia to uterine and cervical cells as the blood supply to the cells is impaired by the stricture of blood vessels. This anoxia may cause pain. As labor progresses and contractions become longer and harder, the ischemia to cells increases, the anoxia increases, and the pain intensifies.

Stretching of the cervix and perineum is also a source of pain. This phenomenon coincides with the phenomenon that causes intestinal pain when intestines are stretched by gas. At the end of the transitional point in labor, when stretching of the cervix is complete and the woman begins to feel like pushing, pain from contractions often magically ends as long as she is pushing.

Additional discomfort in labor may stem from the pressure of the presenting part of the fetus on tissues, including pressure on surrounding organs: the bladder, the urethra, and the lower colon. The pain of delivery is basically pain from stretching of the perineal tissue.

Sensory impulses from the uterus and cervix synapse at the spinal column at the level of T10, T11, T12, and L1. Pain relief for the first stage of labor, therefore, must be either systemic relief or medication that blocks these synapse sites.

Sensory impulses from the perineum are carried by the pudendal nerve to join the spinal column at S2, S3, and S4. Pain relief for delivery, therefore, must be provided either systemically or regionally to block these lower receptor sites. This is an important point to remember when talking to women in labor about pain relief. Some interventions relieve pain for both first *and* second stages of labor; others for first *or* second stage but not for both.

Both analgesia and anesthesia interventions may be used with women in labor. Analgesia refers to the absence or diminished awareness of pain. Anesthesia refers to the complete loss of sensation, regional (loss of sensation just to particular body parts) or general. With general anesthesia, there is accompanying loss of consciousness.

Because most women are not allowed to eat during labor, any medications are generally given by an intramuscular or intravenous route. Exceptions are medications such as barbiturates, which are given so early in labor that they may be ingested orally.

The amount of discomfort a woman experiences

from contractions differs according to her expectations and preparation for labor, the length of her labor, the position of the fetus, the unique character of her labor, and the availability of support people around her. The discomfort experienced with labor becomes compounded when fear and anxiety are also present.

One theory as to why pain is perceived is the *gate-control theory*. This theory suggests that the body can close "gates" at various intervals in the central nervous system, effectively blocking transmission of pain past that point or not allowing the transmission to reach cortical centers where it would register as pain.

Pain apparently is transmitted by small-diameter nerve fibers. These small nerve fibers can be blocked by stimulation (such as rubbing) of large-diameter nerve fibers lying near them. This is why rubbing the skin (an almost involuntary action on your part when you stub a toe or bump a knee) reduces pain. Pain sensation may also be reduced by the use of distraction or by changing the interpretation of pain for that particular person. Prepared childbirth methods incorporate all these methods into plans for reducing pain in labor: gently messaging the abdomen, focusing on a fixed object, and asking for explanations of what is happening so a person can understand clearly what a new pain or a different pain sensation means.

People respond to stress or pain in different ways based on sociocultural expectations and their individual reactions to being themselves. Some people with discomfort want everyone around them to know how uncomfortable they are; others prefer to keep their feelings to themselves. Some women view labor and childbirth as an illness and expect to act "ill" and in distress in labor. Others regard childbirth as a wellness activity and expect to remain quiet and calm throughout the process. Some women are reluctant to show that labor contractions are painful for fear of influencing a young nursing student with them against childbirth!

Pain may be perceived differently by different people not only because of psychosocial responses to pain, but because of physiological ones as well. When pain is perceived by the body, opiate-like substances to reduce pain appear to be produced by the body. The level of these naturally occurring substances or the body's ability to produce and maintain them may influence the amount of pain perceived at any given time.

Evaluate how much discomfort a woman is having in labor by what she voices. Look also for subtle signs of pain such as facial tenseness, flushing or paleness of her face, fisted hands, rapid breathing, or rapid pulse rate. Knowing the extent of the woman's discomfort is a guide to the choice of medication or intervention she needs in labor.

Some women are able to use prepared-childbirth exercises to take the bite or edge off contractions so successfully that no other pain relief measures are needed. Others find that they need some medication to take enough edge off the contraction to begin to breathe effectively and make their prepared-childbirth exercises work.

Women who come into labor believing it will be as horrible as depicted in the stories they have heard are usually surprised afterward to realize that the agony they expected never materialized. Expectations of pain to come, however, make women so tense during labor that the pain of their contractions is worse than it would be if they were relaxed. No one can relax simply because another person tells her to, however. Women in labor relax best if they have a clear understanding that labor contractions are rhythmic in nature: they *come and go, come and go, come and go,* and when a contraction ends, the discomfort ends with it. This seems to be a simple enough explanation to offer patients, who already should be aware of it, since the contractions and the intervals between them are happening to *them*. A woman may not be entirely aware that this is the nature of contractions, however, or she may fear that their nature will change as labor progresses.

The pain of toothaches and severe headaches is unbearable because it is sharp and continuous. But with labor contractions, just knowing that the pain will soon vanish can make it easier to tolerate.

A great deal has been written in nursing literature about calling labor contractions "contractions" and not labor pains. The theory is a sound one, not only because the sensation the woman feels is a contraction but also because the woman who anticipates pain becomes tense, and tension magnifies pain. Remember, nevertheless, that renaming a happening does not change its basic nature. By any name, discomfort accompanies labor. Fortunately, many nursing interventions can help to reduce pain and allow labor to be as fulfilling and rewarding an experience as a woman hopes it will be.

Nursing Interventions to Minimize Discomfort

Careful explanation of what is happening and going to happen during labor goes a long way toward alleviating anxiety and thereby reducing some of the discomfort of labor. When you are a student, the process of explaining everything that is happening seems natural and comfortable, because it is new to you, too, and you appreciate its novelty. After you have cared for the hundredth woman in labor, however, the explanations grow fewer and fewer. You begin to think that surely there is no one in this world who does not know what a delivery room looks like, who is unaware that the rupturing of membranes is painless, that a pink-stained show is normal, that contractions change in character at the second stage of labor. The woman in the labor bed having her first child *does not know*; the woman having her seventh child *does not remember* what it was like the last time or perhaps finds it different enough this time (although still within normal limits) to frighten her. Be certain to give explanations to the woman's husband or other support person as well as to her. It does no good to reassure her that everything is fine when her husband has not been reassured and begins to transmit his anxiety to her.

Anyone can stand a little discomfort from a backache. Anyone can stand being thirsty and having dry lips. Anyone can stand having a leg cramp. Few people can stand feeling all these things at once and experiencing labor contractions in addition.

Use the ordinary comfort measures with labor patients that you would use with all patients. A woman needs ice chips to suck on or a wet cloth to wipe her lips during labor. She needs a cool cloth to wipe perspiration from her forehead. Rubbing or massaging her sacral area often alleviates back pain. Pressing against her sacral area during a contraction may help. Pelvic rocking between contractions may relieve tense back muscles. Think of comfort measures for the woman's support person as well. Is the chair by the side of the bed comfortable? Does he need a stretch or a break? He cannot comfort well if he is uncomfortable himself (Fig. 23-1).

Help the woman find a comfortable position. For many women this is on one side or the other. For some it may be on their back. Other women like to lie flat; still others like the head of the bed raised. In early labor, before membranes have ruptured, the mother may find either sitting in a chair or walking about her most comfortable position. After membranes have ruptured, if the fetal head is not engaged, there is a danger in walking about; the cord might prolapse and fetal circulation might be impaired.

Mothers who choose a back-lying position in labor need to be observed closely for *supine hypotensive syndrome*. This occurs because pressure from the

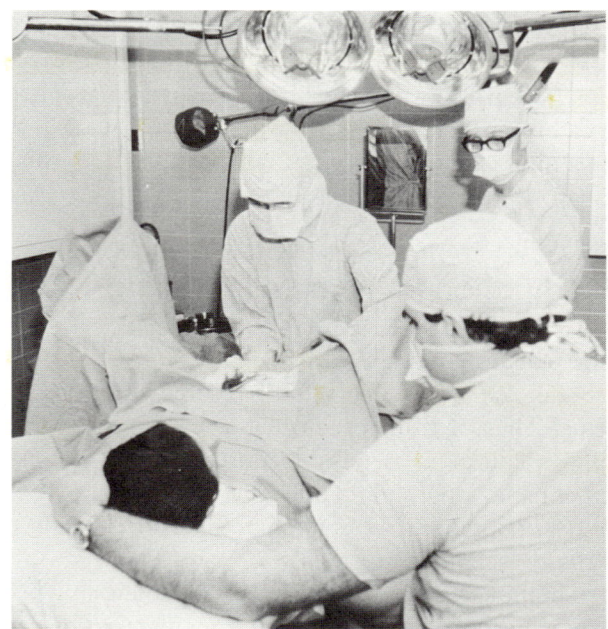

Fig. 23-1. Having a support person present during labor has a great influence on decreasing pain in labor. Here a husband sits with his wife moments before birth. (Courtesy of the Department of Medical Photography, Children's Hospital, Buffalo, N. Y.)

heavy uterus obstructs the flow of blood returning from the vena cava to the heart. The woman suddenly feels faint and breathless; her blood pressure will be low, and her pulse may be rapid and weak. Her facial expression is one of apprehension, as she is frightened by this sudden feeling of helplessness and shortness of breath. Turning her on her side (perhaps administering oxygen for a few minutes) will relieve symptoms. Turning her to her side lifts the weight of the uterus away from the vena cava and allows blood return to flow freely again.

Be aware of what is happening to the woman's bedclothes. Wrinkles form rapidly if she is uncomfortable and moving about a great deal. The waterproof pad under her buttocks, soiled with vaginal secretions, becomes hot and sticky. Her hospital gown becomes wrinkled and sticks to her because she is sweating. Change the waterproof pad frequently. Never use sanitary pads in labor. Although they absorb vaginal secretions well, they tend to move and may carry pathogens from the rectal area forward to the vaginal opening. Halfway through the first stage of labor, clean sheets and a clean gown give a woman a fresh, ready-to-go-again feeling.

Giving good explanations and providing simple comforts are basic nursing skills, and they constitute a form of analgesia to women in labor.

Prepared Childbirth Exercises

A woman's best analgesia for labor is breathing exercises. Help the woman who is prepared to use her breathing patterns. Teach the unprepared woman a breathing pattern such as abdominal breathing. (See Chap. 19.)

Medication for Pain Relief During Labor

For practical purposes, all medication given during labor crosses the placenta and has some effect on the fetus. Thus, it is important that a woman receive as little medication as possible during labor. On the other hand, labor should not test a woman to the limit of her endurance. She is in labor to be a mother, not a martyr.

The history of pain relief in labor is interesting because the pattern of intervention for pain relief has swung from a feeling that none was necessary to a feeling that too much was necessary to a modern-day approach of individual consideration for a woman's needs and preferences. For centuries, offering pain relief in labor was thought to be amoral because, according to the biblical account, God commanded Eve, "I will greatly multiply thy sorrow and thy conception; in sorrow thou shalt bring forth children . . ." (Genesis 3:16). In the witch-burning period of American history, the concept that childbirth should be painful was so strong that women were burned as witches for providing comfort to women in labor.

With the discovery of ether and chloroform in the 1800s it became apparent that childbirth could be managed completely pain-free. Unfortunately, this goal was achieved by means of complete anesthesia or unconsciousness during labor and delivery. In an account describing the first time a woman was delivered under chloroform by Sir James Simpson, in 1847, he wrote, "Shortly after her infant was brought in by the nurse from the adjoining room, it was a matter of no small difficulty to convince the astonished mother that labor was entirely over and the child presented to her was really her own living baby" [10]. Aside from the physiological risk to women from general anesthesia, this inability to accept the event of birth, to change from "being pregnant" to "being a mother" is a major disadvantage of general anesthetics or too much intervention in childbirth.

A suitable medication for use during labor must relax the woman and relieve her pain, yet have minimal effect on her systemically, on uterine contractions, and on the fetus. If a drug causes a systemic response such as hypotension in the woman, there will be a decreased PO_2 gradient across the placenta and fetal hypoxia. If it causes confusion or disorientation in the woman, she will not be able to work effectively with labor and labor may be prolonged. If a medication causes changes in the fetus such as a decreased heart rate or central nervous system (CNS) depression so that it is difficult for the newborn infant to initiate respirations, he will be severely compromised in his important first minutes of life.

Once labor is well under way, medication to relieve discomfort tends to speed labor progress because the woman is better able to work with, not against, contractions. Medication given too early tends to slow or even stop labor contractions. A rule of thumb is to give an analgesic to a primipara only when she is dilated at least 3 cm; a multipara should be dilated 4 cm before receiving analgesia.

Unfortunately, there is no perfect analgesic agent for labor or delivery that has no effect on labor, the mother, and the fetus.

Medications used during labor vary from hospital to hospital, and the efficacy of new drugs is constantly being explored. Thus, it is impractical to memorize a list of drugs that are safe. It is better to remember the criteria that a drug must fulfill to be used in labor and expand the rule of basic medication administration from "Never give any drug unless you know it is safe for your individual patient" to "Never give a drug in labor without knowing it is safe for both your patients, the mother and the fetus." A timetable for administration of analgesics and anesthetics in labor is shown in Table 23-1.

NARCOTICS

Narcotics are given in labor because of their potent analgesic effect. As a category, all these drugs cause fetal CNS depression and should be questioned when ordered for a woman in premature labor. A premature infant may have extreme difficulty standing the added insult of respiratory depression.

Morphine sulfate is an example of a narcotic formerly used a great deal in labor. It is less popular today because of its tendency to reduce maternal respiratory rates and to cause severe respiratory depression in the infant.

Meperidine hydrochloride (Demerol) is a synthetic narcotic commonly used today. Demerol is advantageous because it not only is an analgesic but has sedative and antispasmodic action as well. Thus it is effective in relieving pain and also helps to relax the cervix and give a feeling of euphoria and well-being. Demerol may be given either intramuscularly or intravenously. The dose is 25 to 100 mg depending

Table 23-1. Timetable of Administration Analgesics and Anesthetics in Labor

Preparatory Division	Dilatational Division	Pelvic Division	
Early (1–3 cm dilatation)	Mid (4–8 cm dilatation)	Late (8–10 cm transition) or Deceleration	Second Stage
Independent nursing interventions (back rub, clean bedding, etc.)	Analgesics such as Demerol →	Narcotic antagonists such as Narcan	
Barbiturates alone (to induce relaxation and sleep) →	Analgesics such as Demerol and a tranquilizer such as Sparine in combination →		
Tranquilizers alone (to induce relaxation and to reduce apprehension) →	Analgesics such as Demerol and an amnesic such as scopolamine in combination →		
	Paracervical blocks ——————————————————→		
	Epidural blocks ——————————————————————→		
	Gas analgesic such as Trilene		Pudendal block ————→
			Saddle block
			General anesthesia

on the body weight of the woman. Action begins in about 30 minutes; duration of action is 2 to 3 hours. Since Demerol crosses the placenta, it may cause depression in the fetus. The drug crosses the placenta minutes after being administered to the mother. The fetal liver takes 2 to 3 hours, however, to activate the drug in the fetal system, so the effect will not be registered in the fetus for 2 to 3 hours after administration. For this reason Demerol is given when the mother is more than 3 hours away from delivery (thus the peak action time of the drug in the fetus will have passed by the time of delivery). It is often a paradox to see a sleepy baby delivered to a woman who was given Demerol 2 hours before delivery, a wide-awake baby delivered to a woman who had Demerol within 1 hour of delivery. In the second instance the peak action or peak effect had not yet been reached in the infant.

Alphaprodine (Nisentil) is a narcotic with a shorter onset of action and longer duration than Demerol. Since the maximum fetal drug concentration is unpredictable with Nisentil, neonatal depression may occur even if the drug was administered more than an hour away from delivery. For this reason Nisentil is a less popular medication in labor than previously.

Women who are addicted to narcotics may be given methadone in labor. Care of the narcotic-addicted woman is discussed in Chap. 33.

Whenever a narcotic is given during labor, a narcotic antagonist, such as naloxone (Narcan), should be available for administration to the infant at birth. If severe infant respiratory depression is suspected, Narcan can be given to the mother just before delivery. It crosses the placenta readily and may increase the chance for spontaneous respiratory activity. Narcan is preferable as a narcotic antagonist to nalorphine (Nalline) or levallorphan (Lorfan); the latter two products tend to have depressant effects on neonates in themselves.

SYNTHETIC ANALGESICS

Pentazocine lactate (Talwin) is a comparatively new synthetic agent that appears to alleviate pain as effectively as Demerol. It is usually administered as a single dose of 30 mg given intramuscularly. Its effect begins in 15 to 20 minutes.

BARBITURATES

Occasionally, a woman's most pressing need in labor is not pain relief but sleep. She comes to the hospital in the middle of the night in early labor because she is worried that she will deliver at home. Her contractions, although perhaps frequent, are not strong. Little dilatation has occurred. A short-acting barbiturate such as sodium secobarbital (Seconal) allows the woman to sleep until contractions become stronger and more effective. The usual dose of Seconal is 100 to 200 mg given orally. Barbiturates used in labor must be short-acting and should never be given close to delivery; they cross the placenta readily and cause respiratory depression in the newborn. Narcotic antagonists are not effective in reducing oversedation from barbiturates.

TRANQUILIZERS

Tranquilizers are given as adjunctive therapy in labor because they reduce apprehension and complement narcotics and barbiturates to such an extent that lower doses of narcotics or barbiturates can sometimes be used.

Diazepam (Valium) is a tranquilizer that should be used with caution in a woman in premature labor. Its sodium benzoate base may compete with bilirubin binding sites in the fetal circulation and therefore increase the risk of kernicterus (brain damage from high bilirubin levels) in the newborn. Promethazine (Phenergan), promazine (Sparine), and hydroxyzine pamoate (Vistaril) are frequently used with labor patients. Phenergan has a long effect (up to 8 hours) and so must not be repeated at more frequent time intervals during labor.

AMNESICS

Sixty years ago, a medication combining scopolamine, an alkaloid of belladonna, and morphine sulfate was introduced for use in labor. The anesthesia and amnesia effected by this combination caused the woman to be in deep sleep all during labor (thus the term *twilight sleep*). Although the woman shrieked and thrashed with each labor contraction, she reported afterward that she felt little or no pain. Unfortunately, she also reported that she did not remember anything that happened; it was difficult for her to believe that she had delivered a baby. In addition, the medication induced narcosis and apnea in the infant.

Small doses of scopolamine (0.4 mg) are sometimes used today in conjunction with Demerol, not to induce twilight sleep but to complement the action of Demerol. Scopolamine causes a vascular flush (most noticeable in the face) shortly after administration. It is wise to caution the woman that this may happen, lest she or her husband become concerned when it does. Scopolamine may cause abnormal fetal heart rate patterns (reduced beat-to-beat variability) on a fetal monitoring device; it may reduce the fetal heart rate. The antagonist for scopolamine is physostigmine. It could be administered intravenously to counteract the effect of scopolamine.

Scopolamine should not be given without an accompanying analgesic, or the woman may experience excitement, hallucinations, or delirium if she is then exposed to pain (and in labor she is bound to be exposed to pain). Because scopolamine is an amnesic, a woman who has received even small doses during labor will remember little of what happened during labor. Since it causes the woman to sleep or doze during contractions, its use creates a problem for the woman who wants to use her breathing exercises with her contractions. It is a drug little used today.

GAS ANESTHESIA

Trichloroethylene (Trilene) is a liquid that vaporizes readily. It may be used for pain relief during the latter part of the first stage of labor or during the second stage of labor. Trilene is administered by a specially designed mask strapped to the woman's wrist. When she feels she needs pain relief, such as at the peak of a contraction, she takes a deep breath of the gas. She feels giddy, the pain fades, and her arm falls away from her face. She repeats the action again with the next contraction if necessary.

Although self-administered analgesia seems ideal, it is not totally satisfactory in actual practice. Women under stress think less clearly and make decisions less easily than those free of stress. People under stress enjoy having decisions made for them and having help given to them, rather than actively helping themselves. For this reason, self-administered Trilene may be an unsatisfactory method of pain relief for some women.

It is highly unlikely that a woman will receive too much Trilene when it is used as described and for inducing analgesia. However, there is always a possibility that her hand will not fall away but will remain close to her nostrils, with inhalation of the gas continuing until she becomes anesthetized. Thus, constant attention is required while a Trilene mask is in place. Trilene should not be administered for more than 4 hours during the course of labor as prolonged administration may lead to fetal depression.

Methoxyflurane is a second inhalant that may be self-administered during labor. As with Trilene, there is no significant neonatal depression when the inhalant is used at analgesic levels. Neither of these gases interferes with uterine tone, as may happen with other inhalation agents such as ether or chloroform. With extensive use (more than 15 ml of liquid) renal toxicity may occur with methoxyflurane.

REGIONAL ANESTHESIA

Because regional anesthetics are not introduced into the maternal circulation, it was once believed that they had no effect on the fetus. Now it has been demonstrated that there is some uptake of these drugs by the fetus. Effects on the fetus are minimal compared to those of systemic anesthetic agents, however, and the woman is allowed to be completely awake and aware of what is happening during delivery. Since regional anesthetics do not depress uterine tone, they leave the uterus capable of optimal contraction following delivery, which is an important concern in the prevention of postpartal hemorrhage. Depending on the region anesthetized, the woman may or may not continue to feel contractions following administration of such anesthesia. Injection sites of various regional anesthetic procedures are shown in Fig. 23-2.

Epidural Blocks

The spinal nerves in the cord are protected by a number of layers of tissue. The pia mater is the membrane adhering to the nerve fibers; surrounding this is the cerebral spinal fluid (CSF); next come the arachnoid membrane and the dura mater. Outside the dura mater is a rather vacant space (the epidural space), and beyond it is the ligamentum flavum, yet another protective shield to the vulnerable spinal cord.

If an anesthetic agent is introduced into the area of the CSF (the subarachnoid space), this is a spinal injection or spinal anesthesia. If the anesthetic is placed just inside the ligamentum flavum, it is in the epidural space and is an epidural anesthetic or block.

Anesthetic agents placed in this space block not only spinal nerve roots in the space but also the sympathetic nerve fibers that travel with them. Such a block will provide pain relief for both labor and delivery. Anatomy of the spinal canal illustrating these spaces is shown in Fig. 23-3.

The two anesthetic agents of choice for this type of regional anesthesia are chloroprocaine (Nesacaine 1.5%) and bupivacaine (Marcaine 0.25 to 0.5%). These agents appear to have the least effect on the newborn.

Women will not have "spinal headaches" following epidural anesthesia because those headaches are caused by leakage of CSF and the CSF space is not entered.

As with all regional anesthesia, rapid absorption or toxic reactions to the anesthetic agents may lead to symptoms of drowsiness, loss of coordination, and slurred speech. In extreme reactions, convulsions and loss of consciousness can ensue. Women who begin such reactions need to be provided with an airway and oxygen administration. If hypotension occurs, intravenous fluid and vasopressors may be necessary to stabilize cardiovascular status. Small amounts of short-acting barbiturates or diazepam (Valium) will control convulsions. Such reactions are very rare but should be kept in mind when you are working with

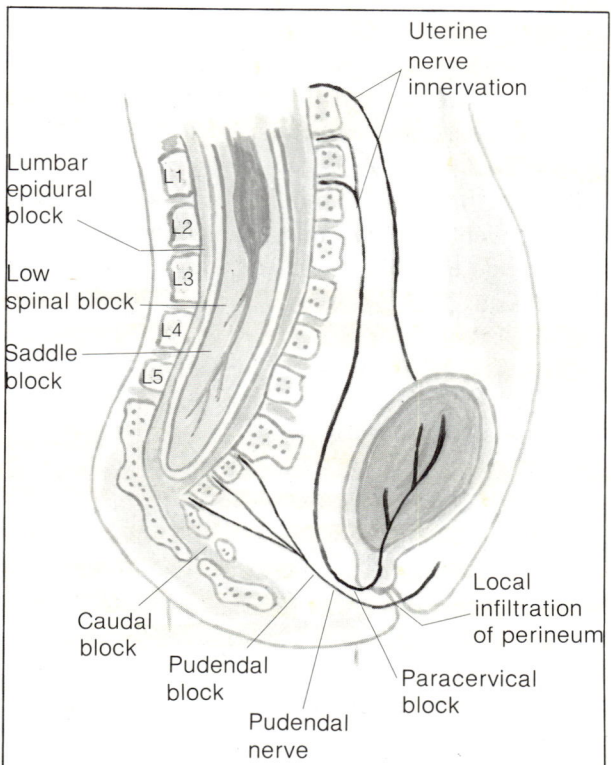

Fig. 23-2. Sites of injection for regional anesthesia for labor and delivery.

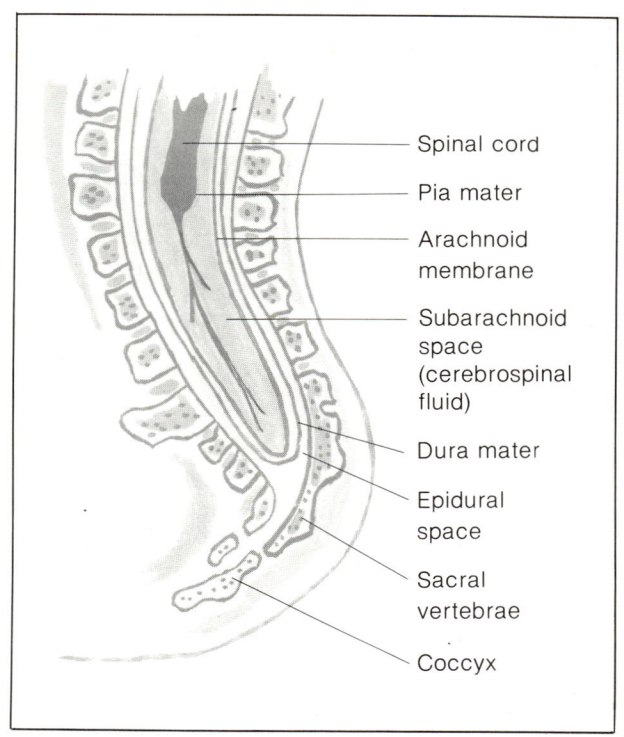

Fig. 23-3. Anatomy of the spinal canal.

persons receiving large amounts of regional anesthetics, as are used with women in labor.

Epidural blocks are advantageous for women with heart disease, pulmonary disease, diabetes, and sometimes severe pregnancy-induced hypertension. They make labor virtually pain-free, and stress from the discomfort of labor minimal. They are acceptable for use in premature labor because the drug has scant effect on the fetus. They allow for a controlled and gentle delivery with less trauma to an immature skull.

The second stage of labor may be prolonged by the use of an epidural block because the woman is unaware of contractions and therefore does not push with them. Relaxation of the levator muscle may impede rotation of the fetal head and further slow labor.

CAUDAL ANESTHESIA. The epidural space at the base of the spinal cord is termed the *caudal canal*. Injection of a local anesthetic into the caudal canal (the space level with the last sacral vertebra) acts by locally blocking the low sacral nerves that leave the caudal canal at this point.

Caudal anesthesia is begun when the cervix is dilated 3 to 4 cm. The woman is turned on her side in a lateral Sims's position. The sacral and coccygeal areas of her back are cleansed with an antiseptic solution. A local anesthetic is injected into the skin to form a wheal over the last sacral vertebra. A 3- to 5-inch needle is then passed through the nonclosure space of this vertebra (the sacral hiatus) down into the caudal space (Fig. 23-4). A physician may want a glove at this point to palpate the woman's rectum to be certain that the needle has not penetrated forward into the rectum. Following needle placement, a polyethylene catheter is passed through the needle into the space and the needle is withdrawn, leaving the catheter to be taped in place. A closed system (a syringe is attached) is established to prevent infection.

A test dose of 2 to 4 ml of a local anesthetic solution is injected through the catheter. Five minutes later, the woman's legs are inspected for flushing and warmness, evidence that the anesthetic is in the caudal space. A rectal examination checks for sphincter relaxation, another good indication that the anesthetic is beginning to work. The woman is asked to demonstrate that she can move her legs and that she has sensory perception or can feel a pinprick in her legs. If she does, this is further evidence that the catheter is indeed in the caudal space and has not been accidentally placed in the fluid of the spinal canal. If it were in the spinal canal, she would feel numbness and not be able to move her legs. An initial dose of about 15 to 20 ml of anesthetic is then given by the catheter. This produces anesthesia up to the level of the umbilicus. The effect of the anesthetic is short-lived (about 40 minutes). Every 40 minutes, therefore, another 20 ml of anesthetic must be administered to keep the woman free from discomfort.

As mentioned, caudal anesthesia tends to prolong the second stage of labor, since pushing with contractions is impaired by lack of uterine sensation. Forceps are usually needed for delivery.

The chief problem with caudal anesthesia is its tendency to induce hypotension in the woman. This is due to sympathetic blockage. When it occurs, there is decreased peripheral resistance in the woman's circulatory system; blood flows freely into peripheral vessels and a pseudohypovolemia registered as hypotension occurs.

Because this complication is seen in about 20 percent of patients, a nurse must be in continuous attendance when a caudal anesthetic is given. To detect hypotension, blood pressure should be taken every minute for the first 15 minutes after each new injection of anesthetic. Blood pressure should be monitored throughout the time the anesthetic is in effect.

Hypotension may be corrected by prompt elevation of the woman's legs (to increase blood flow in upper body areas), by turning her to her left side (to free the vena cava from the pressure of the uterus and increase blood flow), or by the administration of a vasopressor such as ephedrine. Oxygen administration by a face mask will decrease the possibility of hypoxia in the fetus.

Because of the risk of infecting the caudal canal, a caudal anesthetic should not be used if the woman has an old pilonidal sinus or any infection over the

Fig. 23-4. Administration of caudal anesthesia.

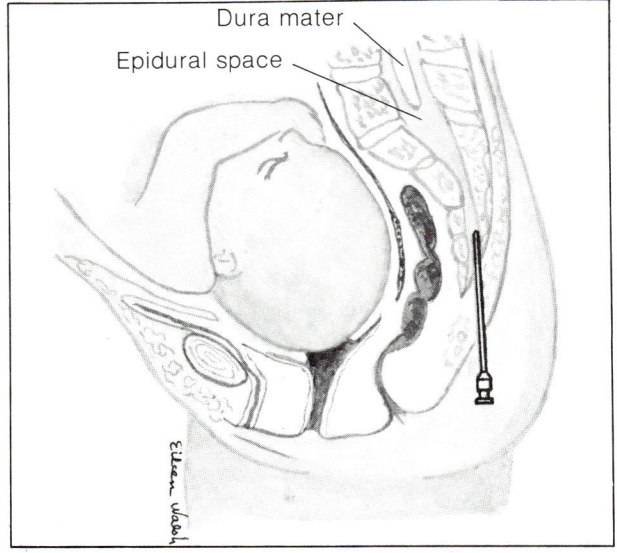

sacral area. Its use should be questioned with women who already have a lowered blood pressure such as would occur with the woman who has had a hemorrhage.

Do not attempt to supervise a woman undergoing epidural anesthesia unless you have a clear understanding of the measures you are to institute if hypotension occurs (usually defined as a systolic pressure below 100 mm Hg or a decrease of 20 mm Hg in a hypertensive woman). The magnitude of the drop may be life-threatening to the fetus unless prompt, effective corrective measures are undertaken. If such measures are instituted quickly, fetal outcome will not be compromised by the event.

LUMBAR EPIDURAL BLOCK. Invading the epidural space through a lumbar approach is technically easier and hence is the epidural block approach most often used today. The mother is turned to her side for the injection; the puncture site is the L3 to L4 or L2 to L3 spinous interspace. A catheter is inserted for continuous injection to provide anesthesia for both labor and delivery. Contraindications and complications of lumbar epidural anesthesia are the same as for caudal epidural anesthesia.

Paracervical Block

In a paracervical block, an anesthetic solution such as bupivacaine (Marcaine) is injected through the vagina into the cervical fornices at the 4- and 8-o'clock positions (Fig. 23-5). This blocks the sympathetic nerve pathway from the uterus, but not the pudendal nerve. It is therefore used as a regional anesthetic for labor, but not for delivery. It is done at 4 to 6 cm dilatation. If the fetal head is at a plus station, paracervical blocks are very difficult to perform.

The woman should void prior to insertion of the drug to allow the anesthesiologist maximum vaginal space available for positioning the needle. She should be on her back with her knees flexed as she would be for a vaginal examination. A paracervical needle is long and may be frightening if the mother is not warned that it is long in order to reach its destination, not long because it is going to be injected that far into her.

Following injection, pain relief occurs within 5 minutes. Local anesthetics are short-acting, and, as with an epidural block, repeated injections may be needed during a lengthy labor. In a woman who receives a paracervical block, a fetal heart monitor should be continuously in place. There is an increased incidence of fetal bradycardia following administration of the medication due to a depressant effect on the fetal myocardium. Fetal heart rates

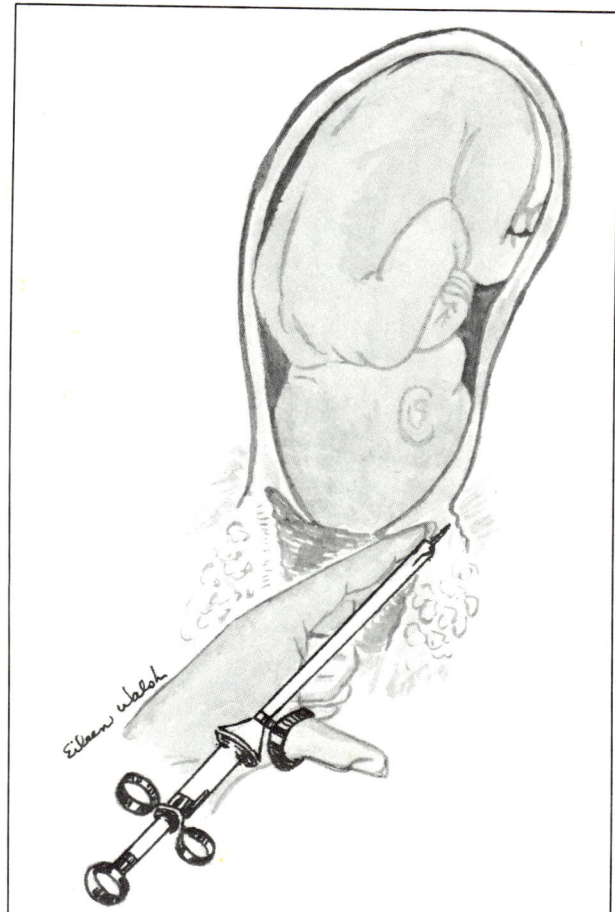

Fig. 23-5. Paracervical block.

sometimes fall as low as 90 per minute from this effect. If a fetal monitor is not available, fetal heart rate must be assessed frequently (every minute for the first 5 minutes after the injection). Fortunately, the bradycardia is usually transitory, and the fetal heart rate returns to normal (120 to 160 per minute) in a few minutes.

A paracervical block gives good pain relief during labor. Coupled with a local anesthetic, such as a pudendal block given in the delivery room, it can produce the always-hoped-for "painless childbirth." It is being used less frequently today, however, because of the risk of fetal bradycardia.

Hypnosis

Hypnosis is another method of achieving pain relief during labor and delivery. However, only one in four people is capable of responding to hypnotic suggestion. If she is in this category, prior to delivery the woman makes a number of visits to her obstetrician or the person who will perform the hypnosis. The hypnotist either gives her a posthypnotic suggestion during a visit, so that when she enters labor she will be unaware of the pain of contractions, or he arranges to meet her when she is in active labor to give her the suggestion at the time.

A woman under hypnosis will go through labor and delivery without feeling pain. The concept seems ideal, except that the effect of hypnosis is like that of twilight sleep: the woman is not aware of anything that went on following her entry into hypnosis. Thus she is uninvolved in the process of birth, and the entire process may not seem real to her afterward. The child she holds in her arms does not feel like "hers." Until she can convince herself that labor and delivery are over and accept a new phase of her life, she is not ready to be a mother.

Medication for Pain Relief During Delivery

NATURAL ANESTHESIA

The simplest form of pain relief for delivery is the pressure anesthesia that results when the fetal head presses against the stretching perineum. This natural anesthesia is adequate to allow the physician to perform an episiotomy without concern that the woman will feel the cut. The pain she experiences as the fetal head is delivered, though intense and hot, is not particularly unpleasant, occurs suddenly, and is quickly over. After the hours of hard contractions the woman has come through, this flash of pain seems almost too easy to be real. However, if the physician wishes to use forceps for better control of the fetal head, the woman will have to be given an anesthetic.

LOW SPINAL ANESTHESIA

In spinal anesthesia, a local anesthetic is injected into the spinal fluid in the subarachnoid space of the spinal column. Spinal injection for childbirth is usually at the L3 or L4 level. Anesthesia up to the umbilicus and including both legs is achieved.

There are many scare stories about women whose legs were paralyzed after spinal anesthesia or who had "bad backs" or continuous headaches ever afterward. Possibly once someone did suffer paralysis following a spinal anesthetic, but with current administration techniques this is a remote possibility because of the anatomical relationship of the spinal column and the space into which the anesthetic is injected. The spinal cord ends at the first or second lumbar vertebra. However, the dural cavity with spinal fluid continues downward to the fourth or fifth lumbar vertebra, where the injection is made into the subarachnoid space. It is almost as if the vertebral column were designed to include a place for lumbar puncture or spinal anesthesia injections. It is good practice to explain this natural phenomenon to women and their husbands during labor if they show the slightest apprehension about a spinal anesthetic or bring up one of the scare stories that are so prevalent.

Some mothers do experience "spinal headaches" following this type of anesthesia. The accepted theory to account for them is that there is leakage of spinal fluid from the point of needle insertion. The incidence of such headaches is reduced if a small-gauge needle is used and the woman remains flat in bed for 8 to 12 hours following delivery and drinks a quantity of fluid. This reduces cerebral irritation from the lack of fluid until new fluid can be replaced.

If a woman is to receive a low spinal anesthetic, she either turns on her side on the delivery table with her back flexed or sits up on the side of the table. The anesthesiologist locates the proper vertebra and, after testing to determine that the needle is in the canal (return of clear fluid through the needle), injects the anesthetic. The effect is almost immediate. No more contractions will be felt. The woman's legs become insensitive to feeling almost at once, and motor control to lower extremities is lost.

The woman should use a pillow on the delivery room table following administration of a spinal anesthetic to prevent the anesthetic from rising too high in the vertebral canal. The anesthetic normally reaches the level of T10. If it rises above T7 the motor nerves of the uterus will be blocked, and uterine contractions will cease. If it rises above T4 respiratory function in the woman will cease. The anesthesiologist protects against the anesthetic's rising in the spinal fluid canal by mixing or "loading" the anesthetic with a heavy glucose solution. This causes the anesthetic to sink in the CSF rather than rise.

Severe hypotension may occur with the administration of spinal anesthesia due to vasodilatation secondary to sympathetic blocking. If this happens, placental blood perfusion is suddenly compromised. The woman needs to be turned on her left side to reduce vena caval compression. The anesthesiologist will quickly administer intravenous fluid to increase blood volume; a vasopressor such as ephedrine and oxygen may be given.

The effect of hypotension may be limited if the woman is well hydrated prior to spinal anesthesia administration (which is why a woman who will receive a spinal anesthetic for delivery may have intravenous fluid begun during labor).

Low or outlet forceps are generally needed for delivery following a spinal anesthetic. Since the woman does not feel contractions, coordinated second-stage pushing is difficult.

SADDLE BLOCK ANESTHESIA

The terms *low spinal anesthesia* and *saddle block anesthesia* are often used interchangeably. In the strict sense saddle block anesthesia is injection of an anesthetic into a low lumbar space. It causes anesthesia of the parts of the body that would be in contact with a saddle: the perineum, the upper thighs, and the lower pelvis—or anesthesia only to the L1 to L5 and S1 to S4 levels. Saddle block anesthesia is administered to the woman while she is sitting on the side of the delivery room table (Fig. 23-6). This position ensures that the anesthetic will not rise high in the spinal canal. When a woman sits up on the side of the delivery table, you must support her in that position or, unbalanced (front-heavy because of her pregnancy), she might fall. Let her lean forward against you and rest her head on your shoulder. Thus she is not only supported but presents the widest expanse between vertebrae for easy injection of the anesthetic.

LOCAL ANESTHETICS

Pudendal Nerve Block

A pudendal nerve block (Fig. 23-7) is the injection of a local anesthetic into the pudendal nerve at the level of the ischial spines. The injection is made through

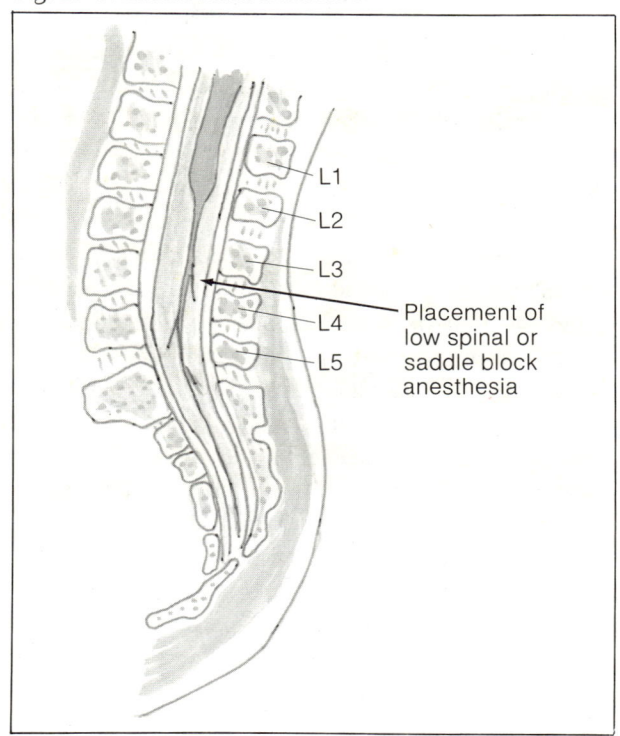

Fig. 23-6. Saddle block anesthesia.

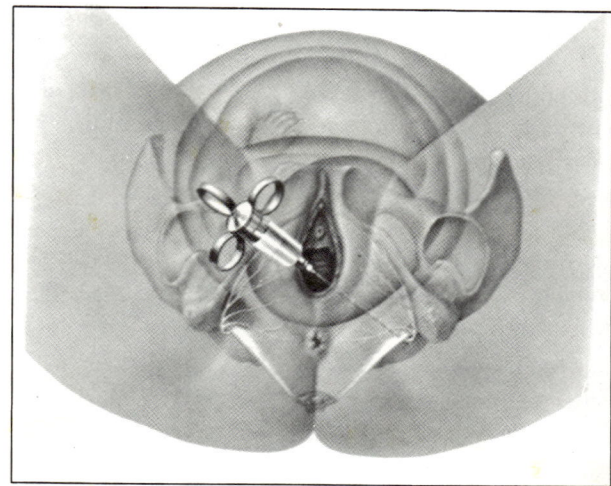

Fig. 23-7. Pudendal block. (From Clinical Education Aid, No. 17, Ross Laboratories, Columbus, Ohio, 1971.)

the vagina with the woman in a lithotomy position to allow for relief of perineal pain during delivery. Anesthesia achieved with this method is sufficiently deep to allow for the use of low forceps during delivery and an episiotomy repair.

Local Infiltration

Local infiltration is the injection of an anesthetic such as Xylocaine into the superficial nerves of the perineum by the placement of the anesthetic along the borders of the vulva. Local infiltration is used for episiotomy incision and repair.

GAS ANESTHESIA

There are a number of volatile gases that give pain relief for delivery. All present some hazard and should, like regional anesthetics, be given only by skilled anesthetists or anesthesiologists.

Nitrous Oxide

Nitrous oxide ("laughing gas") may be administered to the woman as soon as full dilatation is achieved. When she begins to feel a contraction, a mask is placed on her face and she is asked to take three good breaths of a mixture of nitrous oxide and oxygen. The mixture is effective for taking the edge off contractions up to crowning, when for adequate perineal relaxation another anesthetic may have to be substituted. Nitrous oxide should never be used by unskilled operators; if the concentration of oxygen in the gas is less than 50 percent, fetal hypoxia and possible fetal damage may result. Mothers who receive nitrous oxide require close observation in the postpartum period for hemorrhage as nitrous oxide is a potent uterine relaxant.

Cyclopropane

Cyclopropane is a narcotic gas that allows for rapid induction of anesthesia. Being highly explosive, it is administered with a closed system. It is useful as an anesthetic in emergency situations, such as fetal distress, because of its rapid action, but it has a tendency to cause excessive uterine bleeding due to uterine atony. Women who have had this gas during delivery need special observation in the immediate postpartum period.

Ether

Ether is a volatile gas that is best given by a closed system. Once a frequently used gas in obstetrics, it is rarely employed today except in emergencies. The important rule to remember when ether is administered is that a person cannot breathe only ether; air or oxygen must be provided to prevent hypoxia in both woman and fetus.

Ether causes marked uterine atony. Mothers who receive ether for delivery must be observed closely in the postpartum period for hemorrhage.

Chloroform

At one time chloroform was a widely used gas for delivery. Queen Victoria received chloroform anesthesia for the birth of her son, Prince Leopold, in 1853, advancing chloroform's popularity and resulting in its being called "queens' anesthesia." Chloroform is little used today. Prolonged administration may cause necrosis of the liver lobules, resulting in death. It may lead to postpartum bleeding due to uterine relaxation.

Halothane

Halothane is a gas that offers rapid induction. It may be used when rapid delivery of the fetus is imperative. Uterine relaxation is extensive; the woman must be observed closely following delivery for uterine atony.

INTRAVENOUS ANESTHESIA

For complete anesthesia during childbirth, sodium thiopental (Pentothal), a short-acting barbiturate, is usually the drug of choice. Pentothal causes rapid induction of anesthesia and minimal postpartal bleeding. Its short action makes it readily controllable. Following induction with Pentothal, the woman is intubated and anesthesia is then generally maintained by nitrous oxide and oxygen.

Pentothal crosses the placenta rapidly. Infants born of a woman anesthetized by this method, therefore, may be slow to respond at birth and may need resuscitation. However, in view of the degree of barbiturate intoxication demonstrable in the infant, his ability to respond and his alertness at birth are always surprising.

Preparation for the Safe Administration of Anesthetics

The analgesics and anesthetic preparations frequently used in labor and delivery are shown in Table 23-2. Women should be well prepared for the type of anesthetic they will receive during labor and delivery. Some physicians discuss the anesthetic they will use with women during pregnancy visits; others leave this kind of information until women are in the hospital in labor. In any event, prior to the actual administration or injection of the anesthetic, the mother needs a review of how the anesthetic will be administered (you'll need to lie on your back; sit up on the side of the delivery table; etc.) and what she can expect to happen following the medication (not only will you no longer be able to feel pain but your legs will feel numb too; or whatever). Women in labor are under stress, and surprising body sensations happening to them because of lack of preparation can be very frightening and the "straw" that defeats their coping mechanisms. To be struggling against anesthetic administration because one does not understand what is going on adds to the risk of anesthesia.

The delivery room or birthing room should be checked before every delivery to be certain that adequate equipment is available for the safe delivery and safe administration of anesthetic agents.

The anesthesiologist needs a minimum of six drugs readily available in front of him: ephedrine (to use in the event blood pressure falls after regional anesthetic administration), atropine sulfate (to dry oral and respiratory secretions to prevent aspiration), sodium thiopental (for rapid induction of a general anesthetic in an emergency), succinylcholine (to achieve laryngeal relaxation for intubation in an emergency), diazepam (to control convulsions, a possible reaction to regional anesthetics), and isoproterenol (to reduce bronchospasm if aspiration should occur). In addition to these medications, an adult laryngoscope, endotracheal tubes, a breathing bag with a source of 100% oxygen, and a suction catheter and suction source should be at hand.

Although the anesthesiologist checks these supplies himself, they are such important safeguards of the mother's health—particularly the suction and oxygen sources—that checking that they are present is a nursing responsibility too.

ASPIRATION OF VOMITUS

Anesthesia is the fifth most common cause of death in childbirth (hemorrhage, infection, pregnancy-induced hypertension, and heart disease are the first four causes). Half the obstetrical deaths due to anesthesia are attributed to the inhalation of vomitus.

Women should be cautioned during prenatal visits against eating once labor begins. The stomach should be as empty as possible at delivery in case an emergency arises and a general anesthetic is necessary. Regional anesthetics are safer than general anesthesia and should be used whenever possible. When a general anesthetic is chosen, the woman must be treated as a surgical patient and anesthesia induced only by a skilled anesthesiologist.

The woman should be intubated with a cuffed endotracheal tube after a rapid induction period. In order to prevent gastric reflux and aspiration before intubation is achieved, cricoid pressure (which seals off the esophagus by compressing it between the cricoid cartilage and the cervical vertebrae) must be applied. Pregnant women are particularly prone to gastric reflux because of increased stomach pressure from the pressure of the full uterus beneath it. The gastroesophageal valve may be displaced also and so may not be functioning properly.

Some anesthesiologists may order an antacid to be given to the woman before general anesthesia is administered to reduce the level of acid in stomach contents in case aspiration does occur. Explaining to the woman why she is receiving this is often difficult (you have told her not to drink anything and now you are offering her something to drink). Explain briefly that you know this seems to be a contradiction of what you have said but reducing the acidity of gastric secretions prior to anesthesia is important.

The moments of induction of general anesthesia before the endotracheal tube is safely in place are critical ones for the anesthesiologist. Respect his necessity to concentrate on the task at hand until this is achieved. Some women may comment afterward that their throat feels raw or sore. This is from the insertion of the endotracheal tube and is normal. Sipping cold liquids (as soon as this is safe after general anesthesia) relieves the discomfort.

Inhalation of vomitus may be fatal because of occlusion of the woman's airway due to the foreign matter. Also, stomach content has an acid pH and so causes chemical burns and secondary infection of the respiratory tract.

If aspiration of vomitus occurs in the delivery room, prompt attention is essential. The trachea is suctioned by the anesthesiologist to remove as much foreign material as possible; the woman is intubated and given 100% oxygen. She will be given a medication such as isoproterenol intravenously to reduce bronchospasm and a corticosteroid intravenously to reduce an inflammatory reaction. Positive pressure ventilation may be started. A chest x-ray picture will be taken.

The woman will be kept on mechanical ventilation until the chest x-ray films, blood gases, and her overall clinical condition improve. She is critically ill at the time of aspiration and often will be transferred to an intensive care unit for the special care she requires to survive this occurrence.

She needs to be kept informed of her baby's progress and if possible allowed to see the baby. She can thus be assured that, although she is ill, the baby was delivered and is doing well (if that is the circumstance). If she is transferred to another section of the hospital (to the intensive care unit) and taking the baby to her is not practical, being able to see a Polaroid snapshot of her infant is very helpful.

At one time many women asked to be fully anesthetized for delivery. However, the required medication may cause not only aspiration in the mother but also narcosis in the infant. In addition, it may impair the establishment of an early mother-child relationship. All during pregnancy, it is hard for the woman to believe the pregnancy is really happening. The proof that it is real, that she is a mother, that she has a baby is given at the moment of birth, but if she is fully anesthetized at this time she may continue to have difficulty accepting the reality. Being told when she regains consciousness that she has delivered a baby makes the child no more real than did being told she was pregnant. Even later, when she holds the infant in her arms, he may still seem like a stranger. If she believed she carried a boy and hours after delivery she is handed a girl, she may wonder whether it is hers. If she pictured a plump little girl with black, curly hair (like her own in her baby pictures) and is handed a stringy, bald-headed boy instead, she may think someone has made a terrible mistake. Suppose the child has a congenital defect. How can she be sure this is the same child she carried inside her? Thoughts of this kind hamper effective mother-child interaction.

If a difficult birth is anticipated, a general anesthetic may be the method of choice to achieve a safe outcome for both mother and child. However, general anesthesia should never be considered routine in childbirth because of the risk to the fetus if he does not

Table 23-2. Analgesics and Anesthetics Commonly Used in Labor and Delivery

Type	Drug	Usual Dose	Effect on Mother
Narcotic analgesic	Meperidine (Demerol)	25 mg IV, 50–100 mg IM q3–4h	Effective analgesic Feeling of well-being
	Alphaprodine (Nisentil)	10 mg IV, 20–40 mg SQ q3–4h	Effective analgesic
	Morphine sulfate	8–15 mg IM q4–5h	Effective analgesic Slows respiratory rate Can be constipating
Sedative hypnotics	Secobarbital (Seconal)	100–200 mg IM or PO, 50 mg IV	Reduce apprehension Induce lethargy and sleep (Used early in labor to encourage rest)
	Pentobarbital (Nembutal)	100–200 mg IM or PO, 50 mg IV	Same as secobarbital
Tranquilizers	Diazepam (Valium)	5–10 mg IV, IM or PO	Reduce apprehension Induce relaxation (When used with a narcotic analgesic, less analgesic is needed for effect) May cause hypotension that responds poorly to vasopressors
	Promethazine (Phenergan)	25–50 mg IM or PO	
	Promazine (Sparine)	25 mg IM or PO	
	Hydroxyzine pamoate (Vistaril)	5–15 mg IM or PO	
Amnesic	Hyoscine (scopolamine)	0.2–0.6 mg	Flushing of the face Woman will become excited and delirious with pain (use in combination with an analgesic) Woman will have no memory for events of labor afterward
Gas analgesics	Trichloroethylene (Trilene)	Self-administered by taking a breath of gas at peak of contraction	Effective pain relief for first and second stages of labor Some dizziness or light-headedness Some increase in respirations
	Methoxyflurane (Penthrane)	Self-administered by taking a breath of gas at peak of contraction (as with Trilene, only safe when self-administered; should not be given by support person)	May cause hypotension, slowed respirations Effective pain relief for first and second stages of labor
Regional anesthetics Saddle block	Local anesthetic such as mepivacaine	Administered for delivery with mother in sitting position; given between contractions Injection at L3–L4 or L4–L5 into CSF	Rapid onset in minutes Lasts about 2 hours Numbness and loss of sensation in perineum and thighs Loss of pushing sensation Maternal hypotension Postpartum headache
Caudal block	Local anesthetic	Administered for first stage of labor With continuous caudal, anesthesia will last through delivery Injected into epidural space at caudal hiatus	Rapid onset in minutes Lasts 60–90 minutes Loss of pain perception for labor contractions and delivery Maternal hypotension
Lumbar epidural block	Local anesthetic	Administered for first stage of labor With continuous block, anesthesia will last through delivery Injected into epidural space at L3–L4	Rapid onset in minutes Lasts 60–90 minutes Loss of pain perception for labor contractions and delivery Maternal hypotension

Effect on Labor Progress	Effect on Fetus or Newborn
Relaxation may aid progress as cervical relaxation occurs Will halt labor contractions if given too early	Should be given 3 hours away from delivery to avoid respiratory depression in newborn
May weaken contractions for short period Used in women with irregular contractions sometimes to reduce uterine irritability Minimal effect if used in early labor Large doses may impair strength of contractions	Causes serious respiratory distress in newborn Should be given 3 hours away from delivery to avoid respiratory depression Sleepiness for first 48 hours
None apparent	Valium may interfere with bilirubin binding in susceptible infants All tranquilizers may cause slight delay in onset of newborn respirations
None apparent	None apparent
None apparent	Not depressant when used in analgesic proportions Can become depressant if used over 3–4 hours
None apparent	Not depressant when used in analgesic proportions
Progress halts (used just prior to delivery, and delivery managed with outlet forceps)	None apparent
Loss of need to push with contractions; can be coached to push with contraction or delivery will be managed by low forceps May slow labor if given too early	May cause transient behavior changes in newborn for first few days of life
Will slow labor if given too early Obliterates pushing feeling so second stage may be prolonged	May be some differences in response in first few days of life

Analgesia and Anesthesia in Labor and Delivery

Table 23-2 (Continued)

Type	Drug	Usual Dose	Effect on Mother
Paracervical block	Local anesthetic	Administered for first stage of labor Injected into vaginal fornices	Rapid onset in minutes Lasts 60–90 minutes Possible hypotension
Local anesthetics Pudendal block	Local anesthetic	Administered just prior to delivery for perineal anesthesia Injected through vagina	Rapid anesthesia of perineum
Local infiltration of perineum	Local anesthetic	Injected just prior to delivery for episiotomy incision and repair	Anesthesia of perineum almost immediately
Gas anesthetics	Ether	Administered by open-drip method for delivery	Irritating to respiratory tract May be vomiting in recovery period Good relaxation
	Cyclopropane	Administered by closed system Highly inflammable	Rapid anesthesia, so is used in emergency situations May cause cardiac arrhythmias
	Halothane	Administered just prior to delivery by closed system	Rapid anesthesia, so is used in emergency situations
	Nitrous oxide	Administered just prior to delivery by allowing mother to take a few breaths at a time	Good analgesic; light anesthesia. Both induction and recovery are rapid

breathe spontaneously and needs resuscitation, the resultant threat to the mother-infant relationship, and the risk to the mother's life from laryngeal spasm or aspiration.

The Risk of Anesthesia

The risk of anesthesia correlates with the amount and the length of time anesthesia is used. Because of possible aspiration of vomitus, a general anesthetic during delivery carries a much greater risk to both mother and infant than does regional anesthesia such as a pudendal block.

It became customary to rely heavily on the use of analgesia during labor and anesthesia during delivery because it was felt that keeping women quiet and sedated would prevent them from "fighting" procedures and interfering with a safe delivery.

When anesthesia was first used for deliveries in hospitals, women were deprived of their own support persons in labor and delivery. The woman was surrounded by nurses who were technically skilled but not prepared to handle her feelings of fright and loneliness. She was left alone in labor. Since her physician came to the hospital only when it was time for delivery, not before, he provided no support. Is it any wonder that women screamed and fought procedures? A woman protects her body from intrusive or hurtful procedures all during pregnancy. This protective reaction does not stop until after delivery, when it shifts to the body of the newborn. When contrasted with the familiar scene of a woman screaming and thrashing during delivery, general anesthesia seemed like a panacea.

However, when nurses are educated to offer psychological support to patients in labor, a great deal of the fear and fright of childbirth can be handled by words and supportive actions rather than by medication. With a woman's fear controlled, with her lying alert and cooperative on a delivery room table, the risks of general anesthesia begin to outweigh its good points.

Nevertheless, a good deal of anesthesia during childbirth continues to be used because nurses as health care personnel have little say in the formulation of policies governing hospital units. Nurses are often intimidated in decision making because of the pervading atmosphere of "the doctor knows best." Nurses can contribute enormously to making childbirth safer than it currently is. If they would use all the professional skills of nursing to ensure that women who come into delivery rooms are cooperative and "pushing" women, women who feel secure because skilled persons are concerned about and looking after their best interests, the number of deliveries by saddle block or pudendal block could increase

Effect on Labor Progress	Effect on Fetus or Newborn
Effect varies widely; sometimes labor slowed, other times shortened	Fetal bradycardia may result If bradycardia is persistent (over 15 minutes), rapid delivery of the fetus may be considered
None apparent	None apparent
None apparent	None apparent
Extreme uterine relaxation Uterine contractions will be decreased with complete anesthesia Uterine atony will persist into third stage	If deep anesthesia achieved, there is depression of the newborn
Extreme uterine relaxation Allows for rapid intrauterine manipulation Uterine atony will persist into third stage	If baby is born within 8 minutes after administration, there is minimal newborn depression (it takes over 8 minutes for fetal concentrations to reach those of mother)
Extreme uterine relaxation Allows for rapid intrauterine manipulation Uterine atony will persist into the third stage	Some neonatal depression
Uterine relaxation not enough to perform uterine manipulations	If nitrous oxide used in conjunction with 20% oxygen, newborn depression is minimal

dramatically. The concomitant decrease in the use of general anesthetics would bring about a decline in maternal and fetal mortality. Remember that despite all the technical knowledge at our command today, maternal and fetal mortality in the United States is far from the lowest in the world. This is a challenge that nurses have an obligation to meet if they deserve to be called professionals.

Even more serious than nurses' traditional acceptance of the large amounts of anesthesia use in childbirth is their active participation in anesthetic administration. The administration of such agents is beyond the scope of professional nursing unless additional training in anesthesia is undertaken. Far too often, nurses are the "patsies" of the health professions, engaging in tasks below the level of their expertise, or above it, simply because no other person is available for the job. It is difficult to criticize a nurse who does an aide's work for the day because the aide is ill. She does it for the sake of patient welfare. However, it is impossible not to criticize a nurse who does the anesthesiologist's work, either because he or she is not there or because no specialists in anesthesia are on the hospital staff. Taking on such duties is not in the patient's interest. On the contrary, it constitutes a risk to the patient.

True, emergencies do arise in an obstetrics unit, and in an emergency situation many people find themselves doing tasks they do not ordinarily perform. But such emergencies should be anticipated and a plan of action devised that will provide coverage by a professional trained in anesthesia administration.

Problem-oriented Recording: Progress Notes

Christine McFadden
15 years
Para 0, gravida 1

Problem: Comfort in labor; admission assessment

> S. States, "Put me to sleep; I don't want to know anything until this is over." Describes contractions as "really hard. I never felt anything like this before." Asking for something for pain if she can't just go to sleep. Last ate 4 hours ago.
> O. Lies in labor bed very stiffly; tenses with contractions.
> A. Primipara who would benefit from pain relief to help her accept discomfort of contractions.

Goals: a. Pain reduction through use of medication to make labor a more tolerable time.
b. Conclude labor with increased ability to handle stress situations.
c. Conclude labor with increased self-esteem in being able to control variables.

P. 1. Provide support person from nursing personnel.
2. Teach about breathing exercises to help her manage contractions.
3. Review normal labor and delivery so tenseness over unknown can be relieved.
4. Explain advantages of being awake during labor for both her and baby.
5. Ask for early pain relief order (only 2 cm dilated now).
6. Keep NPO in event general anesthetic is necessary for delivery.

Problem: Comfort in labor; 10:00 A.M. interim assessment

S. States, "Can't stand it if labor pain gets any worse."
O. Continues to tense and scream with contractions despite receiving 50 mg Demerol 45 minutes ago.
A. Relief of discomfort inadequate.
P. 1. Continue presence of support person.
2. Continue to encourage breathing pattern.
3. Give encouragement that dilatation is beginning so although labor is uncomfortable it is accomplishing something.
4. Alert medical personnel to continued discomfort.

Problem: Comfort in labor; 11:00 A.M. interim assessment

S. Told that c-section was going to be necessary. States, "It can't happen too soon for me."
O. Appears relieved by c-section decision.
A. Primipara with extreme discomfort from labor. Needs to be familiarized with cesarean section anesthesia.

P. 1. Review sensation of anesthesia with her.
2. Establish fluid line per orders.
3. Prepare for waking in recovery room.
4. Support person from health personnel to remain with her until anesthetic has taken effect.
5. Assess maternal-child relationship in postpartal period due to c-section and general anesthetic delivery.

Problem-oriented Recording: Progress Notes

Mary Kraft
22 years
Para 0, gravida 2

Problem: Comfort in labor; admission assessment

S. States, "I don't want any drug for labor or delivery." Last ate 15 minutes ago (eggs, bacon, and orange juice) so "no one can give me any anesthesia." Has lollipops with her to suck on. Knowledgeable of Lamaze method for control of discomfort in labor; husband will be support person and coach.
O. Using breathing exercises with contractions. Husband is effective coach.
A. Para 0, gravida 2 using Lamaze breathing patterns effectively; no further pain relief necessary.

Goal: Complete labor and delivery without medication or anesthetic intervention.

P. 1. Reassure that her wishes will be respected as to the amount of medication desired.
2. Support breathing pattern efforts as needed.
3. Offer husband relief as desired from position as coach.

Problem: Comfort in labor; 1:00 P.M. interim assessment

S. States, "This system [breathing exercises] really works."

O. Continuing to use breathing techniques with contractions. Focuses on photo at foot of bed for distraction. Husband appears very helpful, effective in coaching role.
A. Comfort in labor adequate.
P. 1. Respect necessity to focus during contractions (do not block vision).
   2. Offer relief to husband as needed (none necessary yet).

Problem: Comfort in labor; 3:00 P.M. interim assessment: beginning second stage of labor

S. States, "It feels good to push. Don't give me any anesthetic."
O. Pushing effectively with contractions; not as prepared for this stage as first stage of labor; husband continues to be supportive but also not as knowledgeable.
A. No need for additional comfort measures for delivery per request.
P. 1. Continue to support pushing efforts.
   2. Support decision to have no delivery anesthetic.

Problem-oriented Recording: Progress Notes

Angie Baco
42 years
Para 6, gravida 7

Problem: Comfort in labor; admission assessment

S. Asking questions about what will happen in terms of analgesia and anesthesia. Wants "a shot for pain, but no spinal." Had severe spinal headache following last delivery 7 years ago. States it made the entire labor experience "just one big headache." Last ate 4 hours ago. Attended no preparation-for-labor classes.
O. Most comfortable on left side; uses short frequent breaths with contractions (learned this last time while in labor). Husband appears supportive but not well informed about labor. Physician has spoken to her about having an epidural block as blood pressure is slightly high (130/90) and he does not want her uncomfortable.
A. Multipara who could benefit from pain relief to allow her to use her breathing exercises more effectively; if epidural will be given, needs good support to accept procedure.

Goals: a. Pain reduction through use of medication or regional block to make labor a more tolerable time.
       b. Increase knowledge of ways to cope with pain in labor.

P. 1. Observe closely for hyperventilation (short catchy breaths make her prone to this).
   2. Keep NPO in case general anesthesia is necessary (high risk for cesarean section as she is a gestational diabetic).
   3. Educate as necessary as soon as method of pain relief is established.
   4. Support husband as necessary and keep him informed of progress. (Patient relies on him to be calm.)
   5. Explain that at her early stage of labor (2 cm dilated) it is too soon to give medication for pain relief.

Problem: Comfort in labor; 4:00 P.M. interim assessment

S. States, "I don't feel a thing. Is anything happening?"
O. Lumbar epidural block begun at 3:30 P.M. for pain relief. Response to test dose of anesthetic was adequate; full anesthetic dose given at 3:35 by Dr. B. No hypotension noted. Flow sheet blood pressures have maintained at 130/88.
A. Lumbar epidural anesthetic effective for comfort.
P. 1. BP, P, and R q15min as epidural procedure protocol.
   2. Encourage to lie on left side to minimize possible supine hypotensive syndrome.
   3. Maintain NPO although epidural is expected to be delivery anesthetic as well.

> 4. Assure that dilatation is progressing even though she is now unaware of contractions.

Problem: Comfort in labor; 5:30 P.M. interim assessment: second stage of labor

> S. Patient growing anxious because this labor has been so different from others on account of epidural block. Voices fear of baby being "stuck" inside her because she does not feel pushing sensations.
> O. Appears noticeably tense; biting fingernails; startles at sound of young girl in next labor room crying.
> A. Although comfortable, needs assurance that this comfort is good for her and her infant.
> P. 1. Assure again that an epidural block is not harming baby or her.
>   2. Continue nursing support in delivery room.
>   3. Husband has decided to view delivery; support for husband as this is new experience for him and patient relies on him to calm her.

References

1. Beazley, J. M., et al. Perineal pain after epidural analgesia in labor. *Midwives Chron.* 91:204, 1978.
2. Beck, W. W. Prevention of the spinal headache. *Am. J. Obstet. Gynecol.* 115:345, 1973.
3. Burdin, C. P. Pain Relief Via Drugs During Labor and Delivery. In J. S. Malinowski, et al. *Nursing Care of the Labor Patient.* Philadelphia: Davis, 1978.
4. Ettinger, B. B., and McCart, D. F. Effects of drugs on the fetal heart rate during labor. *J.O.G.N. Nurs.* 5:41, 1976.
5. Falconer, M. W., et al. *The Drug, the Nurse, the Patient.* Philadelphia: Saunders, 1978.
6. Grad, R. K., and Woodside, J. Obstetrical analgesics and anesthesia: Methods of relief for the patient in labor. *Am. J. Nurs.* 77:242, 1977.
7. Johnson, J. M. Teaching self-hypnosis in pregnancy, labor and delivery. *M.C.N.* 5:98, 1980.
8. Knuppel, R. A. Recognizing teratogenic effects of drugs and radiation. *Contemp. Obstet. Gynecol.* 15:171, 1980.
9. Lanahan, C. C. Variables Affecting Pain Perception During Labor. In L. K. McNall and J. T. Galeener (Eds.), *Current Practice in Obstetrics and Gynecologic Nursing.* St. Louis: Mosby, 1978.
10. Lichtiger, M., and Moya, F. *Introduction to the Practice of Anesthesia* (2nd ed.). New York: Harper & Row, 1978.
11. McAllister, R. G. Obstetric anesthesia—a two-way street. *J.O.G.N. Nurs.* 5:9, 1976.
12. McDonald, J. S. Preanesthetic and intrapartal medications. *Clin. Obstet. Gynecol.* 20:447, 1977.
13. McDonald, J. S. Obstetric anesthesia. *Clin. Obstet. Gynecol.* 21:489, 1978.
14. Mozingo, J. N. Pain in labor: A conceptual model for intervention. *J.O.G.N. Nurs.* 7:47, 1978.
15. Scanlon, J. W. Obstetric anesthesia as a neonatal risk factor in normal labor and delivery. *Clin. Perinatol.* 1:465, 1974.
16. Sciarra, J. J., and Gerbie, A. B. *Gynecology and Obstetrics.* New York: Harper & Row, 1978.
17. Tronick, F., et al. Regional obstetric anesthesia and newborn behavior: Effect over the first ten days of life. *Pediatrics* 58:94, 1976.

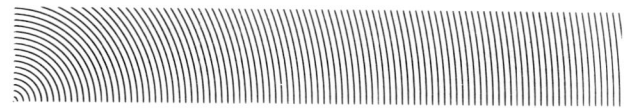

Unit IV. Utilizing Nursing Process: Questions for Review

1. Mrs. A. is admitted to a labor unit in active labor. Which of the following assessments would make you worry she might have difficulty accepting this child?
   a. She says she hates being pregnant.
   b. She says she hasn't slept well lately.
   c. She says she wants a boy.
   d. She says she is exhausted.

2. The major factor that differentiates false labor from true labor is
   a. Contractions becoming increasingly regular
   b. Progressive cervical dilatation
   c. Contractions changing from abdominal to back contractions
   d. Presence of "show"

3. Leopold's maneuvers in labor are used to
   a. Aid in delivery of the child's head
   b. Assess the presentation and position of the fetus
   c. Aid in restoring carbon dioxide level after hyperventilation
   d. None of the above

4. If a fetus is at a plus 1 station, it implies the fetus is
   a. At the pelvic inlet
   b. Engaged
   c. 1 cm above the ischial spines
   d. 1 cm below the ischial spines

5. Most women are allowed only ice chips during labor because
   a. Stomach digestion slows during labor
   b. The woman cannot push effectively with a full stomach
   c. The intestines become gas-filled if food is allowed
   d. Solid food can lead to an air embolus

6. Mrs. A. asks what effacement means. Basically, this is
   a. The reverse of dilatation
   b. An increase in size of the cervical os
   c. Contraction of perineal muscles
   d. A thinning of the cervical canal

7. At the second stage of labor (pelvic stage) a woman generally
   a. Cannot tell the difference in contractions
   b. Is frightened by the change in contractions
   c. Falls asleep from exhaustion
   d. Enjoys the new feel of decrescendo-crescendo contractions

8. During the second stage of labor a woman is generally
   a. Very aware of activities around her
   b. Anxious to have people around her
   c. No longer in need of a support person
   d. Turning inward to concentrate on body sensations

9. The maneuvers a fetus must undergo to complete birth are
   a. Descent, flexion, internal rotation, extension, external rotation
   b. Internal rotation, flexion, descent, extension, external rotation
   c. Flexion, internal rotation, descent, external rotation, expulsion
   d. Descent, internal flexion, expulsion, external flexion

10. The second stage of labor
    a. Is the longest stage
    b. Is from the birth of the infant until the placenta is ready to deliver
    c. Is from delivery of the placenta until 1 hour afterward
    d. Is from full cervical dilatation to birth of the child

11. The preparatory division of labor is from
    a. The first contraction until birth of the child
    b. The first strong contraction until after delivery of the placenta
    c. The beginning of contractions until cervical dilatation is 4 cm
    d. The beginning of "show" until the child's head is delivered

12. Which of the following assessments in labor would cause you to alert a physician immediately?
    a. FHR 130; pink-tinged show; history of ruptured membranes
    b. Contractions 80 seconds in length during the latent phase of labor; FHR 120
    c. Fetal position ROA; FHR 140; contractions 30 seconds in length
    d. Rupture of membranes at beginning of second stage; FHR 125

13. Mrs. A. is to have a paracervical nerve block for pain relief in labor. Which of the following would *not* be part of your preprocedure preparation?
    a. Explain that the method will provide pain relief for both labor and delivery.
    b. Explain that the needle looks long but the injection will be almost painless.
    c. Explain that the injection will be made from the vagina.
    d. Explain that the woman will lie on her back for the injection.

14. You take an injection of Nisentil in to Mrs. B. for pain relief during labor. As you are about to give it, she asks you for a bedpan because she has to move her bowels. Your best action would be to
    a. Give the injection, then offer the bedpan; abdominal comfort will help her move her bowels.
    b. Hold the injection until you evaluate her labor progress.
    c. Give the injection first, then offer the bedpan because you always do clean procedures before contaminated ones.
    d. Give the bedpan before you give the injection as Nisentil is constipating.

15. Following a lumbar epidural block, Mrs. C.'s blood pressure suddenly falls to 90/50. Your *first* action would be to
    a. Raise the head of the bed.
    b. Ask her to inhale deeply at least five times.
    c. Administer oxygen by face mask.
    d. Turn her onto her left side.

16. Mrs. D. refuses to have a caudal epidural block because she does not want to have a spinal headache after delivery. Your best response to her would be to say
    a. The anesthesiologist will do his best to avoid this.
    b. The pain relief offered by the procedure will compensate for the discomfort afterward.
    c. Spinal headache is not a complication of epidural blocks.
    d. Her doctor knows what is best for her.

17. Mrs. E. states that she does not want any medication for pain relief during labor. Her doctor has approved this for her. Your best statement to her concerning this would be
    a. That's wonderful; medication during labor is not good for fetal well-being.
    b. Your doctor [a man] has never been in labor; he may be underestimating the pain you will have.
    c. I respect your preference whether it is to have medication or not.
    d. Let me get you something for relaxation if you don't want anything for pain.

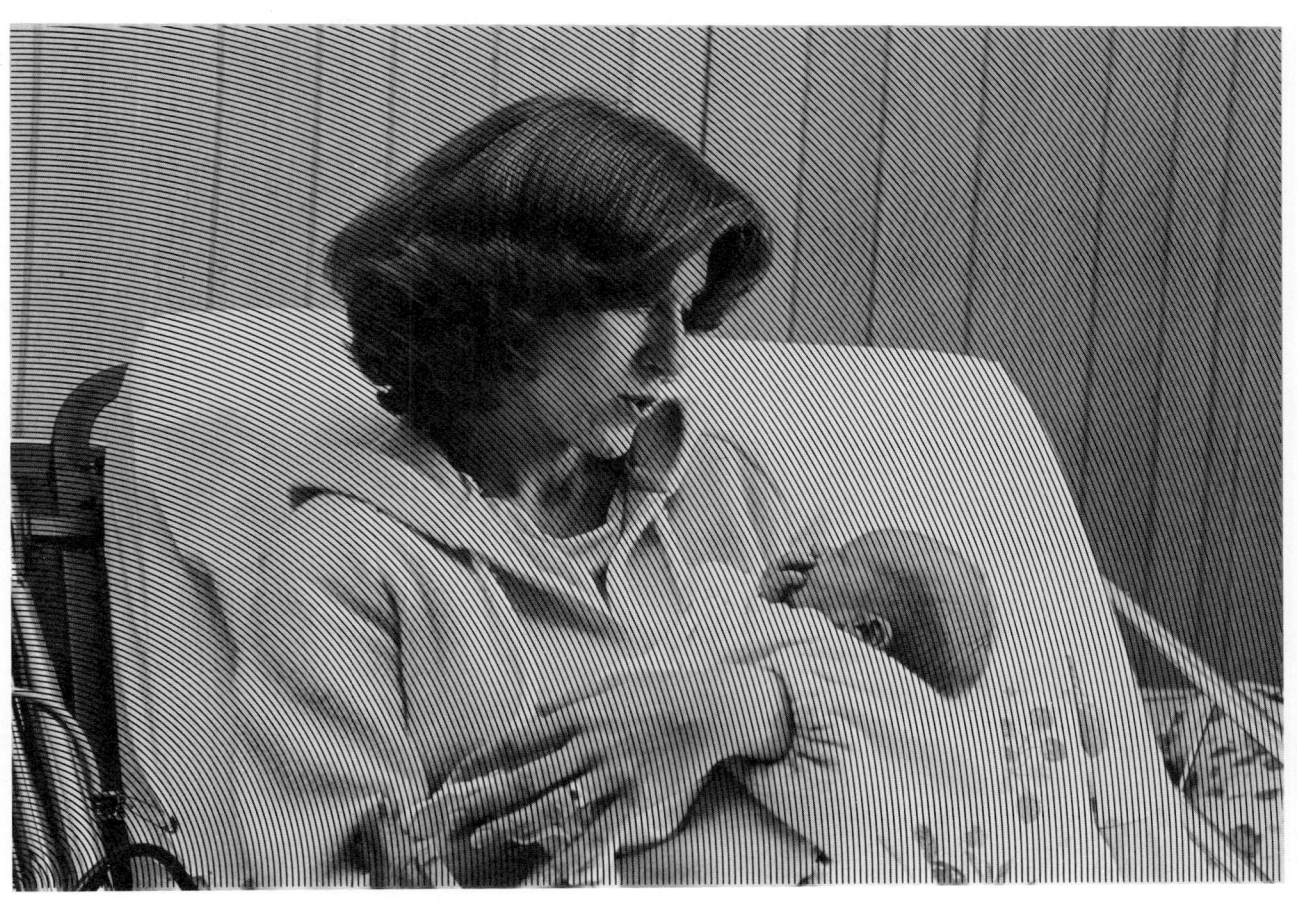

V. The Postpartal Period: Parenthood

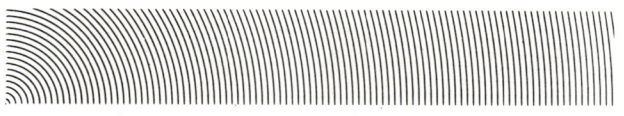

24. Psychosocial Aspects of the Postpartal Period

The term *puerperium* is from the Latin *puer*, "child," and *parere*, "to bring forth." It refers to the six-week period following the birth of the baby and delivery of the placenta and membranes. This six-week puerperium, or postpartal period, is a time of retrogressive changes, when the uterus, vagina, and ovaries return to the nonpregnant state. It is also a period of progressive change, since the normal reproductive cycle is restored and breast tissue is prepared for milk production (lactation). Psychological changes occur too as the woman begins to experience her new role as a mother.

Nursing care during the puerperium has long been considered a routine type of care, and postpartal mothers have been regarded as women with many complaints and small care problems. In fact, the contrary of each of these two propositions is true. The wonder is how *little* the new mother complains, in view of everything that is happening to her. The tremendous psychological and physiological events of this period demand nursing care that is anything but routine.

For every mother, whether this was her first or her tenth child, whether the child was wanted or unwanted, something in the experience has unique meaning. She wants the personnel who care for her to feel the same level of excitement, the same passion, she feels. To a large extent, how she reacts to her new child—tenderly, compassionately, or routinely—will mimic the way hospital personnel react to her during this time.

The physical care the mother receives post partum can influence her health for the rest of her life. The emotional support she receives can influence the mental health of her child or be felt in the next generation.

Parental Love

Every woman worries during pregnancy and, when she finally holds a newborn in her arms, about her ability to be a "good" mother. Some women seem able to recognize a newborn's needs immediately and to care for him with confident understanding right from the start. More often, a woman enters into a relationship with her newborn tentatively and with qualms and conflicts that she has to correct before the relationship can be meaningful.

Fathers may have even more difficulty than mothers in "claiming" an infant or feeling fatherly toward the child. This is especially true if hospital rules do not allow the father to touch and spend time with his new child in the first few days of life.

Maternal love is only partly instinctive. A major portion of it develops gradually, in stages: planning the pregnancy, hearing the pregnancy confirmed, feeling the child move in utero, birth, seeing the baby, touching the baby, finally, caring for the baby. Many women work through these steps slowly and do not have maternal feelings for their infants for days or even weeks after giving birth. Some fathers admit they do not feel love until as late as three months or so after birth, when the child can smile or coo and interact with them.

Forming a strong bond with a child is not a problem only for first-time mothers; experienced mothers can have just as much difficulty. A mother knows she loves 4-year-old Johnny and 2-year-old Sue at home. She worries that her heart may not be big enough to love this new child also.

You need to provide an environment free of stringent rules if good mother-child relationships are to develop. To help parents sort out their feelings about being a mother or father and about their new responsibility, you need to provide a supportive presence and be able to offer anticipatory guidance where necessary.

Before a mother can begin to concentrate on her child, she requires adequate rest and sleep and concerned attention to the relief of her physical discomfort. The more she is ministered to during this period, the easier it seems for her to minister to her new child. The more she is touched and nourished, the more readily she seems to reach out and touch and nourish her infant.

Few mothers show genuine warmth the first time their infants are brought to them. Even though the mother carried the infant inside her for nine months, she approaches the child as she would a stranger. The first time he is shown to her in the delivery room or brought to her in her postpartal room she may decline to touch him. She may hold him so she touches only the blanket and never makes physical contact with him. If she unfolds the blanket to examine the baby or count his fingers or toes, she touches him only with her fingertips, as strangers accidentally touch each other on a crowded elevator and immediately apologize and draw back (Fig. 24-1).

Gradually, as the mother holds the child more and more, she begins to warm toward him. She touches the child with the palm of her hand rather than with her fingertips. She holds him tighter, in a more

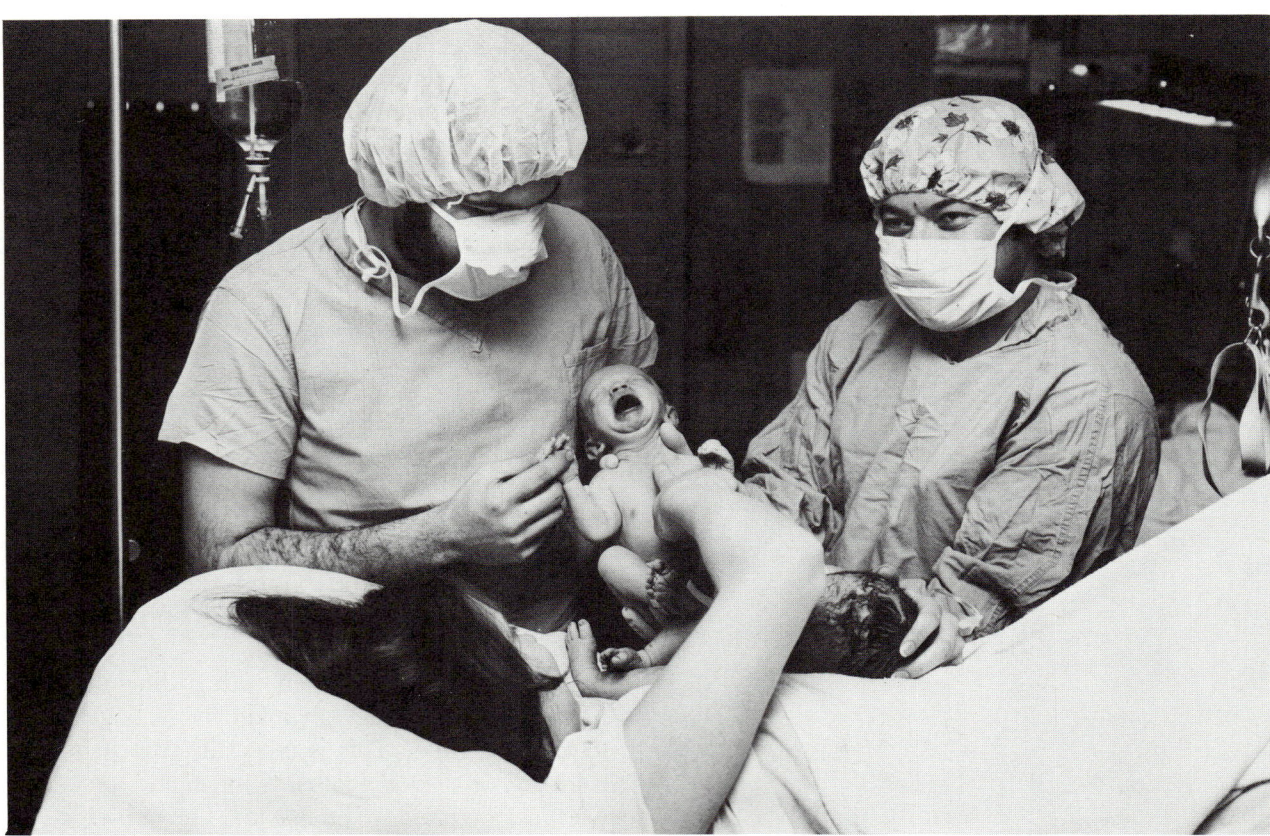

Fig. 24-1. A mother beginning interaction with her twins in the delivery room. Note the way she touches with only a fingertip. (Courtesy of the Department of Medical Photography, Children's Hospital, Buffalo, N.Y.)

motherly way. She smooths his hair, brushes his cheek, plays with his toes, lets his fingers clasp hers, as sweethearts might on a date. Soon, she feels comfortable enough with the baby to press her cheek against his or kiss his nose or mouth; she has become a mother tending to her child. This identification process is termed *claiming*, or *binding-in*, *her child* [16]. Another term is *bonding* [10]. The length of time a mother takes to bond her child depends on the circumstances of the pregnancy and delivery; the wellness and ability of the child to meet the parents' expectations, and the opportunities the mother has to interact with her child. That a mother looks directly at her newborn's face, meeting his eyes directly, is a sign that she is beginning effective interaction with him.

If you are to be a help to the mother, it is important for you to determine how much the mother knows and understands about babies. Many new mothers today have never held an infant. They have no younger family members, and their baby-sitting was confined to caring for toddlers and older children. They read everything on child care they could find during their pregnancy, but now that they actually have a baby, the many child-rearing theories they have read only confuse them.

A mother who is unfamiliar with newborns may be disappointed because her baby does not smile or laugh at her or tends to lose her moving finger with his eyes. She may not understand why he spits up on her or why he cries when she holds him. All these things may lead her to believe that the baby does not respond to her, that she is not a "good" mother.

You may notice that a mother who is uncertain with her newborn is always in the bathroom or talking on the telephone when it is time to care for her baby. It is easy to assume that this mother is not interested in her child. In reality, she may be too *frightened* to care for him. It is easier for her to be "busy" than to reveal how little she knows about holding and soothing babies.

You need to assure a mother that the things her baby is doing are normal. Here, anticipatory guidance would involve instructing the mother in the fundamentals of normal infant development. It is a fallacy to equate the level of formal education a mother has achieved with her ability to give good child care. A mother may have graduated from college and have several advanced degrees, yet know nothing about babies. She may have gone only through grade school, yet have a feeling for children's needs. You have to evaluate each mother individually and adjust your teaching accordingly.

Teaching in the postpartal unit does not have to be formal. You can teach without lecturing by making such comments as: "Notice how large all newborns' heads seem" while you are bathing the baby, or "Babies like to be bundled firmly" while you are dressing the child, or "Notice how uneven newborn respirations are" when the mother is observing the baby. This kind of instruction will save the mother many anxious moments when she is at home.

JEALOUSY

Most new mothers, if given the opportunity, admit to feeling abandoned following delivery. Only hours before, the mother was the center of attention. Everyone asked about her health and her well-being. Suddenly, her baby is the chief interest. Everyone asks how the baby is. The gifts are all for the baby. Even her obstetrician, who made her feel so important for the last nine months, may ask when he visits her, "How's that healthy 8-pound boy?" She feels confused by a sensation very close to jealousy. How can a "good" mother be *jealous* of her own baby?

You can help the mother by verbalizing the problem. "How things have changed! Everyone's asking about the baby today and not about you, aren't they? How strange, even uncomfortable, that must make you feel." These are welcome words for a mother to hear. It is reassuring to know the sensation she is experiencing is normal.

When the newborn comes home, the father may have much the same feelings. He may become resentful over the time his wife has to spend with the infant. Perhaps the two used to sit at the table after dinner discussing the day or the future. Now she hurries away to feed the baby. She used to watch the late show with him at night. Now she goes to bed earlier because she knows she will be up again at 2:00 A.M.

This is a good subject to discuss with new parents. Both motherhood and fatherhood involve some compromising of interests in favor of the baby's. Examination of feelings such as those described should start during pregnancy or early in the postpartal period.

DISAPPOINTMENT

Another common feeling a mother may experience is disappointment in her baby. All during pregnancy she pictured a chubby-cheeked, curly-haired, smiling girl. She finds she is handed a skinny boy, without any hair, who is crying instead.

If the mother is conscious during the delivery and sees the baby being born, the realization that her baby does not meet her expectations is easier to accept than if she was under anesthesia during the delivery. In the latter case the mother may feel that a mistake has been made and wonder if babies were accidentally switched in the nursery. It may take her as long as three or four days to stop referring to the child by the wrong sex.

It is a loss of face for a mother to deliver a child who does not meet her expectations. Even though she objectively understands that the father is responsible for determining the sex of the child, subjectively she feels it is her fault. This myth is perpetuated largely by the media. For example, when a Middle East potentate rejects his wife because she did not "give him a son," the papers report this without comment. If the child is scrawny-looking and definitely not as cute as the infant in the next crib, the mother may remember her adolescence, when she felt gangly and unattractive, and she may experience the inadequacy she felt then all over again.

You can never hope to change the size or sex of the child, but in the three or four days that you care for a postpartal mother and her child, you can change the mother's feelings about the infant's sex and appearance. Handle the child as if you find him satisfactory or even special. Comment on the child's good points: long fingers, lovely eyes, good appetite, and so on. Childbearing is a crisis, and during periods of crisis it is possible for a key person to offer support that can tip the scale toward acceptance, or at least help the persons involved to take a clearer look at their situation and begin to cope with the new circumstances.

The Neonatal Perception Inventory

The Neonatal Perception Inventory is a rating scale designed by Broussard [3] as an early case-finding tool to detect potential disturbances in a child's developmental course and to promote the mental health of both a newborn and his mother.

The mother's background—how she feels about herself, the quality of mothering that she received, her total life experiences, and her cultural values—influences how she perceives her new baby. An infant who is not perceived as being better than average by his mother is at much higher risk for the development of subsequent emotional difficulties than the infant who is viewed as better than average. Broussard has shown that 46.5 percent of mothers rate their babies as above average on the first or second day post partum. Rating a baby under average may reflect lowered self-esteem in the mother or may indicate her lack of knowledge of newborns (situations that can be aided by nursing interventions).

The rating scales used for the Neonatal Perception Inventory are shown in Figs. 24-2 and 24-3. Six behavior items—crying, spitting up, feeding, elimination, sleeping, and predictability—are rated.

The form shown in Fig. 24-2A is given to a new mother on her first or second day post partum with an explanation such as: "We are interested in learning more about the experiences of mothers and their babies during the first few weeks after delivery. The more we can learn about mothers and their babies, the better we will be able to help other mothers with their babies. We would appreciate it if you would help us by answering a few questions. Although this is your first baby, you probably have some ideas of what most little babies are like. Will you please check the blank you *think* best describes what *most* little babies are like."

When the mother has completed the first form, she is given the second (Fig. 24-2B) and told, "While it is not possible to know for certain what your baby will be like, you probably have some ideas of what your baby might be like. Please check the blank that you think best describes what *your* baby will be like."

When the mother has completed both forms, they are scored. Each item on the scale is scored on a five-point basis. "A great deal" equals 5, "a good bit" equals 4, "a moderate amount" equals 3, "very little" equals 2, and "none" equals 1. Each form is scored separately. Then the total score of the *Your Baby* form is subtracted from the total score of the *Average Baby* form (Figs. 24-2A and 24-2B). A plus or positive score indicates that the mother sees her baby favorably; a minus or negative score suggests that the mother sees her baby as less than average.

At 1 month of age, the Neonatal Perception Inventory may be used again (Figs. 24-3A and 24-3B) to determine whether the mother's perceptions have changed. The mother receives the same instructions for the first form. To acquaint her with the second form, it is explained, "You have had a chance to live with your baby for a month now. Please check the blank you think best describes your baby."

At 1 month of age, the third form, Degree of Bother Inventory (Fig. 24-4), may also be given, with something like the following explanation: "Listed below are some of the things that have sometimes bothered other mothers in caring for their babies. We would like to know whether you were bothered by any of these. Please place a check in the blank that best describes how much you were bothered by your baby's behavior in regard to these."

The Neonatal Perception Inventory is a simple tool that can be used on postpartal units to try to identify mothers with unreal expectations of newborns or mothers who lack knowledge of newborns. Effective

NEONATAL PERCEPTION INVENTORY I

AVERAGE BABY

How much crying do you think the average baby does?

| a great deal | a good bit | moderate amount | very little | none |

How much trouble do you think the average baby has in feeding?

| a great deal | a good bit | moderate amount | very little | none |

How much spitting up or vomiting do you think the average baby does?

| a great deal | a good bit | moderate amount | very little | none |

How much difficulty do you think the average baby has in sleeping?

| a great deal | a good bit | moderate amount | very little | none |

How much difficulty does the average baby have with bowel movements?

| a great deal | a good bit | moderate amount | very little | none |

How much trouble do you think the average baby has in settling down to a predictable pattern of eating and sleeping?

| a great deal | a good bit | moderate amount | very little | none |

A

NEONATAL PERCEPTION INVENTORY I

YOUR BABY

How much crying do you think your baby will do?

| a great deal | a good bit | moderate amount | very little | none |

How much trouble do you think your baby will have feeding?

| a great deal | a good bit | moderate amount | very little | none |

How much spitting up or vomiting do you think your baby will do?

| a great deal | a good bit | moderate amount | very little | none |

How much difficulty do you think your baby will have sleeping?

| a great deal | a good bit | moderate amount | very little | none |

How much difficulty do you expect your baby to have with bowel movements?

| a great deal | a good bit | moderate amount | very little | none |

How much trouble do you think that your baby will have settling down to a predictable pattern of eating and sleeping?

| a great deal | a good bit | moderate amount | very little | none |

B

Fig. 24-2. Neonatal Perception Inventory I. A. Average baby. B. Your baby. (From E. R. Broussard and M. S. Hartner. Further Considerations Regarding Maternal Perception of the First Born. In J. Hellmuth [Ed.], Exceptional Infant: Studies in Abnormalities, vol. 2. New York: Brunner/Mazel, Inc.)

NEONATAL PERCEPTION INVENTORY II

AVERAGE BABY

How much crying do you think the average baby does?

| a great deal | a good bit | moderate amount | very little | none |

How much trouble do you think the average baby has in feeding?

| a great deal | a good bit | moderate amount | very little | none |

How much spitting up or vomiting do you think the average baby does?

| a great deal | a good bit | moderate amount | very little | none |

How much difficulty do you think the average baby has in sleeping?

| a great deal | a good bit | moderate amount | very little | none |

How much difficulty does the average baby have with bowel movements?

| a great deal | a good bit | moderate amount | very little | none |

How much trouble do you think the average baby has in settling down to a predictable pattern of eating and sleeping?

| a great deal | a good bit | moderate amount | very little | none |

A

NEONATAL PERCEPTION INVENTORY II

YOUR BABY

How much crying has your baby done?

| a great deal | a good bit | moderate amount | very little | none |

How much trouble has your baby had feeding?

| a great deal | a good bit | moderate amount | very little | none |

How much spitting up or vomiting has your baby done?

| a great deal | a good bit | moderate amount | very little | none |

How much difficulty has your baby had in sleeping?

| a great deal | a good bit | moderate amount | very little | none |

How much difficulty has your baby had with bowel movements?

| a great deal | a good bit | moderate amount | very little | none |

How much trouble has your baby had in settling down to a predictable pattern of eating and sleeping?

| a great deal | a good bit | moderate amount | very little | none |

B

Fig. 24-3. Neonatal Perception Inventory II. A. Average baby. B. Your baby. (From E. R. Broussard and M. S. Hartner. Further Considerations Regarding Maternal Perception of the First Born. In J. Hellmuth [Ed.], Exceptional Infant: Studies in Abnormalities, vol. 2. New York: Brunner/Mazel, Inc.)

DEGREE OF BOTHER INVENTORY

Crying	a great deal	somewhat	very little	none
Spitting up or vomiting	a great deal	somewhat	very little	none
Sleeping	a great deal	somewhat	very little	none
Feeding	a great deal	somewhat	very little	none
Elimination	a great deal	somewhat	very little	none
Lack of a predictable schedule	a great deal	somewhat	very little	none
Other (specify):				
_____	a great deal	somewhat	very little	none
_____	a great deal	somewhat	very little	none
_____	a great deal	somewhat	very little	none
_____	a great deal	somewhat	very little	none

Fig. 24-4. Degree of Bother Inventory. (From E. R. Broussard and M. S. Hartner. Further Considerations Regarding Maternal Perception of the First Born. In J. Hellmuth [Ed.], Exceptional Infant: Studies in Abnormalities, vol. 2. New York: Brunner/Mazel, Inc.)

nursing interventions can then be structured to attempt to correct these situations and promote better mother-infant relationships. It is a helpful tool for community health nurses who make newborn referrals.

Phases of the Puerperium
TAKING-IN PHASE

In terms of physical and psychological happenings, the puerperium may be divided into two separate phases. The first of these encompasses the first two or three days and is the *taking-in* phase [16].

The taking-in phase is a time of reflection for the woman. During this period she is largely passive. She relies on the nurse to initiate action. She prefers having the nurse minister to her, to get her a bath towel or a clean nightgown, arrange flowers for her, and make decisions for her rather than doing these things herself. This dependence is due partly to her physical discomfort from the perineal stitches, afterpains (see Chap. 25), or hemorrhoids, partly to her uncertainty in caring for a newborn, and partly to the extreme exhaustion that follows delivery.

As a part of thinking and pondering her new role, the mother usually wants to talk about her pregnancy and especially about her labor and delivery. She was pregnant for so long, looked forward to her baby's birth for so long, and imagined the baby being born for so long that now that the baby is actually here, it seems almost impossible to believe. She holds the child with a sense of wonder. The birth seems almost anticlimactic next to her visions of it. Can this child really be hers? Is delivery really over? She needs time to rest to regain her physical strength and time to right her swirling thoughts.

TAKING-HOLD PHASE

Following the two or three days of passive dependence, the woman begins to initiate action herself. She prefers to get her own washcloth, to make her own decisions, and may even walk to the nursery to get her baby.

Some women seem overly concerned with their bodily functions during these days, worrying about bladder and bowel control, for example. This is a part of normal taking-hold, since bowel and bladder control is necessary for independence. The woman may express impatience with perineal stitches that still feel uncomfortable or breast tissue that still feels tender. She wants to be doing things for her newborn. She wants to go home and is impatient because she does not feel physically strong enough to do so.

During the taking-in period the mother may have

expressed no great interest in caring for her child. In this second phase she begins to take a strong interest in caring for her baby. She realizes she has only a short time to learn and wants all the practice she can get. It is frustrating for her to watch a nurse change, feed, and bubble her baby while she merely watches. It is better if the mother is given brief demonstrations of baby care and then allowed to care for the child herself—with watchful guidance.

Even though the mother's actions indicate strong independence, she often feels insecure about her ability to care for her child. She needs praise for the things she does well: supporting the baby's head, feeding the correct amount of fluid, bubbling, and so on. Before she leaves the hospital she needs to be confident of her ability to care for and make decisions for her baby (Fig. 24-5).

Neither rush the mother through the phase of taking-in nor prevent her from taking-hold during the last days of her hospitalization. For many young mothers, learning to make decisions about their child's welfare is one of the most difficult phases of motherhood. A mother needs practice in making such decisions in a sheltered setting rather than first taking on the responsibility when she is on her own.

Rooming-In

The more time the mother has to spend with her baby, the faster a mother-child relationship can develop. Because the average postpartal hospital stay is no more than three days, a mother today has very little time to become acquainted with her newborn before she takes him home. If the infant stays in the room with her rather than in a central nursery (rooming-in), she can become better acquainted with the infant and begin to feel more confidence in her ability to care for him after discharge.

Complete rooming-in implies that the mother and child are together 24 hours a day. In partial rooming-in, the infant remains in the mother's room for part of the time, perhaps from 10:00 A.M. to 9:00 P.M., after which he is taken to a small nursery near the mother's room or returned to a central nursery.

With both complete and partial rooming-in, times are provided when the father, after washing and donning a hospital gown, can hold and feed his infant.

Many new mothers find complete rooming-in too great a strain both physically and psychologically. Every time the baby stirs or hiccups or takes a deeper-than-usual respiration they are out of bed peering at him. They do not sleep soundly at night because they are trying to remain alert in case the baby cries. At a time when they need to receive comfort, to take rather than to give, they feel overwhelmed by the degree of responsibility the hospital is giving them.

Many hospitals have tried complete rooming-in, found that mothers were unhappy with it, and returned to a central nursery concept, with the infants brought to the mothers only for a half hour every 4 hours for feeding.

Partial rooming-in seems to incorporate the best of the two systems. The mother can be with her baby during the day and yet can sleep soundly at night, knowing he is being looked after. The father is allowed to share in the first days of his infant's life as well. On discharge the mother is more confident and more comfortable at home with her new infant than if she had seen him only briefly a few times a day.

Not only does rooming-in allow a mother-child and father-child relationship to develop more rapidly, but anticipatory guidance and instructions in newborn care seem to be retained better when the nurse demonstrates bathing, feeding, changing, and so forth

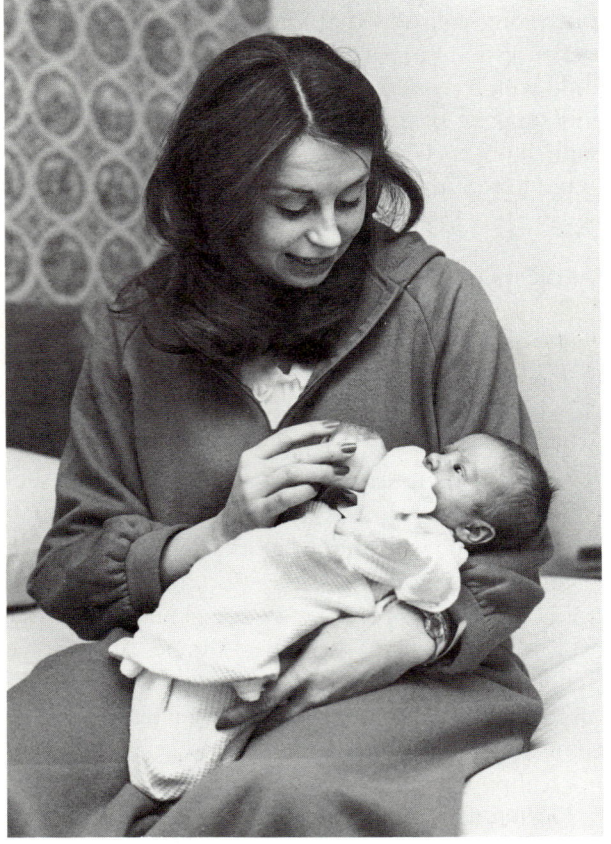

Fig. 24-5. *Mothering a new baby is a responsibility. It takes time and exposure to each other for mother-child interaction to be effective. (Courtesy of the Department of Medical Photography, Children's Hospital, Buffalo, N.Y.)*

on the mother's own child. Anxious calls from a mother concerning child care after she has returned home are fewer if she is discharged feeling confident in her ability to care for her baby and more comfortable with him because she has been allowed to have him with her during most of her hospital stay. Klaus and Kennell [10] have demonstrated that extra hours of mother-infant contact affect mother-infant bonding positively.

That a mother is not adapting well to caring for her infant is often evident by observing her and talking to her about her infant. Signs of poor mother-child adaptation are as follows [2]:

Speaks of infant as ugly and unattractive
Upset by vomiting, drooling, etc.
Doesn't hold baby warmly
Doesn't make eye contact
Juggles and plays roughly
Picks up baby without warning
Thinks that the infant doesn't love her
Thinks that the infant judges her
Concerned that the infant has a defect even though this has been ruled out
Cannot find any physical or psychological attribute to admire
Cannot discriminate between signs of hunger, sleep, etc.

Concerns of the Postpartal Period

Traditionally, it has been assumed that most of a mother's concerns in the postpartal period are with care of her infant. Classes in the postpartal period have centered around teaching how to prepare formula and bathe infants. Although these are concerns for many mothers, they are not necessarily their chief problems. A woman has come through a tremendous psychological experience during pregnancy and birth of a child. She has made a complete role change from being a daughter to being a mother. It is only to be expected, then, that some of her attention and some of her interest during this time will be with herself as she tries to view herself in this role.

Gruis [7] asked mothers to identify their chief concerns in the postpartal period. Each mother in this study delivered a normal infant who was discharged from the hospital with her. She had no complication that required an extended hospital stay and was living with the father of the child at the time of the study. The findings of this study are given in Table 24-1.

Notice that 95 percent of mothers were concerned about the return of their figure to normal. It is

Table 24-1. Percentages of Mothers Noting Specific Concerns During the Puerperium

Area of Concern	Percent of Mothers Concerned		
	Degree of Concern		
	Minor	Major	Total
Return of figure to normal	30	65	95
Regulating demands of husband, housework, children	42	48	90
Emotional tension	48	40	88
Fatigue	28	55	83
Infant behavior	47	33	80
Finding time for self	45	33	78
Sexual relations	53	20	73
Diet	33	40	73
Feelings of isolation; being tied down	42	28	70
Infant's growth and development	45	25	70
Family planning	25	43	68
Exercise	23	45	68
Infant feeding	43	25	68
Changes in relationship with husband	35	25	60
Physical care of infant	45	13	58
Infant safety	33	25	58
Discomfort of stitches	33	20	53
Breast care	40	10	50
Constipation	35	15	50
Setting limits for visitors	27	23	50
Interpreting infant's behavior	27	23	50
Breast soreness	35	13	48
Hemorrhoids	25	23	48
Labor and delivery experience	28	20	48
Father's role with baby	22	23	45
Lochia	35	5	40
Other children jealous of baby	27	13	40
Other children's behavior	25	15	40
Infant's appearance	18	20	38
Traveling with baby	27	8	35
Clothing for baby	20	10	30
Feeling comfortable handling baby	15	8	23

Source. M. Gruis, Beyond maternity: Postpartum concerns of mothers. M.C.N. 2:182, 1977.

difficult to begin a new role if you do not feel at your best. Notice how many were concerned about finding time for themselves (78 percent). Mothers are interested in learning newborn care during this period. They also are interested in having someone appreciate that this is not an easy step in life. There is responsibility involved here. They need time for introspection so as to begin to think through their new role and find constructive ways to deal with their new life.

POSTPARTAL BLUES

During the puerperium, most women experience some feelings of overwhelming sadness that they cannot account for. They burst into tears easily and are irritable over trifles. This temporary feeling after birth has long been known as the *baby blues.*

The postpartal blues are probably largely the result of a let-down feeling, an "after-the-prom" feeling. The mother looked forward to the birth of the baby so long that the actual event seems anticlimactic as compared with her expectations. The blues may also be due to hormonal changes, particularly the decrease in estrogen and progesterone that occurs with the delivery of the placenta. For some women it may be a response to dependence caused by hospitalization. Certainly, exhaustion, being away from home, physical discomfort, and the tension engendered by assuming a new role play their part also.

The woman needs assurance that her sudden crying jags are normal; otherwise, she will not understand what is happening to her. Her husband also needs such assurance or he may think that his wife is unhappy with him or with the baby or is keeping some terrible secret about the baby from him.

Individualized nursing attention, or making certain that the mother is treated as if she, not the child, is the important patient, helps to alleviate postpartal blues. It is also important to give the mother a chance to verbalize her feelings: "There's absolutely no reason for me to be crying but I cannot stop." Some mothers are given tranquilizers or mood elevators during this time to help them through the period.

Not all women crying on a postpartal unit have the baby blues. A woman sometimes has real reasons to feel sad during this time. Perhaps problems at home have become overwhelming. Her husband may have been laid off just when they most need the money. Her mother may be ill, a child at home may be ill, and so on. Open lines of communication with postpartal mothers are important to help you differentiate problems that respond best to discussion and concerned understanding from problems that should be referred to the hospital social service department or to a community health agency.

Occasionally, serious depression that requires psychiatric care occurs during the postpartal period. This is postpartal psychosis and is discussed in Chap. 36.

SEXUAL RELATIONS

At one time, women were cautioned not to resume sexual relations after birth of a baby until their check-up at six weeks. Many physicians still like their patients to observe this rule. Others encourage them to begin sexual relations as soon as lochia serosa (the uterine discharge after birth) has stopped—about two weeks after delivery.

Sex may be painful if begun this early; tissue at the episiotomy site may be sensitive. Exhaustion and concern for her new infant, fear of waking him, may make a woman less receptive to sexual arousal than before.

A little forewarning that problems in this area may occur is helpful in preventing them.

The Unwed Mother

The average unwed woman on a maternity service today is planning on keeping and rearing her child or she would not have allowed the pregnancy to come to completion. For some young couples, conceiving children without marriage is a definite, planned part of their life-style. For other couples, the pregnancy was not planned, but by the end of pregnancy, they are certain they will raise the child.

The unwed woman may need more postpartal teaching than her married counterpart because her network of support people is apt to be less secure. Ask, Where will she be living after discharge? Who will actually be caring for the baby? What will be the source of finances? If the mother will be returning to school or taking a full-time job, who will care for the baby during these times?

Very young girls enjoy having you look at their baby with them and point out features or care points with them. They have none of the experience of older women with babies; they need a lot of help to determine what is "normal" and what is not.

Unwed women need visitors during the postpartal period the same as anyone. If the father of the child wants to visit and hold his newborn, he should be allowed this privilege; his self-esteem is important too. If the father of the child is not going to visit the mother, then another person, either the girl's mother or father or some other person who is important to her should be allowed to come instead.

Investigate the availability of a strong support person. If the woman does not seem to have such a person, help her make contact with a health care center (a well-child conference, a community health nurse, a pediatrician, a community clinic) so she has a resource person to call upon when she has questions about baby care in the first few days or weeks of her baby's life.

The Unwed Father

Many unwed fathers serve as support people in labor and delivery for the child's mother. They enjoy holding and feeding and getting acquainted with their newborn in the postpartal period. They plan on visiting as much as a married father would during this time.

Other fathers are not interested in talking with the child's mother or even in holding the infant, but do want to see the child at least once. There is self-esteem in knowing that you have had a healthy child. Unwed fathers need the assurance that although they will never father this child they are the father of a healthy child.

The Mother Who Chooses Not To Keep Her Child

It is difficult for many nurses to accept the fact that some children are not wanted.

The availability of birth control information and the increasing number of abortions that are being performed have reduced the number of unwanted children. Nonetheless, some children are still unwanted.

There are many reasons for this. The mother may be unmarried or her marriage may be failing, and she has no wish to raise a child alone. The woman may feel her family is already complete. The child may have been wanted if it had been a girl, or if it had been a boy. The woman feels too old to have more children, or she expected to finish school first, or she would like to follow a career—the reasons are endless.

During pregnancy, most women decide whether or not they will keep their child. During labor, they express confidence in their decision, but with the birth of the child, they often find that their resolve wavers. A woman who was certain she was going to surrender her child for adoption may begin to feel she would prefer to keep him. A woman who was certain she was going to keep her child becomes aware of the responsibility involved and decides that the best course for the child will be to surrender him for adoption. In either event, the mother's feelings become confused.

The wait in the delivery room for completion of perineal repair and preparations for transfer of the baby to a nursery is unusually long for the woman who chooses not to keep her child. She is usually alone, with no husband, no father of the child, to accompany her to the delivery room.

It is always a question whether the mother who is going to surrender her child for adoption should see him after delivery. There is a saying that if she holds him once, she will never give him up. Any decision to surrender a child that can be changed this easily is never a firm one and probably would be changed in any event.

Every mother has a right to see her child, to hold him, and to feed him if she wishes. The mother who is not going to keep her child may find a great source of pride in her ability to produce a healthy child. Knowing that the baby is strong and healthy adds to her self-esteem. She cannot be "all bad," as members of her family may have said, if she can produce a beautiful and perfect child. This realization may give her a foundation to build a sounder future. It may make her feel truly a whole woman for the first time.

Do not attempt to persuade her to keep her child or to place her child for adoption while she is in the delivery room. She is extremely vulnerable to suggestion at this time, and such decisions are too long-range, too important to be made at such an emotional moment. Her earlier conclusion that she would not be able to be a good mother to the child may be a sounder one.

During the taking-in phase of the puerperium be especially careful that you do not influence the mother's decision making. Women enjoy having decisions made for them during this time and may ask you what you think is best.

A mother who chooses to place her child for adoption may have been lacking in discretion so that she became pregnant. You have no reason to think she is lacking in her ability to love this child. It is not uncommon for mothers who surrender their infants for adoption to experience grief reactions like those of mothers whose children have died.

If the mother decides to surrender her child for adoption, be certain that she is referred to an official adoption agency. An official agency gives the mother the best assurance that the parents chosen for her child will be the right parents for him. This will help to relieve any misgivings or guilt the mother has about surrendering the child and should reduce the moments of doubt that can come in future years: Is my child well cared for? Is he getting everything I could have given him?

Some mothers do not voice openly a wish not to keep their child, but they do show you by their actions that they feel little attachment to the child. The average mother approaches her newborn tentatively; this mother makes contact even more slowly. By the third or fourth postpartal day she is still barely touching the child and asking few questions about his care. She needs concrete help.

The hospital social service department can be of assistance in discussing and helping to plan the child's future. A married couple, as well as a single woman, may place an infant for adoption. More probably, family counseling is the mother's and family's need.

It is a fallacy to assume that everything will work out once the mother and infant get home. The number of battered children seen in hospital emergency rooms is the proof of this.

The foundation of a firm mother-child relationship is laid in the first days of the infant's life. The mother who seems incapable of beginning to build this foundation should be able to rely on the professional nurse to recognize her problem and to offer her an avenue to a solution.

Sibling Visitation

Whether a child grows up feeling loved or not is influenced by how his older siblings feel about him. Waiting at home separated from mother, listening only to telephone reports of what a new brother or sister looks like, is very difficult for children. They may picture the new baby as much older than he is. "He is eating well" may produce an image of a child sitting at a table using a fork and spoon. "He is sleeping well" may make them envision a child in a regular bed. "He weighs 7 pounds" is meaningless information. A chance to visit the hospital and see the new baby and mother reduces feelings that mother cares more about the new baby than about them (mother, after all, *is* spending four days with the baby and not with them) and provides a true image of the new family member.

Children should be free of contagious diseases (cold, recent exposure to chickenpox) to visit. In some institutions they are allowed to see the new baby through the glass of the nursery; in others they can see the baby in the mother's room.

Separation from children is often as painful for a mother as for the children. Sibling visitation usually goes a long way toward preventing postpartal depression by relieving some of the impact of separation. A mother needs to be cautioned that preschoolers' opinions of a new brother or sister may not be complimentary. This baby with little hair is not their idea of a "pretty baby." If they thought the new baby would be big enough to play with them, they may not feel he is a "big baby." Seeing the baby, however, even if his appearance is not what they expected, is helpful in terms of establishing strong relationships and is a practice to be encouraged in postpartal units.

Problem-oriented Recording: Progress Notes

Christine McFadden
15 years
Para 1, gravida 1

Problem: mother-child interaction, day 1 post partum

> S. States, "I thought I'd have a girl. I thought I could tell he was a girl. I can't trade him, can I?" (laughing)
> O. Holds baby to bottle-feed but does not pick him up unless someone hands him to her. Handed him back as he started to cry after she was through feeding. Lets maternal grandmother give care while she is visiting.
> A. Bonding inadequate as yet because of unplanned pregnancy and disappointment in sex of child.
>
> Goals: a. Form an effective mother-child relationship.
> b. Able to use maternal grandmother as advice and support person, but able to give care herself.
> c. Able to perform safe newborn care by hospital discharge (10 days).
>
> P. 1. Provide time to talk about baby and effect of having a boy instead of a girl.
> 2. Provide adequate rest so patient feels well enough for baby care (postcesarean section).

3. Provide time to hold baby with no obligation to give care, just hold and get acquainted.
4. Beginning third day, begin to teach aspects of baby care.

Problem-oriented Recording: Progress Notes

Mary Kraft
22 years
Para 1, gravida 2

Problem: Mother-child interaction, day 1 post partum

S. States, "He's so tiny." Asking, "When will he smile back at me?" Father asking, "Will this spot [mongolian spot] on his arm go away?"
O. Breast-feeding successfully. Mother smiles and studies baby's face. Father visits often, holds baby during visit.
A. Good parent-child interaction.

Goals: a. Form a parent-child relationship.
b. Able to think of child as well and eager to please because of increased knowledge of normal newborns.
c. Comfortable in giving safe care to child by discharge (24 to 48 hours).

P. 1. Review characteristics of normal newborns.
2. Provide discussion time for questions or anticipated problems at home.
3. Help to identify support person to use as reference for small problems of child rearing.
4. Watch demonstration from mother of ability to give safe and responsible care to newborn; teach additional facts as necessary.

Problem-oriented Recording: Progress Notes

Angie Baco
42 years
Para 7, gravida 7

Problem: mother-child interaction, day 2 post partum

S. States, "I can't believe how beautiful she is. Look at her eyes and her nose. My boys were so plain when they were born. She's beautiful." Is concerned that 7-year-old at home (child with learning disability) stole some money from teacher's desk in school yesterday. Asking for suggestions to help 7-year-old accept new baby better.
O. Always holds child warmly; comforts her easily. Appears tired; crying over action of older child. Father has not visited since recovery room, because of work and care of other children.
A. Mother-child interaction good. Concerns with other children may interfere unless problems are solved in that area.

Goals: a. Form a positive parent-child relationship.
b. Able to integrate new baby into present family.

P. 1. Urge contact with other children through visiting or telephone.
2. Provide time for discussion of how she will divide her time at home with other children.
3. Provide suggestions for 7-year-old management (special time each day).
4. Urge to get sufficient rest so exhaustion does not compound home problems.

References

1. Atkinson, L. D. Is family centered care a myth? *M.C.N.* 1:256, 1976.
2. Bishop, B. A guide to assessing parenting capabilities. *Am. J. Nurs.* 76:1784, 1976.
3. Broussard, E. R., and Sturgeon, M. S. Maternal perception of the neonate as related to development. *Child Psychiatry Hum. Dev.* 1:16, 1970.

4. Brown, M. S., et al. Mothering the mother. *Am. J. Nurs.* 77:438, 1977.
5. Freeman, M. H. Giving family life a good start in the hospital. *M.C.N.* 4:51, 1979.
6. Gallober, M. A comment on the need for father-infant post partum interaction. *J.O.G.N. Nurs.* 5:17, 1976.
7. Gruis, M. Beyond maternity: Post partum concerns of mothers. *M.C.N.* 2:182, 1977.
8. Horowitz, J. A., and Perdue, B. J. Single-parent families. *Nurs. Clin. North Am.* 12:503, 1977.
9. Kiernan, B., and Scoloveno, M. A. Fathering. *Nurs. Clin. North Am.* 12:481, 1977.
10. Klaus, M. H., and Kennell, J. H. *Maternal-infant Bonding.* St. Louis: Mosby, 1976.
11. Kontos, D. A study of the effects of extended maternal-infant contact on maternal behavior at one and three months. *Birth Fam. J.* 5:133, 1978.
12. Kyndely, K. The sexuality of women in pregnancy and post partum. *J.O.G.N. Nurs.* 7:28, 1978.
13. Perdue, B. J., et al. Mothering. *Nurs. Clin. North Am.* 12:491, 1977.
14. Peterson, G. H., et al. Some determinants of maternal attachment. *Am. J. Psychiatry* 135:1168, 1978.
15. Ritchie, C. A. Depression following childbirth. *Nurse Pract.* 2:14, 1977.
16. Rubin, R. Binding-in in the post partum period. *Matern. Child Nurs. J.* 6:67, 1977.
17. Sumner, G., and Fritsch, J. Post natal parental concerns: The first 6 weeks of life. *J.O.G.N. Nurs.* 6:27, 1977.
18. Swanson, J. Nursing intervention to facilitate maternal-infant attachment. *J.O.G.N. Nurs.* 7:35, 1978.
19. Webster-Stratton, C., and Kogan, K. Helping parents parent. *Am. J. Nurs.* 80:240, 1980.
20. Westbrook, M. T. The reaction to child-bearing and early maternal experience of women with differing marital relationships. *Br. J. Med. Psychol.* 51:191, 1978.
21. Wuerger, M. The young adult—stepping into parenthood. *Am. J. Nurs.* 76:1283, 1976.

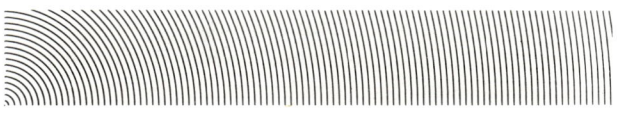

25. Physiology of the Postpartal Period

The six-week period after birth includes physiological changes that are retrogressive in nature (the involution of the uterus and vagina) and some that are progressive in nature (the production of milk for lactation and the restoration of the normal menstrual cycle).

Involution

Involution is the process whereby the reproductive organs return to their nonpregnant state.

THE UTERUS

Involution of the uterus involves two main processes. First, the area where the placenta was implanted is sealed off, and bleeding is therefore prevented. Second, the organ is reduced to its approximate pregestational size (Fig. 25-1).

The sealing of the placental site is accomplished by rapid contraction of the uterus immediately following the delivery of the placenta. The contraction pinches the blood vessels entering the 7-cm-wide area left denuded by the placenta and controls bleeding. With time, thrombi form within the uterine sinuses and permanently seal the area. Eventually, endometrial tissue undermines the site and obliterates the organized thrombi, completely covering and healing the area. This process leaves no scar tissue within the uterus and does not compromise future implantation sites.

The same contraction process reduces the bulk of the uterus. Freed of the placenta and the membranes, the walls of the uterus thicken and contract, reducing the uterus from the size of a container large enough to hold a 7-pound fetus to the size of a grapefruit. Uterine contraction can be compared to a rubber band that has been stretched for many months and now is regaining its normal contour. None of the rubber band is destroyed; the shape is simply altered. A small number of cells of the uterine wall are broken down by an autolytic process into their protein components, and these components are then absorbed by the bloodstream and excreted by the body in urine. However, the main mechanism that reduces the bulk of the uterus is contraction. This is the reason the postpartal period, like pregnancy, is not a period of illness, of necrosing cells being evacuated, but primarily a period of healthy change.

The uterus will never completely return to its virginal state, but the reduction in its size is dramatic. Immediately after delivery the uterus weighs about 1,000 gm. At the end of the first week, it weighs 500 gm. By the time involution is complete (six weeks) it will weigh approximately 50 gm.

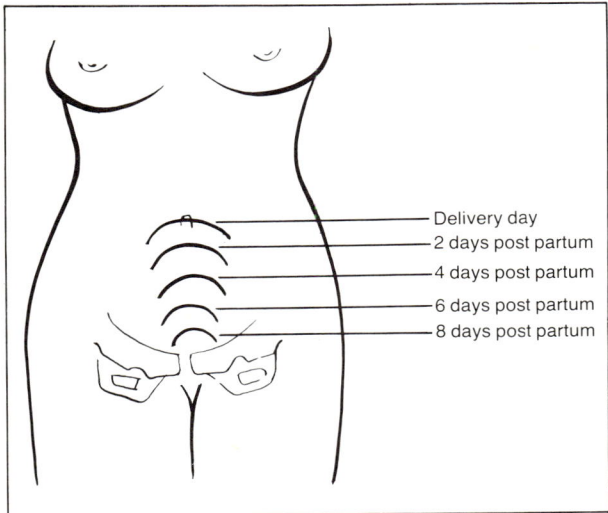

Fig. 25-1. Uterine involution. The uterus decreases in size at a predictable rate during the postpartal period. After 10 days, it recedes under the pubic bone and is no longer palpable.

In the first minutes following delivery of the placenta, as contraction takes place, the fundus of the uterus may be palpated through the abdominal wall halfway between the umbilicus and the symphysis pubis. By an hour after delivery it has risen to the level of the umbilicus, where it remains for approximately the next 24 hours. From then on it will decrease a fingerbreadth (1 cm) a day in size. Thus, on the first postpartal day the fundus of the uterus will be palpable 1 fingerbreadth below the umbilicus; on the second, 2 fingerbreadths below the umbilicus; and so on. In the average woman the uterus will have contracted so much by the ninth or tenth day and be so far withdrawn into the pelvis that it can no longer be detected by abdominal palpation.

The fundus can usually be felt in the midline of the abdomen, although occasionally it is found slightly to the right because the bulk of the sigmoid colon forced it to the right during pregnancy and it tends to remain in that position. Measurements of the height of the fundus should be made shortly after the woman's bladder has been emptied, because a full bladder will keep the uterus from contracting, push it upward, and give a false reading.

An estimation of the consistency of the postpartal uterus is as important as measurement of its height. A well-contracted fundus feels firm. It can be compared with a grapefruit not only in size but also in tenseness, or consistency. Whenever the fundus feels soft or flabby, it is not as contracted as it should be, despite its position in the abdomen.

The first hour post partum is potentially the most dangerous time for the newly delivered woman. If the uterus should become relaxed during this time so the placental site is no longer well sealed, the woman will lose blood very rapidly, because no permanent thrombi have yet formed at the placental site. Hemorrhage is the commonest cause of maternal morbidity and mortality in childbirth, and this is a critical point at which it may occur.

Afterpains

In some women the contraction of the uterus after delivery causes cramps similar to those accompanying a menstrual period. These are afterpains. They occur more frequently in multiparas than primiparas, in mothers who have delivered large babies, and in mothers who are breast-feeding. In the latter, the infant's sucking causes a release of oxytocin from the posterior pituitary, which increases contractions and thus the uncomfortable sensation in the mother's abdomen.

Abdominal Wall

The abdominal wall and the ligaments that support the uterus are obviously stretched during pregnancy and usually require the full six weeks of the puerperium to return to their former state. Any striae that are present on the abdomen gradually become less noticeable as they fade from a reddish color to a silvery white. If a diastasis (an actual separation of muscle fiber) had occurred, this portion of the abdominal wall will probably always remain noticeable as a dark narrow groove.

Lochia

The separation of the placenta and membranes occurs in the spongy layer or outer portion of the decidua basalis. By the second day following delivery the layer of decidua remaining under the placental site (an area 7 cm wide) and throughout the uterus differentiates into two distinct layers. The inner layer attached to the muscular wall of the uterus will remain and serve as the foundation from which a new layer of endometrium will be formed. The layer adjacent to the uterine cavity will become necrotic and will be cast off as a uterine discharge similar to a menstrual flow. This uterine flow, consisting of blood, fragments of decidua, white blood cells, mucus, and some bacteria, is known as *lochia*.

The portion of the uterus where the placenta was not attached will be fully cleansed by this sloughing process and will be in a reproductive state in about three weeks. The placental implantation site will take approximately six weeks (the entire postpartal period) to be cleansed and healed.

For the first three days after delivery, the lochia discharge consists almost entirely of blood, with only small particles of decidua and mucus. Because of its red color, it is termed *lochia rubra*. As the amount of blood involved in the cast-off tissue decreases (about the fourth day), and leukocytes begin to invade the area as they do any healing surface, the flow becomes pink or brownish in color (*lochia serosa*). On about the tenth day, the amount of the flow decreases and becomes colorless or white (*lochia alba*). Lochia alba is present in most women until the third week following delivery, although it is not unusual for a lochia flow to last the entire six weeks of the puerperium.

NORMAL CHARACTERISTICS OF LOCHIA. There are several rules for judging whether lochia flow is or is not normal, and you should be familiar with these rules.

1. Lochia should approximate a menstrual flow in amount. Like the amount of menstrual flow, this amount will vary from woman to woman. Two women in adjoining beds may be having very different quantities of lochia discharge, yet each may be normal for that woman. Mothers who breast-feed tend to have less lochial discharge than those who do not, since the natural release of oxytocin during breast-feeding strengthens uterine contractions. Conservation of fluid for lactation may also be a factor. Lochial flow increases on exertion, especially the first few times the woman is out of bed, but decreases again with rest. The woman should be warned of this possibility or she may become unnecessarily alarmed by a sudden heavy flow.
2. Lochia should contain no large clots. Clots may indicate that a portion of the placenta has been retained and is preventing closure of the maternal uterine blood sinuses. In any event, clotting denotes poor uterine contraction, which needs to be corrected.
3. The pattern of lochia (rubra to serosa to alba) should not reverse. A red flow after lochia serosa or alba usually indicates that placental fragments have been retained or that uterine contraction is decreasing and new bleeding is beginning.
4. Lochia should not have an offensive odor. Lochia has the same odor as menstrual blood (sometimes compared with the odor of marigolds). An offensive odor usually indicates that the uterus has become infected. Immediate intervention is needed to halt postpartal infection.
5. Lochia should never be absent. Absence of lochia, like presence of an offensive odor, may indicate postpartal infection. Lochia is scant in amount following cesarean deliveries, but it is never altogether absent. Characteristics of lochia are summarized in Table 25-1.

THE CERVIX

Immediately following delivery the cervix is soft and malleable. Both the internal os and the external os are well open. Like contraction of the fundus of the uterus, retraction of the cervix begins at once. By the end of seven days the external os is narrowed to the size of a pencil opening, and the cervix feels firm and nongravid again.

In contrast to the process of involution in the fundus, in which the changes consist primarily of old cells being returned to their former position by contraction, the process in the cervix involves the formation of new muscle cells. Like the fundus, the cervix does not return exactly to its virginal state. The internal os will close as before, but, assuming that the delivery was vaginal, the external os will usually remain slightly open and appear slit-like or stellate where it was round before. Finding this pattern on pelvic examination suggests that childbearing has taken place.

THE VAGINA

Following a vaginal delivery the vagina is soft, and its diameter is considerably greater than normal. It takes the entire postpartal period for it to involute (as in the uterus, by contraction), until it gradually returns ap-

Table 25-1. Characteristics of Lochia

Type of Lochia	Color	Duration	Composition
Lochia rubra	Red	1–3 days	Blood, fragments of decidua and mucus
Lochia serosa	Pink or brown-tinged	3–10 days	Blood, mucus, and invading leukocytes
Lochia alba	White	10–14 days May last for 6 weeks	Largely mucus; leukocyte count high

proximately to its nonpregnant state. Like the cervix, the vaginal outlet will remain slightly more distended than before.

THE PERINEUM

The perineum is put under a great deal of pressure during delivery, to which it responds by the development of edema and generalized tenderness following delivery. Portions of it may show ecchymosis from the rupture of surface capillaries. The labia majora and labia minora typically remain atrophic and softened in a woman who has borne a child.

Systemic Changes

During pregnancy, the blood volume of the body increases 30 to 50 percent. The tendency of the body to retain water in interstitial tissue is also increased.

Beginning with the second day of the puerperium, diuresis and diaphoresis combine to rid the body of these sources of excess fluid.

DIURESIS

In the postpartal period, urine tends to contain more nitrogen than normal. This development is probably due in part to the woman's increased muscle activity during labor and in part to the breakdown of protein in a portion of the uterine muscle that occurs during involution. Levels of lactose in the urine may be the same as during pregnancy. If any urine testing for sugar is done either during pregnancy or post partum, therefore, agents such as Clinistix or Tes-Tape that test only the glucose, not the lactose, component of sugar should be used for testing.

As diuresis begins to take place, the daily output of the postpartal woman is increased greatly. Urinary volume may easily rise to as much as 3,000 ml during the second to fifth day after delivery. This marked increase in urine production causes the bladder to fill rapidly.

During a vaginal delivery, the fetal head exerts a great deal of pressure on the bladder as it passes on the bladder's underside. This pressure may leave the bladder with a transient loss of tone. Thus, even though it fills rapidly and becomes distended, the woman may have no sensation of having to void. The woman who has had a spinal anesthetic or a general anesthetic for delivery feels no sensation in the bladder area until the anesthetic has worn off and so is prone to bladder distention.

To prevent permanent damage to the bladder from overdistention, check the woman's abdomen frequently in the immediate postpartal period to see whether bladder distention is developing. A full bladder is felt as a hard or firm area just above the symphysis pubis. On percussion (placing one finger flat on the woman's abdomen over the bladder and tapping it with the middle finger of the other hand) a full bladder sounds resonant or echoing in contrast to the dull thudding sound of non-fluid-filled tissue. Pressure on this area may make the woman feel as if she has to void, but she is then unable to do so. As the bladder fills, it displaces the uterus; uterine position is thus a good gauge of whether the bladder is full or empty. If the uterus is becoming uncontracted and flabby and is being pushed to the side, the usual cause is an overfilled bladder.

DIAPHORESIS

Diaphoresis (excessive sweating) is another way by which the body rids itself of excess fluid. This is noticeable in women soon after delivery.

WEIGHT LOSS

The rapid diuresis and diaphoresis during the second to fifth day post partum will ordinarily result in a weight loss of an additional 5 pounds over the 12 or so pounds that the woman lost at delivery.

CIRCULATORY CHANGES

The diuresis evident between the second and fifth days post partum acts to reduce the added blood volume the woman acquired during pregnancy. This reduction occurs so rapidly that by the second week post partum the blood volume has returned to its normal level before pregnancy.

If the mother was anemic during pregnancy, she can expect to continue to be anemic post partum, although her hematocrit reading (proportion of red cells to proportion of circulating blood) may rise as extra fluid is lost. On the third day post partum, a hemoglobin assessment is usually done to test for the presence of anemia, either from the pregnancy or from blood loss at delivery. If the hemoglobin is below 10 gm per 100 ml, supplementary iron is usually prescribed.

Women generally continue to have the same high level of blood fibrinogen during the first postpartal week as they did during pregnancy. This is a protective measure against hemorrhage. There is also an increase in the number of leukocytes in the blood. The white cell count may be as high as 30,000, particularly if the woman had a long or difficult labor. This, too, is part of the body's defense system, a defense against infection and an aid to healing.

Take note of the laboratory reports on patients and

make certain that any abnormal finding, such as low hemoglobin, is brought to the attention of the physician. The woman's new responsibility at home will tax her energies enough. She does not need the additional burden of an undetected low hemoglobin level.

VITAL SIGNS

Temperature

Temperatures are always taken orally during the puerperium because of the danger of vaginal contamination and the discomfort involved in rectal intrusion.

The woman may show a slight increase in temperature the first 24 hours of the puerperium because of the period of hydration she underwent during labor. If she receives adequate fluid during the first 24 hours, the temperature will be reduced and should be normal thereafter. As stated, most women are thirsty immediately after delivery and so are eager to drink. Drinking a large quantity of fluid is not a problem unless the woman is nauseated from a delivery anesthetic.

Any woman whose oral temperature rises above 38°C (100.4°F), excluding the first 24-hour period, is considered by criteria of the Joint Commission on Maternal Welfare to be febrile, and a postpartal infection should be suspected.

Occasionally, on the third or fourth day post partum, when milk "comes in," the woman's temperature rises for a period of hours because of the increased vascular activity involved in engorgement. This is sometimes referred to as *milk fever*. However, if the elevation in temperature lasts more than a few hours, infection is a much more likely reason for the fever.

Infection is a major cause of postpartal mortality and morbidity. Any rise in maternal temperature must be considered serious and suspect until proved otherwise.

Pulse

The pulse rate during the postpartal period is generally slightly lower than normal. The decline is due to the increased amount of blood that returns to the circulatory system following delivery of the placenta. This increased volume raises blood pressure. The slowing of the heart is a compensatory mechanism to decrease the pressure in the circulatory system. The pulse rate is reduced to between 60 and 70. As diuresis diminishes, the blood volume and blood pressure drop, and the pulse rate increases accordingly. By the end of the first week, the pulse rate has returned to normal.

Pulse rate should be evaluated carefully in the postpartal period. A rapid and thready pulse, for example, is a possible sign of hemorrhage. Be certain that you are comparing the woman's pulse rate with the normal range in the postpartal period, not with the normal pulse rates in the general population; otherwise, you may misinterpret the finding.

Blood Pressure

Blood pressure should also be monitored during the postpartal period because of the information it gives in regard to the presence of bleeding. A blood pressure reading should be compared with the woman's predelivery level rather than the standard blood pressures, since these vary with the age of the woman.

If the reading is above 140 mm Hg systolic or 90 mm Hg diastolic, it may indicate the development of postpartal pregnancy-induced hypertension, an unusual but serious complication of the puerperium (see Chap. 36).

EXHAUSTION

As soon as delivery is completed, the woman experiences a sense of complete exhaustion. During the later months of pregnancy, worried that she might sleep through labor and have the baby at home, she did not sleep soundly. She was unable to find a comfortable position in bed because of the fetus's activity or the presence of back or leg pain. All during labor she ate nothing and worked very hard, with little or no sleep.

She now has sleep hunger. Sleep hunger makes it difficult for her to cope with new experiences and stand stress situations. It probably adds to the development of postpartal depression.

Progressive Changes

Two physiological changes during the puerperium involve progressive changes or the building of new tissue. For this reason, strict dieting that limits cell-building ability is contraindicated in the first six weeks following childbirth.

LACTATION

The formation of breast milk (lactation) will be initiated in a mother whether or not she plans to breast-feed.

For the first two days post partum the average woman notices little change in her breasts from the way they were during pregnancy (see Chap. 14). Since midway through pregnancy, she has been secreting colostrum, the thin, watery prelactation secretion. She continues to excrete this fluid the first two

Physiology of the Postpartal Period

days post partum. On the third day, her breasts tend to become full and feel tense or tender as milk forms within breast ducts.

Breast milk forms as a result of the fall in estrogen and progesterone levels that follows delivery of the placenta. When the production of milk begins, a great deal of distention tends to occur in the milk ducts. The woman experiences this distention as a feeling of heat or a throbbing breast pain. Breast tissue may appear reddened, its appearance simulating that of an acute inflammatory or infectious process. The distention is not limited to the milk ducts but occurs in the surrounding tissue as well, since blood and lymph enter the area to contribute fluid to the formation of milk. The feeling of tension in the breasts on the third or fourth day post partum is termed *engorgement*, and, although painful, is a welcome sign that breast milk production is starting. Care of breasts post partum and breast-feeding are discussed in Chap. 30.

RETURN OF MENSTRUAL FLOW

If the woman is not breast-feeding, she can expect her menstrual flow to return within eight weeks after delivery. If she is breast-feeding, menstrual flow may not return for three or four months, or, in some women, for the entire lactation period. However, the absence of a menstrual flow does not guarantee that the woman will not conceive during this time. She may be ovulating, with the absence of menstruation being the body's way of conserving fluid.

References

1. Aspy, V. H., et al. Considering patient-centered obstetric nursing care: Why and how? *J.O.G.N. Nurs.* 8:297, 1979.
2. Chiota, B. J., et al. Effects of separation from spouse on pregnancy, labor and delivery and the post partum period. *J.O.G.N. Nurs.* 5:21, 1976.
3. Levine, N. H. A conceptual model for obstetrical nursing. *J.O.G.N. Nurs.* 5:9, 1976.
4. Mehl, L. E. Outcomes of early discharge after normal birth. *Birth Fam. J.* 3:101, 1976.
5. Pritchard, J., and McDonald, P. *Williams Obstetrics* (15th ed.). New York: Appleton-Century-Crofts, 1976.
6. Richardson, A. C., et al. Decreasing post partum sexual abstinence time. *Am. J. Obstet. Gynecol.* 126:416, 1976.
7. Sciarra, J. J. *Gynecology and Obstetrics*. New York: Harper & Row, 1978.
8. Tyson, J. E. Mechanics of puerperal lactation. *Med. Clin. North Am.* 61:153, 1977.
9. Wheeler, L. A. A concept of maternity care. *J.O.G.N. Nurs.* 5:15, 1976.

26. The Postpartal Experience: Nursing Interventions

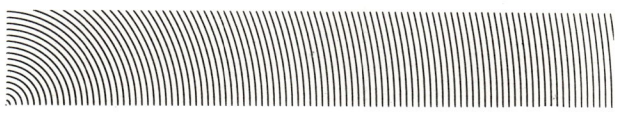

Nursing interventions in the postpartal period are always concerned with two major goals: aiding the physiological changes of the period to occur as spontaneously as possible, and helping strengthen mother-child or parent-child bonding.

Immediate Postpartal Care

Care during the first hour post partum must be done with extreme conscientiousness as the uterus is so prone to hemorrhage at this point. One of the worries with couples delivering at home is that they will not appreciate how dangerous a time this is for the mother and that attention will be focused on the newborn, not on the woman, and postpartal hemorrhage will occur.

REST

After delivery a woman is a paradox. She is excited. She has a baby, something almost impossible to believe, and she wants to hold and be with this new person in her life. She wants to talk to her husband about the experience, their child, their future. At the same time she is exhausted.

This first wish of hers, to have a few minutes with her expanded family, should be granted as soon as possible, ideally in the delivery room immediately after the baby's birth. If the father does not watch the birth, time should be allowed for mother, father, and baby to be together as soon as the mother is taken to the recovery room. The policy in some hospitals is to send the child immediately to a nursery ("infection control," "routine," just "the way things are done"), and this first moment when the family would have a chance to be together is forever lost. Lost with it is a long-to-be-remembered time of pride, fulfillment, and family sharing.

Following a first get-acquainted meeting with the infant, when the mother has a chance to count her child's fingers and toes, she should be encouraged to sleep. All the procedures that must be carried out with the newly delivered mother (blood pressure, pulse, checking of fundal height, and perineal inspection) should be done swiftly and gently, to allow her as much sleep as possible. If she has discomfort from hemorrhoids, perineal stitches, or afterpains, she needs the cause of the discomfort addressed so that she can sleep.

Some women experience a shaking chill immediately after delivery, either as they are being moved from the delivery table or in the recovery room. This is probably due in part to a combination of the exhaustion and the exhilaration they are feeling. In part, it may also be an effect of the pressure changes in the abdomen that occur with reduction in the bulk of the uterus, or of temperature readjustment following the excessive sweating of labor. In any event, shaking chills at this point are commonplace, and the woman needs to be reassured or she may attribute them to a developing cold or infection.

Covering the woman with a warm blanket, offering her a warm drink if she is not nauseated from an anesthetic, and assuring her that the occurrence is a normal one is usually enough to make the chill transient and allow her to fall into a sound, much-needed sleep. Most women will then sleep for at least an hour.

Although she may choose any position to sleep in, the woman will enjoy being able to sleep on her stomach as she has not been able to do during pregnancy. The woman who has had a general anesthetic will sleep soundly from the effect of the anesthetic for an hour or more. Because her gag reflex will not be functional until the bulk of the effect of the anesthetic is "blown off," she should be positioned on her side or on her abdomen so saliva will drain from her mouth and she will not aspirate.

Be certain that the woman who had spinal anesthesia does not sit up for the entire first 8 hours. Sitting up following spinal anesthetics causes tension on the meninges and "spinal headache," an intense, boring type of headache that leaves her incapacitated at a time she wants to feel her best so as to care for her new child.

There are many things that generally need to be taught in the postpartal period about self-care and baby care. During the first hour, however, learning these things is not as important as the need to sleep. Sleep hunger blocks out the ability to learn effectively, and teaching done at this time will have to be repeated later.

UTERINE ASSESSMENT

For the first hour after delivery, the height of the woman's fundus and its consistency should be determined by palpation at least every 15 minutes. If the woman received no oxytocic agent following delivery to help her uterus contract, someone should sit with one hand resting on the woman's abdomen, ready to assist the fundus to contract if it should become soft or relaxed during this important first hour.

Because the uterus is a sensitive organ, gentle massage of the fundus usually causes it to contract immediately and become firm to the touch. Massage is a gentle rotating motion of the hand. It is good practice always to place one hand just above the symphysis pubis before massaging with the other hand in order to give adequate support to the uterus (Fig. 26-1). Massage should never be hard or forceful, lest it be painful to the mother and cause the uterus to expend excess energy. A uterus that contracts too forcefully can become fatigued and subsequently unable to maintain contraction; the result will be uterine hemorrhage.

If massage does not seem to be effective in causing the uterus to contract, there may be a clot in the cavity of the uterus. The clot may be expressed from the uterus by gentle pressure on the fundus, *but only after the uterus has been massaged.* If the uterus is totally relaxed, the pressure may cause inversion of the uterus, an extremely serious complication that leads to rapid hemorrhage and may necessitate an emergency hysterectomy to save the woman's life.

Checking for uterine contraction is a painless procedure for the woman, takes only a moment of your time, and is of prime importance in ascertaining whether the uterus is involuting properly.

Fig. 26-1. The nurse supports the bottom of the uterus with her left hand and palpates the fundus of the uterus with her right hand. This fundus is about four fingerbreadths below the umbilicus. Note the striae gravidarum on the mother's abdomen. (Courtesy of the Department of Medical Photography, Children's Hospital, Buffalo, N.Y.)

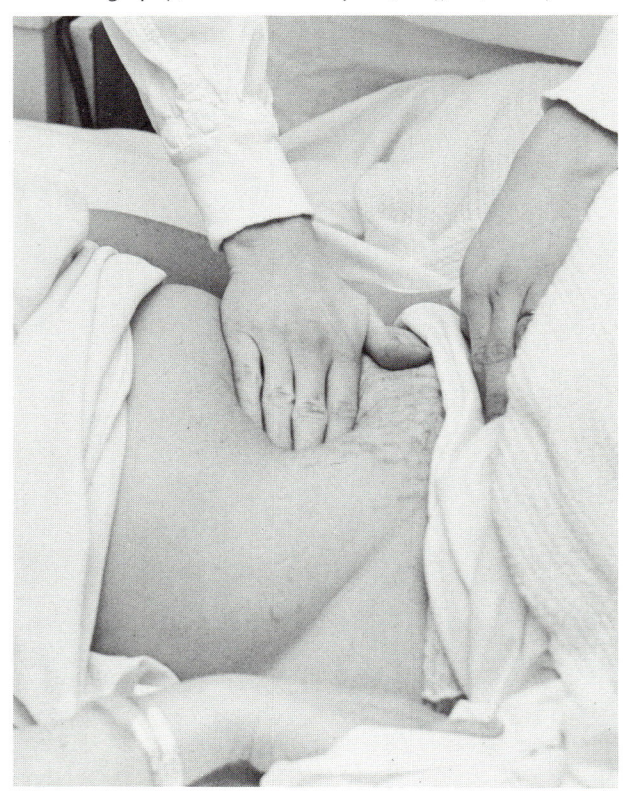

LOCHIA ASSESSMENT

A woman can expect to have a vaginal discharge (lochia) following childbirth for two to six weeks. Characteristics of normal lochia and the change in pattern from red to pink to white are described in Table 25-1.

During the first hour post partum, when the fundus is checked for contraction every 15 minutes, the mother's perineal pad should be removed and the character, amount, and color of the lochia discharge evaluated. In the first hour it will be *lochia rubra*; it may contain small clots. Whether the amount of lochia is normal or not is evaluated against the amount the woman has during a normal menstrual flow. Ask her how often during a normal menstrual flow she changes pads or tampons.

Be certain that you turn the woman and check under her buttocks in order not to miss bleeding that may be pooling below her. If you observe a constant trickle of vaginal flow or the woman is soaking through a pad every 15 minutes, she is losing more than the average amount of blood. She needs to be checked by a physician to be certain that there is no cervical or vaginal tear.

PERINEAL ASSESSMENT

At the time that lochia is evaluated (every 15 minutes for the first hour) the perineum should be inspected. Are any hematomas (blood-filled protruding spheres) forming because surface capillaries were broken? Do the stitches in a suture line appear secure? Applying an ice-bag to the suture line reduces edema and pain and promotes healing and comfort. Many physicians order a soothing analgesic cream or spray to be applied to the suture line. A cortisone-base cream, which helps to decrease inflammation in the area and therefore to decrease tension, is also helpful. Witch hazel preparations, because of their cooling effect, are a mainstay for relief of episiotomy line discomfort.

VITAL SIGNS

Assessment of vital signs may supply the evidence that a woman is bleeding more profusely than desired because of the correlation between changing blood pressure (decreasing) and pulse (increasing) recordings with bleeding. During the first hour post partum, both pulse and blood pressure should be taken and evaluated every 15 minutes.

BLADDER ASSESSMENT

Since the diuresis of the postpartal period begins almost immediately after delivery, the woman's bladder begins filling almost immediately. A full bladder puts pressure on the uterus and may interfere with effective uterine contraction. An overdistended bladder may cause damage to bladder function.

Offer a bedpan at the end of the first hour. Many women still have enough residual effect of epidural, spinal, or pudendal anesthesia at this time so that voiding is painless (later, when the anesthesia has worn off, the acid urine against episiotomy sutures may sting). Other women have too much perineal edema to be able to void this early.

If the woman's bladder is distended, she will need to be catheterized if unable to void at the end of the first hour. Most women, however, do not have this much filling at this time. They must void within 4 to 8 hours after birth, however, or bladder distention will surely have occurred.

BREAST ASSESSMENT

For the first two days post partum, women generally notice little change in breast tissue except perhaps a slight tingling sensation. Palpate the woman's breasts at the end of the first hour post partum as a baseline determination for softness against which later assessments can be compared. During this time breast tissue should feel soft; it may feel slightly tender to the woman.

Suppression of Lactation

If the woman is not going to breast-feed, some intervention to stop the formation of breast milk is helpful in order to increase her comfort on the third or fourth day post partum, when *engorgement* or the first breast milk production takes place.

Breast milk forms in mammary glands stimulated by the pituitary hormone prolactin. Administering either an estrogen or an androgen or both in combination to the woman soon after delivery will prevent prolactin from being produced. Diethylstilbestrol, an estrogenic hormone, or chlorotrianisene (TACE), a synthetic estrogen, is often prescribed for this purpose. Deladumone, which contains testosterone enanthate and estradiol valerate in combination, is an example of a commonly used androgen-containing drug.

To be effective, these lactation-suppressing agents must be started immediately after delivery, usually in the delivery or recovery room or the first hour post partum. They are extremely effective in suppressing lactation but do have some side effects. Women on estrogen compounds may tend to have increased uterine bleeding. Estrogen compounds should be used with caution in women susceptible to thromboembolism (presence of varicosities or family history of thromboembolism) as estrogen tends to lead to increased blood clotting. Androgen compounds are likely to retard menstruation, so a woman who has received one of these drugs should be informed that her first menstrual flow may be delayed more than the normal six or eight weeks after delivery.

MOTHER-CHILD INTERACTION ASSESSMENT

If a woman did not have the opportunity to see her newborn in the delivery room because of a general anesthetic, she should see her infant as soon as she wakes from anesthesia. Having to wait until all babies are brought to mothers is unreasonable. While she waits, she imagines there is something wrong with her baby or why can't she see him? Or what is wrong with the people who work in this hospital that they cannot appreciate her need to see her baby!

Listen to what women say about their newborns in this immediate postpartal period. Do they make positive statements ("I'm glad he's a boy") or negative ones ("I really hoped it would be a girl")? "She's cute" or "She looks like a circus clown with no hair"? First impressions may not be lasting ones, but unless negative comments are identified, so that extra discussion about things such as what it feels like to have four boys can take place, the woman will be discharged with her needs unmet. At home, away from health personnel who are attuned to how disappointment can interfere with mother-child interaction, she may have great difficulty adjusting to and relating to this new child.

Most women appreciate a bath at the end of their initial rest period. They enjoy being ministered to early in their taking-in phase and talking to a nurse about their labor and delivery experience. They enjoy having a nurse with them to serve as a sounding board, a point of reality to use to secure wondering thoughts such as, "I can't believe it's really over. I can't believe the baby's really born."

Following a bath and perineal care the woman can be transferred to a postpartal room. The most dangerous hour for her in childbearing is past.

A timetable for nursing interventions in the first hour post partum is shown in Table 26-1.

Continued Interventions During Hospital Stay

Before World War II, most women stayed in the hospital for 10 or 14 days following childbirth; they expected to rest with little exertion for the first month at home. Changes in postpartal care took place during the war; women then typically stayed only three or four days. Today, with many women giving birth without the use of anesthetics, hospital stays are routinely becoming as short as 24 hours.

Table 26-1. Timetable for Nursing Interventions, First Hour Post Partum

Intervention	Timing
Evaluate fundal height and consistency	q15min
Evaluate color and amount of lochia	q15min
Assess perineum for hematoma or stressed suture line	q15min
Assess bladder distention	At end of hour
Ask woman to void	At end of hour
Take pulse and blood pressure	q15min
Assess breasts	At end of hour
Check to see if lactation suppressant is desired	During first hour
Observe mother-child (parent-child) interaction	At each encounter
Give bath, first perineal care	At end of hour

When hospital stays were long, the nursing role during this time centered around administering care. Now that hospital stays are so much shorter, nursing care centers around *teaching* care. The woman must know how to care for herself to prevent introducing infection to her yet unhealed uterus or suture line. She must be aware of danger signs to look for and know whom to call if she notices any of them. She must understand safe baby care. Every contact with a woman includes some teaching information, therefore, in order to squeeze it all in. At the same time, learning does not take place if a learner is overwhelmed and hurried. Common sense is necessary to determine when it is a time to teach and when it is a time to observe or listen. Observation of mother-child interaction and evaluation of the woman's support system at home are the basis for much of the teaching.

UTERINE ASSESSMENT

Following the first hour after delivery, the uterus may be evaluated for height and consistency less frequently: every hour for the next 8 hours, then once each nursing shift. If a woman is going home before three days, she should be taught to make this assessment herself. Always stress that she put one hand on the lower uterine segment for support before she massages the fundus. By the ninth or tenth day post partum the uterus will have become so small that she will no longer be able to palpate it above the symphysis pubis.

Afterpains

Uterine contractions may cause uterine cramps similar to those accompanying menstrual flows in some women. They are particularly likely to occur in multiparas or women who have had large babies. They almost always occur with breast-feeding as the oxytocin released from the pituitary with breast-feeding increases the firmness of uterine contractions.

Women need to understand that this discomfort is normal and rarely lasts more than three days. If necessary, an analgesic can be prescribed for relief. As with any abdominal pain, heat should never be placed on the abdomen. It may cause relaxation of the uterus and consequent uterine bleeding.

LOCHIA ASSESSMENT

Women should be encouraged to change perineal pads frequently as they begin self-care. Lochia is a medium for bacterial growth, and constantly wet pads against a suture line slow healing.

Be certain that the woman who will be discharged early knows the criteria against which to judge the type and amount of lochia (see Table 25-1).

When she is in the hospital, you need to inspect her lochia discharge once every hour for the first 8 hours, then every 8 hours. Make sure she understands that she must wash her hands after handling pads and must use only her own individual care equipment so that she does not contract or spread infection. Demonstrate good role modeling yourself in terms of hand-washing and equipment use.

PERINEAL ASSESSMENT

A woman who is going to be discharged early and who has perineal sutures should be taught how to lie on her back and view her perineum with a hand-held mirror. Once a day for the next seven days she should inspect for redness or sloughing of sutures or formation of pus at the suture line.

While she is in the hospital you should check her perineum once every 8 hours, examining for any sign of infection or poor healing at a suture line. Ice to the perineum after the first hour is no longer therapeutic, and healing after the first hour takes place faster if blood is encouraged to enter the area through the use of heat, not cold, application.

Perineal Care

In addition to measures to alleviate perineal discomfort, every woman needs attention to perineal cleanliness in the postpartal period. Because the vagina lies in close proximity to the rectum, there is always a danger that bacteria will spread from the rectum to the vagina and cause infection. Lochia allowed to dry and harden on the vulva and perineum furnishes a bed for bacterial growth. Perineal care is thus necessary to prevent infection, but it also promotes healing and provides comfort.

Perineal care should be undertaken as a part of the daily bath and after each voiding or bowel movement or as often as the woman wishes for comfort. While she is on bed rest during her first hours after delivery, you will need to provide the perineal care. As soon as the woman is ambulatory, she can be instructed to carry it out herself.

Perineal care formerly was a sterile procedure, involving sterile gloves, sterile water, and sterile compresses—a complicated business for women to undertake. Most institutions now require only *clean* technique. Women can understand clean technique and can carry it out very well after a minimum of instruction.

Hospitals differ as to the type of cleansing that is done and the articles and solutions used. The solutions may range from warm tap water, which is poured over the vulva from a pitcher or spray can, to soap and water or a mild antiseptic solution applied to the perineum by gauze sponges or disposable washcloths. Cotton balls should not be used for washing the perineum because they stick to the stubble of shaved pubic hair and leave particles behind to invite lochia buildup.

Before beginning perineal care, wash your own hands. More postpartal infection is probably caused and spread by the unclean hands of caregivers than by unclean equipment. With the woman lying in a supine position in bed, remove the perineal pad from the front to back; the direction is important in preventing the portion of the pad that has touched the rectal area from sliding forward to the vaginal opening. A plastic-covered pad should be placed under the woman's buttocks to protect the bed during the procedure.

If actual washing is to be done, use a clean gauze square or a clean portion of the washcloth for each stroke, always washing from front to back, from the pubis toward the rectum. Rinse the area in the same manner and dry.

Be careful that none of the solution enters the vagina, since it might be a source of contamination. The labia normally have a tendency to close and cover the vaginal opening. This will prevent solution from entering if you do not separate the labia but allow them to perform their protective function. If the solution is to be poured or sprayed, with the woman lying on her back the flow will naturally be from front to back because of gravity. Again, the labia should not be separated or the solution will enter the vagina.

The entire perineum is tender, so your touch must be gentle or you will cause pain. Inspect the perineum to detect any stitches that are pulling out or any area that appears inflamed or exceptionally tense (beginning signs of suture-line infection). It may be advantageous to have the woman turn on her side in a Sims's position, so that you fully view the episiotomy area; in some women, better cleansing of the episiotomy area can be done in this position also.

If any cream for the episiotomy area has been ordered, it should be applied after the area has been dried. In unwrapping a new perineal pad to apply it, be careful that you do not grasp the portion of the pad that will touch the perineum; hold it by the bottom side or the ends. In applying the pad, first pin the front side and then the back, so that if it pulls with pinning, a clean part of the pad will lie over a bacteria-prone area, and the part that touched the rectal area will not lie over the vagina. Whether you are unpinning or pinning a perineal pad, the rule is the same: *front first*.

Perineal Self-Care

As soon as the woman is allowed to get up to go to the bathroom (in some health care facilities this may be as early as 1 hour after delivery), she should be instructed how to carry out her own perineal care.

The bathroom of a postpartal room should have a stand or a shelf close to the toilet where the woman can place the equipment she needs for care: the pitcher or basin of solution; the sponges or washcloths; her clean pad; and so forth. She needs instructions on how to remove the soiled perineal pad, where to dispose of it, and how to apply a clean pad. She needs to be told always to work from front to back and to be reminded of the importance of using any cream or medication that has been prescribed. She should be warned not to flush the toilet until she is standing upright; otherwise, the flushing water may spray the perineum.

A woman usually prefers to do her own perineal care. If she is given simple explanations as to why it is important to do it carefully, she usually does it well. However, self-care does not free you from your responsibility of checking the woman's perineum and ascertaining whether or not the suture line is healing and the lochia flow is normal as long as she remains in the hospital. By continuing with these procedures, you remain the woman's first line of defense against postpartal complications.

Episiotomy Care

Episiotomy, the incision of the perineum made at the end of the second stage of labor to avoid laceration of the perineum, is being used more and more as a routine delivery procedure. You can expect many postpartal mothers to have perineal stitches at an episiotomy site. This area is usually 1 or 2 inches long, but if a laceration was involved, the stitches may extend from the vagina back to the rectum. Rarely, they extend forward toward the urethra.

It is easy to inspect an episiotomy incision and think that because of its minimal size it should not cause much discomfort to the mother. However, the perineum is an extremely tender area, and the muscles of the area are involved in many activities (sitting, walking, stooping, squatting, bending, urinating, defecating). Thus, an incision in the area causes a great deal of discomfort.

Most women are not forewarned about the tugging sharpness perineal stitches cause. Women expect the pain of labor to be excruciating and are usually pleasantly surprised to find that it is not nearly so bad as they feared. However, they usually do not expect to have this unexplained pulling pain in the postpartal period. They are distracted by it when they want to pay attention to you talking about baby care. It interferes with their rest and sleep, with eating, and with being able to sit and hold the baby comfortably.

Do not underestimate the physical discomfort experienced by women following episiotomy and make every effort to alleviate this discomfort. Despite the greater frankness today, many women are embarrassed to discuss pain in this part of the body even with nurses. Unless you are alert and observant enough to mention the problem, some women may prefer to put up with the discomfort rather than to point it out themselves.

The woman needs an explanation that this discomfort is normal and fortunately does not usually last more than five or six days, since the perineal area heals rapidly. A woman may worry about additional discomfort when, as she supposes, the episiotomy sutures are removed. Explain to her that episiotomy sutures do not need to be removed; they are made of an absorbable material and are absorbed within 10 days.

Perineal Comfort

MEDICATIONS. Most women require an analgesic to relieve their perineal discomfort. Be certain the woman understands how to use any cream or suture-line spray ordered for her. Some women doubt the efficiency of suture-line medications or worry that applying the cream will hurt more than not applying it, so do not use these helpful aids unless urged to give them a trial.

PERINEAL EXERCISES. Some women find that carrying out a perineal exercise three or four times a day greatly relieves their discomfort. The exercise consists in contracting and relaxing the muscles of the perineum five times in succession as if trying to stop a voiding (Kegal's exercise). This improves circulation to the area and so helps decrease edema. It is only one of a number of postpartal exercises that can help the woman regain her prepregnant muscle tone and form. Others will be discussed later.

Because a normal sitting position stretches the perineal muscles, the woman needs to learn to sit a little differently until the perineum is healed. Before attempting to sit, she should squeeze her buttocks together and sit with them in that position. This seems like a small matter, but it can be most helpful to the mother who is attending classes in formula making or infant bathing and wants to pay attention to the instructor and not be distracted by the physical discomfort of sitting.

HEAT LAMPS. Exposing the perineum to dry heat in the form of a perineal heat lamp is another means of increasing circulation to the area and thereby reducing edema, promoting healing, and providing comfort. The woman lies in a supine position in bed with her legs spread in a lithotomy position to expose the perineum. A heat lamp is placed on a clean sheet on her bed. It is positioned between her legs, about 12 inches from the perineum. She should then be covered by a draw sheet or a bath blanket during the procedure so that she will not remain exposed.

The heat lamp should be left in place for 20 minutes and then removed. If it is left in place any longer, the woman will feel discomfort because of her position, and a heat burn of the healing tissue may occur. After the procedure, which may be repeated three or four times a day, to prevent the possible spread of infection, the washable parts of the lamp should be wiped with an appropriate antiseptic solution before it is returned to a storage area or used with another patient.

SITZ BATHS. A sitz bath is a small portable basin that fits on a toilet seat with water constantly swirling in it. The movement of water is soothing to healing tissue, decreases inflammation, and therefore is effective in reducing discomfort.

Be certain that the water in the sitz bath is not too hot before you help the woman to use it. The woman herself will not be sensitive to the temperature because healing surfaces are not good indicators of heat and cold. This caution applies particularly to the woman who is using an analgesic cream or spray on the perineum or has a great deal of generalized perineal edema. Both these situations make her very prone to burns from scalding water unless you act to protect her.

Like a heat lamp treatment, a sitz bath should not last more than 20 minutes and may be repeated three or four times a day. Because of the soothing effect of the warm water and the sitting position, the woman may feel extremely tired and unsteady on her feet after using a sitz bath and may need help in getting back to bed.

K-PADS. K-pads are yet another means of bringing soothing warmth to the perineal area. These are rubber pads similar in appearance to hot-water bottles except that they are long and narrow, shaped to conform to the perineal area. The K-pad is attached to a pump that circulates warm water through it in much the same way as water circulates in a hypothermia blanket. You must be familiar with the instructions that come with the pump before you attempt to use it or the temperature of the circulating water can become too hot. To prevent chafing, the rubber pad should be covered by gauze or linen before being placed on the perineum. As with other heat treatments, 20 minutes achieves the desired effect, and the treatment should then be discontinued. Few hospitals have enough K-pads for each woman to have her own; therefore, the pad should be washed with an antiseptic solution after each use and before another patient uses it, as with all other postpartal equipment.

BREAST ASSESSMENT

During pregnancy, estrogen and progesterone stimulate mammary glands to grow and begin a secretory function (formation of colostrum). With delivery of the placenta and the sudden reduction of the level of body progesterone, *prolactin,* a pituitary hormone, increases and initiates the production of breast milk. Whether women are going to breast-feed or not, when the placenta is delivered the events that will lead to milk production begin unless a milk suppressant was given.

For the first two days post partum, women generally notice a slight tingling sensation in their breasts. Colostrum secretion is present. On the third day, breasts become full and feel tense and strained as breast milk forms in breast ducts. They may appear reddened as if an acute inflammatory or infectious process were beginning. The woman may experience a sensation of heat or pain from the influx of blood and lymph into the area to contribute fluid to the formation of milk.

Breast tissue feels soft on palpation the first and second day; on the third day, it feels hard and warm to your hand. This change in breast consistency is termed *engorgement*. Although painful, it is a welcome announcement that breast milk is forming.

Breast Care

If the woman is breast-feeding, the sucking of the infant is the main treatment for relief of the tenderness and soreness of primary engorgement. (The techniques of breast-feeding are discussed in Chap. 30.) In addition, the woman may need a firm supporting bra to eliminate tugging sensations and possibly synthetic oxytocic (Syntocinon) nasal spray used just prior to breast-feeding. The nasal spray is absorbed across the mucous membrane of the nose and helps bring milk forward in the breast ducts, reducing engorgement. She may find the application of hot or cold compresses beneficial. An analgesic is usually also helpful. The woman who is breast-feeding needs reassurance that primary engorgement is a normal finding three or four days after delivery, so that she does not view it as a result of something she is doing wrong with breast-feeding. Engorgement with breast-feeding lasts about 24 hours.

The woman who is not breast-feeding experiences similar discomfort. However, when little or no milk is removed from the breasts, the accumulation of milk inhibits further milk formation, and so engorgement will subside in about two days. Hot or cold compresses applied to the breasts three or four times a day during the period of engorgement, or an analgesic, provide relief. There are old wives' tales that restriction of fluid, tight binding, and pumping milk from the breasts aid in relieving discomfort. None of these things are truly effective, and all are to some degree harmful and so should be avoided.

Breast Hygiene

Further breast care during the postpartal period is directed toward cleanliness and support. These are basically the same whether or not the woman is breast-feeding.

The woman should wash her breasts daily at the time of her bath or shower. If she is breast-feeding, she should not use soap, since soap tends to dry and crack nipples and may lead to fissures and possible breast abscess. It is not necessary for women to wash their breasts more often than this even if they are breast-feeding. Excessive washing means unnecessary manipulation, making the process of breast-feeding more complicated than it should be.

To wash her breasts, a woman should never use cleaning products like those that come individually wrapped in foil packets. These products invariably have an alcohol base and are extremely drying to nipples.

Breast Support

A woman should wear some type of breast support for at least the first week after delivery. Breast-feeding women need breast support throughout the period of lactation. As lactation begins, the breasts increase in weight and feel heavy. Good support offers a degree of relief from the resultant pulling sensation and prevents unnecessary strain on the supporting muscles of the breasts, preserving muscle tone. A good support also positions the breasts in good alignment and diminishes the amount of engorgement caused by blocked milk ducts. Support is provided best by a bra. It should give both support and uplift for best alignment. If the woman has not packed one in her suitcase, she can usually arrange to have one brought from home.

A woman who has a considerable discharge of colostrum or milk from her breasts (breast-feeding or not) should insert clean gauze squares in her bra to absorb the moisture. These should be changed as often as necessary to keep the nipples dry. If nipples remain wet for any length of time, fissures may form and lead to infection.

Some women find that a breast binder makes them comfortable, although more and more women are reacting negatively to the bulkiness of this device. A breast binder is simply a straight binder brought around the chest and pinned from the bottom up to ensure uplift. A binder rarely gives the uplift of a good bra, however, and if engorgement is marked, it becomes very tight, and eventually wrinkled and uncomfortable.

Breast Self-Examination

All women should know how to examine their breasts in order that they can check them routinely for signs of breast carcinoma. This procedure can be taught during pregnancy, but many women are not interested in hearing about cancer preventive measures at that time—the possibility of their developing cancer seems far removed from what they are doing during pregnancy: creating life. In the postpartal period they are very conscious that they must remain well in order to raise this new child to maturity. They are receptive to having you review with them or teach them for the first time the technique for breast self-examination.

A week after her menstrual period is the best time of the month for breast self-examination. During a menstrual period or just prior to it, breasts may be tender and the examination uncomfortable. The woman who is breast-feeding may not have a menstrual flow for three or four months. She should pick a day, say the first day of every month, to do the examination until menstrual flow "markers" return.

The first thing she does is stand in front of a mirror and, with her arms at her sides, inspect her breasts for any swelling, dimpling, or change in breast or nipple contour. Many women have asymmetrical breasts (one larger than the other) and they can be assured they are normal and typical. Next she raises her arms over her head and inspects her breasts the same way. Then she places the palms of her hands on her hips and presses in firmly so her chest muscles flex. She inspects again for dimpling, swelling, or any indication of a protruding lump.

She then lies down and places a folded towel under her right shoulder. She puts her right hand under her head. These two measures distribute, or thin out, breast tissue on that side and make any finding in the breast more noticeable. With her left hand, fingers flat, she presses gently in a circular motion around the periphery of her right breast. It is easiest for her to remember to cover all of the breast if she thinks of it as a clock face and begins at 12 o'clock and works her way around past 3, past 6, and so forth, back to 12. She then performs the same motion at about an inch from the periphery of the breast and next does the same with the nipple area. Lastly, she squeezes the nipple to see whether there is any discharge. She repeats the procedure on the left side.

Caution women that they have a rim of supportive tissue in the lower half of each breast so they do not think they are feeling something abnormal when they discover this. If they are very slim, they may be able to palpate ribs through the breast tissue. These also are normal structures. The breast-feeding woman will, of course, have a milk discharge when she squeezes the nipples. She may occasionally discover a distended milk gland that feels very much like a cyst or tumor. She should not worry about such lumps unless they persist beyond two breast-feedings.

Remind women that if they do find a lump or have nipple discharge in their breast by self-examination they should telephone their doctor about the finding but should not worry. Most lumps found in breasts are benign. Many women do not examine their breasts because they are afraid they will find something; other women find something but are then afraid to tell anyone about it. Breast carcinoma discovered early and treated promptly has an excellent cure rate. "Ostrich philosophy" or "what you don't know won't hurt you," leaves the woman with little chance at all.

BLADDER ASSESSMENT

Many women need help to accomplish voiding in the first few hours after delivery. Like all patients, they have difficulty using bedpans. The position of the bedpan makes their perineal stitches hurt and, combined with the awkwardness of using a bedpan, renders voiding impossible. Better results are obtained by helping the mother up to a bedside commode or to a nearby bathroom. You can be of further assistance by providing privacy (but remaining in close proximity, since the woman may become dizzy if this is her first time out of bed), running water at the sink, or offering the woman a drink of water. Pouring warm tap water over the vulva, if that is consistent with the hospital's policy of perineal care, may also help.

If these methods do not induce the woman to void, the physician may order a medication such as bethanechol chloride (Urecholine) to aid bladder contraction and emptying. If the medication does not help, the physician will usually order catheterization.

Because the perineum is usually edematous following delivery, the vulva in postpartal women appears out of proportion, and it is usually difficult to locate the urinary urethra for catheterization. Be certain that in catheterization you do not invade the vagina by mistake and by so doing carry contamination to the denuded uterus.

Occasionally, because of poor tone, the bladder in some women retains large amounts of residual urine following voidings. This urine harbors bacteria, which may cause bladder infection. Also, permanent loss of bladder tone can result if the distended condition is allowed to persist for any length of time.

The first voiding after delivery should be measured to detect urinary retention. Measurement of voidings can be accomplished by having the woman void into a commode or into a bedpan placed on the toilet in the bathroom. The bedpan placed on the toilet in the bathroom this way is still a bedpan, but the situation gives the woman a feeling of normalcy and helps her to void more easily. Whether or not the bladder is emptying may also be judged by fundal height and position (a full bladder pushes the fundus up or to the side) or by palpating or percussing bladder prominence in the lower abdomen.

If the woman is voiding less than 100 ml at a time

or has a displaced uterus or a palpable bladder, the physician may order catheterization for residual urine following a voiding. If the voiding of residual urine is over 150 ml, the physician will probably want the catheter left in place for 12 to 24 hours to give the bladder time to regain its normal tone and to begin to function efficiently.

This is an example of why professional judgment is necessary in nursing. A woman may report that she is out of bed and using the bathroom to void. Only a person with knowledge of the extent of the diuresis being accomplished and the amount that should be voided during this time is able to estimate whether bladder function is adequate.

Fortunately, for most women who must be catheterized the procedure need be done only once following delivery. After another 6 to 8 hours have passed and the bladder has filled again, some of the perineal edema has subsided, the bladder has achieved better tone, and the woman is able to void by herself if helped to the bathroom.

Catheterization in the postpartal period should not be used indiscriminately. On the other hand, it should be done before the woman's bladder is decompensated or the uterus is displaced and uncontracted and bleeding results.

DIAPHORESIS AND COMFORT

Newly delivered women often complain that their hospital rooms are being kept too warm, and to prove it they point out how heavily they are perspiring. Postpartal rooms often *are* too warm because they are located close to the nurseries, but the profuse perspiration normally comes more from the body's attempt to regulate fluid than from the heat.

The woman needs to be reassured that sweating not only is a normal postpartal event but is helping to bring her body back to its prepregnant state. She should be cautioned against becoming chilled during this time and perhaps contracting an upper respiratory infection. If she has soaking sweats, particularly at night, she usually prefers a hospital gown to one of her own. She needs gown changes often to be comfortable.

ABDOMINAL WALL ASSESSMENT

Following childbirth, the abdominal wall and the uterine ligaments are stretched. The abdomen pouches forward. The woman may feel fat and unattractive.

Wearing an abdominal binder or a girdle may make her more comfortable during the first few weeks post partum but does not aid, and may actually hinder, the strengthening of the tone of the abdominal wall. If a scultetus binder is applied for comfort in the postpartal period, it should always be put on from the top down, so that it pushes the uterus down, not up, and uterine contraction is not hampered.

The woman can best help her abdominal wall to return to good tone by good body mechanics and posture, adequate rest, and prescribed exercises.

Constipation

Many women have difficulty moving their bowels during the first week of the puerperium, and in most instances this worries them more than is necessary. If they have had an enema with labor, there is little solid waste in their intestines to be evacuated for the first two or three days.

Constipation tends to occur because of the relaxed condition of the abdominal wall and the intestine now that it is no longer pushed by the bulky uterus. For a bowel movement, the abdominal wall must exert pressure; in its relaxed state, the pressure is not strong enough to be effective. Also, if hemorrhoids or perineal stitches are present, the woman may decline to try to move her bowels for fear of pain until she becomes constipated.

To prevent constipation, many physicians order a stool softener for their postpartal patients beginning with the first day after delivery. If the woman has not moved her bowels by the third day, a mild laxative or cathartic may be ordered for her. There is a danger in giving cathartics before the third day; the increase in intestinal activity may also cause increased activity in the uterus and lead to insufficient contraction.

Early ambulation, a good diet and adequate roughage, and an adequate fluid intake all aid in correcting the problem of constipation.

Hemorrhoids

The pressure of the fetal head on the rectal veins during delivery tends to aggravate hemorrhoids. Some women find that the discomfort from distended hemorrhoidal tissue is their chief discomfort in the first few days following delivery. The discomfort can be relieved by sitz baths, anesthetic sprays, and witch hazel preparations. Assuming a Sims's position several times a day aids in good venous return of the rectal area and also reduces discomfort.

POSTPARTAL EXERCISES

Exercises to strengthen the abdominal and pelvic muscles may be started with the physician's consent as early as the first day after delivery. The woman begins with easy exercises and gradually progresses to more difficult ones. She should continue these exercises until the end of the puerperium if she is to derive the maximum benefit from them.

Abdominal Breathing
Abdominal breathing may be started on the first day post partum, since it is a relatively easy exercise. Lying flat on her back, the woman should breathe slowly and deeply in and out five times, using her abdominal muscles. If she used this method of breathing as a labor exercise, she will be very familiar with it and will do it well. The woman who has never used it before needs some coaching to be certain she is using abdominal, not chest, muscles.

Chin to Chest
The chin-to-chest exercise is excellent for the second day. Lying on her back with no pillow, the woman raises her head and bends her chin forward on her chest without moving any other part of her body (Fig. 26-2). She should start this gradually, repeating it no more than five times the first time and then increasing to 10 or 15 times in succession. The exercise can be done three or four times a day. She will feel her abdominal muscles pull and tighten if she is doing it correctly.

Perineal Contraction
If the woman is not already using this exercise as a means of alleviating perineal discomfort, it is a good exercise to add on the third day. She should tighten and relax her perineal muscles five times in succession as if she were trying to stop voiding. She will feel her perineal muscles working if she is doing it correctly.

Fig. 26-2. Postpartal exercises: chin to chest. From a supine position (left) *the woman raises her chin and touches it to her chest* (right). *This exercise strengthens abdominal muscles.*

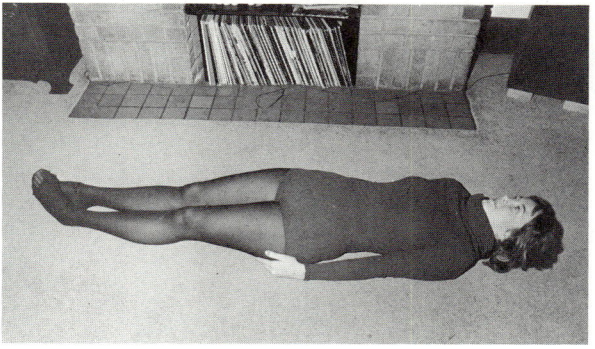
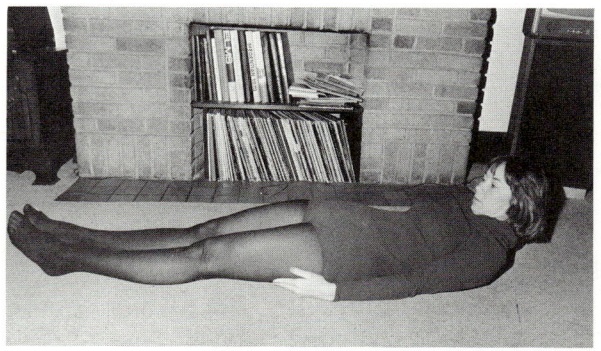

Arm Raising
Arm raising helps both the breasts and the abdomen return to good tone and is a good exercise to add on the fourth day. Lying on her back, arms at her sides, the woman moves them out from her sides until they are perpendicular to her body (Fig. 26-3). She then raises them over her body until her hands touch and lowers them slowly to her sides. She should rest a moment, then repeat the exercise five times.

Knee to Abdomen
The woman should wait until the perineum has healed, at least until the seventh day after delivery, before attempting the knee-to-abdomen exercise. Lying flat on her back, she bends one leg at a time at the knee and brings it up to touch her abdomen (Fig. 26-4). She lowers her foot to touch her buttock, straightens her leg, and lowers it. This exercise strengthens both abdominal and gluteal muscles.

Sit-ups
It is well to wait until the tenth or twelfth day after delivery before attempting sit-ups. Lying flat on her back, the woman folds her arms across her chest and raises herself to a sitting position, keeping her knees outstretched and unbent. This exercise expends a great deal of effort and tires a postpartal woman easily. She should be cautioned to begin it very gradually and work up slowly to doing it 10 times in a row.

Sleeping Position
All during the postpartal period, lying on the abdomen gives support to abdominal muscles and aids involution, since it tips the uterus into its natural forward position. Most women welcome being able to lie on their abdomens after so many months when they could not lie this way and are anxious to assume this position. If it puts too much pressure on sore breasts, a small pillow under the woman's stomach usually solves the problem.

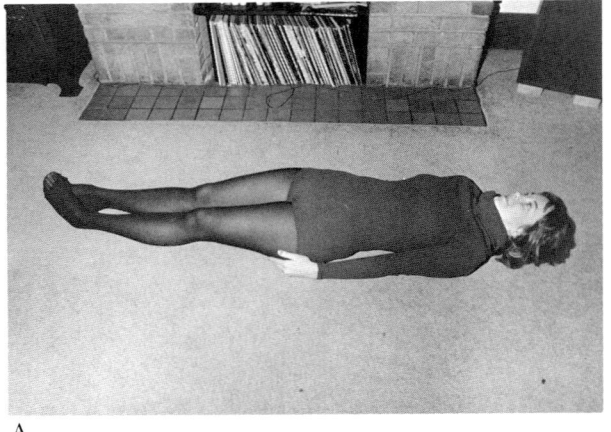
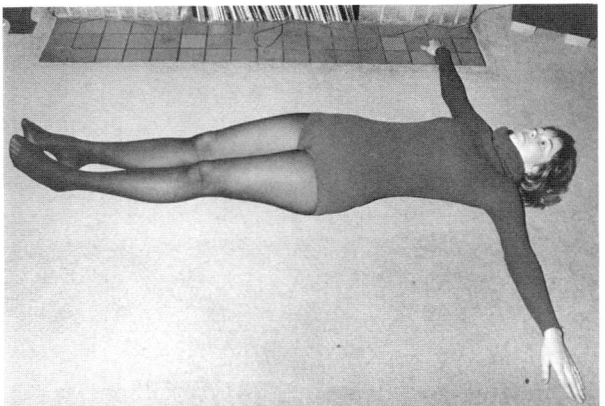
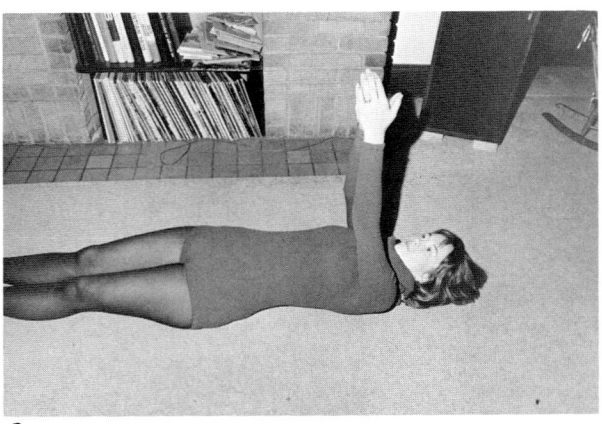
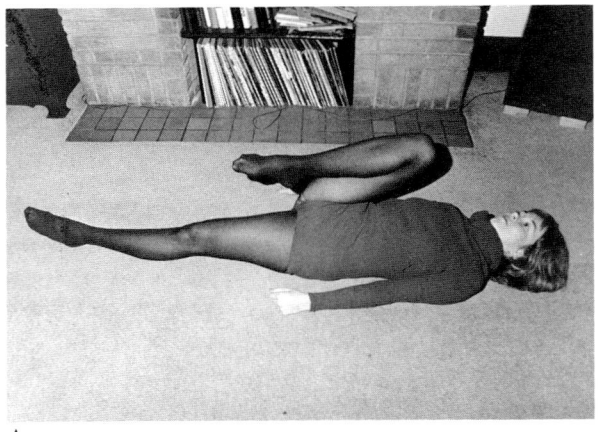
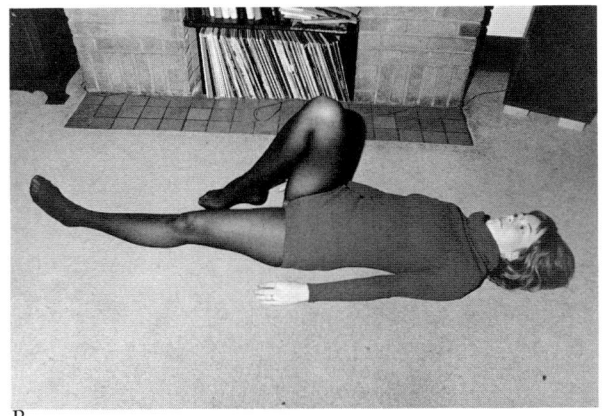
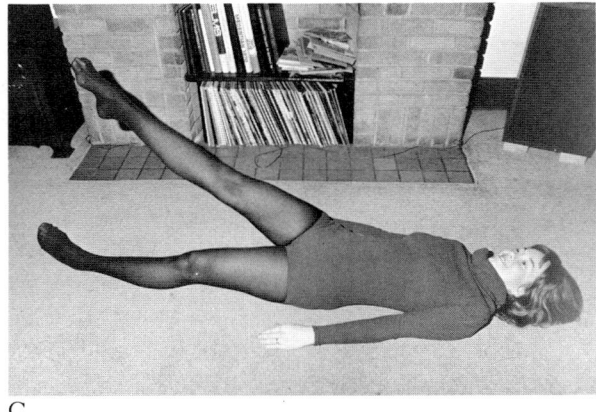

Fig. 26-3. Postpartal exercises: arm raising. A. The woman begins the exercise with her arms at her sides. B. She moves them out until they are perpendicular to her body. C. She raises them over her body until her hands touch, then lowers them slowly to her sides to finish. This exercise strengthens both breast and abdominal tone.

Fig. 26-4. Postpartal exercises: knee to abdomen. A. The woman bends one leg at a time at the knee and brings it up to touch her abdomen. B and C. She then lowers the foot to touch her buttock, straightens her leg, and slowly lowers it. This exercise strengthens both abdominal and gluteal muscles.

Knee-Chest Position

A knee-chest position is dangerous for the woman to assume until at least the third week post partum. In a knee-chest position, the vagina tends to open. Because the cervical os remains open to some extent until the third week, there is a danger that air will enter the vagina and the open cervix, penetrate the open blood sinuses inside the uterus, enter the circulatory system, and cause an air embolism.

It is therefore a good practice for a woman to avoid this position until she returns for a postpartal examination and is assured her cervix has closed properly. Women who have used a knee-chest position during pregnancy to relieve the pressure of hemorrhoids need to be instructed that a modified Sims's position, such as they used for a rest position during pregnancy, is best for them now.

BATHING

Because of increased perspiration, most women enjoy a daily shower or bath. The first time a woman is allowed up to take a shower or tub bath she must have someone accompany her. Warm water tends to make many people light-headed, and they become unsteady on their feet as they return to bed.

Formerly, women were not allowed to take tub baths following delivery for fear bacteria from the bath water would enter the vagina and cause infection. There appears to be little evidence that this is a real danger. The sitz bath has long been used for postpartal women, and this is no less a bath than a regular tub bath. Some women feel that baths are the only way of getting really clean, and the warm water in contact with the perineum gives them the secondary benefit of a sitz bath, namely, relief from perineal discomfort.

WEIGHT LOSS

The rapid diuresis and diaphoresis during the second to fifth day post partum will ordinarily result in a weight loss of an additional 5 pounds over the 12 or so pounds that the woman lost at delivery.

The woman often feels thirsty during this period of rapid fluid loss and wants additional fluid. It seems a paradox that while the body is ridding itself of unwanted fluid it should also demand fluid. Part of this paradox stems from the woman's having very little to drink during a part of her labor. She may say immediately following delivery, "I don't think I'll ever get enough to drink again." Some of her thirst results from the medications used in labor. Atropine and scopolamine both leave mucous membranes feeling dry and cottony. Part of the need for fluid stems from the increased amount of nitrogen being released from catabolized uterine cells. The woman needs to increase her fluid intake in order to rid her body of these wastes.

Some women need to be urged to drink adequate fluid in the first few days post partum because they are restricting fluid themselves in the hope of preventing their breasts from becoming engorged. Others are beginning diets that they hope will bring their bodies more quickly back to their nonpregnant slim state. As mentioned previously, fluid restriction does little to thwart breast engorgement, and unless the woman is extremely obese, this is not a good time for dieting. The postpartal period is a time of rebuilding and readjusting, for which a woman needs both ample nourishment and adequate fluid intake. She should drink three to four 8-ounce glasses of fluid a day.

DIET

A postpartal diet should contain between 2500 and 2600 calories daily and should be high in protein and the vitamins and minerals needed for good tissue repair. It should have an adequate supply of roughage to help restore the peristaltic action of the bowel. The woman who is breast-feeding needs an additional 500 calories and an additional 500 ml of fluid (these may be from the same source) in her diet to encourage the production of high-quality breast milk. Most mothers are hungry during the immediate postpartal period and consume an adequate diet without urging.

On discharge the woman needs to be instructed to continue to eat a nutritious diet after she returns home. Some mothers become too fatigued during their first weeks at home to prepare adequate meals. Thus, neglecting to eat properly leads to more fatigue and so to an even less nutritious diet.

If the woman has any prenatal vitamins or supplementary iron preparations left over from pregnancy, she should, as a rule, continue to take them until her supply is used up. If she needs further supplements, her physician will order them for her either on discharge or when she returns for her postpartum checkup.

REST

The importance of rest throughout the puerperium cannot be stressed too much. Throughout the woman's hospital stay, time for naps (shoes off, feet up) should be provided. Discharge instructions should include a firm statement encouraging the woman to continue to get adequate rest when she is home. This will not be easy for her; she has a newborn who wakes at least twice a night, and relatives and friends come to see the baby during the day.

When families were closely knit and neighborhoods were smaller than they are today, every new mother had someone in her family or neighborhood to call on to look after the baby while she napped. Today, a young couple is likely to live in an apartment building and may have no family or close friends nearby to call on. If the parents have not thought through this problem before delivery, you can help them to look at their situation and see what aid is available to them. Perhaps the wife's or husband's mother could come and stay with them for the first week. Perhaps the husband could take a week off from work or school to help out at home. Perhaps a friend at school or work could take part of the strain of the first week from the mother's shoulders. If none of these solutions seems appropriate, the couple might appreciate being given the name of a community service agency that supplies homemakers on a short-term basis; or you might make a referral to a community health agency, urging an early home visit.

The woman does not have an auspicious start for her role—being a mother instead of a daughter, a mother as well as a wife, a mother of three, not two—if she is so overcome by sleep hunger that her judgment and her senses are blurred.

EARLY AMBULATION

Getting the mother out of bed and assisting her to be ambulatory shortly after delivery seems inconsistent in the face of the mother's exhaustion and need for rest. Those who ambulate quickly, however, in the fourth to eighth hour after delivery, have fewer bowel and bladder complications and fewer circulatory complications, and they feel stronger and healthier by the end of their first week than do those who remain in bed during this time.

The first time the woman is out of bed, she can expect to feel dizzy and wobbly. Before assisting her to ambulate, it is important that you be aware if she was given an anesthetic for delivery. A woman who has had a spinal anesthetic should remain flat in bed for at least 8 hours after delivery; earlier ambulation tends to cause spinal headaches, which are excruciating and difficult to relieve and often continue to recur for days or weeks.

The woman should be allowed to dangle her legs on the edge of the bed for a few minutes the first time she is up. Then assist her as needed for the few steps to a chair or a nearby bathroom. Remain with her the first time she is up; some women are extremely unsteady on their feet and discover that a seemingly easy task like walking across the room becomes overwhelmingly difficult when one is exhausted.

Once the woman has been out of bed with your assistance, she may be up on her own as she wishes. She can begin to care for her own needs, including perineal care after instruction in good technique. However, it is important that she not be left with the impression during this time that because she is able to do these things she is now strictly on her own. She needs continued attention, to give her a feeling that people are concerned about her and enjoy caring for her. She needs professional attention to her physical well-being. She needs to be urged to rest every afternoon and to get a full night's sleep (some women who ambulate early will overdo).

A complication that may occur postpartally in women who do not ambulate early is thrombophlebitis of pelvic or leg veins.

Homans' sign (pain in the calf on dorsiflexion of the foot) is a simple test that reveals the presence of thrombophlebitis in leg veins. Simply flex the woman's leg, slightly dorsiflex her foot, and palpate her calf. If there is pain in the calf of her leg a thrombophlebitis is beginning. Do not massage the area; massaging a thrombophlebitis may cause circulatory emboli.

This test should be done once each nursing shift or every 8 hours during the woman's hospital stay.

A timetable for continued nursing interventions is given in Table 26-2.

Preparation for Discharge

CHILD CARE INSTRUCTION

Many women attend classes in newborn care during their pregnancies. They remember many points from these classes but when they actually have a newborn become worried that they will not remember enough. Many mothers say child care did not seem real during pregnancy, that now is the time when they need the information that was taught earlier. The postpartal period is therefore a time for teaching, reteaching, and offering anticipatory guidance to help in the new situations the family can expect to arise when mother and baby go home.

During the taking-in phase of the puerperium, the woman may not show much interest in learning; she is more in need of the comfort of being taken care of. As she enters her taking-hold period, she grows increasingly receptive to advice and looks to you for the information she needs. Some nurses assume that multiparas will react negatively to child care sug-

Table 26-2. Timetable for Continued Nursing Interventions

Intervention	Timing 2 to 8 Hours Post Partum	1 to 4 Days Post Partum
Evaluate fundal height and consistency	q1h	q8h
Evaluate color and amount of lochia	q1h	q8h
Assess perineum for hematoma or stressed suture line	q1h	q8h
Assess bladder distention	q2–4h	q4–8h
Take pulse and blood pressure	q2h	q4h
Take temperature	q4h	q4h
Assess breasts	q8h	q8h
Observe mother-child (parent-child) interaction	At each encounter	At each encounter
Assess Homans' sign for thrombophlebitis	q8h	q8h

gestions. Multiparas are, after all, veterans of child care. If you listen carefully to the multipara, however, you will discover that a mother of three girls feels insecure about the care of a boy. A mother whose next youngest child is 5 years old admits that in five years she has completely forgotten how small newborns are. She yearns to have a nurse who is comfortable with such small human beings reassure her that she is holding her new baby correctly and giving him the proper care. All mothers, whether primiparas or grand multiparas, need to be evaluated individually and helped at that point where you find they need guidance.

Group Classes

Many hospitals provide group classes in bathing infants, preparing formula, breast-feeding techniques, problems of minimizing jealousy in older children, and maintaining health in the newborn and infant. These classes are helpful to mothers if a time for questions and answers is allowed, so that the mother can apply what she is being taught to her individual circumstances. Maternity services that are truly family-centered open these classes to fathers as well.

Individual Instruction

Every mother needs some individual instruction in how to care for her infant and how to care for herself after discharge. Rooming-in, in which the mother spends at least a portion of the day with her baby, is an ideal setup for letting you observe and work with the mother and her baby. Even if the hospital does not have rooming-in units, you should provide some time each day for the mother to handle her infant and ask any questions she has about child care. How to bathe and feed the baby, how to care for the infant's cord and circumcision, a review of how much infants sleep during 24 hours, and how to fit a newborn into the family's pattern of living are topics that mothers like to have discussed with them. As with formal classes, the father should be included in these sessions. The problems that arise with newborn care are by their nature family problems, and every effort should be made by nursing personnel to help both parents prepare to deal with them. (Home care of the newborn is discussed in Chap. 31.)

DISCHARGE INSTRUCTIONS

Before the mother is discharged, she will be given instructions by her physician concerning her care at home. These instructions differ from physician to physician, but all have points in common, which are as follows:

1. All women should avoid heavy work for at least the first three weeks at home. Women differ in their concepts of heavy work, and it is a good idea to explore with the woman what she considers heavy work. If she plans to do too much, you can perhaps help her to modify her definition of heavy work.
2. The woman should plan at least one rest period a day and try to get a good night's sleep. She can rest during the day when her newborn is sleeping unless she has other children or an aged parent to care for. If she has others dependent on her, as mentioned before, explore with her the possibility that a neighbor, another family member, or a person from a community agency will be able to come in to relieve her.
3. The woman should limit the number of stairs she climbs to one flight a day for the first week at home. Beginning the second week, if her lochia discharge is normal, she may start to expand this activity. This limitation will involve some planning on her part, especially if her washing machine is in the basement and she must wash diapers every day; or if she must go up and down stairs to check on the baby. It is probably better to arrange for places for the baby to sleep downstairs

as well as upstairs, so that he has to be taken upstairs only at bedtime.

4. The woman may take either tub baths or showers. She should continue to apply any cream or ointment ordered for the perineal area and remember to continue to cleanse herself from front to back. Any perineal stitches will be absorbed within 10 days.
5. The woman should not take vaginal douches until she returns for her six-weeks' checkup. Some physicians restrict sexual intercourse until this time also. This restraint is to prevent infection and trauma to areas that have just healed; in the case of intercourse, it is also to prevent possible conception until the organs of reproduction are ready for another pregnancy. This restriction of intercourse may seem unrealistic to many couples today. It is unrealistic to assume that all couples will follow this advice. Just make certain that the couple is aware of the danger of infection and informed about a contraceptive measure (if that is the parents' choice) before the mother is discharged from the hospital.
6. The woman should notify her physician if she notices an increase, not a decrease, in lochial discharge, or if lochia serosa or lochia alba becomes lochia rubra. Delayed postpartal hemorrhage can occur in women who become extremely fatigued. Getting adequate rest during her first weeks at home will do much to prevent the possibility of this complication.
7. Six weeks after birth, the woman should return to her physician or clinic for an examination. Family planning can be discussed with the mother at this time if it was not discussed earlier, before discharge from the hospital.

Prior to discharge from the hospital the woman should also receive instructions on child health care. Just as she herself must return for an examination six weeks after delivery, she must make an appointment to take her baby to a pediatrician, family physician, or well-child clinic for an examination at about four weeks.

It is important that discharge instructions be written for the family. The business of getting ready to go home, dressing the baby, seeing him in his new clothes for the first time, experiencing the thrill of realizing the baby is really theirs to take home is so exciting that your oral instructions may go unheard (Fig. 26-5). On the other hand, the mother should not simply be handed a list of instructions. They

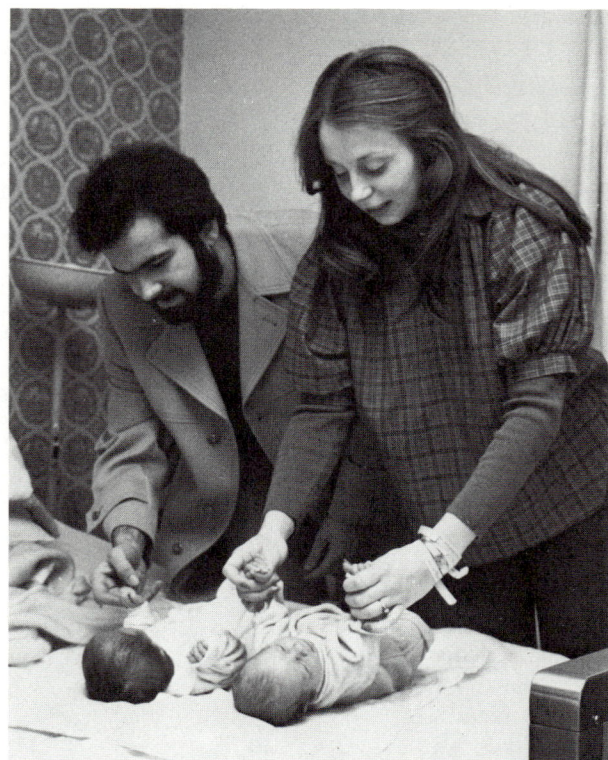

Fig. 26-5. Parents dress their twins to take them home. In the exciting minutes of discharge, instructions are easily forgotten unless they are written. (Courtesy of the Department of Medical Photography, Children's Hospital, Buffalo, N.Y.)

should be reviewed with her to make certain that she understands them.

The hospital should have on its staff a community-hospital liaison person, ideally a nurse, to answer calls from mothers who lose their instructions or are unable to interpret them after they have returned home. It is comforting to have a familiar person one trusts to turn to in the first few days a new baby is at home.

POSTPARTAL EXAMINATION

Every woman should have a checkup by her physician at the end of the six-weeks' postpartal period to assure herself and the physician that she is in good health and has no residual problems from childbearing.

During this examination her abdominal wall will be inspected for tone. Her breasts will be inspected to see that they have returned to their nonpregnant state if she is not breast-feeding, and to see that they are unfissured and free of complications in the breast-feeding mother. Most important, a thorough internal examination is performed to see that involution is complete, that the ligaments and the pelvic muscle supports have returned to good functional alignment, and that any lacerations sustained during birth have healed.

If the woman does not have an adequate rubella antibody titer and anticipates further pregnancies, she may receive a rubella immunization. If she has hemorrhoids or varicosities as a result of the pregnancy, her physician will discuss with her whether further management of these conditions is necessary. You should discuss breast self-examination with her, as well as the necessity for a Papanicolaou smear every 3 years as a means of preventing cervical cancer. The postpartal examination should also be a time for the woman to discuss with you or the physician any problems she had with childbearing and any she now has with child rearing, since these are a continuum. Moreover, it should be a time to discuss a form of future family planning if that is the family's wish and it was not discussed in the immediate postpartal period.

Problem-oriented Recording: Progress Notes

Mary Kraft
22 years
Para 1, gravida 2

Problem: Involution, day 1 post partum

> S. No afterpains. Dislikes heat lamp treatment. Refusing to use heat lamp even though she has "pulling pain" from episiotomy sutures.
> O. Fundal height: 1 F under umbilicus and firm; moderate lochia rubra flow, no foul odor. Doing own perineal care; dried lochia present on suture site. Voiding without difficulty; no BM as yet but not uncomfortable. Suture line intact; no erythema, no separation.
> A. Involution appropriate for 1st day post partum; perineal self-care needs reviewed.
> Goals: a. Early discharge from hospital (24 to 48 hours).
> b. Uterine involution progresses effectively.
> c. Perineal pain reduced so she can manage at home.
> d. Vital signs remain within normal postpartal limits.
> e. Able to describe care at home for self by early discharge date.
> P. 1. Review perineal care so suture line remains cleaner.
> 2. Ask M.D. for sitz bath order in place of heat lamp.
> 3. Teach fundal, lochial, and perineal assessment to be ready for discharge.

Problem: Involution, day 2 post partum

> S. States sitz bath treatment "feels good." Will continue to do at home. Able to describe difference between normal and abnormal lochial discharge and correct fundal consistency.
> O. Fundal height: 2 F under umbilicus and firm. Moderate lochia rubra, no foul odor. Suture line clean, no erythema, no separation. Temperature 98.8.
> A. Uterine involution appropriate for 2nd day post partum. Knowlege of self-care adequate for discharge.
> P. 1. Ask for final questions regarding care.
> 2. Give self-care booklet for reference.
> 3. Remind of necessity for 6-week postpartal visit.
> 4. Remind of nursing liaison number to call if questions regarding self-care arise.
> 5. Review physician's instructions on rest, exercise, douching, sexual abstinence, and provide with written list if not given by M.D.

Problem-oriented Recording: Progress Notes

Angie Baco
42 years
Para 7, gravida 7

Problem: Involution, day 1 post partum

> S. Acute afterpains; feels "as if my stomach is falling out" when she ambulates; suture line painful; relief from sitz bath most effective.
> O. Abdominal muscles weak. Fundus ½ F under umbilicus. Large amount lochia

rubra (2 pads every 2½ hours). Sitz baths every 4 hours being taken by self. Afterpains relieved with Tylenol gr 10 every 4 hours. Suture line intact; no erythema, no separation. Voiding adequate amount.

A. Involution adequate for 1st day post partum. Abdominal musculature weakened from large baby and past pregnancies.

Goals: a. Uterine involution progresses effectively.
      b. Afterpains relieved by use of analgesic.
      c. Suture-line pain relieved by analgesics or sitz baths.
      d. Suture line heals without difficulty by 7th day.
      e. Vital signs remain within normal postpartal limits.
      f. Able to describe self-care in hospital.

P. 1. Teach and help practice abdominal strengthening exercises.
   2. Continue sitz baths as comfort measures.
   3. Check lochia flow q2h until flow is less.
   4. Check vital signs q2h until lochia flow is less.

References

1. Bird, I. S. Breast-feeding classes on the post partum unit. *Am. J. Nurs.* 75:456, 1975.
2. Campbell, S. Post partum assessment guide. *Am. J. Nurs.* 77:1179, 1977.
3. Carlson, S. E. The irreality of postpartum: Observations on the subjective experience. *J.O.G.N. Nurs.* 5:28, 1976.
4. Donaldson, N. E. Fourth trimester follow-up. *Am. J. Nurs.* 77:1176, 1977.
5. Edgar, W. M., et al. Rubella vaccination and anti-D immunoglobulin administration in the puerperium. *Br. J. Obstet. Gynecol.* 84:754, 1977.
6. Foster, R. S. How to encourage breast self-examination. *Female Patient* 5:36, 1980.
7. Gorrie, T. M. A post partum evaluation tool. *J.O.G.N. Nurs.* 8:41, 1979.
8. Jones, D. Home early after delivery. *Am. J. Nurs.* 78:1378, 1978.
9. Malinowski, J. Bladder assessment in the post partum patient. *J.O.G.N. Nurs.* 7:14, 1978.
10. O'Connor, S., et al. The effect of extended post partum contact on problems with parenting. *Birth Fam. J.* 5:231, 1978.
11. Swanson, J. Nursing intervention to facilitate maternal-infant attachment. *J.O.G.N. Nurs.* 7:35, 1978.
12. Wallace, J. P. Exercise during pregnancy and post partum. *Female Patient* 4:78, 1979.

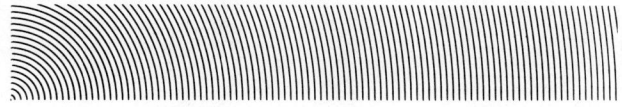

Unit V. Utilizing Nursing Process: Questions for Review

1. Mrs. A. has chosen a rooming-in unit for postpartal care. Rooming-in serves the purpose of
   a. Allowing mothers to spend increased time with their babies
   b. Reducing costs by decreasing number of bassinets needed
   c. Forcing mothers to be ambulatory after delivery
   d. None of the above

2. During the first hour post partum, Mrs. A. seems to want to do nothing but sleep. This attitude probably reflects
   a. Disappointment in her newborn
   b. Reluctance to begin her mothering role
   c. Exhaustion from delivery
   d. Unfamiliarity with hospital rules that say she can be ambulatory

3. You check Mrs. A.'s fundal height every 15 minutes during the first hour post partum. The height of her fundus during this hour should be
   a. Two fingerbreadths under the umbilicus
   b. One fingerbreadth under the umbilicus
   c. At the umbilicus
   d. Two fingerbreadths above the symphysis pubis

4. Mrs. A. is a 35-year-old woman with varicosities. Following her last pregnancy she had a mild thrombophlebitis. Which of the following procedures would you question before carrying it out for her?
   a. Administering aspirin for "afterpains"
   b. Encouraging her to begin perineal exercises
   c. Administering diethylstilbestrol as a milk suppressant
   d. Encouraging her to drink all the fluid on her tray

5. Mrs. B. has a shaking chill as she lies on the delivery room table following delivery. A chill of this nature results from
   a. Decreased fluid intake during labor
   b. Excessive analgesia administered during labor
   c. Legs elevated too long in a lithotomy position
   d. Exhaustion and pressure changes in the abdomen

6. Lochia discharge typically changes from rubra to serosa on which day post partum?
   a. The first day
   b. The third day
   c. The seventh day
   d. The tenth day

7. Mrs. B. is going to breast-feed. Breast care for Mrs. B. should include
   a. Washing breasts with soap and water at the time of her daily bath
   b. Washing breasts with alcohol to toughen nipples for feeding
   c. Washing breasts with clear water once daily
   d. Washing breasts with soap and water prior to each feeding

8. Mrs. C. has difficulty voiding following delivery. You explain to her the reason:
   a. Excessive medication during labor leads to poor bladder function.
   b. She is not trying hard enough.
   c. She must have a cervical tear, reducing bladder sensation.
   d. Perineal edema makes voiding difficult.

9. Mrs. C. stated during labor that she did not want a baby. A sign that she is not adapting well to her baby might be:
   a. She calls her baby J. J. instead of John Joseph.
   b. She says she does not want to breast-feed.
   c. She undressed her baby and checked him thoroughly the first time she saw him.
   d. She does not look at her baby's face.

10. Which of the following observations would make you concerned at the amount of blood Mrs. C. is losing postpartally?
    a. Her pulse rate is only 74.
    b. She feels light-headed the first time she is out of bed.
    c. She is perspiring profusely and is extremely thirsty.
    d. None of the above.

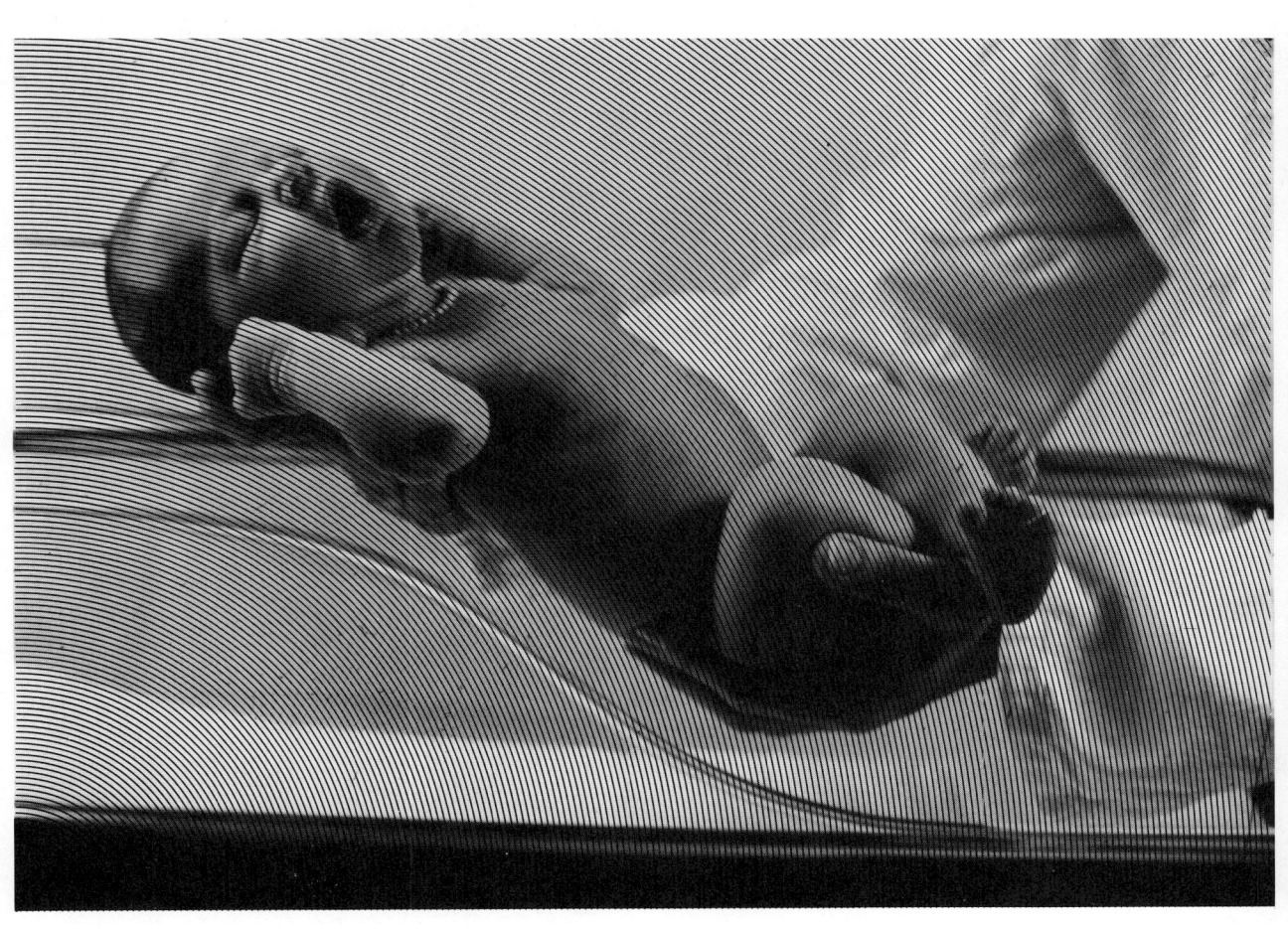

VI. The Newborn

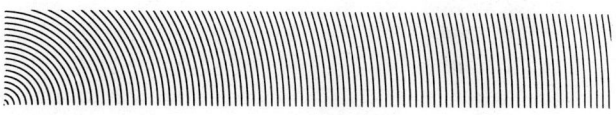

27. Personality Development in the Newborn

Infants are not, as some people assume, passive, parasitic creatures who take and take and never give back. They are alert, participating individuals who are interested in interacting with people around them, particularly the person who gives them primary care (Fig. 27-1).

Infants are people-oriented—how much so can be demonstrated by their reaction to people versus objects. A baby will recognize his mother's face by 4 months of age but will not recognize his bottle until he is 5 months old. He will cry at 4 months if a person who was playing with him leaves him, but not until 5 months will he cry when a toy is taken away from him.

The classic experiments of the Harlows (Harlow and Zimmerman [10]) with newborn monkeys demonstrated how baby monkeys yearn for something more from a mother than physical nourishment. The experimenters fed one group of newborn monkeys from a bottle attached to a wire mesh "mother." A second group was fed from a bottle attached to a soft terrycloth "mother." When the monkeys were frightened, all of them clung to the terrycloth "mother," even those who had not been fed by "her."

A human baby demonstrates this same behavior, enjoying being cuddled, held tightly, and mothered. He reciprocates very soon by cooing and smiling in response to his mother's face.

Newborn Tasks

A newborn has certain developmental tasks that he must master to mature and adjust to his environment. Duvall [5] has isolated a number of these. The infant has to

1. Achieve physiological equilibrium following birth. This involves learning to sleep and be active at appropriate times, so that he receives enough nourishment and has enough exercise to remain physiologically sound.
2. Learn to take foods satisfactorily; sucking is not as instinctive for some infants as others. Developing a taste for new textures and foods is more difficult for some infants than for others.
3. Achieve controlled elimination and not be frightened by his own body urges.
4. Learn to manage his own body. This involves developing coordination, the ability to move about, assurance, and competence.
5. Learn to adjust to other people.
6. Learn systems of communication. This involves both verbal and nonverbal learning.

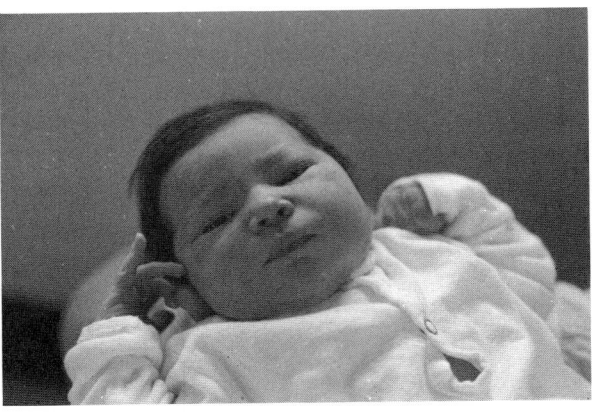

Fig. 27-1. Personality is apparent in a newborn from the start. Note the alert, searching interest.

7. Learn to express and control feelings.
8. Lay the foundations of self-awareness. This involves seeing oneself as a separate entity and finding personal fulfillment both with and without others.
9. Learn to love and be loved.

The greatest task of a new mother is to conceive of her newborn as a separate individual with his own needs and to rely on what his behavior tells her (to be able to interpret his cues). By 2 months of age, most infants can indicate by their cry whether they are feeling cold, hungry, wet, or lonesome. Since the mother spends a great deal of time with the infant in these first months, she has an opportunity to recognize his nonverbal cues and to be aware of his individual needs.

Developmental Task: Trust Versus Distrust

A developmental task is one that is best achieved at a particular time in life so that the individual can proceed to the next step of maturity.

Erikson [6] proposes that the personality developmental task of the infant period is to form a sense of trust. When the infant is hungry, the mother feeds and makes him comfortable again; he is wet, and the mother changes him and makes him comfortable again; he is cold, and the mother holds and warms him and makes him comfortable again. By this process, he learns to trust that when he has a need, or is in distress, a person will come to take care of him.

A synonym for *trust* in this connotation might be *love*. By the way that the infant is handled, fed, talked to, and held, he learns to love and be loved. The infant who has a variety of caretakers, who sometimes is fed on a rigid schedule and sometimes when he is hungry, who sometimes is treated roughly and sometimes gently, has difficulty learning to trust anyone. If a person cannot trust people, he cannot enjoy deeply satisfying interactions with people. If he cannot trust others, he has difficulty trusting himself or feeling self-esteem. Children who are raised in an orphanage or a kibbutz with many caretakers may have difficulty establishing close relationships as adults.

The importance of establishing this ability to love or trust early becomes evident when development is thought of sequentially. If the first developmental step is inadequate, this inadequacy will pervade all future steps. The end result will be an adult who is unable to form deep relationships with others. Such adults are unable to instill a sense of trust in their own children, and thus the inadequacy is perpetuated from generation to generation.

How does a mother encourage a sense of trust in her infant? Trust arises out of a sense of confidence that one knows what is coming next. This does not mean that a mother should set up a rigid schedule of care for her child. It does imply that she should establish *some* schedule: breakfast, bath, playtime, nap, lunch, walk outside, quiet playtime, dinner, story, bedtime, for example. This gentle rhythm of care gives the infant a sense of being able to predict what is going to happen, to feel that life has some consistency. All little children thrive on routine: the same story read over and over again, the same bedtime routine over and over, the same spoon every day for lunch. The newborn period is not too early for the child to learn family traditions that will help him to feel secure in his world as he grows. Some mothers have difficulty seeing this as important. They are so tired of work routines that they want to raise their child as a "free spirit." Do not discourage this philosophy altogether. However, it may be helpful to suggest a few modifications to try to instill a little order into the infant's life.

As important as a rhythm of care is that the care is given largely by one person. This person can be the mother, a grandmother, a conscientious baby-sitter, a foster mother, the father, or anyone who can give consistent care. A mother who must work during the first year of her baby's life should try to arrange for one person to care for her child while she is away from home rather than arranging for care in a day-care center with a multitude of workers. She should discuss her method of child care with baby-sitters, so that changes in baby-sitters do not disrupt the routine of care.

The person who gives an infant constant care must actively interact with the child in order to provide a sense of trust. Passively caring for an infant, never talking to him or stroking him while feeding and changing him, is the same as not being with him at all. Some mothers feel self-conscious talking to a baby who does not talk back. Or they think such interaction can wait until the child is older. The rule that parents should not talk baby talk to the baby is a good one, because children will not learn the correct pronunciation of words from baby talk. Be sure, however, that a mother is not interpreting the rule as "don't talk to babies."

Pointing out to a mother the importance of interacting with her child helps her to include this form of stimulation as she cares for the baby's physical needs.

Rooming-in helps a mother to feel secure about caring for her baby before she is discharged from the hospital. Looking at the baby with her, pointing out that such things as the faint red marks over the eyebrows are normal in newborns, or that the irregular manner that newborns use to breathe is normal, helps her begin to interact with the baby. Even if the mother does not choose rooming-in, she needs to have extra time with her baby. She needs to do more for him during her hospital stay than just feed him and then quickly return him to the nursery again.

If a woman is going to have a short hospital stay or delivers at an alternate birth center, she should spend as much time as possible with her baby during this time. Unfortunately, she may be so exhausted following delivery or still be in a taking-in phase of recovery from childbirth that she is not able to use the time with her baby effectively. Try to identify a support person in her family or among her friends whom she will be able to use when she is at home to answer the questions about her baby that would have been answered by nurses if she had stayed in the hospital longer.

Classes on Mothering

Most hospitals provide instruction in formula making, bathing infants, and breast-feeding, all of which are physical aspects of care. Nurses who are involved in giving the courses should have enough expertise (or realize the need is great enough to secure someone from the community with enough expertise) to include good mothering concepts, discussions of infant temperament, and personality development in these programs.

Sensory Stimulation

Because small infants react strongly to sensory stimuli, the sensory stimulation the mother intends to give her baby is a good area to explore.

HEARING

An infant appears to enjoy soft, musical sounds or soft, cooing voices; he starts at the sound of harsh, raucous rattles or loud bangs. A mother should choose first toys in terms of the sounds they make. They should not be chosen because they appeal to her, but according to their suitability for an infant who is just being introduced into the modern world of high-intensity sound.

SIGHT

Babies appear to enjoy watching their mothers' faces more than any toy. A mother should make a point of initiating eye-to-eye contact with her newborn right from the beginning. Most mothers are aware that infants also enjoy mobiles. Occasionally, a mother overdoes the amount of visual stimulation she gives her child. He has so many patterns around him, so many dangling objects over his head as he lies in his crib, that he must feel overwhelmed. Again, mothers should consider how all these trappings appear from the child's view.

TASTE

Mealtime every day is a time for fostering trust. Feedings should be at the infant's pace, and the amounts should fit his needs, not the mother's idea of what he should eat. Again, he should not be overwhelmed by too many stimuli. New foods should be introduced one at a time, so that the child can accustom himself to a new taste before another new one is introduced. The temperature of formula or food should be neither too hot nor too cold. An infant should be held while he is fed, so that he feels secure; he should have adequate sucking pleasure over and above that necessary for feeding.

TOUCH

An infant needs to be touched, to experience skin-to-skin contact. His clothes should feel comfortable: soft rather than rough; dry rather than wet diapers. He needs to be handled with assurance and gentleness. Some mothers handle their sons roughly, trying not to make them "sissies." Such mothers need reminding that right now their sons are babies; later on, they will have time enough to become men.

It is interesting to explore with new mothers how much they appreciate the benefits or meaning of touch. Sometimes one observes a mother at a social gathering who brings her baby in an infant carrier, leaves him there all during the visit, and takes him out to the car in the carrier when she leaves. The mother has avoided touching by always interposing a plastic barrier between her and her child. Such a mother is not necessarily cold or distant. Probably, no nurse ever took the time to talk to her about the psychological aspects of infant care.

Infant Development

Most mothers ask a number of questions relating to a baby's development: When will he be able to sit up? When will he be able to turn over? When can I expect him to begin to talk? It is good for a mother not to expect these milestones of development to occur before they normally do or she will fear that her infant is retarded. Furthermore, it is dangerous when she believes that certain capabilities develop later than they actually do. If she thinks her child is too young to move to the edge of a bed, she may leave him there unattended, setting the scene for a fall.

You should be familiar with the developmental milestones of infancy in order to be able to answer the mother's questions intelligently. Be sure that mothers understand that babies all proceed through developmental stages, but at different rates. The fact that an older child walked at 12 months does not mean his new brother or sister will walk this early. Some babies walk as late as at 22 months and are still within the normal limits of development. An older child may not have turned over until he was 4 months old; the new baby may flip over at 3 months. The ages at which milestones have been found to occur are averages only.

A guide such as the developmental screening items devised by Provence [16] is a helpful reference to use in discussing development in the first 24 months of life. This is shown in Table 27-1.

Temperament

Temperament is not a characteristic that arises during childhood or in adult life. Infants are born with temperament, which can be defined as characteristic reaction patterns to situations. It is important to explore this concept with new mothers. Awareness that infants are not all alike, that some adapt quickly to new situations, others adapt slowly, some react intensely, some passively, helps the new mother to understand her child better, to learn more quickly the cues her child is giving her, and therefore to deal with him more constructively (Fig. 27-2).

Thomas et al. [19] have identified nine different reaction patterns in infants.

ACTIVITY LEVEL

Some infants have a high level of motor activity and are rarely quiet. They wiggle and squirm in their crib as early as 2 weeks of age. The mother puts such a child to sleep in one end of the crib and finds him in another corner of the crib an hour later. The child will not stay seated in his bathtub. He refuses to be controlled by a playpen. He is constantly "on the go." Other babies move very little, stay where they are placed, appear to take in their environment in a quieter, more docile way. Both patterns are normal; they merely reflect the extremes of the scale of motor activity, which is one characteristic of temperament.

RHYTHMICITY

Some infants manifest a regular rhythm in their physiological functions. They tend to awake at the same time each morning. They appear hungry at regular 4-hour periods. They nap the same time every day, have a bowel movement the same time every day. They are predictable, easy-to-care-for infants in that the mother learns early what to expect from them. On the other end of the scale are infants with an irregular rhythmicity. They rarely awake at the same time two days in a row. They may go a long time without eating one day and the next day appear hungry almost immediately after a feeding. Such a child is difficult to care for because the mother cannot easily plan a schedule for him. She must constantly adapt her daily schedule to the infant's.

APPROACH

Approach refers to the child's response on initial contact with a new stimulus. Some infants approach new situations in an unruffled manner. They smile and "talk" to strangers, and will accept new food without any spitting out or fussing. They explore new toys without apprehension. Other infants demonstrate *withdrawal* rather than approach. They cry at the sight of strangers, new toys, new foods, the first time a tub bath is introduced. They are difficult children to take on vacation because they react so fearfully to new situations.

ADAPTABILITY

Adaptability is the infant's ability to change his reaction to stimuli over a period of time. The infant who

Table 27-1. Items for Developmental Screening, Ages 1 to 24 Months

Age (Months)	Posturing and Gross Motor Development	Grasping Patterns	Play and Use of Toys	Speech	Reactions to Others and Staff
1	Asymmetrical postures predominant	Hands fisted or partially open Grasps voluntarily when toy is placed *in* hand	Follows visually Holds rattle briefly (not reflexively)	Makes small throaty noises Vocalizes responsively to people (musical cooing)	Looks at face of adult Smiles responsively
3	Lifts head high in prone position Rolls prone to supine				Follows moving person visually Distinguishes mother from others
5	No head lag when pulled to sit Rolls supine to prone	Grasps toy when held *near* hand Palmarwise grasp of block	Shows interest in playthings Shows displeasure at loss of toy	Vocalizes spontaneously to self and to toys Localizes sounds	*Initiates* contact by smiling or vocalizing Plays with own foot
7	Sits with trunk erect with support Sits alone	Transfers object from hand to hand Grasps block with thumb and index	Looks briefly for toy that disappears	Vocalizes "da, ba, ha"	Reacts to strangers Pushes away examiner's hand
9	Belly crawl Creeps on all fours		Plays with 2 toys simultaneously	Vocalizes "dada, mama" (*non*specific)	Plays pat-a-cake, so-big, bye-bye
11	Pulls to a stand	Grasps pellet with pincer grasp (index and thumb)	Shows preference for one toy over another	Vocalizes "mama, dada" (specific)	Cooperates in dressing (e.g., pushes arm with sleeve)
13	Walks a few steps alone		Enjoys "putting in and taking out" games	Two words (besides *mama, dada*)	Finger-feeds Rolls ball to adult with pleasure
15	Walks well alone Starts and stops with control			Uses 1–6 words, including names Uses jargon	Hugs and gives kiss to parent
18	Climbs into adult chair		Piles 3–4 blocks Looks at picture book Explores drawers and cabinets	Names 1 or 2 common objects	Identifies parts of own body (e.g., eye, nose)
21	Squats and returns to standing position Runs well		Pushes small cars, etc., about	Combines 2–3 words spontaneously Vocabulary of 20–50 words	Feeds self with spoon
24	Walks up and down stairs alone		Beginning fantasy play: takes care of doll or teddy bear; "goes to store"; etc.	Begins to use pronouns, *I, you, me* Uses 3-word sentences	Imitates parents in domestic activities (dusts, sweeps, puts on father's hat, etc.)

Source. Provence, S. Developmental History. In R. Cooke and S. Levin (Eds.), *The Biologic Basis of Pediatric Practice.* New York: McGraw-Hill, 1968. Vol. 2, p. 1738. Copyright © 1968 by McGraw-Hill Book Company. Used with permission.

is adaptable changes his first reaction to situations without exhibiting extreme distress. The first time he was placed in a bathtub he protested loudly, but by the third time he is happily sitting in it splashing. This contrasts with the infant who cries for months whenever he is put into the bathtub or who cannot seem to accustom himself to a new bed, a new playpen, or a new caretaker.

INTENSITY OF REACTION

Some infants react to situations with their whole being. They cry loudly when their diapers are wet, when they are hungry, when their mother leaves them. Others rarely fuss over irritations such as wet diapers. They wait for their mother to prepare food, and they have a mild or low-intensity reaction to stress.

DISTRACTIBILITY

An infant who is easily distracted is easily managed. A pacifier diverts and calms him. If he is crying over the loss of a toy, he can be appeased by the offer of a new one. Other infants are nondistractible. No offer will distract them from the object they want. The mother of such an infant may describe him as "bullheaded" or unwilling to compromise.

ATTENTION SPAN AND PERSISTENCE

Attention span in infants is variable. One infant will play in a playpen by himself with one toy for an hour;

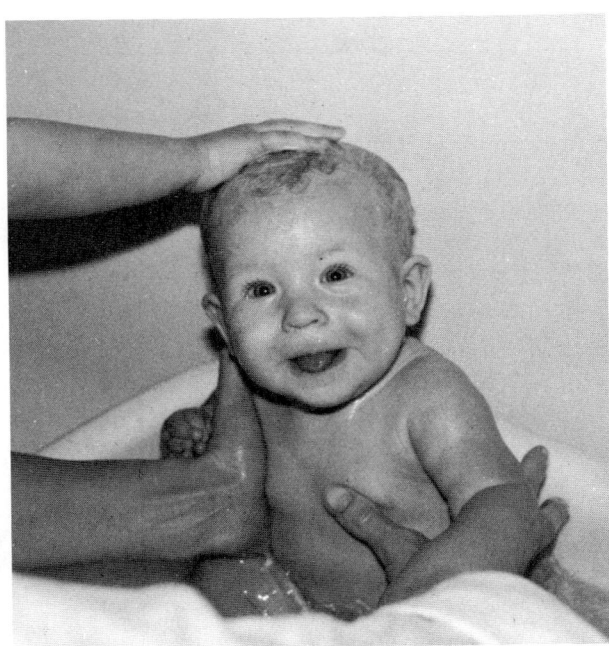

Fig. 27-2. Temperament makes infants respond to new experiences in different ways. Here an infant demonstrates good adaptability to a new situation, a tub bath.

another will spend no more than a minute or two with each toy. Degree of persistence is also variable. Some infants will keep trying to perform an activity even when they fail time after time; others stop trying after one unsuccessful attempt.

THRESHOLD OF RESPONSIVENESS

Threshold of responsiveness is the intensity level of stimulation that is necessary to evoke a response. Infants with a low threshold of responsiveness need very little stimulation to evoke a reaction. Infants with a high threshold level do not react to mild stimuli; they need intense stimulation before they demonstrate a change in behavior.

MOOD QUALITY

The infant who is "always happy, always laughing" can be categorized as having a positive mood quality. The infant whose mother describes him as "always fussy, always cranky" has a negative mood quality. Obviously, the baby's mood pattern can make a major difference in the mother's enjoyment of the baby, and a mother who has fun with her baby is bound to spend more time with him than one whose baby reacts negatively.

Infants who have a normal activity level, a regular rhythmicity, who approach and adapt easily, who have a long attention span, high level of persistence, and a positive mood quality are "ideal" babies to care for. Much harder for new mothers to learn to care for are the highly active infants, especially if they demonstrate irregular physiological rhythms, withdraw rather than approach, and are nonadaptable.

It is good to talk to a mother about her child's reaction patterns, since these patterns tend to persist, and the way the child will react in the future depends a great deal on his present performance. The child who withdraws rather than approaches in breast-feeding may approach toilet training or starting school the same way. The mother will have to focus more on preparing the child for new activities than will the mother whose child approaches new situations easily. The mother who is aware that her baby shies away from new experiences, such as baths and new foods, will take it in her stride when he is slow in adapting to nursery school at age 4, knowing that this is her child's way.

It was in the natural course of events to notice such reaction patterns in children when extended families were common. Grandmothers, with their more objective view, observed and reported consistent nonadaptability or withdrawal patterns that busy mothers, involved in everyday care, did not have time to notice. Mothers are likely to remain unaware of these patterns unless nurses bring them to their attention before they take their babies home. Nurses who do so are giving good anticipatory guidance. If a new mother has difficulties with her new baby, she is likely to assume that it is her fault. If she is aware of temperamental differences in infants, some of the burden of guilt will be lifted. She will be able to accept her infant as being hard to manage. Understanding is the beginning of acceptance and respect for a child as an individual and is essential for successful child rearing.

References

1. Anderson, G. C. The mother and her newborn—mutual caregivers. *J.O.G.N. Nurs.* 6:50, 1977.
2. Brown, J. B. Infant temperament: A clue to childbearing for parents and nurses. *M.C.N.* 2:228, 1977.
3. Carey, W. A simplified method for measuring infant temperament. *J. Pediatr.* 77:188, 1970.
4. deChateau, P. The influence of early contact on maternal and infant behavior in primiparae. *Birth Fam. J.* 4:149, 1977.
5. Duvall, E. M. *Family Development* (4th ed.). Philadelphia: Lippincott, 1971.
6. Erikson, E. *Childhood and Society* (2nd ed.). New York: Norton, 1963.
7. Giovanetti, A. Parenting: Impact on the firstborn. *Compr. Pediatr. Nurs.* 2:1, 1977.

8. Gollober, M. A comment on the need for postpartal father-infant interaction. *J.O.G.N. Nurs.* 5:17, 1977.
9. Grimes, D. A. Routine circumcision reconsidered. *Am. J. Nurs.* 80:108, 1980.
10. Harlow, H. F., and Zimmerman, R. Affectional Responses in the Infant Monkey. In P. Mussen, J. Conger, and J. Kagan (Eds.), *Readings in Child Development and Personality* (2nd ed.). New York: Harper & Row, 1970.
11. Klaus, M. H., et al. Human maternal behavior at the first contact with her young. *Pediatrics* 46:187, 1970.
12. Klaus, M. H., et al. Maternal attachment: Importance of the first post-partum days. *N. Engl. J. Med.* 286:460, 1972.
13. Klaus, M. H., and Kennell, J. H. Mothers separated from their newborn infants. *Pediatr. Clin. North Am.* 17:1015, 1970.
14. Klaus, M. H., and Kennell, J. H. *Maternal-Infant Bonding*. St. Louis: Mosby, 1976.
15. Oliver, C. M., et al. Gentle birth: Its safety and its effect on neonatal behavior. *J.O.G.N. Nurs.* 7:35, 1978.
16. Provence, S. Developmental History. In R. Cooke and S. Levin (Eds.), *The Biologic Basis of Pediatric Practice*, Vol. 2. New York: McGraw-Hill, 1968.
17. Ringler, N. M., et al. Mother-to-child speech at two years—effects of early postnatal contact. *J. Pediatr.* 86:143, 1975.
18. Snyder, C., et al. New findings about mother's antenatal expectations and the relationship to infant development. *M.C.N.* 4:358, 1979.
19. Thomas, A., et al. *Behavioral Individuality in Early Childhood*. New York: New York University Press, 1971.

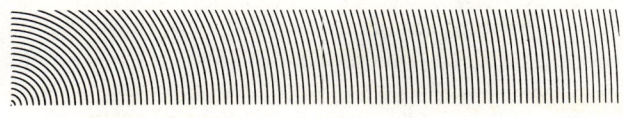

28. Physiological Development in the Newborn

A newborn undergoes profound physiological changes at the moment of birth and probably psychological changes as well. He is released from a warm, snug, darkened, liquid-filled environment in which all his basic needs were met. Suddenly he is in a chilly, glaring, unbounded, gravity-based outside world.

Within minutes of being plunged into this strange environment, the newborn's body must initiate respirations and accommodate the circulatory system to extrauterine oxygenation. Within 24 hours his neurological, renal, endocrine, gastrointestinal, and metabolic functions must be operating competently in order for his life to be sustained.

How well the newborn can achieve these major adjustments will depend on his genetic endowment, the competency of his intrauterine environment, the concern and management he received during the labor and delivery period, and the concern and management he receives as a neonate. Nursing has a major contribution to make at all these stages.

The neonatal period is usually defined as the time from birth through the first 28 days of life.

Half of the neonatal deaths occur in the first 24 hours after birth, an indication of how hazardous a time this is for the infant and the close observation for indications of distress he needs at this time. During the first 24 hours, nursing care has a number of important goals.

1. It should meet the newborn's physiological and psychological needs. This purpose includes initiating and maintaining effective respirations, adequate nutrition, and provision of a feeling of being loved and secure. This aim is best met by including and encouraging the mother in the infant's care.
2. It should aim toward keeping the newborn safe from environmental harm such as chilling or infection.
3. It should include a physical assessment of the newborn to help determine his true gestation age, the general state of his health, and the presence of any congenital anomalies or birth injuries, and to establish a baseline for further estimation of health.
4. It should include assisting the mother or parents of the child to adjust to her or their new roles and teaching the parents how to care for their child after discharge from the hospital.
5. It should aim to lay a foundation of good health concepts that the developing family will assimilate and continue to follow through the coming years.

A Newborn Profile

It is not unusual to hear the comment that "all newborns are alike" from people viewing a nursery full of babies. In actuality, every child is born with individual physical and personality characteristics that make him unique right from the start.

Some infants are born stocky and short, some large and bony, some thin and rangy. Some have a temperament that causes them to feed greedily, protest procedures loudly, and perhaps respond to their mother's inexperienced handling with restlessness and spitting up. Other infants appear to protest little, to sleep soundly, to accept passively this new step in life.

As you gain experience in working with newborns, it becomes easier to differentiate infants who are merely demonstrating the extremes of normal newborn characteristics from those whose behavior or appearance indicates a need for more skilled care than is available in normal nursery surroundings.

WEIGHT

The birth weight of newborn infants differs, depending on the racial, nutritional, intrauterine, and genetic factors that were present during conception and pregnancy. The weight in relation to the gestation age should be plotted on a standard neonatal graph like the one shown in Fig. 28-1, so that it can be interpreted meaningfully. Plotting in this manner helps to identify infants at risk and to separate those who

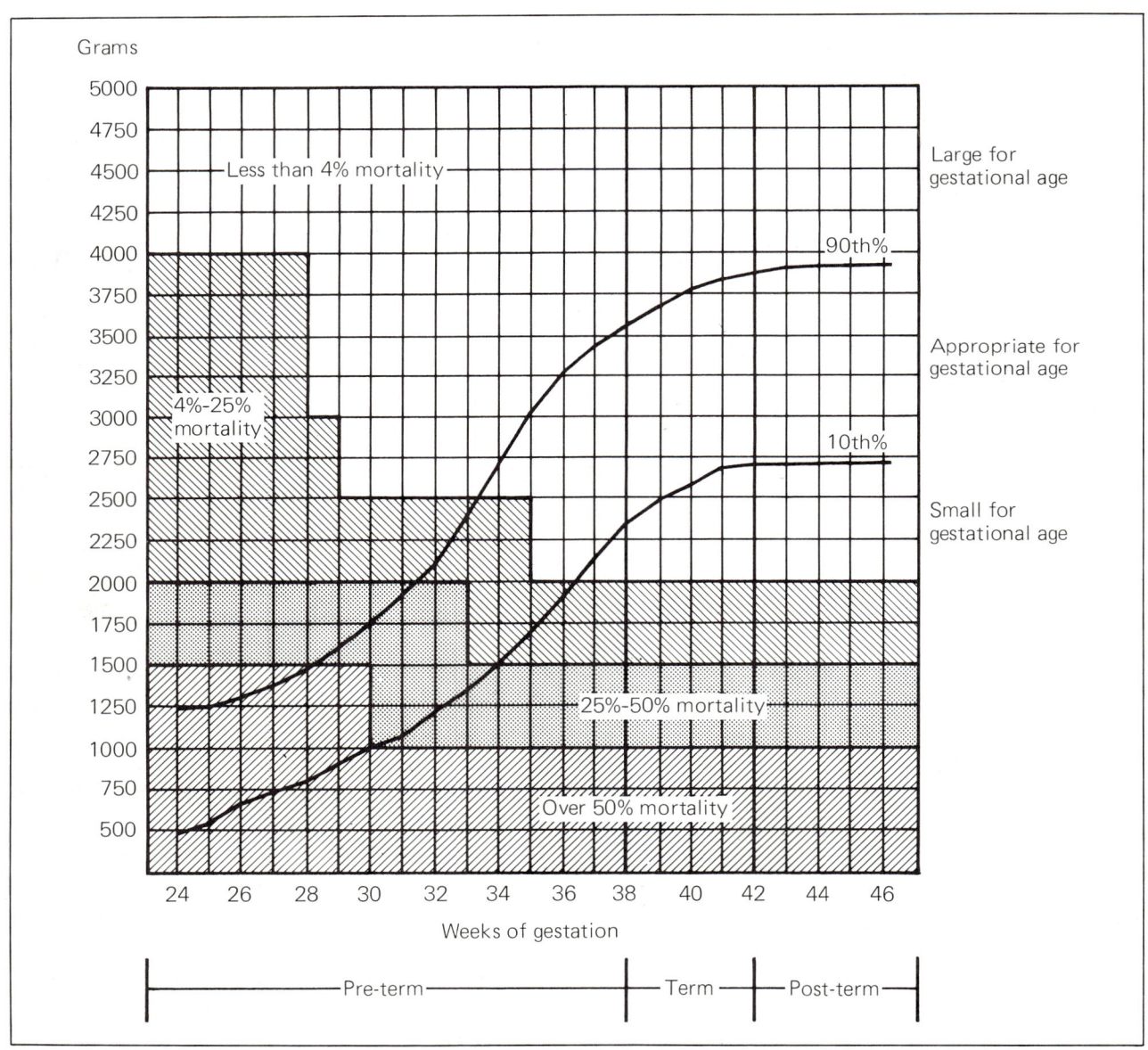

Fig. 28-1. Classification of newborns by birth weight and gestation age and by neonatal mortality risk. (From F. C. Battaglia and L. O. Lubchenco, J. Pediatr. 71:161, 1967.)

are small for their gestation age (children who have suffered intrauterine growth retardation) from low-birth-weight infants (infants who are a good weight for their gestation age, formerly termed *premature*). These first measurements also serve to establish a baseline for future measurements.

A reason for plotting weight, height, and head circumference is to point out disproportionate measurements. All three of these measurements should fall close to the same percentile for the same child. An infant who falls within the 50th percentile for height and weight and whose head circumference is in the 90th percentile may have abnormal head growth. A newborn who is in the 50th percentile for weight and head circumference but in the 3rd percentile for height may have a growth problem such as achondroplastic dwarfism.

As a rule of thumb, Caucasian newborns generally weigh approximately a half pound more than children of other races (probably because of better nutrition in the mother during pregnancy). Second children generally weigh more than firstborns; weight continues to increase with each succeeding child in a family.

The average birth weight (the 50th percentile) for a white mature female newborn is 3.4 kg (7.5 pounds) and for a white mature male newborn, 3.5 kg (7.7 pounds). The arbitrary lower limit of normal is 2.5 kg (5.5 pounds). Under this weight the child is termed a low-birth-weight infant and is given high-risk priority. Birth weight exceeding 4.7 kg (10 pounds) is unusual, but weights as high as 7.7 kg (17 pounds) have been documented. When an infant over 4.7 kg is born, a maternal illness such as diabetes mellitus must be suspected.

The newborn loses 5 to 10 percent of his birth weight (6 to 10 ounces) during the first few days after birth. This weight loss occurs because the infant is no longer under the influence of maternal hormones (which are salt- and fluid-retaining); he voids and passes stools; and his intake until about the third day of life is limited by the relatively low caloric content of colostrum, the fluid preceding breast milk (or feeding of glucose water if he is bottle-fed), and he may have beginning difficulty in establishing sucking.

Following this initial loss of weight, the newborn has one day of stable weight and then will begin to gain about 2 pounds a month (6 to 8 ounces weekly) for the first six months of life.

LENGTH

The average birth length (the 50th percentile) of a white mature infant female is 53 cm (20.9 inches). For white mature males it is 54 cm (21.3 inches). The lower limit of normal length is arbitrarily set at 46 cm (18 inches). Below this limit the child is considered to be preterm. Babies with a length as great as 57.5 cm (23 inches) have been reported.

HEAD CIRCUMFERENCE

The head circumference is 34 to 35 cm (13.5 to 14.01 inches) in a mature newborn. A mature newborn with a head circumference greater than 37 cm or less than 33 cm (14.8 or 13.2 inches) should be carefully investigated for neurological damage, although occasionally a newborn will fall within these limits and still be perfectly normal. Head circumference is measured with a tape measure drawn across the center of the forehead and the most prominent portion of the posterior head (the occiput) (Fig. 28-2).

CHEST CIRCUMFERENCE

The chest circumference in a newborn is about 2 cm (¾ to 1 inch) less than head circumference. It is measured at the level of the nipples. If a large amount of breast tissue or edema of the breast is present, this measurement will not be accurate until the initial edema has subsided.

Vital Signs
TEMPERATURE

The temperature of a newborn is about 37.2°C (99°F) at the moment of birth because he has been confined

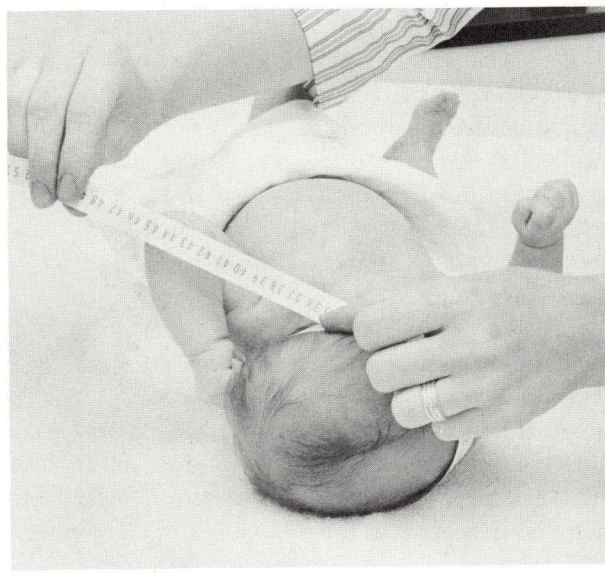

Fig. 28-2. Head circumference is measured between points just above the eyebrows to the protuberant point of the occiput. (Courtesy of the Department of Medical Photography, Children's Hospital, Buffalo, N.Y.)

in an internal body organ. His temperature falls almost immediately to below normal because of (1) heat loss, (2) his immature temperature-regulating mechanisms, (3) the 21° to 22°C (68° to 72°F) temperature of most delivery rooms. Newborns lose heat by four separate mechanisms: convection, conduction, radiation, and evaporation.

Convection is the flow of heat from the body surface to cooler surrounding air. The effectiveness of convection depends on the velocity of the flow (a current of air cools faster than nonmoving air). Being certain that there are no drafts from windows or air conditioners reduces convection heat loss.

Conduction is the transfer of body heat to a cooler solid object in contact with the baby. If the baby were laid on a cold counter, for example, or on the cold base of a warming unit, he would quickly lose heat to the colder metal surface.

Radiation is the transfer of body heat to a cooler solid object *not* in contact with the baby. A baby can lose heat by radiation to cold objects such as a cold window surface or an air conditioner across the room from him.

Evaporation is loss of heat through conversion of a liquid to a vapor. A newborn is wet; he loses a great deal of heat as the amniotic fluid on his skin evaporates. To prevent this rapid loss of heat, he should be dried immediately. Remember to dry his face; the head is a large surface area in an infant.

A newborn not only can lose heat easily by the above means but has difficulty conserving heat under any circumstances. Insulation, an efficient means of conserving heat in adults, is not effective in newborns as they have little subcutaneous fat to provide insulation. Shivering, a means of increasing metabolism and thereby providing heat, is rarely seen in newborns.

Newborns can conserve heat by constricting blood vessels. Brown fat, a special tissue found at no other period of life, apparently helps to conserve or produce body heat. Brown fat is found in greatest proportion in the intrascapular region, the thorax, and the perirenal area. It is thought to aid in the control of temperature in the neonate in much the same way it does in the hibernating animal.

Because newborns have difficulty conserving body heat, exposure to cold can be extremely detrimental at this time of life.

An infant exposed to cool air will kick and cry to increase his metabolic rate to produce more heat. This reaction, however, also increases his respiratory rate; the immature infant with poor lung development will have trouble making such an adjustment. An infant who cannot increase his respiratory rate in response to increased needs will be unable to deliver sufficient oxygen to his system. The resultant anaerobic catabolism of body cells releases acid. Every newborn is born slightly acidotic, and any new buildup of acid may lead to severe, life-threatening acidosis. The infant also becomes fatigued, and additional strain is thus placed on his already stressed cardiovascular system.

Drying and wrapping the newborn and placing him in a warmed crib or drying him and placing him under a radiant heat source are the best mechanical measures to help him conserve heat. All infant care should be done speedily to avoid exposing the infant unnecessarily. Any procedure during which the infant must be uncovered (e.g., resuscitation, circumcision) should be done under a radiant heat source to prevent damaging heat loss. If chilling is prevented, the newborn's temperature stabilizes at 37°C (98.6°F) within 4 hours after birth.

A few newborns run a transient fever between the second and fourth days of life; the temperature may rise as high as 40°C (104°F). The infant's skin will be dry, the fontanelles may be sunken, and urinary output may be decreased. This reaction tends to occur in infants who do not suck well or who for other reasons receive a lower-than-normal fluid intake during the first few days of life. The lowered intake, along with normal water loss, leads to a physiological fever. The condition can be relieved by increasing the amount of formula or giving water between regular milk feedings. If oral intake is a problem, intravenous fluid may be given. With the increase in fluid, the dehydration and symptomatic fever disappear.

A newborn who has a bacterial infection may, in contrast to an adult, run a subnormal temperature. Therefore, when a neonate's temperature does not stabilize shortly after birth, the cause should be investigated so that corrective measures can be taken.

PULSE

The heart rate in utero averages 120 to 160 beats per minute. Immediately after birth, as the newborn struggles to initiate respirations, the heart rate may be as rapid as 180 beats per minute. Within an hour after birth, as the infant settles down to sleep, the heart rate falls to an average of 120 to 140 beats per minute, where it stabilizes.

The heart rate of a neonate is often irregular because of immaturity of the cardiac regulatory center in the medulla. Transient murmurs may be due to the incomplete closure of fetal circulation shunts. During crying, the rate may rise again to 180 beats per minute.

The femoral pulses can be felt readily in a newborn, but the radial and temporal pulses are more difficult to palpate with any degree of accuracy. Thus, a newborn's heart rate should always be determined by listening for an apical heartbeat for a full minute. It is important that the femoral pulses be palpated, since their absence suggests possible coarctation (narrowing) of the aorta.

RESPIRATIONS

The respiratory rate of a newborn at birth may be as high as 80 respirations per minute. As respiratory activity is established and maintained, the rate settles to an average of 30 to 60 per minute when the child is at rest. Respiratory depth, rate, and rhythm are likely to be irregular, and the short periods of apnea (without cyanosis) that may occur are normal. Respirations can be observed most easily by watching the movement of the abdomen, since breathing primarily involves the use of the diaphragm and abdominal muscles.

The coughing and sneezing reflexes present at birth clear the airway. Neonates are nose-breathers and show signs of acute distress if the nostrils become obstructed. Short periods of crying increase the depth of respirations and aid in aerating deep portions of the lungs and so are beneficial to the newborn. Long periods of crying exhaust the cardiovascular system and have no purpose. This is an important fact for the mother to know.

BLOOD PRESSURE

The blood pressure of a newborn is approximately 80/46 mm Hg at birth. By the tenth day it rises to about 100/50 mm Hg. Blood pressure is not routinely measured in newborns unless certain cardiac anomalies are suspected. The blood pressure tends to increase with crying (and a newborn cries when disturbed and manipulated by such procedures as taking blood pressure). Thus blood pressure readings in the newborn are somewhat inaccurate. The cuff width used must be no more than two-thirds the length of the upper arm or thigh for any degree of accuracy to be achieved.

A flush method may be used to take blood pressures in infants: Apply a blood pressure cuff to the child's upper arm or the thigh. Wrap the portion of the extremity distal to the cuff with an Ace bandage. Inflate the blood pressure cuff to about 200 mm Hg of pressure; remove the Ace bandage. The skin distal to the cuff will appear pale. Release pressure in the cuff slowly until the distal portion of the extremity flushes (becomes pink). Read the manometer at this point. Flush pressure is about halfway between systolic and diastolic blood pressure. If the newborn's blood pressure is 80/40, for example, the flush pressure will be about 60 (Fig. 28-3).

Newer ultrasonic or Doppler methods of taking blood pressure are effective with newborns and more accurate than traditional measuring.

Cardiovascular System

Changes in the cardiovascular system are necessary at birth because the blood was formerly oxygenated by the placenta and now must be oxygenated by the lungs. When the cord is clamped, the newborn is forced to take in oxygen through the lungs. As the lungs are inflated for the first time, pressure in the chest in general and particularly in the artery leading to the lungs (pulmonary artery) is greatly decreased. This decrease in pressure in the pulmonary artery plays a role in causing the ductus arteriosus to close. As pressure increases in the left side of the heart from increased blood volume, the foramen ovale closes on account of the pressure against the lip of the structure. Since the remaining fetal circulatory structures —the umbilical vein, two umbilical arteries, and the ductus venosus—are no longer receiving blood, the blood within them clots, and the vessels atrophy.

Figure 28-4 shows the respiratory and cardiovascular changes at birth. These changes in the cardiovascular system begin to occur with the first breath. Table 28-1 shows the timetable of obliteration of fetal cardiovascular structures.

TOTAL BLOOD VOLUME

As the uterus contracts after the birth of the baby, an additional 50 to 125 ml of blood is pushed into the umbilical cord and into the newborn's circulation. The cord pulsates. If the cord is cut before the pulsating ceases, the newborn will not receive this additional blood.

On balance, additional blood appears to be helpful to most newborns. It increases the infant's store of hemoglobin for the months ahead when iron intake will be low because of a diet that is predominantly milk. However, the additional blood may be harmful to infants who are Rh-sensitized, since it loads them with even more maternal antibodies. Further, because infants are already polycythemic, the additional blood

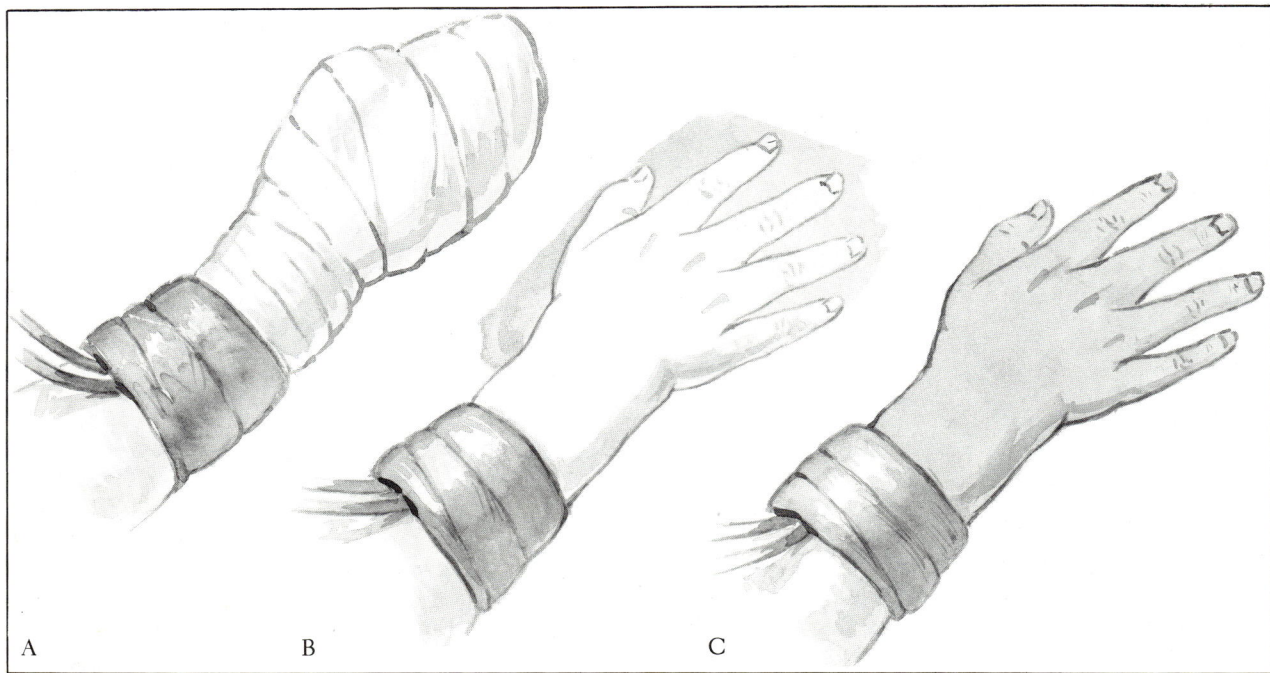

Fig. 28-3. Technique for measuring flush blood pressure. A. A blood pressure cuff is applied. The distal extremity is wrapped snugly with an Ace bandage. B. The blood pressure cuff is inflated; the Ace bandage is removed. C. As pressure in the cuff is released, the pressure at which the distal extremity "flushes" or pinkens is the flush blood pressure. (Courtesy of the Department of Medical Illustration, State University of New York at Buffalo.)

may lead to pulmonary edema from an overload of circulating blood. Finally, pulmonary rales and transient cyanosis appear to be associated with late clamping of the cord in some infants.

The peripheral circulation of the newborn remains sluggish for at least the first 24 hours. It is not uncommon to observe cyanosis in the feet and hands and for the feet to feel cold to the touch for this period of time (acrocyanosis).

BLOOD VALUES

Because of the nature of fetal circulation, a baby is born with a high erythrocyte count, around 6 million per cubic millimeter. The newborn's hemoglobin level averages 17 to 18 gm per 100 ml of blood. Hematocrit is about 52%. Once proper lung oxygenation is established, the need for the high erythrocyte count diminishes. Therefore, within a matter of days, the erythrocyte count begins to fall. The decrease reaches its lowest level at 3 months of age (the life span of red blood cells), when the hemoglobin level may be as low as 11 or 12 gm per 100 ml of blood. Although this is a normal decrease, an iron supplement should be added early to an infant's diet to keep the decline at a minimum.

A newborn has an equally high white blood count at birth, about 15,000 to 45,000 cells per cubic millimeter. Polymorphonuclear cells (neutrophils) account for a large part of this leukocytosis, but by the end of the first month, lymphocytes become the predominant type. It should be remembered that this leukocytosis is a response to the trauma of birth and is nonpathogenic; an increased white cell count should not be taken as evidence of infection. On the other hand, although the high white cell count makes infection difficult to prove in a newborn, infection must not be dismissed as a possibility if other signs of infection (e.g., pallor, respiratory difficulty, or cyanosis) are present.

Blood values in the newborn are summarized in Table 28-2.

BLOOD COAGULATION

The majority of newborns are born with a prolonged coagulation or prothrombin time because their blood levels of vitamin K are lower than normal. Vitamin K is synthesized through the action of intestinal flora and is necessary for the formation of Factor VII (proconvertin), Factor IX (plasma thromboplastin component), and Factor X (Stuart-Prower factor). A newborn intestine is sterile at birth unless membranes were ruptured more than 24 hours before delivery. Flora must therefore accumulate before vitamin K can be synthesized. Because almost all newborns have

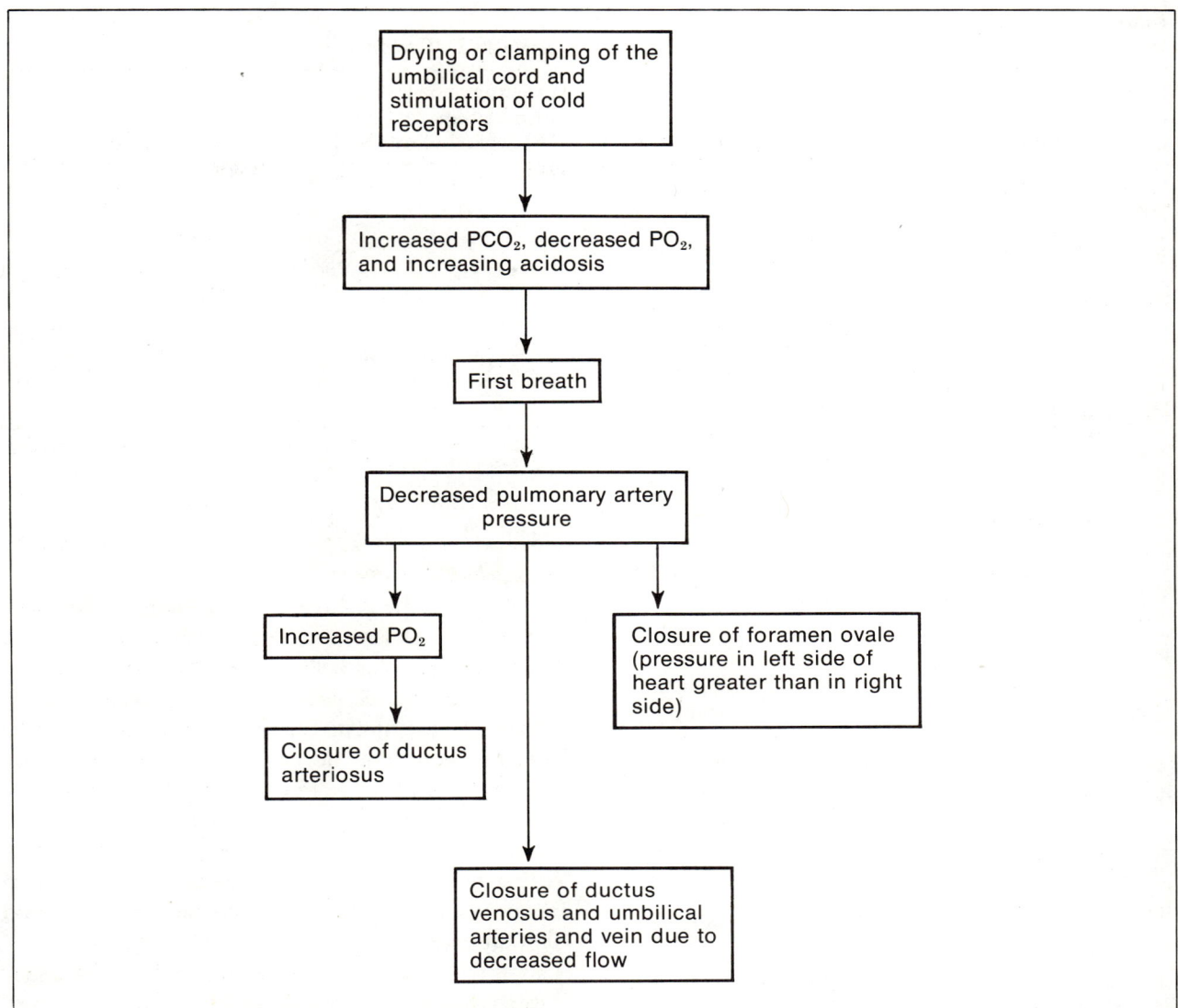

Fig. 28-4. Circulatory events at birth.

Table 28-1. Changes in the Cardiovascular System at Birth

Structure	Approximate Time of Obliteration	Structure Remaining
Foramen ovale	1 year (probe patent)	Fossa ovalis
Ductus arteriosus	1 month	Ligamentum arteriosum
Ductus venosus	2 months	Ligamentum venosum
Umbilical arteries	2–3 months	Lateral umbilical ligament Interior iliac artery
Umbilical vein	2–3 months	Ligamentum teres (round ligament of liver)

Source: Adapted from M. L. Moore, *The Newborn and the Nurse*. Philadelphia: Saunders, 1972.

poor blood coagulation, vitamin K (AquaMEPHYTON) is given routinely to newborns in most hospital delivery rooms.

Respiratory System

The first breath of an infant is initiated by a combination of cold receptors, a lowered PO_2, and an increased PCO_2. A first breath requires a tremendous amount of energy to pull in. A pressure of about 40 to 70 cm H_2O is required. The presence of lung fluid is a mechanism that makes the first breath easier than if dry alveolar walls had to be pulled apart to inflate alveoli. Lung fluid is quickly absorbed by lung blood vessels and lymphatics.

Breaths following the first one are easier, requiring only about 6 to 8 cm H_2O of pressure. Within 10 minutes of birth, an infant has established a good re-

Table 28-2. Hematology Values in Newborns, Neonates, and Infants

Determination (Whole Blood Unless Otherwise Indicated)	Normal Value
Hematocrit (vol %)	
Newborn	44–64%
Neonate	35–49%
Infant	30–40%
Hemoglobin	
Newborn	14–24 gm/100 ml
Neonate	11–20 gm/100 ml
Infant	10–15 gm/100 ml
Hemoglobin, fetal (Hb F)	
Newborn	40–70% of total
Neonate	20–40% of total
Infant	2–10% of total
Nucleated red blood cells	
Cord	250–500/mm^3
Day 1	200–300/mm^3
Day 2	20–30/mm^3
Thereafter	0
Platelet count	
Premature	100–300,000/mm^3
Newborn	140–300,000/mm^3
Neonate	150–390,000/mm^3
Infant	200–473,000/mm^3
Red blood cell count (RBC)	
Newborn	4.8–7.1 million/mm^3
Neonate	4.1–6.4 million/mm^3
Infant	3.8–5.5 million/mm^3
Blood indexes	
Mean corpuscular hemoglobin (MCH)	
Newborn	32–34 $\mu\mu$g
Thereafter	27–31 $\mu\mu$g
Mean corpuscular volume (MCV)	
Newborn	96–108 μ^3
Thereafter	82–91 μ^3
Mean corpuscular hemoglobin concentration (MCHC)	
Newborn	32–33%
Thereafter	32–36%
Reticulocyte count	
Newborn	2.5–6.5% total RBC
Neonate	0.1–1.5% total RBC
Infant	0.5–3.1% total RBC
Erythrocyte sedimentation rate (ESR) (uncorrected)	
Newborn	0–2 mm/hr
Neonate and infant	3–13 mm/hr
White blood cell count (WBC)	
Newborn, total	9,000–30,000/mm^3
% neutrophils	61%
% lymphocytes	31%
1 week, total	5,000–21,000/mm^3
% neutrophils	45%
% lymphocytes	41%
4 weeks, total	5,000–19,500/mm^3
% neutrophils	35%
% lymphocytes	56%
6–12 months, total	6,000–17,500/mm^3
% neutrophils	32%
% lymphocytes	61%

Source: V. C. Vaughan, III, and R. J. McKay (Eds.), *Textbook of Pediatrics*. Philadelphia: Saunders, 1975. Pp. 1792–1793.

sidual volume. By 10 to 12 hours of age, vital capacity is established at infant proportions.

An infant who is delivered by cesarean section does not have as much lung fluid expelled at birth as a baby delivered vaginally. He is therefore likely to have more difficulty with establishing effective respirations. An infant who is immature and whose alveoli collapse each time he exhales (lack of pulmonary surfactant) has trouble in establishing an effective residual capacity and so in establishing effective respirations. If alveoli do not open well, the infant's cardiac system is compromised as closure of the foramen ovale and ductus arteriosus depends on free blood flow through the pulmonary artery and good oxygenation of blood. An infant who has difficulty establishing respirations at birth should be examined closely in the postpartal period for a cardiac murmur or indication that he still has patent cardiac structures that did not close.

Gastrointestinal System

Although the gastrointestinal tract is usually sterile at birth, bacteria may be cultured from the intestinal tract in most babies within 5 hours after birth; at 24 hours of life they can be cultured from all babies. Bacteria enter the tract via the infant's mouth. Some mouth bacteria are airborne; others may come from vaginal secretions at the time of birth, from hospital bedding, and from contact at the breast. Accumulation of bacteria in the gastrointestinal tract is necessary for digestion as well as for the synthesis of vitamin K. Since milk, the infant's main diet for the first year, is low in vitamin K, this intestinal synthesis is necessary.

The newborn has limited ability to digest fat and

starch because the pancreatic enzymes lipase and amylase are deficient for the first few months of life.

STOOLS

The first stool of the newborn is usually passed within 24 hours after birth and consists of meconium, a sticky, tar-like, blackish green, odorless material formed from mucus, vernix, lanugo, hormones, and carbohydrates that have accumulated during intrauterine life. An infant who does not pass a meconium stool by 24 hours after birth should be examined for the possibility of meconium ileus, imperforate anus, or bowel obstruction.

About the second or third day of life, in response to the feeding pattern, the newborn stool changes in color and consistency, becoming green and loose. This is termed a *transitional stool*, which may resemble diarrhea to the untrained eye. By the fourth day of life, breast-fed infants pass three or four light yellow stools per day. These are sweet-smelling, because breast milk is high in lactic acid, which reduces the amount of putrefactive organisms in the stool. An infant who receives formula usually passes two to three bright yellow stools a day. These have a slightly more noticeable odor than do breast-fed babies' stools.

When solid foods are introduced into the infant's diet, the stools again change, gradually becoming like the brown, odorous stools of adults. An infant placed under phototherapy lights to be treated for jaundice will have bright green stools because of increased bilirubin excretion.

Make a habit of inspecting newborn stools and recording their color, consistency (soft, hard), and size (small, medium, large). If mucus is mixed with the stool, milk allergy or some other irritant factor should be suspected. Newborns with obstruction of the bile ducts will have clay-colored (gray) stools because the bile pigments do not enter the intestinal tract. If the stools remain black or tarry, intestinal bleeding should be suspected. Blood-flecked stools usually indicate an anal fissure. Occasionally, a newborn swallows some maternal blood during delivery and will either vomit fresh blood immediately after birth or pass a tarry stool in two or more days. Maternal blood may be differentiated from fetal blood by an Apt test.

Urinary System

The newborn should void within 24 hours after birth. The first voiding may be pink or dusky because of uric acid crystals that were formed in the bladder in utero. An infant who is not fed for 12 to 16 hours after birth may take a little longer to void, but the 24-hour cutoff point is a good rule of thumb. Infants who do not void within this time should be examined. Possible causes are urethral stenosis and absent kidneys or ureters.

The presence of obstruction in the urinary tract can be tested by observing the force of the urinary stream in both male and female infants. Male newborns should void forcefully, so that urine forms a small projected arc. Female newborns should void with enough force so that the urine forms a stream, and voiding is not just continuous dribbling. Urine that is projected farther than normal may also be a sign of urethral obstruction. A normal urine stream is evidence that there is no major constriction of the urinary tract and is an indication of good kidney function.

The kidneys of newborns do not concentrate urine well, and thus the urine is usually light in color and odorless. The infant is about 6 weeks of age before much control over reabsorption of fluid in tubules is evident.

The daily urinary output for the first one or two days is about 30 to 60 ml total. By one week, total volume has risen to about 200 ml. A small amount of protein may be present in voidings the first few days of life until kidney glomeruli more fully mature.

Autoimmune System

The newborn infant has difficulty forming antibodies against invading antigens until he reaches 2 months of age. This is the reason immunizations against childhood diseases are not given to babies less than 2 months old. However, the infant at birth has antibodies (IgG) from his mother that have crossed the placenta—in most instances antibodies against poliomyelitis, measles, diphtheria, pertussis, rubella, and tetanus. There is little natural immunity transmitted against varicella (chickenpox) or herpes simplex. Hospital personnel with herpes simplex eruptions (cold sores) should not be allowed to work near newborns. Herpes simplex II virus becomes systemic in the newborn, a rapidly fatal form of the disease.

Neuromuscular System

A mature newborn demonstrates general neuromuscular function by moving his extremities and attempting to control head movement. Limpness or total absence of a muscular response to manipulation is never normal and suggests narcosis, shock, or cerebral injury. The newborn occasionally makes twitching or flailing movements of his extremities in the absence of a stimulus because of the immaturity of his nervous system.

REFLEXES

A multitude of reflexes are present and can be tested in a newborn infant. Those that can be elicited with consistency by using simple maneuvers will be discussed briefly.

Blink Reflex

A blink reflex in a newborn serves the same purpose as it does in an adult, that is, to protect the eye from any object coming near it by rapid eyelid closure. It may be elicited by shining a strong light such as a flashlight or otoscope light on the eye. It can rarely be elicited by a sudden movement toward the eye.

Rooting Reflex

If a newborn's cheek is brushed or stroked near the corner of his mouth, the child will turn his head in that direction. This reflex serves to help the baby find food. As the mother holds the child and allows her breast to brush the baby's cheek, the baby will turn toward the breast. The reflex disappears about the sixth week of life. At about this time, the eyes focus steadily and a food source can be seen. Thus the reflex is no longer needed.

Sucking Reflex

When the infant's lips are touched, he makes a sucking motion. Thus, as his lips touch the mother's breast or a bottle, he sucks and so takes in food. The sucking reflex begins to diminish at about 6 months of age. It disappears immediately if it is never stimulated—for example, in a newborn with a tracheoesophageal fistula who is not allowed to take oral fluids. It can be maintained in such an infant by offering the child a pacifier after the fistula has been corrected by surgery and until he can take oral feedings normally.

Swallowing Reflex

The swallowing reflex in the newborn and in the adult is the same phenomenon. Food that reaches the posterior portion of the tongue will be automatically swallowed. (Gag, cough, and sneeze reflexes are also present in order to maintain a clear airway in the event that normal swallowing does not keep the pharynx free of obstructing mucus.)

Extrusion Reflex

If any substance is placed on the anterior portion of the infant's tongue, he will extrude it. This is a protective reflex to prevent him from swallowing inedible substances. The reflex disappears at about 4 months of age. Until then the infant may seem to be spitting out or refusing solid food placed in his mouth.

Palmar Grasp Reflex

When an object is placed in a newborn's palm, the child will grasp it by closing his fingers on it (Fig. 28-5). The mature newborn grasps so strongly that he can actually be raised from a supine position and be suspended momentarily from the examiner's fingers. The reflex disappears at about age 6 weeks to 3 months. The baby begins to grasp meaningfully at about 3 months of age.

Plantar Grasp Reflex

When an object touches the sole of the newborn's foot at the base of the toes, his toes grasp in the same manner as his fingers do. The reflex disappears at about 8 to 9 months of age in preparation for walking although it may be present in sleep for a longer period of time.

Step (Walk)-in-Place Reflex

When a newborn is held in a vertical position and his feet touch a hard surface, he will take a few quick alternating steps (Fig. 28-6). This reflex disappears by 3 months of age. By 4 months of age, the baby can bear a good portion of his weight unhindered by this reflex.

Placing Reflex

The placing reflex is similar to the step-in-place reflex, except it is elicited by touching the anterior surface of the newborn's leg against the edge of the

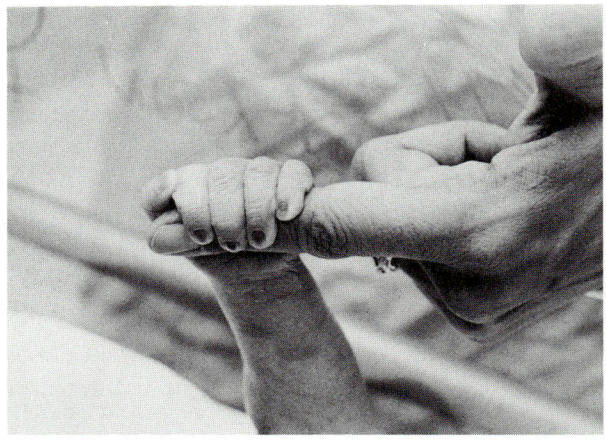

Fig. 28-5. Palmar grasp reflex. (Courtesy of the Department of Medical Photography, Children's Hospital, Buffalo, N.Y.)

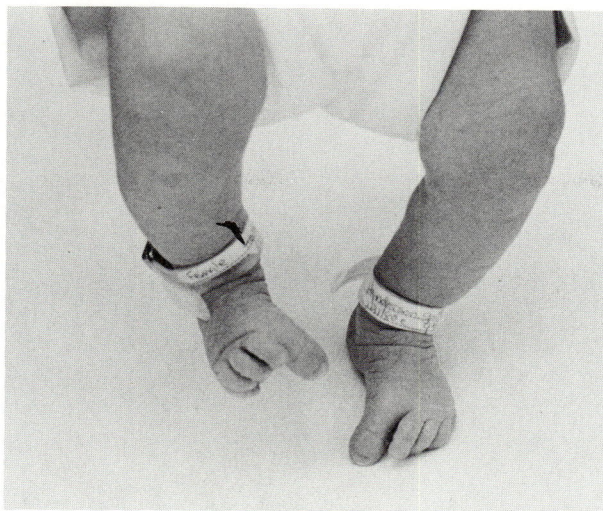

Fig. 28-6. Step-in-place reflex. (Courtesy of the Department of Medical Photography, Children's Hospital, Buffalo, N.Y.)

bassinet or table. The newborn will make a few quick lifting motions as if to step up on the table.

Tonic Neck Reflex

When an infant lies on his back, his head usually turns to one side or the other. The arm and the leg on the side to which his head turns extend, and the opposite arm and leg contract (Fig. 28-7). If you turn his head to the opposite side, he will often change the extension and contraction of his legs and arms accordingly. The movement is most evident in the arms, but should also be observed in the legs. This reflex is also called a *boxer* or *fencing reflex* because the infant's position simulates that of someone preparing to box or fence. Unlike many other reflexes, the tonic neck reflex does not appear to have a function. However, it does stimulate eye coordination, since the extended arm moves in front of the face. It may signify handedness. The reflex disappears between the second and third months of life.

Moro Reflex

A Moro (startle) reflex (Fig. 28-8) can be initiated by startling the infant by a loud noise or by jarring his bassinet. The most accurate method of eliciting the reflex is to hold the infant in a supine position and allow his head to drop backward an inch or so. He abducts and extends his arms and legs. His fingers assume a typical C position. He then brings his arms into an embrace position and pulls up his legs against his abdomen (adduction). The reflex simulates the

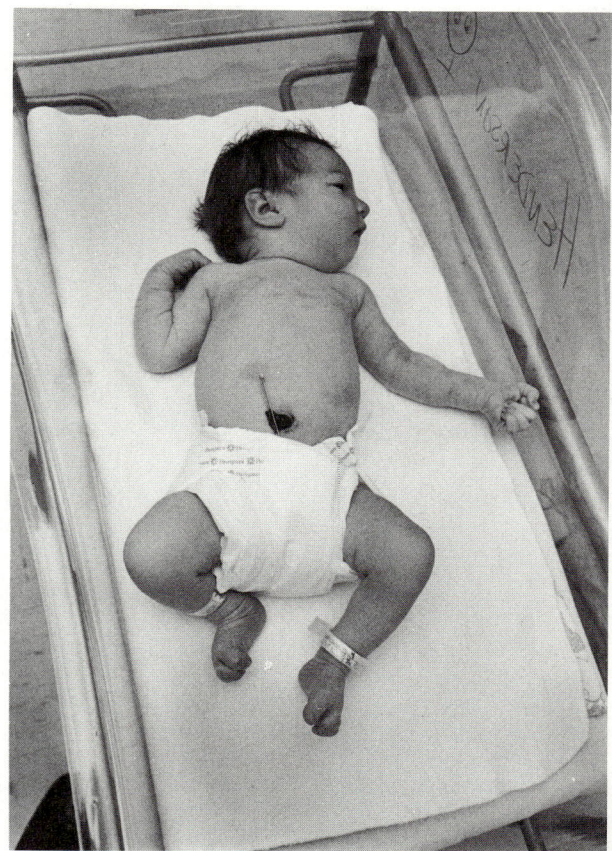

Fig. 28-7. Tonic neck reflex. (Courtesy of the Department of Medical Photography, Children's Hospital, Buffalo, N.Y.)

action of someone trying to ward off an attacker, then covering up to protect himself. The reflex is strong for the first eight weeks of life. It fades by the end of the fourth or fifth month, when the infant can roll away from danger.

Babinski Reflex

When the side of the sole of a newborn's foot is stroked in a J curve from the heel upward, the newborn fans his toes (positive Babinski sign) in contrast to the adult, who flexes his toes. This reaction occurs because of the immature stage of nervous system development. It remains positive (toes fan) until at least 3 months of age, when it is supplanted by the downgoing or flexing adult response.

Magnet Reflex

If pressure is applied to the soles of the feet of an infant lying in a supine position, he pushes back against the pressure. This and the two following reflexes are tests of spinal cord integrity.

Physiological Development in the Newborn

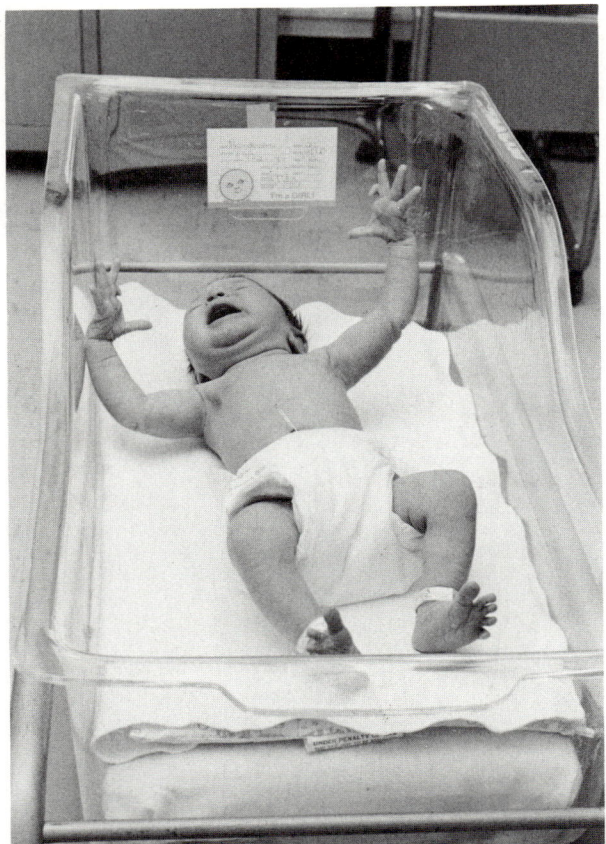

Fig. 28-8. Moro reflex. (Courtesy of the Department of Medical Photography, Children's Hospital, Buffalo, N.Y.)

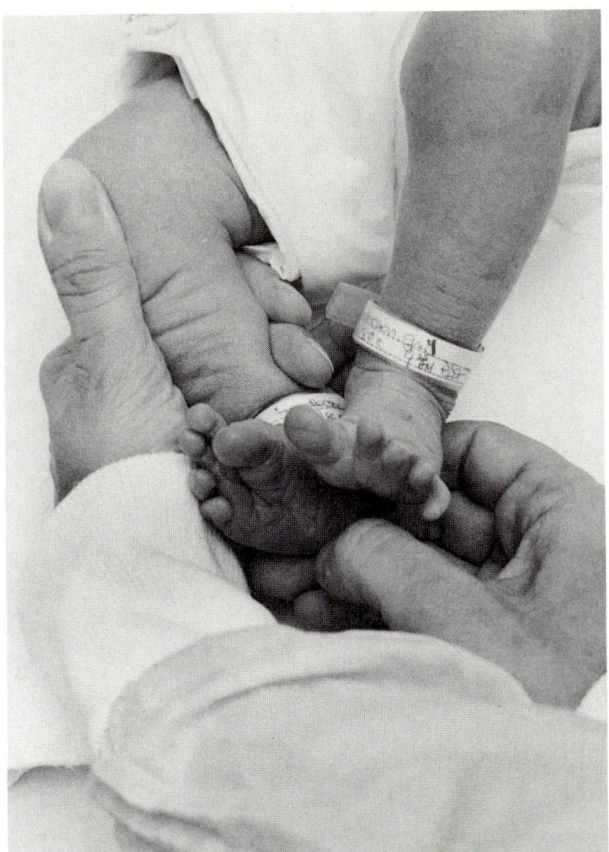

Fig. 28-9. Crossed extension reflex. When the sole of the foot is irritated, the newborn makes an attempt to push away the irritating object. (Courtesy of the Department of Medical Photography, Children's Hospital, Buffalo, N.Y.)

Crossed Extension Reflex

If one leg of a newborn lying supine is extended and the sole of that foot is irritated by being rubbed with a sharp object such as a thumbnail, the newborn will raise the other leg and extend it as if trying to push away the hand irritating the first leg (Fig. 28-9).

Trunk Incurvation Reflex

When the newborn lies in a prone position and is touched along the paravertebral area by a probing finger, he will flex his trunk and swing his pelvis toward the touch (Fig. 28-10). This is an easy reflex to elicit and is another test of spinal cord integrity.

Landau Reflex

When a newborn is held in a prone position with a hand underneath him supporting his trunk, he should demonstrate some muscle tone. While he may not be able to lift his head or arch his back (as he will at 3 months of age), neither should he sag into an inverted U position. The latter response indicates extremely poor muscle tone, and such an infant needs referral for further investigation as to its cause.

SPECIAL SENSES

Recent investigation seems to show that special senses are much better developed than was previously believed.

Hearing

The newborn can hear as soon as amniotic fluid drains from or is absorbed from the middle ear by way of the eustachian tube—within hours after birth. The newborn appears to have difficulty locating sound (or at least may not turn toward a sound). Perhaps he must learn to interpret small differences between sounds arriving at his two ears at different times. He responds to a sound such as a bell ringing a short distance from his ear by generalized activity. If he is actively crying at the time the bell is rung, he will stop crying and seem to attend. Similarly, he calms in response to a soothing or motherly voice and startles at loud noises.

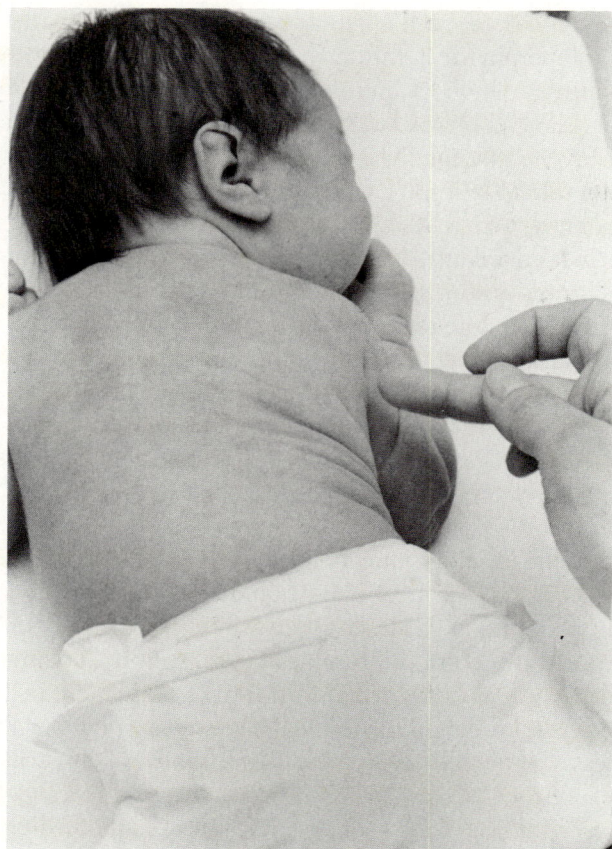

Fig. 28-10. Trunk incurvation reflex. When the paravertebral area is irritated, the newborn flexes his trunk. (Courtesy of the Department of Medical Photography, Children's Hospital, Buffalo, N.Y.)

Vision

Newborns see as soon as they are born and possibly have been "seeing" in utero for months. As the uterus and the abdominal wall stretch at the end of pregnancy, the fetus may be able to distinguish shadowy light and dark images. The newborn demonstrates sight at birth by blinking at a strong light (blink reflex) or following a bright light or toy a short distance with his eyes. Because he cannot follow past the midline of vision, he loses track of objects easily, so it is sometimes reported that he cannot see. His sight converges with accuracy at 6 to 8 weeks of age, and then he begins to follow objects well; at 3 months he can follow past the midline. A pupillary reflex is present from birth.

Touch

The sense of touch is well developed at birth. The infant demonstrates this ability by quieting at a soothing touch and by the presence of sucking and rooting reflexes, which are elicited by touch. He reacts to painful stimuli.

Taste

Taste buds are developed and functioning before birth to such an extent that the newborn has discriminatory ability. A fetus in utero will swallow amniotic fluid more rapidly than usual if glucose is added to sweeten its taste; the swallowing will decrease in amount if a bitter flavor is added. A newborn will turn away from a bitter taste such as salt but will readily accept the sweet taste of milk or glucose water.

Smell

The sense of smell is present in the newborn as soon as the nose is clear of mucus and amniotic fluid. A newborn turns toward his mother's breast partly out of his recognition of the smell of breast milk and partly as a manifestation of the rooting reflex.

Appearance of the Newborn

SKIN

Inspection of the skin of the newborn reveals many findings that are characteristic of the newborn period.

Color

Most mature newborns have a ruddy complexion because of the increased concentration of red blood cells in blood vessels and the decrease in the amount of subcutaneous fat, which makes the blood vessels more visible.

CYANOSIS. Localized cyanosis may occur because of immature peripheral circulation. The infant's lips, hands, and feet are very likely to appear cyanotic. Acrocyanosis is so prominent in some infants that a line seems to be drawn across the wrist or ankle, with pink skin on one side and blue on the other, as if some stricture were cutting off circulation. However, this is a normal phenomenon in the first 24 to 48 hours after birth.

Generalized mottling of the skin is common. Generalized cyanosis is always a cause for concern, since it usually indicates an underlying disease state.

It is important to observe the infant in both a quiet and a crying state. A newborn with atelectasis may be cyanotic when he is quiet and grow pink when he cries and aerates a larger number of alveoli. Infants with congenital heart disease, on the other hand, usually demonstrate the opposite pattern. Such an infant has normal color when he is quiet but becomes cyanotic when the activity of crying demands better oxygen transport than his damaged heart is able to supply.

Newborns are nose-breathers. Any infant whose posterior nares are obstructed by membrane or bone (bilateral choanal atresia) will be cyanotic, the degree of cyanosis depending on the extent of obstruction. You can help diagnose the cause of this form of cyanosis by holding a wisp of cotton in front of one of the nares (after compressing the opposite naris and closing the infant's mouth) and observing the cotton for movement on inspiration and expiration. Obstruction can also be detected by the infant's discomfort or by holding a stethoscope diaphragm next to the nares and listening for the sound of moving air.

Mucus obstructing the respiratory tract will cause sudden cyanosis and apnea in a newborn who had previously had a good color. Suctioning the mucus relieves the condition. Suctioning may be performed through the mouth if there appears to be a large amount of mucus at the back of the throat, but the nose should be suctioned as well because in the infant this is the chief conduit for air.

Cyanosis may result because of damage to the infant's central nervous system at birth. However, if such damage is the cause, the infant usually has other manifestations of damage as well: a very rigid or floppy muscle tone, a poor Apgar score, absence of a strong Moro reflex, or perhaps a high-pitched cry.

PALLOR. Pallor in newborns is usually the result of anemia. Anemia may be due to the following: excessive blood loss at the time the cord was cut; inadequate flow of blood from the cord into the infant at birth; fetal-maternal transfusion; low iron stores caused by poor maternal nutrition during pregnancy; or blood incompatibility in which a large number of red blood cells were hemolyzed in utero. It may be the result of internal bleeding (the baby should be watched closely for signs of blood in the stools or vomitus). Infants with central nervous system damage may appear pale as well as cyanotic. A gray color in newborns is generally indicative of infection. Twins may be born with a twin transfusion phenomenon, in which one twin is larger and has good color and the smaller twin has pallor.

JAUNDICE. Jaundice appears in about 50 percent of all newborns as a normal process of the breakdown of fetal red blood cells (physiological jaundice). The infant's skin and sclera of his eyes become yellow in color.

A fetus has a high red blood cell count to provide for more efficient oxygen and CO_2 transport while in utero. As red blood cells are destroyed (the high hemoglobin level immediately begins to be reduced), heme and globin are released. Globin is a protein component that is reused by the body and so is not a factor in the developing jaundice. Heme is further broken down into iron (which is also reused and so is not involved in the jaundice) and protoporphyrin. Protoporphyrin is further broken down into indirect bilirubin. Indirect bilirubin is fat-soluble and cannot be excreted by the kidneys in this state. It is therefore converted by the liver enzyme glucuronyl transferase into direct bilirubin, which is water-soluble, is incorporated into stool, and excreted in feces. In many newborn infants, liver function is so immature that the conversion to direct bilirubin cannot be made, and it therefore remains bilirubin in the indirect form. When the level of indirect bilirubin rises above 7 mg per 100 ml, bilirubin permeates tissue outside the circulatory system, and the infant begins to appear jaundiced. As long as the bilirubin remains in the circulatory system, the red of the red blood cells obscures its color.

If the level of indirect bilirubin rises above 10 to 12 mg per 100 ml, treatment should be considered. It is important that the level not rise above 20 mg per 100 ml. At this point, bilirubin interferes with the chemical synthesis of brain cells and causes permanent cell damage, a condition termed *kernicterus*, which will leave permanent neurological effects and possibly will cause mental retardation. If treatment for physiological jaundice in newborns is necessary, early feeding (to speed passage of feces through the intestine and prevent reabsorption of bilirubin from the bowel) and phototherapy (exposure of the infant to light to initiate maturation of liver enzymes) are the means generally instituted (see Chap. 38).

Some breast-fed babies have more difficulty in converting indirect bilirubin to direct bilirubin than do formula-fed babies because breast milk contains pregnanediol (a metabolite of progesterone), which depresses the action of glucuronyl transferase. Although stopping nursing in the first week of life must never be a decision taken lightly, if the level of indirect bilirubin rises above 10 mg per 100 ml, breast-feeding is usually halted for one to two days until the level falls again. If the mother expresses her milk manually for the few days that she is not breast-feeding, so that her milk supply does not decline, high indirect bilirubin is not a contraindication to breast-feeding.

Physiological jaundice generally occurs on the second or third day of life. Jaundice occurring in an infant under 24 hours old is usually a result of a blood incompatibility reaction. The old rule that jaundice is serious in an infant under 24 hours of age but not in one over 24 hours old is not an adequate assessment standard. No matter what the cause of jaundice, the level of indirect bilirubin must not be allowed to rise to damaging heights if the well-being and mental ca-

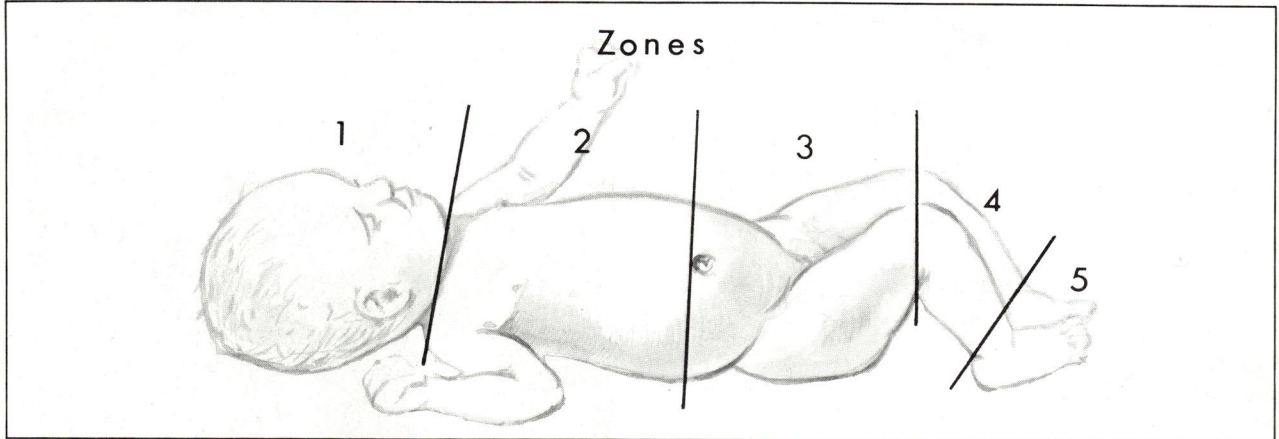

Fig. 28-11. Jaundice may be estimated to some degree by the zone on the child that it has reached. The indirect bilirubin level of zone 1 is 4 to 8 mg/100 ml; of zone 2, 5 to 12 mg/100 ml; of zone 3, 8 to 16 mg/100 ml; of zone 4, 11 to 18 mg/100 ml; of zone 5, 15 mg/100 ml. (Based on data from L. I. Kramer, Advancement of dermal icterus in the jaundiced newborn. Am. J. Dis. Child. 118:454, 1969.)

pabilities of the child are to be protected. Jaundice can be assessed grossly by inspection. Discoloration from jaundice begins in the head and is evident in the trunk and lower extremities only when it is extensive (Fig. 28-11).

Many hospital laboratories do not report indirect bilirubin levels; they report only the total bilirubin and the direct bilirubin level. To reveal the indirect level, you subtract the direct level from the total level report.

HARLEQUIN SIGN. Occasionally, because of immature circulation, an infant who has been lying on his side will appear red on the dependent side of his body and pale on the upper side, as if a line had been drawn down the center of his body. This is a transient phenomenon and, although startling, of no clinical significance. The odd coloring fades immediately if the newborn's position is changed or he kicks or cries vigorously.

Birthmarks

A number of commonly occurring birthmarks can be identified in newborns.

HEMANGIOMAS. The hemangiomas are vascular tumors of the skin. Three separate types are found.

Nevus flammeus (Fig. 28-12) is a macular purple or dark-red lesion (sometimes termed *port-wine* stain because of its deep color) that is present at birth. The lesions generally appear on the face, although they are often found on the thighs as well. Lesions above the bridge of the nose tend to fade; the others are less likely to. Because they are level with the skin surface (macular), they can be covered by a cosmetic preparation later in life or can be removed surgically.

Nevus flammeus lesions also occur as a lighter, pink patch, usually seen on the eyelids or at the nape of the neck (termed a *stork's beak mark*) (Fig. 28-13). These lighter nevus flammeus lesions do not fade but are covered by the hairline and so are of no consequence.

Strawberry hemangiomas are elevated areas formed by immature capillaries and endothelial cells (Fig. 28-14). Most are present at birth, although they may appear up to two weeks following birth. They may continue to enlarge from their original size up to 1

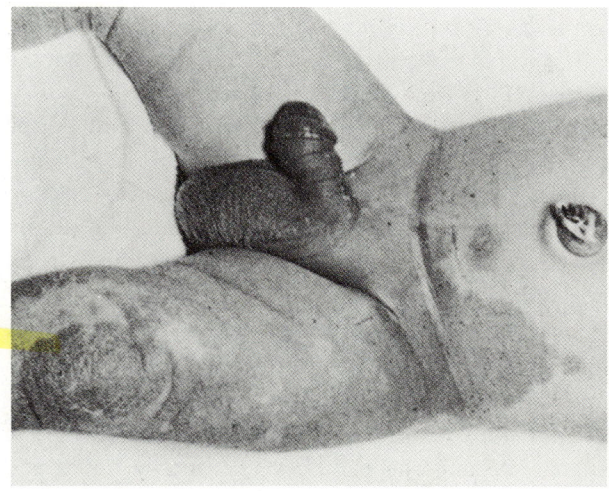

Fig. 28-12. Nevus flammeus (port-wine stain) formed of a plexus of newly formed capillaries in the papillary layer of the corium. It is deep red to purple, does not blanch on pressure, and does not fade with age. (Reproduced with permission of Mead Johnson & Company, Evansville, Ind.)

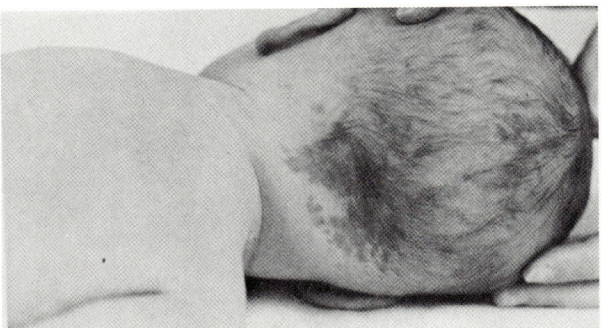

Fig. 28-13. Stork's beak mark, commonly occurring on nape of neck. It blanches on pressure and fades before the end of the first year or is covered by hair. (Reproduced with permission of Mead Johnson & Company, Evansville, Ind.)

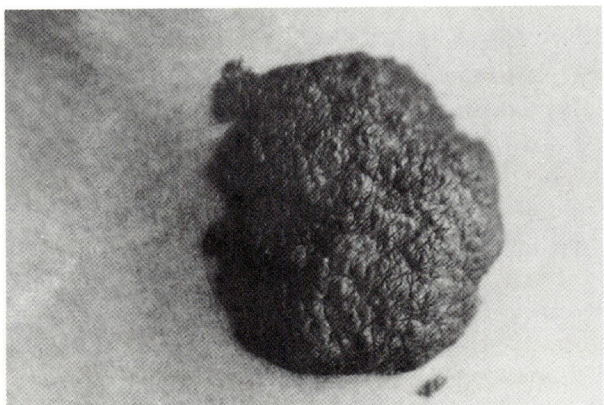

Fig. 28-14. Strawberry hemangiomas consist of dilated capillaries in entire dermal and subdermal layers. They continue to enlarge after birth but usually disappear by age 10 years. (Reproduced with permission of Mead Johnson & Company, Evansville, Ind.)

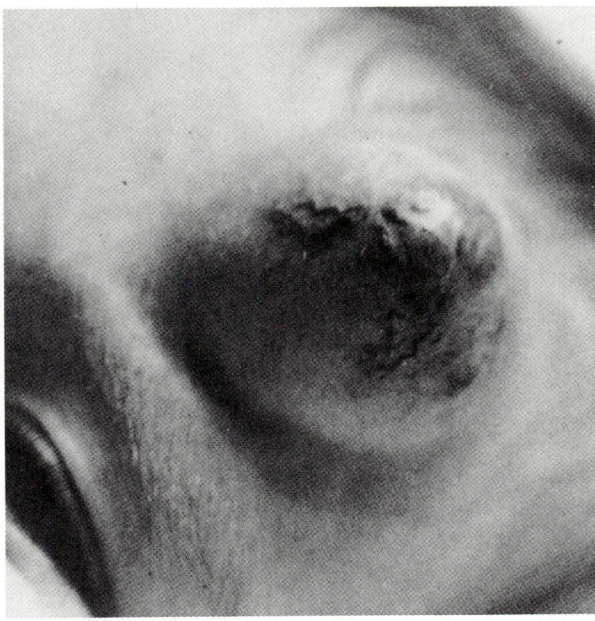

Fig. 28-15. Cavernous hemangiomas consist of a communicating network of venules in subcutaneous tissue and do not fade with age. (Reproduced with permission of Mead Johnson & Company, Evansville, Ind.)

year of age. After the first year they tend to be absorbed and shrink in size. By the time the child is 7 years old, 50 to 75 percent of these lesions have disappeared. A child may be 10 years old before the absorption is complete.

It is important for the mother to understand that the mark may grow; otherwise she may confuse it with cancer (a skin lesion increasing in size is one of the seven danger signals of cancer). She should also understand that the mark will disappear. This second concept keeps her from thinking of her child as imperfect or disfigured. Strawberry hemangiomas clear up best if they are left untreated and are not fussed over. Surgery to remove them may lead to secondary infection, leaving scarring and permanent disfigurement.

Cavernous hemangiomas (Fig. 28-15) are formed of dilated vascular spaces. They are usually raised and resemble a strawberry hemangioma in appearance. They do not disappear. They can be removed surgically. Cavernous hemangiomas may bleed internally, leading to hyperbilirubinemia or anemia. Children who have one obvious skin lesion may have additional lesions on internal organs. Blows to the abdomen such as occur in childhood games, therefore, can cause bleeding from internal hemangiomas.

It is important to learn to differentiate the various types of hemangiomas so that you neither give false reassurances to parents nor worry them unnecessarily about these lesions.

MONGOLIAN SPOTS. Mongolian spots are slate-gray patches seen across the sacrum or buttocks and consist of a collection of pigment cells (melanocytes). They tend to occur in children of Asian, southern European, or African extraction. They disappear by school age without treatment. The mother should be told that they are not bruises, since she may be concerned that her baby has a "weak back" or has sustained a birth injury.

Vernix Caseosa

Vernix caseosa, the white cream-cheese-like substance that serves as a skin lubricant, is usually noticeable on a newborn's skin, at least in the skin folds, for the first two or three days of life. The color of the vernix should be carefully noted, since it takes on the color of the amniotic fluid. If it is yellow, the amniotic fluid was yellow from bilirubin; if it is green, meconium in the amniotic fluid is indicated. In most cases, the color of the amniotic fluid is noted in the labor room or delivery room. However, if the membranes ruptured while the mother was at home, so that the color of the amniotic fluid was not observed, the color of the vernix may provide this information. It is important information to have because the color of the amniotic fluid may suggest the presence of erythroblastosis neonatorum or fetal distress (see Chap. 38).

Vernix caseosa is gradually absorbed by the newborn's skin, and part of it is washed away with each bath. Whether it should be washed away or not is controversial. Although it protects delicate skin from abrasions, it may be a breeding ground for bacteria. For cosmetic reasons, mothers usually prefer that it be washed off, particularly if it is blood-stained from the delivery. Harsh rubbing should never be employed, however, because the newborn's skin is tender, and breaks in the skin from too vigorous attempts to remove the vernix may open portals of entry for bacteria.

Lanugo

Lanugo is the fine downy hair that covers a newborn's shoulders, back, and upper arms. The immature child (37 to 39 weeks gestation age) has more lanugo than the mature infant; postmature infants rarely have lanugo. Most mothers are familiar with lanugo, but occasionally a mother may worry because her small baby girl has thick, almost gorilla-like hair on her arms. Lanugo is rubbed away by the friction of bedding and clothes against the newborn's skin. By age 2 weeks it has disappeared, never to return.

Desquamation

Within 24 hours of birth, the skin of most newborns has become extremely dry. The dryness is particularly evident on the palms of the hands and the soles of the feet. It may result in areas of peeling similar to those following a sunburn. This is normal and needs no treatment. If the mother wishes, she may apply some hand or body lotion to lubricate the dry areas.

Infants who are postmature or have suffered intrauterine malnutrition have extremely dry skin with a leathery appearance and cracking in the skin folds. This should be differentiated from normal desquamation.

Milia

Newborn sebaceous glands are immature. At least one pinpoint white papule (a plugged or unopened

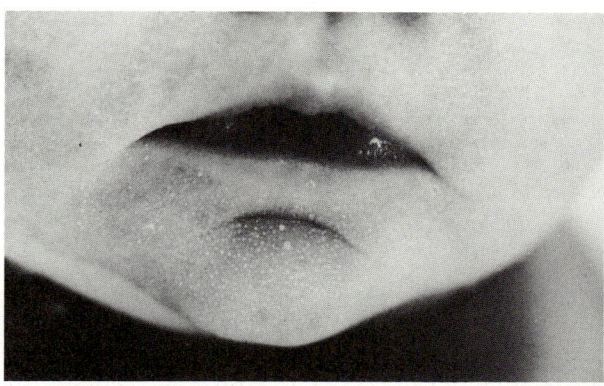

Fig. 28-16. Milia are unopened sebaceous glands frequently found on the nose, chin, or cheeks of a newborn. They disappear spontaneously in a few weeks' time. (Reproduced with permission of Mead Johnson & Company, Evansville, Ind.)

sebaceous gland) can be found on the cheek or across the bridge of the nose of every newborn. Such lesions, termed *milia* (Fig. 28-16), disappear by 2 to 4 weeks of age as the sebaceous glands mature and drain. Mothers need to be told that the lesions are not acne or some other skin disease but are normal in newborns.

Erythema Toxicum

In 30 to 70 percent of normal mature infants, a newborn rash, erythema toxicum, is observed (Fig. 28-17). It usually appears in the first to fourth day of life but may appear in infants up to 2 weeks of age. It begins with a papule, increases in severity to become erythema by the second day, then disappears by the third day. It is sometimes called *flea-bite rash* because the lesions are so minuscule. One of the chief

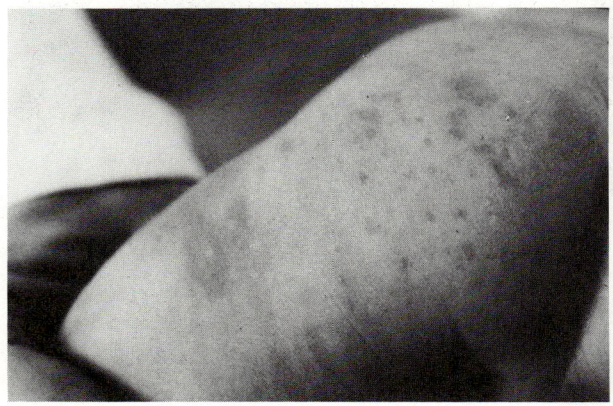

Fig. 28-17. Erythema toxicum is found on almost all newborns. The reddish rash consists of sporadic pinpoint papules on an erythematous base. It fades spontaneously in a few days. (Reproduced with permission of Mead Johnson & Company, Evansville, Ind.)

characteristics of the rash is its lack of pattern. It occurs sporadically and unpredictably as to time and place on skin surfaces. It may last a matter of hours rather than days. It is probably a response to irritation of the infant's skin by sheets and clothes. It needs no treatment.

Forceps Marks

If forceps were used for delivery, there may be a circular or linear contusion matching the rim of the blade of the forceps on the infant's cheek (Fig. 28-18). This mark disappears in two to three days along with the edema that accompanies it. The mark is the result of normal forceps usage and does not denote unskilled or too vigorous application of forceps.

Skin Turgor

Newborn skin should feel resilient if the underlying tissue is well hydrated. If a fold of the skin is grasped between the thumb and fingers, it should feel elastic. When it is released, it should fall back to form a smooth surface. If severe dehydration is present, the skin will not smooth out again but will remain as an elevated ridge. This is seen in infants who suffered malnutrition in utero, who have taken no fluid for a long time after birth, or who have certain metabolic disorders such as adrenogenital syndrome.

HEAD

A newborn's head is disproportionately large, about one-fourth of his total length; in an adult, the head is one-eighth of total height. The forehead of the newborn is large and prominent. The chin appears to be receding, and it quivers easily if the infant is startled or cries.

Fontanelles

The fontanelles are the spaces or openings where the skull bones join. The anterior fontanelle is at the junction of the two parietal bones and the two fused frontal bones. It is diamond-shaped and measures 2 to 3 cm (0.8 to 1.2 inches) in width and 3 to 4 cm (1.2 to 1.6 inches) in length. The posterior fontanelle is at the junction of the parietal bones and the occipital bone. It is triangular and measures about 1 cm (0.5 inch) in length.

The anterior fontanelle will be felt as a soft spot. It should not appear indented (a sign of dehydration) or bulging (a sign of increased intracranial pressure). The fontanelle may bulge if the newborn strains to pass a stool or cries vigorously, and with vigorous crying, a pulse may sometimes be seen in the fontanelle. The posterior fontanelle is so small in some newborns that it is not readily felt. The anterior fontanelle normally closes at 12 to 18 months of age. The posterior fontanelle closes by the end of the second month.

Sutures

The skull sutures, the separating lines of the skull, may override at birth because of the extreme pressure exerted by passage through the birth canal. Overriding is a normal, transient phenomenon. When the sagittal suture between the parietal bones overrides, the fontanelles will be less perceptible than usual. Suture lines should never appear separated in newborns. Separation denotes increased intracranial pressure from either abnormal brain formation, abnormal accumulation of cerebrospinal fluid in the cranium (hydrocephalus), or an accumulation of blood from a birth injury such as subdural hemorrhage.

Molding

The part of the infant's head (usually the vertex) that engages the cervix is molded to fit the cervix contours and appears prominent and asymmetrical; it may be so extreme in the baby of a primiparous woman that it looks like a dunce cap (Fig. 28-19). This is a normal finding, although worrisome to mothers. The head is restored to its normal shape within a few days of birth.

Caput Succedaneum

Caput succedaneum (Fig. 28-20A) is edema of the scalp at the presenting part of the head. It may involve wide areas of the head or may be the size of a goose egg. The edema will gradually be absorbed and disappear about the third day of life. It needs no treatment.

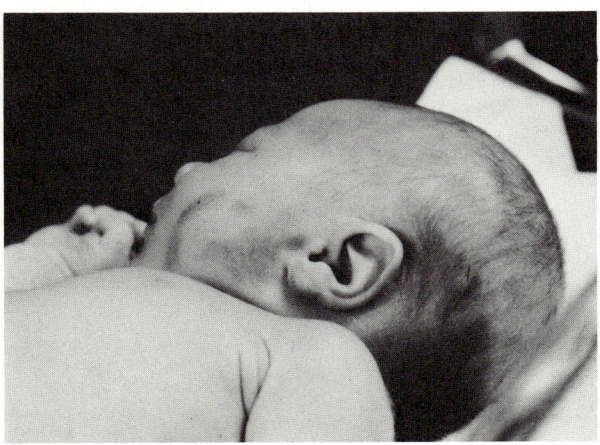

Fig. 28-18. Forceps marks are commonly found in infants delivered by forceps. Such marks are transient and disappear in a day or two. (Reproduced with permission of Mead Johnson & Company, Evansville, Ind.)

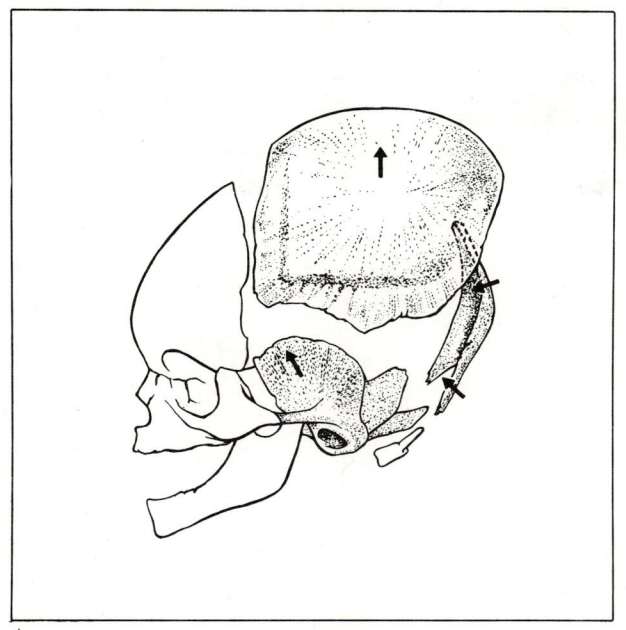
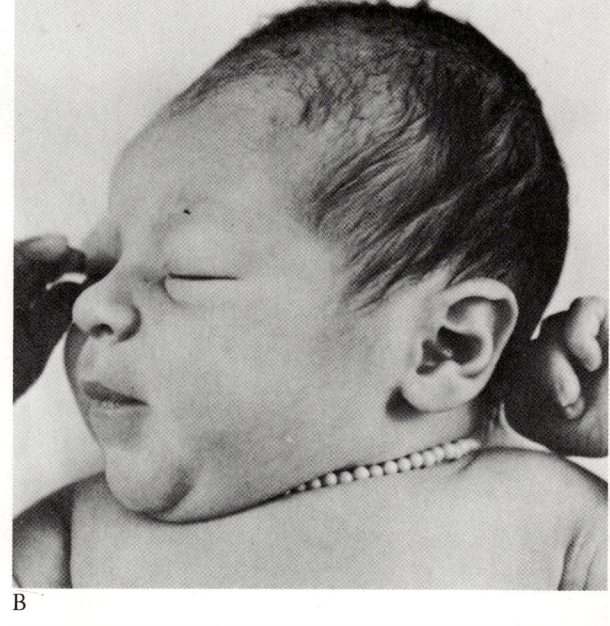
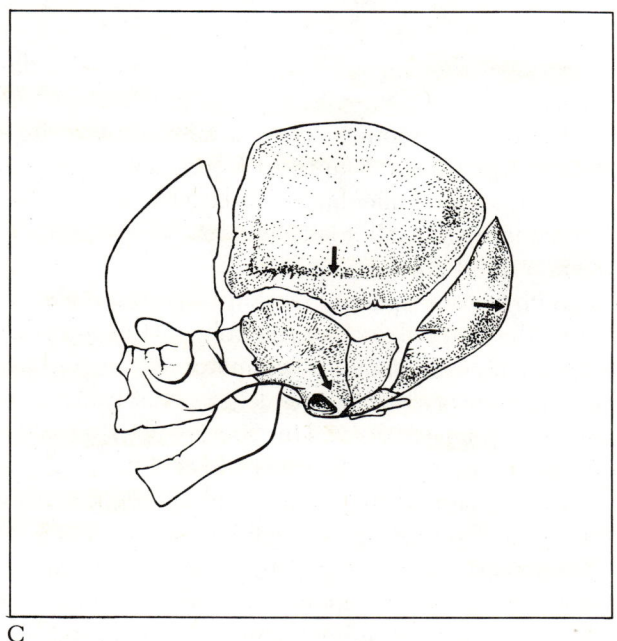
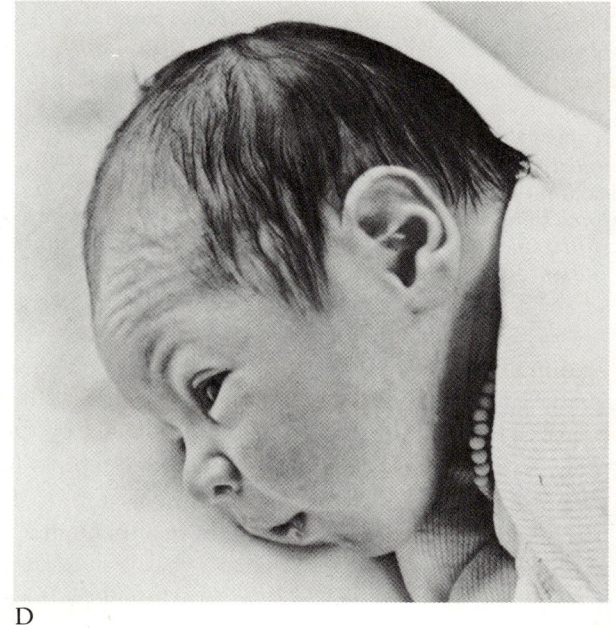

Fig. 28-19. Molding. The infant head molds to fit the birth canal more easily (A, B). On palpation, the skull sutures will be felt to be overriding. The head shape returns to normal within 1 week (C, D). (Reproduced with permission of Mead Johnson & Company, Evansville, Ind.)

Cephalhematoma

A cephalhematoma is a collection of blood between the periosteum of the skull bone and the bone itself caused by rupture of a periosteum capillary due to the pressure of birth (Fig. 28-20B). The blood loss is negligible, but the swelling is generally severe and is well outlined as an egg. It may be discolored (black and blue) because of the presence of coagulated blood. A caput succedaneum may involve both hemispheres of the head, but a cephalhematoma is confined to an individual bone, so that the associated swelling stops at the bone's suture line.

It takes weeks for a cephalhematoma to be absorbed. It might appear that the blood could be aspirated to relieve the condition. However, this procedure would introduce the risk of infection, an unnecessary intrusion since the condition will subside by itself. As the blood captured in the space is broken down, a great deal of indirect bilirubin may be released, leading to jaundice.

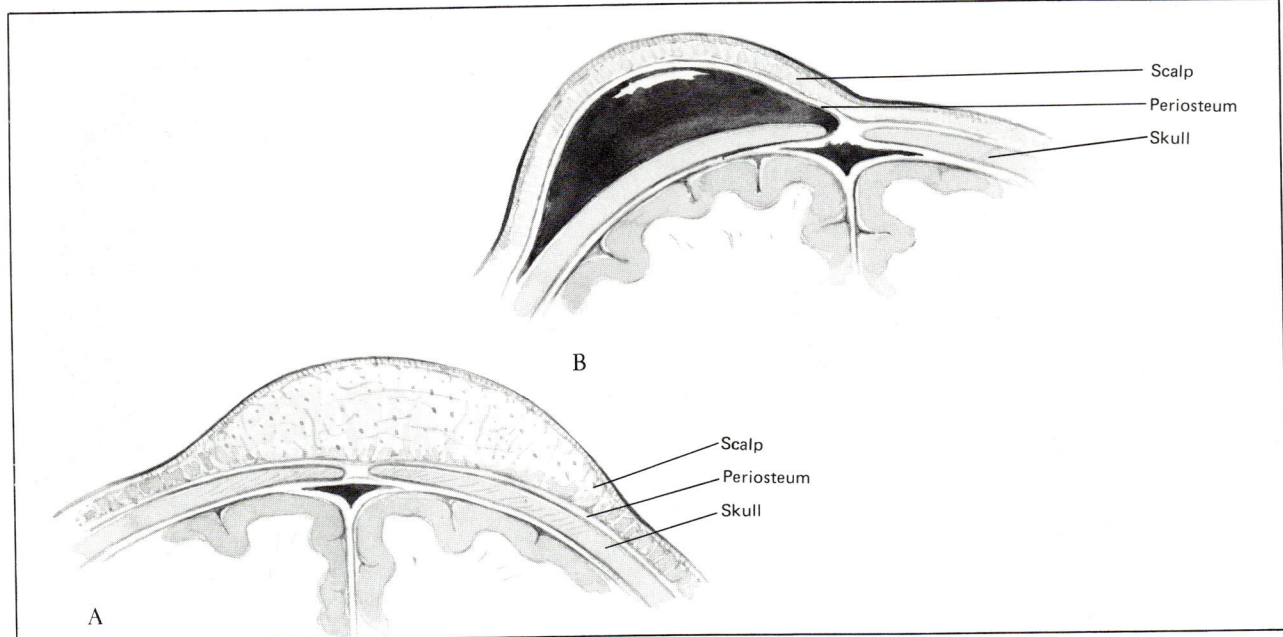

Fig. 28-20. A. *Caput succedaneum*. From pressure of the birth canal, an edematous area is present beneath the scalp. Note how it crosses the midline of the skull. B. *Cephalhematoma*. A small capillary beneath the periosteum of the skull bone has ruptured, and blood has collected under the periosteum of the bone. Note how the swelling now stops at the midline. Since the blood is contained under the periosteum, it is necessarily stopped by a suture line. (Courtesy of the Department of Medical Illustration, State University of New York at Buffalo.)

Craniotabes

Craniotabes is a localized softening of the cranial bones. The bone is so soft it can be indented by the pressure of an examining finger. The bone returns to its normal contour when the pressure is removed. The condition corrects itself without treatment after a matter of months.

Craniotabes is probably due to pressure of the fetal skull against the mother's pelvic bone in utero. It is more common in firstborn infants than in infants born later because of the lower position of the head in the pelvis the last two weeks of pregnancy in primiparous women. It is an example of a condition that is normal in a newborn but is pathological if found in an older child (probably the result of faulty metabolism or kidney dysfunction).

EYES

Almost without exception the irises of the eyes of newborns are gray or blue. They do not assume their permanent color until the child is about 3 months of age.

The eyes should appear clear, without redness or a purulent discharge. Occasionally, a purulent discharge is seen if silver nitrate drops were administered in the delivery room to prevent ophthalmia neonatorum (gonorrheal conjunctivitis). Irritation present for only 24 hours after birth may be attributed to silver nitrate instillation. If it lasts longer than 24 hours, infection should be suspected.

With few exceptions, newborns cry tearlessly because the lacrimal ducts are not fully mature at birth.

Sometimes a small subconjunctival hemorrhage results from pressure during delivery that causes rupture of a small capillary. This appears as a red spot on the sclera, usually on the inner aspect of the eye, or as a red ring around the cornea. The bleeding is slight and needs no treatment. It will be absorbed in two to three weeks, with no evidence that it ever existed. However, the baby's mother should be assured that the hemorrhage is unimportant. Otherwise, she may assume that the baby is bleeding from within the eye and that his vision will be impaired.

Edema is often present around the orbit or on the eyelids. It will remain for the first two or three days until the newborn's kidneys are capable of evacuating fluid efficiently.

The cornea of the eye should be round and proportionate in size to that of an adult eye. A cornea that is larger than usual may be the result of congenital glaucoma. An irregularly shaped pupil, such as one with a keyhole shape (a portion of the iris is missing), is termed a *coloboma*. This may be an isolated finding but must be further investigated because the retina and the child's eyesight may be involved (Fig. 28-21).

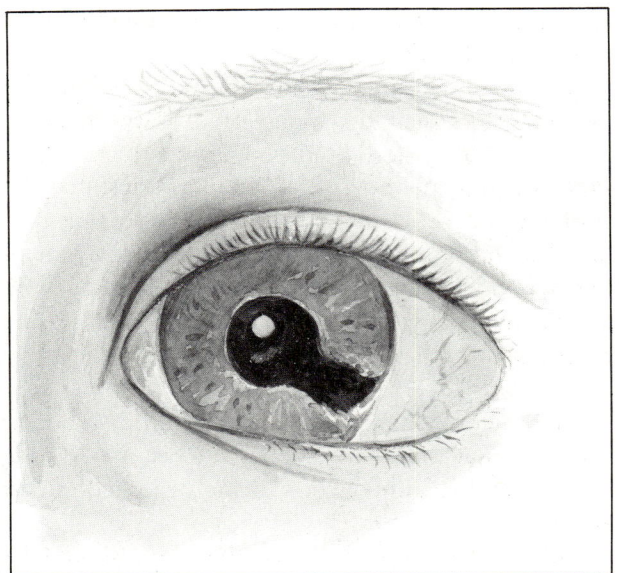

Fig. 28-21. Coloboma. The inferior portion of the iris is incompletely formed, leaving a "keyhole" pupil. (Courtesy of the Department of Medical Illustration, State University of New York at Buffalo.)

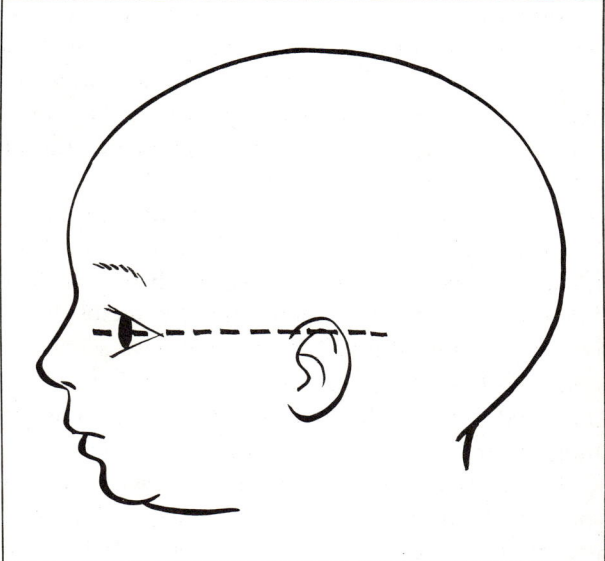

Fig. 28-22. Estimating height of the ears. If a line is drawn from the inner and outer canthus of the eye, it touches the pinna of the ear if the ears are normally set. This is an important determination to make, since low-set ears may be indicative of chromosomal abnormalities.

The pupil should be observed for any whiteness or opacities, which indicate congenital cataract. This should be especially watched for in infants whose mother had a history of rubella during pregnancy or if cytomegalic inclusion disease or galactosemia is suspected.

EARS

The newborn's external ear is still not as completely formed as it will be eventually, and the pinna tends to bend easily. When putting an infant on his side after feeding, be sure that you place the ear in good alignment. If you allow the infant to sleep on his ear in a deformed position, it tends to assume that position permanently.

The level of the top part of the external ear should be on a line drawn from the inner canthus to the outer canthus of the eye and back across the side of the head (Fig. 28-22). Ears that are set lower than this are found in infants with certain chromosomal abnormalities, particularly trisomy 18 and trisomy 13, syndromes in which low-set ears and other physical defects are coupled with mental retardation.

Small tags of skin are sometimes found just in front of the ear. Although they may be associated with chromosomal abnormalities, they are generally isolated findings and are of no consequence. They can be removed by ligation when the child is a few months of age. Directly in front of the ear is a common place for a dermal sinus to be present. The area should be inspected for a pinpoint-size opening. The sinus is usually small and can be removed without consequence when the child is near school age.

NOSE

A newborn's nose may appear large for his face. As he grows, the rest of his face will grow more than the nose, and the discrepancy will disappear. One or two milia are usually present on the tip or bridge of the nose.

MOUTH

A newborn's mouth should open evenly when the baby cries. If one side of the mouth moves more than the other, cranial nerve injury may be indicated. A newborn's tongue appears large and prominent in his mouth. Since the tongue is short, the frenulum membrane is attached close to the tip of the tongue, creating the impression in some mothers that the infant is "tongue-tied." At one time it was almost routine to snip a newborn's frenulum membrane to lengthen it. Now this procedure is regarded as harmful, since it leaves a portal of entry for infection, risks hemorrhage because of the low level of vitamin K in most newborns, and causes feeding difficulties by making the tongue sore and irritated.

The palate of the newborn should be intact. Occasionally, one or two small, round, glistening, well-circumscribed cysts (Epstein's pearls) are present on the palate, a result of the extra load of calcium that is deposited in utero. They are of no significance and need no treatment since they disappear spontaneously in a week's time. The mother may be concerned about them, mistaking them for thrush. Thrush, a Candida infection, usually appears on the tongue and sides of the cheeks as white or gray patches.

All newborns have some mucus in their mouths. If the baby is placed on his side, the mucus drains from his mouth and gives him no distress. If his mouth is filled with so much mucus that he seems to be blowing bubbles through it, he may have a tracheoesophageal fistula. This must be determined before the child is fed or he will aspirate formula into his lungs from the inadequately formed esophagus.

It is unusual for the newborn to have teeth, but sometimes one or two will have erupted. Any teeth present must be evaluated for stability. If they are loose, they should be extracted, lest they be aspirated with a feeding. Small white epithelial pearls (inclusion cysts) may be present on the gum margins.

NECK

The neck of the newborn is short and often chubby. It is creased with skin folds. The head should rotate freely on the neck. It should flex forward and back. If there is rigidity of the neck, congenital torticollis from injury to the sternocleidomastoid muscle during birth should be considered. In infants whose membranes were ruptured more than 24 hours prior to birth nuchal rigidity suggests meningitis.

The neck is not strong enough to support the total weight of the head, but in a sitting position the infant should make a momentary effort at head control. When lying prone, the newborn can raise his head slightly, usually enough to lift it out of mucus or spit-up formula. If he is pulled to a sitting position from a supine position, his head will lag behind considerably; however, again, he should make some effort to control and steady it as he reaches the sitting position.

The trachea may be prominent on the front of the neck. The thymus gland may be enlarged because of the rapid growth of glandular tissue in comparison with other body tissues. The thymus gland triples in size by 3 years of age; it remains at that size until the child is about 10 years old. After that, its size begins to decrease. Although the thymus may appear to be bulging in the newborn, it is rarely a cause of respiratory difficulty as was previously believed.

CHEST

The chest in some infants looks small because the infant's head is so large in proportion. Not until the child is 2 years of age does the chest measurement exceed that of the head.

In both female and male infants, the breasts may be engorged. Occasionally, the breasts of newborn babies secrete a thin, watery fluid popularly termed witch's milk. Engorgement occurs in utero as a result of the influence of the mother's hormones. As soon as they are cleared from the infant's system, the engorgement and any fluid present subsides (about a week). Fluid should never be expressed from infant breasts. The manipulation may introduce bacteria and lead to mastitis.

The clavicles should be straight. A lump on one or the other may indicate that a fracture occurred during delivery and calcium is now being deposited at that point.

Overall, the appearance of the chest should be symmetrical. Respirations are normally rapid (30 to 50 per minute) but not distressed.

Retraction (the chest wall drawn in with inspiration) should not be present. An infant retracting is an infant who has to use such strong force to pull air into his respiratory tract that he sucks in the anterior chest muscles. Retraction is shown in Fig. 28-23.

ABDOMEN

The contour of the newborn abdomen is slightly protuberant. A scaphoid or sunken appearance may be indicative of missing abdominal contents.

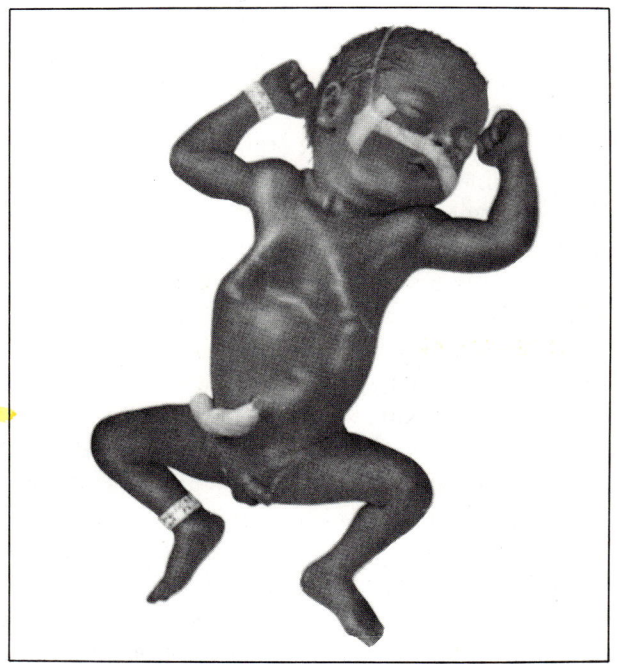

Fig. 28-23. Sternal retraction in a newborn. Retraction indicates labored and difficult breathing. (From Clinical Education Aid, No. 5, Ross Laboratories, Columbus, Ohio, 1960.)

For the first hour after birth, the umbilical cord appears as a white gelatinous structure marked with the red and blue streaks of the umbilical vein and arteries. The vein and arteries should be counted when the cord is first cut in the delivery room to be certain they are present. In 0.5 percent of deliveries (3.5 percent of twin deliveries) [9], there is only a single umbilical artery, and in a third of such infants this single artery is associated with a congenital anomaly. Since the anomaly may not be readily apparent, any child with a single umbilical artery needs close observation and assessment until all anomalies are ruled out.

After the first hour of life, the cord begins to dry up, shrink, and become discolored like the dead end of a vine. By the second or third day it has turned black. It sloughs by the sixth to tenth day, leaving a granulating area a few centimeters across that heals during the following week.

There should be no bleeding at the cord site. Bleeding suggests that the cord clamp has been loosened or the cord has been tugged loose by the friction of the bedclothes. The base of the cord should appear dry. A moist or odorous cord suggests infection. If present, infection should receive immediate treatment or it may enter the newborn's bloodstream and cause septicemia. Moistness at the base of the cord may also indicate a patent urachus (connection between the bladder and the umbilicus), with urine draining at the cord site.

The base of the cord should also be inspected to be certain there is no defect in the abdominal wall (umbilical hernia). If there is a fascial (abdominal wall) defect less than 2 cm wide, it will generally close by itself by school age; a defect more than 2 cm wide will probably require surgical correction. Taping or putting buttons or coins on the abdomen is an old wives' remedy and does not help such defects to close. Heavy taping may in fact worsen the condition by preventing the development of good muscle tone in the abdominal wall. The tape also tends to keep the cord moist and make infection more likely than when the cord is dry.

ANOGENITAL AREA

The anus of the newborn must be inspected to be certain that it is patent and not covered by a membrane (imperforate anus). This condition is best determined by inserting a rectal thermometer into the rectum for the length of the bulb or by inserting the tip of a lubricated little finger. The time after birth that the infant first passes meconium should be noted. If he does not do so in the first 24 hours, the suspicion of imperforate anus or meconium ileus is aroused.

MALE GENITALIA

The scrotum in most male infants is edematous. It may be deeply pigmented in black or dark-skinned infants. Rugae should be evident in the mature infant.

Both testes should be present in the scrotum. Male infants who do not have one or both testes in the scrotum (cryptorchidism) need further referral to establish the extent of the problem. It could be due to agenesis (absence of an organ), ectopic testes (the testes cannot enter the scrotum because the opening to the scrotal sac is closed), or undescended testes (the vas deferens or artery is too short to allow them to descend). Infants with agenesis of the testes are usually referred for investigation of other anomalies. Since the testes arise from the same germ tissue as the kidney, agenesis of the testes may indicate agenesis of a kidney also.

The penis of newborns is usually small. It should be inspected to see that the urethral opening is at the tip of the glans, not on the dorsal surface (epispadias) or the ventral surface (hypospadias).

The prepuce (foreskin) of the penis should be examined to be certain it is not stenosed. In most newborns it slides back poorly from the meatal opening. Although today most male infants are circumcised, the necessity for this operation can be questioned. It is rare to find an infant who physically requires it (with a foreskin so constricting that it interferes with voiding or circulation), and surgery this early in life poses the risk of hemorrhage and infection. Circumcision should not be done if hypospadias or epispadias is present; the plastic surgeon may want to use the foreskin as tissue in the repair of these conditions.

FEMALE GENITALIA

The vulva in female newborns may be swollen because of the action of maternal hormones. Since many male physicians are reluctant, because of their upbringing, to examine the genitalia of a female infant with more than a cursory glance, you should make this inspection your responsibility.

In some infants a mucous vaginal secretion is present, which is sometimes blood-tinged. Again, this is due to the action of maternal hormones, and the discharge will disappear as soon as the infant's system has cleared the hormones. The discharge should not be mistaken for an infection or taken as an indication that a trauma has occurred.

BACK

A newborn should be turned to a prone position and his back observed to determine whether or not his spine is straight. The spine appears flat in the lumbar and sacral areas; the curves seen in the adult appear only when the child is able to sit and walk. The base of the spine should be inspected carefully to be certain no dermal sinus is present there. This looks like a pinpoint opening in the skin.

A newborn normally assumes the position he maintained in utero, in which, typically, the back is rounded and the arms and legs are flexed on the abdomen and chest. A child who was born in a frank breech position will tend to straighten his legs at the knee and bring them up next to his face. The position of a baby delivered by a face presentation sometimes simulates opisthotonos because the curve of the back is deeply concave.

EXTREMITIES

The arms and legs of the newborn are short. The hands are plump and clenched into fists. Newborn fingernails are soft and smooth and are usually long enough to extend over the fingertips.

The arms and legs should move symmetrically (unless the infant is demonstrating a tonic neck reflex). An arm that hangs limp and unmoving suggests injury to the clavicle or the brachial or cervical plexus or fracture of a long bone, all of which are possible birth injuries.

The legs are bowed as well as short. The sole of the foot appears to be flat because of an extra pad of fat in

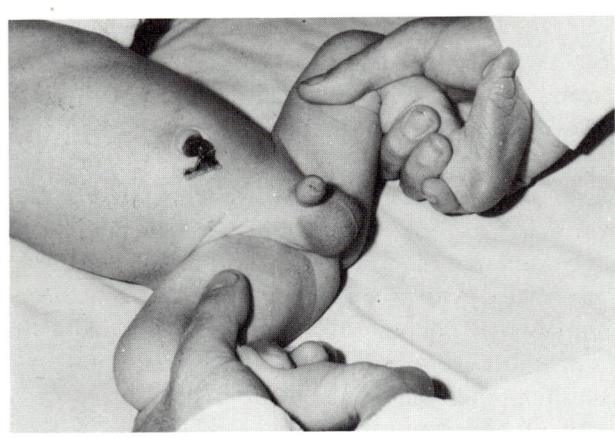

Fig. 28-24. Hip abduction. In a newborn, both hips should abduct so completely they lie almost flat against the mattress (180 degrees). (Reproduced with permission of Mead Johnson & Company, Evansville, Ind.)

the longitudinal arch. In the mature infant there are many crisscrossed lines on the sole of the foot. Absence of such marks usually indicates immaturity.

The feet of many newborns turn in (varus deviation) because of intrauterine position. This simple deviation needs no correction if the feet can be brought to the midline position by easy manipulation; when the infant begins to bear weight, they will align themselves. If a foot does not align readily or will not turn to a definite midline position, a talipes deformity

Table 28-3. Periods of Reactivity: Normal Adjustment to Extrauterine Life

Assessment	First Period (First 15 to 30 Minutes)	Second Period (30 Minutes to 120 Minutes)	Third Period (2 Hours to 6 Hours)
Color	Acrocyanosis	Color stabilizing; pink all over	Quick color changes occur with movement or crying
Temperature	Baby's temperature begins to fall from intrauterine temp. of 100.6°F	Temperature stabilizes at about 99°F	Temperature increases to 99.8°F
Heart rate	Rapid, as much as 180 per minute while crying	Slowing to between 120 and 140 per minute	Wide swings in rate with activity
Respirations	Irregular; 30–90 per minute while crying; some nasal flaring, occasional retraction may be present	Slows to 30–50 per minute; barreling of chest occurs	Respirations become irregular again with activity
Activity	Alert; watching	Sleeps	Awakes
Ability to respond to stimulation	Reacts vigorously	Difficult to rouse	Becoming responsive again
Mucus	Visible in mouth	Small amount present while sleeping	Mouth full of mucus causing gagging
Bowel sounds	Able to be heard after first 15 minutes	Present	Often has first meconium stool

Source: M. N. Desmond et al., The clinical behavior of the newly born: The term baby. *J. Pediatr.* 62:307, 1963.

(clubfoot) may be present. The condition needs investigation, since congenital problems of this kind are best treated in the newborn period.

With the newborn in a supine position, both legs can be flexed and abducted to such an extent that they touch or nearly touch the surface of the bed (Fig. 28-24). If the hip joint seems to lock short of this distance (160 to 170 degrees) hip subluxation (a shallow and poorly formed acetabulum) is suggested; a click heard as the femur head strikes the acetabulum is another indication of this. Subluxated hip may be bilateral but is usually unilateral. It is important that hip subluxation be discovered as early as possible, since correction, as in correction of talipes deformities, is most successful if initiated early.

When lying on his abdomen, a newborn is capable of bringing his arms and legs underneath him and raising his stomach off the bed enough for a hand to be slipped underneath him. This ability helps to prevent pressure or rubbing at the cord site because in this position the cord site does not actually touch the bedding. The immature infant does not have this ability, and thus its presence or absence is an indication of maturity.

Physiological Adjustment to Extrauterine Life

All infants seem to move through a period of irregular adjustment in the first 6 hours of life before their body systems stabilize. This has been described as a transition period [7]. The first phase lasts about half an hour. During this time the baby is alert and exhibits exploring, searching activity; he often makes sucking sounds. His heartbeat and respiratory rate are rapid. This is called the *first period of reactivity*.

Next comes a quiet, resting period. Heartbeat and respiratory rate slow; the infant generally sleeps for about 90 minutes.

The third period, between 2 and 6 hours of life, is the *second period of reactivity*. The infant wakes, often gagging and choking on mucus that has accumulated in his mouth. He is again alert and responsive and interested in his surroundings.

These three periods are summarized in Table 28-3. Infants who are ill or who had difficulty at birth do not pass through these typical stages; they may never have periods of alertness or periods of quiet. Their vital signs may not fall and rise again, but remain rapid; their temperature may remain subnormal. Exhibition of this typical pattern, therefore, is an indication that the infant is well and adjusting well to extrauterine life.

References

1. Baldwin, W., and Cain, V. S. The children of teenage parents. *Fam. Plann. Perspect.* 12:34, 1980.
2. Black, M. Assessment of weight and gestational age. *Nurs. Clin. North Am.* 13:13, 1978.
3. Brazelton, T. B. The remarkable talents of the newborn. *Birth Fam. J.* 5:187, 1978.
4. Brazelton, T. B. Behavioral competence of the newborn infant. *Semin. Perinatol.* 3:35, 1979.
5. Coyner, A. B. Meeting developmental needs of neonates. *Fam. Community Health* 1:79, 1978.
6. Curry, M. A. Contact during the first hour with the wrapped or naked newborn: Effect on maternal attachment behaviors at 36 hours and 3 months. *Birth Fam. J.* 6:227, 1979.
7. Desmond, M. N., et al. The clinical behavior of the newly born: The term baby. *J. Pediatr.* 62:307, 1963.
8. Erickson, M. P. Trends in assessing the newborn and his parents. *M.C.N.* 3:99, 1978.
9. Moore, M. L. *The Newborn and the Nurse*. Philadelphia: Saunders, 1972.
10. Porth, C. M., et al. Temperature regulation in the newborn. *Am. J. Nurs.* 78:1691, 1978.
11. Simkin, P., et al. Physiological jaundice of the newborn. *Birth Fam. J.* 6:23, 1979.
12. Stern, L. Clinical aspects of thermoregulation in the newborn. *Contemp. Obstet. Gynecol.* 13:109, 1979.
13. Sullivan, R., et al. Determining a newborn's gestational age. *M.C.N.* 4:38, 1979.

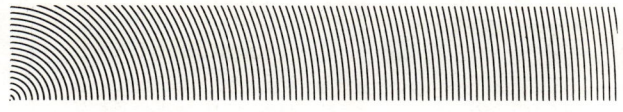

29. Health Assessment of the Newborn

Newborn assessment is an important role of the maternal-newborn nurse. You might use the role doing initial delivery room or birthing room examinations, initial nursery admission examinations, or discharge examinations. A community health nurse or a nurse in a pediatrician's office might visit a new mother in her home before her baby's first visit to a health care agency. You might also use the skills of newborn health assessment doing monthly well-child assessments in a physician's office or child care clinic.

Health assessment of a newborn involves three phases: assessment of the pregnancy, labor, and delivery by reference to the records and by history taking; physical assessment of the infant; and assessment of the maternal-newborn interaction.

All three phases are equally important. The nine months the infant spent in utero and the circumstances of his delivery can have as much effect on his health as anything that comes after birth. For the infant to thrive, he needs not only to be physically healthy but to have someone to take good care of him and interact with him. The three phases in newborn assessment overlap and intertwine.

History Taking

Some information on the pregnancy and delivery can be obtained from the hospital charts of the mother and infant. Part of it must be gained from interviewing the mother.

For a pregnancy history, you need to know the para and gravida number applying to the mother, the date of the last menstrual period, and the predicted date of confinement for this pregnancy. Double-check the date of confinement by Nägele's rule. Is there any suspicion the infant is immature or postmature?

When did the mother go for medical supervision during this pregnancy? Did she keep appointments? What was her nutritional state and her general health during the pregnancy? Did the milestones of pregnancy occur on schedule (e.g., cessation of nausea and vomiting by 4 months, quickening of the fetus at 4½ to 5 months)? Were there any complications during pregnancy such as spotting or beginning hypertension? Did the mother take vitamins, iron, and folic acid during the pregnancy? Did she take any other medication? Were there any injuries such as falls or car accidents? Were any x-ray films made? Does she have any chronic illness such as heart or kidney disease?

If you have access to the mother's hospital admission record, examine it to determine whether she entered the hospital in good health. Was her blood pressure within normal limits? Did she have any signs of infection that could spread to the newborn and impair his health?

Examine the mother's labor and delivery room record for the length and type of her labor, the type of delivery, kind of analgesia or anesthetic used, problems in delivering the child or the placenta. Examine the infant's delivery room record for presentation, position, the time the membranes ruptured, whether or not aseptic technique was broken during delivery, fetal heart rate during labor and delivery, time in which breathing was established after birth, weight (plotted on a neonatal estimation of gestation age chart—see Fig. 28-1), and Apgar score. Check to be certain eye prophylaxis was done and vitamin K was administered (see Chap. 31).

Following examination of the delivery room chart, the infant's nursery chart should be studied for further points of history. The time the infant first passed a stool and first voided will be important in assessing the functioning of the intestinal and urinary systems. The child's response to feeding and his tolerance of feedings provide a clue not only to the state of health of his gastrointestinal system but also to his overall maturity and well-being.

If you do not have the mother's chart, ask her to tell you about her pregnancy, labor, and delivery and the condition of the infant at birth. Ask specifically if the infant cried right away; if there was any cyanosis or jaundice (ask "turn blue or yellow?" with most women); if any special equipment was used with the baby. A mother who was awake in the delivery room had a keen interest in the baby at that time and so is generally an excellent informant on his condition immediately after birth.

What was the outcome of previous pregnancies? Are all previous children healthy? Were there any complications at delivery or in the newborn period with these children? Are there any familial diseases?

Physical Assessment of the Newborn

In the physical assessment of adults and older children, the sequence of assessment is usually overall inspection, then detailed assessment of the body parts from head to toe, including certain neurological components. Many examiners find it more satisfactory to examine infants under 1 year of age by beginning with an overall inspection and then assessing body parts, proceeding from *toe to head*, finishing with the neurological evaluation. This method has the advantage of a gentle and untraumatic beginning and postpones the parts of the examination that are certain to upset the infant and cause him to cry, particularly examination of the mouth and throat. Because it is necessary for the infant to be relaxed and not crying while his chest and abdomen are examined, many examiners start with these body parts after the initial inspection and then proceed from the feet upward. Since it is unrealistic to expect the infant to cooperate in any way during the assessment, this third method appears to have the most merit and is the order of assessment presented here.

INSPECTION

Body proportion is an important observation to make before the newborn is disturbed. Are the infant's proportions typical newborn proportions? Is his head about one-fourth of his overall height? Is the head circumference slightly larger than the chest circumference? Are the legs and arms short in proportion to the trunk? Although the arms appear to be short, fingertips should reach to midthigh. Does the child have gross anomalies? What position does he assume? Is it consistent with his delivery presentation? With his gestation age? Breech-born babies ordinarily assume their delivery position, possibly with legs extended. Vertex-born babies are typically lightly flexed. Brow-born babies often arch their backs. Immature babies do not flex well (they frogleg). Are the arms and legs positioned symmetrically (as they should be unless the infant is exhibiting a tonic neck reflex)? (See p. 427.)

If lying in a prone position, does he exhibit good muscle tone by pulling his knees well under himself and raising his abdomen off the bedding? Does he make sucking movements with his lips? Are his respirations easy or labored? Is the chest retracting while at rest? (Occasional retractions—inward movement of the sternum with inspiration—in a mature infant are normal; persistent retraction is a sign of respiratory distress.) What is his color? Ruddy? Pale? Cyanotic? Jaundiced?

All of these observations are important to make initially since they become increasingly difficult to make once the infant has become upset.

ASSESSMENT OF THE CHEST

Examination of the chest follows the general procedure of all examination: inspection, palpation, percussion, and auscultation. Note the size and contour of the chest. It should appear to be almost as large in the anteroposterior diameter as in width. Inspect the respiratory movements. If retractions are present, are they intercostal or subcostal? Are they constant or occasional? What is the rate of respirations? Is the chest symmetrical? (An enlarged heart may make the left side of the chest appear larger; a diaphragmatic hernia in the right side of the chest may make that side appear larger.) Do both sides of the chest move with respirations? Is the number of ribs even on each side? Are the clavicles smooth and straight?

Inspect the breasts for inflammation (possible infection), presence of breast tissue (the presence of palpable breast tissue is a sign of maturity), drainage, and the presence of supernumerary nipples (usually found below and in line with the normal nipples). Note whether or not the point of maximum impulse of the heart is visible on inspection, as is normal in newborns.

Begin palpating the chest in a systematic order from the top down or from side to side. Do the ribs feel smooth? Examine the clavicles for intactness. A crepitant feeling denotes fracture. A bony prominence on the clavicle may mean that the clavicle was fractured at delivery and callus formation is beginning. Palpate the anterior chest to ascertain the point of maximum intensity of the heartbeat. Can you feel a thrill radiating from that point (thrills suggest heart disease)? Palpate the breast tissue for engorgement; estimate the size of engorgement in centimeters. Palpate the supraclavicular and the axillary lymph nodes for any enlargement.

Chest percussion in a newborn does not always produce meaningful findings, although total lack of resonance on one side of the chest in comparison with the other side might suggest that primary atelectasis or a diaphragmatic hernia is occluding chest space. You should be able to locate the left lateral aspect of the heart by percussion. Lung tissue sounds resonant; as your finger moves over the heart, the sound dulls.

Auscultate heart sounds. Begin at the point of maximum intensity (the heart apex). What is the heart rate? How about the rhythm (listen long enough to be certain that you have heard the rhythm through both inhalation and exhalation)—is it even? Are the sounds clear and distinct? Are there any extra sounds? Do you hear a murmur? Do you hear a splitting of the heart sounds? Is it a fixed or a changing split? The first heart sound is caused by closure of the tricuspid and mitral valves; the second sound, by closure of the pulmonary and aortic valves. Splitting (the sound of *l-lub* instead of *lub*; *d-dub* instead of *dub*) implies that a valve is closing after its mate, not at the same time. (Physiological splitting of the second heart sound widens on inspiration; pathological splitting caused by delayed closure of the pulmonary valve is fixed—that is, it does not change with inspiration or expiration.)

Auscultate at "listening posts" for the sounds of the different valves—that is, at the fourth or fifth left interspace of the ribs for the mitral valve, the second interspace at the left of the sternum for the pulmonary valve, the second interspace on the right of the sternum for the aortic valve, and at the junction of the sternum and xiphoid for the tricuspid valve. Auscultate below the left axilla for radiating sounds. Listening posts for heart sounds are shown in Fig. 29-1.

After you have a good mental picture of the heart sounds, auscultate the chest for breath sounds. Listen to the anterior upper left chest, anterior upper right chest, lower left chest, middle and lower right chest (everyone has two lung lobes on the left side, three lobes or spots to listen to on the right side).

Because the newborn's alveoli open slowly over the first 24 to 48 hours to full capacity and the baby invariably has mucus in the back of his throat, listening to lung sounds often reveals the sounds of rhonchi and perhaps transient other findings. Respiratory rate in a newborn should be between 30 and 50 when he is quiet; as he stirs and cries, it rises to 50 to 80. Adventitious chest sounds are summarized in Table 29-1.

Lastly, turn the baby on his abdomen and listen in the four posterior chest quadrants for radiating heart sounds and for breath sounds.

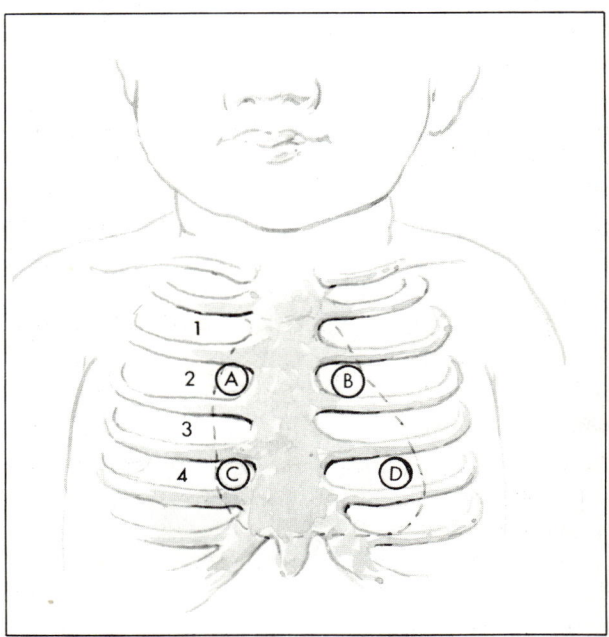

Fig. 29-1. Listening posts for heart sounds. Heart valves are not at these points, but these are the points to which the sounds radiate best. A = aortic valve, B = pulmonary valve, C = tricuspid valve, D = mitral valve. (Courtesy of the Department of Medical Illustration, State University of New York at Buffalo.)

Health Assessment of the Newborn

Table 29-1. Adventitious Chest Sounds in Newborns

Term	Source of Sound	Description	Importance
Rhonchi	Air passing through mucus in a major air passage	A coarse, snoring sound	Little importance in newborns as mucus in the back of the throat causes transmitted sound
Rales	Air passing through fluid in alveoli	Simulates the crackle of cellophane	Should be investigated. Can be the sound of unabsorbed lung fluid; also can be a sign of pneumonia
Stridor	Air being pulled through a narrowed airway, often caused by immature trachea cartilage	A high crowing (rooster-like) sound heard on inspiration	Should be investigated. May be beginning sign of tracheal obstruction
Wheezing	Air being pushed through narrowed bronchioles	A whistling heard on expiration	Should be investigated. May be a beginning sign of obstruction
Grunting	Air being pushed through a partially closed epiglottis	A "grunt" heard on expiration	Should be investigated. Infants with respiratory distress syndrome (hyaline membrane disease) typically grunt to maintain pressure in alveoli
Absent or diminished breath sounds	If air is not entering a lung or lobe of a lung on one side, breath sounds are absent or quieter on that side	Soft, difficult-to-hear breath sounds	Should be investigated. Suggests lack of aeration such as occurs with atelectasis

ASSESSMENT OF THE ABDOMEN

Assessment of the abdomen proceeds from inspection to auscultation, palpation, and percussion. Inspect the skin carefully for color and the presence of superficial veins (superficial veins are generally present in a newborn). Inspect the umbilical area to determine whether the cord is free from drainage. Inspect the cord clamp to be certain it is secure. If the infant is only a few hours old, it may be possible to count the number of umbilical vessels. A newborn's abdomen is slightly protuberant. A depressed abdomen suggests missing organs.

It is good practice to auscultate the abdomen before palpating or percussing it; abdominal pressure will shift intestinal contents and lessen the already low intensity of bowel sounds. These are tinkling sounds, and if they are not present, bowel obstruction is suggested. You have to listen for at least a minute to detect bowel sounds, since they occur at a rate of perhaps only two to five per minute.

Begin palpation by testing the skin of the abdomen for turgor. Grasp the skin between your thumb and index finger to raise it, then release it and note whether or not it returns to its former position. With good hydration, the crease disappears immediately; if the raised portion of skin remains raised, poor turgor or poor hydration is indicated.

First palpate the abdomen superficially, then deeply. Follow a systematic order so that no quadrant is inadvertently overlooked. Begin in any quadrant and palpate clockwise back to the first quadrant. The edge of the liver is usually palpable in newborns at 1 to 2 cm below the right costal margin. The edge of the spleen may be palpable 1 to 2 cm below the left costal margin. Be certain you palpate from the lower to the upper quadrants to detect the liver and spleen, so that your fingertips bump against their lower edges. Otherwise, your fingertips will be on top of the organs and you will not detect their presence.

No areas of weakness or hernias of muscle should be discernible on palpation; no tenderness should be present. Tenderness is difficult to determine in a newborn, but if it is extreme, the infant will cry or thrash about or possibly tense his abdominal muscles to protect his abdomen as you palpate it.

Attempt to identify the presence of kidneys by deep palpation. The right kidney can usually be palpated (at least its lower pole), since it is lower than the left kidney; the latter is more difficult to locate because the intestine is bulkier on the left side, and the left kidney is higher in the retroperitoneal space. Nonetheless, you should try to locate it; the child's voiding only demonstrates that he has at least one kidney, not that he has two. Attempt to evaluate kidney size. Are the kidneys normal in size (about the size of a walnut)? If a kidney is enlarged, a polycystic kidney or pooling of urine from a ureteral obstruction is suggested. Be certain your fingernails are clipped close to your fingertips before you undertake kidney palpation. Otherwise, you will cut the baby's abdominal skin.

Palpate the umbilical ring. Is it open or closed? If open, how wide is the opening? A fascial ring more than 2 cm in diameter is generally accepted as wider than one that will close spontaneously.

Last, percuss the abdomen to determine resonance and to confirm the location of the inferior margin of the liver and spleen and the superior margin of the bladder.

Elicit the abdominal reflex. Stroking each quadrant of the abdomen will cause the umbilicus to move or "wink" in that direction. This superficial abdominal reflex is a test of spinal nerves T-8 through T-10. The reflex may not be demonstrable in newborns until the tenth day of life.

ASSESSMENT OF THE LOWER EXTREMITIES

Begin with the feet and inspect one foot at a time. Inspect for color. Separate the toes and count them. Watch for webbing (syndactyly), extra toes (polydactyly), or unusual spacing of toes, particularly between the big toes and the others (a finding in certain chromosomal disorders, although also a normal finding in some families). Test to see whether the toenails become blanched on pressure.

Observe the foot for position. Feet tend to turn in (varus deviation) because of intrauterine position, and they tend to turn out (valgus deviation) in infants who consistently sleep in a prone position. Check to see that the foot aligns with the ankle. Put the ankle through a range of motion to evaluate whether or not the heel cord is unusually tight. Check for ankle clonus by supporting the lower leg in the left hand and dorsiflexing the foot sharply two or three times by pressure on the sole of the foot. Following the dorsiflexion, one or two continued movements are normal; rapid alternating contraction and relaxation (clonus) is abnormal.

The skin of the legs should be inspected for color and tested for warmth. The skin of the thigh should be tested for turgor. Align the legs and examine for an abnormal degree of bowing (tibial torsion). Flex and extend the knee joint. Check the muscle tone of the lower extremities by extending them, then releasing them and observing the action. The mature newborn will immediately flex them again, but the immature infant will not make a motion this strong.

Inspect the posterior thighs for asymmetrical skin folds as are seen in hip dysplasia. Check further for hip dysplasia by flexing the hips and knees and attempting to abduct the hips. With good joint function, the hips should abduct 160 to 170 degrees. The presence of hip subluxation is further supported by feeling the joint slip in your hands or hearing a click as the head of the femur strikes the ridge of the acetabulum.

The thighs should flex on the abdomen with the knee in a flexed position. Inability of the infant to extend his leg from this position is a sign of meningitis (Kernig's sign), which is rare in a newborn but possible when the membranes ruptured early.

Palpate the inguinal area in both male and female infants for unusual masses that would suggest hernia or enlarged lymph nodes. Palpate the femoral pulses (at the inguinal ligament) and compare their strength.

ASSESSMENT OF THE GENITALIA AND RECTUM

The foreskin of the uncircumcised male infant should be retracted to visualize the urethral opening. Normally, the foreskin retracts far enough for you to locate the meatus; it does not retract over the entire glans.

A few adhesions of the prepuce may be present in newborns but are of no consequence unless they cause obstruction of the urinary meatus.

The urinary meatus should be inspected for appearance and to determine that it is located at the end of the penis (ruling out epispadias or hypospadias). If the opening is round rather than slit-like, scar tissue formation from infection should be suspected.

The scrotum should be inspected for normal asymmetry (the left side is invariably slightly larger). The testes should be palpated to be certain they are descended. Make a practice of pressing your left hand against the inguinal ring before palpating for the testes, so that they do not slip upward out of the scrotal sac as you palpate. Note whether or not rugae are present on the scrotum (a sign of maturity).

The cremasteric reflex is elicited by stroking the internal side of the thigh. As the skin is stroked, the testis on that side moves perceptibly upward. This is a test of the integrity of spinal nerves T-8 through T-10. The response may be absent in newborns less than about 10 days old.

Inspect the genitalia of the female newborn for gross structures: labia majora and minora (often enlarged), clitoris (also often enlarged), and the urethral and vaginal openings. In most newborns, vulvar edema is so severe that locating the urethral and vaginal openings is difficult. Vaginal secretions are present in most newborn females, and they are sometimes blood-tinged.

In both sexes, it is important to observe the stream of urine. It should be forceful and especially in males should curve upward in an arc. Observation of a urine stream is usually possible during the course of physical assessment, since the infant voids with crying; further, his abdomen is chilled, contracting the bladder slightly.

A rectal examination, done by inserting your little finger (encased in a fingercot) into the child's rectum, should be a part of newborn assessment. Patency of the rectum and anus is thus determined.

ASSESSMENT OF THE UPPER EXTREMITIES

Observe the infant for the position of the arms, which should be held flexed at the elbow. The hands are held clenched. Inspect the skin for color, warmth, and turgor. Test the upper extremities for muscle tone by unflexing the arms for approximately 5 seconds. When you release the arm, it should return immediately to its flexed position. Hold the arms down by the sides and note their length. The fingertips should cover the proximal thigh. Unusually short arms may signify achondroplastic dwarfism.

Examine the fingernails for color and blanching of the nails. Separate the fingers and count them. Observe for webbing between fingers. Observe for unusual curvature of the little finger and inspect the palm for a simian crease (a single palmar crease in contrast to the three creases normally seen in a palm). Both simian creases and inward-curved little fingers are signs of Down's syndrome, although curved fingers and simian creases may also occur normally. Test the wrist for range of motion. It should rotate laterally and medially and flex and extend. Palpate the radial pulses and estimate for symmetrical strength. Palpate the long bones for possible fracture.

A scarf sign is a test for movement of the shoulder and an indication of muscle tone and therefore of muscle maturity. With the infant lying on his back and with his chin in the midline, an arm is brought across his chest toward the opposite shoulder and thus up against the chin in the manner of a scarf. In the mature newborn, the hand should reach to the acromion process but no farther. If the hand goes past the acromion process, muscle tone may be lax, indicating immaturity. This is shown in Fig. 29-6D.

ASSESSMENT OF THE NECK

Inspect the neck for good body alignment. Does the infant hold his head straight, or is it tipped to one side, as happens with torticollis (a torn sternocleidomastoid muscle)?

Observe the infant in a prone position. Does he make an attempt to lift his head? Pull the infant to a sitting position from a supine position and observe for head control. A newborn will have complete head lag until he reaches the sitting position, when he will make a momentary attempt at head support. After this momentary effort, his head will fall forward in a lax manner.

Palpate the sides of the neck for the posterior and anterior cervical, submental, postauricular, and occipital lymph nodes (Fig. 29-2). Palpate the sternocleidomastoid muscle for masses (a hematoma

Fig. 29-2. Lymph nodes of the head and neck.

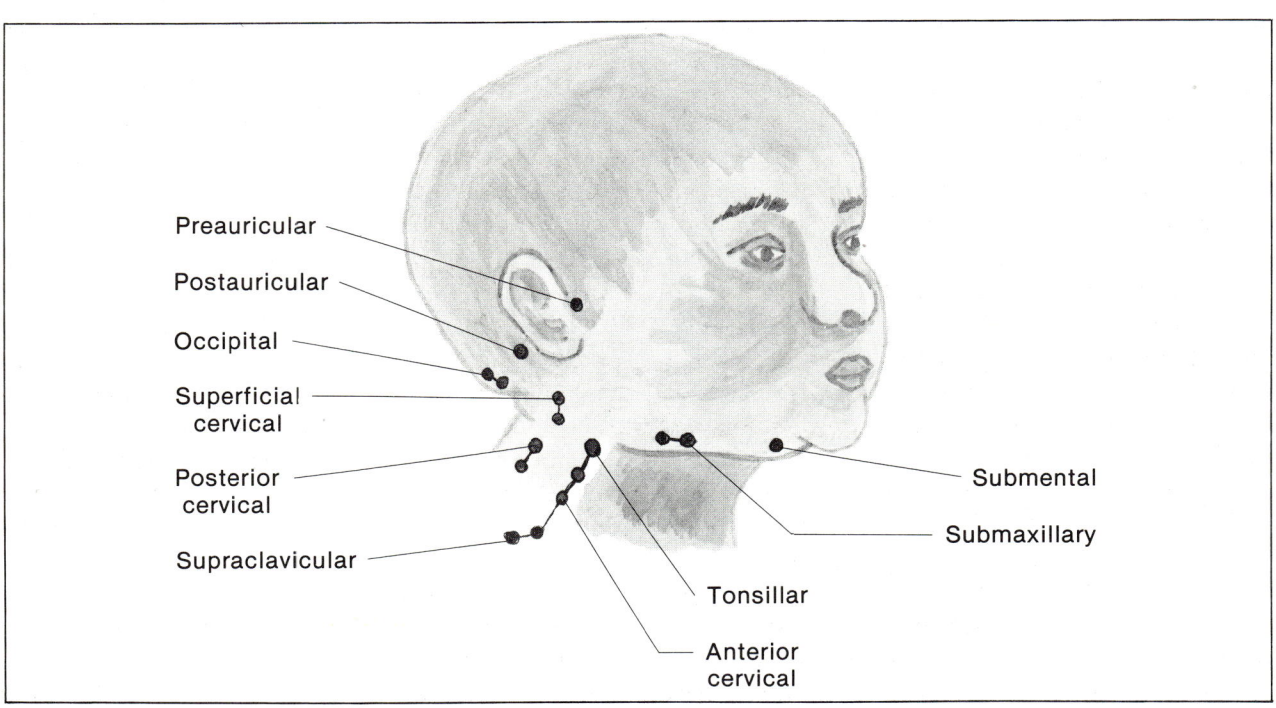

forming from birth injury). Palpate the trachea to be certain that it is in the midline and that the thyroid gland on its lateral aspects is not enlarged.

Turn the infant's head from side to side. Extend it and flex it. Observe for crying or signs of pain when you flex the neck (a test for meningeal irritation). Inspect the anterior neck closely for a dermal sinus, since this is a common opening point for such sinuses.

ASSESSMENT OF THE HEAD

Observe the head and face for symmetry. Observe the infant while he is crying or smiling to see whether both sides of his mouth move in the same direction. Observe the distance between the eyes to detect hypotelorism or hypertelorism (narrowly or widely set eyes).

Inspect the head for molding and the presence of caput succedaneum or cephalhematoma. With the infant in a sitting position, locate and palpate the fontanelles for size and tension. Tension of the fontanelles is deceptive if the infant's head is lowered. Palpate the suture lines for overriding or wide spacing. Feel the hair for texture. Well-nourished newborns have crisp hair; poorly nourished or immature infants have stringy, lifeless hair.

ASSESSMENT OF THE EYES

With the infant in a supine position, lift his head. This maneuver usually causes him to open his eyes. Observe the eyes for periorbital edema (indicated by a bulging of the eye globe) or a sunken appearance (a sign of dehydration). Note any subconjunctival hemorrhage (small hemorrhagic areas on the eye sclera). Check for the presence of strabismus by observing whether or not a light shown in the eyes strikes the same place on both corneas (Fig. 29-3). Transitory strabismus is common in newborns. Test for a blink reflex by shining a light on the eye (a blink reflex is not readily elicited in a newborn by an object moving toward the eye).

Test for pupillary constriction by shining the otoscope light first in one eye and then in the other. Bring the light downward from the forehead or in from the side of the eye, so that the pupil must make an immediate adjustment to the sudden bright light; if you bring the light gradually toward the eye, pupillary constriction will occur so gradually that it is easy to miss. Note whether the corneas are the same size and color. Look for haziness (possible cataract) or an irregular shape such as a coloboma (keyhole pupil) (see Fig. 28-21).

Test for the red reflex by bringing an otoscope light

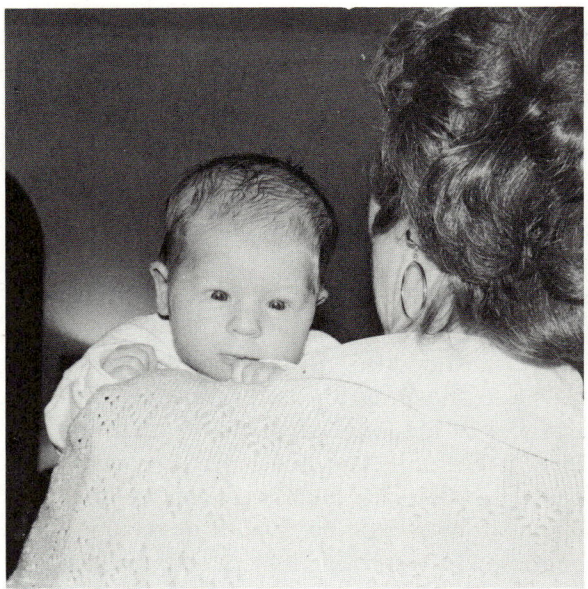

Fig. 29-3. Hirschbrung's test. When a light is shown on a newborn's eyes, the light reflex should strike the pupils equally if they are in good alignment.

up to about 6 inches from the eye. The retina will be visualized as a red disk. Such visualization demonstrates that the cornea, the lens, and the liquid of the eye are clear enough to be seen through and is a gross indication that the retina is intact. The retina and the red reflex are better revealed by use of the ophthalmoscope head of the otoscope.

ASSESSMENT OF THE EARS

Inspect the outer ear for size, shape, and position (the upper portion of the pinna should be on a line drawn backward from the lateral canthus of the eye) (see Fig. 28-22). Inspect the skin immediately in front of the ear for a dermal sinus.

Visualizing the tympanic membrane in a newborn is difficult and generally is not attempted because amniotic fluid and flecks of vernix fill the canal and obliterate the drum and its accompanying landmarks.

It is good practice to test the newborn's hearing by ringing a bell held about 6 inches from each ear. If he is crying, the infant who can hear will stop momentarily; if he is quiet, the newborn will blink his eyes, appear to attend to the sound, and may startle. This method of testing is not highly accurate. A negative response should be noted, however, and the child should be retested at a later time.

ASSESSMENT OF THE NOSE

Inspect the nose for general appearance. Is it unusually broad? Is any ecchymosis present? Are the nares flaring as in an infant with respiratory distress? Shine the otoscope light into the nose to note whether the septum is straight and to attempt to view the turbinates (the cartilage processes on the sides).

Test for choanal atresia by closing the newborn's mouth and compressing one naris at a time with your fingers. Note any discomfort or distress.

ASSESSMENT OF THE MOUTH AND THROAT

Inspect the lips for symmetry. Note any tendency toward a cleft. Introduce a tongue blade into the mouth and inspect the gums for the presence of teeth or a cleft. Look at the tongue and buccal membrane for evidence of thrush (rare under 4 or 5 days of age). Thrush, a monilian infection, appears as white patches on the tongue or mucous membrane. Note the movement of the tongue. Does the infant hold it in the midline or does it deviate to one side?

Inspect the palate for intactness or an unusually high arch; the latter is associated with chromosomal abnormalities. Note any Epstein's pearls (calcium deposits) on the palate or inclusion cysts on the gums.

Introduce the tongue blade farther into the mouth. Using a good light source, gag the newborn by pressing on the base of the tongue with the tongue blade. Note whether the gag reflex is present. Observe in the fleeting instant that the posterior pharynx is visible whether or not the uvula is in the midline and the posterior wall of the pharynx is free of a pharyngeal cyst.

Because newborns have a large quantity of mucus in the back of their throats, turn the infant on his stomach or turn his head to the side following elicitation of a gag reflex so mucus can drain.

ASSESSMENT OF THE BACK

Because you want to leave the newborn in a prone position for a few minutes after eliciting the gag reflex, to be certain he is not choking on secretions, this is a good time to examine his back.

Lanugo is usually evident across the shoulders of newborns. The spine, particularly in the sacral area, should be inspected carefully for any tuft of hair or indentation that would reveal spina bifida occulta.

Inspect the scapulae for symmetry. Inspect the coccygeal area for a pilodermal sinus.

ASSESSMENT OF NEUROLOGICAL FUNCTION

Stroke the newborn's back to calm or quiet him before attempting to elicit any reflexes.

These reflexes should be elicited: rooting, sucking, palmar grasp, plantar grasp, step-in-place, placing, trunk incurvation, magnet, crossed extension. Landau, Babinski, tonic neck, and Moro. The techniques for eliciting these reflexes are discussed in the preceding chapter.

Two deep tendon reflexes should be included in the examination: the patellar and the biceps. A patellar reflex can be elicited in a newborn by tapping the patellar tendon with the tip of a finger; in older children or adults a percussion hammer is needed to demonstrate this reflex. The lower leg will move perceptibly if the child has a mature reflex. A biceps reflex is difficult to elicit in a newborn. To demonstrate this reflex, place the thumb of your left hand on the tendon of the biceps muscle on the inner surface of the elbow. Tap the thumb as it rests on the tendon. You are more likely to feel the tendon contract than to observe movement. A biceps reflex is a test for spinal nerves C-5 and C-6; a patellar reflex is a test for spinal nerves L-2 through L-4.

ASSESSING THE INFANT'S CRY

Assessing a newborn's health is a complex task because of the multitude of normal variations present and because many subtle changes occur as newborns recover from the birth process and establish respirations and other body functions.

If he did not cry during the physical assessment, irritate the soles of his feet or pinch a leg and make him cry. Evaluate the sound of his cry for loudness and pitch. A brain-injured newborn has a high, shrill cry; an immature infant has a weak cry; a child with laryngeal stridor has a hoarse cry.

MEASUREMENTS

Securing accurate measurements of the head, chest, abdominal circumferences, and length is part of a newborn assessment. It is good to leave these measurements to the last so that the newborn is not tired out by them before the neurological assessment. The measurements must be plotted on a growth chart such as that shown in Fig. 28-1 in order to be interpreted meaningfully.

Assessment of Gestation Age

The best way of judging whether a newborn is a term infant is not by the due date but by the specific findings of the physical assessment.

There are many indexes of maturity. Usher [11] has proposed the five criteria given in Table 29-2 as a basis for evaluating gestational maturity. These are easy, quick criteria to use for assessment of all newborns.

Table 29-2. Clinical Criteria for Gestational Assessment

Finding	Gestation Age (Weeks)		
	0–36	37–38	39 and Over
Sole creases	Anterior transverse crease only	Occasional creases in anterior two-thirds	Sole covered with creases
Breast nodule diameter	2 mm	4 mm	7 mm
Scalp hair	Fine and fuzzy	Fine and fuzzy	Coarse and silky
Earlobe	Pliable; no cartilage	Some cartilage	Stiffened by thick cartilage
Testes and scrotum	Testes in lower canal; scrotum small; few rugae	Intermediate	Testes pendulous; scrotum full; extensive rugae

Source. R. Usher et al., Judgment of fetal age. *Pediatr. Clin. North Am.* 13:835, 1966.

DUBOWITZ MATURITY SCALE

Dubowitz [5] has devised a gestational rating scale whereby newborns can be observed and tested and rated as to maturity level based on much more extensive criteria.

All newborns that appear to be immature by Usher's criteria or who are light in weight at birth or early by date should be assessed by means of the more definitive criteria. Although completing a Dubowitz assessment takes practice, it is a tool that can be used successfully by nurses. Alone in a small community hospital nursery, debating whether the infant just delivered needs immediate medical intervention or can wait until morning for care, the nurse who can do a Dubowitz examination and report a standardized gestation age report may make the difference in the physician's actions.

The Dubowitz scale has been modified by Ballard [2] to an assessment that can be completed in 3 to 4 minutes. The assessment consists of two portions (Figs. 29-4 and 29-5). The first is a series of observations about such things as skin texture and color, lanugo, foot creases, and genital, ear, and breast maturity. The body part is inspected and given a score of 0 to 5 as described in Fig. 29-4. This observation scoring should be done as soon as possible after birth as skin assessment becomes much less reliable after 24 hours.

To complete the second half of the examination, you observe or position the baby as shown in Fig. 29-5. Again, the child is given numerical scores from 0 to 5. Examples of reflexes or tests of maturity are shown in Fig. 29-6.

To establish the child's gestation age, the total score obtained (on both sections) is compared to the rating scale in Fig. 29-7. As can be seen by this scale, an infant with a total score of 5 is at 26 weeks' gestation age; a total score of 10 reveals a gestation age of about 28 weeks; a score of 40 total points is found in infants at term or 40 weeks' gestation.

Using such a standard method of rating maturity is helpful in detecting infants who are small for gestation age (they are light in weight but the neuromuscular and physical observation scales will be adequate for their weeks in utero) and those who are immature because of a miscalculated due date. An infant who is found to be at a lower gestation age than was predicted by the mother's calculation of due date needs careful observation in the neonatal period and should not be admitted to routine nursery care.

Fig. 29-4. Physical maturity assessment criteria. (From J. L. Ballard et al., A simplified assessment of gestational age. Pediatr. Res. 11:374, 1977.)

	0	1	2	3	4	5
SKIN	gelatinous red, transparent	smooth pink, visible veins	superficial peeling &/or rash, few veins	cracking pale area, rare veins	parchment, deep cracking, no vessels	leathery, cracked, wrinkled
LANUGO	none	abundant	thinning	bald areas	mostly bald	
PLANTAR CREASES	no crease	faint red marks	anterior transverse crease only	creases ant. 2/3	creases cover entire sole	
BREAST	barely percept.	flat areola, no bud	stippled areola, 1–2 mm bud	raised areola, 3–4 mm bud	full areola, 5–10 mm bud	
EAR	pinna flat, stays folded	sl. curved pinna, soft with slow recoil	well-curv. pinna, soft but ready recoil	formed & firm with instant recoil	thick cartilage, ear stiff	
GENITALS Male	scrotum empty, no rugae		testes descending, few rugae	testes down, good rugae	testes pendulous, deep rugae	
GENITALS Female	prominent clitoris & labia minora		majora & minora equally prominent	majora large, minora small	clitoris & minora completely covered	

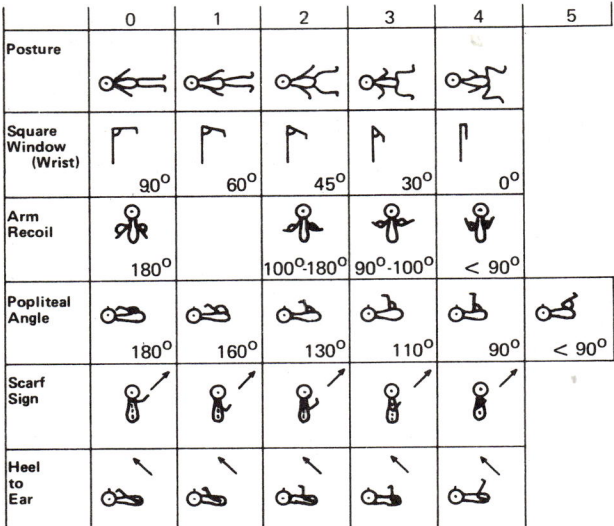

Fig. 29-5. Neuromuscular maturity assessment criteria. Posture: *With infant supine and quiet, score as follows: arms and legs extended = 0; slight or moderate flexion of hips and knees = 1; moderate to strong flexion of hips and knees = 2; legs flexed and abducted, arms slightly flexed = 3; full flexion of arms and legs = 4.* Square window: *Flex hand at the wrist. Exert pressure sufficient to get as much flexion as possible. The angle between hypothenar eminence and anterior aspect of forearm is measured and scored. Do not rotate wrist.* Arm recoil: *With infant supine, fully flex forearm for 5 seconds, then fully extend by pulling the hands and release. Score as follows: remain extended or random movements = 0; incomplete or partial flexion = 2; brisk return to full flexion = 4.* Popliteal angle: *With infant supine and pelvis flat on examining surface, flex leg on thigh and fully flex thigh with one hand. With the other hand extend leg and score the angle attained according to the chart.* Scarf sign: *With infant supine, draw infant's hand across the neck and as far across the opposite shoulder as possible. Assistance to elbow is permissible by lifting it across the body. Score according to location of the elbow: elbow reaches opposite anterior axillary line = 0; elbow between opposite anterior axillary line and midline of thorax = 1; elbow at midline of thorax = 3; elbow does not reach midline of thorax = 4.* Heel to ear: *With infant supine, hold infant's foot with one hand and move it as near to the head as possible without forcing it. Keep pelvis flat on examining surface.* (From J. L. Ballard et al., A simplified assessment of gestational age. Pediatr. Res. 11:374, 1977.)

THE BRAZELTON NEONATAL BEHAVIORAL ASSESSMENT SCALE

The Brazelton Neonatal Behavioral Assessment Scale is a rating scale devised by Brazelton [4] to evaluate the newborn's behavioral capacity or his ability to respond to set stimuli. Six major categories of behavior—habituation, orientation, motor maturity, variation, self-quieting ability, and social behavior—are assessed. These terms are defined in Table 29-3.

It is important that one have a wealth of experience with newborns before utilizing a Brazelton Neonatal Behavioral Assessment Scale. Performing an assessment by use of the scale may be done by a nurse but requires training in the different techniques so that it is used consistently from one individual to another.

There are 27 behavioral items (Table 29-4) that are evaluated on a score of 1 to 9 and 20 elicited responses or reflexes scored on a 3 point scale. An "average" baby scores about the midpoint on each scale. Since many infants have uncoordinated behavior for the first 48 hours after delivery, it is suggested that the infant be evaluated on the third day of life. Unlike many assessment scales, the infant is scored on his *best* performance rather than on his average performance.

Table 29-3. Categories on a Brazelton Neonatal Behavioral Assessment Scale

Category	Description
Habituation	A newborn is capable of diminishing his response to stimuli such as light, sound, and a pinprick to his heel. When first stimulated this way, he may startle, his respirations become more rapid, he may blink rapidly. Gradually, he "shuts out" the stimulus and does not respond to it. This is habituation
Orientation	When a newborn is given an auditory or visual stimulus (bell or bright light), he looks or turns toward the stimulus or at least indicates by a change of respirations that he is aware of the new experience being presented to him
Motor maturity	The organization of the newborn's motor coordination and the degree of that coordination are assessed throughout the examination by his ability to respond to the examiner's interventions
Variation	Infants have variable degrees of peaks of excitement, general activity, color, and periods of alertness and sleep
Self-quieting ability	When disturbed, a newborn uses interventions to console himself: putting his hand to his mouth, sucking on his fist or tongue, etc.
Social behavior	A newborn naturally responds to being held closely by cuddling; despite many unbelievers, he can smile

Source. T. B. Brazelton, *Neonatal Behavioral Assessment Scale. Clinics in Developmental Medicine*, Vol. 50. Philadelphia: Lippincott, 1973.

Table 29-4. Behavioral Items Assessed (Brazelton Neonatal Behavioral Assessment Scale)

1. Response decrement to repeated visual stimuli.
2. Response decrement to rattle.
3. Response decrement to bell.
4. Response decrement to pinprick.
5. Orienting response to inanimate visual stimuli.
6. Orienting response to inanimate auditory stimuli.
7. Orienting response to animate visual—examiner's face.
8. Orienting response to animate auditory—examiner's voice.
9. Orienting responses to animate visual and auditory stimuli.
10. Quality and duration of alert periods.
11. General muscle tone—in resting and in response to being handled.
12. Motor maturity.
13. Traction responses as he is pulled to sit.
14. Cuddliness—responses to being cuddled by the examiner.
15. Defensive movements—reactions to a cloth over his face.
16. Consolability with intervention by examiner.
17. Peak of excitement and his capacity to control himself.
18. Rapidity of build-up to crying state.
19. Irritability during the examination.
20. General assessment of kind and degree of activity.
21. Tremulousness.
22. Amount of startling.
23. Lability of skin color.
24. Lability of states during entire examination.
25. Self-quieting activity—attempts to console self and control state.
26. Hand-to-mouth activity.
27. Smiling.

Source. T. B. Brazelton, *Neonatal Behavioral Assessment Scale. Clinics in Developmental Medicine*, Vol. 50. Philadelphia: Lippincott, 1973.

The total evaluation takes 20 to 30 minutes to complete.

Throughout the testing, the infant's state of consciousness will affect his ability to perform. Prior to any stimulation activity, therefore, the infant is rated as to his "state" as follows:

Sleep states:
1. Deep sleep with regular breathing, eyes closed, no spontaneous activity except startles or jerky movements at quiet regular intervals; external stimuli produce startles with some delay; suppression of startles is rapid, and state changes are less likely than from other states. No eye movements are present.
2. Light sleep with eyes closed; rapid eye movements can be observed under closed lids; low activity level, with random movements and startles or startle equivalents; movements are likely to be smoother and more monitored than in state 1; responds to internal and external stimuli with startle equivalents, often with a resulting change of state. Respirations are irregular, sucking movements occur off and on.

Awake states:
1. Drowsy or semidozing; eyes may be open or closed, eyelids fluttering; activity level variable, with interspersed, mild startles from time to time; reactive to sensory stimuli, but response often delayed; state change after stimulation frequently noted. Movements are usually smooth.
2. Alert, with bright look; seems to focus attention on source of stimulation, such as an object to be sucked or a visual or auditory stimulus; impinging stimuli may break through, but with some delay in response. Motor activity is at a minimum.
3. Eyes open; considerable motor activity, with thrusting movements of the extremities, and even a few spontaneous startles; reactive to external stimulation with increase in startles or motor activity, but discrete reactions difficult to distinguish because of generally high activity level.
4. Crying; characterized by intense crying that is difficult to break through with stimulation.

A typical item that is scored in the assessment is the infant's response to being held in the cuddled position against an examiner's chest or shoulder. This typical item (cuddliness) is scored as follows:

1. Actively resists being held, continuously pushing away, thrashing, or stiffening.
2. Resists being held most but not all of the time.
3. Does not resist but does not participate either, lies passively in arms and against shoulder (like a sack of meal).
4. Eventually molds into arms, but after a lot of nestling and cuddling by examiner.
5. Usually molds and relaxes when first held; nestles head in crook of neck or elbow of examiner. Turns toward examiner's body when held horizontally; on shoulder, seems to lean forward.
6. Always molds initially with above activities.
7. Always molds initially with nestling, and turns toward examiner's body and leans forward.
8. In addition to molding and relaxing, baby nestles and turns head, leans forward on shoulder, fits feet into cavity of other arm; all of body participates.
9. All of the above, and baby grasps hold of the examiner to cling to him/her.

Premature Infant   *Full-term Infant*

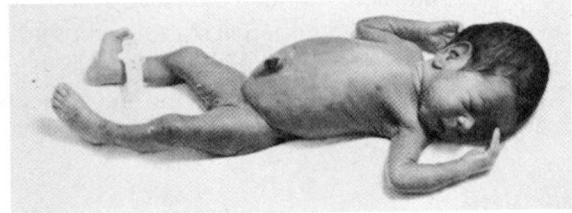 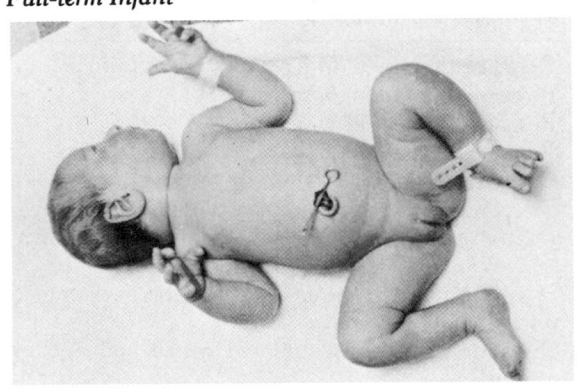

RESTING POSTURE *The premature infant is characterized by very little, if any, flexion in the upper extremities and only partial flexion of the lower extremities. The full-term infant exhibits flexion in all four extremities.*

A

Premature Infant, 28–32 Weeks   *Full-term Infant*

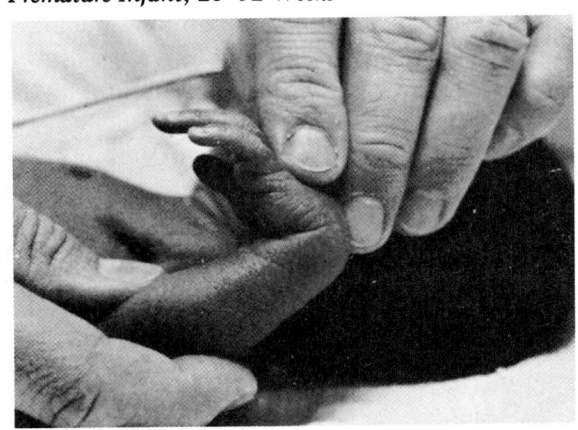 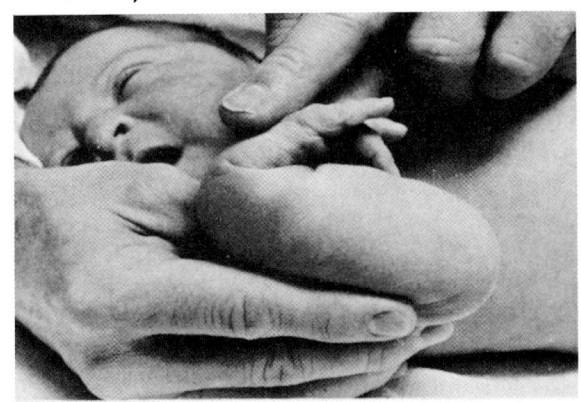

WRIST FLEXION *The wrist is flexed, applying enough pressure to get the hand as close to the forearm as possible. The angle between the hypothenar eminence and the ventral aspect of the forearm is measured. (Care must be taken not to rotate the infant's wrist.) The premature infant at 28–32 weeks' gestation will exhibit a 90° angle. With the full-term infant it is possible to flex the hand onto the arm.*

B

Fig. 29-6. Examples of reflexes or tests used to judge gestation age. A. Posture. B. Square window. C. Recoil of extremities. D. Scarf sign. E. Heel to ear. F. Plantar creases. G. Breast tissue. H. Ear. I. Male genitals. J. Female genitals. (From R. Sullivan et al., Determining a newborn's gestational age. M.C.N. 4:38, 1979. Original source: R. L. Schreiner [Ed.], Care of the Newborn. Indianapolis: Indiana University Press, 1978.)

Flex Extremities and Hold

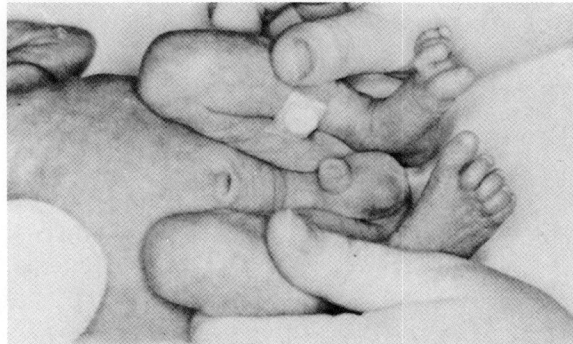

Response in Premature Infant

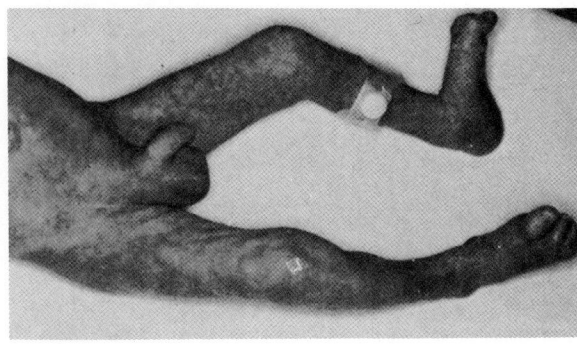

Extend

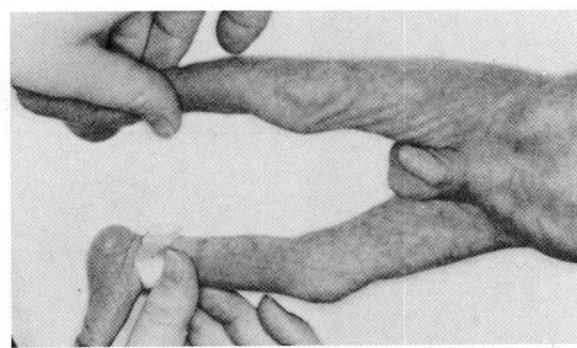

Response in Full-term Infant

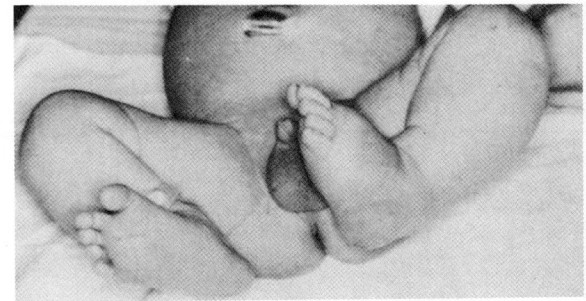

RECOIL OF EXTREMITIES *Place the infant supine. To test recoil of the legs (1) flex the legs and knees fully and hold for five seconds, (2) extend by pulling on the feet, (3) release. To test the arms, flex forearms and follow same procedure. In the premature infant response is minimal or absent; in the full-term infant extremities return briskly to full flexion.*

C

Premature Infant

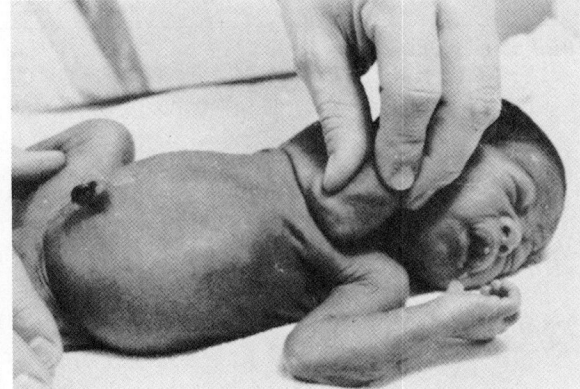

Full-term Infant

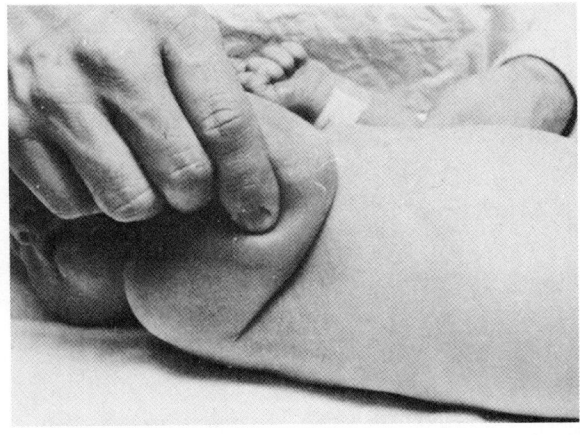

SCARF SIGN *Hold the baby supine, take his hand, and try to place it around his neck and above the opposite shoulder as far posteriorly as possible. Assist this maneuver by lifting the elbow across the body. See how far across the chest the elbow will go. In the premature infant the elbow will reach near or across the midline. In the full-term infant the elbow will not reach the midline.*

D

Health Assessment of the Newborn

Premature Infant

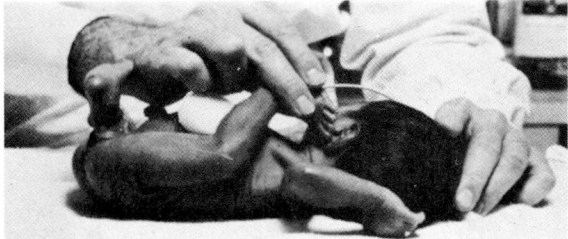

Full-term Infant

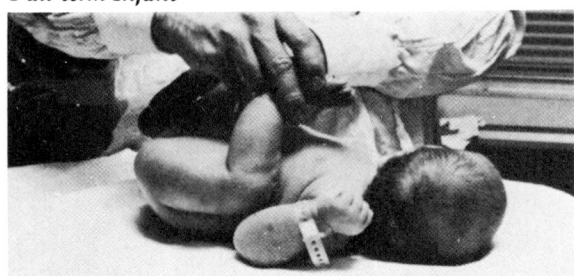

HEEL TO EAR *With the baby supine and his hips positioned flat on the bed, draw the baby's foot as near to his ear as it will go without forcing it. Observe the distance between the foot and head as well as the degree of extension at the knee. In the premature infant very little resistance will be met. In the full-term infant there will be marked resistance; it will be impossible to draw the baby's foot to his ear.*

E

Premature Infant

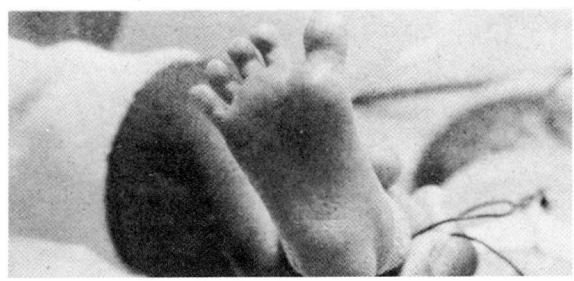

Full-term Infant

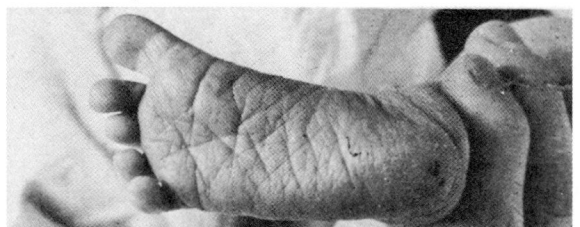

SOLE CREASES *The sole of the premature infant has very few or no creases. With the increasing gestation age, the number and depth of sole creases multiply, so that the full-term baby has creases involving the heel. (Wrinkles that occur after 24 hours of age can sometimes be confused with true creases.)*

F

Premature Infant

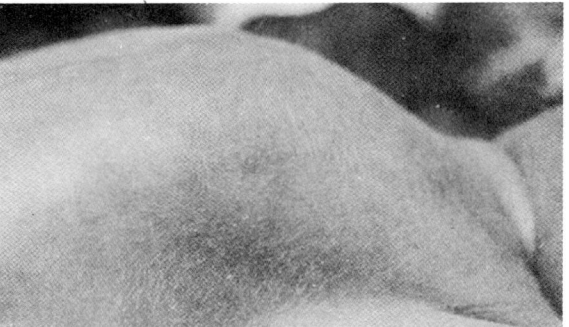

Full-term Infant

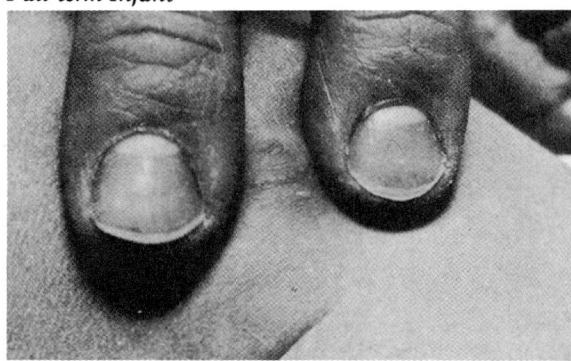

NIPPLES AND BREAST *In infants younger than 34 weeks' gestation the areola and nipple are barely visible. After 34 weeks the areola becomes raised. Also, the infant of less than 36 weeks' gestation has no breast tissue. Breast tissue arises with increasing gestation age due to maternal hormonal stimulation. Thus, an infant of 39–40 weeks will have 5–6 mm of breast tissue, and this amount will increase with age.*

G

EARS At less than 34 weeks' gestation infants have very flat, relatively shapeless ears. Shape develops over time so that an infant between 34 and 36 weeks has a slight incurving of the superior part of the ear; the term infant is characterized by incurving of two-thirds of the pinna; and in an infant older than 39 weeks the incurving continues to the lobe. If the extremely premature infant's ear is folded over, it will stay folded. Cartilage begins to appear at approximately 32 weeks so that the ear returns slowly to its original position. In an infant of more than 40 weeks' gestation, there is enough ear cartilage so that the ear stands erect away from the head and returns quickly when folded. (When folding the ear over during examination be certain that the surrounding area is wiped clean or the ear may adhere to the vernix.)

Premature Infant, 34–36 Weeks

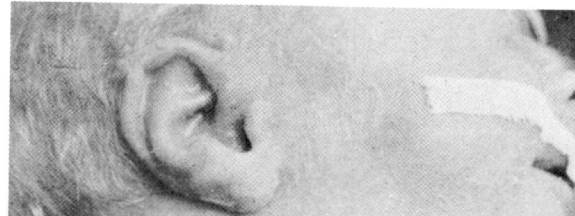

Full-term Infant

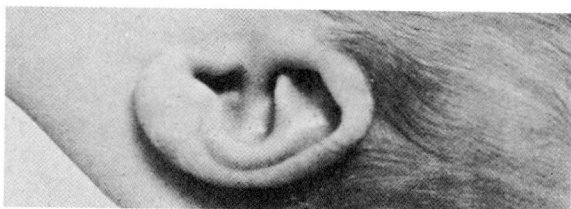

H

Premature Male

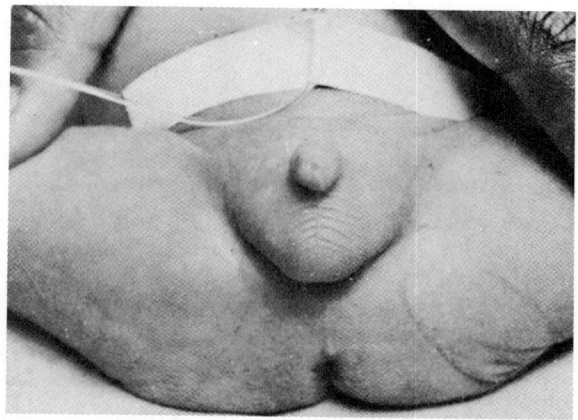

Full-term Male

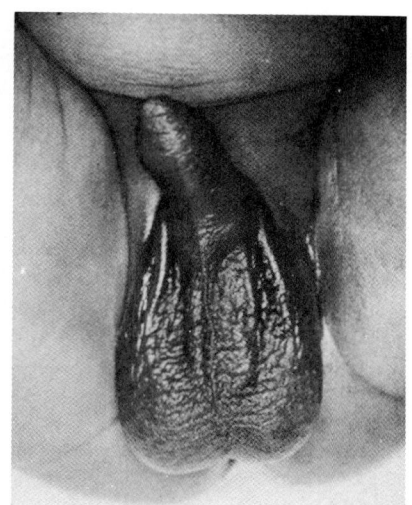

MALE GENITALIA In the premature male the testes are very high in the inguinal canal and there are very few rugae on the scrotum. The full-term infant's testes are lower in the scrotum and many rugae have developed.

I

Premature Female

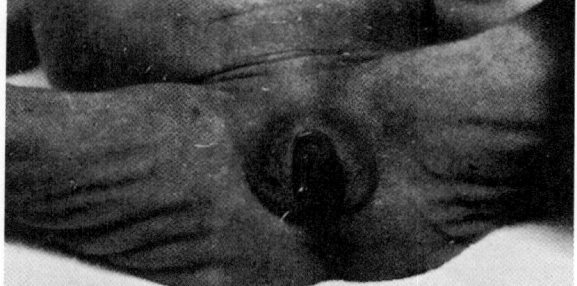

Full-term Female

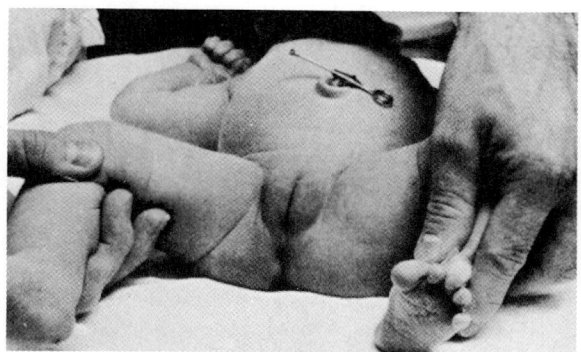

FEMALE GENITALIA When the premature female is positioned on her back with hips abducted, the clitoris is very prominent and the labia majora are very small and widely separated. The labia minora and the clitoris are covered by the labia majora in the full-term infant.

J

Score	Wks
5	26
10	28
15	30
20	32
25	34
30	36
35	38
40	40
45	42
50	44

Fig. 29-7. Scoring for a Ballard assessment scale. The point total arrived at by assessment is compared to the left column. The matching number in the right column reveals the infant's age in gestation weeks.

Following the detailed scoring of items using the test form, a descriptive paragraph relating particular characteristics of the infant is written. Examples of such descriptive paragraphs follow:

This was a well-muscled, well-proportioned, active, responsive boy with an alert, inquisitive face, big dark eyes, and a shock of black hair. He gave the appearance of being "older" and of "looking right through you." As one played with him, he became more alert, and on several occasions seemed to smile as he alerted. He was not fat, but was muscular and square in appearance. There were no signs of dehydration or undernutrition, and he showed remarkable autonomic stability (skin color changes) even after he was undressed for a long period. He maintained steady states of alertness for long periods. His main feature was the maturity of motor responsiveness that he could command. As one set off a tonic-neck response, he quickly used it to help him bring his hand up to his mouth. After a Moro and the usual cry, he turned his head to one side, brought his hand up to his mouth to quiet himself. Even as he responded to visual and auditory stimulation with rapid alerting and continuous responses, one felt that he had himself under control. A mother would feel that this was a mature, exciting boy, but she might also feel that he could manage pretty well by himself. Striking about him was his maturity, resourcefulness, and his capacity to respond and master stimulation both from within and without. One would predict a rapid, smooth, developmental course for him. [4]

This thin, wiry boy weighed 6 lbs. 10 oz. He was stringy and long in appearance, had a tense look and tense musculature with little subcutaneous fat. His arms and legs seemed constantly in motion when he was awake. He had been in deep sleep when he was first approached, but he waked up screaming. His changes of state were characteristically rapid, and there was little opportunity to reach him as he moved from sleeping to crying or back again. In order to quiet him, the E[xaminer] had to swaddle him or hold him tightly or provide him with a pacifier and rock him. When a rattle, voice or sudden movement was presented, he startled, and began to cry. He made little effort to quiet himself. This over-reaction to stimuli seemed to interfere with his ability to attend to auditory and visual stimuli for when he was successfully restrained, he could look around and alert to the face or a red ball, or to alert and turn to the voice or a rattle. As soon as the E[xaminer] realized this, his performance changed from that of an overreactive, hyperactive one to that of an alert, responsive baby. But the restraint of interfering motor reactions and the abrupt state changes which went with them was a prerequisite to finding this ability to attend to stimuli.

A kind of autonomic instability when he was undressed and unrestrained went along with this reactivity. As soon as he was uncovered, he turned red then bluish, but when he was covered again, his good color returned. We felt he was a kind of baby who could be very difficult for a mother who was not aware of the need for a calming, restraining environment in which to offer cues from the outside. [4]

For nurses, the most significant information supplied by use of this scale is the concrete evidence that newborns are not passive, nonhearing, unseeing, unresponsive, or all alike. They can see and hear; they are able to respond to stimuli presented to them and after a time shut out the stimulus so it no longer affects them. They are able to quiet themselves after crying. They are individual in their responses to the happenings around them.

Pointing out to the parents many of the items tested on the assessment scale, such as how the infant alerts (eyes widen, head held as if listening) or orients himself to sound (turns toward the direction of his mother's voice or appears to listen to the sound of her voice), how he follows objects (carefully, he loses them at the midline), how he naturally cuddles when held next to his mother, are excellent examples of newborn behaviors to point out to parents. If parents perceive a newborn as just someone passive and unresponsive, they are likely to talk to him very little, to look at him very little. If they see that right from the beginning he is capable of interacting with them, they are more responsive. The more they know about their baby, the more they will be able to understand his cues and determine and meet his needs.

The descriptive paragraph on each baby is invaluable for helping everyone involved in the infant's care come to know him as an individual and be more able to meet his newborn needs.

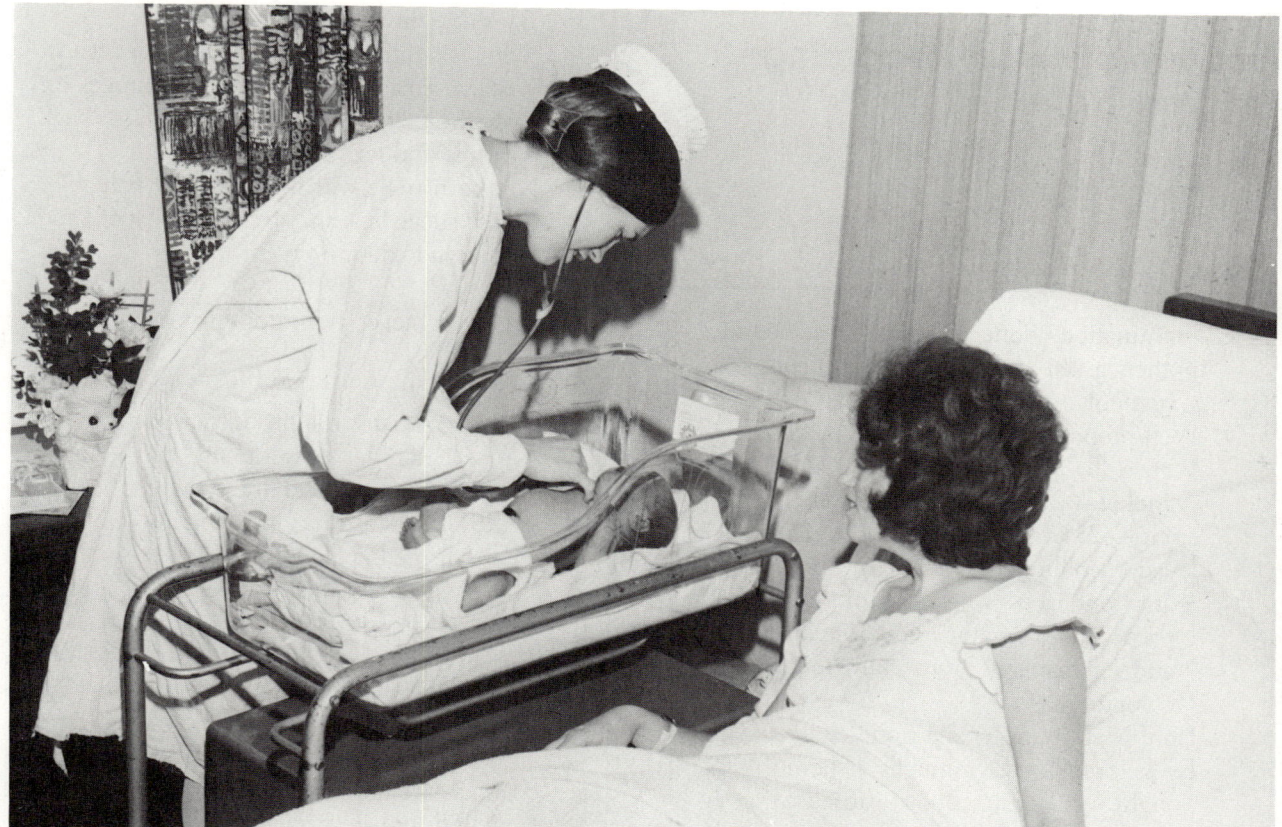

Fig. 29-8. A nurse examining a newborn. Doing a physical assessment by the bedside allows the mother an opportunity to ask questions about her child's development or care. (Courtesy of the Department of Medical Photography, Children's Hospital, Buffalo, N.Y.)

Assessment of the Maternal-Newborn Interaction

The manner in which a new mother handles her infant is the result of several factors: her expectations of a newborn baby, her familiarity with newborns, her perception of herself as a mother, and the events occurring during pregnancy. To assure yourself that this mother and child will be able to establish a good mother-child relationship, you need to observe the mother handling her child and to discuss with her the significant events of her pregnancy and her plans for her child.

It is helpful to know whether or not the pregnancy was planned. If it was not, how did the woman feel when she first suspected that she was pregnant? When pregnancy was confirmed? At quickening? During labor? At delivery? When she first saw or held the child?

Most women can name a point in pregnancy when they knew they wanted the baby. Such a point may not have been reached during pregnancy; it may not have been reached until delivery or until the mother first fed the baby. Some mothers are unable to say that they know they want this child until he has been home for a number of weeks.

In the hospital, it is important to ask the mother to try to identify this point. If she cannot do so by the time she leaves the hospital, she is still within the normal time period of response. The physician who will be caring for the infant or the community health nurse who will be visiting the child should be informed, however, that maternal-child interaction is still incomplete, so that they can be alert to the need for counseling if interaction does not improve in the coming months.

Chapter 24 describes the pattern of initial maternal contact. Be certain that you handle the newborn with the mother present; seeing you in action may speed up the process of learning how to handle her baby. Performing a physical assessment at the mother's bedside (Fig. 29-8) gives her an opportunity to watch skilled newborn handling and to ask questions about her newborn. Further, as you note your findings on the newborn's reflexes, vaginal discharge, caput succedaneum, and so on, you can immediately assure the mother that these are normal newborn findings.

Health Assessment of the Newborn

Problem-oriented Recording: Progress Notes

Baby Kraft (John Joseph)
Day 1

Problem: Health assessment

> S. Examination done by mother's bedside; mother asked questions about breast engorgement.
> O. Well-proportioned, black male newborn.
> Wgt: 6 lb. 5 oz.—10% (AGA). Hgt: 19½ inches—25%. Head circumference: 34 cm—25%.
> Head: Molding at vertex still prominent; ant. font.: 3 × 4 cm and soft; post. font.: pinpoint. Edematous raised area on right and left parietal 3 cm diameter, no discoloration.
> Hair: Mature in thickness and character.
> Eyes: Small subconjunctival hemorrhage right eye. Extraocular muscles grossly intact. Follow both sides to midline. Edema on eyelids present; mild inflammatory response on conjunctiva present.
> Ears: Normal alignment; apparent patent canal meatus; firm cartilage, no discharge. Pinpoint dermal sinus in front of right ear, not inflamed, no discharge.
> Nose: Midline septum, no discharge, patent.
> Mouth: Midline uvula, palate intact, no teeth; 2 epithelial cysts on soft palate; gag reflex intact.
> Neck: Midline trachea, no dermal sinuses, supple, no nodes palpable. Clavicles intact.
> Heart: Rate 130, normal tones, no murmur heard.
> Lungs: Air exchange all lobes, rate 30; rhonchi heard in both upper lobes.
> Chest: Symmetrical, no retractions, breast tissue palpable 2 cm; no discharge.
> Abdomen: Soft, no masses. Liver palpable 1 cm, spleen not palpable, 2 kidneys palpable.
> Genitalia: Urinary meatus present; left testis not palpable; scant rugae on left scrotum.
> Extremities: Full range of motion; hips abduct to 180 degrees.
> Back: No dimples, hair tufts visible.
> Skin: Slate gray 2 × 3 cm macular area in sacral area; scattered pinpoint papules on erythematous base on abdomen, back arms, and legs.
> A. Newborn male with left testis not palpable. Caput succedaneum, mongolian spot, and erythema toxicum present.
>
> Goals: a. Achieve transition to extrauterine life.
> b. Mother to become familiar with normal variations in newborn.
> c. Testicular abnormality to be confirmed or ruled out by M.D.
> d. If testicular abnormality is confirmed, plan of care to be outlined for parents before discharge.
>
> P. 1. Parents not told of undescended testis—wait for M.D. confirmation.
> 2. Discuss mongolian spot, caput, and newborn rash with mother and assure her these are normal.
> 3. Notify private pediatrician. Parents want early discharge, 24–48 hours if possible.

References

1. Alexander, M., and Brown, M. S. *Pediatric Physical Diagnosis for Nurses*. New York: McGraw-Hill, 1977.
2. Ballard, J. L., et al. A simplified assessment of gestational age. *Pediatr. Res.* 11:374, 1977.
3. Bellig, L. L. The expanded nursing role in the neonatal intensive care unit. *Clin. Perinatol.* 7:159, 1980.
4. Brazelton, T. B. *Neonatal Behavioral Assessment Scale. Clinics in Developmental Medicine*, Vol. 50. Philadelphia: Lippincott, 1973.
5. Dubowitz, L., et al. Clinical assessment of gestational age in the newborn infant. *J. Pediatr.* 77:1, 1970.
6. Erickson, M. P. Trends in assessing the newborn and parents. *M.C.N.* 3:99, 1978.
7. Kiergis, C. A., et al. Predicting infant Apgar scores. *Nurs. Res.* 26:439, 1977.
8. O'Doherty, N. Characteristics of the normal infant at term. *Midwives Chron.* 90:120, 1977.
9. Schweitzer, B. The pediatric nurse practitioner and the normal neonate. *Pediatr. Nurs.* 3:43, 1977.
10. Sullivan, R., et al. Determining a newborn's gestational age. *M.C.N.* 4:38, 1979.
11. Usher, R., et al. Judgment of fetal age. *Pediatr. Clin. North Am.* 13:835, 1966.

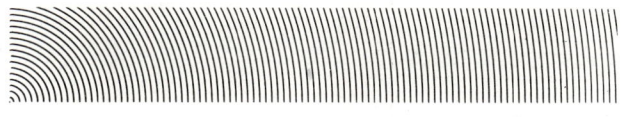

30. Nutritional Needs of the Newborn

Because proper nutrition is essential for optimal growth and development, knowledge of good infant nutrition is a fundamental requirement for persons involved in the health supervision of newborns. In no other area of nutrition, with the possible exception of weight control or diabetes, is the nurse asked more questions than she is asked about the process of infant feeding.

Nutritional Allowances for the Newborn

Although breast-feeding is for many reasons the method of choice for feeding human infants, a mother should be urged to choose for herself the method of infant feeding, breast or bottle, that will be most satisfying and convenient for her. No matter which method she chooses, the end result must meet the nutritional and psychological needs of her infant.

Nutrition is extremely important in the early months of life, because brain growth is proceeding at a rapid rate during this time. Infants in whom kwashiorkor (a protein depletion disease) develops when they are 3 to 6 months old may have permanent stunting of physical growth and may fail to reach their full intellectual or psychological development. Mental retardation has been observed in infant rats when their caloric intake is inadequate. Rats, piglets, and puppies fed a diet adequate in calories but deficient in protein show signs of degenerative changes in nerve cells [23].

As important in terms of growth is the maternal stimulation or love the infant receives. This is directly related to feeding, since the mother is close to her infant during feeding time and he will be particularly sensitive to her demonstration of affection or to her lack of warmth. An infant who does not experience a warm relationship with his mother may fail to thrive as surely as one denied sufficient protein or calories.

CALORIC REQUIREMENT

Growth in the neonatal period and early infancy is more rapid than at any other period of life. Therefore, the caloric requirements exceed those at any other age. A newborn and an infant up to 2 months of age require 120 calories per kilogram of body weight (50 to 55 calories per pound) every 24 hours to provide an adequate amount of food for maintenance and allow for growth as well. After 2 months of age, the amount gradually declines until the requirement at 1 year is down to 100 calories per kilogram, or 45 calories per pound per day. In adults, the requirement is 42 calories per kilogram, or 20 calories per pound per day.

The actual caloric requirement, of course, depends on the activity of the baby and the rate of his growth. An active infant, one who cries frequently and squirms constantly, will need more calories than one who is more passive and is content to spend long hours playing quietly or just studying his environment.

A large number of mothers tend to feed their babies more calories than they physiologically need (especially extra quantities of milk), believing that a chubby-cheeked baby with fat legs is a healthy one. This is not necessarily the case; an overweight baby is more likely to become an overweight adult than one whose weight is within the usual range during the first year of life. The fat cells in the overweight infant appear to increase in size and remain large, so that he tends to be obese ever afterward. Unusually rapid weight gain in the early months of life of a term infant is related to obesity and overweight in later childhood [9].

A formula should contain about 9 to 12 percent of the calories as protein and 45 to 55 percent of the calories as lactose carbohydrate. The balance should be fat, of which about 10 percent (4 percent of the calories) should be linoleic acid [15].

PROTEIN REQUIREMENT

Because of the extremely rapid growth during infancy and because protein is necessary for the formation of new cells and the maturation and maintenance of existing cells, protein requirements are high during the newborn and infancy period. The nutritional allowance of protein for the first two months of life is 2.2 gm per kilogram of body weight; for ages 2 to 6 months it is 2.0 gm per kilogram; for ages 6 months to 1 year it is 1.8 gm per kilogram. Both human milk and cow's milk provide all the essential amino acids. Histidine, an amino acid that appears to be essential for infant growth but is not necessary for adult growth, is found in both forms of milk.

Cow's milk contains about 16 percent of its calories as protein; human milk, about 8 percent. Thus the milk in a formula containing cow's milk must be diluted. Undiluted cow's milk creates such a rich solute load (the amount of urea and electrolytes that must be excreted in the urine) that newborn kidneys are overwhelmed. The protein in cow's milk differs from that in human milk in composition as well as in amount. The main protein in human milk is lactalbumin; the main protein in cow's milk is casein. The curd tension in milk is related to the amount of casein present. Thus, the curd in cow's milk is large, tough, and difficult to digest; in human milk, the curd is softer and easier to digest.

FAT REQUIREMENTS

Linoleic acid is an essential fatty acid necessary for growth and skin integrity in infants. It is found in both human and cow's milk, but human milk contains about three times as much. Infants fed on skimmed milk for long periods of time (when other sources of food are not being offered) may be deficient in linoleic acid. Therefore feeding skimmed milk is not the answer to controlling obesity in young infants. In addition, skimmed milk does not contain sufficient calories (only about half as many).

CARBOHYDRATE REQUIREMENTS

Lactose, the disaccharide found in human milk, appears to be the most easily digested of the carbohydrates. It improves calcium absorption and aids in nitrogen retention, both of which are positive factors. When included in a formula, it produces stools most like those of a breast-fed baby, in which gram-positive rather than gram-negative bacteria predominate, another positive factor. An adequate carbohydrate level in a formula allows protein to be used for building new cells rather than for calories, encouraging normal water balance, and preventing abnormal metabolism of fat.

Cow's milk contains about 29 percent of its calories as carbohydrate; human milk, 37 percent. Cow's milk formulas need added carbohydrate to bring their carbohydrate content up to that of human milk.

FLUID REQUIREMENTS

Maintaining a sufficient fluid intake in newborns is important because their metabolic rate is high and metabolism requires water. An adult utilizes 25 to 30 calories per kilogram of body weight in 24 hours for metabolism. In the same period, a newborn utilizes 45 to 50 calories per kilogram. This high rate of metabolism requires a large amount of water. In addition, the surface area of the newborn is large in relation to his body mass. Thus, he loses a larger amount of water by evaporation than does an adult.

Water is distributed differently in the newborn than in the adult. In an adult, about 20 percent of body weight is extracellular fluid; in a newborn, 30 to 35 percent of body weight is extracellular fluid. Consequently, loss of fluid or inadequate fluid intake, which depletes the extracellular water supply, can affect as much as 35 percent of the newborn's fluid component. Because the kidneys of a newborn are not yet capable of fully concentrating urine, the newborn cannot conserve body water by this mechanism and must have an adequate fluid intake to prevent dehydration.

The fluid requirement for a newborn is 160 to 200 ml per kilogram (2.5 to 3.0 ounces per pound) per 24 hours.

MINERAL REQUIREMENT—CALCIUM

Calcium is an important mineral because of its contribution to bone growth. Calcium levels tend to fall after birth, and phosphate levels tend to rise. Since milk is high in calcium, tetany from a low calcium level seldom occurs in infants who suck well, whether taking human milk or cow's milk formula. Milk contains more calcium than phosphorus, but the ratio is higher in human milk than in cow's milk (2 : 1 versus 1.2 : 1.0).

IRON REQUIREMENT

The infant of a mother who had an adequate iron intake during pregnancy will be born with iron stores that, theoretically, will last for the first three months of life, until he begins to produce adult hemoglobin. Because not all mothers' diets are iron-rich during pregnancy (and socioeconomic level is not a good criterion for judging the quality of a diet), the American Academy of Pediatrics recommends that an iron supplement be given to formula-fed infants for the entire first year of life [6].

FLUORIDE REQUIREMENT

Fluoride is essential for building sound teeth and for resistance to tooth decay. When the infant's teeth are first forming during pregnancy, it is important for mothers to drink fluoridated water. The lactating mother should continue drinking fluoridated water (although fluoride does not pass in great amounts in breast milk), and formulas should be prepared with flouridated water. This is an essential point to remember, because a mother may think she is helping her child by using bottled "natural" water in the formula rather than the chlorinated (but fluoridated) water from a tap.

If the mother is breast-feeding or a source of fluoridated water is not available (the family drinks well or spring water or bottled water, or the tap water is not fluoridated), it is recommended that a fluoride supplement be given: 0.25 mg daily [11].

VITAMIN REQUIREMENTS

Vitamin additives are necessary for the bottle-fed infant.

Formerly, vitamin C was introduced by adding orange juice to the diet and vitamin D by adding cod liver oil. Orange juice causes colic or skin rashes in some infants, and it is a rare infant who takes cod liver oil well. Therefore, as with iron, the American Academy of Pediatrics recommends supplemental multivitamins (A, C, and D) for the entire first year of life. Infants taking commercially prepared formulas do not need additional vitamins because such formulas already contain them.

Breast-Feeding

All women should be asked during pregnancy if they have thought yet about whether they plan to breast-feed or formula-feed their newborn.

Some physicians recommend that mothers who expect to breast-feed practice a few simple techniques toward the end of pregnancy to improve milk production and ease of feeding. Nipple rolling—that is, holding the nipple between the thumb and finger and rolling it gently to cause it to protrude—done two or three times a day, is helpful in releasing adhesions at the base of the nipple and in making it more protuberant.

Practicing breast massage to move the milk forward in the milk ducts (manual expression of milk) is helpful. This allows the woman who may feel diffident about handling her breasts to grow accustomed to it and will enable her to assist with milk production in the first few days after birth. Manual expression consists in supporting the breast firmly, then placing the thumbs on the areolar margin and pushing inward and backward toward the chest wall until secretion begins to flow (Fig. 30-1). During the last months of pregnancy and immediately following birth, the fluid obtained will be colostrum. By the third day of life, milk will be obtained.

A woman should avoid using any soap on her breasts during pregnancy because soap tends to dry and crack nipples. The use of creams or lotions does not help in any way and may overstimulate the nipples because of too much handling, leading to nipple fissures and soreness.

PHYSIOLOGY OF BREAST-FEEDING

Milk is formed in the acinar or alveolar cells of the mammary glands. (Internal breast anatomy is shown graphically in Fig. 30-2.) Colostrum, a thin, watery, high-protein fluid, has been secreted by these cells since the 4th month of pregnancy. With the delivery of the placenta, the level of progesterone in the mother's body falls dramatically, stimulating the production of prolactin, an anterior pituitary hor-

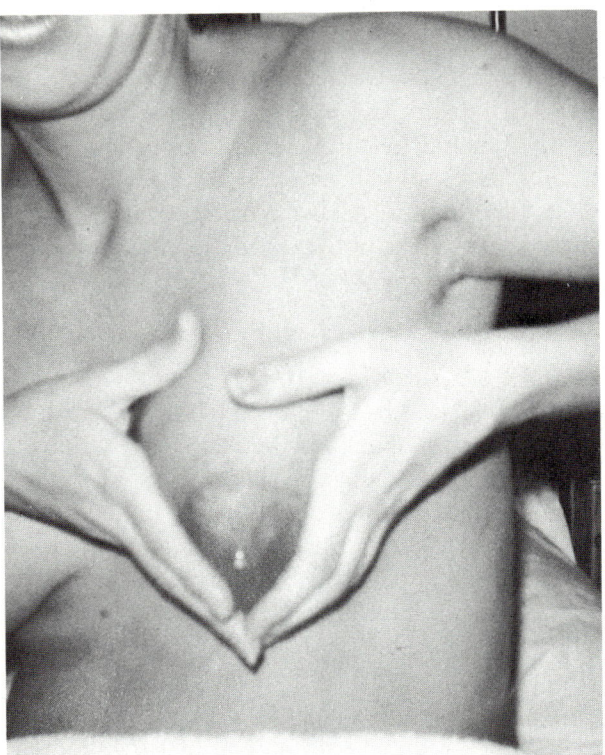

Fig. 30-1. Manual expression of milk. The breast is supported firmly and the thumbs are pushed back firmly until breast milk begins to flow. (From Sr. A. Murdaugh and L. E. Miller, Helping the breast-feeding mother. Am. J. Nurs. 72:1420, 1972.)

Fig. 30-2. Breast anatomy. A. Nonpregnant. B. Pregnant. C. During lactation.

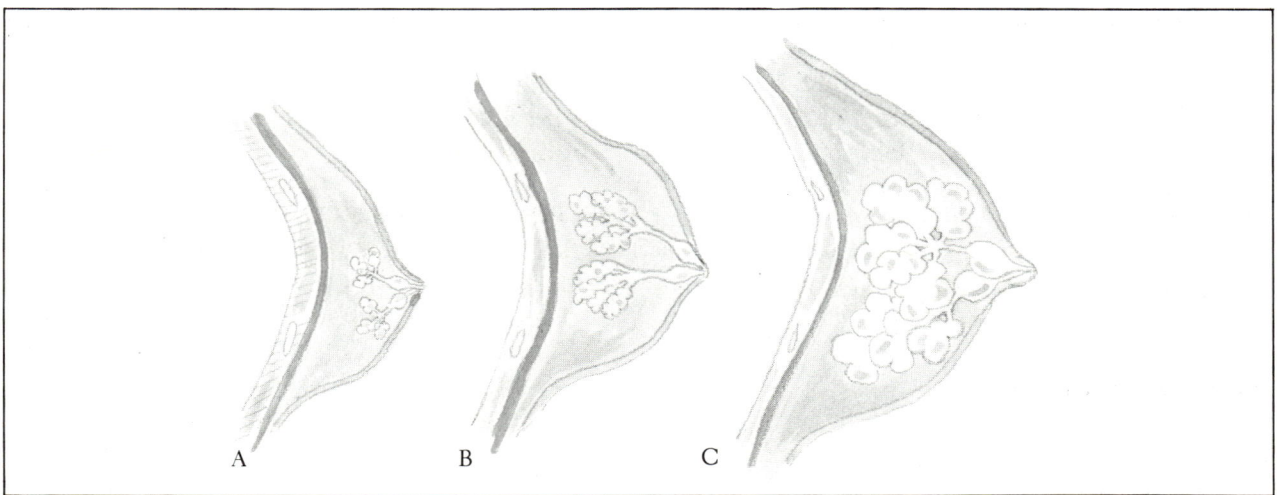

mone. Prolactin acts on the acinar cells of the mammary glands to stimulate the production of milk. Moreover, when an infant sucks at the breast, nerve impulses travel from the nipple to the hypothalamus to stimulate the production of prolactin-releasing factor. This factor then passes to the pituitary and stimulates further active production of prolactin. Other anterior pituitary hormones such as ACTH, TSH, and growth hormone probably also play a role in growth of the mammary glands and their ability to secrete milk.

Milk flows from alveolar cells through small tubules to reservoirs for milk, *lactiferous sinuses*, behind the nipple. This constantly forming milk is termed *foremilk*. Its availability depends very little on the infant's sucking at the breast. Foremilk is produced in all mothers three to four days after delivery.

A second result of an infant's sucking at the breast is release of oxytocin from the posterior pituitary. Oxytocin causes smooth muscle to contract. It also stimulates the uterus to contract, and the breast-feeding mother will feel a small tugging or cramping in her lower pelvis during the first few days of breast-feeding. Oxytocin causes the collecting sinuses of the mammary glands to contract too, forcing milk forward through the nipple and making it readily available for the baby. This action is termed the *let-down reflex*. In addition, new milk, termed *hind milk*, is formed after the let-down reflex. Hind milk tends to be higher in fat than foremilk and is the milk that will make the breast-fed infant grow most rapidly.

COLOSTRUM

Colostrum is the thin, slightly yellow fluid that is the antecedent of milk production. Colostrum is composed of protein, sugar, fat, water, minerals, vitamins, and maternal antibodies. It is high in protein and fairly low in sugar and fat. Its low fat content makes it easy to digest.

PHYSIOLOGICAL ADVANTAGES OF BREAST-FEEDING

The advantages and disadvantages of breast-feeding are a popular subject. Everyone seems to feel compelled to take a position on one side or the other.

The easiest way for a woman to decide whether to breast-feed is to ask herself what would please her most and make her most comfortable. If she is comfortable and pleased with what she is doing, her infant will be comfortable and pleased, will enjoy being fed, and will thrive. The choice is that simple.

Advantages for the Mother

There are a number of physiological benefits to the woman from breast-feeding.

1. The incidence of breast cancer in women who breast-feed appears to be lower than in those who do not. In a study in Boston [22], mothers who breast-fed for more than 3 months had a significantly lower incidence of breast cancer than did those who did not breast-feed or who breast-fed for less than 3 months.
2. The release of oxytocin from the posterior pituitary aids uterine involution.
3. Women in whom varicosities develop during pregnancy are prone to thrombophlebitis following delivery. If such women breast-feed and thus are not given diethylstilbestrol to suppress lactation, they are not subjected to the increased risk of thromboembolic complications with administration of this drug.

Many mothers feel that breast-feeding will give them the best chance of forming a true symbiotic bond with their child. This is not necessarily true. A mother who holds her baby to bottle-feed can form this bond equally well. Many mothers feel that breast-feeding is a foolproof contraceptive technique. Again, they are incorrect. Among mothers who breast-feed, 50 percent start ovulating by the fourth week post partum [7]. Thus by the sixth week after delivery, by the time they come in for a postpartal checkup these mothers have no contraceptive protection from lactation.

Some mothers are reluctant to breast-feed because they fear it will tie them down to have to be available to feed the baby every 3 or 4 hours. In reality, their situation is no different from that of the mother who is bottle-feeding; she also has to be available every 4 hours. Both breast-feeding and bottle-feeding mothers should have time away from their babies occasionally. Both can prepare bottles of formula for the baby-sitter or father to use while they are away.

Advantages for the Baby

Breast-feeding has certain physiological advantages for the baby. Breast milk contains secretory immunoglobulin A (IgA), which binds large molecules of foreign proteins including viruses and bacteria and keeps them from being absorbed through the gastrointestinal tract into the infant. Lactoferrin is an iron-binding protein that binds iron in such a way that pathogenic bacteria that require iron for growth cannot utilize it. This decreases the growth of such bacteria. Lysozyme is an enzyme that apparently actively destroys bacteria by lysing (dissolving) their cell membranes. It may increase the effectiveness of antibodies. Leukocytes are present in breast milk and provide protection against infectious invaders. Macrophages are responsible for producing *interferon*, which interferes with virus growth. The *bifidus factor* is a specific growth-promoting factor that the bacteria *Lactobacillus bifidus* needs in order to grow. The presence of *Lactobacillus bifidus* interferes with colonization of the gastrointestinal tract by pathogenic bacteria.

In addition to these anti-infection properties, breast milk contains the ideal electrolyte and mineral composition for human infant growth. Breast milk is higher in lactose than is cow's milk. Lactose is a readily digested sugar that provides ready glucose for rapid brain growth. The ratio of cysteine to methionine (two amino acids) in breast milk also appears to favor rapid brain growth in early months. Although the protein content of breast milk is less than that of cow's milk, it is more readily digested by the infant and therefore the infant may actually receive more. Breast milk contains nitrogen in compounds other than protein and so the infant receives cell-building materials from sources other than just protein. Breast milk contains more linoleic acid, an essential amino acid for skin integrity, than does cow's milk. It contains less sodium, potassium, calcium, and phosphorus than do many formulas. These lower levels are enough to supply infant needs, and they spare the infant's kidneys from having to process a high renal solute load of unused nutrients. Breast milk also has a better balance of trace elements such as zinc than do formulas.

Babies on breast milk appear to have less difficulty with regulation of calcium-phosphorus levels than those who are bottle-fed. Cow's milk formulas contain a high level of phosphorus. As the phosphorus level in the infant's bloodstream rises, his calcium level falls because of the inverse relationship between phosphorus and calcium. Decreased calcium levels in the newborn lead to tetany. The increased concentration of fatty acid in commercial formulas may bind calcium in the gastrointestinal tract and further increase the danger of tetany.

There is a great deal of discussion about the benefits of breast-feeding from the standpoint of the formation of the dental arch. Babies suck differently from a breast and from a bottle (Fig. 30-3). An infant pulls his tongue backward as he sucks from a breast; he thrusts it forward to suck from a rubber nipple. Tongue thrusting may lead to malformation of the dental arch.

Mothers who have a familial history of allergy are usually encouraged to breast-feed and thus eliminate the possibility of exposing the infant to cow's milk protein, which is allergenic.

BEGINNING BREAST-FEEDING

Breast-feeding should begin as soon after delivery as possible. Ideally, the first breast-feeding should begin while the mother is still on the delivery room table and the infant is in the first reactivity period. The release of oxytocin from breast-feeding at this time not only gets the production of milk off to an early start but stimulates uterine contraction as well. If the mother is fatigued—and it is a rare mother who is not—adding this new skill of child care at this point may only convince her that breast-feeding is not for her, however, so when to initiate breast-feeding should be individually considered.

The infant should be fed by 4 to 8 hours after delivery if he is not fed at birth, provided his color, respirations, and temperature are normal. It is important that the infant grasp the areola of the nipple, as well as the nipple itself, when he sucks. This gives him an effective sucking action and helps to empty the col-

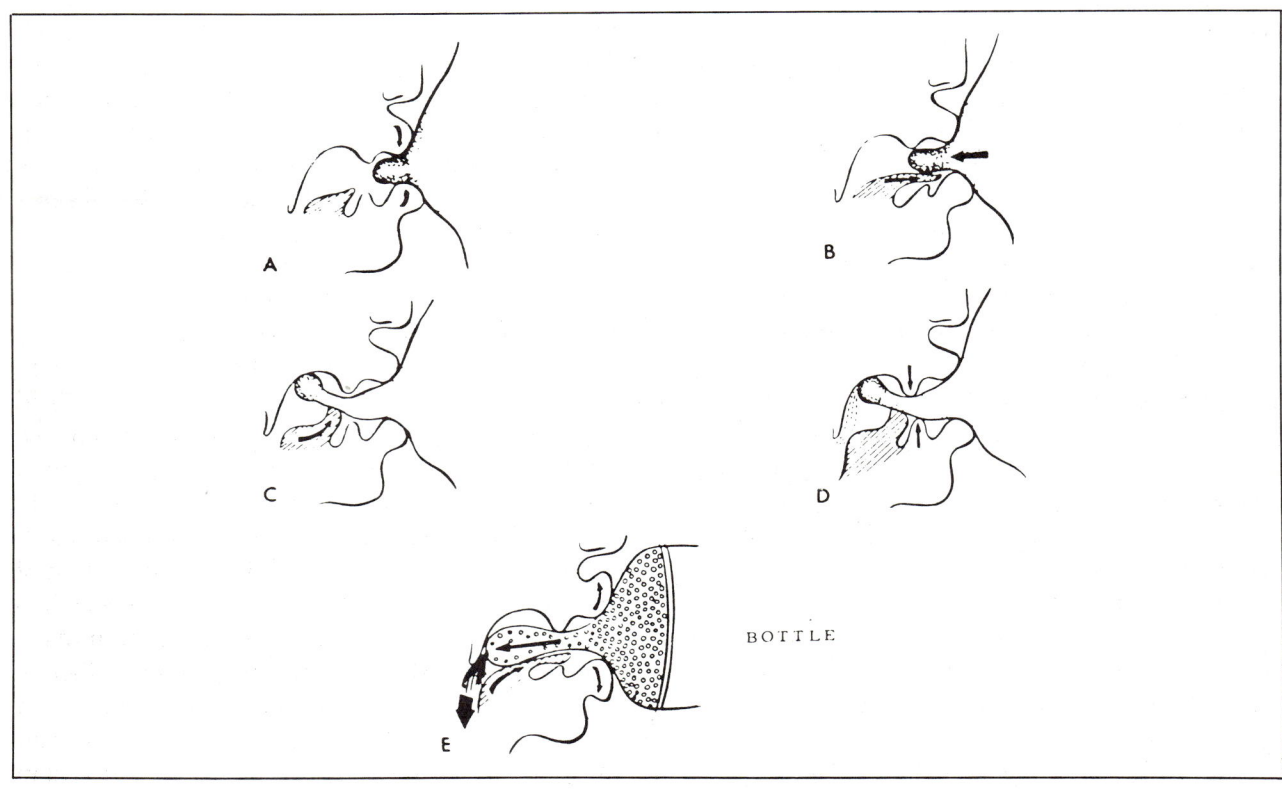

Fig. 30-3. Sucking mechanism at the breast (A–D) and bottle (E). A. The lips of the infant clamp in a C shape at the concave junction of nipple and areola, fitting like a glove. The cheek muscles contract. B. The tongue thrusts forward to grasp nipple and areola. C. The nipple is brought against the hard palate as the tongue pulls backward, bringing the areola into the mouth. Negative pressure is created by action of tongue and cheeks against the nipple, and the result is a true sucking motion. D. The gums compress the areola, squeezing milk into the back of the throat. Milk flows against the hard palate from the high-pressure system of the breast to the area of negative pressure at the back of the throat. E. In contrast, the large rubber nipple of a bottle strikes the soft palate (causing gagging) and interferes with the action of the tongue. The tongue moves forward against the gum to control the overflow of milk into the esophagus. (From R. M. Applebaum, The modern management of successful breast feeding. Pediatr. Clin. North Am. 17:203, 1970.)

lecting sinuses completely. To prevent nipples from becoming sore and cracked, the infant should be fed for only 5 minutes at each breast at each feeding the first day. The time at each breast is increased 1 minute per day until, by the sixth day, he is nursing for 10 minutes at each breast at each feeding. This schedule also keeps the infant from becoming fatigued. At each feeding, the infant should be placed first at the breast he fed at last in the previous feeding. Thus each breast is completely emptied at every other feeding.

Milk forms to the extent that it is used. If the breasts are completely emptied, they completely fill again. If half-emptied, they only half-fill, and after a time, milk production will be insufficient for proper nourishment.

As important as making certain that the infant is grasping the areola of the breast is helping him to break away from the suction of the breast when he is through feeding. This can be done by inserting a finger in the corner of his mouth or by pulling his chin down (see Fig. 30-4). Otherwise he may pull too hard on the nipple and cause cracking or soreness.

Breast-feeding is, in more simple cultures, the method of feeding babies that is used by all mothers; the technique is learned early. In the United States most mothers must be shown the technique because they have had few, if any, opportunities to observe the process. One of the first things a mother needs to learn to do before she will be a successful breast-feeder is relax. If she is tense and anxious, she will not achieve a good let-down reflex, and her infant will have difficulty getting adequate milk. She will become more tense and anxious because her infant does not seem content, the infant will have more difficulty, and shortly she will stop breast-feeding.

Relaxing is not easy when you are a new mother because stitches hurt (and never underestimate the sharpness and the pain of stitches) and the baby is so small and looks so helpless and dependent.

Lying on her side with a pillow under her head is a good position for the mother to assume when she is first attempting breast-feeding (Fig. 30-5). It is comfortable for her and allows the infant to rest on the bed, a comfortable position for him, too. Figure 30-6 shows an alternative position for breast-feeding. The mother should wash her hands before breast-feeding as she would if she were bottle-feeding, to be sure they are free of pathogens picked up from handling

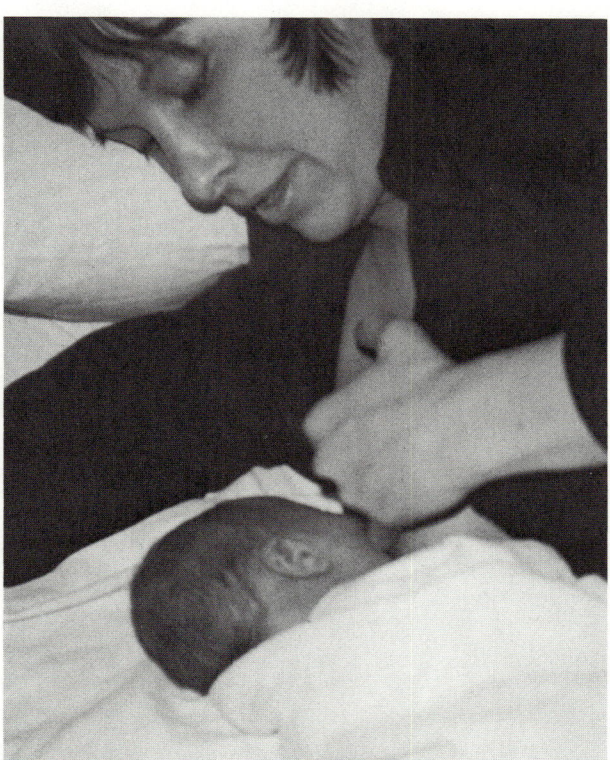

Fig. 30-4. Pressing a finger against the corner of the baby's jaw to release suction. (From Sr. A. Murdaugh and L. E. Miller, Helping the breast-feeding mother. Am. J. Nurs. 72:1420, 1972.)

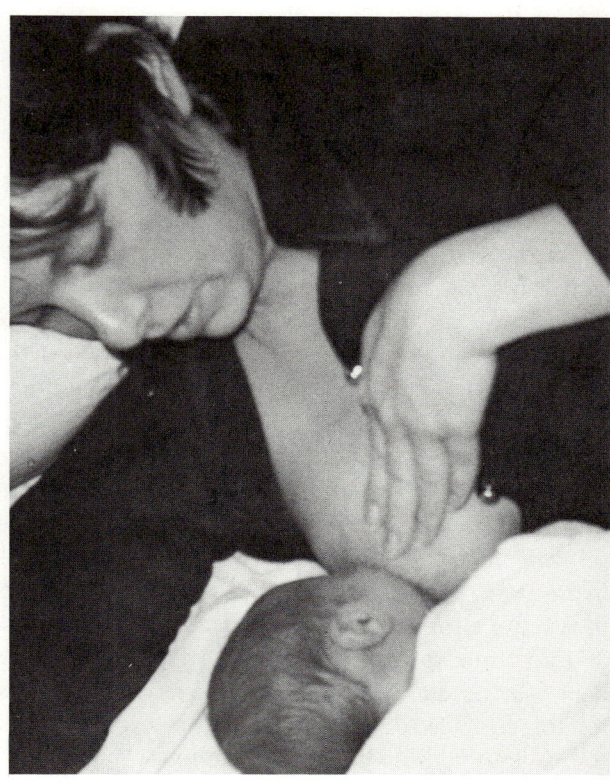

Fig. 30-5. Side-lying position for breast-feeding. Notice how the mother holds the bulk of breast tissue away from the infant's nose. (From Sr. A. Murdaugh and L. E. Miller, Helping the breast-feeding mother. Am. J. Nurs. 72:1420, 1972.)

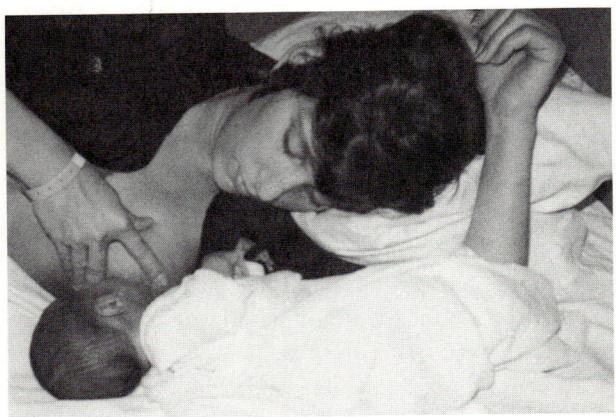

Fig. 30-6. Reversing the baby's position to ease sore nipples. (From Sr. A. Murdaugh and L. E. Miller, Helping the breast-feeding mother. Am. J. Nurs. 72:1420, 1972.)

perineal pads. She need not wash her breasts before feeding unless she notices a lot of caked colostrum on the nipple.

If the mother brushes the infant's cheek with her nipple, he will turn toward the breast (rooting reflex). Be careful that *you* do not initiate a rooting reflex by trying to press the baby's face against the mother's breast and causing him to turn *away* from the mother. Such a move may make her think her baby does not like breast-feeding.

If a mother has large breasts, the infant may have trouble breathing as he nurses and breast tissue presses against his nose. The mother may prevent this by grasping the areolar margin between her thumb and forefinger, holding the bulk of the breast supported. The nipple is thus made more protuberant as well.

The breasts will secrete only colostrum the first one or two days. On the third or fourth day, milk will form. The infant should be put to the breast and encouraged to suck during the first two days since the stimulation of sucking aids the formation of breast milk. Breast milk looks like skimmed milk; it is thin and almost blue-tinged in color. Many mothers need assurance that the color and consistency are normal for breast milk. Otherwise, they think their milk is not nutritious enough for their infants.

A baby should be fed as often as he is hungry the first few days of life, because he is receiving only colostrum and so needs the nutrients and fluid obtained by frequent sucking. Further, the more often the breasts are emptied, the more efficiently they will fill and continue to maintain a good supply of milk. A baby may need to be fed as often as every 2 or 3 hours for the first few days rather than the every-4-hours schedule some hospital nurseries follow.

A newborn being breast-fed will often drop off to sleep during the first few feedings, as bottle-fed infants do. In order for milk production to be effectively stimulated, and to ensure an adequate fluid intake, the infant should be kept awake and urged to suck. The mother can prevent his falling asleep by waking him up well before feeding by handling him and stroking his back, changing his position during feeding, or rubbing his arms and chest. Tickling the bottom of a baby's feet wakes him up effectively, but most mothers are unwilling to cause their newborns discomfort in order to keep them awake. This may be the first sign that the mother is transferring the protectiveness she felt all during pregnancy toward her own body to that of her newborn and is therefore a positive rather than a negative reaction.

If the infant seems to tire easily or is too affected by the delivery anesthetic to suck vigorously, the mother can massage her breasts to increase the flow of milk while the infant sucks (Fig. 30-7). This is the same breast massage she practiced during pregnancy. If the infant is sucking strongly and effectively, and sucking is well paced, she should not attempt breast massage. Massage will increase the flow of milk to such an extent that the infant will begin to choke or aspirate.

Fig. 30-7. Sitting position for breast-feeding. (From Sr. A. Murdaugh and L. E. Miller, Helping the breast-feeding mother. Am. J. Nurs. 72:1420, 1972.)

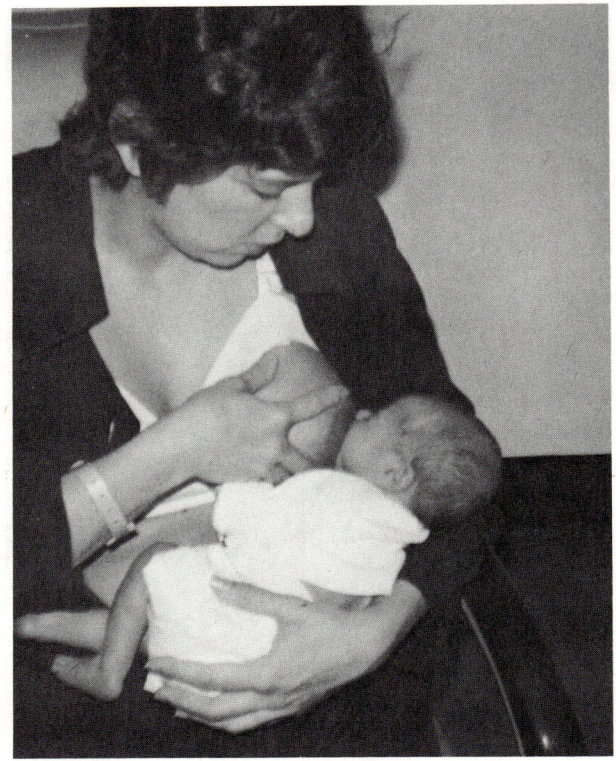

If the infant is not sucking well at all, the mother can use breast massage following the first feedings to empty her breasts manually. This will ensure good milk production for the time when the infant is ready to suck.

An infant who is taking in little breast milk because of poor sucking or insufficient nipple projection, which makes it difficult for him to grasp the nipple and suck effectively, needs some fluid supplementation. Many people believe that additional fluid should not be given in a bottle, since the infant may become accustomed to a bottle rather than to the breast. They recommend that the extra fluid be given by spoon or medicine dropper. However, the infant needs this additional fluid only for the first three or four days of life. After that, the mother's breast milk has formed, the infant is free of the effects of anesthesia, and he will obtain adequate fluid without supplementation. Further, the infant will be offered a bottle of glucose water for only a very short time, and the danger of aspiration rises with medicine-dropper, spoon, or cup feedings. Finally, some mothers are ready to stop breast-feeding at the slightest sign of trouble, and having to give supplementary feedings by medicine dropper may precipitate their rejection of breast-feeding. Thus, the advantages of giving supplemental fluid by bottle seem to outweigh its disadvantages.

COMMON PROBLEMS WITH BREAST-FEEDING

The common problems that arise with breast-feeding, if handled intelligently by the health care personnel advising the mother, will pass and be as nothing to her. Handled wrongly, or overemphasized, they may so complicate breast-feeding that the mother is discouraged from continuing it. It is bizarre that complications should deter a mother from using the most natural and least complicated of all infant feeding methods.

Engorgement

On the third or fourth day, when breast milk comes in, the mother may notice swelling, hardness, tenderness, and perhaps heat in her breasts. The skin may appear red, tense, and shiny. This is engorgement and is caused by vascular and lymphatic congestion arising from an increase in the blood and lymph supply to the breasts. An infant has difficulty sucking on engorged breasts because the areola is too hard to grasp (Fig. 30-8). The mother has difficulty with nursing because her breasts are extremely painful, and the baby's sucking accentuates the discomfort.

The primary method of relief for engorgement is

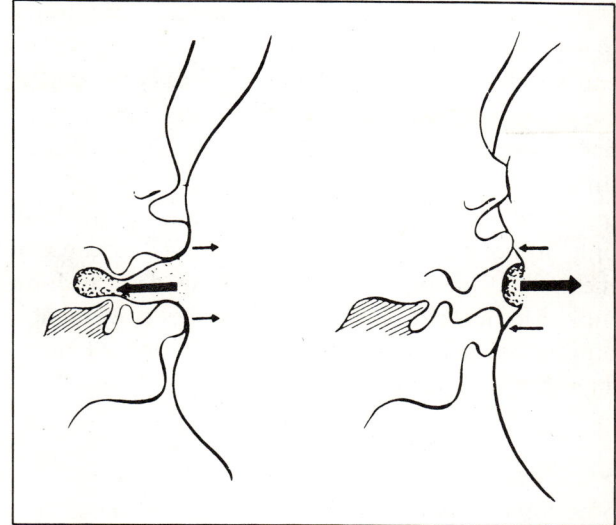

Fig. 30-8. The relationship of breast engorgement and sore nipples. Left, when an infant sucks at a normal breast, his lips compress the areola and fit neatly against the concave nipple-areola junction. He also has room to breathe. Right, if the breast is engorged, the nipple-areola junction becomes convex. The infant attempts to suck the inverted nipple, causing soreness and damaging the nipple epithelium. Furthermore, normal breathing space does not exist. Preventing engorgement will prevent sore nipples by allowing the infant a proper grasp. (From R. M. Applebaum, The modern management of successful breast feeding. Pediatr. Clin. North Am. 17:203, 1970.)

emptying the breasts of milk by having the infant suck more often than previously, or at least continuing to suck as much as he did before. Unfortunately, the breasts are so sore that it is difficult for the mother to continue to breast-feed unless she is given something to alleviate the pain. An analgesic may be necessary, but some mothers find that ice packs applied for 20 minutes at a time give relief. Others find that hot packs applied for a comparable length of time afford the most relief. In addition, good breast support from a firm-fitting bra prevents the pulling feeling.

If the infant cannot grasp the nipple to suck strongly, hot packs applied to both breasts for a few minutes before feeding will often facilitate drainage and promote softness so that he can suck. Synthetic oxytocin (Syntocinon) nasal spray used for a few minutes prior to feeding may also be effective. Syntocinon is absorbed across the nasal mucosa and acts to contract milk ducts and bring milk forward. Manual expression or the use of a hand breast pump to complete emptying of the breasts after the baby has nursed is helpful in maintaining or promoting a good milk supply during the period of engorgement.

Engorgement is a transient problem. Unfortunately, it occurs just as the mother feels she is becoming skilled at breast-feeding. Suddenly her breasts are swollen, hot, and painful. She may worry that she has an infection or that the baby is not getting enough milk.

Mothers need to be assured that engorgement not only is normal but is to be welcomed because it means that breast cells are actively working to form milk. Mothers also should be told that engorgement is only temporary and will begin to subside 24 hours after it becomes apparent.

Sore Nipples

Sore nipples may result from improper sucking, that is, from the infant's not grasping the areola as well as the nipple; from forcefully pulling the infant from the breast; from the infant's sucking too long a time at a breast because the mother places the infant on the same breast where he nursed last at the previous feeding; or from the nipple's remaining wet from leaking of milk.

Nipples feel sore because they are cracked or fissured. Healing a fissure here is the same as healing irritated skin anywhere else on the body. Exposing the nipples to air by leaving the bra unsnapped for 10 to 15 minutes after feeding is often sufficient to clear up the problem. The mother should avoid using the plastic liners that come with nursing bras, so that air is always circulating around her breasts. Application of a lanolin-based cream following air exposure may toughen the nipple and prevent further irritation.

If normal air-drying is not effective, simultaneous exposure to a 20-watt bulb in a gooseneck lamp two or three times a day may be helpful. The light should be 12 to 18 inches away from the breasts to prevent burns, and it should be left in place about 10 minutes.

Sore nipples, like engorgement, are not a contraindication to breast-feeding. They are enough to discourage a mother, however, if she does not realize that they are a temporary result of adjustment to nursing, both hers and her baby's. If her nipples are so sore that she cannot nurse, the baby should be given supplemental formula for a day or two, and the breast milk should be expelled manually until the nipples have had a chance to heal. Do not use a hand pump with sore nipples, or fissures will worsen.

If the baby's sucking patterns are corrected, and if the mother uses air exposure following feedings and returns to nursing again by gradually increasing the time the baby sucks at each feeding, the problem of sore nipples is unlikely to become acute again.

Assessing Amount of Milk Taken

Many mothers who are breast-feeding wonder whether the infant is getting enough to eat. They watch a woman bottle-feeding and listen to her report, "She took 3 ounces this feeding," and wish they could tell as surely that their infant is getting an adequate intake.

They can be assured that the ultimate test of whether a baby, either breast-fed or bottle-fed, is getting enough to eat is whether he seems content between feedings and is gaining weight. Although the bottle-feeding mother uses measuring the amount of formula as a way of determining this in the early weeks, very soon she too is using the alternative criteria: her baby is happy and growing larger.

At one time breast-fed babies were weighed before each feeding and then again after each feeding. The difference in weight gave a gross estimate of the amount of breast milk they had taken. If a mother is particularly worried that her infant is not getting anything to eat, he can be weighed for a few feedings to assure her that the infant is taking in milk. The practice should not become routine, however. It is better to help the mother begin to use the criteria she will use at home. That way she will develop confidence in her judgment to evaluate her child's health, a role that will be hers for the next 18 years.

ADVICE ON GOING HOME

Some mothers do well with breast-feeding while they are in the hospital but after going home grow discouraged with the process and stop.

A mother must regard breast-feeding time as a time in which she is devoting herself only to feeding the baby. If she approaches it with an attitude such as "I'll get this over as quickly as possible so I can get to something else," her let-down reflex will be affected, and she will discover that she no longer has adequate milk. If milk remains in her breasts, either because it did not move forward as it should have (weak let-down reflex) or because the infant sucked poorly or not at all, the tension created inhibits subsequent milk production.

Mothers who do not remember to begin nursing the baby at the breast he finished on the last time may find their milk supply decreasing. It is easy to remember this in the hospital, but the many distractions at home may make the sequence hard to keep in mind. Pinning a safety pin to the bra strap on the correct side is a useful aid to memory.

Another problem of mothers after they return home is fatigue. The mother needs to realize that she cannot expect to feed a baby, by any method, attend many social functions, and be a perfect housekeeper and gourmet cook. Adequate rest periods during the day are essential. Sitting relaxed in a comfortable chair with her feet elevated, feeding her baby and enjoying it, is an excellent way to rest.

The mother must take in adequate fluid to maintain an adequate milk supply. In the hospital fluid intake is supervised by the health care personnel. When she is at home and involved in other things, she may neglect to take adequate fluids. Sometimes a mother will deliberately limit fluid intake after she returns home in the hope of shedding the pounds she put on during pregnancy.

Mothers who are breast-feeding should drink at least four 8-ounce glasses of fluid a day; many women need to drink six glasses. A daily diet plan for a lactating mother compared with her intake during and before pregnancy is given in Table 30-1.

At one time mothers were given a list of foods not to eat while they were breast-feeding because they tend to cause diarrhea, constipation, or colic in infants. Today there are no rules other than to use common sense. The mother can eat anything during lactation that agrees with her and is taken in moderation. She should not eat foods to which she is allergic or that cause gastrointestinal upsets. But then such foods should be avoided whether or not she is lactating.

Many mothers stop breast-feeding after they return home because they have no one to talk to about their problems or to give them support. A nurse who works as a hospital-community liaision person receives countless calls from breast-feeding mothers asking for support or advice. The community health nurse is another person to whom mothers turn for help.

Mothers should be made aware of the La Leche League, an international organization of breast-feeding mothers that has chapters in most major cities. The most helpful service the League offers is its hot line, through which a breast-feeding mother who is discouraged or is having difficulty can contact a member and ask for advice. *The Womanly Art of Breastfeeding* [18], published by the La Leche League, is a comprehensive and readable book for mothers. Like any organization, it can attract a number of hard-liners. Some of these are women who feel that breast-feeding is the ultimate in infant feeding and that any woman who does not breast-feed or stops breast-feeding is not a good mother. You need to be available to offer middle-of-the-road advice: that the method to choose is the one with which the mother will feel most comfortable.

DRUGS AND BREAST MILK

For years people talked about a placental "barrier," which theoretically protected the fetus from drugs taken by the mother. A similar protection was postulated for breast milk. Today it can be shown that the fetus is very susceptible to drugs ingested by the mother. The same is true of breast-fed infants. Almost any drug may cross into the acinar cells and be secreted with breast milk.

Drugs that should be avoided by breast-feeding mothers because of their harmful effect on the infant are shown in Table 30-2.

The rule that the mother followed all during preg-

Table 30-1. Quantities of Food Necessary During Pregnancy and Lactation

Food Group	Active Nonpregnant Woman	Pregnant Woman	Lactating Woman
Meat	2 servings of meat, fowl, or fish daily; 3–5 eggs per week	3 servings of meat, fowl, or fish daily; 1 egg per day	3–4 servings of meat, fowl, or fish daily; 1 egg per day
Vegetables			
Dark green or deep yellow	1 serving (at least 3 times per week)	2 servings per day	2 servings per day
Other vegetables	2 or more servings per day	1 serving per day	1 serving per day
Fruits			
Citrus, melon, strawberry, tomato	1 serving per day	1 or more servings per day	2 or more servings per day
Other fruits	1 serving per day	1 serving per day	2 servings per day
Bread and cereals	4 or more servings per day	4 servings per day	4 servings per day
Milk	1 pint (two 8-oz glasses) per day	1 quart (four 8-oz glasses) per day	Four–six 8-oz glasses per day
Additional fluid	Ad lib	At least two glasses per day	At least two glasses per day

Table 30-2. Drug Excretion in Breast Milk and Effect on the Infant

Drug	Excreted	Implications
Analgesics		
Acetaminophen (Datril, Tylenol)	Yes	No significant effect on infant from therapeutic doses
Acetylsalicylic acid (aspirin)*	Yes	Tendency toward bleeding noted; if given to nursing mother, should be given after nursing; check infant for adequate sources of vitamin K
Codeine	Yes	No significant effect on infant reported from therapeutic doses
Heroin†	Yes	Controversial reports as to the long-term effect on infant; usually goes through withdrawal depending on maternal dose
Meperidine hydrochloride (Demerol)	Yes	No significant effect on infant from therapeutic doses
Methadone*	Yes	Controversial as to whether user should breast-feed; if she does, the daily dose should be given after the feeding, and the next feeding should be by bottle
Morphine	Yes	No significant effects on infant from therapeutic doses
Pentazocine (Talwin)	No	
Phenylbutazone* (Azolid, Butazolidin)	Yes	Drug should be used judiciously; manufacturer states that it is excreted in cord blood and breast milk; infant should be monitored; may increase kernicterus—highly protein-bound
Propoxyphene hydrochloride (Darvon)	Yes	No significant effect on infant from therapeutic doses
Anticoagulants		Differing opinions as to whether mother on anticoagulants should nurse; all agree that if she does, infant should be monitored with the mother
Bishydroxycoumarin* (Dicumarol)	Yes	May cause hypoprothrombinemia in infant; monitor infant
Ethyl biscoumacetate* (Pelentan, Tromexan)	Yes	No significant effect on infant from therapeutic doses, but monitor infant; do not use if infant suffered any birth injury such as cephalhematoma, or forceps damage resulting in vascular injury
Heparin	No	
Phenindione† (Dindevan, Hedulin)	Yes	May cause hypoprothrombinemia; one incident of massive hematoma in infant whose mother received it
Warfarin sodium* (Coumadin)	Yes	May cause hypoprothrombinemia; monitor infant
Anticonvulsants		
Phenytoin* (Dilantin)	Yes	Methemoglobinemia in breast-fed infant; enzyme induction may occur
Primidone† (Mysoline)	Yes	Manufacturer recommends breast-feeding be avoided, since substantial amounts found in breast milk; drowsiness may occur in newborn
Antidiabetics		
Chlorpropamide (Diabinese)	Yes	No significant effect on infant from therapeutic doses
Insulin	Yes	Destroyed in the infant's GI tract
Tolbutamide (Dolipol, Mobenol, Orinase, Tolbutol)	Yes	No significant effects on infant from therapeutic doses
Tolazamide (Tolinase)	?	Has not been completely evaluated; 6.7 times more potent than tolbutamide
Antihistamines		
Chlorpheniramine maleate (Chlor-Trimeton)	Yes	May cause drowsiness in the infant
Diphenhydramine (Benadryl, Benhydril)	Yes	No adverse effects on infant from therapeutic doses

Table 30-2. (Continued)

Drug	Excreted	Implications
Promethazine hydrochloride (Phenergan)	Yes	No significant effects on infant from therapeutic doses
Trimeprazine tartrate (Temaril)	Yes	No significant effects on infant from therapeutic doses
Anticholinergics		
Atropine sulfate†	Yes	May inhibit lactation and may cause atropine intoxication in infant; although documentation scarce, best avoided until further research available
Scopolamine	Yes	No significant effects on infant from therapeutic doses
Antihypertensives—Diuretics		
Acetazolamide* (Diamox)	Yes	Infant may develop idiosyncratic reaction to this sulfonamide diuretic
Furosemide (Lasix)	No	Women ill enough to receive Lasix should not breast-feed
Hexamethonium	Yes	Rarely used drug; very toxic
Reserpine† (Serpasil)	Yes	May cause nasal stuffiness, drowsiness, and diarrhea in infant, galactorrhea in mother
Spironolactone (Aldactone)	No	Watch for potassium deficiency and dehydration in mother
Thiazides†	Yes	Manufacturer suggests avoiding; watch fluid, electrolyte balance
Anti-infectives		With all anti-infectives that cross into breast milk, the possibility of sensitization of the infant must be considered
Amantadine hydrochloride† (Symmetrel)	Yes	May cause skin rash and vomiting; manufacturer suggests avoiding
Aminoglycosides*	Yes	Should be reserved for severe infection; avoid in high G-6-PD-deficient populations, as hemolysis may occur
Ampicillin	Yes	No significant effects on infant from therapeutic doses
Chloramphenicol* (Chloromycetin)	Yes	May affect infant's bone marrow; avoid use, particularly during the first 2 weeks of life
Erythromycin* (E-Mycin, Erythrocin, Ilosone, Ilotycin)	Yes	Appears in breast milk in concentrations higher than that of maternal plasma; sensitization possible; estolate form (Ilosone) may cause jaundice
Isoniazid†	Yes	If possible, avoid use during lactation; if given, infant must be monitored for toxicity
Mandelic acid†	Yes	Probably best avoided during lactation; for this urinary antiseptic to be effective, urine must be strongly acid and fluids must be limited
Metronidazole† (Flagyl)	Yes	No adverse oral or GI effects noted in infants, but some authors feel that because of possible carcinogenicity it would be best to avoid, as long-term effects are not known
Nalidixic acid† (NegGram)	Yes	Hemolytic anemia, especially in G-6-PD populations
Novobiocin†	Yes	May cause kernicterus in large doses
Penicillin	Yes	Possibility of sensitization; may alter intestinal flora of infant
Quinine	Not in clinically significant amounts	In very high maternal doses, thrombocytopenia in infants
Sulfonamides*	Yes	Avoid in high G-6-PD populations; high doses for long-term use is questionable; may cause kernicterus; avoid in the first 2 weeks of life
Tetracyclines†	Yes	Slows bone growth and deposits in bones and teeth
Cancer-Chemotherapeutic Agents†		Breast-feeding is generally considered ill-advised in patients receiving chemotherapy

Nutritional Needs of the Newborn

Table 30-2. (Continued)

Drug	Excreted	Implications
Hormones		
Estrogen, progestogen, androgens†	Yes	Breast-feeding not indicated if mother is on oral contraceptives; may alter the composition of breast milk (decreasing the amounts of protein, fats, and minerals); long-term effects on infants have not been adequately determined
Corticosteroids†	Yes	Should be avoided by the nursing mother, as they may interfere with normal function and cause growth suppression
Laxatives		
Aloe*	Yes	Conflicting evidence regarding catharsis in infants; avoid in high doses
Cascara†	Yes	Thought to cause diarrhea in infants
Danthron† (Dorbane, Dorbantyl, Doxan, Doxidan)	Yes	Conflicting reports regarding the cathartic effect of these drugs; probably best avoided
Dioctyl sodium sulfosuccinate (Colace)		No reports of having caused any problems in the infant
Milk of magnesia	No	No adverse reactions noted
Phenolphthalein (Evac-U-Lax, Ex-Lax, other nonprescription drugs)	Yes	No significant effects noted in usual doses
Psyllium hydrophilic mucilloid (Metamucil)	Yes	No adverse reactions noted
Senna compounds*	Yes	Controversial reports with moderate doses; high doses may cause diarrhea in infants
Muscle Relaxants		
Carisoprodol† (Rela, Soma)	Yes	According to manufacturer, two to four times more concentrated in breast milk than in maternal blood plasma; infant may experience CNS depression and GI upset
Methocarbamol (Robaxin)	Yes	No significant effects on infant from therapeutic doses
Oxytocics		
Ergot preparations†	Yes	May suppress lactation by blocking the release of prolactin; symptoms in the infant may include vomiting, diarrhea, cardiovascular changes
Oxytocin	Yes	Oxytocin nasal spray used prior to breast-feeding appears to increase the volume of milk produced; may be used for hemorrhaging mother; very short half-life
Psychotropics–Psychotherapeutics		
Butyrophenones, haloperidol* (Haldol)		Manufacturer recommends that benefits must outweigh risks in the use of these drugs, since their safe use in pregnancy and lactation has not been established
Chlordiazepoxide* (Librium)	Yes	No significant effects on infant from therapeutic doses; some authors suggest using caution
Diazepam* (Valium)	Yes	May cause weight loss, lethargy, jaundice in the infant; some authors feel that breast-feeding should be discontinued if high doses are given to mother
Imipramine* (Tofranil)	Yes	Safe use during lactation has not been established
Lithium carbonate† (Lithonate, Lithane)	Yes	May alter electrolyte balance; most authors state that indications for its use should be unequivocal; long-term effect on infant unknown; best avoided until further evidence available
Phenothiazines* (Compazine, Thorazine, etc.)	Yes	All phenothiazines are excreted in breast milk, and except for reported jaundice in the infant and galactorrhea, no other effects are known at this time

Table 30-2. (Continued)

Drug	Excreted	Implications
Sedatives–Hypnotics		
Barbiturates†	Yes	May increase the activity of hepatic drug metabolizing enzymes; high single dose may cause more drowsiness than small, multiple doses
Bromides† (ingredient in many nonprescription sleeping medications)	Yes	May cause rash and drowsiness in infant; difficulty in feeding, lethargy, hypotonia or hypertonia
Chloral hydrate (Noctec, Somnos)	Yes	Drowsiness in infant
Chloroform†	Yes	Anesthetic effect in infant
Glutethimide* (Doriden)	Yes	May cause drowsiness in infant; one author suggests avoiding during lactation; manufacturer suggests caution during lactation
Meprobamate† (Equanil, Miltown)	Yes	Very high level in milk (two to four times maternal plasma); alternate drug advised; if given, infant should be monitored for signs of meprobamate toxication
Thyroid and Antithyroid Preparations		
Carbimazole† (Neo-Mercazole)	Yes	May cause goiter in infant
Methimazole† (Tapazole)	Yes	Manufacturer recommends that user not breast-feed
Thiouracil† (+ derivatives)	Yes	Excreted in high levels (3 to 12 times maternal plasma levels); may cause goiter or agranulocytosis
Thyroid	Yes	No significant effects on infant with therapeutic doses
Thyroxine sodium† (Choloxin)	Yes	Manufacturer states that use in pregnancy and lactation is contraindicated
Iodides		
^{131}I† (radioactive)	Yes	All radioactive agents should be avoided in the breast-feeding mother
Iodides† (contained in many nonprescription cough preparations)	Yes	Infant's thyroid functioning may be affected; avoid taking large or frequent doses of iodide-containing cough preparations; may have thyrotropic effect on infant or cause rash
Vitamins, Minerals, Food Products		
Vitamins B_1 (thiamine)	Yes	Mothers with severe deficiency (beriberi) should not nurse because of excretion of toxic substances, sodium pyruvate and methylglyoxal, which have caused infant death
B_6 (pyridoxine)	Yes	Some authors report that it successfully suppressed lactation in doses of 150–200 mg po tid
B_{12} (cyanocobalamin)	Yes	No effect with therapeutic doses
D (calciferol)	Yes	High doses may cause hypercalcemia in infant
K	Yes	No significant effects on infant with therapeutic doses
Caffeine* (many nonprescription drugs contain caffeine: Awake, 100 mg; No-Doz, 100 mg; Sta-Alert, 100 mg; Vivarin, 200 mg; and coffee and tea, 100–150 mg per cup)	Yes	Unless large amount ingested, no significant effect on infant; ingestion of large quantities of tea or coffee can cause irritability and poor sleeping patterns in infants
Carrots	Yes	In large quantity, may cause yellow discoloration of skin
Egg protein	Yes	Allergic sensitization possible
Fava bean	Yes	In G-6-PD-deficient infants, hemolysis has occurred
Fluoride (toothpaste, water supply, tablets)	Yes	Not significant in usual quantities; excess may affect tooth enamel; La Leche League advises either *not* breast-feeding or to stop taking fluoride tablets; may cause GI upsets, rash in infants

Table 30-2. (Continued)

Drug	Excreted	Implications
Vaccines–Immunosuppressives		
DPT	Yes	Probably no immunity transfer to baby
Poliovirus	Yes	If infant is immunized after 6 weeks, probably negligible effect on antibody titer
Rh_0 (D) immune globulin (human) (Gamulin Rh, RhoGAM)	No	
Rubella	No	Probably no transfer of live virus to infant
Other		
Alcohol (ethyl alcohol)	Yes	No significant effect in moderate amount; prolonged ingestion of large amounts may intoxicate infant; large doses may also inhibit the milk ejection reflex, whereas small amount of alcohol prior to nursing may enhance the milk "let-down"
Clomiphene citrate (Clomid)		May suppress lactation
Dihydrotachysterol* (DHT)	Yes	May cause hypercalcemia in infant (osteoporosis, bone dysgenesis)
L-dopa		May suppress lactation by inhibiting prolactin secretion
Lead†		Caution against the use of lead acetate ointment in breast creams, as it may lead to encephalitis
Marijuana†	Yes	May interfere with DNA and RNA formation
Mercury†	Yes	In cases of mercury contamination in the environment, watch infant for CNS symptoms and mercury intoxication
Nicotine*	Yes	Probably very little effect on infant with moderate use (20 cigarettes per day or less); may decrease milk production; one recorded case of nicotine intoxication in infant (restlessness, vomiting, diarrhea, insomnia, circulatory disruptions)—mother smoked 20 cigarettes per day; infants of smoking mothers absorb smoke through GI tract, respiratory tract, and skin as well

* Use with caution in nursing mother.
†Avoid drug whenever possible.
Source: E. J. Dickason, et al., *Maternal and Infant Drugs and Nursing Intervention.* New York: McGraw-Hill, 1978. Copyright © 1978 McGraw-Hill Book Company. Used with the permission of McGraw-Hill Book Company.

nancy, that she should take no drug unless prescribed or approved by her physician, continues to apply during lactation.

PROLONGED JAUNDICE IN BREAST-FED INFANTS

Physiological jaundice may persist for a longer time in breast-fed than in bottle-fed infants because the pregnanediol (a breakdown product of progesterone) in breast milk depresses the action of glucuronyl transferase enzyme. Discontinuing breast-feeding for a day or two usually corrects this problem, causing the indirect level of bilirubin to drop and the jaundice to clear. The mother should pump her breasts manually during this time to protect her supply of breast milk. Prolonged jaundice is not a reason to discontinue breast-feeding permanently.

If the jaundice progresses, the mother should be referred to a health care facility. She may be reporting a rise in direct bilirubin level caused by obstruction of the bile ducts.

SUPPLEMENTAL FEEDINGS

A breast-feeding mother may leave her child during the day or evening in the care of a baby-sitter, just as a bottle-feeding mother may. She needs to express breast milk manually and leave it bottled in the refrigerator or prepare a single bottle of formula for the time she is away. If she chooses to use formula, one of the commercial formulas is best, because these formulas so closely resemble breast milk. Buying the prepackaged and prepared type is the most convenient; the mother need only take a bottle of it down from a shelf, and it is ready. If cost is a problem, the powdered type is probably the next best solution. The powder can be stored for long periods, and one bottle at a time can be prepared.

The mother may notice breast discomfort if she is away from her baby at feeding time. After breast-feeding has been established, missing one feeding will not affect the production of milk enough to make a difference at the next feeding. Thus, there is no need for her to express milk manually to safeguard a milk supply, although she may prefer to do so to reduce the tension and discomfort that she feels.

BURPING THE BREAST-FED BABY

Some infants seem to swallow very little air when they breast-feed; others swallow a great deal. As a rule, it is helpful to bubble the baby after he has emptied the first breast and after the total feeding.

WEANING

Mothers who breast-feed do so for varying lengths of time. Some breast-feed for one, two, or three months, then wean the child from breast to bottle. Other mothers breast-feed until the child is 6 to 12 months of age and then wean directly to a small cup or glass. Discontinuing breast-feeding should be done gradually to prevent engorgement and pain in the breasts. The woman should first omit one breast-feeding a day, substituting a bottle-feeding or milk from a glass or cup. Then she should omit two breast-feedings, then three, and so on, until the child is feeding entirely from a bottle, glass, or cup. If the breasts are not emptied, the resulting pressure leads to milk suppression and natural, gradual discontinuance of breast milk secretion.

Common problems mothers may experience with breast-feeding are summarized in Table 30-3.

Formula-Feeding

There is little controversy over the proposition that breast-feeding is the best method of feeding human infants—except when the mother does not want to breast-feed. A mother (or her husband) who feels that breasts are "dirty," that breast-feeding is a form of promiscuity, or who is uncomfortable with the thought of exposing her body in this way, cannot hold a baby warmly and gently and cannot enjoy feeding her infant. Mothers who plan to return to work or who have older children to watch may choose not to breast-feed. Mothers who develop a breast abscess may be advised not to breast-feed. Formulas that closely resemble human milk and are safe for infant feeding are available for the infant who will be bottle-fed.

Table 30-3. Common Problems of Breast-Feeding

Problem	Cause	Nursing Interventions
Engorgement	Lymphatic filling as milk production begins	Engorgement subsides best if infant can be encouraged to suck normally; warm packs to breasts prior to feeding may help soften breast tissue; oxytocin nasal spray prior to feeding may aid the let-down reflex
Sore nipples	Infant not gripping entire areola Nipple kept wet	Help infant to grasp nipple correctly; expose nipple to air between feedings; lanolin cream afterward to help harden nipple; possible heat lamp treatments
Mother worried about amount of milk being taken	Mother cannot see the amount taken	Assure mother that the best way to judge amount taken is to note if infant is gaining weight and appears content between feedings
Infant does not suck well	Possible effect of anesthesia Infant brought to mother when not hungry Infant exhausted by crying from hunger	Adjust feeding pattern to child's need; assure mother that effect of anesthesia is temporary
Mother reports infant's stools are loose and thin	Stools are normally looser and lighter in color than in formula-fed babies	Examine stool; assure and explain normal stool pattern
Mother tired	Exhaustion is a common postpartal finding due to psychosocial and physiological adjustments of time	Help mother to plan rest times; assess diet and fluid intake

COMMERCIAL FORMULAS

Commercial formulas are designed to simulate breast milk as closely as possible in terms of protein, carbohydrate, fat, mineral, and vitamin content. Commercial formulas contain 20 calories per ounce when diluted according to directions.

There are four separate forms of commercial formulas: a powder that the mother combines with water; a condensed liquid type that she dilutes with an equal amount of water; a ready-to-pour type, which requires no dilution; and individually prepackaged and prepared bottles of formula.

The powder is the least expensive type but the most difficult for the mother to prepare. It does not dissolve well and must be beaten with a hand beater to remove lumps. The prepackaged type has the advantage of never needing refrigeration or preparation (take off a bottle cap and it is ready), but it is the most expensive. The ready-to-pour type is convenient but also expensive. Many mothers are not aware of the existence of the liquid condensed type and need to be informed that it is available and is convenient and economical. The cost is as much as 50¢ to $2 a day less than that of the ready-to-pour or prepackaged types, which amounts to a saving of $15 to $60 a month.

Commercial formulas may be purchased with added iron, so that iron supplementation is not necessary. As indicated, they also contain added sufficient vitamins.

You should be familiar with all four types of commercial formula in order to discuss their advantages and disadvantages with mothers. Cost should not be the only basis for a choice. Acceptance by the infant and convenience for the mother are also important factors to consider.

Calculation of a Formula

The calculation of a newborn formula is not, and should not be, a complicated procedure. There are only a few rules of thumb to learn.

1. The total fluid used for 24 hours must be sufficient to meet the child's fluid needs; 2.5 to 3.0 ounces of fluid per pound of body weight per day (160 to 200 ml per kilogram) is needed.
2. The protein requirement is 1 gm per pound of body weight per day (2.2 gm per kilogram).
3. The number of calories required per day is 50 to 55 per pound of body weight (100 to 120 per kilogram).

If an infant is going to be discharged on a commercial formula, total fluid is all that needs to be calculated. The 7-pound infant needs 17.5 to 21.0 ounces (7 × 2.5 to 3.0 ounces) of formula per day. As commercial formula contains 20 calories per ounce, this supplies 350 to 420 calories per day, which can be divided into six feedings of 3.0 to 3.5 ounces each. The 9-pound infant needs 22.5 to 27.0 ounces of fluid per day, which supplies 450 to 540 calories.

A rule of thumb to determine how much an infant usually takes at a feeding is to add 2 or 3 to the infant's age in months. A newborn (0 age) takes 2 to 3 ounces each feeding; a 3-month-old infant, 5 to 6 ounces; and a 6-month-old infant, 8 ounces per feeding. As the infant changes from six to five feedings a day (at about 4 months of age), he begins to take more at each feeding to keep his total intake the same.

You should be able to calculate formulas and, using the minimum requirements of fluid and calories per day, evaluate the adequacy of an infant's intake.

PREPARED FORMULAS

If a mother is not going to use a commercially prepared formula, she must prepare one herself, with milk, added carbohydrate, and water. Babies cannot digest cow's milk for at least 4 months and it should not be used before then (and preferably not until the infant is 1 year of age).

Types of Milk

EVAPORATED MILK. Evaporated milk is whole milk from which 60 percent of the water has been removed. Because the solution is concentrated, its caloric content and its protein content are almost twice as high as those of whole milk (44 calories, usually considered as 40 calories for calculation, and 2 gm protein per ounce). Evaporated milk is sterile, and it is inexpensive. It has other advantages: It can be stored without refrigeration as long as the can is unopened; it has a fine curd, both because it is homogenized and because the casein curd is reduced in size in the evaporating process. Before using evaporated milk you must first dilute it with at least an equal part of water to restore the water removed in its processing. There is a possibility that evaporated milk may contain a fairly high lead content from leaching of the metal can into the milk during storage.

CONDENSED MILK. It is important for you to be able to differentiate condensed milk from evaporated milk. Some mothers use the terms interchangeably, but they are two different products and cannot be interchanged in formulas. Condensed milk is evaporated milk to which sugar has been added. It contains about

100 calories per ounce and is intended for use in rich desserts and puddings. It is too rich for infant feeding, and the additional sugar will usually cause intestinal upset and diarrhea. Make certain you know which product the mother is talking about when she tells you what milk she is using.

SKIMMED MILK. Skimmed milk is milk from which the bulk of the fat has been removed. Whole milk has about 3.5 gm of fat per 100 ml of milk; skimmed milk has 0.2 to 1.0 gm; 2 percent skimmed milk has 2 gm per 100 ml of milk. Thus the caloric content is reduced from the 20 calories per ounce of whole milk to 10 to 12 calories. Skimmed milk is not appropriate for continuous long-term feeding in infants (as long as this is the only food source) because of its low caloric and low fat content.

DRIED MILK. Dried milk is whole or skimmed milk from which the water has been completely evaporated. A fine curd is produced by the drying process. The powder can be stored for indefinite periods without refrigeration. Each brand has its own directions for reconstitution, and the mother should follow them accurately. The milk appears pale after reconstitution, and occasionally a mother will try to make it more nutritious by adding less water than specified. This will not result in a more nutritious mixture but in a stronger mixture that is less easy to digest and may be vomited.

GOAT'S MILK. In the United States, in contrast to some other countries, goat's milk is rarely used in preference to cow's milk, but in certain rural areas its use is widespread. The curd tension of goat's milk is lower than that of cow's milk, so an infant may do well on a goat's milk formula. Another advantage is that goats rarely contract tuberculosis; however, they are susceptible to brucellosis. Goat's milk is not recommended over a long period of time for infants because it is deficient in folic acid.

Types of Carbohydrate

Commercial formulas are self-contained and need no added carbohydrate. A whole- or evaporated-milk formula will need additional carbohydrate. Sugar additives all contain 120 calories per ounce. Sugar may be added in the form of Dextri-Maltose, Karo syrup, or sucrose (table sugar).

DEXTRI-MALTOSE. Dextri-Maltose is a commercial preparation that consists of maltose and dextrin, carbohydrates that are easily broken down into monosaccharides. It is frequently recommended for infant formulas. Because the powder is light and fluffy in texture, 4 tablespoons are required to make an ounce (120 calories).

KARO SYRUP. Karo syrup (a corn syrup) is easily digested and is inexpensive. It is important to remember that because Karo syrup is thick and heavy only 2 tablespoons are required to make an ounce (120 calories). A mother may switch from one to another of these carbohydrates (a neighbor suggests that Karo is less expensive, or the mother is out of Dextri-Maltose and uses the Karo she has on hand). When she switches to Karo, she must remember to add only half as much Karo as she did Dextri-Maltose.

If a baby who is on an evaporated-milk formula has diarrhea, it is a good idea to explore with the mother the amount of corn syrup being used.

SUCROSE. Sucrose is table sugar, and it may be used in formulas. Since it tends to taste very sweet, however, and is difficult to dissolve, it is not used often. Two tablespoons contain 120 calories.

Calculation of Prepared Formulas

In addition to a familiarity with fluid, caloric, and protein requirements, a few additional rules of thumb are necessary to know for calculating adequate prepared infant formulas.

1. Carbohydrate must be added to bring the caloric content of home-prepared formulas up to an adequate level for infant growth.
2. Evaporated milk is the milk of choice for prepared formulas and is prescribed (undiluted) in the proportion of 1 ounce to 1 pound of body weight (30 ml per 2.2 kg).
3. A formula that meets the preceding requirements (sufficient milk, carbohydrate, total fluid, and calories) will be adequate in minerals, but iron and possibly fluoride, as well as vitamin C, must be added.

Following these principles, a discharge formula for a 7-pound newborn whose mother will be using evaporated milk would be as follows:

Total amount of fluid required:
7×3 ounces = 21 ounces

Total amount of calories required:
$7 \times 50–55 = 350–385$ calories

Total amount of evaporated milk needed:
7×1 ounce = 7 ounces

The amount of evaporated milk needed (7 ounces) will provide 280 calories (7×40 calories). The mother will need to add 2 tablespoons (1 ounce) of corn syrup or 4 tablespoons of Dextri-Maltose (1 ounce) to make 120 additional calories and bring the total caloric value up to 400 calories. The total fluid needed is 21 ounces, so the mother will need to add about 14 ounces of water. The formula, then, contains 7 ounces of evaporated milk, 14 ounces of water, and 2 tablespoons of corn syrup or 4 tablespoons of Dextri-Maltose. This formula provides approximately 20 calories per ounce.

The formula could be divided into six feedings of 3.5 ounces each.

A discharge formula for a 9-pound infant would be the following:

Total fluid required: 9×3 ounces = 27 ounces
Total calories required:
$\qquad 9 \times 50\text{--}55$ calories = 450–495 calories
Total evaporated milk needed:
$\qquad 9 \times 1$ ounce = 9 ounces

The amount of evaporated milk needed (9 ounces) will provide 360 calories (9×40 calories). The mother will need to add 2 tablespoons of corn syrup (1 ounce) or 4 tablespoons Dextri-Maltose (1 ounce) to make 120 additional calories and bring the total calories up to 480. The total fluid need is 27 ounces, so the mother will need to add 18 ounces of water. The formula, then, is 9 ounces of evaporated milk, 18 ounces of water, and 2 tablespoons of corn syrup (or 4 tablespoons of Dextri-Maltose). The formula could be divided into six feedings of 4.5 ounces each. It provides approximately 18 to 19 calories per ounce.

SUPPLIES FOR FORMULA-FEEDING
Bottles
To prepare a full day's formula, a mother needs eight bottles. Only six are actually required for 24 hours, but the two additional bottles will take care of the first two feedings on the next day, giving her a chance to prepare formula for that day a little ahead of time. She may select a type of bottle from any of those available, all of which have advantages and disadvantages. If she is going to sterilize the formula, she should be guided into buying glass rather than plastic bottles, since plastic eventually deteriorates from being exposed to high heat. A newer form of bottle is available that is actually an empty shell into which a disposable plastic bag is inserted. The advantages of this type of bottle are that only the nipples and bottle caps need be washed and that many babies feeding from it suck less air, reducing the chance of colic. The disadvantages are that terminal sterilization cannot be used and that the mother must continue to purchase the disposable liners.

Nipples
An infant should have a nipple firm enough so that he will suck on it vigorously. A soft, flabby nipple allows him to suck in milk too rapidly and does not fulfill his need for sucking. Nipples come in two forms: the crosscut nipple (which has a slit across the top) and the standard single-hole nipple. A mother has to decide after experimentation which is best for her baby. She should buy single-hole nipples first; if they are not satisfactory, she can enlarge the hole by pressing a red-hot needle into the hole, or she can purchase crosscut nipples. If an infant finishes a feeding in 20 minutes, the nipple hole is probably adequate as is.

A way to judge a nipple's adequacy is to hold the bottle of milk with nipple attached upside down. The milk should drop through the nipple at a rate of about one drop a second.

Many mothers are too eager to enlarge nipple holes, so that "the baby doesn't tire" or because "the baby works so hard at sucking that he perspires." Babies do perspire when they suck, but sucking is a pleasurable and needed activity for them.

Bottle Caps
A bottle cap is necessary after preparation of the formula to keep the nipple clean until it is used. If the mother is feeding the baby outdoors or anywhere there are flies about, she should cover the nipple with a bottle cap while she stops feeding to bubble the baby.

PREPARATION OF FORMULA
Infant formulas must be prepared with careful attention to cleanliness and accuracy. The American Academy of Pediatrics states that if a mother is using chlorinated water and pasteurized milk, proceeds with clean technique, then refrigerates the formula until it is ready to be used, she does not need to sterilize the formula. Sterilization is necessary, however, if any of these conditions cannot be met—that is, if the mother uses unchlorinated well or spring water, unpasteurized milk, or a technique that is not absolutely clean.

All mothers, whether or not they are going to sterilize, need to begin preparation of the formula with clean equipment. Bottles, nipples, and bottle caps need to be washed with warm, soapy water or detergent. Water should be squeezed through the nipple holes to be certain they are patent and not clogged with milk. The bottles, caps, and nipples should be rinsed well to remove all soap.

If the mother is not going to sterilize, but is using

presterilized formula, she need only do the following to prepare a full day's supply of formula: wash off the top of the can with warm soapy water and rinse; open the can; pour the desired amount of formula and water into each bottle; put on the nipples, with care not to handle the nipple projection. Finally, she puts on the bottle caps and refrigerates the bottles.

Aseptic Method of Sterilization

In addition to thoroughly washed bottles, caps, and nipples, the mother needs the following: a large pan with a cover, a small pan with a cover, measuring cup (calibrated), measuring tablespoon, can opener, long-handled spoon, funnel (optional), tongs, teakettle or pan for boiling water, and a bowl or pitcher in which to mix ingredients.

The steps for preparing formula by the aseptic method are as follows:

1. Place all equipment except the nipples in the large covered pan and boil in water for 10 minutes.
2. Place the nipples in the small pan and boil them for 3 minutes. Boiling them too long makes the rubber soft and the nipples useless.
3. Boil the amount of water required for the formula in the teakettle or pan for 5 minutes.
4. Drain the water from the pan of equipment and let the pan stand for a minute until the equipment is cool enough to touch. Remove the measuring cup by the handle; do not touch the inside. From the teakettle, pour the correct amount of boiled water required for the formula into the measuring cup. Pour the water into the pitcher or bowl.
5. Measure the required amount of sugar or syrup into the boiled tablespoon. Add to the water in the bowl or pitcher, and stir until dissolved.
6. If evaporated milk or a commercial formula that requires dilution is going to be used, wash the top of the can with soap and water, rinse with water as hot as available. Open the can with the boiled can opener.
7. Pour the required amount of milk or commercial formula into the boiled measuring cup and pour into the pitcher along with the water-sugar mixture. Stir with the long-handled spoon.
8. Pour the formula into sterile bottles (may have to use boiled funnel), put on the nipples, touching only the edges, and cover with bottle caps.
9. Refrigerate the formula until needed.

Aseptic sterilization is the form to use with disposable bottles, since these cannot be sterilized by the other method. With disposable bottles, the following changes are made: In step 1, omit boiling the bottles, since they have been sterilized. In step 3, be sure to allow the water to cool for at least 15 minutes before proceeding, since formula that is too hot will melt some brands of disposable bottles.

Terminal Sterilization

Terminal sterilization is the safest, most efficient form of sterilization, since it eliminates any contamination of the bottles that may have occurred during preparation of the formula, and equipment does not have to be boiled separately. The disadvantage of terminal sterilization is the long cooling period required before the formula can be used (about 2 hours). Thus, the mother must prepare and sterilize formula at least 2 hours before she needs it. Further, some brands of disposable bottles cannot be terminally sterilized, because they will usually melt and leak if exposed to high heat.

1. Wash the bottles, nipples, and caps. Prepare the formula, using a clean (not sterilized) bowl, spoon, and can opener. Fill the bottles, and put on the nipples and caps. The caps should not be screwed absolutely tight or the pressure inside from the steam as they boil will break the bottles. A good idea is to tighten the caps to the limit and then loosen them half a turn.
2. Place the bottles in a bottle sterilizer or a large Dutch oven. The rack on the bottom of the sterilizer or pan must be in place; the heat will make the bottles crack if they rest directly on the pan bottom. A high Dutch oven (covered) can be used for sterilizing as long as it is high enough for the bottles to stand upright in it. To protect the bottles from cracking, either a metal pie pan punched with holes (to simulate a rack) or a dishcloth should be placed on the bottom of the pan. Fill the sterilizer up to the line marked on the sterilizer, or up to the shoulders of the bottles, place on the stove to boil, and boil for 25 minutes after boiling starts, determined by listening to the sound of the boiling water and the gentle jiggling of the bottles. The lid should not be lifted to check for boiling, since pressure in the bottles from steam will force milk up into the nipples and clog the holes.
3. After 25 minutes, turn off the stove and move the sterilizer to a cool burner. Do not lift the lid until the sides are cool enough to be touched with bare hands. If the lid is lifted before that, milk will be

forced up into the nipples and will clog them. The sterilizer takes about 2 hours to cool. When it is cool enough to touch, remove the bottles, tighten the caps, and refrigerate the bottles.

Preparing Individual Bottles

Many women today do not prepare a whole day's formula at one time but make up individual bottles as needed. Mothers who are breast-feeding and using supplemental bottles do the same thing.

If the mother is using ready-to-pour formula, she merely cleans the bottle, nipple, and cap, pours the desired amount of formula into the bottle, and puts on the nipple and cap. If she is using a condensed formula that needs to be diluted, she adds the correct amount of formula and an equal amount of water.

TECHNIQUES OF BOTTLE-FEEDING

To warm or not to warm the formula is up to the mother, since studies have shown that infants who are fed cooled formula directly from the refrigerator thrive as well as infants who are fed warmed formula. Most mothers feel uncomfortable giving cool formula, however, and choose to warm it. The bottle can be removed from the refrigerator about an hour before feeding time and allowed to come up to room temperature gradually. Or it can be put into a pan of hot water or warmed up in a pan of water on the stove.

Heating it on the stove is the quickest method, and if the baby is hungry and crying, this is often the method chosen. The mother should be certain she does not allow the pan to boil dry or the bottle of milk will burst (this happens to every mother at least once, usually with the last bottle of formula on hand). She also must be sure to check the temperature of the formula by allowing a drop or two to fall onto the inside of her wrist, so that it will not burn the baby's mouth. She should not heat disposable bottles on the stove; they tend to melt and then leak during feeding.

Once a bottle has been used, any contents remaining should be thrown away. It should never be stored and reused. As the infant sucks, he exchanges a small amount of saliva with the milk. Because milk is a good growth medium for bacteria and the baby's mouth harbors many bacteria, the bacteria content in reused formula is likely to be high.

Feeding an infant is a skill that, like all skills, has to be learned. A mother needs a comfortable chair (and so does a nurse who feeds babies) and adequate time (at least half an hour) to enjoy the process of feeding and not to rush the baby. The baby is held with his head slightly elevated, to reduce the danger of aspiration and retention of bubbles. The mother should be sure that the nipple is filled with milk as the baby sucks, that he is sucking milk, not air. You can tell that a baby is sucking effectively if small bubbles rise in the bottle as he sucks.

Babies in the early weeks should be bubbled after every ounce of fluid taken. A mother may place the baby over her shoulder and gently pat or stroke his back. This position is not always satisfactory for small infants, since their head control is poor, and the mother may not be able to support the baby's head and pat his back at the same time.

Holding the baby in a sitting position on her lap, leaning him forward against one hand, with the index finger and thumb supporting the head, is the best position to use for bubbling because it provides head support and yet leaves the other hand free to pat the baby's back (Fig. 30-9). Mothers usually have to be shown this method. It does not seem as natural as putting the baby against the shoulder.

Some nurses are taught to feed babies by holding them in a supine position on their knees, not cradled

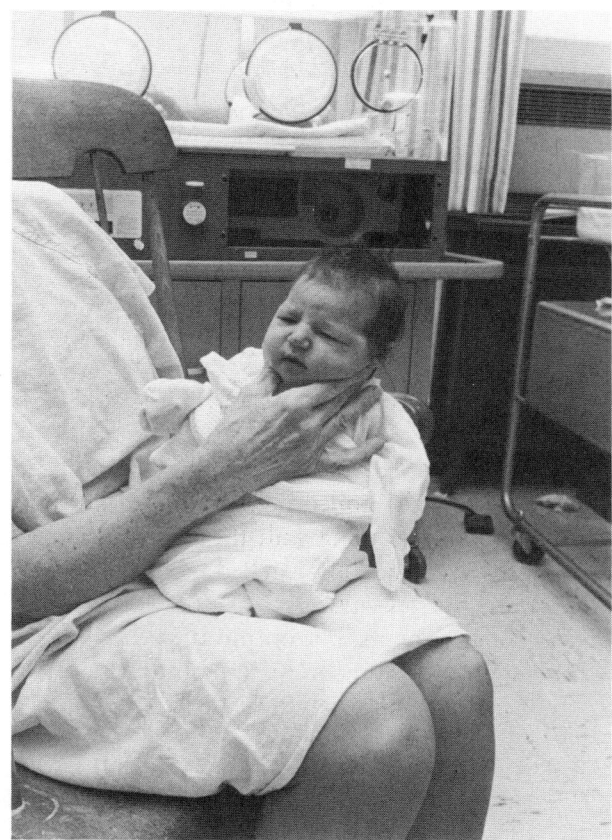

Fig. 30-9. A sitting position for burping a newborn. The infant's head is well supported by the anterior hand. (Courtesy of the Department of Medical Photography, Children's Hospital, Buffalo, N.Y.)

in their arms in a motherly fashion. Theoretically, this position gives you a better view of the infant's face, so that you will see any signs of distress in the infant immediately. It also keeps the infant away from your clothes and hair, which are possible sources of infection. In practice, you can see the infant's face as clearly in a motherly position as this other. Your gown should be clean, and in a newborn nursery, your hair should be short or controlled.

It is foolish to try to teach mothers to hold their babies warmly and comfortably if they are watching nurses holding and feeding infants in a cold, "clinical" manner.

Mothers need to be reminded not to prop up bottles. A mother whose infant spits up following feedings may feel that propping will relieve spitting up because it will reduce the amount of handling involved. Others prop up bottles because it allows them to feed the baby and do something else at the same time, such as preparing dinner. Babies who spit up actually need to be held more than babies who do not, because they are in greater danger of aspiration. Mothers might have to shift their usual dinner time to some other hour to coincide with their newborn's stomach clock. This is not an easy adjustment to make because husbands and older children have stomach clocks as well. Many a father enjoys feeding the baby while his wife prepares dinner or simply relaxes. The mother who appreciates what it means to her baby to be held and made to feel secure will more readily make sitting down for feedings a top priority and will prop up very few bottles.

The mother should be cautioned that her infant may not eat well his first day home from the hospital because of the change in environment and the increase in activity and stimulation; for the same reason, he might not eat well when traveling. However, some infants eat as if they are starved on their first day home, probably on account of the increase in activity. Common problems with formula-feeding are summarized in Table 30-4.

Introducing Solid Foods

The time to introduce solids to an infant's diet depends on a variety of factors: the baby's temperament and his ability to accept new experiences, the mother's readiness to introduce solids (most mothers are too eager to do so), the degree of development of the musculature of the jaw that enables the baby to bite, the maturity of digestive enzymes, and the fading of the extrusion reflex.

In order to digest the complex structure of solid food, the infant needs salivary enzymes. These are not present until he is 2 to 3 months of age. The extrusion reflex lasts until 3 or 4 months of age. Biting is an accomplishment that becomes possible at about 6 months of age.

Nutritionally, an infant does not appear to need solid food until he is 5 or 6 months of age, as long as he is breast-feeding and receives a daily supplement of fluoride or is taking an iron-fortified commercial formula and receives a daily supplement of fluoride.

Table 30-4. Common Problems of Formula-Feeding

Problem	Cause	Nursing Interventions
Infant sucks for a few minutes, then stops and cries	Either nipple is blocked and infant is unable to get milk or flow is too fast and he has choking sensation	Show mother how to test flow of milk from the nipple (hold bottle upside down); milk should flow from nipple at about rate of 1 drop per second
Infant does not "bubble" well after feeding	Some infants swallow little air with feeding. Mother may be handling infant too tentatively	Observe baby feeding and mother's technique of handling him; rubbing a newborn's back may be more effective than patting it
Mother reports loose stools	Bowel movements from formula-fed infants are not quite as loose as those from a breast-fed infant but so different from adult stools that a mother may be concerned	Examine stool; assure and explain normal stool pattern
Mother tired	Exhaustion is a common postpartal finding due to psychosocial and physiological adjustments of time	Help mother to plan rest times; assess diet intake

Problem-oriented Recording: Progress Notes

Baby Kraft (John Joseph)
Day 1

Problem: Nutrition

> S. Mother states, "I thought breast-feeding would be hard. It's easier than it looks."
> O. Infant breast-feeding q2h; 6 minutes each breast. Sucks eagerly; content between feedings. Voiding qs; no meconium stool yet. Skin turgor good, mucous membranes moist.
> Weight: Birth weight minus 2 oz.
> A. Breast-feeding established well at day 1 level.
>
> Goals: a. Breast-feeding to be viewed as an enjoyable experience by both infant and parents.
> b. Mother is knowledgeable of breast-feeding technique by discharge (24–48 hours).
> c. Mother to use hospital liaison nurse as reference person for breast-feeding concerns when at home. (No community or family support person identified.)
> d. Breast milk to be entire nutritional pattern for 6 months.
>
> P. 1. Review physiology of engorgement with mother as she will be at home by 3rd day post partum.
> 2. Review care of engorgement (warm compresses prior to feeding; encourage infant to suck).
> 3. Review practice of checking with M.D. before beginning any medication while breast-feeding.
> 4. Review need for rest and adequate fluid intake while at home.
> 5. Review availability of hospital liaison nurse for consultation while at home.

Problem-oriented Recording: Progress Notes

Baby McFadden (no name yet)
Day 2

Problem: Nutrition

> S. Mother (15 years old) asking to feed baby but unable to hold her for entire feeding because of "pain from c-section incision." Grew concerned when baby spit up some mucus; asking when she will be old enough to feed by spoon.
> O. Infant taking about 2 oz 20 cal/oz formula q4h. Sucks readily; voiding qs; meconium stool ×2. Skin turgor good; mucous membranes moist.
> Weight: Birth weight minus 3 oz.
> A. Nutrition adequate for day 2.
>
> Goals: a. Both mother and infant to view formula-feeding as enjoyable experience.
> b. Mother to increase feeding time as physical condition improves.
> c. Maternal grandmother to serve as resource person at home for nutrition problems.
> d. Formula to be entire nutritional basis for 6 months.
>
> P. 1. Observe mother-infant interaction at each contact.
> 2. Encourage mother to feed infant so she grows accustomed to spitting up and handling infant.
> 3. Review adequacy of formula for infant and why there is no need for solid food.
> 4. Review feeding technique (holding, milk in nipple, burping, etc.)

References

1. Afrin-Slater, R. B., and Jelliffe, D. Nutritional requirements with specific references to infancy. *Pediatr. Clin. North Am.* 24:3, 1977.
2. Anderson, T. A. Commercial infant foods: Content and composition. *Pediatr. Clin. North Am.* 24:37, 1977.
3. Appel, J. A., and King, J. C. Energy needs during pregnancy and lactation. *Nutr. Health Promotion* 1:7, 1979.
4. Applebaum, R. M. The modern management of successful breast feeding. *Pediatr. Clin. North Am.* 17:203, 1970.
5. Catz, C., and Giacoia, G. Drugs and breast milk. *Pediatr. Clin. North Am.* 19:151, 1972.
6. Committee on Nutrition, American Academy of Pediatrics. Iron balance and requirements in infancy. *Pediatrics* 43:134, 1969.
7. Cronin, T. J. Influence of lactation upon ovulation. *Lancet* 2:422, 1968.
8. Dickman, S. R. Breast feeding and infant nutrition. *Nutr. Health Promotion* 1:19, 1979.
9. Eid, E. E. Follow-up study of physical growth of children who had excessive weight gain in the first 6 months of life. *Br. Med. J.* 2:74, 1970.
10. Foman, S. J. What are infants fed in the United States? *Pediatrics* 56:350, 1975.
11. Foman, S. J., et al. Recommendations for feeding normal infants. *Pediatrics* 63:52, 1979.
12. Frantz, K. B., et al. Breastfeeding works for cesareans, too. *R.N.* 42:38, 1979.
13. Grassley, J., and Davis, K. Common concerns of mothers who breast-feed. *M.C.N.* 3:347, 1978.
14. Hambraeus, L. Proprietary milk versus human breast milk in infant feeding. *Pediatr. Clin. North Am.* 24:17, 1977.
15. Hansen, A. E., et al. Role of linoleic acid in infant nutrition. *Pediatrics* 31:171, 1963.
16. Jackson, R. L. Long term consequences of suboptimal nutritional practices in early life. *Pediatr. Clin. North Am.* 24:63, 1977.
17. Johnson, N. Breast feeding at one hour of age. *M.C.N.* 1:12, 1976.
18. La Leche League International. *The Womanly Art of Breastfeeding* (13th ed.). Danville, Ill.: Interstate Printers and Publishers, 1971.
19. Lamm, E., et al. Economy in the feeding of infants. *Pediatr. Clin. North Am.* 24:71, 1977.
20. Lawson, B. Perceptions of degrees of support for the breast-feeding mother. *Birth Fam. J.* 3:67, 1976.
21. Markesbery, B. A., and Wong, W. M. Watching baby's diet: A professional and parental guide. *M.C.N.* 4:177, 1979.
22. Moore, F. D., et al. Carcinoma of the breast. *N. Engl. J. Med.* 277:293, 1967.
23. Nelson, G. K., and Dean, R. F. A. The electroencephalogram in African children: Effects of kwashiorkor and a note on the newborn. *Bull. W.H.O.* 21:779, 1959.
24. Neumann, C. G., et al. Birthweight doubling time: A fresh look. *Pediatrics* 57:469, 1976.
25. Nichols, M. G. Effective help for the nursing mother. *J.O.G.N. Nurs.* 7:22, 1978.
26. Tyson, J. E. Mechanisms of puerperal lactation. *Med. Clin. North Am.* 61:153, 1977.
27. Webster-Stratton, C., and Kogan, K. Helping parents parent. *Am. J. Nurs.* 80:240, 1980.
28. Woodruff, C. Iron deficiency in infancy and childhood. *Pediatr. Clin. North Am.* 24:85, 1977.

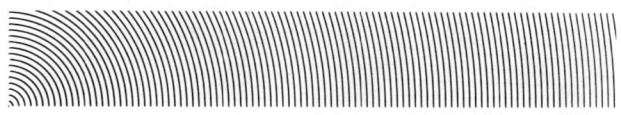

31. Newborn Care: Nursing Interventions

Nursing care of the newborn is a continuation of the care the fetus received during pregnancy and during labor and delivery.

Delivery Room Care

An island for newborn care should be provided in the delivery room or birthing room apart from the equipment needed for the mother's care. A radiant heat table, a warm bassinet, a warm soft blanket, and equipment for oxygen administration, resuscitation, suction, eye care, identification, and weighing the newborn must be provided.

In most hospital delivery rooms, the delivering physician hands the newborn to the delivery room nurse moments after birth so she can begin her care. You should wash your hands thoroughly with an appropriate antiseptic solution, then, holding a warm sterile blanket, grasp the infant through the blanket by placing one hand under his back and the other around a leg. Newborns are slippery because they are wet from amniotic fluid and vernix caseosa.

Rub the infant dry so that no body heat is lost by evaporation. Then swaddle him loosely with the blanket so that respiratory effort is not compromised, and lay him on his side in a warmed bassinet or unwrapped on a radiant heat table. The bassinet should be tipped to a 30-degree Trendelenburg position to allow mucus or fluid to drain from the mouth. The tilt should not be exaggerated or the infant's abdominal contents will be pressed against the diaphragm, interfering with lung expansion.

EVALUATION OF RESPIRATIONS

Good respiratory function obviously has the highest priority. A Silverman and Andersen index [14] can be used to estimate degrees of respiratory distress in infants. The newborn is observed once and scored on the items listed in Table 31-1. As shown, each item is given a value of 0, 1, or 2. These values are then added. A total score of 0 indicates no respiratory distress. Scores of 4 to 6 indicate moderate distress. Scores of 7 to 10 indicate severe distress. Note that this index's scores are opposite those of the Apgar. In an Apgar score, a value of 7 to 10 denotes a well infant. On a Silverman and Andersen score, a value of 7 to 10 denotes a seriously distressed infant.

Suctioning

Mucus should be suctioned from a newborn's mouth by a bulb syringe as soon as the head is delivered. As soon as the infant is born, he should be held for a few seconds with his head slightly lowered for further

Table 31-1. Evaluation of Respiratory Status

Feature Observed	Score		
	0	1	2
Chest movement	Synchronized respirations	Lag on inspiration	Seesaw respirations
Intercostal retraction	None	Just visible	Marked
Xiphoid retraction	None	Just visible	Marked
Nares dilatation	None	Minimal	Marked
Expiratory grunt	None	Audible by stethoscope only	Audible by unaided ear

Source. W. A. Silverman and D. H. Andersen, A controlled clinical trial of effects of water mist on obstructive respiratory signs, death rate and necroscopy findings among premature infants. *Pediatrics* 17:1, 1956. Copyright American Academy of Pediatrics 1956.

drainage of secretions. Mucus must be removed from the mouth and pharynx before the first breath to prevent aspiration of the secretions. If the infant continues to have an accumulation of mucus in his mouth or nose following these first steps, you may need to suction further when he is placed in the bassinet (Fig. 31-1). Use a bulb syringe or a soft small (No. 10 or 12) catheter. With a De Lee glass trap between the catheter and the suction tubing, the mucus obtained can be observed for color, consistency, and the presence of any blood. Vigorous suctioning should never be employed. It irritates the mucous membrane and leaves portals of entry for infection. Brisk suctioning has also been associated with bradycardia in newborns. If a bulb syringe is used, the bulb should be decompressed before being inserted in the infant's mouth or the force of decompression will force the secretions back into the pharynx or bronchi. When an infant is born with meconium-stained amniotic fluid, it is important that the infant be not only suctioned but intubated so that deep tracheal suction can be accomplished before the first breath. This action prevents meconium, which is very irritating to lung tissue, from being drawn into the lungs with the first breath.

Recording First Cry

A crying infant is a breathing infant because the sound of crying is made by a current of air passing over the larynx. The more lusty the cry, the more assurance there is that the newborn is breathing deeply and forcefully. Vigorous crying also helps to "blow

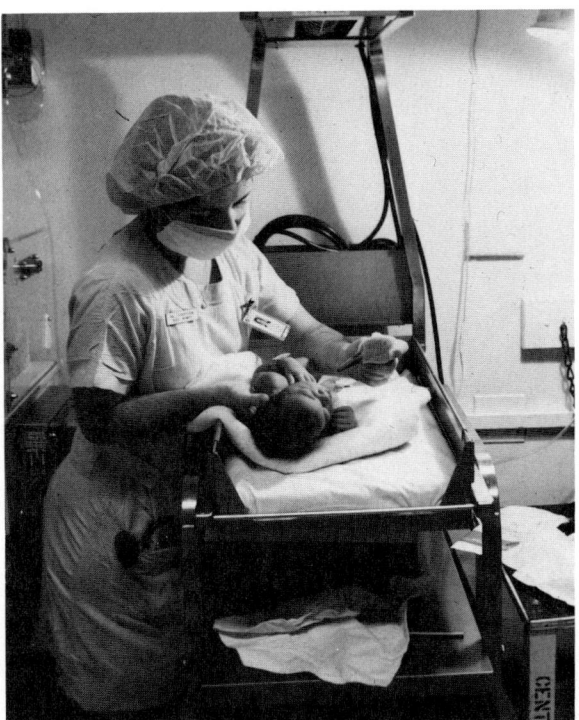

Fig. 31-1. Suctioning the newborn. A newborn is suctioned by means of a bulb syringe to remove mucus from his mouth. His head-down-and-to-the-side position facilitates drainage. Care is given with the infant under a radiant heat source. (From J. E. Roberts, Suctioning the newborn. Am. J. Nurs. 73:63, 1973.)

off" the extra CO_2 that makes all newborns slightly acidotic and thus helps to correct this condition. Although gentleness is necessary to make the infant's transition from intrauterine life to extrauterine life as untraumatic as possible, most people believe you should not be so motherly in handling a newborn in the delivery room that you rock or jiggle him to completely stop this initial crying.

It is important to note what time after birth the child first gasped and cried and whether or not he was able to maintain respirations unaided. The newborn who does not breathe spontaneously, or who takes a few quick gasping breaths but is unable to maintain respirations, needs resuscitation as an emergency measure (see Chap. 38).

CONTROL OF BODY TEMPERATURE

As discussed in Chap. 28, a newborn has difficulty in regulating his body temperature. He tends to become chilled in the delivery room because his body is wet and the temperature of the room is low. Nursing care should be accomplished as quickly as possible, with minimum exposure of the child to chilling. Any extensive procedures such as circumcision or resuscitation should be done under a radiant heat source to reduce heat loss. There is no need for the infant to be removed immediately from the delivery room in order to prevent chilling. This is an important time for his parents to have an opportunity to see him. Newborns are very alert (first period of activity) and respond well to their parents' first tentative touches or interaction with them. Although the temperature of newborns who are dried and wrapped and held by their parents in the delivery room apparently falls slightly lower than that of infants placed in heated cribs, their rectal temperature does not fall below safe limits [12].

APGAR SCORING

At 1 minute and 5 minutes after birth, the newborn must be observed and rated according to the Apgar score [1]. As shown in Table 31-2, heart rate, respiratory effort, muscle tone, reflex irritability, and color are rated 0, 1, or 2; all five scores are then added. An infant whose total score is under 4 is in serious danger and needs resuscitation. A score of 4 to 6 means that his condition is "guarded" and he may need clearing of the airway and supplementary oxygen. A score of 7 to 10 is considered a good Apgar rating, indicating that the infant scored as high as do 70 to 90 percent of infants at 1 and 5 minutes after birth (10 is the highest score possible). The Apgar score standardizes infant evaluation and serves as a baseline for future evaluations. There is a high correlation between low 5-minute Apgar scores and mortality and morbidity, particularly neurological morbidity.

An Apgar rating is most accurate when it is done by a nurse. (Obstetricians tend to rate high; pediatricians tend to rate low.) For this reason you should be very familiar with how the rating is carried out. The following points should be considered in obtaining an Apgar rating.

Heart Rate

Auscultating the newborn chest with a stethoscope is the best way of determining heart rate. However, heart rate may also be obtained by observing and counting the pulsations of the cord at the abdomen if the cord is still uncut at 1 minute after birth. The newborn's heart rate ranges between 150 and 180 beats per minute immediately after birth as he struggles to begin respirations.

Respiratory Effort

A mature newborn usually cries spontaneously at about 30 seconds after birth. By 1 minute he is maintaining regular, although rapid, respirations. Difficulty might be anticipated in a newborn whose mother received large amounts of analgesics or a general anesthetic during labor or delivery.

Muscle Tone

A mature newborn holds his extremities tightly flexed, simulating his intrauterine position. He should resist any effort to extend his extremities.

Reflex Irritability

One of two possible cues is used to evaluate reflex irritability, *either* the newborn's response to a suction catheter in his nostrils *or* his response to having the soles of his feet slapped. A baby whose mother was heavily sedated will tend to have a low score in this category.

Color

All infants appear cyanotic at the moment of birth. They grow pink with or shortly after the first breath. The color of the newborn thus corresponds to how well he is breathing. Acrocyanosis (cyanosis of the hands and feet) is so common in newborns that a score of 1 in this category can be thought of as normal.

Table 31-2. Apgar Scoring Chart

Sign	Score 0	Score 1	Score 2
Heart rate	Absent	Slow (below 100)	Over 100
Respiratory effort	Absent	Slow, irregular; weak cry	Good; strong cry
Muscle tone	Flaccid	Some flexion of extremities	Well flexed
Reflex irritability Response to catheter in nostril or	No response	Grimace	Cough or sneeze
Slap to sole of foot	No response	Grimace	Cry and withdrawal of foot
Color	Blue, pale	Body pink, extremities blue	Completely pink

Source. V. Apgar, et al., Evaluation of the newborn infant—second report. J.A.M.A. 168:1985, 1958. Copyright © 1958, American Medical Association.

CARE OF THE UMBILICAL CORD

The umbilical cord pulsates for a moment after the infant is born as a last flow of blood passes from the placenta into the infant. Two Kelly clamps are applied to the cord about 8 inches from the infant's abdomen, and the cord is cut between the clamps. It is then clamped again by a cord clamp, such as a Hazeltine or a Kane clamp, or tied with cord string or umbilical tape before the Kelly clamp is released. If a string is used, it should be tied in a square knot gently but firmly, so that the hands do not slip and tear the cord in the process of tying. The Kelly clamp on the maternal end of the cord should not be released following cord cutting; otherwise, blood still remaining in the placenta will leak out. This loss is not important since the mother's circulation does not connect to the placenta. It is messy, however, and that is why the clamp is left in place.

Inspect the infant's cord to be certain it is clamped or tied securely. If the clamp loosens before thrombosis obliterates the umbilical vessels, hemorrhage will result. As previously mentioned, the number of cord vessels should be counted and noted while the infant is in the delivery or birthing room. Cords begin to dry almost immediately, and by the time of the infant's first thorough physical examination in the nursery, the vessels will be obscured.

CARE OF THE EYES

Although the practice may shortly become obsolete (it is in Europe), every state requires that newborns receive prophylactic treatment against gonorrheal conjunctivitis of the newborn. Such infections are acquired from the mother as the infant passes through the birth canal. Silver nitrate is the drug most commonly used for prophylaxis although tetracycline and erythromycin ointments are becoming popular. Silver nitrate comes prepared in wax ampules that are opened by puncturing one end with a pin supplied by the manufacturer. The face of the newborn should be dried first with a soft gauze square, so that the skin is not slippery. It is difficult to open a newborn's eyes. The best procedure is to shade the eyes from the overhead light and open one eye at a time by pressure on the lower and upper lids. Two drops of a 1% solution of silver nitrate are dropped one drop at a time into the conjunctival sac. Be careful not to drop any on the infant's cheek, since it may stain the skin a brown color. This is a transient phenomenon, but it causes needless worry to the parents. Do not drop the solution directly on the eye cornea or it will cause excessive pain. Silver nitrate should *not* be washed away with saline after instillation. A chemical conjunctivitis, characterized by inflammation, edema, and a purulent discharge, will result from silver nitrate instillation. Chemical conjunctivitis is confusing in the newborn period because it simulates an infectious process and makes the diagnosis of a true infection difficult. The antibiotic ointments eliminate the conjunctivitis and are easy to instill (simply squeeze a line of ointment into the lower conjunctival sac).

Prophylaxis against gonorrheal conjunctivitis was first proposed by Credé, a German gynecologist, in 1884. For this reason, it is often referred to as the Credé treatment and may be listed that way on the hospital delivery form. Penicillin ophthalmic ointment or drops may be used for eye prophylaxis. This is effective against most gonorrheal strains, but its use is generally discouraged because of the dangers of introducing penicillin sensitivity at an early age.

Babies born outside hospitals (in taxicabs, for example) must have the prophylactic treatment administered on admission to the hospital. Because it is a delivery room routine it is easy to forget in infants who are born elsewhere.

VITAMIN K ADMINISTRATION

All newborns should receive an injection of 1 mg of water-soluble vitamin K (AquaMEPHYTON) in the delivery room. Higher doses may lead to hyperbilirubinemia and should not be given. Vitamin K is administered intramuscularly, usually into the lateral anterior thigh, the preferred site for all injections in the newborn (Fig. 31-2).

IDENTIFICATION

Some form of identification must be attached to all newborns before they are removed from the delivery room. One traditional form is a plastic bracelet or bead necklace with permanent locks that need to be cut to be removed. A number that corresponds to the mother's hospital number, the mother's full name, the date and time of birth, and the sex of the baby compose the information necessary for identification. If the identification band is attached to a newborn's arm or leg, two bands should be used. A newborn's wrist and hand, as well as his ankle and his foot, are not very different in width, so bands tend to slide off with very little movement.

Following the attachment of the identification band or bands, the infant's footprints may be taken (Fig. 31-3) and thereafter kept with his chart for permanent identification. Because footprints will be part of the permanent record and are important for

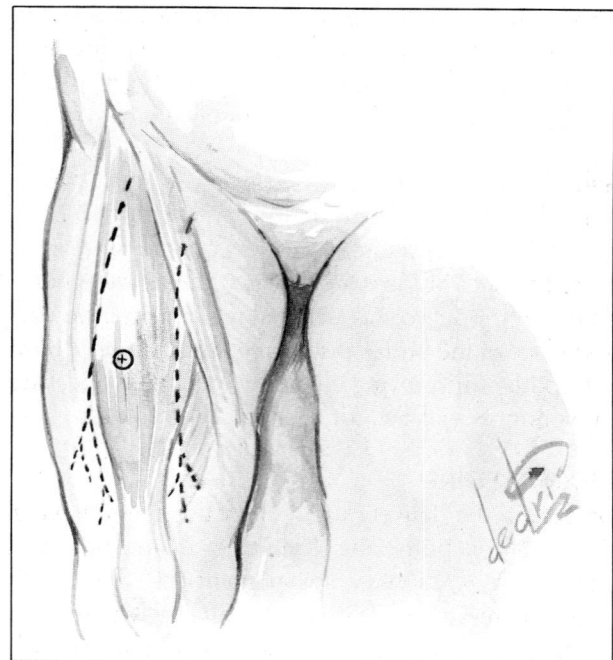

Fig. 31-2. Preferred site for intramuscular injection in a newborn: lateral aspect of the anterior thigh. (Courtesy of the Department of Medical Illustration, State University of New York at Buffalo.)

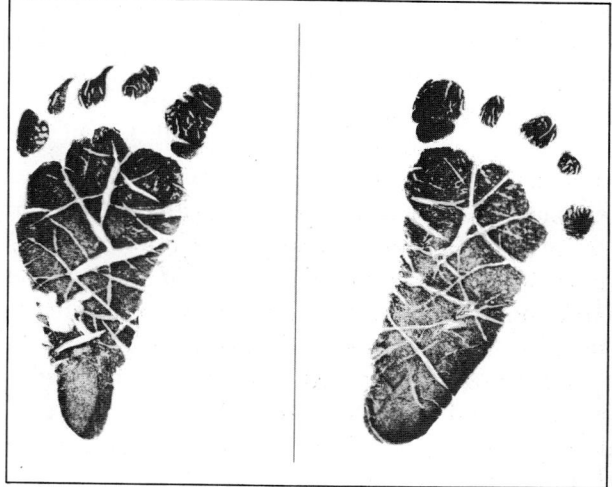

Fig. 31-3. Newborn footprints. (Courtesy of the Department of Medical Photography, Children's Hospital, Buffalo, N.Y.)

identification, care should be taken in securing them. Gleason [5] suggests the following procedure for obtaining accurate and identifiable prints.

1. Proper equipment must be used, including a disposable footprinter ink plate and high-gloss paper.
2. As soon as the infant is wrapped in a warm blanket, his foot should be wiped clean. Vernix caseosa is thus prevented from drying on it and it is easier to clean when the actual footprinting is done.
3. After respiratory and circulatory functions have been established, but before the baby is taken from the delivery room, the foot should be cleansed gently but thoroughly. Scrubbing too vigorously makes a newborn's skin peel. The foot should be dried. Flex the baby's knee so that his knee is close to his abdomen, and grasp the ankle between your thumb and middle finger. Next, press your index finger on the upper surface of the foot just behind the newborn's toes to prevent his toes from curling. Press the footprinter gently against the sole of the foot.
4. The footprint paper, attached to a hard surface such as a clipboard, should be pressed gently against the inked foot. The heel should be pressed on the chart first, then the foot "walked" onto the chart with a heel-to-toe motion. The foot should not be rolled back and forth in the hope of making a better print; the result will only be a blurry print.
5. Any excess ink should be wiped from the infant's foot. The baby should then be well swaddled to prevent chilling. The mother's index fingerprint or thumbprint is commonly placed on the same paper, along with the mother's and child's number.

Footprinting should be done in the same way on babies who are born outside the hospital when they are admitted to the newborn nursery for follow-up care.

MEASUREMENTS

The newborn should be weighed nude and without his blanket in the delivery room. His height and his head, chest, and abdominal circumferences should be measured in the newborn or transitional nursery. Doing these measurements in the delivery room only exposes the newborn unnecessarily.

ASSESSMENT

The newborn is given a preliminary physical examination in the delivery room to detect such grossly observable conditions as meningocele, cleft lip and palate, hydrocephalus, birthmarks, imperforate anus, tracheoesophageal atresia, and bowel obstruction. This assessment may be the responsibility of the delivering physician, the anesthesiologist, a pediatrician, or the delivery room nurse using extended assessment skills. The health assessment must be done rapidly, so that the newborn is not exposed for a long period of time, yet it must not be done so swiftly that important findings are overlooked.

The delivery room appraisal should include auscultation of the chest for heart and respiratory sounds (perhaps already done as a part of Apgar scoring). Van Leeuwen and Glenn [17] suggest a number of procedures that can be performed to rule out the common birth anomalies. These procedures and their screening importance are shown in Table 31-3.

A thorough generalized inspection and tentative gestation age determination should be included in the delivery room appraisal in addition to the procedures that have been described.

MOTHER-CHILD INTERACTION

As mentioned in Chap. 22, the mother or parents should be allowed some time to be with the child before he is removed from the delivery room (unless he is in distress). Except for the few moments allowed for inspection of fingers, toes, and sex, the infant should be kept wrapped during the visit so that he does not become chilled and have his respiratory function compromised. If the mother wishes to begin breast-feeding in the delivery room, she may do so.

BIRTH REGISTRATION

The physician who delivered the infant must be certain a birth registration is filed with the Bureau of Vital Statistics of the state in which the infant is born. The infant's name, his parents' names, and the date and place of the birth must be recorded. Proof of birth is important in proving eligibility for school and later for voting, Social Security benefits, and so on.

RECORD-KEEPING

Be certain the delivery room chart lists the following: the time of birth; the time the infant breathed; whether respirations were spontaneous; the child's Apgar score at 1 and 5 minutes of life; whether eye prophylaxis was given; whether vitamin K was administered; the general condition of the infant; the number of vessels in the umbilical cord; whether cultures were taken (they are taken if at some point sterile delivery technique was broken); and whether the infant (1) voided and (2) passed a stool (the latter items are helpful if, later on, the diagnosis of bowel obstruction or absence of a kidney is considered).

GENTLENESS IN CARE

The philosophy of caring health care providers has always been that newborns should be handled as gently at birth as they are at any other time. The image of the obstetrician holding the newborn up by his heels and spanking him to make him breathe has existed only in Hollywood movies. It has long been accepted that holding a baby by his feet and letting his back extend fully is probably painful after his months in a flexed position in utero; a measure such as spanking is not as effective in helping a newborn to breathe as is gentle stimulation such as rubbing the back.

Leboyer [8], a French obstetrician, has stressed in recent years that gentleness at birth should be a prime priority of care. In addition to the accepted measures mentioned, he advises dimming the delivery room lights to reduce the pain of sudden exposure to light and immersing the newborn in a tub of warm water shortly after birth.

Gentleness in delivery room care must extend to nursing interventions in order for the concept to be complete in all situations, whether specific Leboyer interventions are carried out or not.

Table 31-3. Congenital Anomaly Appraisal

Procedure	Abnormalities Considered
Inquire for hydramnios	Presence of hydramnios suggests congenital gastrointestinal or genitourinary obstruction or extreme prematurity
Appearance of abdomen	Distended abdomen suggests ascites or tumor. Empty abdomen suggests diaphragmatic hernia
Passage of nasogastric tube (No. 8 feeding catheter)	Failure to pass nasogastric tube through nares on either side establishes choanal atresia. Failure to pass it into the stomach confirms presence of esophageal atresia
Aspiration of stomach with recording of color and amount of fluid	With excess of 20 ml of fluid, or yellow fluid, duodenal or ileal atresia is suspected
Insertion of rectal catheter	Failure to obtain meconium suggests imperforate anus or higher obstruction
Counting of umbilical arteries	The presence of one artery suggests possible congenital urinary anomalies or chromosomal trisomy (if other portions of examination are consistent)

Source. G. Van Leeuwen and L. Glenn, Screening for hidden congenital anomalies. *Pediatrics* 41:147, 1968. Copyright American Academy of Pediatrics 1968.

Care of the Newborn in the Hospital
GENERAL PRINCIPLES

A newborn should be kept in either a birthing room or a careful-watch nursery (Fig. 31-4) for optimal safety for the first few hours of life. This nursery functions as a recovery room and provides a space where intensive care can be given during the first crucial period of life.

Following careful-watch time, there are three main types of hospital nursery care. One is a central care system, in which babies remain in units with about 12 bassinets each, are taken to the mothers every 4 hours for feeding, and then are returned to the nursery. A second type is a rooming-in system, in which each baby stays in a bassinet in the mother's room or in a small nursery adjacent to her room. In a third system, the central nursery and rooming-in concepts are combined; the baby remains in the mother's room during the day and is returned to the central nursery at night or when the mother wants to nap.

No matter which system of nursery care is used, certain general principles always apply:

Fig. 31-4. An observation nursery. Following delivery, newborns need at least an hour of "careful watch" care either in a birthing room or a special nursery before they are transferred to a regular nursery or the mother's rooming-in unit. (Courtesy of the Department of Medical Photography, Children's Hospital, Buffalo, N.Y.)

1. Infants should be housed in close proximity to the postpartal unit. The nurseries and the postpartal unit should, in fact, be a continuous service, so that the mother and child are thought of as one unit.
2. Each infant should have his own bassinet (Fig. 31-5). Compartments in the bassinet should hold a supply of diapers, shirts, gowns, and individual equipment for bathing and temperature taking. The sharing of equipment leads to the spread of infection.
3. The temperature of the baby's environment should be about 75°F (24°C). When procedures that require undressing the infant for an extended period of time are being done (e.g., circumcision), a radiant heat source should be used.
4. Areas where babies are housed should be well lighted for the easy detection of jaundice and cyanosis. Nonglossy white or pale beige walls are best.
5. An oxygen source and emergency call lights should be readily accessible.
6. Personnel, parents, or siblings caring for newborns should wash their hands and arms to the elbows thoroughly with an antiseptic solution before handling infants. Personnel should wear cover gowns or nursery uniforms.

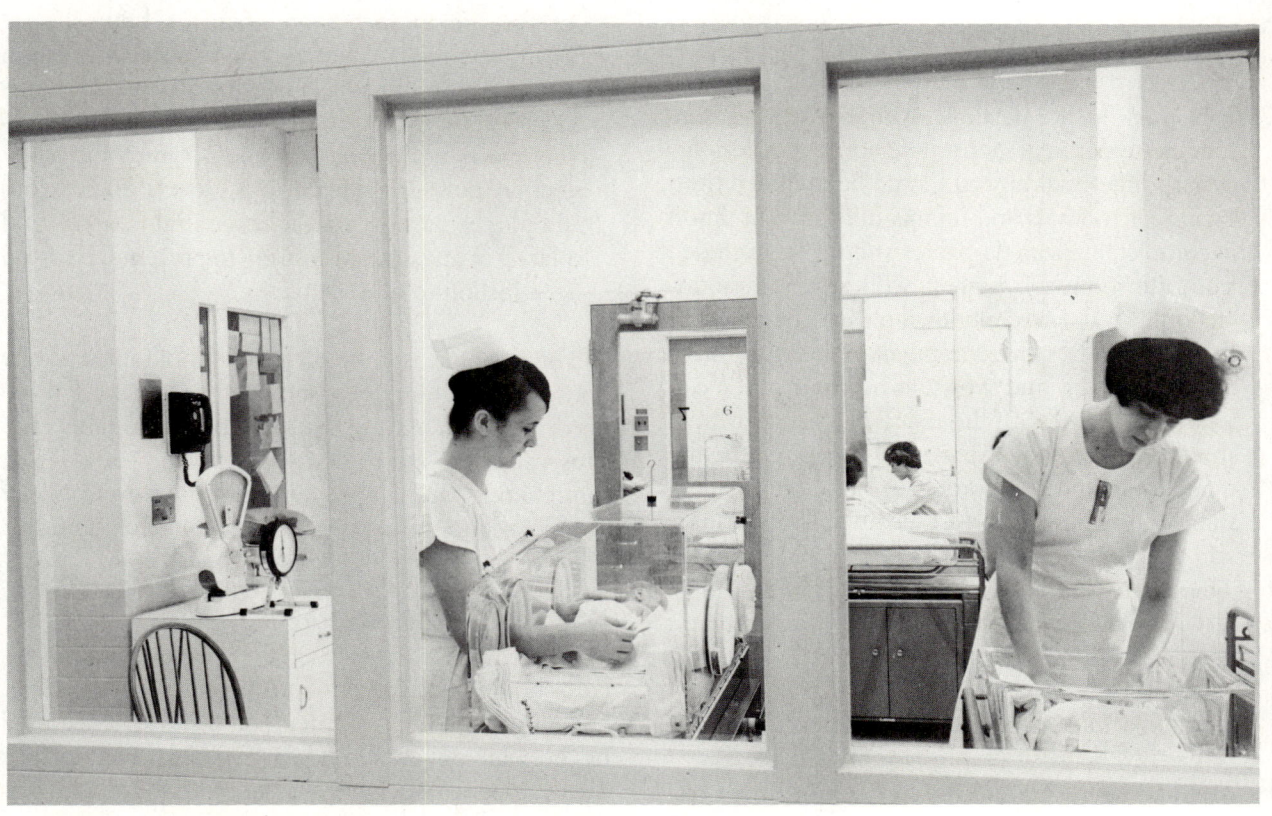

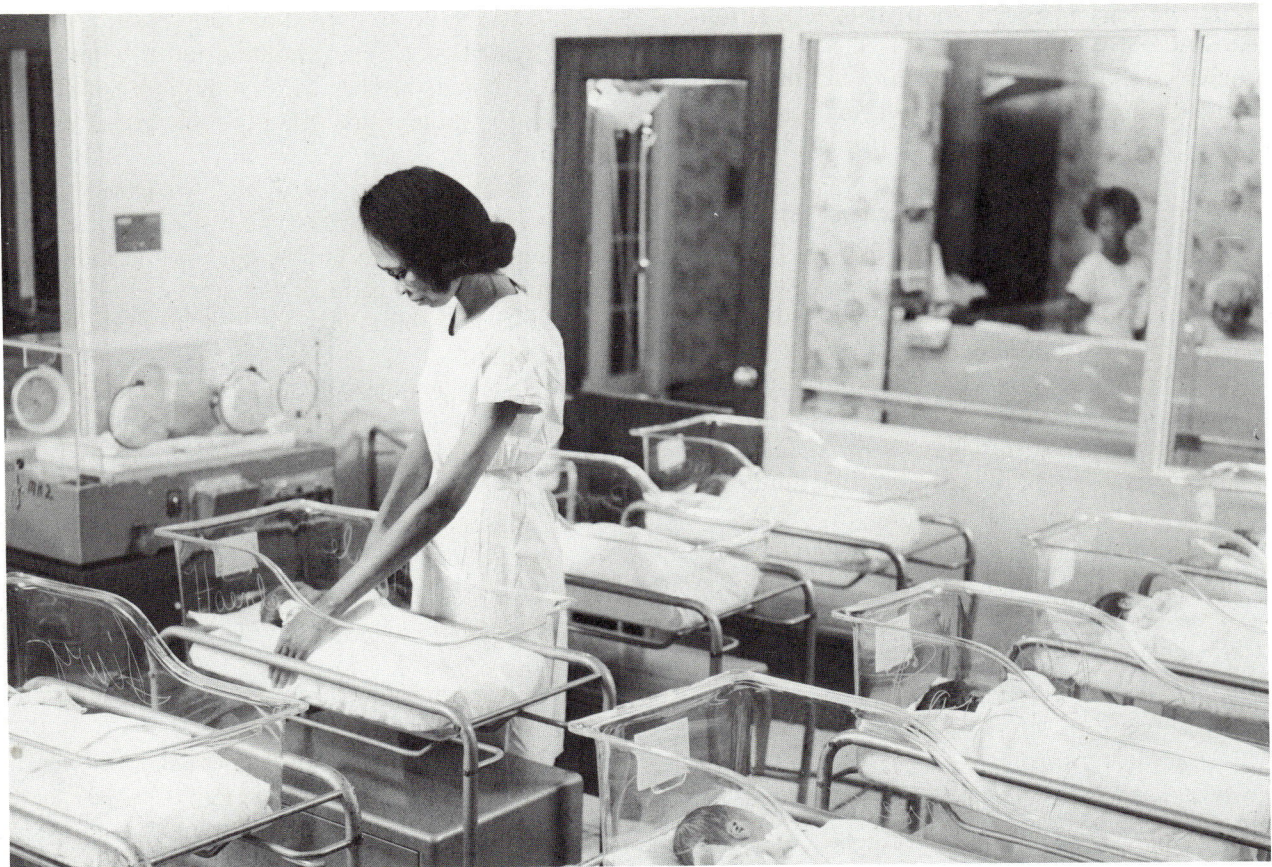

Fig. 31-5. A newborn nursery. Each infant has a self-contained unit for care. (Courtesy of the Department of Medical Photography, Children's Hospital, Buffalo, N.Y.)

7. Personnel with infections (herpes simplex, sore throats, upper respiratory infections, skin lesions, or gastrointestinal upsets) should be excluded from caring for mothers and infants until the condition is completely cleared. Babies should be excluded from the rooms of mothers with any of these infections. A Polaroid photograph can be taken or the baby can be carried to the door of the mother's room, however, and shown to her, so that she can follow his progress. If the infant is breast-fed, milk should be manually expressed during the time the infant is excluded in order to maintain the milk supply and allow for breast-feeding as soon as it is safe.

8. The number of babies housed together in a nursery should not exceed 16. Then, if an infection occurs, it will spread to no more than 16 babies. It is best if nurseries are limited to six newborns and are used on a rotating basis, so that each one can be cleaned between each group of six babies.

9. Any baby born outside the hospital or under circumstances conducive to infection (e.g., rupture of the membranes more than 24 hours before birth) should be admitted to a special isolation nursery or a closed Isolette for at least 24 hours until negative cultures show that he is free of infection. Any newborn in whom symptoms of infection develop (skin lesions, fever, and so on) should be removed from a central nursery and placed in an isolation nursery to prevent the spread of infection to other babies.

There is no reason for the mother not to visit a baby housed in isolation care. She may, in fact, have more need to hold her baby than the average mother, because she has an extra reason to be worried that something is wrong with her child. However, as staff members do, she must use isolation techniques at these visits.

ADMISSION TO THE NURSERY

When the newborn arrives at the recovery nursery, his cord should be checked for any possibility of bleeding, and any antibiotic ointment or triple dye required by hospital policy should be applied. The infant's measurements—height, weight, and head circumference—should be taken and recorded. Color and respirations should be noted. Be sure that the infant's identification band or necklace is in place. He should be reswaddled in a warm blanket and placed in a bassinet or in his mother's arms, or placed nude except for a diaper in a heated Isolette. He should be laid on his side.

During the first hour of life he should be observed closely for changes in color or respiratory effort. Leaving him on his side allows mucus to drain from his mouth. Some physicians prefer newborns to rest with the foot of the bassinet elevated at a 15- to 20-degree angle. This position obviously aids the drainage of mucus, but some physicians believe that it also unnecessarily increases intracranial pressure.

At the end of the first hour of life, the newborn's temperature should be taken. If it is subnormal and he is in a bassinet, he should be placed in an Isolette for additional heat. If his temperature is normal, he can be bathed quickly to remove excess vernix caseosa and any blood. Then he should be dressed in a shirt and diaper, reswaddled in a snug blanket or sheet (to give him a feeling of the tight confines of the uterus he is so used to), and placed in a bassinet or returned to his mother's side. If a mother is going to keep her baby with her during this time, she needs close observation. She is more tired than she realizes and may fall asleep easily.

When a newborn awakes or is awakened from his first period of sleep, he usually appears hyperreactive to stimuli. His cry will be vigorous and his reflexes active. Mucus may have been pooling in his mouth during sleep; now, with activity, he gags and chokes. This may be the body's way of ensuring good circulation and lung expansion during this time. In any event, the infant's temperament should not be judged by these actions. They are not necessarily typical of his behavior thereafter.

Occasionally, a child remains groggy when awakened. His extremities are floppy and his head control lags behind normal. He is probably still affected by analgesia or anesthesia; however, he may be demonstrating the first signs of increased intracranial pressure or infection. In either event, he should be watched closely for respiratory difficulty. Either he is a candidate for a special care nursery or he will need to remain in the admitting nursery longer than the average child, until the grogginess passes.

NEWBORN ASSESSMENT

Following an hour of undisturbed rest, the newborn should have a thorough physical assessment, the details of which are discussed in Chapter 29. In addition, he should have a heel-stick hematocrit or hemoglobin determination and a Dextrostix test for hypoglycemia. Both hematocrit and Dextrostix determinations require a minimum of blood and can be obtained by nurses.

Newborn anemia is difficult to detect by clinical observation. Anemia may have been caused by hypovolemia due to bleeding from placenta previa or abruptio placentae, or perhaps from a cesarean section that involved incision into the placenta. As dangerous to the newborn as anemia is the presence of an excess of red cells (polycythemia), probably caused by excessive flow of blood into the infant from the umbilical cord.

Heel-stick hematocrits reveal both of these conditions, and treatment can be instituted. The mean hematocrit at 1 hour of life is about 62%. If the hematocrit is below 40%, the infant will probably be transfused with fresh whole blood. Newborns with a hematocrit over 75% will probably have a modified exchange transfusion with low-hematocrit blood to reduce the hemocrit value.

If the Dextrostix reading is less than 45 mg per 100 ml of blood, the physician will probably order 10% dextrose in water or infant formula given orally immediately. Treating hypoglycemia is important, because excessive hypoglycemia leads to brain damage. If the infant is showing the symptoms of hypoglycemia (see Chap. 38), intravenous glucose will be administered.

MOTHER-CHILD INTERACTION

If the mother was not awake for the delivery, the baby should be taken to her room for at least a short visiting period as soon as she is awake and the baby's first hour of rest is over. The mother who delivered under a general anesthetic has a harder time believing that the pregnancy is over and that her child has been born than does the mother who was wide awake during delivery. Making her wait to see her baby until the first routine feeding time, which may be as late as 12 hours after birth, is unfair to her and harms her relationship with the baby.

FIRST FEEDING

A mature newborn who will be breast-fed may be breast-fed in the delivery room. A baby who will be formula-fed receives a first feeding at 6 to 12 hours of age. This is a test feeding, to be certain that the infant can swallow without gagging and aspirating and to rule out the presence of a tracheoesophageal fistula connecting the esophagus and trachea and causing the infant to aspirate the feeding.

A first feeding is traditionally given by the nursery

nurse, but there is no reason why the mother cannot give this feeding if the nurse remains in attendance. One approach to first feedings is for the nurse to take the newborn to the mother for a visiting period and then bring him back to the nursery for his first feeding. This method serves several purposes. It allows the mother some time with her infant, assures you that the infant swallows properly, and protects the mother from possibly having to see her baby choking and spitting, which is frightening to a first-time mother, who wants and needs to do everything perfectly.

A first feeding consists of about an ounce of sterile water. Glucose water, which used to be the traditional first feeding fluid, if aspirated, has proved to be almost as irritating to the lungs as aspirated formula. Some physicians prefer that a baby who will be breast-fed also be given a test feeding of sterile water. This feeding can follow the initial delivery room breast-feeding experience because babies do not obtain much fluid at this first feeding, since only colostrum is present in the mother's breast. It is mainly a time to give both mother and baby practice in being together and getting used to each other, which is important to the success of breast-feeding.

Following an initial feeding of water, the formula-fed infant will be placed on an every-4-hour schedule or a demand schedule. If he is to be bottle-fed, the next three or four feedings will be glucose water (Fig. 31-6), and then formula-feeding will be started. Breast-fed infants do best on a demand schedule. They may receive supplemental glucose water after each feeding for the first two or three days to prevent hypoglycemia. Infant feeding is discussed in detail in Chap. 30.

DAILY CARE

The routines of a newborn's daily care may be carried out largely by the nursery staff or by the parents, depending on the policy of the particular hospital and the wishes of the parents.

Temperature

During the first day of life, the newborn's temperature is usually taken every 4 hours. Thereafter, unless the temperature is elevated or subnormal, or the infant appears to be in distress, once a day is often enough for temperature to be recorded during his hospital stay. It is better to take axillary temperatures in the newborn period to avoid injury to the rectal mucosa. If an axillary temperature is being recorded, the thermometer must be held firmly in the axilla with the child's arm pressed against it for 5 minutes (Fig. 31-7). Electronic thermometers are ideal for use with

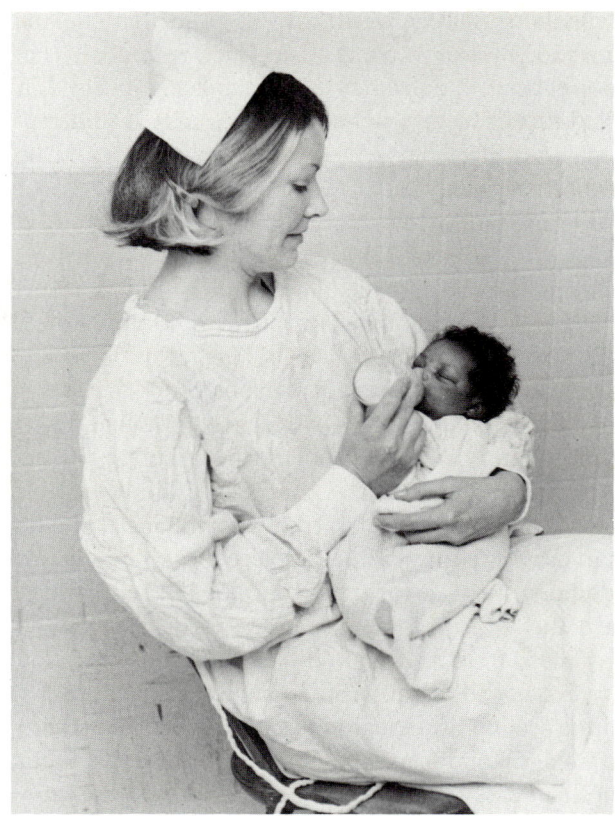

Fig. 31-6. A newborn receives a bottle feeding. Notice the motherly position the nurse uses to feed him. (Courtesy of the Department of Medical Photography, Children's Hospital, Buffalo, N.Y.)

newborn infants since they register the temperature almost instantaneously and minimize the amount of manipulation necessary.

Weight

The newborn should be weighed on the delivery room scale at birth and on the nursery scale when he is admitted to the nursery (to establish a baseline weight against which all others will be compared). Thereafter, he should be weighed nude once a day at approximately the same time every day. More frequent weighing subjects the infant to unnecessary manipulation. The weight each day should be compared with the preceding day's weight to be certain that the infant is not losing more than the normal physiological weight loss (5 to 10 percent of birth weight). Too often, the daily weighing of newborns is regarded as busywork by nurses rather than the health assessment tool that it is. The first indication that newborns have an inborn error of metabolism, such as adrenogenital syndrome (salt-dumping type), or that dehydration is occurring, may be an abnormal loss of weight. Weighing the baby every day is only

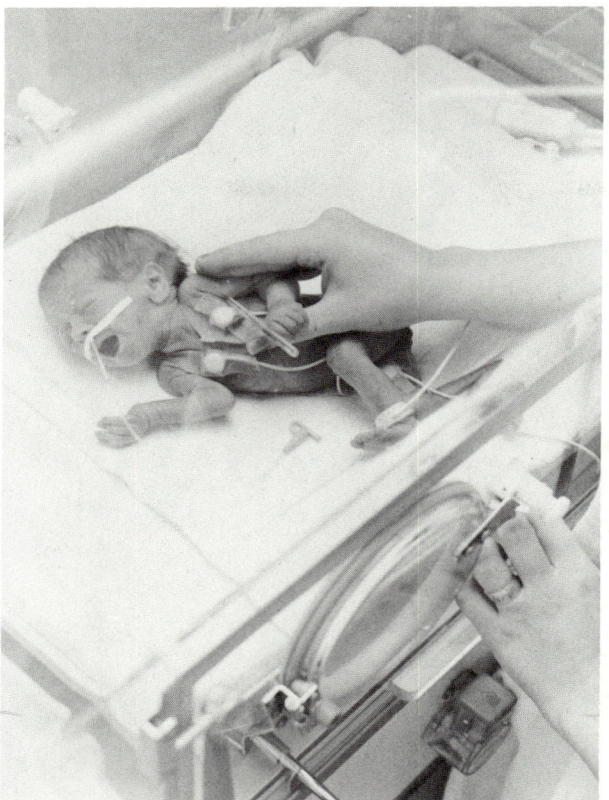

Fig. 31-7. Taking an axillary temperature. Notice how the infant's arm is held snugly against the thermometer tip. An immature infant, he has an indwelling gavage tube and cardiac monitor leads in place. (Courtesy of the Department of Medical Photography, Children's Hospital, Buffalo, N.Y.)

half the task. Comparing this day's weight to the weight of the day before and interpreting the two figures meaningfully is a nursing assessment.

An individual scale liner should be used with each baby to prevent the spread of infection from infant to infant. A baby should never be left alone on a scale and he should be protected by a sheltering hand during the weighing procedure (Fig. 31-8). Even a newborn can twist and turn enough to fall from a scale if left alone.

Bathing

In most hospitals the newborn is bathed once a day, although the routine may vary to include a full bath one day and a partial one the next. Bathing may be done by you in the nursery or by you or one of the parents at the mother's bedside. The room should be warm (about 75°F, 24°C) to prevent chilling during bath time. Bathwater should be around 98° to 100°F (37° to 38°C), a temperature that feels pleasantly warm to the elbows or wrist. The soap used should be mild and without a hexachlorophene base. Bathing should take place prior to, not after, a feeding, to prevent spitting up or vomiting and possible aspiration.

The equipment for the bath consists of a basin of water, soap, a washcloth and towel, a comb, and clean diaper and shirt. It should be assembled beforehand, so the baby is not left exposed while the bather goes for more equipment.

Until a newborn's cord falls off, at about the seventh to tenth day of life, he should be sponge-bathed, not immersed in a tub. It is best if a bath proceeds from the cleanest to the most soiled areas of the body, that is, from the eyes and face to the trunk and extremities and last to the diaper area. The eyes should be wiped with clear water, and a clean portion of the washcloth should be used for each eye to prevent spread of any infection present to the other eye. The face should also be washed in clear water to avoid skin irritation by soap, but soap may be used on the rest of the body.

Hair is washed daily with the bath. The easiest way to wash a newborn's hair is first to soap it with the baby lying in the bassinet, then hold the infant in one arm over the basin of water as you would a football (Fig. 31-9), and then splash water from the basin against his head to rinse the hair. Dry the hair well to prevent chilling.

Each portion of the baby's body should be washed, and each portion should be rinsed, so that no soap is left on the skin (soap is drying and newborns are prone to desquamation), and then dried. The skin around the cord should be washed, with care taken not to soak the cord. A wet cord remains in place longer than a dry one and furnishes a breeding ground for bacteria. Particular care should be given to the creases of skin, where milk tends to collect if the child spits up after feedings.

In male infants, the foreskin of the uncircumcised penis generally does not retract. It should not be forced back or constriction of the penis may result. The vulva of female infants should be washed with the bath, wiping from front to back to prevent rectal contamination of the vagina or urethra.

Most hospitals do not apply powder or lotion to newborns because some infants are allergic to these products. Many adult talcum powders contain zinc stearate, which is irritating to the respiratory tract; they should always be avoided. If the newborn's skin seems extremely dry, so dry it is cracking and portals for infection are becoming apparent, a lubricant such as Nivea oil added to the bathwater or applied directly to the baby's skin should relieve the excessive dryness. Because vernix caseosa may serve a protective func-

Newborn Care: Nursing Interventions 497

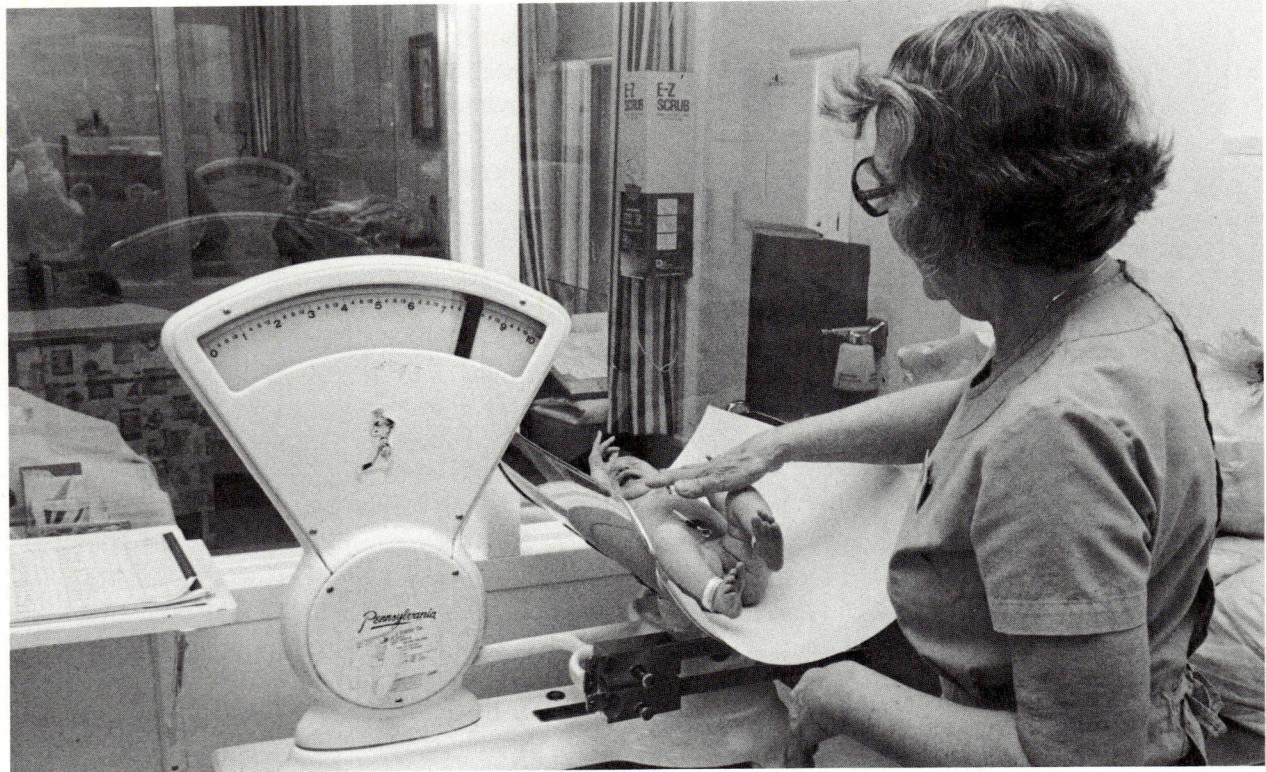

Fig. 31-8. Weighing a newborn. Notice the protective hand held over the infant. (Courtesy of the Department of Medical Photography, Children's Hospital, Buffalo, N.Y.)

Fig. 31-9. A football hold. Such a position supports the infant's head and back and leaves the nurse's or mother's other hand free for assembling or using equipment. (Courtesy of the Department of Medical Photography, Children's Hospital, Buffalo, N.Y.)

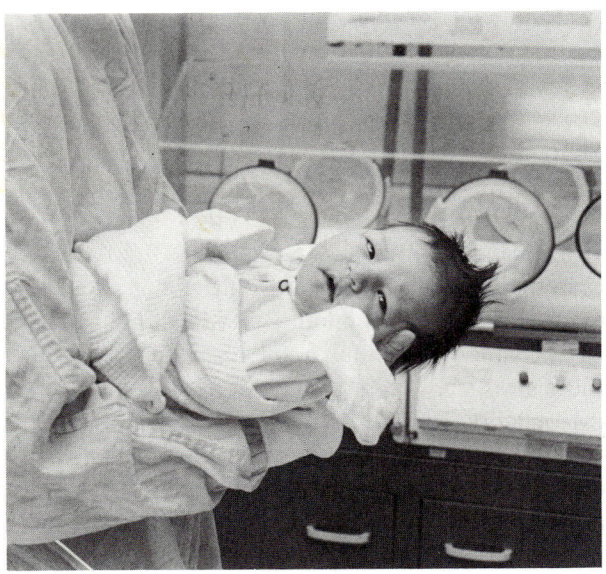

tion, some people recommend that newborn babies not be bathed, except for the washing away of meconium from the rectal area or blood-streaked vernix from the face.

Diaper-Area Care

With each change of diapers, the baby's diaper area should be washed with clear water and dried. Thus one prevents the ammonia in urine from irritating the infant's skin and causing diaper rash. Following the cleaning, an ointment such as Vaseline or A and D may be applied to the buttocks. The ointment keeps ammonia away from the skin and also facilitates the removal of meconium, which is very sticky and tarry in consistency.

Rest

The newborn should be allowed to sleep with a minimum of disturbance between feedings. A newborn may sleep as much as 20 out of 24 hours, although the time varies widely depending on the activity or temperament of the infant. The infant should be positioned on alternate sides following feedings, to keep respiratory secretions or mucus from collecting or pooling in one lung or the other and to prevent flattening of one side of his head. A healthy newborn has enough head control to move his head up out of

498 The Newborn

spit-up milk on a sheet, so he may safely sleep on his stomach; some infants are unable to sleep in *any other* position. In infants who sleep constantly on the abdomen, however, a valgus deviation of the foot may develop. For this reason, changing the infant's sleeping position, from side to side and occasionally onto his abdomen, seems to have merit.

Identification

The identification bands of the infant should be checked to see that they are in place when he is bathed and before he is removed from his bassinet or Isolette or from the nursery for any reason. When he is taken to the mother for feeding, the number on his band should be checked with hers before he is handed to her or left with her. On discharge, it is extremely important that the number of the baby's band be checked to see that it corresponds with the number of the mother. Otherwise, a baby could be accidentally discharged with the wrong mother.

CONTINUING PARENT-CHILD RELATIONSHIP

Every attempt should be made during the infant's hospital stay to promote a good parent-child relationship. The mother should be encouraged to hold and get acquainted with her infant not only at feeding time but at other times as well. Encourage her to think of the infant as an individual, not just an extension of herself. Encourage her to talk to her baby. She will be surprised how intently the infant listens to the sound of her voice and how he responds to her—how from the very beginning he seems to be saying that he is a new, wholly unique person and that his mother should listen and pay attention to his needs. When a father visits, he may need some encouragement to hold his child if he feels self-conscious. Siblings need an opportunity to interact with the new baby as well (Fig. 31-10).

The mother should have infant care demonstrated to her (Fig. 31-11), and before discharge she should have a chance to care for her baby enough to be comfortable handling him. She should spend some time just watching him sleep, to become accustomed to the sucking and twitching movements that are characteristic of sleeping infants. She should feed and bubble her baby often enough to have confidence in the feeding method she has chosen and not to be

Fig. 31-10. Sibling visitation allows an older child to gain a realistic view of the new baby. Here, a 3-year-old sees a new brother for the first time. (Courtesy of the Department of Medical Photography, Children's Hospital, Buffalo, N.Y.)

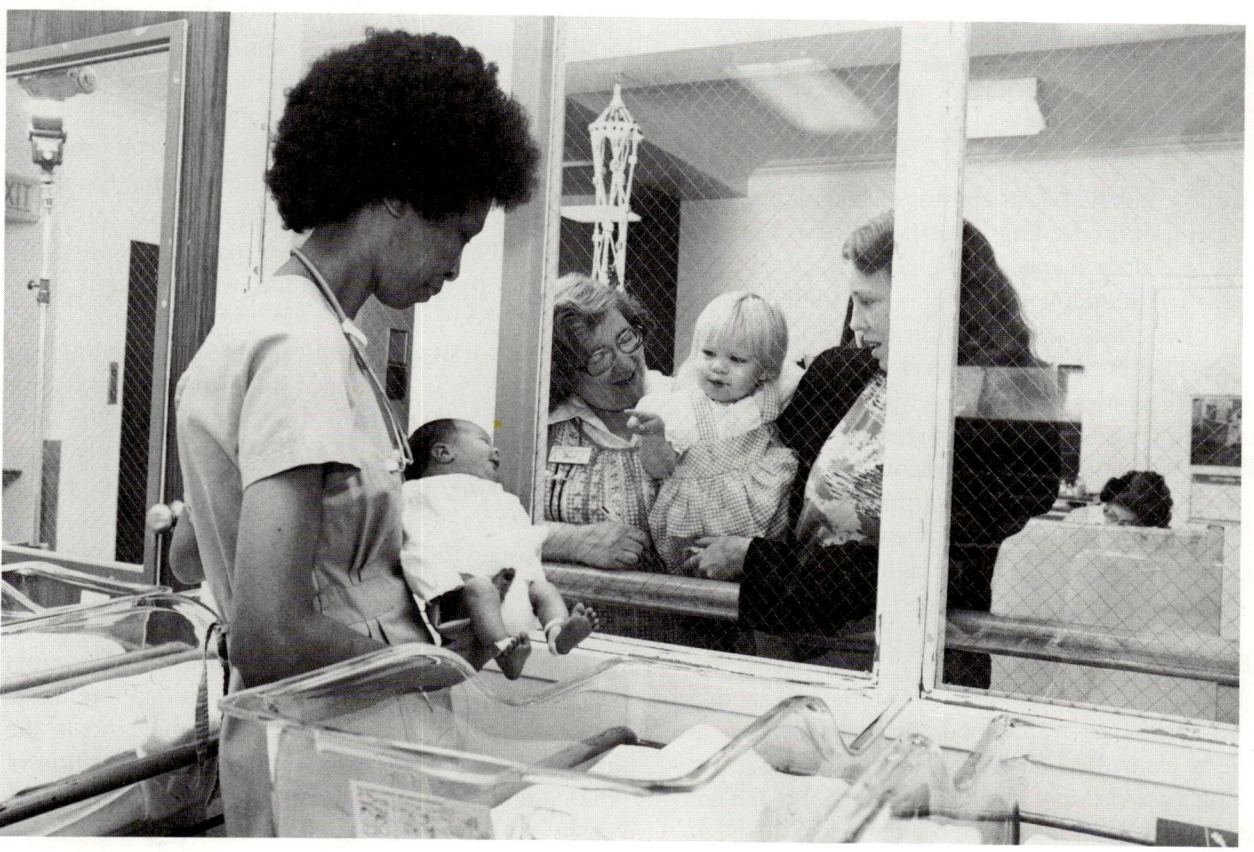

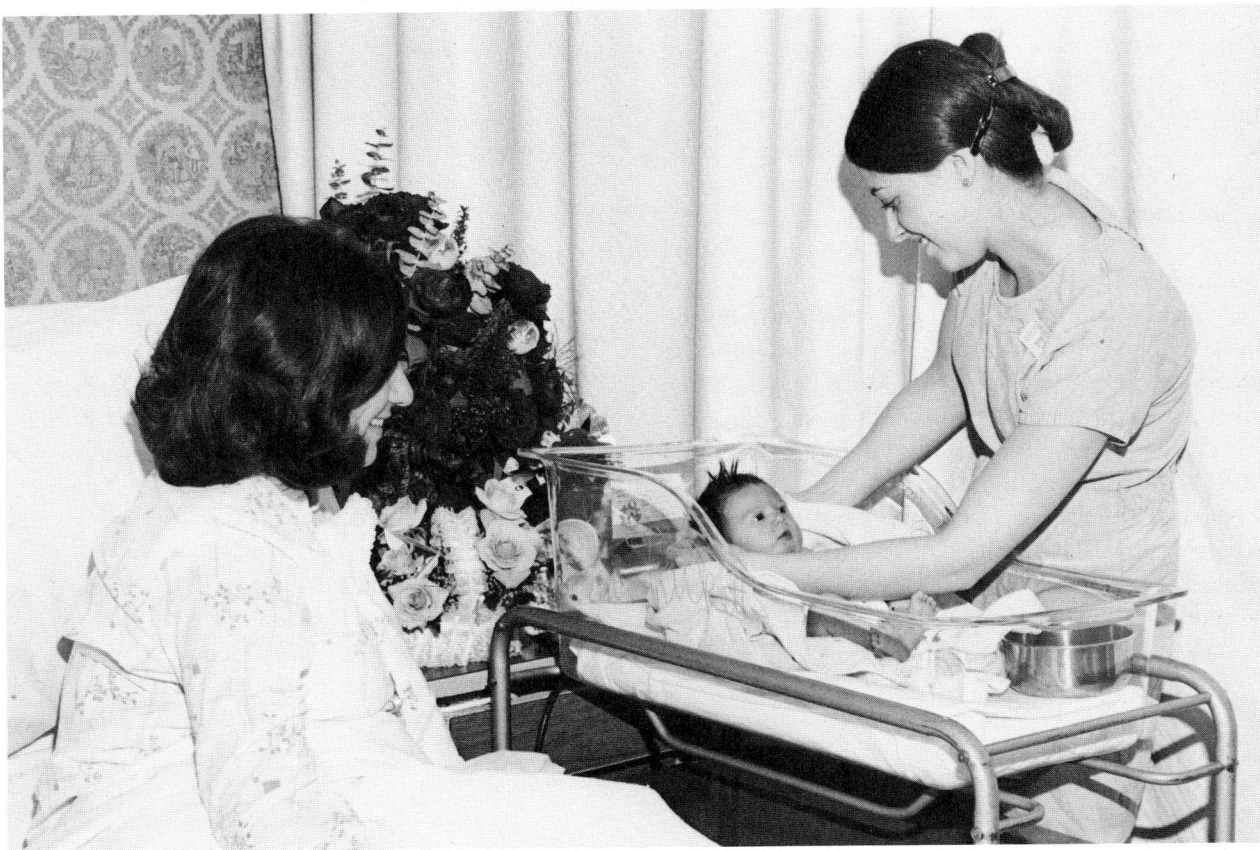

Fig. 31-11. Rooming-in unit. In a rooming-in unit, the mother has her child with her for a greater part of the day, and mother-child interaction is thus increased. Here, the nurse is demonstrating a newborn bath by the mother's bedside. (Courtesy of the Department of Medical Photography, Children's Hospital, Buffalo, N.Y.)

upset if no bubble is forthcoming or the infant spits up at the end of the feeding. She should have an opportunity to change diapers enough so that she can grow skilled at it (handling diaper pins and folding diapers to the correct size is difficult at first). She also needs to change diapers to observe bowel movements. Many new mothers assume that a newborn's stools will be brown and firm and are surprised at their black or yellow color and loose consistency. A new mother needs the opportunity to be surprised at these things while she is in the hospital, where there are knowledgeable people around her, rather than at home, where she might become alarmed.

PHENYLKETONURIA TESTING

Every infant, by state law, must be screened for phenylketonuria by a blood test before he is discharged from the hospital. This is a simple test requiring three drops of blood from the heel of the baby dropped onto a special piece of filter paper. The baby must have been on milk for two days or must have had an intake of phenylalanine (an essential amino acid found in milk) before the test will be accurate. Previously, such testing was done by a physician or technician, but it is becoming more and more a nursing routine. Be certain you check that the infant has received adequate milk before taking the blood sample. Otherwise, the results may be false-negative (a child with phenylketonuria will test as if he is normal). Many institutions are beginning other metabolic tests at birth (such as screening for hypothyroidism) that need filter paper blood tests taken also. If the baby is discharged before the third day of life, the mother must be made aware that they were not done so she will remind her primary health care provider to obtain the blood sample at a first health supervision visit.

RECORD-KEEPING

A daily log of the baby's progress in the nursery should be kept, including the number of voidings; the number, consistency, and color of bowel movements; the infant's color and degree of activity; the condition of the cord and skin; and the general feeding adaptation of the infant.

In hospitals where patient charts are put on microfilm after a period of time, special provision should be made to preserve the footprint record, so that it is available for later identification.

DISCHARGE OF THE NEWBORN

Before the newborn is discharged, a thorough physical assessment should be performed. Its purpose is to determine whether or not some congenital defect or birth injury is present that has not been detected up to this point and to discover any condition that may have developed in the preceding three or four days.

Be certain that the mother has thought through child care at home. Try to anticipate problems she may have, so that they can be averted or solved. An important aspect to discuss with a mother who is not going to breast-feed is what she will use to feed the baby for the next 24 hours until she has had time to prepare formula. Most hospitals supply or sell a discharge formula kit to mothers to tide them over until they can prepare formula at home.

Be sure the mother understands when and where she is to take her newborn for health supervision. The identification bands should be checked one final time with her identification band before the infant is discharged to her.

Care of the Newborn at Home

The day a newborn comes home from the hospital is an important day in the life of most families. Taking a long-wished-for baby home after a normal pregnancy and delivery is a time of happiness. Parents are strongly aware of their responsibility for the new child or perhaps frightened because they feel unable to cope with their new life situation.

Talking with a mother about her plans for home care of her child will help her make more realistic plans.

HOUSING

The physical environment of the home to which the child will be discharged is a good subject to explore with parents. Is it an apartment or a house? How many flights of stairs will the mother have to climb when she takes the baby home? When she takes the baby out in his carriage? To go back and forth to the baby's room? How many other people live in the home? Are there grandparents who will visit or help care for the child? Does the mother have anyone to turn to if she has questions about the baby? If she is unmarried, is she returning to her family's home or her own apartment? Will the baby be sleeping in a room by himself or with older children? Will the mother be the primary caregiver to the child?

Does she have a bed for the baby? Is there a refrigerator in which formula can be stored? Is there adequate heat? An infant needs a temperature of 70° to 75°F during the day and 60° to 65°F at night. Are the windows draft-free? Are they screened to keep out insects? Is there a danger that rats might attack the baby?

Does the mother or do the parents have a source of income? If not, what sort of referral should be made so that money can be provided to care for this child?

These are not prying questions but are a means of ascertaining whether the home that will receive the child is adequate and safe for him. All the good prenatal and postnatal care is wasted if an infant contracts pneumonia his first week home because no one at the hospital took the time to ask the right questions about his home environment.

DAILY CARE

Infants thrive on a gentle rhythm of care, a sense of being able to anticipate what is to come next. Most mothers have questions to ask concerning the kinds of care a newborn baby needs and how the care should be scheduled.

Every mother should decide what is the best daily at-home routine for her and her child. There are no fixed rules for infant schedules. There is no set time an infant must be bathed every day. There is not even a rule that he must have a bath every day. There is no rule that all infants must be in bed for the night by eight o'clock. If the father works evenings, it may be important for the family to have the baby awake at midnight when he comes home from work, so that he has some time to spend with the baby.

Your aim in helping a mother plan her schedule of care is to arrive at one that (1) offers a degree of consistency (a mother cannot expect an infant to stay awake until midnight five nights a week, then go to sleep at seven o'clock the next two nights); (2) appears to satisfy the infant; and (3) satisfies the parents, giving them a sense of well-being, a sense of contentment with their child.

Help the mother to realize that her infant is a real person with individual needs. Although physically he is a part of his mother and father, he is still an individual in his own right, and the schedule should respect his individuality. Some parents have difficulty with newborns because they do not appreciate this simple fact. They may be upset when they find their baby wants to be fed at six o'clock at night, just when they usually have their dinner; that he has needs he insists be met on his terms. They are surprised to find their infant is a real person who coos and "talks" and smiles at them, having assumed that he was going to be passive in his relationship to them for a long time.

Babies enjoy the gentle motion of a rocking chair. Mothers need to include a rocking chair in their budget as part of basic baby equipment (as should hospitals as part of basic nursery equipment).

As the mother cares for the baby, urge her to "discuss" things with her baby. It does not matter whether she talks about day-to-day happenings or about all her future hopes and aspirations for her child. The important thing is that she begin communicating with her child and establish a closeness that can continue all the years of the child's growing up. Talking to a baby is also necessary for his speech development.

BATHING

Most mothers today are overly concerned with the technique of bathing their newborns, as if it were a complicated procedure that must be done just one way. In reality, there are only a few simple guidelines to follow in giving a baby a bath. In warm weather it is refreshing for the infant to have a daily bath. It is not necessary to bathe the baby if the house is chilly or if the mother feels that she is too tired or that she would not enjoy it. Washing the infant's face and neck (to wash away formula spills) and his diaper area (to avoid rash from ammonia irritation) is sufficient in lieu of a bath in these instances. In some infants, however, the hair needs to be washed as frequently as every other day in order to keep dry, scaling patches (cradle cap, or seborrheic dermatitis) from forming. Bath time should be fun for both mother and baby. It is a good time for mother-child interaction and is perhaps the first project they accomplish together.

The major piece of equipment needed for bathing babies at home is a baby bathtub placed on a table or counter of comfortable height so the mother does not have to stretch or bend. If the mother does not own a baby bathtub, there is really nothing wrong with bathing an infant in the kitchen sink. As soon as the baby begins to have good back support (at 5 or 6 months), he can be bathed in the family bathtub. Until this time, he is too slippery to be held firmly in an adult tub by a mother who has to stretch to reach him at all.

Water for bathing should be pleasantly warm. There is no need for the mother to take the temperature of the water, but she should feel it with her wrist or elbow to judge that it is pleasantly warm.

Additional bath articles she will require are a towel and washcloth, clean from the laundry basket or linen closet (there is no need to buy high-priced infant towels); hand soap (whatever type the rest of the family uses, but one cake should be used just for the baby); and a comb or hairbrush. No lotion or oil is necessary for routine use on babies. If the infant's skin appears dry, the mother may use a mild hand lotion or baby oil on the dry areas if she wishes. If the baby tends to have diaper rash, she may routinely use an ointment such as A and D on the diaper area after the bath and after each diaper change. Powders, like oils, are unnecessary. They create a pleasant "baby" smell, however, so many mothers enjoy using them; but if powder is used too liberally, the infant will inhale it.

Babies should have only sponge baths until the cord comes off, at about the seventh to tenth day of life. Mothers need to be reminded that the fontanelles can be washed. Otherwise, they will wash around them.

When the baby is ready for a tub bath, the mother should place him on a soft towel on the tabletop and wash his eyes first, using clear water and different portions of the washcloth for each eye, to prevent the spread of any infection present to the other eye. Next, the face is washed in clear water. The hair is lathered, and then the infant is held over the bathtub in a football position (see Fig. 31-9) and the soap is washed away.

The easiest way to complete the bath after the hair is washed is to lay the infant on his back on the tabletop and lather his front, then turn him on his abdomen and lather his back. Then pick him up and, slowly and gradually, holding his back supported, lower him into the bathwater to rinse him off.

Some babies take readily to bathing and enjoy it from the start. Others are furious at being exposed to this new sensation and take a month or more before they begin to smile and splash as they are washed. It helps to accustom these "slow-to-adapt" infants to bathing if the mother uses a gentle, soothing touch and speaks calmly. If the infant reacts strongly to being submerged in water, the mother can continue to give sponge baths for a longer time than usual. The guideline on bathing is that infants *may* be submerged once the cord comes off, not that the infant *must* be submerged once the cord is off.

CORD CARE

It is important to remind the mother to keep the cord dry until it falls off. She should fold diapers down in front so that a wet diaper will not touch the cord area. If the mother uses plastic pants on the baby, she should be certain that these are folded down below the cord as well.

The use of creams, lotions, and oils on the cord should be avoided since they tend to slow drying of the cord and invite infection. Some physicians like the mother to dab rubbing alcohol onto the cord once or twice a day to hasten drying; others prefer that the cord be left strictly alone.

The first day the cord falls off, a small, pink granulating area about a quarter of an inch in diameter may remain. This should also be left clean and dry until it has healed (about 24 or 48 more hours). If it remains as long as a week, it may require cautery with silver nitrate to speed healing.

CLOTHING

A mother invariably dresses her infant too warmly. She should use only enough clothing to keep him comfortably warm. The less clothing the baby wears, the easier it is to dress him and the greater his freedom to move and exercise. A mother can judge how much clothing is enough by how much she needs to put on herself. If she needs a sweater, her infant does also; if she is warm, her infant does not need a sweater. On very hot days, just a diaper will be enough clothing. The mother has to learn to trust her own judgment and not be swayed by friends who constantly tell her to put more clothing on the infant.

CIRCUMCISION

Most male infants today are circumcised (have the foreskin of the penis removed surgically). There is little reason for the procedure as only a few men have such a tight prepuce that it interferes with voiding. Most mothers prefer to have it done because uncircumcised males have to include cleaning under the foreskin as part of routine bathing in order to avoid infection from accumulated secretions whereas circumcised males do not. Another reason is that, since most boys are circumcised, being circumcised makes a boy appear like his classmates in school. Jewish children, of course, are circumcized as an important religious ceremony.

In many agencies, circumcision is completed as part of delivery room care. This policy has some disadvantages: The infant probably has a prolonged clotting time at birth (lowered amount of vitamin K), and he is exposed unnecessarily to the cold of the delivery room. It also prevents the parents from enjoying the wide awake phase of the infant at birth.

Circumcision, then, is probably best done during the first or second day of life rather than in the delivery room. It is unfair to mothers to have the procedure done on the day of discharge from the hospital. Infants may bleed following the circumcision, and this timing puts the responsibility for observing bleeding on the new mother rather than on experienced nursing personnel.

Circumcision is theoretically a painless procedure. The infant is immobilized, either by restraining hands or by a special restraining board. The penile area is prepared and draped. A specially designed clamp is fitted over the end of the penis, stretching the foreskin taut. The stretching inhibits sensory conduction to the foreskin. Under sterile conditions, the skin is then quickly cut with a sharp scalpel and removed. The area is covered by sterile petrolatum gauze to keep the diaper from rubbing against it. The infant should be checked for bleeding at the circumcision site every 15 minutes for the first hour, then every 30 minutes for the next 4 hours. At every diaper change, a notation as to the state of healing should be recorded. The petrolatum gauze should remain in place for 24 hours unless it is soiled by stool. After 24 hours, application of a petroleum jelly (Vaseline) to the site seems comforting for another 48 hours until healing is complete. Keeping the diaper pinned firmly helps to reduce bleeding and prevents the diaper from rubbing against the site.

Circumcision sites appear red and sore but should never have a strong odor or a discharge. A thin yellow exudate forms over the healing surface within 24 hours of the procedure (similar to a scab). Do not confuse this with an infectious exudate or attempt to wash it away.

If infants cry while being circumcised, it is theoretically not from the pain of the procedure but from the manipulation of being restrained. A few infants appear to be fussy for the first hour following the procedure as if they are uncomfortable. However, when circumcision is done in the delivery room, the reaction may be more the result of their first period of reactivity than of the procedure itself.

At discharge, the circumcised infant seems most comfortable if the healing site is kept covered by an ointment such as Vaseline for four to five days. This prevents the diaper from touching and clinging to the healing tissue and causing bleeding with diaper changes. The mother should observe the site daily and report to her physician any redness, foul odor, or discharge that suggests infection.

Health Problems in the Newborn

Mothers who have private physicians call them for advice on health problems in their newborns. In many hospitals, mothers who do not have private physicians are urged to phone the hospital after discharge if they are concerned about some aspect of care or health and it is not yet time for them to take the infant for his clinic visit. A high proportion of newborn problems can be managed successfully by advice given on the telephone by a nurse in consultation with a physician.

Many child care problems that arise with newborns are simply the result of the mother's misinterpretation of the child's reactions or are problems of the child's adjustment to his new world and the new stimuli around him, which takes a little time. Mothers ask questions about cord care, bathing, and feeding, and they often call about the common illnesses of infancy.

CONSTIPATION

Constipation is rare in breast-fed infants because their stools tend to be loose. Rarely, constipation may occur with bottle-fed infants if the diet is too deficient in fluid. Some infants on iron-fortified commercial formula tend toward constipation. The problem can be corrected by adding more fluid or carbohydrate to the diet. Some babies need a formula change because they have grown since the formula was prescribed and now have a greater fluid requirement. Offering a bottle of water with a teaspoon of Karo syrup added may be helpful.

Some mothers misinterpret the normal pushing movements of a newborn as constipation—infants do make faces, get red in the face, and make small grunting noises when passing stools. As long as the stool is not hard and no fresh blood is on the stool (as might occur with a rectal fissure), this is not constipation but an example of a new mother's misinterpreting her infant's behavior.

If the infant is constipated, and the problem persists beyond a few months of age, the addition of bulky foods such as fruits or vegetables generally relieves it. One-half to 1 ounce of prune juice daily may be given as a temporary measure. It is better not to give prune juice over a long period of time (mothers often believe that if a little is good for the baby, a lot will be even better), since too much of it will cause diarrhea.

All infants with a history of constipation for more than a week should be examined for an anal fissure or a tight anal sphincter. Softening the hard stools by means of an oral stool softener, and therefore alleviating the pain of defecation, often solves the problem and helps an anal fissure to heal. If the infant has an unusually tight anal sphincter, the mother will be given instructions to dilate the sphincter two or three times daily until it stretches sufficiently to eliminate the obstipation. Hirschsprung's disease (congenital aganglionic megacolon) may be manifested early in life as constipation. If no stool is found on rectal examination of a constipated infant, congenital aganglionic megacolon is suggested.

LOOSE STOOLS

Many new mothers report loose stools in their infants as a problem because they are unfamiliar with the consistency of the normal newborn's stools. Every mother needs to handle and care for her newborn enough in the hospital before discharge to be familiar with what a newborn's stools are like before she goes home.

When talking to a mother about the problem of loose stools, you need to investigate the duration of the condition, the number of stools per day, their color and consistency, and the presence of any mucus or blood. Is there associated fever, cramping, vomiting? Does the infant continue to eat well? Does the infant appear well? Is the infant thriving?

The infant of a mother who is mixing formula inaccurately, adding too much sugar, or not diluting formula properly will have loose stools. Correcting the problem, of course, is simply a matter of correcting the error in formula preparation. Occasionally, loose stools begin with the introduction of solid food. In this instance, food sensitivity is suggested. Ask exactly what foods the baby is being fed. Malabsorption syndrome may be the cause, since it may manifest itself first by loose stools.

As previously mentioned, stools of breast-fed infants are usually softer than those of formula-fed infants. Further, a laxative taken by the mother while breast-feeding may cause the infant to have loose stools.

Infants who have loose stools and associated symptoms (fever, cramping, vomiting, loss of appetite, loss of weight) should be seen by a physician. Dehydration occurs rapidly in a small infant who is not eating and is losing body water in loose stools.

COLIC

Colic is paroxysmal abdominal pain. It generally occurs in infants under 3 months of age. The discomfort appears abruptly. The infant cries loudly and pulls his legs up against his abdomen. His face is red and flushed, his fists clench, and his abdomen is tense. If offered a bottle, the infant will suck vigorously for a few minutes as if he were starved, then stop when another wave of intestinal pain overwhelms him.

The cause of colic is unclear. It may occur in susceptible infants from overfeeding, from swallowing too much air while feeding, or from being on a formula too high in carbohydrate. Its occurrence is associated with a tense and unsure mother. Women who fear that their infant will have congenital abnormalities tend to have infants with colic more than do women who do not have this concern.

Colic should not be dismissed lightly as an unimportant disease of infancy. It is a major problem for the mother because it is so frightening. The infant appears to be in acute pain and distress. Since colic persists for hours and usually in the middle of the night, neither mother nor child gets adequate rest. This is a bad beginning to a mother-child relationship, which needs to be strong and binding for the mother to enjoy mothering and for the infant to thrive in her care. Prevention of colic or the relieving of colic may do as much for the future mental health of the child as it does for his temporary pain and discomfort.

A thorough history should be taken on infants with the symptoms of colic, since intestinal obstruction or infection may mimic an attack of colic and will be misinterpreted by the casual interviewer. Ask how long the problem has been going on and about the frequency and time of attacks (colic usually occurs at bedtime). Ask for a description of what happens just prior to the attack and what the attack of colic is like. Ask for associated symptoms. It is important to know the number of bowel movements associated with the condition, since bowel movements are not abnormal with colic. Constipated stools or narrowed "ribbon" stools suggest other complicating problems. Ask about the family medical history. Allergy to milk may simulate colic.

The mother of a baby with colic should be asked the type of formula the infant is being fed and how she is preparing it. Explore with her how she is feeding the baby and whether she is bubbling him adequately. While feeding the baby, the mother should hold him in as upright a position as possible, so that air bubbles can rise. Both bottle-fed and breast-fed babies should be bubbled thoroughly after feeding. After feeding, many babies with colic are more comfortable sleeping on their abdomens than on their side or back. A towel rolled under the abdomen for a little extra pressure is often helpful.

Many mothers feel uneasy placing a baby under 3 months of age on his stomach to sleep. This creates no problem in a well newborn (and a baby with true colic is a well baby), who will have no difficulty in lifting his head to clear the airway. Some persons recommend placing a hot-water bottle under the infant's stomach, but this should be discouraged as a common practice; a basic rule in dealing with any abdominal discomfort is to avoid heat because the pain may be symptomatic of appendicitis. Such a diagnosis is highly unlikely in an infant, but the mother will remember that a hot-water bottle was recommended for her infant's abdominal pain and may use one with an older child whose pain may be due to appendicitis.

Changing to a commercially prepared formula from an evaporated milk formula may alleviate colic. Changing the type of bottle to one with a disposable bag that collapses as the baby sucks and reduces the amount of air swallowed may be helpful.

Occasionally, a colicky baby needs sedation to relieve his pain and to give him and his mother some rest. It is important to think of colic as a problem for two people, the infant and the mother, or a vicious circle begins. The infant cries and the mother becomes tense and unsure of herself. The colic worsens because the infant senses her tenseness. He cries more, the mother becomes even more unsure, and so on.

Colic almost magically disappears at 3 months of age. If the mother can be supported until this milestone arrives, she will discover that despite the colic her infant has grown during this time. *Support* is the prime word in colic. Three months of living with a fussy, crying, unappeasable infant seems like three years.

SLEEPING PATTERNS

Mothers who call about their infant's sleeping patterns may be concerned because they think the baby is sleeping too much or because he appears to be sleeping too little.

A baby sleeps an average of 16 hours out of every 24 in his first week home and sleeps an average of 4 hours at a time. By 4 months of age he sleeps an average of 15 hours out of 24 hours and 8 hours at a time (through the night).

Mothers try various devices to induce the baby to sleep through the night much earlier than at 4 months of age. One approach is introducing solids (particularly cereal) early, in the first week of life, on the theory that the cereal's bulk will fill up the infant's stomach for the night, and therefore he will not wake up crying to be fed. Actually, there is no correlation between the age at which solid food is introduced and the baby's capability for sustained sleep. A baby wakes every 4, 5, 6, or 8 hours for feeding because of physiological need for fluid. It is, of course, exhausting for mothers who are already tired from the experience of labor and delivery to have to wake at night and feed a newborn. It is a rare husband who can feed a newborn at night without waking his wife to ask her whether he is doing everything correctly. Thus, having a husband say he will take over at night may not really help.

Be certain that the mother who is troubled about

her baby's waking at night is describing a newborn who is healthy in every way: taking a sufficient amount of formula or spending enough time at the breast every day, sleeping well during the day, having normal bowel movements, and being normally active. You should have a total picture before blindly assuring a mother of anything. But once you are satisfied that the mother is simply describing a normal baby waking at night for a feeding, assure her that he is normal and that there is no reason to try to eliminate this feeding. Knowing that her baby is not sick, that you are concerned with her problem and willing to listen to her, and that every other mother of a newborn is also up at night does not solve her difficulty, but it is a help. Being assured that a baby's behavior is normal is always welcome news to parents.

CRYING

Many new mothers are not prepared by their experience in the hospital for the amount of time a newborn spends in crying. Whenever the mother saw the baby, he was sleeping. She woke him up to feed him, and he immediately went back to sleep. It is not uncommon to hear a mother say on leaving the hospital with a newborn, "I'm sure he's going to be a good baby. I've never heard him cry."

Brazelton [3] reports that infants cry an average of 2¼ hours out of every 24 for the first seven weeks of life. The incidence of crying seems to peak at age 6 or 7 weeks and then taper off.

Almost all infants have a period during the day when they are wide awake and invariably fussy. Each new mother needs to recognize this period as normal and not concern herself that her child is ill because once a day he seems out of sorts. She might use this fussy time for bathing him or playing with him, arranging her schedule to cope with his wakefulness. The most typical time for wakefulness to occur is between 6:00 and 11:00 P.M., which unfortunately is a time when the mother is tired and least able to tolerate crying.

SPITTING UP

Almost all babies do some spitting up; formula-fed more than breast-fed babies. A mother who does not handle her infant very much in the hospital may, in the first week home, interpret spitting up as vomiting or as a sign of infection.

Ask the mother to describe carefully what she means by spitting up. How long has the baby been doing it? How frequently does he do it? What is the appearance of the spit-up milk? Almost all milk that is spit up smells sour, but it should not contain blood or bile. What is the intensity of the spitting? Does the baby spit out forcefully, or is the mother just describing a mouthful of milk rolling down his chin? Are there any associated symptoms (diarrhea, abdominal cramps, fever, cough, cold, inactivity)? What has she tried as a remedy?

If the mother describes associated symptoms, the child should be seen by a physician, because she is describing an ill child. If he is spitting up so forcefully that the milk is projected 3 or 4 feet away, she may be describing beginning pyloric stenosis (obstruction of the pyloric opening from the stomach). This requires medical or surgical intervention.

If she is describing an infant who two or three times a day (or sometimes after every feeding) spits up or allows a mouthful of milk to roll down his chin, she is describing the normal spitting up of early infancy.

Ask her to describe how she bubbles the baby; thorough bubbling often reduces spitting up. Changing formulas (which she will probably suggest as a solution) generally has little effect. Spitting up decreases in amount as the baby better coordinates his swallowing and digestive processes and possibly because as he grows older he is more often in an upright position, and gravity corrects the problem.

COLDS

Upper respiratory infections are infrequent in children under 1 month of age. A mother sometimes reports that her newborn has a stuffy nose, or makes "snoring noises" in his sleep, or sneezes occasionally. Most newborns continue to have some mucus in the upper respiratory tract and posterior pharynx for about two weeks after birth, and it is this, not a cold, that causes the snoring noise. Infants also breathe irregularly for about the first month. A new mother who did not room in with her child at the hospital may wake at night, notice this breathing pattern, and become alarmed that her child is in respiratory distress.

Ask the mother about the exact duration, nature, frequency, and intensity of the symptoms she is reporting. Is she describing normal newborn breathing? A head cold with rhinitis? A cold in which bronchial and lung areas are involved? Ask for associated symptoms such as fever, vomiting, and diarrhea. Ask what action she has taken to relieve the symptoms. Ask for a careful description of what sound the baby is making. Stridor is a harsh, vibrating, high-pitched, shrill, or crowing noise that is marked on inspiration. It is a sign of respiratory obstruction.

If the mother is describing normal newborn breathing, she needs to be reassured about its normality. If there is no fever (ask her if she has actually taken the baby's temperature or is judging fever by touch), but the baby has symptoms of congestion and rhinitis, the physician may wish her to purchase a nasal syringe and gently suction secretions from the infant's nose, particularly before feeding. Infants cannot suck and breathe at the same time. An infant with a stuffy nose will constantly stop sucking to breathe. He becomes fatigued, his intake falls, dehydration may occur, and a simple cold becomes complex.

Most physicians prefer to examine a young infant with upper respiratory symptoms to be certain his lungs are clear. If the infant has a fever, he should be examined to determine the reason for the fever.

SKIN PROBLEMS
Diaper Dermatitis
Some newborns have such sensitive skin that diaper rash is a problem from the first few days of life. Diaper rashes have a variety of causes; most commonly irritation from feces, urine, or laundry products creates the problem.

FECES IRRITATION. In an infant whose mother does not change his diapers as frequently as she might, so that feces remain in contact with the skin, dermatitis from fecal contact may result, with the rash involving the perianal area. More frequent changing of diapers and screening the skin from fecal material with an ointment such as Vaseline or A and D ointment is the solution to the problem.

URINE IRRITATION. After a time, the urine in urine-soaked diapers breaks down into ammonia, a chemical that is extremely irritating to infant skin. Ammoniacal dermatitis is usually a problem of the second half of the first year of life, when the infant is producing a larger quantity of urine than he did initially, but in some infants it is a problem from the first week on. Again, frequent diaper changing and application of Vaseline and A and D ointment may be the answer. Some infants may have to sleep without diapers at night in order to relieve the problem. Some need to have plastic pants removed to decrease irritation. Disposable diapers may cause the difficulty; often changing the brand of diapers helps.

Rinsing cloth diapers in a final rinse of methylbenzethonium chloride (Diaparene) helps to discourage the breakdown of urine. Exposing the infant's diaper area two or three times a day to a low-wattage light bulb may also be beneficial. However, when using this heat source, the mother must make sure that the light bulb is at least 12 inches away so it does not touch the infant's buttocks or clothes or the sheets, since they may become dangerously hot. She should not face a male infant toward the light or his urine stream might shatter the bulb.

IRRITATION FROM LAUNDRY PRODUCTS. Any time the entire diaper area is erythematous and irritated, so that the outline of the diaper appears on the skin, the products the mother is using to wash diapers are suspect as the cause of the irritation. Mothers should rinse diapers well, removing all soap and fabric softener. If the mother is washing diapers at a laundromat, paying for an extra rinse cycle may be a problem for her. If she adds up the cost of washing diapers, buying soap and softener, and rinsing adequately, she may find that disposable diapers or diapers from a diaper service are actually more economical for her.

Miliaria
Miliaria (prickly heat) rash occurs most often in warm weather or on babies who are overdressed or sleep in overheated rooms. Clusters of pinpoint-sized, reddened papules with occasional vesicles and pustules and surrounded by erythema ususally first appear on the neck. They may spread upward to around the ears and onto the face or down onto the trunk.

Bathing the infant twice a day during hot weather, particularly if a small amount of baking soda is added to the bathwater, is helpful in clearing up the rash. Eliminating sweating by reducing the amount of clothes on the infant or lowering the room temperature will bring about almost immediate improvement and prevent further eruption.

INFECTION
Oral Candidiasis
Oral candidiasis (thrush) is a *Candida* infection in which numerous small white and gray patches are present on the tongue and buccal membrane. During delivery, the baby contracts the infection from *Candida* organisms in the mother's vagina. Milk curds remaining on the tongue after feeding simulate thrush. Milk curds can be scraped away, but thrush cannot. Infants with thrush need to be referred to a physician, since a prescription antifungal agent (usually nystatin) is necessary for treatment.

Candidiasis
Candidiasis is a *Candida* infection of the diaper area. The anal mucosa and perianal skin appear macerated, and raw red areas spread from the anus outward. The irritation does not respond to the usual measures. The

infant should be seen by a physician, since, again, nystatin is necessary for treatment.

Impetigo

Although it is almost impossible to judge the nature of skin lesions from a telephone account, ask the mother to describe minutely the lesion that concerns her. It may be impetigo, a skin infection most often caused by a streptococcus. The lesions begin as pustules that rupture into thick, honey-colored crusts. Because impetigo is ordinarily due to a streptococcal infection, it must be treated systemically with an antibiotic, usually penicillin, and the infant should be referred to a physician for care.

Seborrheic Dermatitis (Cradle Cap)

Cradle cap is a common scalp condition of early infancy characterized by dirty-looking, adherent, yellow, crusting patches. The skin beneath the patches may be slightly erythematous. Cradle cap can be largely prevented by frequent shampoos (every other day). The patches may be removed by oiling the scalp with mineral oil or Vaseline at night. This softens the crusts, which can then be removed by shampooing the next morning.

Strawberry Hemangiomas

Strawberry hemangiomas may appear for the first time in the first two weeks following birth. Those the child is born with may continue to grow up to 12 months of age. A mother who calls concerning a birthmark usually fears cancer, since she has heard that a skin lesion that is growing is one of the seven danger signals of cancer. She needs assurance that, although strawberry hemangiomas continue to grow, they are benign and they disappear by the time the child is 10 years of age.

Health Maintenance at Home

There is no need for a mother to continue to weigh her infant while he is at home. This practice may only cause her worry, since an infant's weight gains fluctuate. She should learn to judge her infant's state of health in terms not of increases in weight but of overall appearance, eagerness to eat, general activity, and disposition.

The mother should be shown in the hospital how to take the infant's temperature rectally. Then, if she suspects a fever, she can take the temperature before calling her physician for advice.

The mother should know before she leaves the hospital what kind of follow-up care her child is going to have. If she chooses a pediatrician or a general practitioner, he will visit her while she is hospitalized, discuss his philosophy of child care with her, and give her an appointment for a visit to his office in about four weeks. If she chooses a well-child conference, health maintenance organization, or pediatric clinic for care, she should be given the telephone number of the agency, so that she can call for an appointment for her child.

It is important that the mother understand the necessity for follow-up care for her baby. She has been conscientious throughout pregnancy because she wanted to bring a well child into the world. She now needs to begin a health care program that will keep her child well.

Recommendations for preventive health care for the first five years of life are presented in Table 31-4. This is a guide for the care of well children who receive competent parenting, who have not manifested any important health problems, and who are growing and developing satisfactorily. Children with special problems would need more frequent care or different patterns of care.

Newborn Safety

Accidents are the leading cause of death from age 1 month through 24 years and are second only to acute infections as a cause of acute morbidity and as a reason for visits to the physician throughout childhood.

Most accidents in infancy occur because the mother either underestimates or overestimates her child's ability. Helping mothers to get to know their newborn in the hospital, therefore, is important not only in terms of getting a mother-child relationship off to a good start but also for the child's future safety.

PREVENTION OF ASPIRATION

The leading type of fatal accident in the newborn period is aspiration. Explore with the mother who will bottle-feed her baby whether she intends to prop bottles up or hold her baby for feeding. Some mothers prop up an evening bottle in the baby's bed; others prop a bottle up at dinnertime or when they are with older children. Others prop bottles up all the time. All of these mothers are propping bottles up because they do not appreciate what being held and rocked and made to feel secure means to a small infant. Furthermore, they are overestimating the infant's ability to push away the bottle, sit up or turn his head to the side, and cough, or clear his airway if milk should flow too rapidly into his mouth and he begins to aspirate it.

Table 31-4. Recommendations for Preventive Health Care, by Age

Health Supervision Procedure	2–4 Weeks	Months								5–6 Years
		2	4	6	9–12	15	16–19	23–25	35–37	
History	x	x	x	x	x	x	x	x	x	x
Measurements										
Height and weight	x	x	x	x	x	x	x	x	x	x
Head circumference	x	x		x		x		x		
Blood pressure									x	x
Sensory screening										
Sight	x	x		x					x or	x
Hearing				x					x or	x
Developmental appraisal	x	x	x	x	x	x	x	x	x	x
Physical examination	x	x	x	x	x	x	x	x	x	x
Immunizations										
DPT		x	x	x			x			x
Oral polio		x	x	x*			x			x
Combination measles and mumps						x				
Laboratory procedures										
Tuberculin test					x or	x			x	
Hematocrit or hemoglobin					x				x or	x
Urinalysis									x	
Urine culture (girls only)									x	x
Discussion and counseling	x	x	x	x	x	x	x	x	x	x
Dental screening	x	x	x	x	x	x	x	x	x	x
Initial dental examination									x	

*Optional.

If mothers must prop up bottles—and it is unrealistic to think you can persuade all mothers not to do so—be certain the mother understands she must never leave her infant alone with a propped bottle. An infant farther away than arm's reach feeding from a propped-up bottle is an accident waiting to happen.

When final night bottles are propped up, milk is left in contact with the teeth for hours. This leads to a high incidence of decay of deciduous teeth (bedtime-bottle syndrome). If deciduous teeth become so decayed or abscessed that they have to be removed, eruption of the permanent teeth may be adversely affected, since the space for this eruption is not adequate. Exposure to infection is an additional hazard if tooth extraction is necessary.

In other instances of aspiration, the mother has underestimated her baby's ability to grasp and place objects in his mouth. A newborn's grasp and sucking reflexes give him this ability automatically, so from day 1, the mother must be certain that nothing comes within her baby's reach that should not be in his mouth. She should make certain that toys have no small parts that will snap off. She must keep any object painted with lead-base paint out of his reach. Rattles should be checked to make sure that whatever makes the noise cannot come out. The baby's clothes should have no buttons on the front that the child can pull off. Diaper pins should be closed and put well out of the newborn's reach while the mother changes diapers. Even a newborn can wiggle to a new position to touch an attractive object. The safe distance for objects in relation to the baby rapidly expands from an arm's reach to yards away. In a very short time, safety will require objects to be locked in cupboards.

PREVENTION OF FALLS

Falls are a second major cause of infant accidents. A mother underestimates her infant's ability to turn over or crawl. No infant, beginning at birth, should ever be left on a surface unattended. Normal newborn wiggling can easily bring a baby to the edge of a bed or tabletop and over the edge. You will note that many mothers in rooming-in units leave the newborn infant lying on the bed while they answer the telephone or go to the bathroom. They will justify this carelessness by saying that babies do not turn over until they are 3 months old. These mothers are revealing how little they know about a newborn's capabilities or about newborn safety.

CAR SAFETY

Car accidents are a safety problem all during childhood. Infants who are laid on a car seat unprotected by any kind of restraint are at great risk if an accident should occur. The car stops suddenly, and the infant is thrown to the floor, or out of the car, or through the windshield. Infants standing on car seats are in equal danger. Many mothers do not think of an infant car seat as being an essential piece of equipment for a baby. They envision buying one "later on, when the baby sits up." If they are going to be transporting the infant in the car, however, this could be the most important piece of baby equipment they will buy. While the infant is small, a car bed with a safety belt is a good investment. The best type of infant car seat to buy is the model in which the infant's back is placed toward the front of the car. This gives optimal support to the baby in an accident and also places him where the driver, if he or she is alone, can safely glance at the infant's face and make sure he is all right.

OTHER SAFETY MEASURES

Mothers with older children may need to be reminded that children under 5 years of age, as a group, are not responsible enough or knowledgeable enough about newborns to look after their safety. Some preschoolers are so jealous of a new baby that they will harm a baby if left alone with him.

Explore the plans for the infant's sleeping space with the mother. Make sure the baby is not going to sleep in the same bed with his parents. The danger of accidental suffocation by bedding or by the pressure of a 150-pound adult is too great. Caution mothers not to use pillows in cribs or bassinets for the same reason.

THE ROLE OF STRESS IN ACCIDENTS

Time spent talking to mothers about accident prevention is always time well spent because what you are actually doing is helping the mother to know her child better. Anticipatory guidance in this area is not always successful in preventing accidents, however. In some instances the mother may believe that none of these things will happen to her child. In others, stress factors may be operating; these have been shown to play as great a role in accidents as do unsafe conditions. Meyer et al. [9] have identified a number of factors associated with accidental injury in children by comparing the incidence of certain family life events in the families of over 100 preschool children injured seriously enough to require hospitalization with their incidence in a matched control group. The results of the study are shown in Table 31-5.

Mothers in families in which one of these stress factors is operating are particularly in need of accident prevention counseling. If you have conducted a careful admission interview with the mother and have spent time getting acquainted with her on the labor or postpartal unit, you will be aware of many such factors. If a mother appears to have so many life contingencies bearing in on her at this time that she does not seem capable of beginning good infant care, or if she needs extra guidance for any reason, a referral to a community health agency should be made. The agency will arrange for a community health nurse to visit the home to provide guidance and help and to suggest further referral if necessary.

Table 31-5. Factors Associated with Accidental Injuries

Family Factor	Percentage in Which Factor Was Present	
	Accident Group	Comparison Group
Parents unresponsive to child's needs	87	3
Maternal health incapacity	54	2
Disruptive supervisory shift	52	0
Family separated or unstable	44	5
Other family life stress	35	1
Instability in community	16	2

Source. R. J. Meyer et al., Accidental injury to the preschool child. *J. Pediatr.* 63:95, 1963.

Problem-oriented Recording: Progress Notes

Baby Kraft (John Joseph)
Day 1, delivery room

Problem: Physiological adjustment to extrauterine life

S. Mother states, "He's beautiful." Father present at delivery, pleased with sex.
O. Born LOA, breathed at 30 seconds, Apgars 8 and 9. No anesthesia, no forceps.
Catheter inserted through left naris, esophagus, and into stomach; 15 ml stomach contents removed. No gross anomalies, no hydramnios, 3-vessel cord.
Weight: 6 lb. 5 oz.
A. Appropriate for gestation age newborn; no immediate difficulty.

Goals: a. Establish immediate respiratory and cardiovascular extrauterine changes.
b. Maintain body temperature.
c. Effect parent-child interaction.
d. Initiate breast-feeding.

P. 1. Infant to remain in birthing room for 1 hour post partum, then transfer to rooming in, 2nd floor.
2. Footprinting, ID identification; review with parents.
3. Administer vitamin K 1 ml to left thigh.
4. Erythromycin ointment to both eyes following initial parent-child interaction.
5. Initial breast-feeding in birthing room.
6. Encourage mother to hold to maintain temperature.

Problem: Circumcision

S. Permission form signed by both parents.
O. Circumcision done in birthing room by Dr. C. Slight bleeding from surgery site; Vaseline gauze applied. Baseline pulse: 140, regular. Vit. K. administered prior to procedure.
A. Delivery room circumcision; minimal post-procedure bleeding.

Goals: a. Surgery area remains free of infection.
b. Bleeding remains at minimal level; vital signs are stable.
c. Mother learns care of surgery site before discharge.

P. 1. Vaseline gauze for 24 hours, then Vaseline as needed.
2. Check vital signs q15min for 1 hour, then 30 min for 4 hours.
3. Keep diaper snug for pressure; position on side to decrease irritation.
4. Show site to mother and review care and possible symptoms of infection.

References

1. Apgar, V., et al. Evaluation of the newborn infant—second report. *J.A.M.A.* 168:1985, 1958.
2. Aradine, C., et al. Collaborating to foster family attachment. *M.C.N.* 3:92, 1978.
3. Brazelton, T. B. Crying in infancy. *Pediatrics* 29:578, 1962.
4. Dunbar, J. Maternal contact behavior in newborn infants during feeding. *Matern. Child Nurs. J.* 6:209, 1977.
5. Gleason, D. Footprinting for identification of infants. *Pediatrics* 44:302, 1969.
6. Gollober, M. A comment on the need for father-infant post-partum interaction. *J.O.G.N. Nurs.* 5:17, 1976.
7. Haddock, N. Blood pressure monitoring in neonates. *M.C.N.* 5:131, 1980.
8. Leboyer, F. *Childbirth Without Violence.* New York: Knopf, 1974.
9. Meyer, R. J., et al. Accidental injury to the preschool child. *J. Pediatr.* 63:95, 1963.
10. Normand, I. C. Dilemmas in neonatal care. *Midwives Chron.* 91:285, 1978.
11. Oliver, C. M., et al. Gentle birth: Its safety and its effect on neonatal behavior. *J.O.G.N. Nurs.* 7:35, 1978.
12. Phillips, C. R. Neonatal heat loss in heated cribs vs mother's arms. *J.O.G.N. Nurs.* 3:11, 1974.
13. Schmidt, J. Using a teaching guide for better post partum and infant care. *J.O.G.N. Nurs.* 7:23, 1978.
14. Silverman, W. A., and Andersen, D. H. A controlled clinical trial of effects of water mist on obstruc-

tive respiratory signs, death rate and necropsy findings among premature infants. *Pediatrics* 17:1, 1956.
15. Stern, L. Clinical aspects of thermoregulation in the newborn. *Contemp. Obstet. Gynecol.* 13:109, 1979.
16. Swanson, J. Nursing interventions to facilitate maternal infant attachment. *J.O.G.N. Nurs.* 7:35, 1978.
17. Van Leeuwen, G., and Glenn, L. Screening for hidden congenital anomalies. *Pediatrics* 41:147, 1968.
18. Washington, S. Temperature control of the neonate. *Nurs. Clin. North Am.* 13:23, 1978.
19. Whiteside, D. Proper use of radiant warmers. *Am. J. Nurs.* 78:1694, 1978.

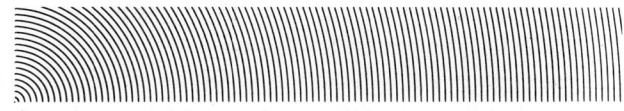

Unit VI. Utilizing Nursing Process: Questions for Review

1. Baby Brown weighs 7 pounds at birth. The nutritional requirement for him for the first six months of life is
   a. 250 cal/24 hours
   b. 300 cal/24 hours
   c. 350 cal/24 hours
   d. 450 cal/24 hours

2. The development task of the newborn period is best encouraged by providing
   a. A variety of experiences for the child
   b. A consistent caregiver
   c. Breast-feeding
   d. A variety of toys

3. Temperament is a factor that
   a. Is learned
   b. Is important only in the newborn period
   c. Determines how the child adapts to new situations
   d. Is not readily apparent in girls

4. When a newborn loses heat to a cold adjoining object, he is losing heat by
   a. Evaporation
   b. Convection
   c. Radiation
   d. Conduction

5. A normal 1-minute Apgar score is
   a. 1–2
   b. 5–9
   c. 7–10
   d. 12–15

6. On an Apgar evaluation, reflex irritability is tested by
   a. Raising the infant's head and letting it fall back
   b. Slapping the sole of a foot
   c. Dorsiflexing the foot against resistance
   d. Tightly flexing the infant's trunk and then releasing him

7. If a newborn lies on his back and turns his head to the right side,
   a. His right arm and leg extend.
   b. His right arm and leg contract.
   c. His left arm and leg extend.
   d. None of the above.

8. Mrs. Brown is breast-feeding. She asks how long a baby should nurse at each breast after she is home. Your best answer would be
   a. No longer than 3 minutes
   b. Until each breast is emptied
   c. At least a half hour to ensure emptying
   d. Forty-five minutes is about average

9. Mrs. Brown has engorgement on the third postpartal day. Which of the following would you recommend to her as a means of alleviating this?
   a. Discontinue breast-feeding for 24 hours.
   b. Decrease her fluid intake to below 500 ml/24 hours.
   c. Encourage her to continue regular breast-feeding.
   d. Have her apply lanolin cream to each breast q2h.

10. Vernix caseosa in a newborn refers to
    a. Edema of the vertex
    b. A collection of blood beneath the skull periosteum
    c. A protective covering to the infant's skin
    d. Fine, downy hairs on the shoulders and back

11. At birth, a newborn's hemoglobin level averages
    a. 2–3 gm/100 ml blood
    b. 12–15 gm/100 ml blood
    c. 14–24 gm/100 ml blood
    d. 25–30 gm/100 ml blood

12. Mrs. Brown asks you whether she should wash her baby's "soft spot" with a bath. Your best advice to her would be
    a. No; this can be harmed by pressure.
    b. No; water can penetrate this fine skin covering.
    c. Yes; the term *soft spot* is misleading in terms of daily care.
    d. Yes, but only after the first month.

13. If Baby Brown is a mature newborn, his sole creases should cover
    a. The entire sole of his feet
    b. Two-thirds the length of the sole
    c. Only to the level of the transverse arch
    d. None of his foot

14. When you examine Baby Brown's umbilical cord, you would want to report which of the following?
    a. A cord at birth that has 2 arteries, 1 vein
    b. A cord with fluid oozing from the base at day 2
    c. A cord that on the third day is black and dried
    d. A cord that is drying without a strong odor

15. In the delivery room, Baby Brown is given vitamin K. The reason for this is
    a. Vitamin K will aid respiratory function.
    b. His liver is too immature to produce vitamin K until 6 days of age.
    c. Vitamin K helps prevent retinal infections.
    d. He has no intestinal flora to synthesize vitamin K at birth.

BUT SOUVENIRS

Daughters may die—but why?
For even daughters can't live with half a heart.

Three days isn't much of a life
But long enough to remember
Thin blue lips
Uneven gasps in incubators
Wracking breaths that caused pain to those who
    watched.
Long enough to remember
I never held her, felt her softness
Counted her toes
Knew the color of her eyes.
Long enough to remember
Death paled hands not quite covered
By the gown she was to go home in;
Moist earthy smells, one small casket, and the tears.

I hold in my hand but souvenirs of an occasion:
    A sheet of paper filled with statistics
    A certificate with smudged footprints
    A tiny bracelet engraved "Girl Smith."

You say that you're sorry, that you know how I feel,
But you can't know because I don't feel—not yet.

By Carrol Nessiage Wilkes (From the *American Journal of Nursing*, 72:1596, 1972. Reprinted by permission.)

VII. The High-Risk Pregnancy

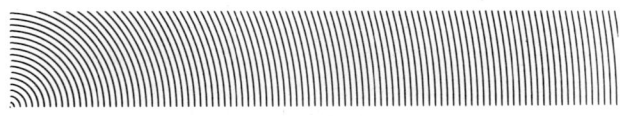

32. The Impact of a High-Risk Pregnancy

A high-risk infant is one who is born with less ability or chance to survive or a greater chance to be left with a permanent handicap, either psychosocial or physiological, than the average child. A *high-risk pregnancy* is one in which some maternal factor, either psychosocial or physiological, will result in the birth of a high-risk infant or in some way harm the woman herself.

Some women enter pregnancy in good health but then develop a complication of pregnancy that causes it to become high-risk. Others enter pregnancy with a chronic illness that, superimposed on the pregnancy, makes it high-risk. Other women's particular circumstances—poverty, lack of support people, genetic inheritance, past history of pregnancy complications—cause the pregnancy to be categorized as high-risk.

In most instances, no single factor causes a pregnancy to be classified this way. The pregnancy of a woman who is a known diabetic, for example, is automatically termed one of greater than normal risk. The fetus growing in utero in an environment in which hyperglycemia is the rule runs increased danger. During the pregnancy, the woman, worrying that something will happen to her baby, fails to begin the "pregnancy work" that she must do so that bonding can take place. At birth, the child is in double jeopardy. Not only may he be born with a handicap but he is high-risk for poor maternal-child attachment as well.

A teenage girl has a low-birth-weight infant. The infant, again, has a double problem. Not only is he immature and must contend with the accompanying dangers; he has an immature mother as well. His risk is compounded.

Remembering that the term *high-risk* rarely refers to just one causative factor will help you plan nursing care. Because high-risk factors are often compounded, nursing care must be multidimensional in scope if it is going to be effective.

Defining the Concept "High-Risk"

The circumstances that can cause a pregnancy to be high-risk are endless when the concept is broadened to include psychosocial aspects.

A high-risk classification system such as Goodwin's Antepartum Fetal Risk Score (see Table 16-1) should be used routinely with all pregnant women to attempt to identify early in pregnancy those who have a physiological interference. Rose's criteria of factors that interfere with mothering attachment (see Table 12-1) should also be used at antenatal visits to try to identify pyschosocial reasons for special care during pregnancy.

Accepting the Pregnancy

The first psychological task the mother has to complete with any pregnancy is accepting the pregnancy. She must get used to the idea that a new cycle of life is beginning. This is difficult when there is a possibility that the pregnancy will not come to term. Many people feel, superstitiously, that if they plan on something, something will go wrong. If they do not plan, proceed as if nothing is happening, everything will then go all right. This was the philosophy of the ancient Greeks, who believed that gods were basically vengeful, spiteful beings. It is the origin of lullabies (singing certain songs over babies kept the god Lilith from knowing a baby was in the house).

This philosophy is healthy in that it protects the woman from being hurt, and if this is the third or fourth or fifth pregnancy that has not come to term, she needs something of this nature to get her through the experience. It is unhealthy, however, in terms of mother-child bonding. It never lets the "pregnancy work" of accepting the pregnancy—or accepting the child—begin.

During her current pregnancy visits, ask a woman with a history of high-risk pregnancies, "Are you starting to feel pregnant yet? Have you made any plans for the baby yet? Have you thought about where this baby is going to sleep yet?" to find out where she is in terms of accepting the pregnancy.

You cannot force her to think about being pregnant. She needs the protection of not thinking for her own mental health. You can, however, document how far along she is in the process of accepting the pregnancy. Then at the birth of her child the extra help she requires to interact effectively with her child will be recognized and can be given.

Accepting the Child

The second psychological step which must be taken in all pregnancies is accepting the child, a change from "I'm pregnant" to "I'm having a baby." This step too is difficult to take when the pregnancy is high-risk and the outcome is guarded. How much a woman wants a child can be measured by the amount of strain, inconvenience, medical visits, laboratory tests, and added expense she is willing to undergo to continue a pregnancy.

Women need support from health personnel during procedures such as oxytocin challenge tests or amniocentesis when they are called for. Some need support when, despite all they have endured, the pregnancy ends without a viable child or with a very damaged one. At some point, in this event, the physician, who has also invested his energy in this pregnancy, and the woman's family support people, who have been with her through the experience, leave. The only person left standing at the end of the bed is you. Knowing what to say, or *not* say, at such a time begins with an appreciation of what high-risk pregnancies mean to women.

Identifying Coping Abilities

The ability to cope with a stressful situation depends on the woman's perception of the event, the support people available, and the woman's ability to cope successfully with stress in the past.

PERCEPTION OF THE EVENT

It is difficult to predict high-risk situations in terms of psychosocial criteria because what is a crisis for one person in this area may not be for another; what one person can cope with easily, another finds overwhelming.

The multiple factors in high-risk pregnancy often make it difficult for the person to perceive clearly the extent of the problem. She might have been able to cope with being hospitalized during the last half of pregnancy (because of pregnancy-induced hypertension, for example) if she were married and had a supportive husband. Being single and still in school makes the forced hospitalization not only financially disabling but career defeating as well.

Timing has a great deal to do with perception of the event. At first, when a physician tells the woman that something is going wrong with this pregnancy, because she cannot see inside herself, she cannot believe that anything is the matter. It is often hard to talk to people during this time of initial diagnosis about the problem because they have not yet admitted there is one. Time, however, forces the woman to accept what is happening. Weeks are passing, but her abdomen is not growing any larger (or her blood pressure is not getting any better and other signs are appearing).

At health care contacts, it is a good habit to explore with women during pregnancy what they know about their situation. At some point, when they have internalized the fact that they have a problem, they are ready to talk about it and what it means to them. It may be four or five weeks from the time they were first told about their situation before they are able to perceive it as what it is and not what they would like it to be.

In order for women to understand what is happening to them, they must have explanations that are at their level of comprehension. The average woman knows very little about the way babies grow in utero. She accepts on faith the concepts that a fetus can live surrounded by water without drowning, that enough nutrients will cross the placenta to sustain him, that labor will not harm him. When something is interfering with these processes she does not understand its importance because she never understood the basic process.

Serving as a factual source of information for mothers with high-risk pregnancies is an important role. The physician with whom you work will undoubtedly reserve the right to tell the woman what her diagnosis is. Check with her that she understood the explanation. Nothing is worse than having a test for fetal well-being done and then waiting days for the results. Check that she was called and told the results. Caution women not to get information on prognosis from their friends at the supermarket; it is invariably wrong because the circumstances their friends are relating were so different. Caution them not to read medical books from the library; new discoveries make statements about prognosis inaccurate very quickly. Advise them to use their physician as their source of medical information. If they are reluctant to ask the physician questions because they are afraid of taking up too much of his or her time, ask the questions for them. People cannot begin to deal with problems until they are aware that they have them. They cannot appreciate the extent of a problem until they understand it.

Women with physical interferences during pregnancy may be referred to specialty clinics or obstetrical specialists for care during their pregnancy. They may be hospitalized for care in specialized units some distance from their home and their support people. Communicating with these new caregivers may be difficult for the woman. Asking questions of specialists may be harder for her than asking questions of her family doctor. Working in high-risk areas, remember how new and strange everything seemed to you your first day there. Women coming for care are rarely comfortable with these strange new settings. Finding a nurse they can talk to, who will intercede for them with people who intimidate them by their importance, is their chief hope when they walk in the door. It is the thing that will keep this experience in perspective for them.

SUPPORT PEOPLE

Someone who is an excellent support person for the tasks of everyday living and who is adequate during a normal pregnancy may be no help at all when a complication of pregnancy occurs. Some women, therefore, have their usual support people cut off from them during a high-risk pregnancy. In many instances they are able to reach out to secondary support people such as members of their church or a community group. Others are left with no one to fill the gap. They do not recognize unless it is pointed out to them that health care personnel are willing and able to serve as support people to them.

Ask at prenatal visits, "How is this affecting everyone at home?" You may discover a woman in the midst of many people but very much alone.

COPING SUCCESS

Ways of coping with situations in the past may not seem relevant or meaningful now because this stress seems so different, so much more serious than anything that happened in the past. Comments such as "We've come through worse things" or "We've had trouble before" are good to hear. They show that the woman is relying on past performance to sustain her in the present crisis.

Immobilizing Reactions to High-Risk Pregnancy

How women react to being told that something about the pregnancy is not going as hoped varies with the individual person and how much she wants the pregnancy or the child. A number of emotions are generally present, however.

FEAR

Although the possibility exists that any woman might die with a pregnancy, it is a light, barely perceived fear for the majority of women, something that flickers once through their mind the day they are diagnosed as pregnant and again when they begin labor.

For the woman with a high-risk pregnancy, fear of dying may remain very real all during pregnancy. The woman with a small pelvis may fear being mutilated at birth or bleeding to death; the woman with hypertension may worry that her cerebral arteries will burst from pressure and leave her dead or paralyzed. Women worry that the child is dying inside them. A child who is part of them, dying inside them, is the same as dying themselves.

Living with fear of this nature for nine months is defeating (Fig. 32-1). The woman cannot make

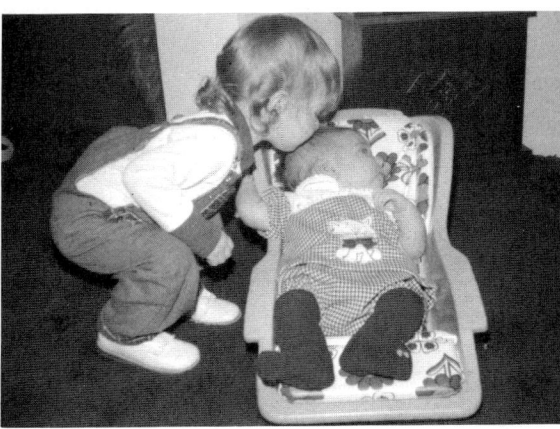

Fig. 32-1. A sibling greets a new sister. This idealistic picture, every mother's hope, may seem a long way off for the woman with a high-risk pregnancy.

plans—to move or not to move, to go back to school or not—because nine months from now she may be dead. She cannot begin to bond with her child. She feels that she will never mother this child because she will die.

She needs reassurance at every step of the way that her condition is not this serious (providing that is true information). At delivery, relief that she is all right, that she has survived the pregnancy intact, may be her chief feeling. She may not be ready to care for her child until the realization that she is really safe has been worked through.

GUILT

Most women accept the responsibility of eating better, not taking medications, and getting more rest as the price to pay for having children. They feel rewarded for their efforts when they see a perfect baby. If something is going wrong with the pregnancy, they search their minds to discover what it was they did or did not do that caused it. Even if what is happening has no documented cause—pregnancy-induced hypertension, for example—they often feel as if they are at fault. If only they were a better person, if only they had not insisted on buying expensive furniture, playing baseball the Sunday before, this would not be happening. It is punishment for their greed, their lack of charity, their selfishness.

A woman who believes she caused the mishap is having difficulty perceiving the event clearly. She cannot utilize her support people because she feels they no longer respect her or care about her (she imagines they hold her as responsible as she holds herself). She has trouble relating the way she dealt with past events to the present because she wishes she had done things differently in the past.

Guilt, therefore, is a destructive emotion during pregnancy. It puts the woman in the worst possible position to cope with what is happening to her. Guilt can never be totally eliminated from her mind, but making certain that she knows the cause of the problem (or that no cause is known) is a help. If the cause *is* unknown—premature labor, for example—it is good to list things that are *not* the cause: running upstairs, picking up a 2-year-old, eating a rich meal. If the woman did do something in pregnancy that is hurting the fetus—smoke heavily, drink heavily, use a street drug—assuring her that people understand she did not mean to hurt the child (or did not realize that she was hurting the child) is a help.

At birth, a woman who feels guilt about what she has done or imagined she has done may have difficulty beginning interaction with her child. She needs some time first to see that the infant responds to her and does not dislike her before she can give herself freely to the relationship.

DEPRESSION

Chronic depression is a numbing state. It blocks out all emotions so that nothing can be felt. If the woman cannot feel, she cannot adapt to her pregnancy or to bonding with her child.

In order to protect themselves from feeling the full shock of learning that their child will be born malformed or has died, women may begin a pattern of *anticipatory grief* after they are first told that something is wrong with the pregnancy. At one time, this reaction was encouraged. People pictured the woman as letting herself down through the stages of grief easily and gently rather than being assaulted with the full blow all at once. It seemed therapeutic. What happened, however, when the child was born normal or did not die? The woman had already mourned for the child; he was already dead in her mind. She could not revive her feelings to reestablish an effective relationship with the child.

Children who cannot be loved because they have already been mourned as dead are termed *vulnerable children* [5]. They tend to have behavior problems as they grow older (they demand to be noticed and loved, to be counted among the living).

Based on a philosophy that preventing anticipatory grief is therapeutic for maternal-child bonding, therefore, the approach to telling high-risk women that their pregnancy is threatened has changed. In the past, a woman who had bleeding at three months' gestation, for instance, was told that bleeding at that point generally meant pregnancy loss. The chance that painless bleeding would go on to cramping and loss of the child was good; better to get prepared for that. Today, with the same symptoms, a woman is told that bleeding all by itself is not a meaningful happening. There is no reason to think yet that the pregnancy is lost.

This change in philosophy does not mean that the woman is not told the basic truth. It means that she is told an optimistic truth: "You have symptoms of pregnancy-induced hypertension, but with rest, we feel sure we can keep them under control and get you the baby you want," not "You have pregnancy-induced hypertension, so prepare for the worst."

It is important that all health personnel in contact with the woman understand the philosophical difference in those two pieces of information. Nothing is worse than being told two stories, or feeling that one is being told less than the truth. A woman must have confidence in health care providers during pregnancy; she is laying her life in their hands.

Signs of Grieving

The grieving or mourning process affects everyone a little differently, but there are enough common signs of grief so that it is possible to identify the woman who is undergoing chronic grief or has begun to grieve for the fetus inside her.

DENIAL. The first step in grief is denial. Denial is a temporary pain reliever and a necessary step on the way to acceptance and the beginning of grief. Although the woman has just been told that the fetus has not grown since the last prenatal visit a month ago, she may want to talk instead about the new color the examining room has been painted. She may want to talk about her sister's children, who are all small. Hiding the knowledge of what is happening or rationalizing the cause reduces the pain of the knowledge.

ANGER. The second step in grief is often anger. A change from thinking, "Surely not me" to "It's not fair that this is happening to me." When a woman is angry about what is happening inside her, she may project her anger inappropriately at people or things. She is angry at the bus she rode to the office; angry at the receptionist for asking her her name; angry at you for tightening a blood pressure cuff too tightly. It is difficult to respond to this kind of anger because it erupts so suddenly and so unfairly. Your first reaction is likely to be anger in return. After all, you applied the blood pressure cuff as you usually do and you are not responsible that the receptionist did not remember the woman's name or the bus was late. A more therapeutic reaction is to accept the anger for what it is—a stage of grief—and respond accordingly: "I'm sorry the cuff felt uncomfortable, but you seem angry about more than the blood pressure. Would it help to talk to me about it?"

BARGAINING. Bargaining is a stage of grief in which the woman tries to "trade off" what is happening to her for something more acceptable. She might say, "If I ever make it through this pregnancy, I'm going to go to nursing school and do things for other people the way you do" (i.e., if God will only let her have a perfect baby, she will spend the rest of her life doing good). A mother may feel very betrayed if after this type of bargaining, the pregnancy is lost.

DEPRESSION. The fourth stage of grief is a change from "It's not fair that this is happening to me" to "Yes, it is happening to me." Crying is the most common sign that this stage has been reached. The woman may ask more questions about the problem than she did previously. She may want to talk more about her hopes and expectations of this pregnancy or child than she did before. She may seem upset by laboratory reports when before she accepted them calmly even though they were equally ominous. On the surface, it seems as if she has taken a step backward. She was managing so well; now she seems so out of control. In reality, this is the first time she has allowed herself to really feel what is happening to her, the first time the laboratory report seemed to be about her.

ACCEPTANCE. The final stage of grief is acceptance. The woman puts herself back together again and goes on with life. It may be as long as six weeks after the first time she was told that something was wrong before she reaches this stage. If the pregnancy is lost, the woman needs to have a return appointment to the health care setting about this time for an evaluation of whether she has worked through a grief process to this stage.

If the pregnancy is not lost, you do not like to see a woman reach this stage. She has completed mourning for a child who is still alive.

LOWERED SELF-ESTEEM

For generations, fertility and the ability to bear and raise children have been regarded as a woman's chief functions. If she has difficulty fulfilling them, she may feel that she is less than other women despite any other achievement she has made. During pregnancy, all women need to be reminded of all the other things they are besides being pregnant so that if a pregnancy is lost, or the outcome of the pregnancy is not perfect, they still retain their self-esteem. Low self-esteem will not allow maternal-child bonding to happen. The woman needs time at birth to get acquainted with her newborn before she can believe that a child would like her and respond to her.

The High-Risk Father

Many women have a hard time understanding what is happening when there is an interference with normal pregnancy. Fathers, who often know less about normal pregnancy than women, understand even less. They receive most of their reports secondhand—not from the physician but from their wife. They may feel reluctant to call and ask questions, to admit that they do not know something. Their perception of the event is likely to be distorted, therefore. They may tell the woman that she misunderstood or did not listen well to the explanation, thus, because they do not understand, they lower her self-esteem further.

Fathers are generally left feeling extremely helpless in their one-person-removed position. They want a child and yet have no control over the pregnancy's outcome. In addition, by wanting this pregnancy, they may have caused the person they love most to be hurt.

Their emotions during the pregnancy, like the wife's, range through fear, depression, guilt, anger. They need careful explanations of what is going on in order to control these feelings. They cannot be support people with overwhelming guilt and doubt about what it is they are expected to be supportive of.

References

1. Aladjem, S. (Ed.). *Perinatal Intensive Care*. St. Louis: Mosby, 1977.
2. D'Angelo, L., and Sokol, R. J. Prematurity: Recognizing patients at risk. *Perinatal Care* 2:16, 1978.
3. Dore, S. L., et al. Catharsis for high-risk antenatal inpatients—patient self help. *M.C.N.* 4:96, 1979.
4. Furman, E. P. The death of the newborn—care of the parents. *Birth Fam. J.* 5:214, 1978.
5. Green, M., and Solnit, A. Reactions to the threatened loss of a child: A vulnerable child syndrome. *Pediatrics* 34:58, 1964.
6. Harper, R. G., et al. The high-risk perinatal registry. A systematic approach for reducing perinatal mortality. *Obstet. Gynecol.* 50:264, 1977.
7. Hobel, C. J. Identification of the Patient at Risk. In R. H. Schwarz and R. J. Bolognese (Eds.), *Perinatal Medicine*. Baltimore: Williams & Wilkins, 1977.
8. Hobel, C. J. Risk assessment in perinatal medicine. *Clin. Obstet. Gynecol.* 21:287, 1978.
9. Ishida, Y. How to deal with grief in childbirth. *Female Patient* 5:74, 1980.
10. Korones, S. B. *High-Risk Newborn Infants—The Basis for Intensive Nursing Care* (2nd ed.). St. Louis: Mosby, 1976.
11. Lubchenco, L. *The High-Risk Infant*. Philadelphia: Saunders, 1976.
12. Pugh, R. E. Perinatal care: Major hazards ahead—unless . . . *Nurs. Mirror* 147:18, 1978.

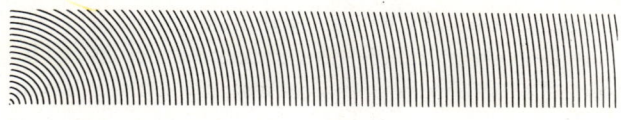

33. Deviations from the Normal in Pregnancy: Nursing Interventions

Some women enter pregnancy with chronic conditions such as heart disease, kidney disease, or hypertension. The course of a normal pregnancy imposed on these disease conditions may cause complications of the disease or of the pregnancy.

Some women enter pregnancy in apparent good health, but, for reasons that are sometimes unexplainable, deviations from the course of normal pregnancy develop and threaten the pregnancy or the woman's health.

If every pregnancy is considered a crisis situation in itself—and it is—it is clear that the advent of a complication can place a very severe burden on the woman and her family. Any woman benefits from the support and the skill of a professional nurse who helps her work through the tasks of pregnancy, accepting it and preparing to become a mother. The support and skill of a professional nurse are essential to a woman who, in addition to the usual tasks of pregnancy, must question whether or not she or her baby will be all right.

The leading causes of maternal death are hemorrhage, infection, hypertension of pregnancy, anesthesia, ectopic pregnancy, heart disease, and thromboembolism.

Bleeding During Pregnancy

Bleeding is a deviation that may occur at any time during pregnancy. It is never normal, and it is always frightening. It may or may not be serious, but it must always be carefully investigated, because if it occurs in sufficient amount or for sufficient cause, it can impair both the outcome of the pregnancy and the woman's life or health. The time during pregnancy at which it occurs is usually a clue to its cause.

FIRST-TRIMESTER BLEEDING: ABORTION

The two most common causes of bleeding during the first trimester of pregnancy are abortion and ectopic pregnancy. An abortion is any interruption of a pregnancy before the fetus is viable. A fetus is said to be viable if the stage of development will enable the fetus to survive outside the uterus. A viable fetus is usually defined as a fetus of at least 20 weeks gestation age (some authorities use 24 weeks) or weighing 400 gm (600 gm at 24 weeks).

An abortion is an early abortion if it occurs prior to the 16th week of pregnancy; a late abortion if it occurs between the 16th and 20th weeks. For the first six weeks of pregnancy, the developing placenta is very tentatively attached to the decidua of the uterus; during the 6th to 12th week a moderate degree of attachment to the myometrium is accomplished. After the 12th week, the attachment is penetrating and deep into the uterine myometrium. Because of the degrees of attachment achieved at different weeks of pregnancy, it is important to try and establish the week of the pregnancy at which bleeding has become apparent. Bleeding before the 6th week is rarely severe; bleeding after the 12th week can be very great in amount. Fortunately, at this time, with such deep placental implantation, the fetus is expelled as in natural childbirth before the placenta separates. Uterine contraction thus helps to control placental bleeding as it does postpartally. For some women, then, the stage of attachment between the 6th and 12th weeks can lead to the most severe bleeding and threat to their life.

Spontaneous Abortion

Spontaneous abortion is abortion that occurs from natural causes. It is popularly known as a miscarriage. Spontaneous abortions occur in about 10 percent of all pregnancies. The presenting symptom is almost always vaginal spotting, which is one of the danger signs of pregnancy. At the first indication of vaginal spotting, the woman should telephone her physician and describe what is happening. If you are working in an office, clinic, or labor unit of a hospital where such calls are received, you need to ask the following:

1. Does she know for certain that she is pregnant (positive pregnancy test or physician confirmation)? A woman who has been pregnant before and states that she is sure she is pregnant is probably right even if she has not yet had confirmation.
2. Duration. How long did the bleeding last? Is it continuing?
3. Intensity. Was it just a few drops? A stream?
4. Description. Was it mixed with amniotic fluid or mucus? Was it bright red (fresh blood) or dark (old blood)? Was it accompanied by tissue fragments? Was it odorous?
5. Frequency. Steady spotting? A single episode?
6. Associated symptoms. Cramping? Sharp pain? Dull pain?
7. Actions. Did anything happen that may have started the bleeding? What did she do about the bleeding?

The woman's actions are important to know about to make certain she has not made an attempt to self-abort. She may prefer not to mention such an attempt, but usually will if asked directly. Ask what she has done about the bleeding to be sure she has not inserted a tampon to stop bleeding and actually has an unknown amount of blood loss, although reporting only slight spotting.

Depending on the symptoms and the description of the bleeding or spotting the woman gives, the physician will make a decision as to whether or not the woman should be seen in the clinic, office, or hospital.

THREATENED SPONTANEOUS ABORTION. Threatened abortion is manifested by vaginal bleeding, usually bright red in color and moderate in amount. There are no associated symptoms such as cramping and no cervical dilatation. Limiting activities for 24 to 48 hours is usually advised; complete bed rest is unnecessary. If the woman is extremely upset (and bleeding, perhaps watching a pregnancy end, and seeing hopes crushed are bound to be upsetting), the physician may prescribe a sedative.

Some women expect health personnel to have a cure for everything. They are disappointed to learn that there is nothing the physician can prescribe for them to "hold the pregnancy." There is no sure evidence that giving estrogen or progesterone at the time of threatened abortion aids in retaining the pregnancy. The administration of diethylstilbestrol (DES) to women in the past at the time of threatened abortion in an attempt to improve pregnancy outlook is an example of overtreatment. The administration of DES did not improve the number of pregnancies that were retained, and daughters born of the DES-aided pregnancies are now in danger of developing vaginal cancer from their intrauterine exposure to DES.

It is important to convey concerned reassurance that abortions happen spontaneously, not because of anything the woman did. Women with threatened abortions look for reasons and never fail to find them: running up a flight of stairs, forgetting to take an iron pill that morning, growing angry at an older child. Being told that none of these things causes abortions will help to free the woman of guilt.

Keep your opinion about the outcome of the pregnancy to cautious optimism. If the spotting is going to stop, it usually does so within 24 to 48 hours of the time the woman began to rest. After that, the woman can gradually resume normal activities. Coitus is usually restricted for two weeks following the bleeding episode to prevent the posibility of infection and in case it might induce further bleeding.

About 50 percent of women with threatened abortion continue the pregnancy; in 50 percent, the threatened abortion changes to imminent abortion.

IMMINENT ABORTION. A threatened abortion becomes imminent if uterine contractions and cervical dilatation occur. With cervical dilatation, the loss of the products of conception is inevitable. A woman who reports cramping or uterine contractions is usually asked to come to the hospital, where she is examined. She should save and bring to the hospital with her any tissue fragments that she has passed. In the hospital, a dilute solution of intravenous oxytocin may be begun to aid the cervix in dilatation and expulsion of the products of conception. The physician may perform a dilation and curettage to ensure that all the products of conception are removed. Any tissue fragments passed in the labor room should be saved, so that they can be examined for an abnormality such as hydatidiform mole or to assure the physician that all the products of conception have been removed from the uterus. Weighing perineal pads before and after use and subtracting the difference is a good way to accurately determine vaginal blood loss.

COMPLETE ABORTION. In a complete abortion, the entire contents of conception are expelled: fetus, membranes, and placenta. There is minimal, self-limiting bleeding.

INCOMPLETE ABORTION. In an incomplete abortion, part of the conceptus (usually the fetus) is expelled, but the membranes or placenta is retained. *Incomplete* is a confusing term to women. They may interpret it as indicating that because the abortion is only partial the pregnancy may continue. Be careful not to encourage false hopes by misinterpreting this term yourself.

In an incomplete abortion, there is a danger of maternal hemorrhage as long as part of the conceptus is retained in the uterus. The physician will usually perform a dilation and curettage to evacuate the remainder of the conceptus. It is important that the woman be informed what is happening, that she know the pregnancy is already lost and that the procedure is being done only to protect her from hemorrhage and infection, not to end the pregnancy.

MISSED ABORTION. In a missed abortion, the fetus dies in utero but is not expelled. Women also find the term *missed* misleading. A missed abortion is usually discovered at a prenatal examination when the fundal height is measured and no increase in size can be demonstrated, or when previously heard fetal heart sounds are absent. The woman may have had symptoms of a threatened abortion (painless vaginal bleeding); she may have had no clinical symptoms.

If there are no symptoms, the woman is usually not told that the fetus appears to be dead (only that he has not grown) because of the psychological impact that can result should she feel overwhelming sorrow or revulsion at carrying a dead child. Within two weeks, the symptoms of abortion usually occur, and the fetus is delivered. If abortion fails to occur after four weeks, most physicians will attempt to induce it; there is a danger that disseminated intravascular coagulation, a coagulation defect, might develop if the dead (and possibly toxic) fetus remains too long in utero. The methods used to induce abortion in these instances are the same as those used with therapeutic abortion, which is discussed later in this chapter.

Most women hope until the moment the abortion is induced that the physician is mistaken, that their baby is alive. They need support in accepting the reality of the situation. They may need counseling in order to accept a future pregnancy, because of fears that whatever force struck silently and strangely in one pregnancy might strike again.

CAUSES OF EARLY SPONTANEOUS ABORTION. The most frequent cause of abortion in the first trimester of pregnancy is abnormal fetal formation, due either to a teratogenic factor or to a chromosomal aberration. About 60 percent of fetuses aborted early have structural abnormalities; 40 percent have grossly observable pathological conditions. Early abortion may be thought of, therefore, as nature's way of preventing the birth of ill or deformed children.

Another common cause of early abortion is an implantation abnormality (about 50 percent of zygotes are never implanted). With inadequate implantation, the placental circulation will not be well established, and fetal formation will be inadequate. Poor implantation may result from inadequate endometrial formation or from an inappropriate site of implantation.

Abortion may occur if the corpus luteum fails to produce enough progesterone to maintain the decidua basalis. Progesterone therapy may be attempted at a time of threatened abortion if this cause is documented.

Abortion may occur following trauma, such as a blow to the woman's abdomen in an automobile accident. The reason for the abortion is probably hemorrhage in the decidua basalis, resulting in fetal detachment. It is always amazing, however, to discover how many women have accidents or falls during pregnancy without aborting. Such pregnancy histories provide good justification for the presence of the amniotic fluid; it truly serves as a buffer against fetal trauma.

There are many stories of women who have suffered abortion following an emotional shock. It is difficult to find documentation for these instances, and they appear to be due to chance. Emotional causes of abortion cannot be totally discredited, however. Severe fright or stress could cause an elevation of maternal epinephrine sufficient to bring about extensive vasoconstriction, possibly leading to necrosis of the decidua basalis. Interference with circulation of the decidua basalis might lead to fetal death.

Infection in the woman may be another cause of abortion. Rubella and poliomyelitis viruses cross the placenta readily and may cause fetal death. *Mycoplasma* infections are implicated in both infertility and early abortion.

Most women want to know the exact reason for a spontaneous abortion. This gives them courage to attempt another pregnancy. Other women, strong believers in the theory that "what I don't know won't hurt me" would rather not know. In many instances, a reason for the abortion is not apparent.

Most couples find comfort in the theory that most early abortions occur because of aberrations in fetal development. However, some couples are so insecure about their ability to reproduce that they are demoralized to learn that they conceived a less-than-perfect child. Each couple and each woman need to be evaluated as individuals before deciding how much information should be given about the loss of a pregnancy.

Illegal Abortion

An illegal abortion is an abortion performed in an uncontrolled setting, usually by a person other than a physician, and without legal sanction. No follow-up care is provided, and unsafe and unsterile practices may be involved. Professional nurses are subject to loss of their nursing licenses if they participate in illegal abortions.

Therapeutic Abortion

A therapeutic abortion is an abortion performed by a physician in a controlled office or hospital setting. It is also referred to as an *induced*, a *medical*, or a *planned abortion*. Nurses employed in a health agency where therapeutic abortions are performed, or by a physician who performs them, are asked to assist with the procedures as a part of their duties.

Therapeutic abortions are done for a number of reasons: to end the pregnancy of a woman whose life is in danger because of the pregnancy (such as a woman with class IV heart disease), to prevent the growth of a fetus who has been found on amniocentesis to have a chromosomal defect, or to accede to the wishes of the woman who chooses not to have a child at this time. The majority of therapeutic abortions are done for the last reason.

In 1973, the United States Supreme Court ruled that therapeutic abortions must be offered in all states as long as the pregnancy is under 12 weeks. Whether abortions are performed after that point in pregnancy has been left to the individual states. Whether an institution allows therapeutic abortions to be done depends on the policy of the institution.

An abortion is a decision reached mutually by the woman and her physician. The husband's consent for the procedure is not necessary. Most midtrimester abortions take place in hospitals, and most hospitals require that the permission of the husband be obtained before the procedure is performed.

Therapeutic abortions involve a number of techniques, depending on the gestation age at the time the abortion is undertaken.

MENSTRUAL EXTRACTION. Menstrual extraction is the simplest of abortion procedures. At four to six weeks following a menstrual period (before pregnancy tests are reliable enough to prove that a pregnancy exists) a polyethylene catheter is introduced through the vagina into the cervix and uterus. By means of a syringe or vacuum extractor, the lining of the uterus that would be shed with a normal menstrual flow is removed. Because menstrual extractions are done before a pregnancy is confirmed, probably some women who have them done do not need them. Menstrual extraction is an outpatient procedure, completed quickly and with a minimum of discomfort. Although some women's groups advocate menstrual extraction as a do-it-yourself procedure, too much risk is associated with it for this to be practical.

DILATION AND CURETTAGE (D & C). If the gestation age is under 12 weeks, dilation and curettage is often used for therapeutic abortions. The woman is admitted to a hospital or clinic for the procedure. If in the hospital, she may receive a general anesthetic, although a regional anesthetic such as a paracervical block works well for pain relief and is used in ambulatory settings. The use of a paracervical block does not completely obliterate pain but limits what the woman experiences to cramping and a feeling of pressure at her cervix.

Following the block, the cervix is dilated by graduated dilators until a sound and a curet can be inserted through the cervical os. The uterus is then scraped clean with the curet.

DILATION AND VACUUM EXTRACTION (D & E). In dilation and vacuum extraction, as with dilation and curettage, a paracervical block is carried out and the cervix is dilated. In some centers, dilation of the cervix is accomplished by having the woman come into the center one day before and inserting a laminaria "tent" into her cervix under sterile conditions. Laminaria is seaweed that has been dried and sterilized. In a moist body part such as a cervix, it begins to absorb fluid and swell in size. Over a 24-hour period, gradually, painlessly and untraumatically, it will dilate the cervix enough for a vacuum extraction tip to be inserted without further dilatation. There is some concern that frequent dilatation of the cervix leads to an incompetent cervix, or one that dilates so easily that it will not remain contracted during pregnancy. This procedure is often chosen for adolescent girls who will perhaps have more than one abortion in their lifetime, to try to safeguard their bodies for later childbearing. Antibiotic prophylaxis may be begun at the time of the laminaria insert to protect against infection. The woman is cautioned not to have sexual relations until the abortion is complete, to reduce the possibility of infection being introduced.

Following either laminaria dilation or dilation by traditional dilators, a suction tip, specially designed, is introduced into the cervix. The negative pressure of a suction pump or vacuum container then gently evacuates the uterine contents. A woman may feel some pressure and some cramps similar to menstrual cramps, but it is not a painful procedure.

After either a dilation and curettage or a vacuum extraction, the woman must remain in the hospital or clinic for a number of hours. She is given the same careful assessment of vital signs and perineal care as a woman in the postpartal period receives. She usually receives an oxytocin medication to ensure firm uterine contraction and minimize bleeding. If there are no complications, she may return home after approximately 4 hours.

SALINE INDUCTION. If the gestation age is between 14 and 16 weeks, a D&E may be used, but the technique generally used is saline or prostaglandin induction. The woman is admitted to the labor unit of the hospital. She should void immediately before the procedure to reduce the size of her bladder so that it will not be accidentally punctured. Her abdominal wall is then prepared with an antiseptic solution and anesthetized by a local anesthetic. For a saline abortion, a sterile spinal needle is inserted into the uterus through the abdominal wall, and 100 to 200 ml of amniotic fluid is removed by a sterile syringe. A 20% hypertonic saline solution is then injected through the same needle in the abdominal wall into the amniotic fluid. The needle is withdrawn. Within 12 to 36 hours, labor contractions begin. Labor may be assisted by administration of a dilute oxytocin intravenous solution. The woman is treated like any woman in labor: She needs frequent explanations of what is happening; she needs her family or a support person with her; she needs medication for discomfort; she may find breathing exercises helpful to minimize discomfort; and she needs to have health care personnel with her.

In most hospitals, women undergoing saline induction complete the abortion in the labor room and are not transferred to the delivery room. Because the products of conception are small, the actual delivery causes only a momentary stinging pain as the perineum is stretched. Women need to be reassured that it will not be dangerous for them to deliver in a labor room. They are not "second-class" patients because they are not being transferred to a delivery room; they simply do not need such a facility.

A serious complication of saline abortions that can occur is hypernatremia from accidental injection of the hypertonic saline solution into a blood vessel within the uterine cavity. The presence of such a concentrated salt solution in the bloodstream will cause body fluid to shift into the blood vessels in an attempt to equalize osmotic pressure. Serious dehydration of tissue will result. This is an intense reaction that occurs at the moment of injection and is manifested by increased pulse rate, flushed face, and severe headache. The injection must be stopped immediately in the event of such a reaction and an intravenous solution of 5% dextrose begun to restore fluid balance.

If large amounts of oxytocin are necessary to induce labor with a saline abortion, the woman must be observed closely for signs of water intoxication, or body fluid accumulating in body tissue. Signs of water intoxication are severe headache, confusion, drowsiness, edema, and decreased urinary output. These symptoms occur subtly at first, then grow in severity. Stopping the oxytocin drip is mandatory. Water intoxication will then decrease as body fluids shift back to normal compartments.

Such complications of saline abortions are unexpected for the woman. She envisioned a simple procedure and is overwhelmed with the amount of pain she is having and the seriousness of the complication. She needs reassurance that, although unexpected, these complications can be dealt with and she will be safe.

Following delivery of the products of conception, it is important that the tissue be examined to determine whether the entire conceptus has been delivered. The woman should be carefully observed for hemorrhage following delivery, just as if she had delivered at term.

PROSTAGLANDIN INJECTION (PGF2a) Second-trimester abortions can be done by the injection of prostaglandin F2a into the uterus through the abdominal wall in place of hypertonic saline. The woman's abdomen is prepared and anesthetized as with a saline injection. Because the amount of prostaglandin administered is small, no amniotic fluid needs to be removed prior to the injection. Uterine contractions begin much sooner after injection than with saline (½ to 1 hour). Generally no oxytocin assist is necessary for delivery to be accomplished.

Although prostaglandin injection is easier and contractions begin sooner, prostaglandins cause extreme nausea, vomiting, and diarrhea in some women and make them feel extremely ill. Their use is contraindicated if the woman has a respiratory disease or hypertension because they also cause vasoconstriction and bronchial constriction. They will induce a severe bronchospasm in women with asthma. The woman should be watched carefully for signs of respiratory distress as the medication is injected. Stopping the injection will fortunately reverse this effect quickly, as the half-life of PGF2a is very short.

A second form of prostaglandin, E2, may be injected intramuscularly to effect uterine contractions and abortion. Newer methods also include transcervical insertion and vaginal suppository instillation. Oral administration, once thought to be the answer to easy administration, appears to cause so much nausea, vomiting, shaking chills, and increased temperature that it is an unacceptable method of administration.

HYSTEROTOMY. If the gestation age is more than 16 to 18 weeks, a hysterotomy is the safest method of abortion. Since the uterus becomes resistant to the effect of oxytocin as it reaches this phase of pregnancy, it may not respond to saline induction or prostaglandin injection even with an oxytocin assist. Further, the chances are great at this gestation age that the uterus will not respond and contract afterward, leading to hemorrhage following a vaginal delivery. The technique for hysterotomy is the same as that for cesarean section.

LABORATORY STUDIES. All women having therapeutic abortions should have laboratory studies performed before the procedure. These usually include a pregnancy test, complete blood count, blood typing (including Rh factor), gonococcal smear, serological test for syphilis, urinalysis, and Papanicolaou smear.

POSTABORTION DANGER SIGNS. All women having therapeutic abortions should be told the danger signs to watch for in the immediate postabortion period, namely, heavy vaginal bleeding (more than two pads saturated in an hour), the passing of clots, abdominal pain or tenderness, and fever over 100.4°F. All women should have a follow-up examination about two to four weeks after the abortion, so that it can be ascertained that the organs of reproduction have returned to their prepregnant state. Sexual relations and douching are generally contraindicated until the time of the postabortion checkup or for two weeks. The woman can expect to have spotting for as long as two weeks and a menstrual flow two to eight weeks following the procedure.

PSYCHOLOGICAL ASPECTS. With the new abortion laws, women of all ages, married or unmarried, with and without previous children, request therapeutic abortions. As mentioned, the majority of women choose to have a therapeutic abortion to end an unwanted pregnancy. Some women who have been exposed to a disease such as rubella have not chosen the abortion willingly, but only as what seems to be the better of two bad alternatives. Others choose abortion because their pregnancy is the result of rape or incest and not of their choosing. These women may find the period of abortion extremely distressful because it may remind them of the original assault and violence.

Most women feel anxious when they appear at the hospital or clinic for an abortion. Some of the anxiety comes from having made a difficult decision to reach this step. A great deal of it comes from having to face the unknown; they have never had an abortion before; they are worried that nurses may not be kind to them.

Women having therapeutic abortions need the same kind of explanations that women in labor receive (often more because women do not share abortion experiences with each other as they share labor experiences, so a woman may know very little about what will happen to her). During the hours when the woman is waiting for labor to begin after a saline injection, she is likely to behave in an introverted manner, perhaps because her progesterone level is beginning to fall, or perhaps because she feels that minimizing interaction with the nursing staff prevents nurses from criticizing her for her decision.

Many nurses find caring for women who elect to have a therapeutic abortion distasteful. They chose maternity nursing because they enjoy seeing children born; they resent caring for women who will not allow their child to be born. However, the goals of maternity care encompass more than helping to ensure the birth of healthy children. A child should not only be born healthy but be born into a loving environment. He will not have this kind of environment if he is born to a mother who does not want him. Therapeu-

Table 33-1. Percentage Distribution of Women Who Used Contraception Prior to Abortion and Four Months Postabortion, by Age and Method

Age	Total	No method		Pill		IUD		Diaphragm	
		Pre	Post	Pre	Post	Pre	Post	Pre	Post
Total	100	41	7	5	60	5	7	5	7
15–17	10	36	9	9	73	0	9	0	0
18–19	17	61	11	0	83	0	0	0	0
20–21	22	52	17	4	52	4	4	4	13
22–29	31	27	3	6	61	9	12	3	6
30–39	9	10	0	0	30	10	10	30	20
Unknown	10	54	0	9	54	0	0	0	0

	Condom, Foam		Rhythm, Withdrawal		Sterilization		Other	
	Pre	Post	Pre	Post	Pre	Post	Pre	Post
Total	22	8	21	2	0	4	3	5
15–17	27	0	27	0	0	0	0	9
18–19	17	5	22	0	0	0	0	0
20–21	4	4	26	0	0	0	4	9
22–29	30	9	21	6	0	3	3	0
30–39	40	20	10	0	0	20	0	0
Unknown	18	18	9	0	0	9	9	18

Source. E. W. Freeman, Abortion: Subjective attitudes and feelings. *Fam. Plann. Perspect.* 10(3):151, 1978. Reprinted with permission.

tic abortions are one way of helping to guarantee parental love and concern to every child born.

To have or not to have an abortion is a value judgment the woman has to make herself. She knows the situation in her home, her feelings, and her capabilities better than you or anyone else does.

Most physicians do not want the woman to know the sex of the child who is therapeutically aborted. A simple "It's too soon to tell" (and often it *will* be too early to tell from gross inspection) satisfies most women and solves the problems. This is to prevent guilt or grief feelings in the future if, for example, the woman who aborts a girl today later on gives birth only to boys (or vice versa). If she never learns the sex of the fetus, her feelings of loss or guilt or grief should be ameliorated.

Women who are Rh-negative should receive an injection of RhoGAM following a therapeutic abortion. If it has not been discussed at the time the abortion decision was made or on admission to the hospital or clinic, counseling on contraception should be done before the woman leaves the hospital. She needs such counseling to avoid having to use abortion as a birth control method in the future.

Freeman [12] has demonstrated that the postabortion period is a time when the woman is ripe for contraception counseling. Table 33-1 contrasts the means of contraception used prior to abortion and after abortion by 106 women.

When women in this same study were asked the open-ended question: What did you learn most about yourself as a result of your abortion experience? Typical answers were "I learned that I could make up my own mind in a difficult situation." "I learned that I'm stronger than I thought." "I learned I can get through difficult times."

The replies of women asked four months after the experience as to how they reacted to the abortion are shown in Table 33-2. Notice that only 15 percent of the women described it as an "ordinary" experience.

Remembering that this is not a decision taken lightly, and one that may be remembered by the woman for a long time to come, plan your nursing care to include interventions aimed at making the abortion as nontraumatic as possible for her.

Complications of Abortion (Spontaneous or Therapeutic)

Abortion itself is a deviation from normal pregnancy, and it may lead to other deviations. In some instances, abortion may cause serious maternal complications. As with term childbirth, hemorrhage and

Table 33-2. Percentage Distribution of 106 Reactions to Abortion 4 Months After the Experience

Reaction	Percent
It was a hard experience but I learned a lot.	42
It was an ordinary experience.	15
The experience still troubles me: I think about it often.	29
The experience was upsetting; I don't like to think about it.	9
It was a hard experience but I learned nothing.	3
No answer	2

Source. E. W. Freeman, Abortion: Subjective attitudes and feelings. *Fam. Plann. Perspect.* 10(3):151, 1978. Reprinted with permission.

infection are the chief complications following abortion. They may occur whether the abortion is therapeutic, spontaneous, or illegal, but they occur most often with illegal abortions because of the lack of quality care and the use of less-than-sterile instrumentation. Some women are admitted to labor units with these complications after having undergone illegal abortions.

HEMORRHAGE. With a complete spontaneous abortion, serious or fatal hemorrhage is rare. With incomplete abortion or in the woman who has an accompanying coagulation defect (usually disseminated intravascular coagulation), major hemorrhage is a possibility. For an immediate measure, the woman needs a dilation and curettage to empty the uterus of the material that is preventing it from contracting and achieving hemostasis. She should have a transfusion to replace blood, and she may require direct replacement of fibrinogen to aid coagulation.

The woman who is being managed at home after a self-limiting complete abortion should telephone the physician's office or clinic daily for the first three or four days following the abortion to report her condition. Ask her about (1) the amount of bleeding she is having (in relation to that in a normal menstrual period), (2) the color (gradually changing to a dark color and then to the color of serous fluid as it does with the postpartal woman), and (3) any unusual odor or passing of clots. If the physician has prescribed an oral medication such as ergonovine maleate to aid with contractions, check to see that she is taking it as prescribed. Some women want to forget the experience as quickly as possible; repression helps them to handle their anger or grief at the loss of the pregnancy most effectively. Be careful that in repressing the experience the woman does not also repress the memory of her medication.

If the woman is hospitalized following an abortion, the same observations, plus careful recording of vital signs, are carried out.

If hemorrhage cannot be controlled by the measures that have been described, ligation of the hypogastric arteries or a hysterectomy may be necessary.

Hysterectomy is an extreme measure and always a difficult one for the woman to accept. Her feelings may range from anger (at the fetus, health care personnel, the child's father, herself, God, a contraceptive device that failed her), to grief (for loss of her body part, for loss of this unborn child and other unborn children), to pity for herself, to fright, bewilderment, and inadequacy. She needs strong support from her family and from the health care personnel around her if she is to weather a complication of this magnitude and put her life back together again.

INFECTION. Infection is a minimal possibility when the loss of the conceptus occurs over a short period of time, bleeding is self-limiting, and instrumentation is limited.

Women should still be observed closely for signs of infection following abortion, including fever, local tenderness, and a foul vaginal discharge. Some women have a transient fever with abortion that is probably due to the period of lowered fluid intake preceding abortion in some instances. In other instances, the fever may be a systemic reaction to the abortion process. All fevers over 100.4°F should be evaluated carefully, however, so that the woman who is contracting an infection will not be overlooked.

Infection tends to occur in women who have lost appreciable amounts of blood, probably on account of the debilitating effect of blood loss. Such women need especially careful observation to rule out this second, possibly fatal, complication.

The organism responsible for infection following abortions is usually *Escherichia coli* (spread from the rectum forward into the vagina). The woman should be cautioned to wipe the perineal area from front to back after voiding and particularly after defecation, to prevent the spread of bacteria from the rectal area. Caution her not to use tampons to control vaginal discharge, since stasis of any body fluid increases the risk of infection. Be careful about statements such as "You'll have some vaginal flow now almost exactly like a menstrual flow." The woman may proceed to treat it as a menstrual flow and use tampons.

Endometritis is the infection that usually occurs following abortion. It may be more extensive, however, and parametritis, peritonitis, thrombophlebitis, and septicemia can occur (see Chap. 36). The management of these infections is the same as if they were occurring post partum, after the safe delivery of a child.

Causes of Recurrent Abortion

In the past, women who had three spontaneous abortions that occurred at the same time in pregnancy were called habitual aborters. They were often advised that they were apparently too "nervous" or that something was so wrong with their hormones that childbearing was not for them. Today, a thorough workup is done in women who lose one or more pregnancies to discover the cause and so to be able to predict more accurately whether or not the woman will be able to bear children.

DEFECTIVE SPERMATOZOA OR OVA. A careful family history may reveal a familial tendency to produce children with defects. The husband's sperm will be examined under a microscope to see whether defective spermatozoa are present. A pathological report on an aborted fetus may reveal a chromosomal abnormality. A chromosomal investigation may be done to see whether aberrant chromosomes can be detected in either the husband's or the wife's karyotype. (Chromosome abnormalities are discussed in Chap. 34.)

HORMONAL INFLUENCES. In women who have recurrent abortions, the progesterone level of the blood may be decreased. If this is suspected as the cause of the abortions, the pregnanediol levels in urine will be monitored during the woman's next pregnancy. Supplemental progesterone therapy might be indicated.

In ordinary pregnancy, the protein-bound iodine (PBI), butanol-extractable iodine (BEI), and globulin-bound iodine (GBI) are elevated. In women with recurrent abortions, these values may be lowered. Thyroid function is checked by determining the woman's basal metabolic rate and by other thyroid function tests. Poor thyroid function is a cause of infertility as well as of abortion. Thus, if the tests indicate poor thyroid function, the woman may be started on therapy to aid in conception as well as to help carry the next pregnancy.

NUTRITIONAL STATUS. Poor nutritional intake may add to the incidence of recurrent abortion. Low levels of vitamins A, B complex, C, D, and E may contribute to fetal loss. A nutritional history should be recorded for any woman with a history of recurrent abortions.

DEVIATIONS OF THE UTERUS. The uterus first forms in utero as an organ with a midseptum. As the organ matures, the septum atrophies and disappears. Occasionally, a woman reaches adulthood with a uterine septum. The blood supply to the septum is not ordinarily as good as that of the endometrium covering the normal walls of the uterus. Placental implantation on the septum may result in an inadequate nutrient supply to the fetus and consequent abortion. The uterus may be only half the normal size because of the dividing septum, so the pregnancy may end prematurely.

A bicornuate uterus is one with sharp poles (horns). This abnormal shape may lead to abortion, although 75 percent of women with bicornuate uteri carry pregnancies to term.

PSYCHOLOGICAL FACTORS. Although certainly not applicable in all women who have recurrent abortions, psychological factors may influence the outcome of pregnancy in some women. Personality factors of basic immaturity and extreme dependence have been found in women who have recurrent abortions. For these women psychiatric counseling and support may be effective in preventing further pregnancy loss.

BLOOD INCOMPATIBILITIES. Rh incompatibilities do not appear to cause abortions, but ABO incompatibilities may play a role in recurrent abortions. This is a factor that should be considered in the overall assessment of a woman having recurrent abortions.

All women who have recurrent abortions should be thoroughly investigated to determine, if possible, the underlying cause. They should not simply have to accept this as their fate, as they have been forced to do in the past.

Isoimmunization and Abortion

When the placenta is dislodged, either by spontaneous delivery or by dilation and curettage at any point in pregnancy, blood from the placental villi (the fetal blood) may enter the maternal circulation. This has implications for the Rh-negative woman. Enough Rh-positive fetal blood may enter her circulation to cause isoimmunization—that is, the production by her immunological system of antibodies against Rh-positive blood. If her next child should have Rh-positive blood, these antibodies would attempt to destroy the red blood cells of the infant during the months he was in utero.

Following an abortion, because the blood type of the conceptus is unknown, all women with Rh-negative blood should receive Rh_o (D antigen) immune globulin (RhoGAM) to prevent the buildup of antibodies in case the conceptus was Rh-positive (see p. 592).

FIRST-TRIMESTER BLEEDING: ECTOPIC PREGNANCY

An ectopic pregnancy is one in which implantation occurs outside the uterine cavity. The implantation may occur on the surface of the ovary, anywhere in the abdominal cavity, or in the cervix, but the most usual site (in about 95 percent of such pregnancies) is in the fallopian tube (Fig. 33-1). About 1 in every 200 pregnancies is ectopic, and ectopic pregnancy is the second most frequent cause of bleeding early in pregnancy.

Fertilization takes place in the distal third of the fallopian tube, and immediately after the union of ovum and spermatozoon the zygote that is formed begins to divide and increase in size. If any obstruction is present, such as adhesions of the fallopian tube from previous infections (chronic salpingitis), congenital formations, scars from tubal surgery, or a uterine tumor pressing on the proximal end of the tube, the zygote may not be able to traverse the course of the tube and will lodge at a site along the tube and be implanted there instead of in the uterus. There is some evidence that intrauterine devices used for contraception may slow the transport of the zygote and lead to tubal or ovarian implantations.

Assessment

There are no unusual symptoms at the time of implantation. The corpus luteum of the ovary continues to function as if the implantation were in the uterus. No menstrual flow occurs, and the woman may experience the nausea and vomiting of early pregnancy.

At the 6th to 12th week of pregnancy (4 to 10 weeks following a missed menstrual period), the growing zygote ruptures the slender tube, or the growing trophoblast cells break through the narrow base of the fallopian tube, with resultant invasion and destruction of the blood vessels. The extent of the bleeding that occurs depends on the number and size of the ruptured vessels. If implantation is in the interstitial portion of the tube (where the tube joins the uterus), rupture will cause severe intraperitoneal bleeding. Fortunately, the incidence of tubal pregnancies is highest in the ampullar area (the distal third), where the blood vessels are smaller and profuse hemorrhage is less likely. However, the bleeding may in time result in a great loss of blood. Ruptured ectopic pregnancy is serious, no matter what the site of implantation.

The amount of bleeding *evident* with ectopic pregnancy is deceptive. The products of conception from the ruptured tube and the blood may be expelled into the pelvic cavity rather than into the uterus and then will not reach the vagina and become evident. The woman usually experiences a sharp, stabbing pain in one of the lower abdominal quandrants and notes a little vaginal spotting. (With placental dislodgment, progesterone secretion stops and the uterine decidua begins to slough, causing this bleeding.) She may experience light-headedness and rapid pulse, which are signs of shock.

The possiblity of ectopic pregnancy is the reason it is important to ask all women when they call the physician's office or the clinic in the first trimester of pregnancy reporting vaginal spotting whether or not there is any associated pain. Any woman with sharp pain and vaginal spotting must be seen, so that ectopic pregnancy can be ruled out.

Occasionally, a woman will move suddenly and pull the round ligament, the anterior uterine support. There will be a sharp, momentary lower-quadrant pain. However, it would be very rare for this phenomenon to be reported in connection with vaginal spotting.

By the time the woman arrives at the hospital or physician's office, she may be in shock, with a rapid, thready pulse, rapid respirations, and falling blood pressure. Her abdomen gradually becomes rigid. If blood is slowly seeping into the peritoneal cavity, the umbilicus may have a bluish tinge (Cullen's sign). She may have extensive vaginal and abdominal pain; movement of the cervix on pelvic examination causes excruciating pain. A tender mass is usually palpable in the cul-de-sac of Douglas. Leukocytosis may be present, not from infection but from the trauma. The temperature is usually normal.

Ectopic pregnancy must be considered an emergency situation. The woman's condition must be evaluated quickly, the amount of blood *evident* being a poor estimate of her actual blood loss. Blood must

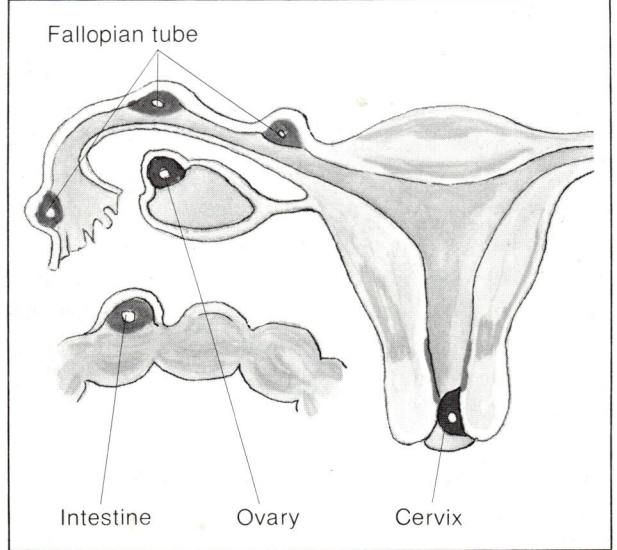

Fig. 33-1. Sites at which an ectopic pregnancy may occur.

be drawn immediately for hemoglobin value, typing, and cross matching. Blood is drawn for serum human chorionic gonadotropin level or a urine sample is usually sent for immediate pregnancy testing (or this is done by you by one of the short-term reporting techniques) if pregnancy has not been confirmed. Intravenous fluid to restore intravascular volume is begun. If the diagnosis of ectopic pregnancy is in doubt, the physician may, under sterile conditions, insert a needle through the postvaginal fornix into the cul-de-sac to see whether blood that has collected there from internal bleeding can be aspirated. Either laparoscopy or culdoscopy can be used to visualize the fallopian tubes if the symptoms alone do not reveal a clear-cut picture of what has happened.

Intervention
The treatment for a ruptured ectopic pregnancy is laparotomy to ligate the bleeding vessels and to remove or repair the damaged fallopian tube. Previously, physicians attempted to "save" ruptured tubes to protect the woman's fertility. Now the ruptured tube is usually removed because a suture line on a fallopian tube may lead to another tubal pregnancy. This rationale should be explained to the patient. Otherwise, she may feel that she has not been given the correct treatment.

Following removal of one tube, the woman is theoretically only 50 percent fertile, since every other month, when she ovulates from the ovary adjoining the removed tube, the sperm cannot reach the ovum on that side. This cannot be counted on as a contraceptive measure, however. It has been shown in rabbits that translocation of ova can occur—that is, an ovum released from the right ovary can pass through the pelvic cavity to the opposite (left) fallopian tube, and vice versa.

A woman who has an ectopic pregnancy not only has grief stages to work through (she has lost a child) but may have problems of diminished self-image to resolve as well. She may believe that she is only half a woman if she equates childbearing with being a woman. She needs to verbalize concerns about future childbearing and concerns that her husband may view her differently now that she is not fully fertile. The process of working through grief and role images takes weeks to months. It should begin in the hospital, where the woman has professional people to help her through the first days and estimate whether she will need counseling.

A woman who has had one ectopic pregnancy is more prone to have a second one than is the average woman because of the nature of ectopic pregnancies. Salpingitis that leaves scarring is usually bilateral. Congenital anomalies such as congenital webbing may also be bilateral. If chronic pelvic inflammatory disease (ordinarily a result of gonorrheal infection) was the reason for the ectopic pregnancy, the woman may feel that having premarital relations caused it, and that she is now being punished for these activities. She needs to verbalize her feelings, so that she does not leave the hospital feeling guilty and unworthy.

Very rarely—so rarely that the instances are difficult to document (although they have occurred)—after rupture, the products of conception will be expelled into the pelvic cavity with a minimum of bleeding. The placenta will continue to grow in the fallopian tube, spreading perhaps into the uterus for a better blood supply; or it may escape into the pelvic cavity and successfully implant on an organ such as an intestine. The fetus will grow in the pelvic cavity (an abdominal pregnancy). It is possible that such a pregnancy would reach term.

As with abortion, women with Rh-negative blood should receive Rh_o (D) immune globulin (RhoGAM) following an ectopic pregnancy for isoimmunization protection in future childbearing.

Abdominal Pregnancy
In abdominal pregnancy, the placenta is usually located posterior to the uterus on the intestines or in the cul-de-sac of Douglas. It may remain in the uterine fundus or the fallopian tubes if the abdominal pregnancy resulted from a surviving fallopian pregnancy.

In an abdominal pregnancy, the fetal outline is not easily palpable. The woman may not be as aware of movements as she would be normally or she may experience painful fetal movements and abdominal cramping with movements.

Past history of the woman may include previous uterine surgery or the sudden pain of ectopic pregnancy earlier in the pregnancy. An x-ray film or a sonogram may be used to reveal the fetus outside the uterus.

The danger of abdominal pregnancy is that the placenta will infiltrate and erode a major blood vessel in the abdomen, leading to hemorrhage. If implanted on the intestine, it may erode so deeply that it causes bowel perforation and a peritonitis. The risk to the fetus is also high. Survival in an abdominal pregnancy is only 20 to 40 percent because of a poor nutrient supply due to abnormal placental implantation. In those infants who do survive there is an increased incidence of fetal deformity.

At term, the infant must be delivered by laparotomy. The placenta is difficult to remove if it is implanted on an abdominal organ such as the intestine. If left in place, it will be absorbed spontaneously in two or three months.

SECOND-TRIMESTER BLEEDING

There are two main causes of bleeding during the second trimester: hydatidiform mole and incompetent cervix.

Hydatidiform Mole

Hydatidiform mole is proliferation and degeneration of the trophoblast villi, which occurs for unknown reasons. As the cells degenerate, they become filled with fluid, appearing as fluid-filled, grape-sized vesicles, and the embryo fails to develop (Fig. 33-2).

ASSESSMENT. The incidence of hydatidiform mole is about 1 in every 2,000 pregnancies. It tends to occur most often in women from low socioeconomic groups who have a low protein intake, in young women (under 18 years), and in women over 35 years of age. Women receiving clomiphene citrate (Clomid) to induce ovulation appear to have a higher number of hydatidiform mole formations than others. Because the proliferation of the trophoblast cells occurs so rapidly, the uterus expands faster than it normally does. The uterus reaches its landmarks (just over the symphysis brim at 12 weeks, at the umbilicus at 20 to 24 weeks) before the usual time. This rapid development is also diagnostic of multiple pregnancy or miscalculated due dates, however, so it must be evaluated carefully. The nausea and vomiting of early pregnancy is usually marked. No fetal heart sounds can be heard. A blood or urine test for pregnancy will be strongly positive in women with hydatidiform mole. Human chorionic gonadotropin (HCG) in the blood or urine is the substance that causes pregnancy tests to be positive. The trophoblast villi produce HCG, so even though there is no fetus present, because villi are growing at many times their normal rate the test results will be strongly positive. Results continue to be strongly positive after the 100th day of pregnancy, when the level normally would begin to decline. This fact must be evaluated carefully also, since highly positive test results are characteristic of multiple pregnancies with more than one placenta. Symptoms of hypertension of pregnancy (hypertension, edema, and proteinuria) are ordinarily not present before the 24th week of pregnancy; with a hydatidiform mole, they may appear before this time. A sonogram will show dense growth (typically a "snowflake pattern") but no fetal growth in the uterus.

At about the 16th week of pregnancy, if the structure was not identified earlier by sonogram, it will identify itself with vaginal bleeding. This may begin as vaginal spotting of dark brown blood or as a profuse fresh flow. As the bleeding progresses, it is accompanied by discharge of the clear fluid-filled vesicles. This is one reason women who begin to abort at home should bring to the hospital with them any clots or tissue they have passed. The presence of clear fluid-filled cysts changes the diagnosis immediately to hydatidiform mole.

INTERVENTIONS. Treatment is therapeutic abortion or dilation and curettage to evacuate the mole. Although HCG levels are usually negative within a week following a normal pregnancy, the level remains high following hydatidiform mole. One-half of women still have a positive reading at three weeks; one-fourth will still have a positive test result at 40 days.

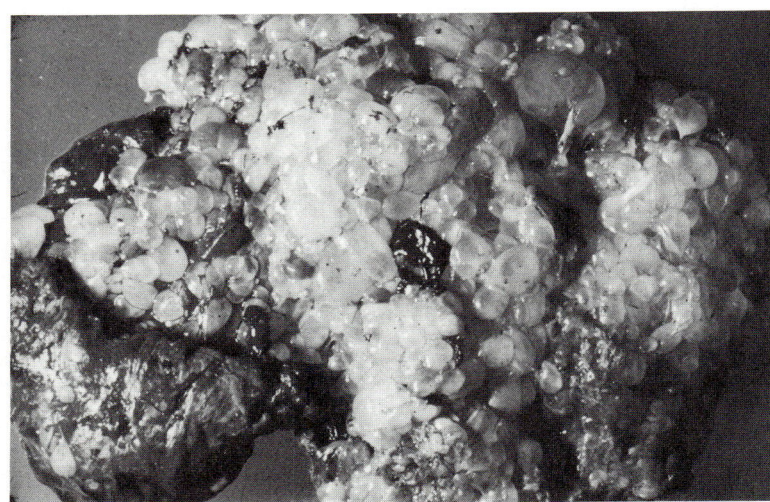

Fig. 33-2. Hydatidiform mole. (From L. Crowley, An Introduction to Clinical Embryology. Copyright © 1974 by Year Book Medical Publishers, Inc., Chicago. Reprinted by permission.)

As a rule, women who still have a positive test result for HCG at 30 days are readmitted to the hospital for a repeat dilation and curettage and biopsy to check for the presence of choriocarcinoma, a malignant uterine cancer, as retained trophoblastic tissue in such instances may convert to this malignancy.

Every woman who has had a hydatidiform mole should have a urine specimen or blood serum tested for HCG every month for a year, so it can be ascertained whether new villi are developing, and she should use contraceptives during the year, so that a positive pregnancy test (the presence of HCG) resulting from a new pregnancy will not be confused with developing malignancy. Some physicians give women who have had a hydatidiform mole a prophylactic course of methotrexate, the drug of choice for choriocarcinoma. Since the drug has side effects that interfere with blood formation, however, the wisdom of prophylaxis must be weighed carefully.

After a year, the woman is theoretically free of complications from the hydatidiform mole if pregnancy test results are still negative at that time.

Although the development of a hydatidiform mole means that a pregnancy never materialized, that a fetus never formed, the woman experiences the same reactions following its evacuation that she does following the loss of a true pregnancy. She did, after all, believe that she was pregnant. On top of losing the pregnancy, she has the added anxiety of being aware that a malignancy may develop. She also must delay her childbearing plans for a full year. If, in addition, she has already put off having a child (so that she or her husband could finish school or they could buy a house), the year may seem to be the longest year of her life.

She needs to express her anger and sense of unfairness. She may also feel very inadequate because something went wrong with her pregnancy. She wonders whether it will happen again, whether she will ever be able to have children. Fortunately, the occurrence of a second hydatidiform mole is rare, and she can be assured of this.

Incompetent Cervix

An incompetent cervix is one that dilates prematurely and therefore cannot hold the fetus until term. The dilatation is usually painless. The first symptom is show (a pink-stained vaginal discharge), which is followed by rupture of the membranes and discharge of the amniotic fluid. Uterine contractions begin, and after a short labor the fetus is born—but unfortunately at about the 20th week of pregnancy, when the fetus is too immature to survive.

It is often difficult to explain in a particular instance what has caused incompetent cervix. Congenital developmental factors or endocrine factors may be responsible. Trauma to the cervix such as might occur with a dilation and curettage is probably often the cause.

Following the loss of one child due to an incompetent cervix, a surgical operation termed *cervical cerclage* can be performed to prevent this from happening again. At about the 14th to 18th week of a new pregnancy, under anesthesia, pursestring sutures are placed in the cervix. This is called a McDonald or a Shirodkar-Barter procedure after the surgeons who perfected it. The sutures serve to strengthen the cervix and prevent it from dilating. With a McDonald procedure, the sutures may be removed at the 38th to 39th week of pregnancy, so that the fetus may deliver vaginally. Sutures may be left in place and the woman delivered by cesarean section following a Shirodkar-Barter procedure, or they may be removed and the delivery allowed to proceed vaginally. The success rate with both of these procedures is between 65 and 80 percent.

It is important with these procedures that the suture be removed before vaginal delivery is attempted. Be certain to ask women who are reporting painless bleeding (the symptoms of spontaneous abortion) whether they have had past cervical operations.

Still newer techniques allow the pursestring sutures to be set before the woman is pregnant. This gives her the added assurance that she will not begin aborting before the 14th week of pregnancy, the earliest time the operation can be done during pregnancy.

Women with incompetent cervixes were formerly included in the category of habitual aborters and told to accept their fate. The cervix was thought simply not strong enough to support a pregnancy. Today, the prognosis in such women is favorable.

THIRD-TRIMESTER BLEEDING

Bleeding during late pregnancy occurs because of either placenta previa, premature separation of the placenta, or premature labor, all of which are serious conditions. Slight spotting late in pregnancy can be caused also by trauma from a pelvic examination, an innocent finding.

Placenta Previa

Placenta previa (Fig. 33-3) is low implantation of the placenta. It occurs in three forms: implantation in the lower rather than in the upper portion of the uterus (low implantation), implantation that occludes a portion of the cervical os (partial placenta previa), im-

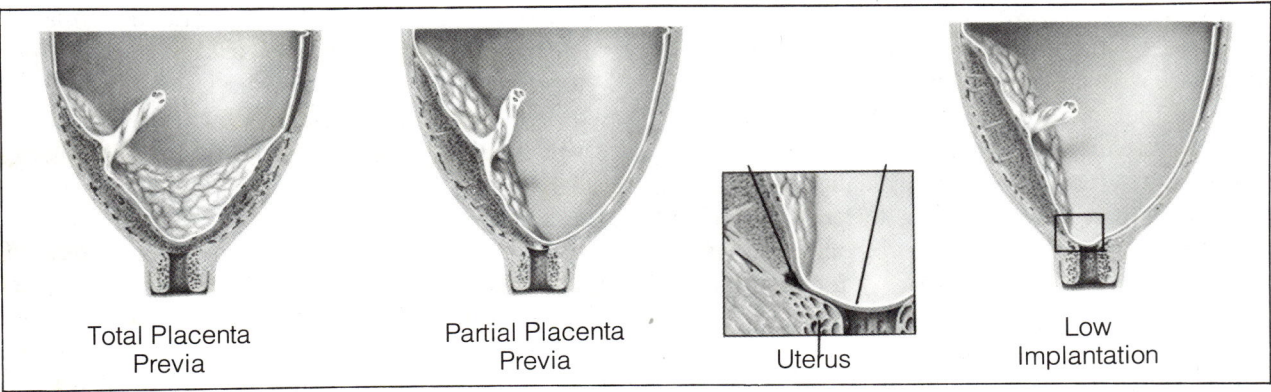

Fig. 33-3. Placenta previa. (From Clinical Education Aid, No. 12, Ross Laboratories, 1963, Columbus, Ohio.)

plantation that totally obstructs the cervical os (total placenta previa). The degree to which the placenta covers the internal cervical os is generally estimated in percentages: 100 percent, 75 percent, 30 percent, and so forth.

Fibroid tumors of the uterus, uterine scars from surgery, or abnormal uterine position or shape might cause placenta previa, but generally the reason for the low implantation is not apparent. It does occur in women with increased parity or age, as if possibly the placenta must spread to seek adequate nutritional sources. The incidence in all pregnancies is about 1 in 200.

BLEEDING. Bleeding with placenta previa occurs when the lower uterine segment begins to differentiate from the upper segment and the cervix begins to dilate. The bleeding is the result of the placenta's inability to stretch to accommodate the differing shape of the lower uterine segment or the cervix. Such bleeding generally occurs after the 7th month of pregnancy. The bleeding is usually abrupt and painless, and it is not associated with increased activity. It may stop as abruptly as it began, so that by the time the woman is seen at the hospital she is no longer bleeding, or it may slacken after the initial hemorrhage but continue as continuous spotting. The bleeding is usually acute and sudden enough to frighten the woman thoroughly. She telephones her physician, who instructs her to come to a hospital. She may arrive by ambulance. In any event, she is frightened for herself and for her baby.

ASSESSMENT. The bleeding of placenta previa, like that of ectopic pregnancy, is an emergency situation. The bleeding is from the uterine decidua (maternal blood), so the mother is in danger from hemorrhage. Because the placenta is loosened, the fetal oxygen supply may be compromised and the fetus be in threat also. Once more it is difficult to evaluate how much blood has been lost or whether bleeding is still occurring, since the blood may pool at the base of the uterus and not be apparent.

The woman requires immediate bed rest. You need to know the following: the time the bleeding began; her estimation of the amount (ask her to estimate in terms of cupfuls or tablespoonfuls—a cup is 240 ml; a tablespoon is 15 ml); whether there was accompanying pain; the color of the blood (the redder the blood, the fresher it is); what she has done for the bleeding (it is important to know that she did not insert a tampon to halt the bleeding, so that there may be hidden bleeding); whether there were prior episodes of bleeding during the pregnancy; and whether she had prior cervical surgery (do not mistake an incompetent cervix for placenta previa). To help determine management, you must know the duration of the pregnancy.

In the labor room, check the perineum for bleeding. Estimate the present rate of blood loss. Weighing perineal pads before and after use and subtracting the difference is a good method to determine vaginal blood loss. *Never attempt a pelvic or rectal examination with bleeding late in pregnancy. Any agitation of the cervix when there is a placenta previa may initiate massive hemorrhage, fatal to both mother and child.* Take vital signs to determine whether symptoms of shock are present and to establish a baseline of information. Attach an external fetal monitor and begin recording fetal heart sounds. Obviously, any type of monitor that requires invasion of the cervix is completely contraindicated. Ascertain whether the uterus is contracting (whether the woman appears to be in labor).

Fetal heart sounds should be monitored continuously; maternal pulse, respirations, and blood pressure should be taken every 15 minutes until it can be ascertained that they are stable. Oxygen equipment should be available in case the fetal heart sounds indicate fetal distress (bradycardia or tachycardia; late deceleration or variable deceleration dips if the woman is in labor). The woman should have blood drawn for typing and cross matching, and an intravenous fluid line for intravascular volume replacement should be begun. Vaginal delivery is always safest for an infant. Therefore, it is essential to locate the placenta as accurately as possible in the hope that its position will make vaginal delivery feasible.

On abdominal examination, the fetal head may be discovered to be nonengaged because of the interfering placenta. However, this finding gives little indication of how much of the placenta is obscuring the os and thus preventing the head from engaging.

The placenta may be located by ultrasound scanning. The woman needs to be reassured that ultrasound waves are not x-rays, and that there is no evidence that ultrasound will harm her baby. The procedure will be painless for her.

If a source of ultrasound is not available, the placenta may be located by x-ray placentography. If the pregnancy is at term, this can be undertaken without risk to the fetus. Other, less used techniques are amniography (instillation of radiopaque dye into the amniotic fluid), isotope injection, and thermography.

The physician may attempt careful speculum examination of the vagina and cervix to rule out a source of bleeding such as ruptured varices or cervical trauma and to establish the percentage of placenta covering the os. If this is under 30 percent, it may be possible for the fetus to be delivered past it. If over 30 percent, and the fetus is mature, the safest delivery method for both mother and baby will be a cesarean section.

Vaginal examinations (actual investigation of dilatation) to determine whether placenta previa exists are done in the operating room only so that, if hemorrhage does occur with the manipulation, the woman may be immediately sectioned to remove the child and the bleeding placenta, contract the uterus, and save both the child and herself. Be careful when reporting the woman's symptoms to her physician on admission that you paint a clear picture of what has happened: "Sudden gush of about 100 ml of red blood, no pain, now a continuous trickle in a woman 32 weeks pregnant" so placenta previa will register quickly in his mind as he skims through the list of potential diagnoses. When you are working with inexperienced house staff, it is not unprofessional to suggest, "Do you want me to set up an operating room so you can do your vaginal exam there?" for the woman's safety.

INTERVENTIONS. Once a tentative diagnosis of placenta previa has been made, the age of the gestation will largely dictate the management. If labor has begun, or bleeding is continuing, or the fetus is being compromised, delivery must be accomplished irrespective of gestation age. If the bleeding has stopped, the fetal heart sounds are of good quality, maternal vital signs are good, and the fetus is not yet 36 weeks of age, the woman is usually managed by expectant watching. About a fourth of all women with bleeding from placenta previa are managed this way.

The woman remains in the hospital for close observation. Careful assessment of fetal heart sounds is required, and daily determination of hemoglobin or hematocrit is necessary for detection of hidden bleeding.

Placenta previa bleeding may involve only one episode of painless bleeding as labor activity begins. If it occurs early in the last trimester of pregnancy, it may involve a number of episodes of progressive painless bleeding.

The woman who has placenta previa bleeding needs a clear explanation of what is happening and what is planned. It is difficult for a woman to wait for a pregnancy to come to term following placenta previa bleeding. She cannot stop wondering whether her infant is all right. She is very aware of fetal movement and may even test movement several times a day by lying in the position in which she usually feels the fetus stir. Listening to fetal heart sounds and being reassured that they are in a healthy range is very helpful. She is afraid that the next bleeding she experiences may kill her, or her infant, or both.

She needs to be able to talk to someone about her fears. She may become so worried about the safety of her child that she begins to think of her child as dead. She might neglect her diet or her supplementary vitamins because "it doesn't matter any more." No matter what her outward appearance is during this time, she is under severe emotional stress.

DELIVERY. As soon as the fetus reaches 36 weeks of age (2,500 gm), an amniocentesis test for maturity shows a positive result, bleeding occurs again, labor begins, or the fetus shows symptoms of distress, the fetus will be delivered. The woman should be told during her weeks or days of waiting that delivery will probably be by cesarean section because of the low implantation of the placenta. She must be told that her baby may have a low birth weight.

On her day of delivery, she needs a great deal of support. It is one thing to talk about being ready for surgery; it is another to be truly ready. She is as frightened as she was the evening her bleeding first began.

If, at the time of the initial bleeding, the pregnancy

is past 36 weeks, a delivery decision will generally be made immediately.

If the placenta previa is found to be total, delivery through the placenta is impossible, and the baby must be delivered by cesarean section. If the placenta previa is partial, the amount of the blood loss, the condition of the fetus, and the woman's parity will influence the delivery decision. When a cesarean section is used in placenta previa, the incision is usually closer to the traditional longitudinal suture line than is the newer transverse (bikini) incision because the uterine cut must be made high, above the low implantation site of the placenta.

Following delivery, whether vaginal or cesarean section, the mother inspects her child very carefully, looking for defects. If the placenta was implanted wrongly, she thinks there must surely be something wrong with her child as well. During the postpartal period, she needs long visiting periods with her child to make certain that he is normal.

Any woman who has had a placenta previa is prone to postpartal hemorrhage because the placental site is in the lower uterine segment, which does not contract as efficiently as the upper segment. Also, because the uterine blood supply is less in the lower segment, the placenta tends to grow larger than it would normally. Thus a larger surface area is denuded when it is removed. The woman is liable to infection, too, because the placental site is close to the cervix, the portal of entry for pathogens.

Premature Separation of the Placenta (Abruptio Placentae)

Unlike placenta previa, in premature separation of the placenta (Fig. 33-4) the placenta appears to have been implanted correctly. Suddenly, however, it begins to separate and bleeding results. By definition, this occurs after the 20th to 24th week of pregnancy; separation occurring earlier would be considered a spontaneous abortion. Although it generally takes place late in pregnancy, it may occur during the first or second stage of labor.

The primary cause of premature separation is unknown, but certain predisposing factors apparently contribute to it: chronic hypertensive disease, hypertension of pregnancy, or direct trauma, as in an automobile accident. Pressure on the vena cava from the enlarging uterus may contribute to the problem. It tends to occur after a woman has had more than five pregnancies.

Premature separation may follow a rapid decrease in uterine volume, as occurs with sudden release of amniotic fluid. Since the fetal head is usually so low in the pelvis that it prevents loss of the total volume of the amniotic fluid at one time, a rapid reduction in amniotic fluid does not occur normally.

ASSESSMENT. Because premature separation of the placenta may occur during an otherwise normal labor, you have to always be alert to the amount and kind of vaginal discharge a woman is having in labor. Listen to her description of the kind of pain she is having to detect this grave complication.

Heavy bleeding usually accompanies premature separation of the placenta, but it may not be readily apparent. There will be external bleeding if the placenta separates first at the edges and blood escapes freely from the cervix. If the center of the placenta separates first, however, blood will pool under the placenta and be hidden from view. Blood may infiltrate the uterine musculature (Couvelaire uterus, or uteroplacental apoplexy), forming a hard, boardlike uterus with no apparent, or minimally apparent, bleeding. Shock usually follows quickly because of

Fig. 33-4. Premature separation of the placenta. (From Clinical Education Aid, No. 12, Ross Laboratories, 1963, Columbus, Ohio.)

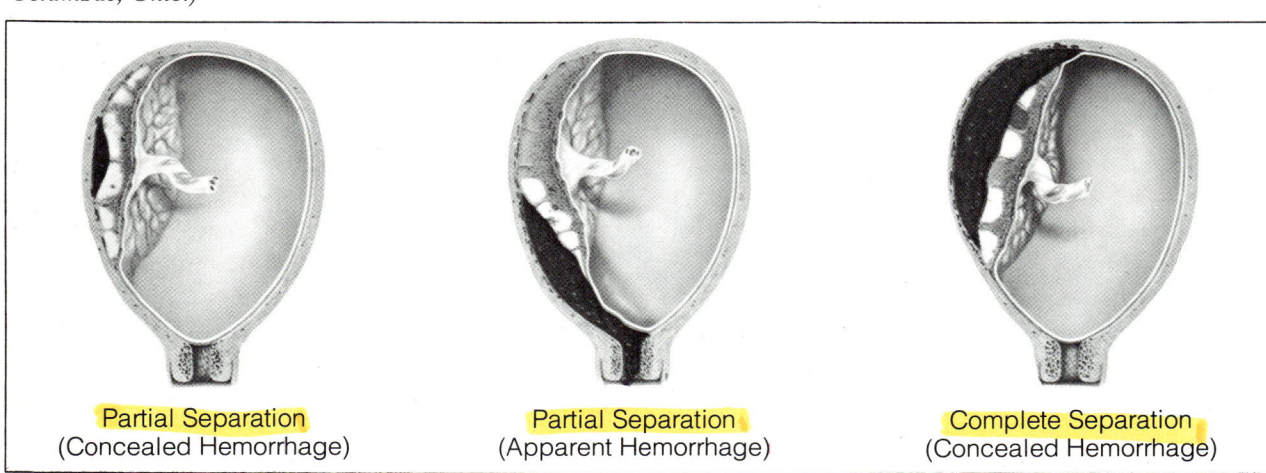

the blood loss, and the uterus becomes tense and rigid to the touch.

The woman may experience a sharp stabbing pain high in the fundus as the initial separation occurs. If labor begins with the separation, each contraction will be accompanied by pain over and above the pain of the contraction. In some women the pain is not evident with contractions but is felt on uterine palpation. If bleeding is extensive, the woman's reserve of blood fibrinogen may be used up in her body's attempt to accomplish effective clot formation. Initial blood work should include not only hemoglobin level, typing, and cross matching but a fibrinogen level to detect the occurrence of disseminated intravascular coagulation syndrome.

If the woman is being admitted after experiencing symptoms at home, you need to know the time the bleeding began, whether or not pain accompanied it, the amount and kind of bleeding, and the woman's actions.

INTERVENTIONS. On her admission to the hospital, give oxygen by mask to the woman to limit fetal anoxia. Fetal heart sounds should be monitored by an external monitor, and maternal vital signs should be recorded to establish baselines and observe progress. The baseline fibrinogen determination is followed by hourly determinations up to delivery. Keep the woman in a lateral, not a supine position to prevent pressure on the vena cava and additional compromising of fetal circulation. Do not do a vaginal or pelvic examination or give an enema in order not to disturb the injured placenta any further.

For better prediction of fetal and maternal outcome, the degrees of placental separation are graded, as shown in Table 33-3.

Unless the separation is minimal (grades 0 and 1) the pregnancy must be terminated. If the premature separation occurs during active labor, rupturing the membranes or assisting labor with intravenous oxytocin may be the method of choice to speed delivery. Rupturing membranes keeps so much blood from being trapped in the myometrium of the uterus wall that it prevents contractions of the uterus. Since membranes are ruptured with just a pinprick opening to allow a slow, steady escape of amniotic fluid, a sudden change in uterine pressure does not encourage more separation. If delivery does not seem imminent, cesarean section is the delivery method of choice.

If the woman has developed disseminated intravascular coagulation, surgery may be a grave risk for her because of the possibility that she will hemorrhage from the surgical incision. Her fibrinogen level must be elevated by the intravenous administration of

Table 33-3. Premature Separation of the Placenta: Degrees of Separation

Grade	Criteria
0	No symptoms of separation were apparent from maternal or fetal signs. The diagnosis that a slight separation did occur is made after delivery when the placenta is examined and a segment of the placenta shows a recent adherent clot on the maternal surface
1	This is minimal separation, but enough to cause vaginal bleeding and changes in the maternal vital signs. No fetal distress or hemorrhagic shock occurs, however
2	This is moderate separation. There is evidence of fetal distress; the uterus is tense and painful on palpatation
3	This is extreme separation. Without immediate interventions, maternal shock and fetal death will result

fibrinogen or cryoprecipitate (which contains fibrinogen). If neither fibrinogen nor cryoprecipitate (cryoprecipitate is the coagulant administered to persons with hemophilia and therefore may not be available in hospitals which do not routinely treat a large number of persons with hemophilia) is at hand, fresh frozen plasma or platelets will aid in restoring clotting function. Administration of heparin (to interfere with clotting at the placenta site and free fibrinogen to take care of systemic clotting needs) may be begun.

Fetal prognosis depends on the extent of the placental separation and the degree of fetal hypoxia. Maternal prognosis depends on how promptly treatment is instituted. Death is caused by massive hemorrhage leading to shock and circulatory collapse or renal failure from the circulatory collapse.

Any woman who has had bleeding prior to delivery is more prone to infection following delivery than the average woman. A woman with a history of premature separation of the placenta needs to be observed closely for the development of infection in the postpartal period.

SHOCK. The process of shock due to blood loss is shown in Fig. 33-5. Note that danger to the fetus occurs not as a last physiological step but at the point the body begins to decrease blood flow to nonessential organs, although the increased blood volume of pregnancy allows more than normal blood loss before hypovolemic shock occurs. It is important to know a baseline blood pressure for pregnant women because it varies so from woman to woman. Women during pregnancy should be told their blood pressure ("Your pressure is 110 over 70—that's normal"; not just

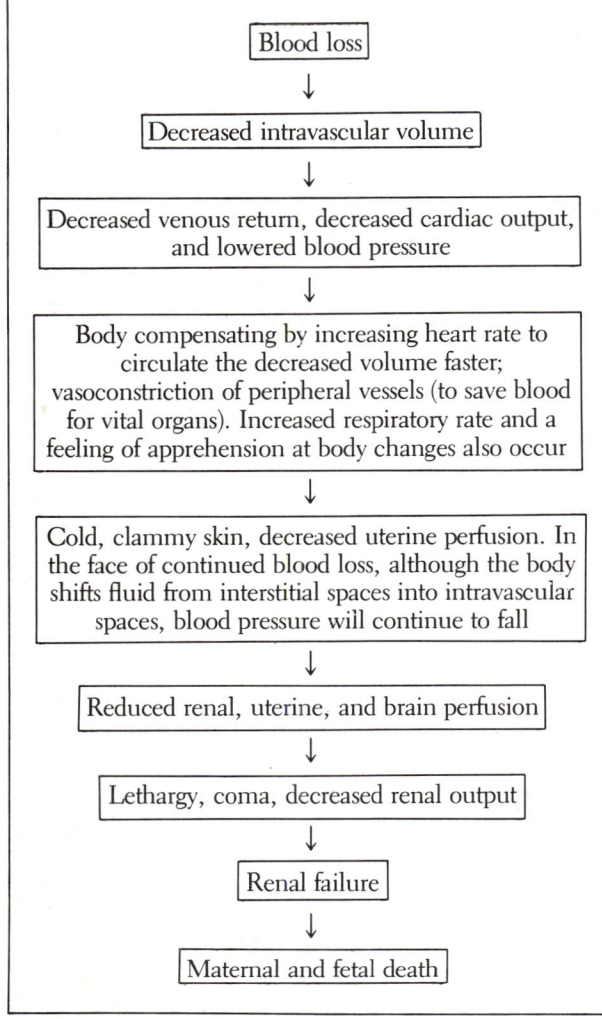

Fig. 33-5. *The process of shock due to blood loss.*

"Your pressure is normal"). Then if blood loss should occur, the woman can be helpful in offering her baseline pressure.

A woman suspected of bleeding should have an intravenous fluid line begun and have a hemoglobin, typing, and cross matching for blood done. She may have a central venous pressure (CVP) catheter inserted. She should never lie on her back but in a lateral position so that there is minimal pressure on the vena cava and as little blood as possible is trapped in the lower extremities. If respirations are rapid, oxygen by mask should be administered and blood gases drawn. Frequent assessments of vital signs and continuous fetal monitoring (by external monitoring device) should be started.

CENTRAL VENOUS PRESSURE. Central venous pressure is an estimate of the pressure or the amount of blood returning to the right atrium of the heart.

A thin polyethylene catheter is inserted at the antecubital fossa into a vein or more directly into the subclavian or internal or external jugular vein. It is threaded forward until it rests in the vena cava just outside the right atrium. The distal end of the catheter is attached to a manometer. This is connected to a bottle and tubing of intravenous fluid (Fig. 33-6). Tape the intravenous tubing and catheter connections securely. If the tubing should come unfastened, the woman could bleed profusely from the site or air could be introduced and form an air embolus. A chest x-ray may be ordered after the insertion to confirm proper catheter placement. Assure the woman that an x-ray is safe for her; be certain the x-ray technician provides a lead screen for her abdomen during the x-ray.

To obtain a CVP reading, ask the woman to lie on her back and lower the bed until it is flat. The 0 marking of the manometer must be at the midaxillary line of the woman's body (a level that is equal to the position of the right atrium). It is a good practice to mark this point on the woman's side with a marking pen so that everyone who will be taking readings uses the same level marker. Next, turn the stopcock on the manometer so intravenous fluid enters the manometer. Fill the manometer to a point over 15 cm H_2O. Next, turn the stopcock so the manometer fluid flows through the catheter into the woman. The fluid in the manometer will fall until it is equal with her central venous pressure. Read the manometer at this point. The column of fluid will never be completely stationary, as it fluctuates with respiratory movements.

Following a reading, change the stopcock position so the intravenous fluid infuses again to prevent the catheter from clotting. Urge the woman to turn onto her side rather than remain on her back so supine hypertension syndrome does not occur.

Normal CVP values range between 5 and 12 cm H_2O. A low reading indicates hypovolemia; a high reading indicates fluid overload or that the right atrium is unable to handle all the blood returning to it. Women admitted with shock from hemorrhage will have a low CVP reading; as they receive a great deal of intravenous fluid to replace blood loss, fluid overload is a possibility.

As important as the fact that the CVP values are within normal limits is the fact that they are not changing. A CVP reading that is gradually changing from 12 cm H_2O to 10 cm H_2O to 7 cm H_2O is still within normal limits. It suggests that bleeding and hypovolemia is occurring, however.

Check the insertion site of a CVP catheter daily to be certain that signs of infection (redness, tenderness)

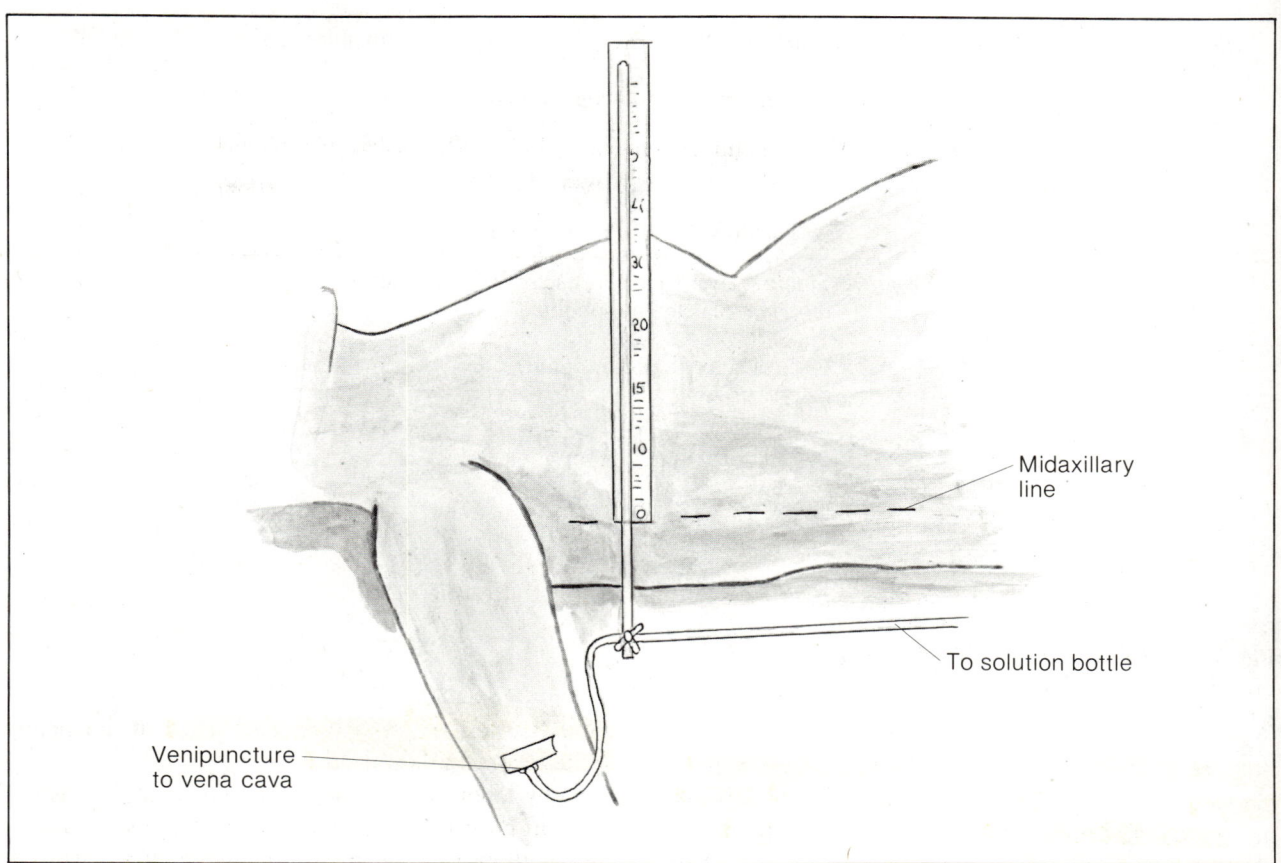

Fig. 33-6. Placement of a central venous pressure catheter. The 0 marking on the manometer should be level with the midaxillary body line.

are not evident. Check connections to be certain that they are secure. If fluid tends to infuse slowly at any time it is generally due to one of two problems: there is a kink in the tubing, or a clot is forming at the catheter tip. Check the tubing for kinking, and rearrange it to a freeflowing position as necessary. If a clot forming appears to be the difficulty, attach a syringe to the catheter and aspirate to draw back the clot. Do not irrigate the catheter, as this might force a clot forward and cause an embolus. In most instances, correcting the hypovolemenia that occurs with bleeding in pregnancy can be accomplished quickly, so these long-term problems of CVP catheters do not usually occur.

DISSEMINATED INTRAVASCULAR COAGULATION. This is an acquired disorder of blood clotting that results from excessive trauma or some similar underlying stimulus. Situations associated with childbirth that may cause it are premature separation of the placenta, hypertension of pregnancy, amniotic fluid embolus, placental retention, septic abortion, retention of a dead fetus, and saline abortion. The mechanism of normal clotting is shown in Fig. 33-7.

Extreme coagulation begins at one point in the circulatory system, depleting the availability of clotting factors from the general circulation. A paradox exists. The person has both a coagulation defect and a bleeding defect at the same time.

Laboratory tests usually show that the platelet count is depressed. The level depends on the rate at which bone marrow is able to replace the platelets. On a blood smear, many of the platelets appear large, evidence of their recent production, and they may appear fragmented from passing through meshes of collecting fibrin. As a rule, both the prothrombin time (PT) and the partial thromboplastin time (PTT) are reduced. Fibrinogen, the final factor necessary to make the clot, will have a markedly low level in serum.

Observe all women with a complication of pregnancy carefully for signs of increased bleeding: skin petechial and oozing from blood drawing sites.

To stop the process of disseminated intravascular coagulation, the underlying insult that began the phenomenon must be halted. When this happens with complications of pregnancy, ending the pregnancy by delivering the fetus and placenta is therefore part of the answer. The marked coagulation can be

```
Factor XII (Hageman factor) + Factor XI (plasma thromboplastin antecedent)
                              ↓
            Factor IX (thrombin thromboplastin component)

Factor IX (thrombin thromboplastin component) + Factor VIII (platelet phospholipid)
            + Factor VIII (antihemophilic factor)
                              ↓
                  Factor X (Stuart-Prower factor)

        Factor X (Stuart-Prower factor) + Factor V (proaccelerin)
                  + platelet phospholipid
                              ↓
                    Factor II (prothrombin)

                           Factor II
                              ↓
                           Thrombin
                              ↓
                          Fibrinogen
                              ↓
                          Fibrin clot
```

Fig. 33-7. The mechanism of blood coagulation.

stopped by the intravenous administration of heparin. Heparin must be given with caution close to delivery or postpartal hemorrhage will occur when the placenta is delivered. Since heparin is one of the few substances that does not cross the placenta, it will not cause coagulation problems in the newborn. Although blood transfusion will be necessary to replace blood loss if bleeding during pregnancy is the beginning stimulus, it may be delayed until after heparin has been administered so that the new blood factors are not also consumed by the coagulation process.

It is bewildering to patients with a disorder such as premature separation of the placenta to have their physician tell them one minute that bleeding is what he is worried about and the next minute hear him order heparin or watch you add heparin to their intravenous line. If they understand the action of heparin—to discourage blood coagulation—it seems as if the physician has ordered exactly the wrong medication (or you are adding exactly the wrong medication). Be certain that the woman and her support person have the whole explanation of what is happening—the woman has an increased risk of hemorrhaging because part of her system has begun coagulation—so that confidence in her caregivers is maintained.

Premature Labor

Labor is premature when it occurs before the 27th week of gestation or before the fetus weighs 2,500 gm. Because babies under 2,500 gm seldom do well in the neonatal period, premature labor accounts for nearly 60 percent of infant deaths.

Why labor begins before the fetus is mature is not clear in most instances. Certain conditions are associated with premature labor. The chance that a woman will deliver prematurely with these conditions is shown in Table 33-4.

Premature labor may begin with rupture of the membranes or *show* from cervical dilatation. Initially the woman may report this as bleeding in pregnancy.

Most women assume that premature labor will be shorter than normal labor. This is not necessarily the case. The first stage of labor, the longest stage, proceeds exactly as it would with a term pregnancy. The second stage of labor *may* be shorter, because a small infant is pushed through the dilated cervix and the birth canal much more easily than one of normal size. Since the second stage takes at most an hour, the difference will be not more than about a half hour to an hour. Unless they have this explanation, women will worry during labor that not only is their labor premature but something is going wrong as well since it is taking so long.

Artificial rupture of membranes is not done as a rule in premature labor until the fetal head is firmly engaged because there is such a potential for prolapse of the cord around the small head. Delaying rupturing of the membranes may prolong the first stage of labor.

Analgesic agents are administered with caution during premature labor. The immature infant will have enough difficulty breathing on his own without

Table 33-4. Risk for Preterm Delivery by Availability of Treatment

Risk Factor	Multiple by Which Risk Is Increased	Estimated Chance That Patient Will Deliver Preterm
Average patient		1 in 15
Prevention possible		
Elective deliveries		
Acute pyelonephritis	3×	1 in 6
Rx may decrease risk		
Twins	5×	1 in 3
Severe preeclampsia	4×	1 in 4
Narcotic use	3×	1 in 5
Low-lying placenta	4×	1 in 4
Partial previa	7×	1 in 2
Total previa	12–13×	1 in 1
Premature rupture of membranes	2–3×	1 in 6
Incompetent cervix	10×	1 in 2
Intensive observation		
Previous stillborn	3×	1 in 5
Previous premature	3×	1 in 5
Previous neonatal death	2–3×	1 in 6
Habitual abortion	3–4×	1 in 4
Vaginal spotting	3–4×	1 in 4

Source. L. D'Angelo and R. J. Sokol, Prematurity: Recognizing patients at risk. *Perinatal Care* 2:16, 1978.

the additional burden of being born sedated. An epidural, spinal, or infiltration anesthetic is preferable because it does not further compromise the infant's ability to initiate respirations at birth. Again, the woman needs to know why a particular method of anesthesia is chosen. She will bear a great deal of pain in the interest of her child's welfare. She will tolerate very little if she feels it is for the convenience of the hospital staff.

Uterine contractions and fetal heart sounds should be monitored during labor. The woman is reassured by the evidence of the monitor screen or graph or the projected sound that, although her infant is likely to be small, his heart tones seem to be of good quality and he is reacting to labor well.

Most women also assume that because the infant's head will be small, an episiotomy will be unnecessary for delivery, and they can therefore escape the discomfort of postpartal stitches. Although the head of a premature infant is smaller than that of a mature infant, it is also more fragile. Excessive pressure might result in a subarachnoid hemorrhage that could be fatal. The woman may therefore need an episiotomy incision larger than normal. Forceps may be used for the same reason at delivery: to reduce pressure on the fetal head.

The cord of the premature infant is usually clamped immediately, rather than after waiting for pulsations to cease. Such an infant has a difficult time excreting the large amount of bilirubin that will be formed if this extra blood is added to the circulation, and the extra amount of blood may overburden his circulatory system.

A woman in premature labor is undergoing an extreme crisis situation. She cannot help asking herself: What did I do to cause this? People who are looking for reasons find them. She may believe that the large meal she ate the night before is responsible because it "crowded out" the fetus. She may remember the old wives' tale that a woman should not raise her hands over her head during pregnancy and associates the premature labor with hanging curtains in the baby's room. She may worry that sexual relations the night before precipitated the premature labor. She needs to be assured that in no way is this her fault. Why labor begins at all is still a mystery. Why it sometimes begins prematurely is even more of a mystery.

Before giving advice or reassurance, it is usually

wise to wait for the woman to bring up the topic first. No one will listen to advice or counsel until she is ready for it. However, reassuring a woman in premature labor that it is not her fault is an exception to the rule. Whether or not the woman is voicing her concern, she is feeling it. While you are taking the initial history or timing contractions, you have an opportunity to bring the concern out in the open. "Did Dr. Smith explain to you that labor sometimes begins early this way without any reason?" "Some women worry that they did something to bring on premature labor. Have you had any thoughts like that?"

Most women in premature labor are anxious to talk to someone who gives them any opening at all. It is true that the child, if too immature, may die. He may have cerebral palsy or some other neurological disorder that low-birth-weight infants are susceptible to. Help the woman to be able to say to herself afterward: I'm sorry this happened. I'd give anything to stop it from happening. I didn't mean for it to happen. *But it was not my fault.*

Be careful, however, that you do not give false reassurances as to the health or weight of the child in your effort to relieve the woman's guilt. On the other hand, do not be overly pessimistic. If she is going to establish a good mother-infant relationship, she needs to perceive her child as viable. Find a middle ground. "The baby's heartbeat is good. Labor is going well. Let's face one thing at a time."

A woman in premature labor needs a support person with her: her husband or the child's father. She is more concerned than the average person about being alone in labor. She imagines that the child will be delivered very easily and worries he may be born in the labor room, so she should have health care personnel with her as well. She feels as if she has disappointed her unborn child, her husband, and herself. She needs frequent assurance during labor that she is breathing well with contractions or just that she is "doing well." She is not mentally prepared for labor; not keyed up to it. During the postpartal period she also needs reassurance that she is doing well. She must rid herself of guilt, in order to be ready to be a mother to her prematurely delivered child.

HALTING PREMATURE LABOR. Until recent years, there were no measures available to halt premature labor. Today, if fetal heart sounds are good, and there is no evidence that bleeding is occurring that will affect maternal or fetal welfare, medical attempts can be made to stop labor.

The first tocolytic agent used with considerable success was ethyl alcohol (ethanol) administered intravenously to the mother. Ethanol apparently blocks the release of oxytocin by the pituitary gland, thereby blocking, or at least delaying, labor contractions. It makes the mother mildly intoxicated, and she may experience light-headedness, vomiting, nausea, or restlessness. Unfortunately, the prescribed level of ethanol must be maintained over a long period of time to halt labor effectively. When administration is discontinued, labor may be initiated again. New knowledge concerning the effect of alcohol on a growing fetus has now made halting labor by the administration of alcohol infusion questionable. An infant delivered while the maternal alcohol level is still elevated may be sleepy and have difficulty initiating respirations. He is more apt to develop respiratory distress syndrome than if the mother's blood alcohol level is allowed to return to normal before delivery.

The fetal heart sounds should be monitored closely while the woman is receiving the infusion, and her contractions should be monitored until they stop. Her vital signs must also be observed closely; a drop in blood pressure or rapid pulse indicates the presence of intrauterine bleeding.

Isoxsuprine hydrochloride (Vasodilan) is an adrenergic substance that acts on beta 2 receptor sites in the uterine myometrium to halt uterine contractions. Unfortunately, isoxsuprine also acts on beta 1 receptor sites in heart muscle causing the adverse cardiovascular side effects of tachycardia and hypotension. If it is administered intravenously, the woman assumes a lateral position to aid blood return to the right side of the heart and minimize hypotension. She is usually well hydrated by an intravenous solution before administration—also to reduce hypotension. Following the initial administration of the drug intravenously, the woman may be maintained on intramuscular or oral forms.

Ritodrine, a muscle relaxant, is similar in action to isoxsuprine but has less beta 1 receptor stimulation. Therefore, it has a milder hypotensive and tachycardiae effect and thus has a wider use than isoxsuprine. After labor has been halted by intravenous administration, women may be maintained contraction-free on oral forms of this drug. Isoxsuprine and ritodrine may both cause hyperglycemia in the mother. An infant born after use of these agents must be observed closely for hypoglycemia in the first hours after birth. Magnesium sulfate may be administered to halt uterine contractions. It appears to interfere with calcium metabolism and therefore makes the uterine muscle less able to contract. For poorly understood reasons, the administration of a corticosteroid to the fetus appears to hurry the formation of lung surfactant. During the time the labor is being chemically halted, therefore, the mother may be given a steroid (bethamethasone) as well to attempt to hurry fetal lung maturity.

If membranes have ruptured or the cervix is over 50 percent effaced and 3 to 4 cm dilated, it is unlikely that labor can be halted. The rupturing of membranes, especially, can be thought of as a point of no return in stopping or delaying labor because of the risk of infection that begins with ruptured membranes.

It is important for the woman to call her physician or the clinic immediately if she begins to experience labor contractions late in pregnancy. Some women wait, unwilling to face the fact that labor contractions have started (an ostrich phenomenon—if I don't think about it, it won't be true). Some diagnose their contractions as nothing more than extremely hard Braxton Hicks contractions and do not seek help until membranes rupture. This is a judgment that the primigravida especially is unable to make. She should call her physician and allow him to make the evaluation. Today, when labor can be delayed until the fetus reaches a level of maturity that will allow him to survive in the outside environment, evaluation and the institution of therapy before membranes rupture is vitally important.

OTHER CAUSES OF BLEEDING DURING PREGNANCY
Coexisting Disease
Cervical or vaginal polyps, vaginal varicosities, carcinoma of the cervix, or blood dyscrasias such as leukemia or decreased platelet levels may cause bleeding during any phase of pregnancy. These are not complications of pregnancy, however, but the reverse: Pregnancy is a complication of the disease entity.

Cervical Ripening
Following a pelvic examination late in pregnancy, a woman may notice some slight vaginal spotting due to the manipulation of the cervix as cervical ripening is occurring. The bleeding should be slight and of short duration if this is the only cause.

Causes of bleeding in pregnancy are summarized in Table 33-5.

Premature Rupture of Membranes
Premature rupture of the membranes is a threat to the fetus, since in most instances labor begins in 24 hours following rupture, and following rupture, infection may occur.

If the fetus is estimated to be mature enough to survive in an extrauterine environment at the time of rupture, and labor does not begin within 24 hours, it is usually induced by intravenous administration of oxytocin. Induction of labor is necessary in this situation because rupture of the membranes destroys the integrity of the uterus, allowing bacteria to enter the uterine cavity through the vagina and infect both mother and fetus. Rupture of the membranes also may permit prolapse of the umbilical cord (extension of the cord out of the uterine cavity into the vagina), particularly if it happens when the fetal head is still too small for a firm cervical fit.

Rupture of the membranes should be ascertained by the history. The woman will usually describe a sudden gush of clear fluid from the vagina, with continued minimal leakage. Amniotic fluid cannot be differentiated from urine by appearance. A nitrazine paper test makes this differentiation, amniotic fluid giving an alkaline reaction and urine an acidic reaction. Occasionally, a woman will mistake urinary incontinence caused by exertion for rupture of the membranes. The nitrazine paper test will reveal the error.

If, after premature rupture of the membranes, labor does not begin, the fetus is too young to survive outside the uterus, and the woman seems capable of following instructions, she is usually allowed to return home. She is instructed to take her temperature twice a day and to report a fever (temperature over 100.4°F) promptly. She should refrain from intercourse and douching because of the danger of introducing infection. The physician may prescribe a prophylactic antibiotic for her in order to prevent infection, although the actual effectiveness of antibiotic prophylaxis is not well documented.

Before the woman is discharged after an initial observation period, be certain that she knows how to read a thermometer (have her demonstrate her knowledge to you) and that she has specific instructions as to what to report. Exactly what degree of temperature should she report? When should she report to her physician for her first checkup?

There are old wives' tales about the agony of labor following premature rupture of the membranes (dry labor). The woman hopes every day that the fetus is at term and that labor will begin, ending the long wait, yet she is afraid to begin labor. She needs a great deal of support for the remainder of the pregnancy and reassurance that because amniotic fluid is always being formed, there is no such thing as a "dry" labor.

Pregnancy-induced Hypertension
Pregnancy-induced hypertension (formerly termed toxemia) occurs in only 5 to 7 percent of all pregnan-

Table 33-5. Summary of Causes of Bleeding During Pregnancy

Time	Type	Cause	Assessment	Cautions
First trimester	Threatened abortion (early—under 16 weeks) (late—16 to 24 weeks)	Unknown; possibly chromosomal, uterine abnormalities	Vaginal spotting, perhaps slight cramping	
	Imminent (inevitable) abortion		Vaginal spotting, cramping, cervical dilatation	
	Missed abortion		Vaginal spotting, perhaps slight cramping; no apparent loss of pregnancy	Disseminated intravascular coagulation associated with missed abortion
	Incomplete abortion		Vaginal spotting, cramping, cervical dilatation, but incomplete expulsion of uterine contents	
	Complete abortion		Vaginal spotting, cramping, cervical dilatation, and complete expulsion of uterine contents	
	Ectopic (tubal) pregnancy	Implantation of zygote at site other than in uterus. Tubal constricture, adhesions associated	Sudden unilateral lower-abdominal-quadrant pain; minimal vaginal bleeding, possible signs of shock or hemorrhage	May have repeat ectopic pregnancy in future if tubal scarring is bilateral
Second trimester	Hydatidiform mole	Abnormal proliferation of trophoblast tissue; unknown cause	Overgrowth of uterus; highly positive HCG test; no fetus present on sonogram; bleeding from vagina of old or fresh blood accompanied by cyst formation	Retained trophoblast tissue may become malignant (choriocarcinoma); follow for 1 year with HCG testing
	Incompetent cervix	Cervix begins to dilate, and pregnancy is lost at about 20 weeks; unknown cause, but cervical trauma from D&C may be associated	Painless bleeding leading to expulsion of fetus	Can have cervical sutures placed to ensure a 2nd pregnancy
Third trimester	Placenta previa	Low implantation of placenta possibly due to uterine abnormality	Painless bleeding at beginning of cervical dilatation	No vaginal exams to minimize placental trauma
	Premature separation of the placenta (abruptio placentae)	Unknown cause; associated with hypertension	Sharp abdominal pain followed by uterine tenderness; vaginal bleeding; signs of maternal shock, fetal distress	Disseminated intravascular coagulation associated with condition
	Premature labor	Unknown cause; increased chance in multiple gestation, maternal illness	"Show"—pink-stained vaginal discharge accompanied by uterine contractions becoming regular and effective	Premature labor may possibly be halted up to the point that membranes rupture

cies in the United States, yet it is the third most frequent cause of maternal mortality, following only hemorrhage and infection. Despite years of research, the cause of hypertensive disease of pregnancy is still unknown. Originally it was called *toxemia* as researchers pictured a toxin of some kind being released by the woman in response to the foreign protein of the growing fetus, the toxin leading to the typical symptoms of hypertension, proteinuria, and edema. No toxin has been identified, however. Poor nutrition (particularly poor protein intake) is strongly correlated with the development of symptoms. A deficiency in pyridoxine (vitamin B_6) has also been suggested as a factor contributing to development of the condition.

A basic cause of the three symptoms is vascular spasm, and why this vascular spasm occurs is difficult to say. As the disorder tends to arise most often in primigravidas and has a high incidence in multiple pregnancy and the pregnancies of women with diabetes mellitus, uterine ischemia due to uterine stretching is a possibility. Normally, blood vessels during pregnancy are very resistant to the effects of pressor substances such as angiotensin and norepinephrine. With hypertension of pregnancy, this reduced responsiveness to blood pressure changes appears to be lost and so blood pressure increases. Whether the change in responsiveness is a primary cause or a secondary result of the vasospasm is still unknown.

The vasospasm reduces the blood supply to organs,

as well as adding to or causing hypertension. This effect is most marked in the kidney, liver, brain, and placenta. Tissue hypoxia may ensue in the maternal vital organs; poor placental perfusion may reduce the fetal nutrient and oxygen supply.

The arterial spasm causes the bulk of the blood volume in the maternal circulation to be pooled in the venous circulation. Measuring hematocrit levels helps to assess the extent of plasma lost to venous volume or the extent of the vasospasm.

The degenerative changes that develop in kidney glomeruli because of the vasospasm lead to increased permeability of the glomerular membrane. This in turn allows the serum proteins albumin and globulin to cross into the urine (proteinuria). The degenerative changes also result in decreased glomerular filtration and lowered urine output. Increased tubular reabsorption of sodium occurs, causing edema. Edema is further increased as more protein is lost, the hydrostatic pressure of the circulating blood falls, and fluid diffuses from the circulatory system into the intracellular spaces to equalize the pressure (edema). Extreme edema will lead to brain edema and convulsions (eclampsia).

ASSESSMENT

Pregnancy-induced hypertension tends to occur more frequently in certain women than in others: in primiparas under 20 years of age; in primiparas over 30 years of age; in women from a low socioeconomic background (perhaps because of poor nutrution); in women who have had five or more pregnancies; in nonwhites; with multiple pregnancy; with underlying disease such as heart disease, diabetes with vessel or renal involvement, and essential hypertension. If symptoms of hypertension of pregnancy are going to develop, they are rarely apparent before the 24th week of pregnancy. With a hydatidiform mole, they appear abnormally early, a clue to the presence of a hydatidiform mole rather than a normal pregnancy.

Any woman who falls into one of these high-risk categories should be considered at high risk for hypertension of pregnancy and should be observed especially carefully for symptoms at prenatal visits. She should be told the symptoms to watch for so that she can call and alert medical personnel if developing symptoms occur between visits.

Classification of Hypertension of Pregnancy

The symptoms of hypertension of pregnancy are divided into three classifications in order that management can be directed toward the correct level.

MILD PREECLAMPSIA. A woman is said to be mildly preeclamptic when her blood pressure rises 30 mm Hg or more systolic or 15 mm Hg or more diastolic above her prepregnancy level, taken on two occasions at least 6 hours apart. The diastolic value of blood pressure is extremely important to note as the rise in diastolic pressure indicates peripheral vascular spasm.

Another method of assessing blood pressure is by recording the mean arterial pressure. By this criterion, a woman is hypertensive when her mean arterial pressure rises 15 mm Hg (taken on two occasions at least 6 hours apart) or is over 100 mm Hg. Mean arterial pressure is one-third of the pulse pressure (the difference between the systolic and diastolic pressure) plus 80. If a blood pressure is 120/70, the mean arterial pressure is $120 - 70 = 50 \div 3 + 80 = 96.6$.

Formerly, a blood pressure of 140/90 was considered the criterion for preeclampsia and it is still a useful "cutoff" point. This general rule for everyone is obviously less meaningful than measuring each woman's blood pressure against her early pregnancy baseline. It is still a rule of thumb to keep in mind, however, if a woman comes for prenatal care for the first time late in pregnancy and there is thus no baseline pressure available for her.

Average blood pressures in American females are shown in Table 14-2. Looking at the average pressure for young Caucasian women, you can see that a woman in the under 20 category could have a blood pressure of 98/61 and still be within normal limits. If her blood pressure were elevated 30 mm Hg systolic and 15 mm Hg diastolic, it would be only 128/76. This is beneath the traditional warning point of 140/90 yet would be hypertension for her.

With mild preeclampsia, in addition to the hypertension the woman has edema in the upper part of the body, rather than just the normal ankle edema of pregnancy, and she has proteinuria (1 or 2+ on a reagent test strip). A gain in weight of more than 2 pounds a week in the second trimester and 1 pound in the last trimester usually indicates tissue fluid retention. This is likely to be the first symptom to appear and is discovered when the woman is weighed at a prenatal visit. Noticeable edema may or may not be present when this sudden increase in weight first occurs.

SEVERE PREECLAMPSIA. A woman has passed from mild to severe preeclampsia when her blood pressure has risen to 160 mm Hg systolic and 110 mm Hg diastolic or above, marked proteinuria is found, and extensive edema is present. Many women show a trace of protein during pregnancy. Proteinuria is said to exist when it registers as at least 1+ or more on a reagent strip. With marked proteinuria, the reading is 3 or 4+.

Occasionally, women have orthotic proteinuria (on long periods of standing, they excrete protein; at bed rest they do not). If a woman has no other signs of hypertension of pregnancy, (no hypertension, no edema) and the urine she offers for testing is not her first morning one, but one she has voided in the physician's office or clinic, asking her to bring in a first morning urine may reveal that this is the problem.

With severe preeclampsia, the extreme edema will be noticeable in the woman's face and hands as "puffiness." It is most readily palpated over bony surfaces, where the sponginess of fluid-filled tissue can best be revealed. Palpating or pressing over the tibia on the anterior leg, the ulnar surface of the forearm, and the cheekbones is a good way to detect edema. Edema is nonpitting if you suspect swelling or puffiness at these points with your palpating finger but you are unable to indent it with your finger. If you are able to indent tissue slightly, this is 1+ edema; moderate indentation is 2+; deep indentation is 3+; indentation so deep it remains as a pit after you remove your finger is 4+ pitting edema.

Further assess edema by asking the woman if she has been aware of any. Most women at the end of pregnancy have edema of the feet at the end of the day. They report this as difficulty fitting into their bedroom slippers or kicking off their shoes at dinnertime and then not being able to put them back on again. This is normal edema. Edema that has progressed to upper extremities or the face is abnormal and what you are listening for. Women report upper-extremity edema as "rings are so tight that I can't get them off"; facial edema as "When I wake in the morning, my eyes are swollen shut" or "I'm unable to talk until I walk around awhile."

Some women have severe epigastric pain and nausea and vomiting possibly due to abdominal edema. Pulmonary edema may cause them to feel short of breath. Cerebral edema will cause visual disturbances such as blurred vision or seeing spots before their eyes. Cerebral edema also gives symptoms of severe headache and marked hyperreflexia. This accumulating edema will reduce their urine output to about 400 to 600 ml per 24 hours.

ECLAMPSIA. This is the severest classification of hypertension of pregnancy. A woman has passed into this third stage when the cerebral edema is so acute that convulsions occur.

At all prenatal visits, all women should be screened for proteinuria, edema, increased blood pressure, and weight. They should be asked too about the symptoms of cerebral and visual disturbance: dizziness, spots before the eyes, or blurring of vision.

Roll-over Test

Roll-over tests should be done routinely on all women at the 28th to 32nd week of pregnancy in an attempt to predict whether hypertension of pregnancy is likely to occur. Have the woman lie on her left side for 15 minutes and establish a baseline diastolic pressure for her (take two readings that have the same diastolic pressure), then have her turn to her back (supine) and measure her blood pressure in that position at 1 and 5 minutes. Use the last heard heart sound for the diastolic reading in both positions. The woman who has an increase of diastolic pressure of 20 mm Hg or more in the supine position will probably develop hypertension of pregnancy. She will need closer follow-up during this pregnancy than will the average woman.

INTERVENTIONS
Mild Preeclampsia

BED REST. If edema is the only symptom present, additional bed rest may be all that is necessary for treatment. Sodium tends to be excreted at a more rapid rate during rest than during activity. The result is lowered levels of plasma sodium, and diuresis occurs.

Rest should always be in a lateral recumbent position to avoid uterine pressure on the vena cava and prevent supine hypotension syndrome. If the woman is able to rest at home, she can remain at home. If there is a question as to her compliance, she may be hospitalized even at this early date. In one study, when nulliparas with beginning signs of preeclampsia were hospitalized to ensure bed rest, the perinatal mortality rate was 9 per 1,000. Among women who left the hospital against advice, the perinatal mortality was 129 per 1,000 [16]. The increased mortality may be due to more than the difference in bed rest, as the reason the women left the hospital may reflect overall poor compliance to medical regimens.

DIET. Because the woman is losing protein in the urine, she needs a high-protein diet. Mild salt restriction (no added salt at the table; no extremely salty foods) may be advised. Stringent restriction of salt may activate the angiotensin system and result in increased blood pressure, compounding the problem.

DIURETICS. For years, diuretics to evacuate fluid and decrease the edema were routinely prescribed in preeclampsia, but their use in this condition is now contraindicated. Diuretics, particularly the thiazides, are effective in decreasing the reabsorption of sodium, thus lowering levels of sodium in the plasma. Fluid then shifts from the extracellular spaces into the circulatory system and is excreted. Edema is thereby reduced, but plasma volume that is already depleted will be depleted even further and poor placental perfusion may result.

Diuretics also stimulate the release of renin. This increases the permeability of glomerular vessels, leads to increased proteinuria, and activates angiotensin, which raises the blood pressure. Diuretics may therefore actually worsen preeclampsia.

EMOTIONAL SUPPORT. It is difficult for a woman to appreciate the potential seriousness of her symptoms because they are so vague at this point. Neither high blood pressure nor protein in urine is something that she can see or feel. She is aware that edema is present, but it seems unrelated to the pregnancy; it is her hands that are swollen, not a body area near her growing child. Many women therefore take instructions such as getting rest at this time rather lightly.

Women are also used to having severe disorders treated with some form of medication, and their physician has given them none here. How can this be really serious? Furthermore, it is not always easy to comply with the instruction to get additional rest during the day. Forty percent of women of childbearing age work outside their home. About half the women you talk to, therefore, are being asked to stop work in order to rest more. Physicians may give that instruction lightly, because they may not view a woman's earnings as adding greatly to a couple's basic income; they are only "frosting" or "egg money." In reality, the contribution of most working women goes not for luxuries but for a good part of the mortgage or rent or car payments. If a woman is not married, her income is probably her sole support. Asking her to stop work, then, when she may be evicted, or have a loan or a house or a car foreclosed because of missed payments, on the basis of a few vague symptoms—a little swelling, a little headache—is asking a great deal.

You cannot solve people's financial problems, but ask enough questions of the woman so that you can be aware of her problem. A question such as "What will it mean to your family if you have to quit work?" brings it out in the open.

People can make arrangements with loan companies or banks to make partial payments or delayed payments during periods of hardship. The couple may have savings they were planning to use for something else that can carry them over during this time. Perhaps they can borrow money or change their living arrangements. In any event, they need to begin to consider what extra rest during pregnancy will mean to them. People cannot begin to solve problems until they are aware of them.

A woman with other children must think through her day and make changes in order to get additional rest. The mother who spends considerable time chauffering school-age children to scouts, dancing lessons, and so forth may have to investigate car pooling. A mother may have to drop being a Brownie leader, or ask children or husband for more help cleaning or cooking. Again, the woman needs to understand that although the symptoms she is experiencing are mild they may be forecasting an extremely serious disorder. Ask, "What will it mean to your other children or your husband if you have to rest?" to allow her to face this problem.

Women with beginning signs of hypertension will be seen about every two weeks now for the remainder of pregnancy. Be certain the woman understands that if symptoms worsen before two weeks she should not wait the two weeks but call for an earlier appointment. There is little cure for eclampsia of pregnancy. Prevention at the early stage is what is important.

Severe Preeclampsia

If the preeclampsia is severe (systolic blood pressure over 160 mm Hg, diastolic blood pressure over 110 mm Hg, or both on two occasions 6 hours apart after the woman has been on bed rest; extensive edema, marked proteinuria—3+ or 4+—cerebral or visual disturbances, or marked hyperreflexia; oliguria—400 ml per 24 hours or less), hospitalization is strongly recommended. If the pregnancy is 36 weeks or more in length, or fetal maturity is confirmed by amniocentesis, induction of labor may be undertaken. If the pregnancy is less than 36 weeks or the amniocentesis reveals immature lung function, interventions will be instituted to attempt to alleviate the symptoms and allow the fetus to come to term.

BED REST. With hospitalization, bed rest can be enforced, and the woman can be observed closely. The woman with severe preeclampsia should be admitted to a private room so she may rest undisturbed by a roommate. She should lie in a left lateral recumbant position as much as possible. She should be away from the sound of women in labor or the crying of infants on a postpartal unit. A loud noise such as a crying baby or a dropped tray of equipment may be sufficient to trigger a convulsion, initiating eclampsia.

The room should be darkened; a bright light can also trigger convulsions. However, the room should not be so dark that you need to use a flashlight. Having to shine a flashlight beam into the woman's eyes is the stimulus you are trying to avoid.

Some physicians order *no visitors* for the woman, but this type of order needs to be evaluated individually. Social visitors should be restricted, but support people (husband, father of the child, mother, or older children) may enable her to rest more readily by assuring her that they are managing at home and are as interested in her continuing the pregnancy as is she.

MATERNAL MONITORING. The woman's blood pressure should be taken at least every 4 hours to detect any increase, which is a warning that her condition is worsening.

A urinary catheter is usually inserted for recording of output and comparison with intake. Urinary output should be over 600 ml per 24 hours; an output lower than this means that oliguria is present. Urinary proteins and specific gravity should be measured and recorded with voidings or hourly by catheter. Urine should be saved for 24-hour protein determinations and possibly for estriol determination to evaluate fetal well-being (see Chap. 13). A woman with mild preeclampsia spills about 0.5 gm of protein every 24 hours (1+ on an individual specimen); a woman with severe preeclampsia spills about 5 gm per 24 hours (3+ or 4+ on individual specimens).

Weight should be measured daily at the same time each day for evaluation of tissue fluid retention. The woman should bring a light duster or bathrobe with her to wear at every weighing, so that any change in weight does not merely reflect a change in the weight of her clothes. A daily hematocrit level should be determined to monitor blood concentration, an index of how well fluid is being retained in the intravascular system. Plasma estriol and electrolyte levels will also be measured frequently. The woman's optic fundus should be assessed daily for signs of arterial spasm, edema, or hemorrhage.

FETAL MONITORING. The fetal heart rate may be assessed by continuous fetal external monitor, but generally simple stethoscope auscultation at about 4-hour intervals is sufficient at this stage of management. The woman may have a nonstress test done once weekly to assess placentouterine sufficiency (see Chap. 13). Urinary estriol levels may be deceptively low in the woman with hypertension of pregnancy because her overall output is decreased and must be assessed in light of this reduced output.

SAFETY. The side rails on the woman's bed should be raised to keep her from falling should she have a convulsion. She needs to be told that the side rails have been raised not to imprison her but for her safety and the safety of her unborn child. With this explanation, a side rail rule is not difficult to enforce, and protection is provided when no nurse is present.

DIET. The woman needs a high-protein, moderate-salt, but not salt-free, diet to compensate for the protein she is losing in the urine.

MEDICATION. To encourage complete bed rest, a barbiturate such as phenobarbital, or a tranquilizer such as diazepam (Valium) may be prescribed. A fluid line to serve as an emergency route for drug administration should be initiated and maintained. It is important that the insertion site be observed carefully for infiltration because if the woman is heavily sedated she may not be aware that the site is swelling; irritation from an infiltrated intravenous site is the sort of irritation that can trigger a convulsion in a severely preeclamptic woman.

A hypotensive drug such as hydralazine (Apresoline) may be prescribed to reduce the hypertension. Apresoline causes peripheral dilatation and hence no interference with placental circulation. Apresoline may cause tachycardia; thus not only blood pressure but pulse as well should be assessed following its administration. Diazoxide (Hyperstat) or cryptenamine (Unitensen) may be used for their ability to produce rapid decreases in blood pressure. Diazoxide is not used for long-term administration as it tends to cause hyperglycemia. If vasopressors are used, diastolic pressure should not be lowered below 90 mm Hg or inadequate placental perfusion may occur.

Despite many new drugs suggested for the treatment of preeclampsia or eclampsia, magnesium sulfate is still the drug of choice in most institutions. Magnesium sulfate is actually a cathartic. It reduces edema by causing a shift in fluid from the extracellular spaces into the intestine. It also has a central nervous system depressant action (it blocks peripheral neuromuscular transmissions) that lessens the possibility of convulsions and a vasodilating effect that lowers blood pressure. Magnesium sulfate may be given intramuscularly or by a slow intravenous infusion.

To effect immediate reduction of the blood pressure, magnesium sulfate may be begun intravenously (a dose of 4 gm [40 ml] of a 10% solution in 100 ml of 5% dextrose in water). Given intravenously, the drug begins to act immediately but the effect lasts only 30 to 60 minutes.

Following the initial reduction of blood pressure, magnesium sulfate is generally administered intramuscularly. The dose is large (5 gm [10 ml] of a 50% solution every 4 hours). This must be given deeply so that absorption can take place. To reduce the pain of the injection, 1% procaine can be added to each injection.

In order for magnesium sulfate to act as an anticonvulsant, blood serum levels are maintained at 4.0 to 7.5 mEq per liter. If serum levels rise to 10 mEq per liter, deep tendon reflexes fade; at 15 mEq per liter, respiratory paralysis occurs; at 25 mEq per liter, total body paralysis takes place.

Urine output must be observed carefully when a woman is receiving magnesium sulfate since magnesium is excreted from the body almost entirely through the urine. If severe oliguria occurs (less than 100 ml in 4 hours), excessively high blood levels of magnesium will be seen. The most evident symptom of overdosage with magnesium sulfate administration is depression of respirations and deep tendon reflexes. Respirations should be above 16 per minute, and deep tendon reflexes should be checked to be certain they are present before the next dose of drug is administered or every hour if a continuous intravenous infusion is being used.

The easiest deep tendon reflex to check is the patellar reflex (knee jerk). With the woman in a supine position, ask her to bend her knee slightly and to then relax her leg. Place your left hand under her knee to support the knee. Locate the patellar tendon in the midline just below the knee cap. Strike it firmly and quickly with a reflex hammer. The technique for eliciting a patellar reflex is shown in Fig. 33-8. The method by which deep tendon reflexes are scored is shown in Table 33-6. If an epidural block has been given you must assess with a biceps reflex.

A third assessment that should be done before further magnesium sulfate is administered is measurement of the urinary output. If this is not over 30 ml per hour (specific gravity 1.018 or better), the dose should be questioned.

Table 33-6. Scoring of Deep Tendon Reflexes

Score	Description
4+	Hyperactive; very brisk; abnormal
3+	Brisker than average but not abnormal
2+	Average response
1+	Somewhat diminished response but not abnormal
0	No response; hypoactive; abnormal

Prevention of overdosing from magnesium sulfate therapy by conscientious checking of urine output and tendon reflexes and respiratory rate is an important nursing responsibility. In addition to these measures, when magnesium sulfate is being given, a solution of 10% calcium gluconate should be kept ready nearby for immediate administration. Calcium is the specific antidote for magnesium toxicity.

At the time of delivery, the anesthesiologist must be alerted to the fact that the woman has been receiving magnesium sulfate. If magnesium sulfate is given intravenously within 2 hours of delivery, the baby may be born severely depressed because the drug crosses the placenta. Since this effect is rarely seen with intramuscular injection, however, that is the method of administration generally used close to delivery. Because magnesium sulfate is a neuromuscular blocking agent, the anesthesiologist must be cautious in administering other neuromuscular blocking agents such as succinylchloride (used to give relaxation for intubation with general anesthesia).

Eclampsia

SYMPTOMS. Degeneration of the woman's condition from severe preeclampsia to eclampsia occurs when edema worsens. Cerebral irritation results from the

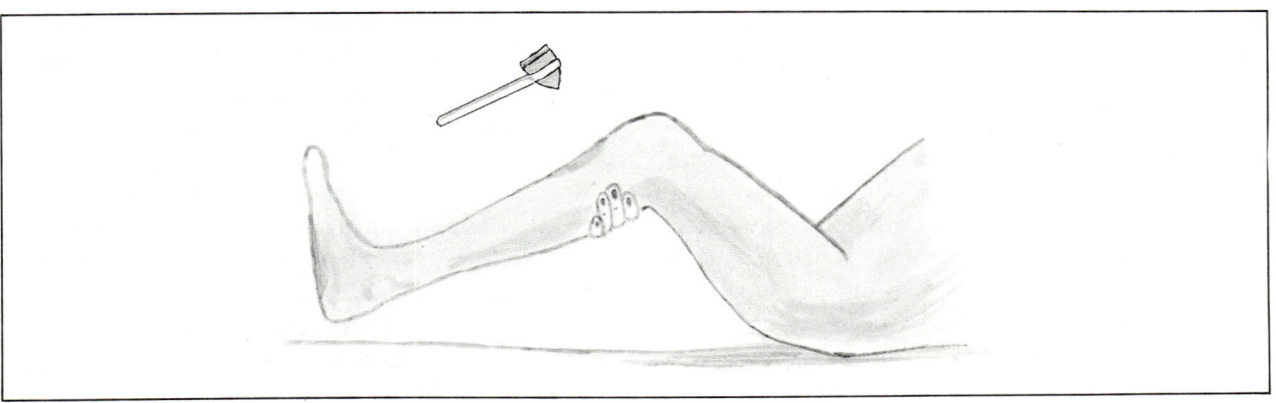

Fig. 33-8. Eliciting a patellar reflex. The patellar tendon is tapped with a percussion hammer.

increasing cerebral edema. This change is usually marked by discernible signals. The woman's temperature may rise sharply, to 39.4° or 40°C (103° or 104°F). Her blood pressure also may rise suddenly. She may notice blurring of vision or severe headache (from the increased cerebral edema). She may have hyperactive reflexes. She may have a premonition that "something is happening." There may be epigastric pain and nausea as a result of vascular congestion of the liver. Urinary output may slacken abruptly, to less than 30 ml per hour.

PHASES AND TREATMENT OF CONVULSIONS. An eclamptic convulsion is a grand mal convulsion. Following the preliminary signals, all the muscles of the woman's body contract. Her back arches, her arms and legs stiffen, and her jaw closes abruptly. She may bite her tongue from the rapid closing of her jaw. Respirations will be halted, since her thoracic muscles are held in contraction. This phase of the convulsion, called the tonic phase, lasts about 20 seconds. It seems longer because the woman may grow cyanotic from the cessation of respiration.

Oxygen administered by face mask may be needed to protect the fetus during this interval. The woman should be turned on her side; or, even though she is almost at term, she can be placed on her abdomen to allow secretions to drain from her mouth. An external fetal heart monitor should be attached if it is not already in place to follow the condition of the fetus. Inserting a tongue blade between the woman's teeth to prevent her from biting her tongue is not recommended. The convulsion occurs suddenly, and thus the action that causes the jaw to clench shut has taken place before you can put a tongue blade between her teeth. Attempting to do so *after* the contraction has occurred rarely has any therapeutic effect and leads to broken teeth, scraped gums, bitten fingers, or broken tongue blades.

Following the tonic phase, all the muscles of the body begin to contract and relax, contract and relax, causing the woman's extremities to flail wildly. She inhales and exhales irregularly as her thoracic muscles contract and relax. She may aspirate the saliva that collected in her mouth during the tonic phase if she was not placed on her side or abdomen. She blows through the collected saliva and any blood that is present in her mouth, causing the "foaming at the mouth" sometimes associated with convulsions. Her bladder and bowel muscles contract and relax; incontinence of urine and feces may occur. Although she begins to breathe during this stage, the breathing is not entirely effective. Her color may remain cyanotic and she may need continued oxygen therapy, not for herself, but for the fetus. This is the clonic stage of a convulsion, and it lasts approximately 1 minute. Magnesium sulfate or diazepam (Valium) may be administered intravenously as an emergency measure at this time.

The third stage is a postictal state. The woman cannot be roused except by painful stimuli for at least an hour and sometimes up to 4 hours. Extremely close observation is as necessary during the postictal stage as it is during the first two stages. Labor may begin during this period, and because the woman is unconscious, she is unable to report the sensation of contractions. Also, the painful stimuli of contractions may initiate another convulsion. Check for contractions by resting your hand on her abdomen and feeling for tenseness. A monitor to record uterine contractions may be attached to obtain this information, provided the device does not appear to irritate the woman. Fetal heart sounds should be continuously monitored. Check for vaginal bleeding every 15 minutes; the convulsions may have caused premature separation of the placenta. Evidence that separation may have occurred will appear first on the fetal heart sound record; vaginal bleeding will strengthen the presumption.

The woman should be regarded as and treated like any comatose patient. She should remain on her side, so that secretions can drain from her mouth. She should be given nothing to eat or drink. Remember that in coma hearing is the last sense lost and the first one regained. Be aware that when you are discussing the woman's condition she may be able to hear you.

TERMINATION OF PREGNANCY. If the gestation age is over 36 weeks, a delivery decision will be made as soon as the woman's condition stabilizes, which is usually about 12 to 24 hours after the convulsion. There is some evidence that the fetus does not continue to grow after eclampsia occurs. Thus, terminating the pregnancy at this point is appropriate for both mother and child. For an unexplained reason, fetal lung maturity appears to advance rapidly with hypertension of pregnancy (possibly from the intrauterine stress), so even though the fetus is younger than 36 weeks, the lecithin-sphingomyelin (L-S) ratio of amniotic fluid may be mature.

The preferred method is vaginal delivery using a pudendal block. Because the vascular system is low in volume, the woman may become very hypotensive with conduction anesthesia such as an epidural block.

Cesarean section is always more hazardous for the fetus, who may already be under sufficient strain. Further, the woman with eclampsia is not a good candidate for general anesthesia and surgery. Rupture of the membranes or induction of labor by intravenous oxytocin may be instituted. If this is not effective and the fetus appears to be in imminent danger, a cesarean section will have to be done.

PROGNOSIS. Eclampsia can result in death of the mother from cerebral hemorrhage, circulatory collapse, or renal failure. Fetal prognosis in eclampsia is poor because of hypoxia and consequent acidosis. If premature separation of the placenta occurs, the prognosis is even graver. If the fetus must be delivered before term, all the risks of the immature infant will be faced. In preeclampsia, perinatal mortality is approximately 10 percent. If eclampsia develops, the mortality increases to about 25 percent.

Pregnancy-induced hypertension may occur up to 10 to 14 days after delivery, although most postpartal hypertension occurs in the first 48 hours following delivery. Women need follow-up care in the postpartal period to detect residual hypertensive or renal disease.

A summary of the classification of hypertension of pregnancy is shown in Table 33-7.

PSYCHOLOGICAL ASPECTS OF CARE. A woman hospitalized with severe hypertension needs almost constant nursing observation. Stress is a stimulus capable of increasing blood pressure and possibly evoking convulsions in the woman with severe preeclampsia. She should receive clear explanations of what is happening and what is planned for her. If she understands the importance of complete bed rest, she will tend not to "cheat" and get out of bed. She will accept the fact that, in the interest of maximal rest and minimal stimulation, visitors must be restricted to just her husband or, if there is no husband, to one other person. She must have opportunities to express how she feels about what is happening, how bewildered she is because the few simple symptoms she noticed two weeks ago (increase in weight, increasing edema) have now developed into a syndrome that may be lethal to her baby and possibly to her. She needs to talk about the things she did during pregnancy that she believes may have brought on her condition. Perhaps the night before her symptoms first became apparent she ate a half box of potato chips. Could that have set off this event? The first three months of the pregnancy she wished she was not pregnant. Could that have been responsible?

The woman may want to discuss the financial impact of the hospitalization. She planned to work until the end of pregnancy. She planned on a three-day hospitalization, and now she may be here for a month. She cannot afford a private room. Where is the money coming from?

Table 33-7. Summary of the Classification of Pregnancy-Induced Hypertension

Classification	Description
Mild preeclampsia	Blood pressure 140/90 or an increase of 30 mm Hg systolic, 15 mm Hg diastolic above pre-pregnancy level
	Proteinuria (1+ or 2+)
	Mild edema in face or upper extremities
	Sudden weight gain due to edema
Severe preeclampsia	Blood pressure of 160/110 mm Hg
	Marked proteinuria (3+ or 4+)
	Extensive edema
Eclampsia	Convulsions have occurred

Perhaps there are other children at home. Who will look after them? Who will remind them to brush their teeth? Who will remember that the youngest is afraid of the dark and the oldest needs help with his math? These are all real problems that prevent a woman from resting.

A woman with severe pregnancy-induced hypertension should not have a telephone in her room, because a ringing phone is a sudden, sharp stimulus, and all such stimuli are to be avoided. She should be encouraged to write short notes to her children unless she is too heavily sedated to do so. Her older children should be encouraged to send her notes or school drawings.

If the woman cannot be freed of these worries even with help, it is a fallacy to think that she is calmly waiting for her pregnancy to come to term.

Chronic Hypertensive Vascular Disease

Women with chronic hypertensive disease come into pregnancy with elevated blood pressure. The hypertension is usually associated with arteriosclerosis or renal disease. It tends to be a problem of the older pregnant woman. Retinal changes may be apparent on physical examination. Deterioration of the renal glomeruli may have occurred, resulting in chronic proteinuria. Fetal well-being may be compromised by poor placental perfusion during the pregnancy.

Usually, the woman who enters pregnancy with slight hypertension will have an additional elevation of blood pressure with pregnancy and is prone to the development of edema and proteinuria. It is difficult to differentiate this increased blood pressure from developing preeclampsia if the woman comes to the clinic or office late in pregnancy for her first prenatal checkup.

Women with chronic hypertensive vascular disease must be followed by an internist during pregnancy, as well as by an obstetrician. If the blood pressure becomes extremely high, complete bed rest for the entire pregnancy may be necessary, and the pregnancy may have to be terminated in order to prevent a cerebral vascular accident. Since women with hypertension are advised not to take birth control pills, contraception may be a problem in the postpartal period. The infants of women with chronic hypertension tend to have retarded fetal growth.

Diabetes and Pregnancy

Unlike most diseases, diabetes in pregnancy is increasing in frequency. The reason is that before insulin was made synthetically (1921), diabetic women either failed to survive to reach childbearing age, or were infertile, or had spontaneous abortions early in pregnancy.

Now that diabetes can be well controlled, three new problems have developed: (1) how to bring a diabetic woman through a pregnancy in good control, (2) how to protect her infant in utero from the adverse effects of the diabetes, and (3) how to care for the infant in the first 24-hour period after birth until his insulin-glucose regulatory mechanism stabilizes. Many women with diabetes cannot take birth control pills because the pills cause problems with glucose level control. Thus, family planning may be a fourth concern in a diabetic woman.

Diabetic complications occur in about 1 in every 200 pregnancies. The perinatal infant mortality for pregnancies complicated by diabetes is between 10 and 30 percent, an inordinately high figure. When diabetic control is poor, the woman is more prone to pregnancy-induced hypertension, hydramnios, and infection than other women. Infants of diabetic women tend to be large (over 9 pounds) on account of overstimulation of pituitary growth hormone during intrauterine life and excessive subcutaneous fat deposits. A large-size infant may cause delivery problems at the end of the pregnancy.

For these reasons, the woman with diabetes should come to the obstetrician for care before she becomes pregnant. He can discuss with her the problems that arise in diabetic women with pregnancy and why early diagnosis of pregnancy and frequent follow-up care during pregnancy are important. He should consult with the woman's family physician to determine the best insulin control program for her during pregnancy.

ASSESSMENT

All women who have a history of large babies (9 pounds or more), unexplained fetal loss, congenital anomalies in previous pregnancies, unexplained natal or neonatal loss, obesity, or a family history of diabetes should be checked for diabetes on every prenatal visit. Such women may have preclinical diabetes or gestational diabetes, that is, diabetes so labile that it becomes clinical only under the stress of pregnancy. Although the diabetes arises with the pregnancy and the symptoms fade again at the end of pregnancy, there is a high incidence of recurrence of diabetes in these women at a later date. True diabetes develops in about 7 percent of such women within six months of delivery; in 28 to 40 percent within 5½ years. Overt juvenile diabetes may occur for the first time during the pregnancy if the woman is very young.

GLUCOSE-INSULIN CHANGES IN PREGNANCY

All women experience a number of changes in the glucose-insulin regulatory system during pregnancy. Glomerular filtration of glucose is increased, causing glycosuria, the rate of insulin secretion is increased, and the fasting blood sugar is lowered. The woman appears to have a decreased insulin sensitivity (that is, insulin does not seem normally effective during pregnancy), a phenomenon that is probably caused by the presence of the hormone human placental lactogen (chorionic somatomammotropin). This resistance to insulin prevents the blood sugar in a normal pregnancy from falling to dangerous limits, despite the increased insulin secretion. It causes difficulty for the pregnant diabetic woman in that she must increase her insulin dosage.

Glucose Tolerance Tests

A 2-hour postprandial or a 1-hour glucose tolerance test may be done in early pregnancy to rule out diabetes. For the 1-hour test, the woman fasts overnight. In the physician's office or clinic she is given an oral 50-gm glucose load, and 60 minutes later a venous blood sample is taken for blood sugar. With both of these tests, if blood sugar is under 150 gm per 100 ml of blood, glucose management is normal. If full laboratory facilities are available, a standard glucose tolerance test with blood drawn at 10, 20, 30, 40, 50, and 60 minutes may be done.

At subsequent visits, urine is tested for glucose by means of a dipstick method, or fasting blood sugar levels are drawn. Late in pregnancy, and during the postpartal period, lactose, the sugar of breast milk, may spill into the urine and cause a positive reaction to Benedicts' solution or Clinitest. Clinistix and Tes-Tape, on the other hand, because they measure only glucose, not all sugars, in urine, give a negative reaction to lactose. Many juvenile diabetic patients are taught to use Clinitest tablets. Thus, during pregnancy, they not only have to change their insulin dosage (a change that brings a feeling of insecurity) but also must change the method of urine testing.

INTERVENTIONS

White [43] has divided diabetes into various categories in order to predict pregnancy outcome. These are shown in Table 33-8. The pregnancy outcome becomes less successful with more diabetic involvement in the mother. In class A, fetal survival is high. Infants of mothers in classes D and E may have a perinatal mortality as high as 25 percent. Class F and class R women may have a perinatal mortality close to 100 percent. Women with diabetes mellitus this severe are generally advised not to become pregnant.

Both women with gestational diabetes and those with overt diabetes need more frequent prenatal visits than the average woman. Those with overt diabetes are usually seen weekly (preferably in a high-risk diabetic clinic, where an internist, an obstetrician, a nurse, and a nutritionist work in combination). Women with gestational diabetes are usually briefly hospitalized to see whether insulin will be necessary early in pregnancy. Then they are followed every week or two during pregnancy.

GESTATIONAL DIABETES

Diabetes all by itself is a stress to a woman. Developing symptoms of diabetes during pregnancy constitutes extreme stress. It is helpful to know what the woman's concept or knowledge of diabetes is. Does anyone in the family have diabetes? How does she perceive this person—as mainly ill or predominantly well? If there is an Aunt Sally in the family who can never come to dinner because she has to have all of her food specially prepared, who cannot drive her car because she is afraid she might faint, who cannot go on vacation because she does not want to be any distance from her doctor, what diabetes means to this woman during pregnancy is totally different from what it means if Aunt Sally holds a full-time job, volunteers in community or political activities, and—oh, by the way—has diabetes. In one instance she has just been told that she has a disease that is a

Table 33-8. Classification of Diabetes Mellitus

Class	Description
Class A	Pregnant woman whose glucose tolerance test is only slightly abnormal. Dietary regulation is minimal; no insulin is required
Class B	Pregnant women whose diabetes is of less than 10 years' duration or whose disease began at age 20 or older. There is no vascular involvement
Class C	Pregnant women whose diabetes began between ages 10 and 19 or whose disease has lasted from 10 to 19 years. There is minimal vascular involvement
Class D	Pregnant women whose diabetes has lasted 20 years or more or whose disease began before age 10. There is greater vascular involvement than in class C
Class E	Pregnant women in whom calcification of the pelvic arteries has been demonstrated on x-ray
Class F	Pregnant women whose diabetes has caused nephropathy
Class R	Pregnant women with active retinitis proliferans

Source. P. White, Pregnancy and Diabetes. In A. Marble et al. (Eds.), *Joslin's Diabetes Mellitus* (11th ed.). Philadelphia: Lea & Febiger, 1971.

minor inconvenience; in the other she has been given a lifelong sentence of disability.

Most women with gestational diabetes are identified because they have a positive glucose urine test at a prenatal visit. A postprandial test or glucose tolerance test is then scheduled, and the diagnosis is established. Be certain that the woman is provided some time to talk about what the diagnosis means to her before she leaves after this. Thinking that a baby who is not even born yet has made one incapacitated is not a healthy beginning to maternal-child bonding.

Dietary management during pregnancy is generally all that is necessary for most women with gestational diabetes, although insulin administration may lower morbidity in the newborn.

The primary problem for the pregnant diabetic woman is control of the balance between insulin and blood glucose in order to prevent acidosis. Acidosis is the chief threat to the fetus.

If insulin amount is insufficient, glucose cannot be utilized by body cells. The cells register their glucose want, and the liver quickly converts stored glycogen to glucose to increase the blood glucose level. Because of the insulin insufficiency, the body cells still cannot use the glucose, and the blood glucose levels continue to rise (hyperglycemia).

When the level of blood sugar of a pregnant woman is 100 to 150 mg per 100 ml, the kidneys begin to excrete quantities of glucose in the urine in an attempt to lower the level (glycosuria). Because of the heavy osmotic action, the increased amount of glucose in the urine reduces fluid absorption in the kidney, and large quantities of fluid are lost in urine (polyuria).

Dehydration begins to occur; the blood becomes concentrated, and the blood volume may fall. Cells do not receive adequate oxygen, and anaerobic metabolic reactions cause large stores of lactic acid to pour out of muscles into the bloodstream. Fat is mobilized from fat stores, metabolized, and poured into the blood as ketone bodies. Ketone bodies are acid (the best example is acetone). These two acid sources affect the pH of the blood. The woman is in metabolic acidosis.

Protein stores are next tapped by the body as it attempts to find a source of energy for body cells. Protein catabolism reduces the supply of protein to body cells. Cell catabolism results in the loss of potassium and sodium from the body.

Diabetes in poor control therefore interferes with the glucose, fat, and protein metabolism of the body. It creates an environment in which there is poor placental perfusion and, because of the acidosis, one that may be toxic to the fetus.

DIET

Dietary control or maintaining an adequate glucose intake so that hypoglycemia does not occur on account of the daily dose of insulin may be extremely difficult early in pregnancy because of nausea and vomiting. A 2200-calorie diet (30 cal per kilogram ideal body weight), divided into three meals and three snacks is a good regimen for a diabetic woman during pregnancy. Keeping calories evenly distributed during the day helps to keep the blood glucose constant.

Even though the woman is overweight, she should not be encouraged to reduce her intake below 1800 calories during pregnancy. A diet too low in carbohydrate causes breakdown of fat, which produces acidosis. In the diabetic woman, the weight of the infant is directly correlated with the weight the woman gained in pregnancy. She must thus be extremely diet-conscious and keep her weight gain to a suitable amount (about 25 pounds), in the hope of limiting the size of her infant and making a vaginal delivery possible.

INSULIN

Because of the change in body metabolism, the woman's insulin dosage may have to be changed during pregnancy. If she has been taking one particular kind of insulin and a specified dosage for a long time before the pregnancy, changing the type and dosage is frightening to her. She has no confidence in other types of insulin and other dosages. She needs to be informed that reregulation is a necessity for pregnancy because of the changes in her metabolism.

Early in pregnancy she may need less insulin because the fetus is taking so much glucose in rapid cell growth; later in pregnancy she will need an increased amount.

The dosage and type of insulin will be specific for each woman. The insulin is usually either a long-acting type or an intermediate type combined with a short-acting insulin. The woman may need combination insulin injected again just before dinner in the evening.

Fasting blood glucose is usually kept between 90 and 100 mg per 100 ml of blood. Oral hypoglycemic agents (aside from being controversial at present for any patient) are not used for regulation because, unlike insulin, they cross the placental barrier.

All diabetic women must test their urine daily for sugar and acetone. Insulin dosage is usually regulated to keep urine 1+ for glucose (negative for acetone). This slight level of hyperglycemia is not harmful and is definitely better than a state of hypoglycemia, a condition that might be present but hidden if the woman's urine showed no glucose on repeated tests. Any finding of acetone should be reported without fail. Acidosis during pregnancy must be prevented because maternal acidosis leads to fetal anoxia. The most frequent time during pregnancy for insulin coma (hyperinsulinism) is the 2nd and 3rd month; for diabetic coma (hypoinsulinism) the 6th month.

TIMING OF DELIVERY

The timing of the delivery is a chief concern with diabetic women. One of the most hazardous times for the infant is the 36th to 40th week of pregnancy. The pregnancy must be terminated early enough to prevent fetal loss from placental insufficiency due to poor perfusion, but not so early that immaturity of the child poses further complications.

Placental Function Tests

To predict placental insufficiency, the woman is asked to collect a 24-hour urine three times a week after the 28th to 32nd week of pregnancy for estriol determination. A sudden drop in estriol in the urine, or a low flat curve, may indicate that the pregnancy must be terminated. It is important to begin these determinations as early as the 28th to 32nd week of pregnancy in order to establish a baseline, since women with diabetes frequently have small placentas, and the amount of estriol secretion may be low-normal from the first test.

Placental functioning may also be established by means of a weekly oxytocin challenge or nonstress test (see Chap. 13). Fetal stress tests are stressful procedures for the woman. Having to wait after each test to hear how the fetus is doing, and having to do this weekly, is something like having to take a final examination every week. The woman feels that it is somehow her fault, her doing, her failure (it is, after all, her diabetes) if the monitor equipment shows fetal distress. The failure may be absolute, for if the distress is acute, the fetus can no longer live in utero. If its gestation age is no more than 34 to 35 weeks, the chances of continuing life outside the uterus are also small.

These tests may take 1 to 3 hours to complete. The time can be used to teach the woman abdominal breathing or used as a short rehearsal time for actual labor. Thus a positive tone is imparted to the test, which may counterbalance the tension the test evokes in some women. A husband is often unable to take off time from work to come to the hospital and be with his wife once or twice a week while she is having this test. The woman needs someone with her to give her emotional support. She needs health care personnel with her who will help her to minimize the feeling that she is all alone.

Sonography to determine the biparietal diameter or L-S ratio by amniocentesis is undertaken by the 36th week of pregnancy to assess fetal maturity. The L-S ratio in pregnancies complicated by diabetes tends to not show maturity as early as in other pregnancies because the synthesis of phosphatidyl glycerol, the compound that stabilizes surfactant, is delayed in diabetes pregnancy. Although it is known that giving corticosteroids to the mother during the last part of pregnancy can hurry lung maturity, corticosteroids may also impair fetal insulin release and perhaps fetal islet development. Therefore, with a fetus who already has a risk at birth from poor glucose control, this is not usually attempted.

DELIVERY

For many years, cesarean section was almost routinely performed in pregnant diabetic women at about 37 weeks' gestation. Delivery was scheduled for this time because the 37th to 40th weeks are the most hazardous for the fetus; placental insufficiency is most likely to occur then. Cesarean section was chosen because it is very difficult to induce labor this early in pregnancy. The cervix is not yet ripe or responsive to labor contractions. Further, babies of diabetic women are invariably large, making vaginal delivery difficult. And finally, a fetus suffering placental dysfunction or insufficiency, which may occur with maternal diabetes, will not do well in labor and may actually be killed. Early cesarean deliveries, however, often resulted in immature infants who died in the neonatal period.

Today, with fetal heart monitoring equipment and the availability of tests for fetal maturity and well-being, the timing for delivery is much more individualized. When it can be demonstrated that fetal lung tissue is still immature and the placenta is still adequate, delivery can be delayed. When placental function appears to be growing inadequate (and, it is hoped, fetal lung tissue will appear to be mature at the same time), delivery can be instituted.

Delivery should be vaginal if this seems at all a possibility. Cesarean section always presents a high risk for the fetus, and because of the difficulty of glucose-level regulation, the fetus of a diabetic mother is already under enough stress. Labor is induced by rupture of the membranes or an oxytocin infusion. Both maternal labor contractions and fetal heart sounds should be monitored during labor, so that placental dysfunction can be detected if it does occur. The woman's glucose level must be regulated during labor, by an intravenous infusion of regular insulin, with blood glucose assessed every hour. Regulating the glucose level carefully during labor reduces the possibility of hypoglycemia in the newborn.

POSTPARTAL ADJUSTMENT

During the postpartal period, a diabetic woman has to undergo another readjustment to insulin regulation. Often, she needs no insulin during the immediate postpartal period. Diabetic women may breast-feed, because insulin is one of the few substances that does not pass into breast milk from the bloodstream. The woman requires careful observation during the immediate postpartal period because, if hydramnios was present during pregnancy, she is at risk of hemorrhage from poor uterine contraction.

EMOTIONAL SUPPORT

Women with diabetes, or those in whom diabetes develops during pregnancy, are a challenge to health care personnel. The obstetrician, internist, and nursing personnel must work together during the pregnancy. At the end of the pregnancy, this basic team must be joined by the anesthesiologist and pediatrician.

It is not easy for a woman to report to a clinic or physician's office every week for nine months. The transportation is expensive, and the visits are time-consuming. Her apprehension for her baby's and her own safety grows as the pregnancy progresses. She needs support from the people closest to her to survive the pregnancy emotionally, and she needs support from the health care personnel. She is investing a great deal in a pregnancy that may end with a less-than-perfect or a stillborn child or in an abortion. In no other instance does one of the ideals of maternal-newborn care—a healthy mother and a healthy baby—come closer to a test than in the management of a diabetic woman during pregnancy. (The infant of a diabetic woman is discussed in Chap. 38.)

Heart Disease and Pregnancy

As more and more congenital heart anomalies are corrected in early infancy, and rheumatic fever is being more actively treated to reduce cardiac damage, the number of women of childbearing age with heart disease is diminishing. Heart disease is still a continuing problem in pregnancy, however, because improved management during pregnancy has enabled women with heart disease to attempt pregnancy when in the past they would never have done so.

The two most frequent heart conditions that affect pregnancy outcome are rheumatic fever with valvular involvement and uncorrected coarctation of the aorta. A rare condition, peripartal heart disease, or heart disease associated with pregnancy, can occur. Women with artificial but well-functioning heart valves can be expected to complete a pregnancy with consistent prenatal and postpartal care.

Pregnancy taxes the circulatory system of every woman, increasing the cardiac volume and output about 30 percent. Most of this increase occurs in the first six months of pregnancy, and the greater blood volume continues to be maintained.

Because of the increased blood flow, heart murmurs are observed in many women during pregnancy. These are functional (innocent) murmurs, which are transient and will disappear on termination of the pregnancy. Heart palpitations on sudden exertion are also normal in pregnancy. Thus, neither is a sign of heart disease, but merely of normal physiological adjustment to pregnancy.

The New York Heart Association classifies heart disease into four categories shown in Table 33-9.

The woman with class I or II heart disease will experience a normal pregnancy and delivery. Women with classes III and IV heart disease are poor candidates for pregnancy.

As with diabetic women, the woman with a heart disease needs a team approach to care during pregnancy, combining the talents of internist, obstetrician, and nursing personnel.

The woman should visit her obstetrician or family physician before conception, so that he can become familiar with her state of health when she is not pregnant and can make a positive evaluation of her heart function. She should begin prenatal care as soon as she suspects she is pregnant (two weeks after the first missed menstrual period), so that close watch on her general condition and circulatory system can be maintained.

RISKS OF PREGNANCY

The dangers of pregnancy in a woman with heart disease are as follows: The cardiac output may become so diminished that the vital organs (including the placenta) are no longer perfused adequately with arterial blood, and their oxygen and nutritional requirements are thus not met. The left side of the heart

Table 33-9. Classification of Heart Disease

Class	Description
I	Patients have no limitation of physical activity. Ordinary physical activity causes no discomfort. They do not have symptoms of cardiac insufficiency and do not have anginal pain
II	Patients have slight limitation of physical activity. Ordinary physical activity causes excessive fatigue, palpitation, and dyspnea or anginal pain
III	Patients have a moderate to marked limitation of physical activity. During less than ordinary activity they experience excessive fatigue, palpitation, dyspnea, or anginal pain
IV	Patients are unable to carry on any physical activity without experiencing discomfort. Even at rest they will experience symptoms of cardiac insufficiency or anginal pain

Source. The Criteria Committee of the New York Heart Association, *Nomenclature and Criteria for Diagnosis of Diseases of the Heart and Blood Vessels* (8th ed.). Boston: Little, Brown, 1979.

may not empty the pulmonary vessels adequately, and they become engorged, resulting in pulmonary hypertension and pulmonary edema. Blood returning to the heart from the venous system may not be handled adequately, so that venous pressure rises, the liver and other organs become congested, and fluid escapes through the walls of engorged capillaries to form edema or ascites.

ASSESSMENT

A woman in whom these conditions are developing will have the same symptoms shown by any person in congestive heart failure: dyspnea (severe at night), peripheral edema, and exhaustion. She may have pulse irregularities or chest pain on exertion. If fluid is retained in the pulmonary system, and pulmonary edema is present, she will usually wake at night, anxious and coughing. She may have cyanosis of the nail beds. As more and more fluid fills the lung tissue, the respirations become noisy and labored, the cough is productive, and the sputum is blood-tinged.

The infants of women with heart disease tend to have low birth weight; there is an increased incidence of premature labor. If the woman has a cyanotic heart disease, the risk of abortion, premature labor, and delivering a low-birth-weight infant rises sharply.

INTERVENTIONS
Rest

A woman with heart disease needs more rest during pregnancy than the average woman to lessen the strain of the increased burden on her heart. Exactly how much rest she is to have should be carefully detailed to her. She may need to discontinue work early in pregnancy rather than work until midpregnancy or the end of pregnancy as the average woman usually plans to do. Exactly how much housework she will be allowed to do should be covered as well. Allowing "normally heavy" housework may mean nothing more strenuous than dusting to some women. To others, it may mean washing windows, turning mattresses, and shoveling snow. Make certain that the woman's definition of heavy work is the same as yours and the physician's.

Many physicians prefer that women with heart disease remain on complete bed rest after the 30th week of pregnancy. The purpose is to ensure that the pregnancy will be carried to term, or at least past the 36th week, so that fetal maturity can be assured. Rest should be in the left lateral recumbent position to prevent hypotension and increased heart effort.

Diet

The woman with heart disease may need closer supervision of her diet than does the average woman. She must gain enough weight to ensure a healthy pregnancy and a healthy baby, but not so much that supplying additional cells with nutrients overburdens her heart and circulatory system.

Medication

A woman who needs digitalis before pregnancy will continue to require it during pregnancy. A woman who was not digitalis-dependent before pregnancy may need such therapy prescribed as pregnancy advances and her cardiac output has to be increased or strengthened. Since anemia adds to the strain on the heart, women with heart disease should be certain to take an iron supplement during pregnancy.

It is often difficult to keep healthy women from taking over-the-counter medicines during pregnancy. It is sometimes as difficult to encourage women who need medicine during pregnancy to take it. They must understand that there are valid exceptions to the rule of "no medicine during pregnancy."

Evaluation of Edema

Evaluation of edema in patients with heart disease must not be taken lightly. You have to ask yourself whether the edema is the normal edema of pregnancy or the edema of heart failure. (Remember that edema of pregnancy-induced hypertension usually begins after the 24th week.) Edema of either pregnancy-induced hypertension or heart failure may begin as ankle edema. If the edema is a sign of heart failure, other symptoms will probably also be present: irregular pulse, rapid or difficult respirations, and perhaps chest pain on exertion. Every woman with heart disease who reports coughing should be seen because pulmonary edema from heart failure may first be manifested as a cough. As a general rule, the woman should report any infection she contracts; even a cold may overtax a system already using all of its reserves.

Emotional Support

A woman with heart disease needs a great deal of support during pregnancy. She is worried, not only for the fetus, but also for herself. In many instances, a well-meaning physician or family member or friend has told her long ago that she would never be able to have children. Much as she would like to believe the obstetrician who is telling her now that she can, the old prediction keeps running through her mind. If she feels that the pregnancy will never reach a good conclusion, it is hard for her to follow instructions;

everything seems more or less in vain. She needs the frequent reinforcement of being told that everything is going well.

It helps some women to look at the pregnancy one day at a time rather than at the entire pregnancy. Today, everything is going well. Let's do everything that is necessary today. Tomorrow we will think about what needs to be done then.

DELIVERY

The anesthetic of choice for delivery in women with heart disease is often an epidural or a caudal anesthetic because this can make both labor and delivery effort-free as well as pain-free. Many women with heart disease should not push with contractions; pushing requires more effort than they should expend.

The period immediately following the delivery may be the most critical time for the woman with heart disease. With delivery of the placenta, the blood that supplied the placenta is now released into the general circulation, and the blood volume increases between 20 to 40 percent. During pregnancy, the rise in blood volume occurred over a six-month period. Following delivery, it takes place within 5 minutes, and the heart must make a rapid and a major adjustment.

The woman should be ambulated early to avoid the formation of emboli; she may need to wear elastic stockings to increase venous return. Many women with heart disease are placed on prophylactic antibiotics prior to delivery and continue to take them during the postpartal period to discourage subacute bacterial endocarditis due to a mild postpartal infection. (Some endometrial infections are caused by streptococci, which are most likely to cause subacute bacterial endocarditis.)

A woman with heart disease is very interested in close inspection of her baby in the delivery room. She needs more assurance than "You have a beautiful baby." She needs to know that her infant does not appear to have a heart defect. Be sure to point out that acrocyanosis is normal, so that she does not interpret her baby's severe peripheral cyanosis as cardiac inadequacy.

In the postpartal period ergot compounds to encourage uterine involution must be used with caution as they tend to increase blood pressure. Estrogen compounds to decrease lactation should also be used cautiously; they may lead to thromboembolus. Sterilization procedures are generally delayed rather than done in the postpartal period to allow for better circulatory stabilization.

PERIPARTAL HEART DISEASE

An extremely rare condition, peripartal heart disease, originates late in pregnancy and is apparently due to the effect of the pregnancy on the circulatory system. Since it occurs most often in women from low socioeconomic areas, the possibility of accompanying protein malnutrition is suggested; it may occur in women with hypertension of pregnancy. Late in pregnancy, the woman develops signs of myocardial failure (shortness of breath, chest pain, edema). Her heart begins to increase in size (cardiomegaly). Activity must be sharply reduced. Many women need diuretic and digitalis therapy. Low-dose heparin may be administered to decrease the risk of thromboembolism.

If the cardiomegaly persists past the postpartal period, it is generally suggested that she not attempt any further pregnancies.

MITRAL STENOSIS

The heart defect that is most likely to occur with rheumatic fever is mitral stenosis. During pregnancy, the increase in heart rate and cardiac output forces an increased flow of blood through the stenosed valve. There is pressure in the left atrium due to the inability of the valve to handle the increased flow. Pulmonary veins become distended. Pressure on lung capillaries causes a transudate of fluid into lung or pulmonary edema.

Management is aimed toward decreasing the flow of blood through the mitral valve. The woman may be placed on oral diuretics to limit plasma volume. Digitalis therapy will reduce the heart rate. If she is taking a diuretic for an extended time, the woman will probably be placed on a potassium supplement as well so as not to become potassium-depleted. Prophylactic penicillin will reduce the possibility of subacute bacterial endocarditis due to the stasis of blood flow at the damaged valve. A woman whose symptoms are becoming so severe that it is evident her heart is failing can undergo cardiac surgery to repair the valve during pregnancy. With this insult to her body and the long period of anesthesia, the fetal risk from the procedure is obviously high.

PULMONARY ARTERY HYPERTENSION

The maternal risk during pregnancy is very high (about 50 percent) if pulmonary artery hypertension exists. A woman might have this from a mitral stenosis or a congenital heart defect. Death may occur at the time of delivery or early in the postpartal period because of the increased blood flow following the delivery of the placenta. Since oxygen inhalation during labor and delivery tends to decrease vascular resistance in the lung, it should be used during this time. Anesthesia that causes hypotension should be avoided (the heart cannot make this adjustment; it is already overtaxed). Blood loss at delivery must be replaced, but very cautiously lest rapid intravenous administration tax the mother's circulatory system further. Following delivery, she will be started on heparin anticoagulant therapy to reduce the chance of pulmonary vascular thrombosis.

ARTIFICIAL VALVE PROSTHESIS

Once women with a heart valve prosthesis were told they should not become pregnant. Today, caring for a woman with a valve prosthesis during pregnancy would not be unusual. Many women with valve prostheses take oral anticoagulants to prevent the formation of clots at the valve site. This kind of medication may increase the risk of congenital anomalies in infants. Women may be placed on heparin therapy to reduce this risk (heparin does not cross the placenta). Subclinical bleeding may cause placental dislodgment, so the woman must be observed closely for signs of premature separation of the placenta. Anticoagulant therapy may be stopped about two weeks prior to delivery to reduce the level in the fetus at birth and prevent his being born with a coagulation defect. Regional block anesthesia into the spinal cord is generally not used at delivery because of the danger of bleeding into the spinal cord from surrounding vessels.

Anemia

Because the blood volume expands during pregnancy slightly ahead of the red cell count, most women have a pseudoanemia of early pregnancy. This is normal and should not be confused with the true anemia that can occur as a complication of pregnancy.

IRON DEFICIENCY ANEMIA

Many women enter pregnancy with an iron deficiency anemia resulting from poor diet, heavy menstrual periods, or unwise weight-reducing programs. When the hemoglobin level is below 11 gm (hematocrit under 35 vol%), iron deficiency is suspected. Women may have erythrocyte indexes done to determine the cause of the low hematocrit level. Iron deficiency anemia is characteristically a microcytic (small-size red blood cell), hypochromic (less hemoglobin than the average red cell) anemia, because when iron is not available for incorporation into red blood cells, they are not as large or as rich in hemoglobin as normally. Mean corpuscular volume (MCV, or the size of the average erythrocyte) and mean corpuscular hemoglobin (MCH, or the amount of hemoglobin in the average erythrocyte) will both be low.

All women should receive an iron supplement during pregnancy as prophylactic therapy against iron deficiency anemia; those with iron deficiency anemia will receive therapeutic levels of medication.

Be certain to ask the woman at prenatal visits whether she is taking her iron supplement. Women do not appreciate the value of iron; it is an over-the-counter medication and therefore it does not seem as urgent or important to take it as to take a prescription drug. Some women who find that iron compounds tend to constipate them stop taking their iron supplement after a few weeks. If this is a problem, a stool softener such as Colace may be prescribed with the iron compound. Aside from limiting the amount of oxygen available for fetal exchange (oxygen is carried in combination with hemoglobin; decreased hemoglobin amount decreases oxygen transportation), the woman will feel chronically tired if she has iron deficiency anemia. Nine months of pregnancy with iron deficiency anemia makes a pregnancy something to be endured, not something that is the beginning step to firm mother-child bonding.

FOLIC ACID DEFICIENCY

Megaloblastic anemia due to low levels of vitamin B_{12} or folic acid also occurs during pregnancy. Folic acid deficiency has serious effects on fetal development and may be responsible for early abortion or abruptio placentae (premature separation of the placenta). For this reason, women should receive a folic acid supplement during pregnancy. Routine vitamin preparations prescribed during pregnancy contain folic acid. Over-the-counter multivitamin preparations generally do not. Ask at prenatal visits whether the woman is taking her prescribed vitamin source. In order to save money, she may not have had the prescription filled and may be using an over-the-counter, less expensive type, not aware of the difference.

Megaloblastic anemia implies that the red blood cells are enlarged. Thus the MCV with folic acid deficiency is elevated, in contrast ot the lowered level seen with iron deficiency anemia.

If there are small children in the house, caution the woman that she must regard iron compounds and pregnancy vitamins as medicine and keep them up away from small hands. Both iron compounds and pregnancy prescribed vitamins, because of the folic acid content, are dangerous if ingested by young children.

Urinary Tract Disorders
URINARY TRACT INFECTION

Urinary tract infection occurs in 1 to 2 percent of pregnancies. Many nonpregnant women have asymptomatic bacteriuria. In the pregnant woman, because of the stasis of urine in the dilated ureters, asymptomatic infections are greatly increased in importance because they lead to pyelonephritis. The organism most commonly responsible for urinary tract infection is *Escherichia coli.*

With pyelonephritis the woman notices pain in the lumbar region (usually on the right side) and perhaps nausea and vomiting, malaise, pain, and frequency of urination. Her temperature may be elevated. The infection usually occurs on the right side because the uterus tends to be pushed to that side by the large bulk of the intestine on the left side. The greater compression on the right ureter creates greater stasis on that side.

A clean-catch urine should be obtained for a culture and a sensitivity test. The sensitivity test report will determine which antibiotic will be prescribed. Ampicillin is effective against most organisms causing urinary tract infection and is a safe antibiotic for pregnancy. Nitrofurantoin (Furadantin) is frequently ordered. The sulfonamides are used early in pregnancy but not so frequently near term as they interfere with protein binding of bilirubin, which leads to hyperbilirubinemia in the newborn. Similarly, tetracyclines are contraindicated in pregnancy; they cause retardation of bone growth and staining of the fetal teeth.

The woman needs to take additional fluid to flush out the infection from the pelvis of the kidney. Never tell her to "push fluids" or "drink lots of water." Tell her a specific amount to drink every day (up to 3 to 4 liters per 24 hours), to make certain that her fluid intake will be sufficiently increased.

The woman can promote urine drainage by assuming a knee-chest position for 15 minutes morning and evening. In this position, the weight of the uterus is shifted forward, freeing the ureter for drainage. Women should assume a knee-chest position twice a day during pregnancy as prophylaxis against urinary tract infection as well as against the development of hemorrhoids and varicosities.

Be sure to ask the woman about any associated symptoms, such as frequency of urination, when she is describing back pain during pregnancy, so that you do not interpret this symptom of developing urinary tract infection as normal backache. An increased incidence of premature labor and fetal loss is associated with pyelonephritis. Many physicians ask the woman for a clean-catch urine specimen at intervals during pregnancy to detect this infection in its earliest stage.

If a woman has one urinary tract infection during pregnancy, the chance that she will develop another late in pregnancy is high. She may therefore be kept on prophylactic antibiotics through the remainder of the pregnancy. Ask the woman at prenatal visits whether she is continuing to take this type of prophylactic medicine. While women have pain and symptoms of urinary frequency, they take medication very well. When they no longer have any clinical evidence that they are sick, their compliance rate begins to fall dramatically. The woman may need to post a chart on her refrigerator door or in her bathroom to remind herself to take this kind of medication. Leaving the medicine on a counter to remind herself to take it is not a good habit to develop. Shortly she will have a new baby in the house. Encourage her to keep medicine out of sight and reach so as to get into the habit of "childproofing" even at this early stage.

CHRONIC RENAL DISEASE

In previous years, children with chronic renal disease did not reach childbearing age or were advised not to have children because of the high risk for them during pregnancy. Today, women with chronic renal disease are having children. As many as 100 children have been born to women who have even had renal transplants.

Pregnancy increases the work load on the kidneys because the woman's kidneys must excrete waste products not only for herself but for the fetus for nine months. Many women with renal disease take corticosteroids (prednisone) at a maintenance level, and they should continue to do so throughout pregnancy. Although reports of animal studies have demonstrated an increased incidence of cleft palate from the taking of corticosteroids during pregnancy, this does not appear to happen in humans.

It is difficult to interpret kidney function during pregnancy. Many women spill a trace of sugar and protein during pregnancy because of increased glomerular permeability. If the woman is told about this possibility, she will understand that it is an expected change of pregnancy, not a forecast of changing kidney function. Her blood pressure level during pregnancy must be compared to prepregnancy levels.

Because the glomerular filtration rate increases

during pregnancy, normally a woman is able to clear waste products for both herself and the fetus from her body with such efficiency that her serum creatinine and blood urea nitrogen (BUN) levels are actually slightly below normal during pregnancy. Normal blood creatinine is 0.7 mg per 100 ml; during pregnancy it is about 0.5 mg per 100 ml. BUN is normally 13 mg per 100 ml; duirng pregnancy it is about 9 mg per 100 ml. Women with kidney disease who normally have an elevated blood creatinine level over 1.7 gm per 100 ml or a BUN over 30 mg per 100 ml probably should not undertake a pregnancy or the increased strain on already damaged kidneys may lead to kidney failure.

Toward the end of pregnancy, fetal well-being may be evaluated by urinary estriol determinations. These findings can be erroneous, however, because of the overall decreased output. They must always be interpreted in light of the woman's kidney-diseased state, not compared to normal values.

Infants of women with chronic renal disease tend to have intrauterine growth retarded. If the mothers are taking steroids, they may be hyperglycemic at birth on account of the suppression of insulin activity by corticosteroids at birth.

Women with kidney transplants should be considered individually as to whether they will be able to carry a pregnancy to term before a pregnancy is initiated. Criteria that should be evaluated are the woman's general health and the time since the transplant (preferably more than two years), whether she has proteinuria, signs of graft rejection, hypertension, level of serum creatinine, and whether she is taking medication to reduce graft rejection. If her drug usage is limited to prednisone and azathioprine (an antimetabolite, but no reports of fetal compromise have been made with this), pregnancy may be possible for her.

Women with renal disease need a great deal of support during pregnancy. They are aware that kidneys are vital for life and that the stress of pregnancy on damaged kidneys may cause them to fail. They are aware that they are risking not only the life of the growing child inside them but their own life.

They need extra time with their infant at birth for bonding as they have had difficulty beginning bonding during pregnancy. They need extra assurance that the baby is well.

Respiratory Disorders

Women who have chronic respiratory disorders have a potential for the disorder's worsening during pregnancy. The rising uterus compresses lung space, and increased lung function is needed to provide adequate oxygen exchange for the fetus as well as herself.

ACUTE NASOPHARYNGITIS

Acute nasopharyngitis (common cold) tends to be more severe during pregnancy than otherwise. With pregnancy there is normally some degree of nasal congestion. With even a minor cold, therefore, the woman finds it difficult to breathe. Women should be cautioned that, unless they have a fever with the cold, taking aspirin is unnecessary. Because common colds are invariably caused by a virus, antibiotic therapy is ineffective except to prevent a secondary infection.

INFLUENZA

Influenza is caused by a virus that has been isolated and identified as type A and type B. It spreads in epidemic form and is accompanied by high fever, extreme prostration, aching pains in the back and extremities, and generally a sore, raw throat. There is some correlation between influenza outbreaks and congenital anomalies in children. During the famous Asian flu epidemic (caused by a variant of type A virus) abortion and premature labor increased.

PNEUMONIA

Pneumonia is a serious complication of pregnancy because fluid collects in alveolar spaces, limiting, at least to some extent, oxygen exchange in the lung. If collection of fluid is extreme, it will limit the oxygen available to the fetus. There is a tendency for women with pneumonia late in pregnancy to begin premature labor. During labor oxygen should be administered so that the fetus has adequate oxygen resources.

ASTHMA

About 1 percent of all pregnant women have asthma. Basically an allergic phenomenon that leads to narrowing of bronchioles due to bronchial spasm, asthma has the potential of reducing the oxygen supply to the fetus if a major attack should occur during pregnancy. Many women find that their asthma is improved during pregnancy by the high circulating levels of corticosteroids at that time. A woman should check with her physician as to the safety of the medications she routinely takes for the disorder to be certain it will be safe to continue them during pregnancy.

PULMONARY TUBERCULOSIS

Tuberculosis is a disease that should have been eradicated in view of the effective treatment now available. However, in some highly populated areas, its incidence is actually increasing. Worldwide, it is one of the leading causes of death.

In high-risk areas, women should be skin-tested with a tine or PPD method at their first prenatal visit. A chest x-ray film can then be taken of women who show positive reactions to skin testing. Women need to be cautioned that a positive reaction does not necessarily mean that they have the disease; it can also mean that they have at some time been exposed to it and so have antibodies in their system. A chest x-ray film confirms the diagnosis.

A woman with tuberculosis shows symptoms of a chronic cough, weight loss, hemoptysis, night sweats, a low-grade fever, and chronic fatigue. Women with active tuberculosis should be treated during pregnancy. Isoniazid (INH), ethambutol hydrochloride, rifampin, streptomycin, and para-aminosalicylic acid (PAS) may all be given without apparent teratogenic effects. Isoniazid may cause hepatitis-like symptoms of nausea, anorexia, malaise, fever, and enlarged liver. It may also result in a peripheral neuritis if the woman does not take supplemental pyridoxine as well. Ethambutol may cause optic nerve involvement (optic atrophy and loss of green color recognition) in the mother. To detect this, the woman can be tested monthly by a Snellen eye chart.

A woman who has had tuberculosis is usually advised to wait a full year, perhaps two years, before attempting to conceive after her tuberculosis becomes inactive.

Tuberculosis lesions never actually disappear; the bacillus is "closed off" by calcium deposits in the lung and therefore made inactive. The woman who has active tuberculosis, or has had it recently, must be especially careful to maintain an adequate level of calcium during pregnancy in order to ensure that tuberculosis pockets form or are not broken down. Recent inactive tuberculosis can become active during pregnancy, because pressure on the diaphragm from below changes the shape of the lung, and a sealed pocket may be broken in this process. Pushing during labor may increase intrapulmonary pressure and cause the same phenomenon. Recently inactive tuberculosis may become active during the postpartal period, as the lung returns to its more vertical pre-pregnant position.

A woman with a recent history of tuberculosis should have at least three negative sputum cultures before she holds or cares for her infant. If they are negative, there is no need to isolate the infant from the mother; she can even breast-feed. If there is active tuberculosis in the home, the infant is generally sent home on prophylactic isoniazid or given a BCG vaccine in early infancy (at age 2 to 4 months). Once an infant has received BCG (Calmette-Guérin bacillus vaccine), a tine or PPD test will always be positive, something the mother should be made aware of. He should not be routinely tested at well-child visits or a large area of sloughing may occur at the test site.

The woman taking rifampin should be cautioned that this medication increases the failure rate of oral contraceptives. She should use some other measure for family planning.

Venereal Disease

If a disease is spread by coitus, it is a venereal disease. Because the two most commonly known venereal diseases (gonorrhea and syphilis) are harmful to fetuses, and syphilis is fatal to the adult if not treated, the term *venereal disease* has come to mean a crippling disease state. It is better, therefore, not to refer to diseases other than gonorrhea and syphilis as venereal diseases when talking to women during pregnancy. If the physician with whom you work uses the term in reference to another disease, be sure to explain the use of the term (he is simply talking about a disease spread by coitus or one that can be transferred from a wife to a husband and back to the wife and so forth, not a disease that is socially unacceptable or can bring harm to her baby).

Common vaginal infections are listed in Table 33-10.

CONDYLOMATA ACUMINATA

Condylomata acuminata are vulvar warts. They may vary in size, are usually multiple, and are probably due to the same virus that causes ordinary skin warts. They tend to be seen frequently on women with a leukorrheal discharge. Like ordinary warts, they have a rough, irregular surface; they are not painful.

The woman needs to be assured that these lesions are a form of common wart so that she does not worry for fear they are a form of tumor or vulvar cancer. Most physicians draw blood for a VDRL (test for syphilis) if vulvar warts are present as it is sometimes difficult to differentiate these growths from the lesion of primary syphilis.

If the lesion is small, it can be painted with a solution that causes lysis of the lesion (20% podophyllin in tincture of benzoin). Large lesions must be surgically removed or removed by electrocoagulation. Unless they are bothersome, they may be left in place during pregnancy and removed during the postpartal period. Their presence appears to have no effect on the fetus.

Table 33-10. Common Vaginal Infections

Causative Agent	Symptoms	Interventions
Candida	Vulvar pruritus Thick, white vaginal discharge	Nystatin suppositories or 1% gentian violet Bathing with dilute sodium bicarbonate solution may relieve pruritus
Trichomonas	Thin, irritating, frothy discharge Strong, putrid odor	Flagyl orally (except in first trimester) Douche with weak vinegar solution
Herpesvirus II	Painful pinpoint vesicles on an erythematous base Possibly a watery vaginal discharge Voiding may be irritating and painful	Bathe with dilute sodium bicarbonate solution to relieve pain Vaseline applied to lesion may reduce pain Analgesic such as aspirin may be necessary for pain relief
Condylomata acuminata	Warty, grayish, irregular raised growths on vulva	Generally not treated during pregnancy Can be removed by electrocoagulation or application of podophyllin in tincture of benzoin
Hemophilus vaginalis	Edema of vulva Reddened vulva	Douche with weak vinegar solution Specific antibiotic therapy
Neisseria gonorrhoeae	May be symptomless May have profuse yellow-green vaginal discharge	Penicillin (procaine penicillin G, 4.8 million units IM in 2 sites on one visit)
Pinworm (*Enterobius vermicularis*)	Itching, especially on rising in the morning Accompanied by rectal pruritus as a rule	Oral administration of an antihelminth.
Treponema pallidum (syphilis)	Painless ulcer on vulva or vagina	Penicillin (benzathine penicillin G, 2.4 million units IM in 2 sites at one visit)

HERPES GENITALIS

Vulvar herpes lesions are caused by infection by herpesvirus type II. The virus is introduced at a time of coitus. Herpes lesions consist of clustered pinpoint vesicles on an erythematous base that are very painful. After about 24 hours, the vesicles break and leave a raw, reddened pinpoint ulcer that persists for about a week before it heals.

Approximately 20 percent of adult women have antibodies to herpesvirus II in their bloodstream, evidence that they have had a type II infection at some time. If the infection occurs during pregnancy, the fetus can be infected. Infection can be spread to the fetus at delivery if herpes lesions are present on the vagina or vulva at that time. Interestingly, about 90 percent of women with carcinoma of the cervix have antibodies against herpes type II virus. This high association has caused researchers to question whether herpes infection may be an etiological factor in the development of cervical cancer. In any event, a woman who has a herpes type II infection should be told that she has the infection in relation to its implication for the pregnancy and that she must be conscientious for the rest of her life in having Pap tests to detect beginning cervical cancer.

There is no effective treatment for vulvar herpes infection. The pain of lesions may be lessened by applying a soothing ointment such as Vaseline. Warm baths may help.

It is important that nurses working in labor units be able to recognize herpesvirus lesions as cesarean section to safeguard the fetus can be anticipated in these women. Herpesvirus II infections become systemic and may be lethal in the newborn.

CANDIDIASIS

The candidal organism is a fungus that thrives on glycogen. About 5 percent of nonpregnant and as many as 20 percent of pregnant women have candidal vaginal infections because of the unusually high content of glycogen in vaginal cells during pregnancy. Since birth control pills produce a pseudopregnancy state, pill users also have frequent vaginal candidal infections. When a woman is being treated with an antibiotic during pregnancy (which kills off normal vaginal flora and lets fungal organisms grow more readily), she is particularly susceptible to these infections.

The woman notices vulvar burning and itching; her vulva generally appears reddened and may even bleed from irritation. The vagina sometimes shows white "patches" on the walls; these are adherent and cannot be scraped away without bleeding.

Candidal infections are diagnosed by scraping a tongue blade against a vaginal wall to remove some discharge. This is placed on a glass slide; 3 or 4 drops of a 20% potassium hydroxide (KOH) solution are then added to the slide, and the mixture is protected by a coverslip. When you look at the slide under a microscope, if *Candida* organisms are present, you may observe typical fungal hyphae (Fig. 33-9).

Immediate relief for pruritus may be provided by vulvar and vaginal application of 1% gentian violet. Caution women that gentian violet stains underclothes permanently. Nystatin suppositories are generally preferred treatment to preclude this staining.

Unfortunately candidal infections are likely to recur as long as the pregnancy lasts. A woman who has frequent recurrences should have her urine tested for glucose as the infections are found frequently in diabetic women. Her male partner may need to be treated for the infection as well or he will tend to reinfect her.

If a candidal infection is present in the vagina at birth, it may cause a candidal infection (thrush) in the newborn.

TRICHOMONIASIS

Trichomonas vaginalis is a single-cell protozoon that is spread by coitus. With a trichomonal infection, the woman will notice vaginal irritation and a frothy white to gray vaginal discharge. The frothiness of the discharge is an important typical finding. The upper vagina is reddened and may have pinpoint petechiae present. Males with the infection rarely show any symptoms.

Fig. 33-9. The appearance of common organisms seen in vaginal infection. A. Candida. B. Trichomonas. C. H. vaginalis.

The infection is diagnosed by scraping and placing a few drops of vaginal discharge on a glass slide, adding a few drops of Ringer's solution, protecting the mixture with a cover slide, and observing the mixture under a microscope. Trichomonads typically appear as rounded, mobile structures (Fig. 33-9).

Flagyl (metronidazole), taken orally, eradicates trichomonal infections in the nonpregnant woman. This should never be given during the first trimester of pregnancy and must be used with caution for the remainder of pregnancy as it can be teratogenic to a growing fetus. Treating the sexual partner will prevent recurrence of the infection. Vaginal douching with a dilute vinegar solution will decrease symptoms until metronidazole can be used.

HEMOPHILUS VAGINALIS INFECTION

Hemophilus vaginalis infection is caused by a gram-negative rod. The organism grows well in the vagina because it prefers areas with reduced oxygen levels. The associated discharge is milk-white and has a fish-like odor. Pruritus may be intense.

A few drops of the vaginal discharge mixed with saline solution on a slide shows gram-negative rods adhering to vaginal epithelial cells.

The treatment is oral ampicillin; the woman's sexual partner should be treated also to prevent recurrence of the infection. Assure the woman that ampicillin is a safe drug to take during pregnancy so that she will take the full prescription.

PINWORMS (ENTEROBIUS VERMICULARIS)

Vaginal irritation may be caused by pinworms, which typically live in the cecum of the bowel. During periods of rest the female worm migrates to the anus and deposits eggs on the perineum. The worms may invade the vagina. The woman notices intense itching when she awakes in the morning from the irritation of the half-inch thread-like worms on the perineum.

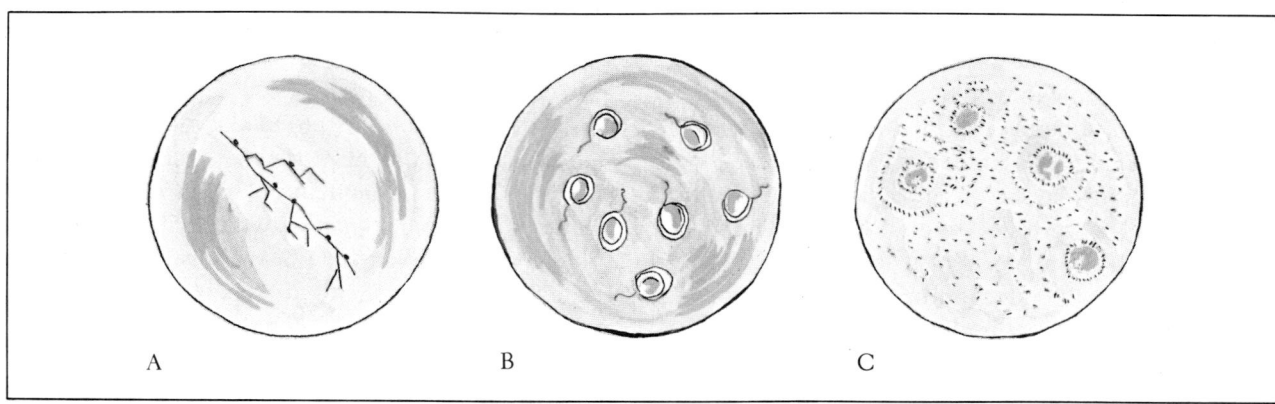

Treatment is with one of the oral common antihelminth drugs available.

Pinworms are often found in children of low socioeconomic families who do not have good handwashing facilities and so tend to become reinfected (the child scratches his rectum, does not wash his hands because there is only cold water to use, and so carries the eggs to his mouth; they hatch in his gastrointestinal tract, and the cycle begins again). Some people therefore equate pinworms with poverty and find it difficult to believe that they could have this disorder. They can be assured that the worms do spread readily and do occur in all socioeconomic levels and among all people.

SYPHILIS

Syphilis is a systemic disease caused by the spirochete *Treponema pallidum*. It is transmitted by sexual contact with a person who has an active spirochete-containing lesion. Following an incubation period of 10 to 90 days, a typical lesion appears, generally on the genitalia although it may be present on the mouth or lips or rectal area. As a rule the lesion is a deep ulcer that is painless despite its size. There is local lymphadenopathy, but this is unlikely to be noticed by the affected individual. In women, the lesion itself is often not noticed, especially if it is located inside the vagina.

In the next stage, the woman may have a generalized macular rash; it is different from many other rashes in that the soles of the feet and the palms of the hands are affected. This is the stage of secondary syphilis. The third stage involves neurological symptoms. A woman is contagious through primary, secondary, and latent stages, a period of about two years.

At the first prenatal visit, blood is drawn routinely for a serological test for syphilis (VDRL). If the result is positive, the woman is treated with large doses of penicillin (benzathine penicillin G, 2.4 million units intramuscularly, in two sites on one visit). Women who are sensitive to penicillin may be treated with erythromycin. Discovering the infection at the first visit (provided the first visit is early in pregnancy) allows time to treat the disease and protect the fetus against the spirochetes of syphilis from the early months of pregnancy, thus preventing congenital abnormalities.

The spirochetes of syphilis can cross the placenta only after the 18th week of pregnancy. Following treatment, the woman is tested monthly for repeat VDRL titers. Since titers take six to eight weeks to return to normal levels, they may not fall to normal during the pregnancy. Unless a titer recedes in amount, however, one may strongly suspect that either the penicillin therapy was not adequate or reinfection has occurred. Sexual contacts of the woman should be identified and treated so that reinfection will not occur. (Congenital syphilis is discussed in Chap. 38.)

Once the woman is free of syphilis, there is no guarantee that she will not contract it again.

GONORRHEA

If a woman has active gonorrhea at the time of delivery, the fetus may contact the organism of gonorrhea, the gram-negative coccus *Neisseria gonorrhoeae*. Women are rarely aware that they have active gonorrhea because they tend to be asymptomatic. Their male partner usually has symptoms of burning on urination, frequency, and a purulent discharge.

In early pregnancy, at the time of the Pap test, most physicians also take a routine culture for gonorrhea or draw blood for gonorrheal antibodies. If a culture is positive, the woman is treated with large doses of penicillin (procaine penicillin G, 4.8 million units intramuscularly, in two sites on one visit, plus probenecid, 1 gm orally one-half hour before the injection of penicillin; probenecid delays urinary excretion of penicillin and maintains high blood levels of penicillin for a sustained time). Women who are sensitive to penicillin may be treated with erythromycin.

Ask at prenatal visits whether the woman has any reason to think that she may have contracted this disease. Women with varied sexual contacts have more chance of having the disease, but if worded correctly the question can be asked of anyone without embarrassment: "Some diseases have almost no symptoms, so we ask every woman if she thinks there is any chance that she may have contracted them since she was here last. Do you think that you could have been exposed to gonorrhea? Syphilis? Tuberculosis?" Included as a routine screening question this way, it does not imply that the woman is being singled out in any special way and allows her to answer without feeling threatened. The fact that a woman is married and has no other sexual partner but her husband does not mean that she is not concerned about the possibility of contracting venereal disease; her husband may not be as selective in choosing his sexual partners as she is. *Clap* is a common name for gonorrhea and may be the term to use to describe the infection the woman is concerned about.

If a fetus is exposed at birth to gonorrhea, the eye infection that can occur, *ophthalmia neonatorum*, is sometimes severe enough to lead to blindness.

Chronic gonorrheal infection can lead to pelvic inflammatory disease and obstruction of the fallopian tubes in the woman.

Collagen Disorders
JUVENILE RHEUMATOID ARTHRITIS
Juvenile rheumatoid arthritis, a disease of connective tissue with joint inflammation and contracture, occurs in women of childbearing age. Symptoms of the disease may improve during pregnancy because of the increased circulating level of corticosteroids in the maternal bloodstream then. During the postpartal period, when the woman's corticosteroid levels fall to normal again, arthritis symptoms will probably recur. Women with juvenile rheumatoid arthritis frequently take corticosteroids and salicylate therapy to prevent joint pain and loss of mobility.

Women who take large amounts of salicylates may have prolonged pregnancies (salicylate interferes with prostaglandin synthesis, which may help initiate labor contractions). The infant may have a bleeding defect due to the high salicylate level. For this reason, the woman is asked to decrease her intake of salicylates about two weeks before term.

She should continue to take corticosteroids during pregnancy if they are necessary to control her symptoms. Despite reports that exposure to corticosteroids during pregnancy leads to increased congenital anomalies in animals, humans do not seem to be affected. Since urinary estriol levels may be decreased in a woman taking prednisone, levels must be evaluated in light of the prednisone therapy. The fetal adrenal output is apparently suppressed and less estrogen is formed.

The woman should not take phenylbutazone or indomethacin to reduce inflammation during pregnancy. These two drugs are known teratogens.

SYSTEMIC LUPUS ERYTHEMATOSUS
Systemic lupus erythematosus is another disease of connective tissue that can occur in women of childbearing age. Thickening of collagen tissue causes obstruction of blood vessels. This is life-threatening to the woman when blood flow to vital organs is compromised, to the fetus when blood flow to the placenta is obstructed. The woman may be taking corticosteroid and salicylate therapy to reduce symptoms of joint pain and inflammation.

The increased circulation of corticosteroids during pregnancy may lessen symptoms in some women. In others, the chief complication of the disorder—acute nephritis—may occur during pregnancy.

With nephritis, the woman's blood pressure will rise. She will have hematuria and decreased urine output. Edema may begin. It is difficult to differentiate these symptoms from the symptoms of pregnancy-induced hypertension except that with the latter there is no hematuria.

Infants of women with systemic lupus erythematosus tend to be small for gestation age. The incidence of abortion and premature birth rises. During the postpartal period there may be an acute exacerbation of symptoms in the woman as corticosteroid levels again fall to normal.

Gastrointestinal Diseases and Pregnancy
HIATAL HERNIA
Hiatal hernia may generate symptoms during pregnancy as the uterus pushes the stomach against the diaphragm and increases the hernia. The woman notices "heartburn" at about the 20th week of pregnancy, which she cannot seem to relieve. She may lose weight because of her inability to eat. If the problem is extreme, she may have hematemesis (vomiting of blood).

That a hiatal hernia is present may be diagnosed by x-ray examination. Following pregnancy, as the uterine pressure is decreased, the symptoms disappear.

PEPTIC ULCER
Women with peptic ulcer can expect symptoms to decrease during pregnancy because of decreased stomach acidity. They should be warned that, following pregnancy, symptoms will probably return to prepregnancy level lest they neglect their diet in the postpartal period.

CHOLECYSTITIS AND CHOLELITHIASIS
Hypercholesterolemia occurs during pregnancy; whether it leads to increased cholecystitis or cholelithiasis (gallbladder inflammation and gallstone formation) during pregnancy is questionable. Symptoms of cholecystitis typically occur following a meal rich in fat. Pain is sharp and peristaltic and located high in the right upper quadrant.

Surgery for gallbladder involvement may be done during pregnancy if the woman's symptoms cannot be controlled by conservative dietary management for the remainder of the pregnancy.

APPENDICITIS
Because appendicitis is a disease of young adults, it can occur in the young pregnant adult. Any woman

with abdominal pain during pregnancy should call her physician (that is one of the basic danger signs of pregnancy). Differentiating the cause of the pain (an acute abdomen) from a disorder that is special to the pregnancy (abruptio placentae, ectopic pregnancy) is often difficult.

Assessment

History taking is important. Appendicitis usually begins with a few hours of nausea (the woman skipped lunch because she just did not feel hungry). An hour or two of generalized abdominal discomfort follows. The woman may have vomiting during this time. Then comes the typical sharp, peristaltic, lower-right-quadrant pain of acute appendicitis.

This is different from the pain of ectopic pregnancy; with ectopic pregnancy there is no nausea and vomiting. In the nonpregnant woman the sharp localized pain of appendicitis appears at McBurney's point (a point halfway between the umbilicus and the iliac crest on the lower right abdomen). If you press at that point, it is not so tender while you are pressing; releasing your hand abruptly, however, causes the abdominal contents to jiggle, and the jiggling of the inflamed appendix brings sharp pain (rebound tenderness). In the pregnant woman the appendix is often displaced upward in the abdomen, and the localized pain may be so high it resembles the pain of gallbladder disease.

The woman should take nothing to eat and no laxatives while she is waiting to be seen by a physician, as increasing peristalsis tends to cause an inflamed appendix to rupture. Blood work will reveal leukocytosis. Her temperature may be elevated. There are typically ketones in the urine.

Interventions

If the woman is near term and there is reason to believe that the fetus is mature, a cesarean section may be done to deliver the baby and then the inflamed appendix is removed. If appendicitis occurs early in pregnancy, an abdominal incision to remove the inflamed appendix can usually be made without disturbing the pregnancy. As long as the anesthesiologist is aware that the woman is pregnant and carefully controls oxygen levels during anesthesia administration, the outcome of the pregnancy will be good.

If the appendix ruptures before surgery, the risk to both mother and fetus increases dramatically. With rupture, infected material is free in the peritoneum. It can spread by the fallopian tubes to the fetus. Generalized peritonitis is such an overwhelming infection it is difficult for the woman's body to combat it effectively and maintain the pregnancy too.

A woman reporting abdominal pain during pregnancy should always be listened to attentively. One of the reasons for abdominal pain in young adults can be acute appendicitis, which calls for immediate physician intervention.

VIRAL HEPATITIS

Hepatitis may occur from invasion of either the A or B virus. Hepatitis A is spread by contact with another person who has the infection or by ingestion of fecally contaminated water or shellfish; it can also be contacted by contamination from a syringe or needle. Hepatitis B virus (serum hepatitis) is spread by transfusion of contaminated blood or blood products.

The woman notices symptoms of nausea and vomiting. Her liver area may feel tender. Jaundice is a late symptom. On physical examination, her liver is found to be enlarged. Her bilirubin level will be elevated, as her liver is unable to complete bilirubin conversion; her liver transaminase value will be increased. Specific antibodies against the A or B virus can be detected in her blood serum.

The woman will be put on bed rest and is encouraged to eat a high caloric diet. Use enteric precautions (wear a cover gown, wash hands well on entering and leaving room, wear gloves to handle articles contaminated with fecal material). If the woman has hepatitis B infection, use precautions with blood samples or blood drawing equipment.

The danger of hepatitis during pregnancy is abortion or premature labor. The fetus may contact hepatitis B virus during the pregnancy or during delivery. Following delivery, the infant should be washed well to remove any maternal blood, and hepatitis B immune globulin (HBIG) will be administered. The infant needs to be observed carefully for symptoms of infection. The mother will be advised not to breast-feed, as hepatitis B antigens can be recovered from breast milk.

Neurological Conditions
RECURRENT CONVULSIONS

Recurrent convulsions (epilepsy) have a number of causes, such as head trauma or meningitis. The majority of instances of recurrent convulsions in children, however, occur for unknown reasons (idiopathic epilepsy).

Before convulsions could be as well controlled as they can be today, recurrent convulsions were so incapacitating that women who suffered them were generally advised not to have children. Today, there is no contraindication to such a woman's having children as long as she is aware that the medication she must take to control the convulsions increases the chance of anomalies in her infant.

In the early months of pregnancy, women with recurrent convulsions often need help with relief of nausea and vomiting. They must not become so nauseated that they are unable to take their seizure control medications. They have to understand that the rule "Do not take medication during pregnancy" does not apply to their seizure control medications.

Women who have taken Dilantin (phenytoin sodium) may have chronic hypertension. A baseline blood pressure should be established early in pregnancy, so that later changes can be interpreted in terms of an already elevated pressure.

Many women wonder what a convulsion during pregnancy might do to their unborn child. Convulsions vary so much from person to person that it is impossible to answer the question. Petit mal convulsions (often just a rapid fluttering of the eyelids, a moment's staring into space) will have no effect on the fetus. Grand mal convulsions (sustained clonic-tonic full-body involvement), because of the anoxia that can occur from the spasm of chest muscles, could conceivably affect the fetus.

If a convulsion should occur, the woman must be evaluated to be certain that it was from her underlying disease, not from eclampsia. Ordinarily, persons having grand mal convulsions do not need oxygen administered to them during a convulsion. In pregnancy, administering oxygen by mask is good prophylaxis to ensure adequate fetal oxygenation.

The woman should be told to alert hospital personnel at the time of delivery to the fact that she has recurrent convulsions and to report the type medication she is taking. An anesthesiologist needs to know about her convulsions before he administers anesthesia; during the excitement phase of anesthesia a convulsion may occur if he is not forewarned to prevent it.

All through pregnancy, the woman requires encouragement and support for the things that she is doing right. Many women with recurrent convulsions have low self-esteem. Despite all the information at hand about most disease, the actual cause of convulsions is still unknown, and they continue to be regarded as a mysterious or "strange" disease. In the past, people with convulsions were thought to be possessed by devils; in witch-burning times, women with convulsions met death at the stake. In many people's mind this is still a "dirty," or unclean, disorder.

A woman will often worry that her child will have convulsions as he grows older. If her convulsions are the result of an acquired disorder—infection, such as meningitis, or head trauma—there is no basis for thinking they will be inherited and she can be assured that her child will have no more tendency toward convulsions than any other child. If the etiology of her convulsions is unknown (idiopathic epilepsy), the chances that her child will have them too are slightly higher than in the normal population. This prediction is only theoretical, however, and cannot be made without a thorough review of the onset and nature of the woman's disorder.

Dilantin, a drug frequently prescribed for the control of grand mal seizures, appears to be teratogenic, resulting in a Dilantin syndrome (mental retardation, and a peculiar facial proportion, not unlike that of the fetal alcohol syndrome). Tridione, a drug often used to control petit mal seizures, is also a known teratogen. The woman is in a "Catch-22" position of having to take drugs to safeguard her own health, but by taking them she may not be safeguarding the health of the fetus.

Multiple Gestation

Multiple gestation is a complication of pregnancy. In addition to the effects of one fetus on the woman's body, her body must adjust to the effects of another fetus, or two others, or more.

Identical (monozygotic) twins begin with a single ovum and spermatozoon. In the process of fusion, or in one of the first cell divisions, the zygote divides into two identical individuals. Single-ovum twins usually have one placenta, one chorion, two amnions, and two umbilical cords. The twins are always of the same sex. Fraternal (dizygotic) (nonidentical) twins are the result of the fertilization of two separate ova by two separate spermatozoa. These twins are actually siblings growing at the same time in utero. Double-ova twins have two placentas, two chorions, two amnions, and two umbilical cords. The twins may be of the same or different sex.

It is sometimes difficult at delivery to discern whether twins are identical or fraternal because the two fraternal placentas may fuse and appear as one large placenta.

Multiple pregnancies of three, four, five, or six children may be single-ovum conceptions, multiple-ova conceptions, or a combination of two types. Multiple pregnancies are more frequent in nonwhites than in whites. The higher a woman's parity and age, the more likely she is to have a multiple gestation. The mother's inheritance appears to play a role in dizygotic twinning; dizygotic twinning has a familial maternal pattern of occurrence.

ASSESSMENT

Multiple gestation is suspected early in pregnancy when the uterus begins to increase in size at a rate faster than usual. A sonogram will reveal multiple gestational sacs. At the time of quickening the woman may report flurries of action at different portions of her abdomen rather than at one consistent spot (where the feet are located). On auscultation of the abdomen, two sets of fetal heart sounds may be heard; but if one twin has his back positioned toward the woman's back, only one set may be heard. Diagnosis may be confirmed at term or after the 28th week by a roentgenogram if sonogram equipment is not available. On occasion, twinning is not discovered until after the birth of the first child when it is found that the uterus is not empty.

Because the woman is carrying a double weight during pregnancy, she notices extreme fatigue and backache. She may have more difficulty resting or sleeping than the average woman because of greater discomfort and increased fetal activity. She may need sedation to encourage rest and sleep. As the growing uterus compresses her stomach, she may find her appetite decreasing and her intake falling. She may need to eat six small meals a day rather than three large ones to maintain adequate nutrition. She must take her iron, folic acid, and vitamin supplement.

Toward the end of pregnancy the woman may have extreme difficulty ambulating because of fatigue and backache. Her abdomen may become so stretched that she feels as if she were going to burst.

INTERVENTIONS

Some physicians routinely put women with multiple pregnancy on bed rest during the last two or three months of pregnancy. This minimizes the number of falls and accidents that occur from body imbalance and increases the possibility that the pregnancy will come to term, or at least pass the 36th week, when the chances for survival of the fetuses rise markedly. The woman is usually urged to refrain from coitus during the last two or three months because the cervix may be dilating prematurely on account of the early onset of labor.

Women with a multiple gestation are more susceptible to such complications of pregnancy as pregnancy-induced hypertension, hydramnios, placenta previa, and anemia than women carrying one fetus, and they are more prone to postpartal bleeding. Since a multiple pregnancy usually ends before the normal term, immaturity of the newborns is a crisis superimposed at birth. The woman will need closer prenatal supervision than the woman with a single gestation.

EMOTIONAL SUPPORT

The woman with a multiple pregnancy has to work through two role changes during pregnancy rather than one. First, she is surprised to find that she is pregnant (pregnancy is almost always a surprise) and must work through to acceptance of being pregnant. By the 20th week of pregnancy, she is beginning to "nest-build" and show signs that she accepts the pregnancy, that she is preparing to become a mother, or the mother of four rather than of three. Suddenly, at a routine office visit, two sets of heart sounds are heard and many small body parts can be palpated. She is told that she has a twin pregnancy. Now, starting late in pregnancy, she has to work through a second role change: becoming a mother of two, not of one; a mother of five, not of four. This is difficult to complete in the four months of pregnancy remaining (possibly three months because multiple pregnancies usually end at 37 to 39 weeks). She may need postpartal follow-up counseling if she is to form a close mother-child relationship with her babies (Fig. 33-10).

In addition to having to rework a role change, the woman with a multiple pregnancy has more reason to fear for her life and the life of her babies than does the average woman. Most women worry at some time during a twin or multiple pregnancy that the infants will be born joined (like the Siamese twins she remembers seeing on an old circus poster). The chances of this event with twin pregnancy are so small that they can be discounted. Every woman has also heard stories about twins being born so prematurely that they did not survive, and about the special danger for the second twin at delivery. If she has not already heard these stories, she will surely hear them before her due date. Unfortunately, they cannot simply be filed away under the heading of "old wives' tales." Both prematurity and high risk to the aftercoming twin are real hazards in multiple gestation. Although you cannot ignore them, you can help the woman to deal with them as positively as possible. You can tell her that there is no indication so far that her babies are in any danger; that right now it is best to continue doing the things that have to be done. If any problems should arise, you and the rest of the health care team and her family will be there to support her.

Sometimes a woman is so fearful that one or both of her twins will not survive that she makes no preparations for the infants or buys clothes and a crib for

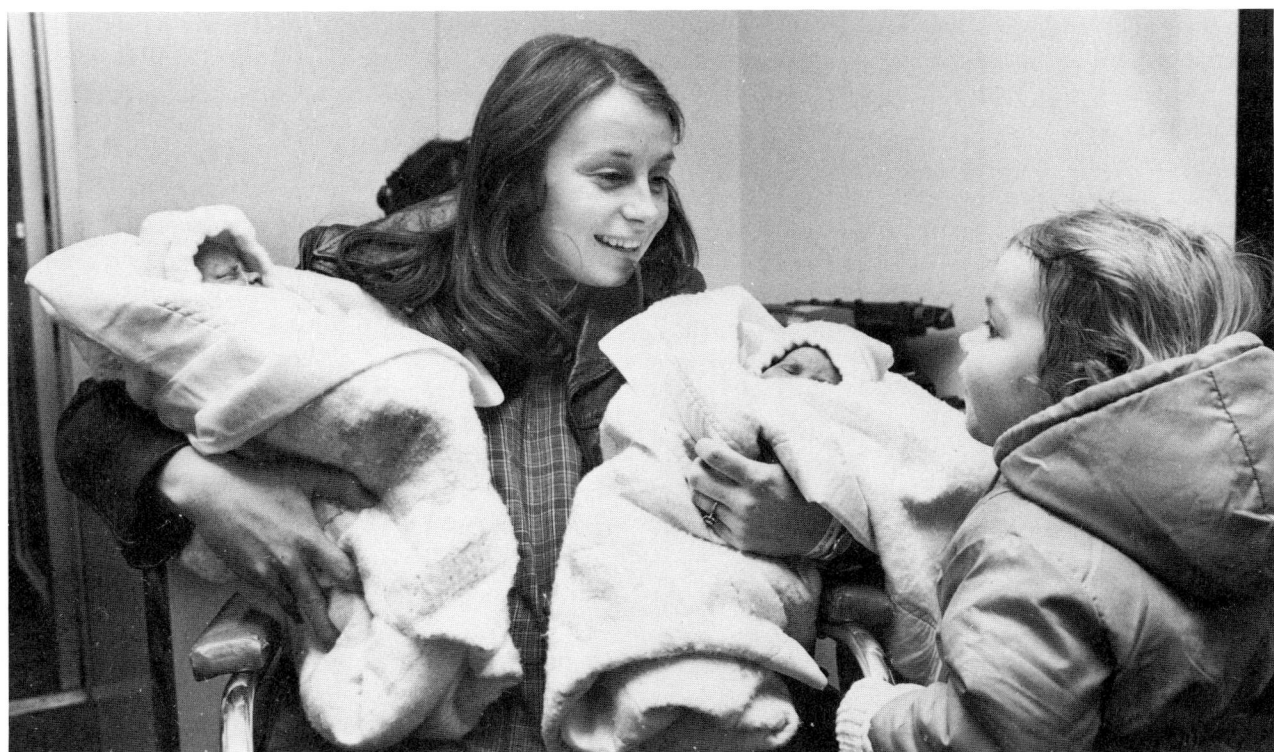

Fig. 33-10. Women need a great deal of support throughout a pregnancy when there are deviations from the normal. Here, a mother shows off twins to an older sibling. (Courtesy of the Department of Medical Photography, Children's Hospital, Buffalo, N.Y.)

only one. This is an indication not so much that she does not accept the second child as that she lacks confidence in herself. She cannot imagine that she will be lucky enough or "good" enough to be able to carry a twin pregnancy to completion. She needs assurance during pregnancy that she is managing well, that she is following instructions well, so that her self-esteem is maintained at as high a level as possible. When her babies are born and both are healthy, the proof she needs that she "deserved" this or was "capable" of it will be present in her arms. Then she will be free to begin interaction with the second child.

The problems that arise at delivery with multiple birth are discussed in Chap. 35.

Hydramnios

Hydramnios is excessive amniotic fluid. Amniotic fluid is usually 500 to 1,000 ml in amount at term. An amount over 2,000 ml is hydramnios.

That hydramnios is occurring will be evidenced by a more rapid enlargement of the uterus than is normal during pregnancy. The small parts of the fetus are difficult to palpate because the uterus is unusually tense. Auscultating fetal heart rate is difficult because of the increased amount of fluid surrounding the fetus.

The woman will begin to notice extreme shortness of breath as the overly distended uterus pushes up against her diaphragm. She may develop lower-extremity varicosities and hemorrhoids because of poor venous return from the extensive uterine pressure. She will have an increased weight gain.

Sonography will generally be ordered in an attempt to discover the reason for the excessive amount of fluid. Amniotic fluid is formed by the cells of the amniotic membrane. It is swallowed by the fetus, absorbed across the intestinal membrane into the fetal bloodstream, and transferred across the placenta. Accumulation of amniotic fluid suggests difficulty with the fetus's ability to swallow or absorb. This occurs in infants who are anencephalic or who have tracheoesophageal fistula with stenosis or intestinal obstruction. It tends to occur in diabetic women.

It is possible to perform an amniocentesis to remove some of the extra fluid to give the woman some relief from the increasing pressure. But since amniotic fluid is replaced rapidly, this is only a temporary measure.

In most instances of hydramnios there is premature rupture of the membranes due to excessive pressure, followed by premature labor. The infant must be appraised carefully in the newborn period for the factors that made him unable to swallow in utero.

The Postmature Pregnancy

A term pregnancy is 38 to 42 weeks long. A pregnancy that exceeds these limits is prolonged, or postmature. The infant of such a pregnancy is postgestational or postmature.

Some pregnancies appear to extend beyond the due date set for them because of a faulty due date. Women who have long menstrual cycles (40 to 45 days) do not ovulate on the 14th day as in a typical menstrual cycle; they ovulate 14 days from the end of their cycle, or on the 26th or 31st day. Thus their child will be "late" by 12 to 17 days.

In other instances the pregnancy is truly overdue. For some reason, the "trigger" that initiates labor did not work. Prolonged pregnancy can occur in a woman on a high dose of salicylates (for severe sinus headaches, rheumatoid arthritis) because salicylate interferes with the synthesis of prostaglandins. Prostaglandins may be responsible for the initiation of labor.

It is dangerous for a fetus to remain in utero more than 2 weeks beyond his time to be born. A placenta seems to have a growth potential for only 40 to 42 weeks. After that it is apparently too old to function adequately. A fetus still in utero will be forced to live with decreased blood perfusion. He may suffer from a lack of oxygen and fluid and nutrients.

At each prenatal visit, the fundal height of a pregnancy is compared to normal standards in an attempt to predict the true gestation age. The gross size of the fetus is palpated to assess whether the infant seems to correlate in size to the month of gestation. If labor has not begun within 42 weeks, the woman may be asked to collect a 24-hour urine for estriol levels. She may have a nonstress test done. If the findings are normal and the physical examination suggests an infant smaller than a normal term infant, perhaps checked by sonogram, the due date is recalculated. If the tests are abnormal or the physical examination or biparietal diameter measured on sonogram suggests that the fetus is term size, the infant will be delivered by inducing labor. The fetal heart rate must be monitored closely during labor to be certain that placental insufficiency is not occurring from aging of the placenta. Problems of the postmature infant are discussed in Chap. 39.

It is difficult for a woman to be pregnant past her due date. The same disappointing reaction occurs when a vacation trip is canceled or it rains on a Fourth of July picnic. She was promised something and now it is being withheld. She knows objectively that her distress is irrational; subjectively she is hurt and angry about what is happening to her.

At birth of the baby, she needs time to examine the child and assure herself that although he did not arrive on the day expected he is well and up to her expectations after all.

The Elderly Primipara

No woman over 35 likes to be referred to as elderly, but women over 35 who are pregnant for the first time are traditionally termed *elderly primiparas*.

A first pregnancy at this age is a high-risk pregnancy from several standpoints. Chromosomal abnormalities are more frequent in the infants of women of this age than in the infants of younger women. The woman is more likely to have hypertension, varicosities, or hemorrhoids prior to pregnancy than a younger woman, and these are conditions that increase in severity during pregnancy and lead to complication. Women over 35 are more prone to pregnancy-induced hypertension than are younger women. The chances are high that an older woman will have a low-gestation-age or low-birth-weight infant. All these factors combined make perinatal mortality in the babies of women over 35 much higher than that in babies of younger women. At delivery, dilatation does not seem to occur as spontaneously in women over 35 as it does in younger women, and uterine inertia (slowing or stopping of uterine contractions during labor) may occur.

Even if the woman has been waiting to become pregnant, she has a major role change to undertake during pregnancy. She is probably well established in a career or has an accustomed routine at home, or in community groups to which she belongs, or both. She needs to discuss how this pregnancy and child rearing are going to fit into her life. She does not have many friends her age who are also having babies; some are close to becoming grandmothers. She does not have access to the daily "shop talk" of other pregnant women, with someone to turn to to ask whether the backache she is experiencing is normal. The only things her friends remember of pregnancy and labor are their highs and lows.

She needs access to health care personnel who can supply her with factual information. She needs a sympathetic ear to listen to her while she works through this role change.

The Pregnant Adolescent

Pregnancy in the adolescent is a high-risk pregnancy from both a psychosocial and a physical standpoint. The psychosocial aspects were discussed in Chap. 12.

The girl under 15 years old who is pregnant is particularly prone to developing pregnancy-induced hypertension and iron deficiency anemia. Vaginal delivery may be difficult, as a cephalopelvic disproportion may exist. Her child is apt to be born prematurely or have a low birth weight. The incidence of stillborn infants is higher in this age group than in the average population.

ASSESSMENT

The adolescent girl needs a detailed health history taken at prenatal visits. It is best to take this history without the girl's mother present. The girl needs practice in being responsible for her own health. Having to account for her health practices during the past month helps her to do this. It also helps prevent her from fabricating the truth so that her mother does not become angry with her.

Adolescents may leave home if their family disapproves of their pregnancy. Trying to manage by themselves, young girls may have tremendous financial difficulties. Ask the girl at prenatal visits where she is living, what the source of her income is, and whom she would call if she suddenly became ill. It is important also to ask her what she had to eat the day before. And you should try to uncover any special problems she is having.

If the mother of the girl accompanies her, ask her separately if she has any concerns she would like to discuss. A young adolescent is very much still a daughter, and her mother is as concerned about her health during this pregnancy as she was at health visits where the girl was being seen for a cold or injury.

Adolescents are prone to pregnancy-induced hypertension. They need a baseline blood pressure determination taken early in pregnancy. Adolescents are often active in a waiting room—walking to get a magazine, returning it, looking out the window—whereas older women tend to accept waiting by seating themselves. Be certain that the girl has 15 minutes of rest before you take a blood pressure or you will measure a false-high recording. Adolescents tend to fail to bring urine specimens with them for their appointments and ask to void for you at the visit. If a girl cannot void, in order not to be criticized, she may return a cupful of water to you for her specimen. If in doubt as to the substance you are testing, check the specific gravity. The specific gravity of water is 1.000. Urine specific gravity ranges from 1.003 to 1.030.

Many adolescents like to weigh themselves at prenatal visits. Weight gain in early pregnancy is one of the ways they have proof that they are pregnant. Because weight gain is such an early indication that pregnancy-induced hypertension is developing, recheck the weight to see that the girl's recording is accurate. It is good practice to make a note of what type of clothing the girl is wearing the first time she is weighed (jeans, a halter top) so later weight determinations can be compared more accurately.

Adolescents may come late for prenatal care because they did not know, or denied, that they were pregnant until the pregnancy was far advanced. They may be unable to drive and may have to depend on other people to transport them to the physician's office or clinic. They may feel so uncomfortable surrounded by the adults in an office or clinic that they come for one visit but never return.

NUTRITION

Good nutrition is a major problem during an adolescent pregnancy. The girl's diet must not only be sufficient to maintain her own health and allow for growth of the fetus but provide for the needs of her own growing body. Protein, iron, and folic acid deficiencies may become acute. Besides eating larger amounts of food than an older woman, the pregnant adolescent must eat the proper foods and abandon the adolescent food fads she has been following. Some girls are so peer-oriented that they balk at substituting a glass of orange juice for a cola beverage because no one else they know drinks orange juice. Many adolescent girls do not know what good nutrition is. They want to eat a good diet but simply do not know what it includes. Some girls have little choice in what foods are prepared at home. To change her dietary pattern you may have to talk to the person who cooks for her.

All adolescents are poor takers of medicine. They need frequent reminders that vitamin and iron supplements during pregnancy not only have to be purchased but have to be swallowed as well.

HEALTH TEACHING

Adolescent girls may respond to health teaching that is directed to their own health more than to that of the fetus inside them: "Eat a high-protein diet because protein makes your hair shiny (or prevents split fingernails)." "Taking the iron supplement should make you feel less tired." These are true statements and appeal to an adolescent's preoccupation with self. This type of health teaching is the only form to which the adolescent who is denying her pregnancy can respond. Be careful about overselling the effects of something in health teaching. Adolescents are suspicious of people in authority. If you are caught in a lie, their suspicions that adults are not to be trusted are confirmed, and they may not return to the office or clinic.

Adolescent girls may not plan enough rest during pregnancy, especially if they are proceeding as if nothing is happening to them.

A young girl often has distorted concepts about her body. Despite all the health information given to children in school, it still is not uncommon to find an adolescent girl who thinks that her baby is growing in her stomach. Such a girl is unwilling to eat large meals during pregnancy (or eat at all) for fear of suffocating the fetus. All adolescent girls need education on the anatomical and physiological events of pregnancy. The pregnant adolescent needs factual information about labor and delivery to counteract all the scare stories her peers have told her. She needs to attend preparation-for-childbirth and motherhood classes as much as do older women.

DELIVERY DECISION

Pelvic measurements should be taken early and accurately in adolescent girls; cephalopelvic disproportion is a very real possibility due to the girl's incomplete pelvic growth. Most girls respond well to the news that their baby will have to be delivered by cesarean section, and many are relieved. Surgery seems controlled and simple when compared with the agonies of labor that they imagine are in store. The decision on the method of delivery should be shared with the girl and her parents when it is reached by the health care team. This is part of being honest with the girl. It cannot be stressed enough that adolescents, for the most part, want to know the truth. They tend to regard the withholding of information, such as that their child must be delivered by surgery, not as a way of protecting them from worry but as an indication that they are being treated like children.

PLANS FOR THE BABY

An adolescent needs additional time at prenatal visits to talk to a good listener concerning her feelings about being pregnant. Scared? Bewildered? Numb? Happy? The plans for the baby should be discussed. Often the girl does not begin to make plans for the baby until very late in pregnancy. She should know the options available to her so that when she is ready to begin planning she knows the alternatives: keeping her baby or placing the baby in a temporary foster home or for adoption. She needs to make some plans for her life after this pregnancy. Will she return to school? Try to get a job? Marry?

It is always amazing how much concerns and problems can be diminished merely by talking about them. Putting a problem or feeling into words puts a fence around it, limits it to a certain size, a certain definite form; and in this size and form, it can be dealt with. One of the most important functions of a nurse in a prenatal clinic or physician's office is being a good listener to an adolescent mother-to-be.

Hyperemesis Gravidarum

Hyperemesis gravidarum (sometimes called *pernicious vomiting*) is nausea and vomiting of pregnancy that are prolonged past the 12th week of pregnancy or are so severe that dehydration, ketonuria, and significant weight loss occur within the first 12 weeks. This condition occurs much less frequently today than formerly. The normal nausea and vomiting of pregnancy are now being treated as entities in themselves and thus rarely progress to hyperemesis gravidarum.

SYMPTOMS

The nausea and vomiting of normal pregnancy follow the rise in human chorionic gonadotropin (HCG), beginning at about the 6th week of pregnancy and declining at about the 12th week. Women with hyperemesis gravidarum have unexplained low HCG levels. Their difficulty may arise from sensitivity to estrogen.

The woman with the normal nausea and vomiting of pregnancy notices the nausea on arising in the morning; she shuns breakfast because she feels that she may vomit; she is likely to vomit once during the morning. By noon the nausea has completely disappeared, and she is suddenly ravenously hungry. In other women (and still within a normal pattern), the nausea and vomiting occur around dinnertime when she begins to prepare food and smell its odors, and also at the times of day when she is most tired. Because normal nausea and vomiting last for only part of the day, the woman's nutrition, even without therapy such as an antiemetic, can be adequately maintained.

ASSESSMENT

With hyperemesis gravidarum, the woman may show an elevated hematocrit or hemoglobin concentration at her monthly prenatal visit, not because her hemoglobin level is so high, but because her inability to retain fluid has resulted in hemoconcentration. Her electrolyte balance may be affected if vomiting is severe during the day or persists for an extended period. Concentrations of sodium, potassium, and chloride may be reduced, and hypokalemic alkalosis may result. In some women, polyneuritis, due to a deficiency of vitamin B, develops. She may be losing weight. Her urine will test positive for ketones, evidence that her body is breaking down stored fat and protein for cell growth.

There may be a number of psychosocial factors involved in the development of pernicious vomiting. A woman with this condition may be ambivalent toward her pregnancy (but then, so are many women who do not have it). She may be psychosexually immature; she may be one of those persons who responds to stress through gastrointestinal symptoms.

Hyperemesis gravidarum must be stopped before starvation occurs and fetal damage results. Ask the woman at prenatal visits whether she is having nausea and vomiting. Determine exactly how much. Ask her to describe the events of the day before if she says it was a typical day. How late into the day did the nausea last? How many times did she vomit? What was the total amount of food she ate? Did she take adequate fluid?

INTERVENTIONS

For treatment of this condition the woman needs to be hospitalized so that her intake, output, and blood chemistries can be monitored and dehydration prevented.

During the first 24 hours of the hospital admission, no food and fluid are allowed by mouth. The woman receives approximately 3,000 ml of an intravenous dextrose solution with added vitamin B. A sedative such as phenobarbital is ordered to encourage rest, and an antiemetic such as Bendectin may be prescribed. Many physicians exclude all visitors for the first 24 hours or until the vomiting has ceased. If there is no vomiting after 24 hours, every 2 or 3 hours small quantities of dry toast, crackers, or cereal are given, and clear fluid (not over 100 ml at a time) is given at hours other than the dry foods. If no vomiting occurs, the woman is gradually advanced to a soft diet, then to a normal diet. If these measures are not effective, tube feeding may be tried. Total parenteral nutrition (hyperalimentation) may be attempted.

The normal nausea and vomiting of pregnancy are precipitated by fatigue and the smell of cooking, and so is pernicious vomiting. The portions of food served should be small, so that the amount does not appear overwhelming. Food should be attractively prepared. Hot foods should be hot and cold foods cold.

Although an emesis basin is an important piece of equipment for the person who is vomiting, put it out of sight, not on the bedside table, so that the woman is not constantly reminded of vomiting. Be sure that food carts smelling of fish, bacon, or coffee are not parked outside her door at mealtimes.

A woman with hyperemesis gravidarum needs the opportunity to express how she feels about the strange thing that is happening to her. She needs to talk about how it feels to be pregnant; how it feels to live with ever-present nausea. In some women, so many psychosocial factors are involved that psychotherapy is required to help them decide either to terminate the pregnancy or to accept it and allow it to go to completion.

Pseudocyesis

In pseudocyesis, nausea and vomiting, amenorrhea, and enlargement of the abdomen occur in a nonpregnant woman. In some women, the abdomen is so enlarged that the woman appears seven or eight months pregnant. This is sometimes called *psychogenic* or *false pregnancy*. It tends to occur in women who are lonely, very desirous of having children, and perhaps infertile. The woman's body responds to her needs with physiological symptoms. On physical examination, it is obvious the woman is not pregnant. Her abdominal wall is enlarged, but her uterus is not. No other signs of pregnancy but the amenorrhea, nausea, and vomiting are present.

The woman needs psychotherapy to learn how to handle her needs on a sound mental health basis.

Drug Dependence

Drug dependence is an increasing problem during pregnancy because it is a growing problem in women of childbearing age.

A drug-dependent person is one who craves a drug for either psychological or physical well-being. The number of drugs that can lead to such a state comprises long lists. They can be categorized as stimulants, depressants, and psychedelics.

Stimulants include drugs such as amphetamines that give a feeling of increased productivity. They are termed *uppers* or *speed*.

Depressants give a feeling of passive, calm well-being. Barbiturates, tranquilizers, narcotics, alcohol, and volatile solvents (airplane glue) are examples. These are termed *downers* and may be alternated with uppers for increased effect.

Psychedelic drugs give a feeling of "spacing out" or being removed from reality. Examples are lysergic acid diethylamide (LSD), phencyclidine hydrochloride (PCP or angel dust), mescaline or cannabis (marihuana). These drugs are termed *trippers* or *hallucinogens*.

THE DRUG-DEPENDENT WOMAN

Typically, drug-abusing women are in the younger age group. They have less standardized life-styles because they spend their money for drugs rather than for home furnishings. Very settled-appearing women may be drug-dependent, however. Use of amphetamines (begun originally as an aid to dieting) is not confined to any one age group. The use of barbiturates and alcohol is an older-age problem.

Carr [4] has identified three characteristics of the typical drug-dependent woman. She is a woman from a disrupted family background (many of these women leave home as adolescents; they have few meaningful support people and few skills or little education to use to support themselves). She is a woman with negative sexual experiences (many drug-dependent women have been victims of incest or rape). They have low self-esteem. They use drugs to ease psychological pain, fill a sense of emptiness, and promote social interaction.

A drug-dependent woman is apt to have difficulty following prenatal instructions. Although they mean to eat well, women addicted to street drugs such as barbiturates or narcotics rarely have enough money for both drugs and food, and their diets during pregnancy are thus often inadequate. Further, they are unlikely to have money for supplemental vitamins or iron preparations.

Abused drugs cross the placenta readily. As a result, the fetus of an addicted mother is exposed to the drug. If a woman uses a drug that she injects, she may well develop hepatitis unless her injection equipment is clean each time. Because a majority of women addicts become prostitutes to earn money for drugs, they are more likely than the average woman to contract venereal diseases, posing an additional threat to the fetus.

The drug-abusing woman may be reluctant to come for prenatal care, afraid that she will be "found out" and reported to legal authorities. She may not have the money to pay for prenatal services or transportation to and from a clinic. If she is using a drug that only sustains her for 4 hours, she cannot wait long for an appointment.

The infants of drug-abusing women tend to be small for gestation age and to have a higher-than-average incidence of congenital anomalies. They will have the same withdrawal symptoms after birth as the mother would if she abruptly stopped taking the drug.

Because the fetus is exposed to drugs that must be processed by the liver during pregnancy, his liver is forced to mature faster than normally. For this reason, newborns of drug-abusing women seem better able to cope with bilirubin at birth than other babies; hyperbilirubinemia is rarely a problem. Fetal lung tissue also appears to mature more rapidly than is normal. Thus even though the infant is born prematurely, the chance that he will develop a condition such as respiratory distress syndrome is less than average.

If at all possible, the narcotic-dependent woman should be enrolled in a methodone maintenance program or a drug withdrawal program during pregnancy. Infants born of a woman on methadone do not escape withdrawal symptoms (some infants appear to have more severe reactions to methadone withdrawal than to heroin withdrawal), but because the woman is being provided drugs legally, the fetus is assured better nutrition, better care, and less exposure to pathogens such as hepatitis virus.

Drug withdrawal symptoms of the newborn are discussed in Chap 38.

Drug-dependent women need your support during pregnancy. They are women of low self-esteem who need reassurance at prenatal visits that everything is going well with the pregnancy. They need anticipatory guidance throughout pregnancy as they have few effective support people to discuss their problems or worries with them or to answer questions about pregnancy for them.

THE ALCOHOL-DEPENDENT WOMAN

Alcohol abuse is a problem of all age groups. Young women may use alcohol to supplement the effect of narcotics or barbiturates. Older women may use it exclusively because it is so readily available and legal and acceptable for their style of life.

Formerly it was believed that alcohol, per se, had no effect on a growing fetus. Its effect during pregnancy was that of malnutrition because the woman spent her money on alcohol rather than food. Now it is evident that alcohol itself has an effect on the growing fetus. Infants of alcohol-dependent women tend to be small for gestation age and have mental retardation and an unusual facial appearance, including a prominent nose or "bird-like face."

All women should be cautioned not to drink alcohol during pregnancy. Ask at prenatal visits, "What is your usual alcohol consumption?" A term such as *social drinker* is meaningless, and you need to ask a woman who uses it to define it. Some social drinkers drink a cocktail every three months; other social drinkers have five cocktails every day.

Deviations from the Normal in Pregnancy: Nursing Interventions 577

Most women who are alcohol-dependent are not aware of their dependency. The only reason they drink so much, they say, is that alcohol is forced on them at parties or that it is necessary as a part of their job to attend luncheons, receptions, and so forth. They are certain they can stop this very afternoon. When a reason for stopping such as pregnancy occurs, they are distressed to find that they cannot stop. They enjoy alcohol and depend on it to make them feel comfortable at social functions or under stress.

Withdrawing from using alcohol, if the woman is dependent, is as complicated as withdrawing from other drugs. Joining Alcoholics Anonymous is very helpful. The woman's support people may have to be involved in helping her avoid situations where she is most likely to feel the need for alcohol.

At a time in life when she needs to have high self-esteem (she is about to have a baby; that involves thousands of decision-making opportunities every day, and effective decision making requires high self-esteem) a woman discovers that she is not even independent enough to control what she drinks or does not drink in a day's time. She needs reassurance that the things she is doing right are right. Many women with a high alcohol consumption are vitamin B–deficient because of the interaction between alcohol and the synthesis of vitamin B. They may need a vitamin B supplement during pregnancy in addition to other vitamins prescribed.

THE CIGARETTE-DEPENDENT WOMAN

Smoking is one form of drug ingestion because nicotine is absorbed in the process of smoking cigarettes. Infants of cigarette-smoking women tend to be small for gestation age. Further, the incidence of prematurity in these women is increased, probably because of constriction of uterine arteries due to the vasoconstriction action of nicotine. Prematurity may result from high carbon monoxide levels in the bloodstream.

Stopping smoking is very difficult; one can be as dependent on cigarettes as on any other drug. If the woman cannot stop, she should be urged to cut back the number of cigarettes smoked to 10 per day. All prenatal offices should have *Please, No Smoking* signs.

Women who quit smoking often express strong desires for snack foods, to have "something in my mouth." Review their diet intake for the last 24 hours with them at prenatal visits to see whether, now that they are not smoking so much, they are taking in more high-carbohydrate food than protein-rich food. They will invariably gain more weight during pregnancy than might otherwise be expected, and they need assurance at prenatal visits that the extra weight gain is a compensation for stopping smoking, not the sudden weight gain of edema from pregnancy-induced hypertension.

Assure the woman that health personnel appreciate the problem she has in reducing smoking. It is preferable that she gain extra pounds for having stopped smoking than that she deliver a premature baby because of smoking.

The Battered Woman

More than a million women in the United States are battered or beaten yearly. This is a problem of all socioeconomic levels. Battered women are seen in prenatal settings because they are unable to resist sexual advances from their abusive partner. The pregnancy may not be wanted; on the other hand, the woman may think that having a child will change the partner and make him a better person.

Women remain with abusive partners because they are afraid to leave, and fear immobilizes them. They often feel that this state of affairs is their fault and if they were better people their partner would not resort to beating them. This guilt further immobilizes them. Since they generally have no access to money and no skills to earn money, they feel that leaving the man would be worse than staying. Even if they have a skill—they were capable secretaries or salesgirls once—their self-esteem has become so low that they no longer believe they can successfully put it to use.

Beatings may increase during pregnancy because stress is often a "trigger" to beatings and pregnancy involves stresses. The woman so nauseated that she cannot cook, so tired that she did not make a bed is liable to be beaten. A husband concerned about the hospital bill can resort to a beating.

A battered woman may come late for pregnancy care because of lack of transportation (her husband controls the use of the car) or because she has tried to pretend that the pregnancy did not exist. "Not rocking the boat," keeping the stress level down, is her best defense against violence.

She may be noticeable in a prenatal setting in that she purchases no clothing especially for the pregnancy (she has no funds for herself, and asking for new clothes may incite violence). She may not go for laboratory tests if going involves transportation or money. She is different from women whose main problem is poverty. Even the poorest family will squeeze out money for one dress that will show off the pregnancy; squeeze out money for laboratory tests if having these done will ensure a successful outcome to the pregnancy.

She may have difficulty following a pregnancy diet (she must cook what her partner wants cooked or she will be beaten). She may leave before the nurse or physician sees her, or she may grow very anxious if her prenatal appointment is running late (she must be home to cook dinner or she will be beaten).

She may dress inappropriately for warm weather, wearing long-sleeved tight-necked blouses to cover up the bruises on her neck or arms. She may call and cancel appointments frequently (or simply not keep appointments) because she has an obvious black eye or a bleeding facial laceration she does not want to reveal.

If undressed for a physical examination, she may have bruises or lacerations on her breasts, her abdomen, or her back that she cannot explain. Her neck may reveal linear bruises from strangulation. Ask any woman with bruises to account for them. Listen to see whether the explanation seems to correlate with the extent and placement of the bruise. The woman may be very anxious to listen to the baby's heartbeat at prenatal visits because her partner recently punched or kicked her abdomen and she is worried that the fetus has been hurt.

It is perplexing to work with battered women because it is hard to understand why they stay in their situation. Remember that fear of the abusive person (if they leave, he may find them and kill them) and the guilt and low self-esteem they feel (he has told them so many times that this is their fault and they deserve to be treated this way that they believe it) immobilize them. They are as paralyzed to do anything about their situation without outside help as if they were totally physically paralyzed. To compound the problem, their low self-esteem leads them to think that no one would *want* to help them.

The woman needs help to make decisions. Support any ability to make constructive decisions that she has left. Be familiar with safe shelters for battered women in your community; help her obtain a restraining order to keep the abusive person from coming near her again if this is necessary.

After the birth of the child, the woman may be depressed to realize how alone she is. She may have unreal expectations of the child, trying to make him smile at her and interact with her more than a newborn is capable of doing. She has a great need to be loved. Try to caution her that her newborn does love her but she has to give him or her time to grow. Show the mother all the things her child can do, such as attend to the sound of her voice, or cuddle against her. Otherwise her unreal expectations may lead to disappointment and an interference with her mothering.

Do not leave a battered woman without a support system after birth of the child. If she was depending on you during pregnancy, you cannot abandon her after the pregnancy until you fill in the gap with another support system. This could be a social agency that deals specifically with battered women in your community; it could be a community health nurse who will be visiting when she returns home. If she is left without a support person, her low self-esteem will not allow her to reach out and seek help. She may decide that suicide or returning to the person who abused her is her only resource.

Battered women need to be identified during pregnancy not only so they can be helped but to help the mental health of the child. A child raised in a home where the mother is battered will learn that this is acceptable conduct, and the battering will extend to yet another generation.

Problem-oriented Recording: Progress Notes

Angie Baco
42 years

Problem: Health assessment, 20th week of pregnancy

> S. States, "I feel dizzy all the time. I'm thirsty all the time. My diabetes has come back, hasn't it?" Patient had gestational diabetes treated by diet alone during last pregnancy 7 years ago. Glucose tolerance test done at 12 weeks of this pregnancy was normal.
> O. Urine (single specimen) 3+ glucose; trace of acetone. SG = 1.020. Hydration adequate by skin turgor.
> A. Evidence of gestational diabetes symptoms present.
>
> Goals: a. Patient understands gestational diabetes disease process and reason for all interventions.
> b. Patient learns to test urine and give own insulin, if necessary, for control.
> c. Patient understands importance of prescribed diet and prepares it for herself.
> d. Fetus is not exposed to acidosis or hypoglycemia during pregnancy.

e. Patient to carry pregnancy to as near term as possible.

P. 1. Schedule for hospital admission for evaluation of diabetes.
   2. Arrangements must be made for 7-year-old child while mother is hospitalized. Husband to call when arrangements are made.

Problem: Gestational diabetes, 22nd week of pregnancy

S. Learned insulin injection technique in hospital. Dosage is 6 units NPH, 3 units regular daily. Husband gives insulin to her.
She "can't learn to get the hang of it," "too awkward."
No referral to community health nurse was made from hospital for further teaching.
Urines testing 1+ for glucose, negative for acetone.
States that she understands urine testing procedure; no difficulty carrying this out.
Is on 2200-calorie diet. Following it "pretty well." Had difficulty getting to clinic today because 7-year-old has extra reading class after school on Tuesdays.
O. Urine (single specimen) 1+, neg.
Weight gain 1 lb since last visit (total weight gain is 18 lbs).
A. Gestational diabetic who needs further information on disease and her responsibilities toward care.
P. 1. Review diet to move compliance closer than "pretty well."
   2. Review motivation for giving own insulin; if truly wants to learn this, make referral for community health nurse to visit and teach.
   3. Review schedule for future clinic appointment times so conflict with older child's schedule will not be a problem.
   4. Capillary blood sugar taken.
   5. Reschedule return appointment in 1 week. Review signs of hypo or hyperglycemia and necessity to call if symptoms occur.

Problem: Gestational diabetes, 30th week of pregnancy

S. Had nonstress test done yesterday; pleased that result was negative.
Insulin dose is now 10 units NPH, 4 units regular daily.
Gives own insulin. Urines test 1+ neg.
No edema other than slight ankle edema; no blurring of vision or headache.
Family has learned to omit some desserts along with her so she can maintain 2200-calorie diet. States that this is good for all of them.
Husband present for visit. Appears to be supportive. Asking if a negative nonstress test means that baby has no congenital defects. (One other child died at birth of congenital heart disease.)
O. Weight gain 1 lb in last week. Total 26 lb.
Urine 1+, neg. for glucose and acetone, Neg. for protein.
Blood pressure 122/80; no edema palpable.
A. Gestational diabetic who is managing illness well.
Derives support from husband and children.
P. 1. Review nonstress test and how it measures placental function.
   2. Schedule nonstress test every week now until delivery.
   3. Explain process for collecting 24-hour estriol collection (to collect once a week from now until delivery).
   4. Review plans for hospitalization and delivery. To take no insulin on day scheduled for hospital admission.

References

1. Ayromlooi, J., et al. Management of the diabetic pregnancy. *Obstet. Gynecol.* 49:137, 1977.
2. Bahr, J. E. Rising perinatal infections: Herpes virus hominis type 2 in women and newborns. *M.C.N.* 3:16, 1978.
3. Bell, W. R. Hematologic abnormalities in pregnancy. *Med. Clin. North Am.* 61:165, 1977.
4. Carr, J. N. Psychological Aspects of Pregnancy, Childbirth and Parenting in Drug-dependent Women. In J. L. Rementeria (Ed.), *Drug Abuse in Pregnancy and Neonatal Effects*. St. Louis: Mosby, 1977.
5. Cates, W. D&E after 12 weeks: Safe or hazardous? *Contemp. Obstet. Gynecol.* 13:23, 1979.
6. Chesley, L. C. Hypertensive disorders in pregnancy. *Drug Ther.* 2:10, 1977.

7. Chung, H. J. Arresting premature labor. *Am. J. Nurs.* 76:810, 1976.
8. Clark, J. Preventing maternal death in advanced abdominal pregnancy. *Contemp. Obstet. Gynecol.* 12:137, 1978.
9. Davison, J. M., et al. Renal disease in pregnant women. *Clin. Obstet. Gynecol.* 21:411, 1978.
10. Dore, S. L., and Davies, B. L. Catharsis for high-risk antenatal patients. *M.C.N.* 4:96, 1979.
11. Duhring, J. Diabetes in Pregnancy. *Female Patient* 5:12, 1980.
12. Freeman, E. W. Abortion: Subjective attitudes and feelings. *Fam. Plann. Perspect.* 10:151, 1978.
13. Fuchs, F. Prevention of premature birth. *Clin. Perinatol.* 7:3, 1980.
14. Gabbe, S. G. Diabetes in pregnancy: Clinical controversies. *Clin. Obstet. Gynecol.* 21:443, 1978.
15. Gabbe, S. G. New ideas on managing the pregnant diabetic patient. *Contemp. Obstet. Gynecol.* 13:109, 1979.
16. Gant, N. F., et al. Clinical management of pregnancy induced hypertension. *Clin. Obstet. Gynecol.* 21:397, 1978.
17. Gordis, E., and Kreek, M. J. Alcoholism and drug addiction in pregnancy. *Curr. Pract. Obstet. Gynecol.* 1:5, 1977.
18. Graf, C. M. Sexually transmitted disease: A new look at an old problem. *Comp. Pediatr. Nurs.* 2:11, 1978.
19. Hendrix, M. J. The battered wife. *Am. J. Nurs.* 78:650, 1978.
20. Hughey, M. J., et al. The effect of fetal monitoring on the incidence of cesarean sections. *Obstet. Gynecol.* 49:513, 1977.
21. Jones, M. B. Hypertension disorders of pregnancy. *J.O.G.N. Nurs.* 8:92, 1979.
22. Knox, G. E. How infection damages the fetus. *Contemp. Obstet. Gynecol.* 12:96, 1978.
23. Leontic, E. A. Respiratory disorders in pregnancy. *Med. Clin. North Am.* 61:111, 1977.
24. Leppert, P. C. Hyperemesis gravidarum. *Nurs. Digest* 3:15, 1975.
25. Lieberknecht, B. A. Helping the battered wife. *Am. J. Nurs.* 78:654, 1978.
26. Linzey, E. M. Controlling diabetes with continuous insulin infusion. *Contemp. Obstet. Gynecol.* 12:43, 1978.
27. Marchant, D. J. Urinary tract infection in pregnancy. *Clin. Obstet. Gynecol.* 21:921, 1978.
28. McGovern, C. Recognizing a tubal pregnancy. *M.C.N.* 3:303, 1978.
29. McKay, S. R. Smoking during the childbearing year. *M.C.N.* 5:46, 1980.
30. Petrella, J. M. The unwed pregnant adolescent: Implications for the professional nurse. *J.O.G.N. Nurs.* 7:22, 1978.
31. Rein, M., and Chapel, R. Trichomoniasis, candidiasis and other minor venereal diseases. *Clin. Obstet. Gynecol.* 18:73, 1975.
32. Richart, R. M. When a renal transplant patient becomes pregnant. *Contemp. Obstet. Gynecol.* 13:153, 1979.
33. Roberts, J. M. When the hypertensive patient becomes pregnant. *Contemp. Obstet. Gynecol.* 13:49, 1979.
34. Rotterdam, H. Vaginal and cervical abnormalities in DES daughters. *Female Patient* 4:22, 1979.
35. Schuler, K. When a pregnant woman is diabetic: Antepartal care. *Am. J. Nurs.* 79:448, 1979.
36. Sonstegard, L. Pregnancy induced hypertension: Prenatal nursing concerns. *M.C.N.* 4:90, 1979.
37. Steinman, M. E. Reaching and helping the adolescent who becomes pregnant. *M.C.N.* 4:35, 1979.
38. Tanzi, F. Tuberculosis in pregnancy: Real threat in urban areas. *Contemp. Obstet. Gynecol.* 12:125, 1978.
39. Tichy, A. M., and Chong, D. Placental function and its role in toxemia. *M.C.N.* 4:84, 1979.
40. Ueland, K. Pregnancy and cardiovascular disease. *Med. Clin. North Am.* 61:17, 1977.
41. Ueland, K. What's the risk when the cardiac patient is pregnant? *Contemp. Obstet. Gynecol.* 13:117, 1979.
42. Welt, S. I., and Crenshaw, M. C. Concurrent hypertension and pregnancy. *Clin. Obstet. Gynecol.* 21:411, 1978.
43. White, P. Pregnancy and Diabetes. In A. Marble et al. (Eds.), *Joslin's Diabetes Mellitus* (11th ed.). Philadelphia: Lea & Febiger, 1971.

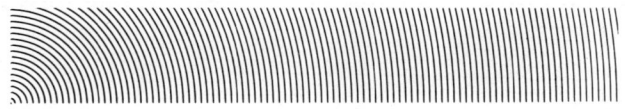

34. Genetic Disorders and Pregnancy

The genetic composition that a couple brings into the formation of a fertilized ovum has implications not only for the successful completion of the pregnancy but for the future of the child.

Chromosomal abnormalities occur in the moment of fusion of the ovum and spermatozoon or, even earlier, in the meiosis division phase of the formation of the gametes (reproductive cells) of the parent. A great many early spontaneous abortions are apparently due to malformations caused by these abnormalities that are so severe that they are incompatible with life. Sometimes the defect does not affect life in utero; only after birth will the abnormality become apparent. As many as 1 in every 150 infants is born with some kind of chromosomal abnormality.

The material of heredity (deoxyribonucleic acid, or DNA) is carried as genes on thread-like intranuclear structures known as chromosomes. In humans, the spermatozoa and ova each carry 23 such chromosomes. For each chromosome in the sperm cell there is a like chromosome in the ovum of similar size and shape and the same type of gene content. The exception to this is the chromosome that determines sex. The female sex chromosome is medium-sized, with arms of equal length (metrocentric); the male sex chromosome is small and has an off-center midpoint (acrocentric).

The individual formed from the union of two gametes has 46 chromosomes in every body cell (44 autosomes and 2 sex chromosomes). If the sex chromosomes are both X (the medium-sized, metrocentric type), the individual is female (Fig. 34-1A); if one is an X and one a Y (the small, acrocentric type), the individual is a male (Fig. 34-1B).

Mendelian Inheritance: Dominant and Recessive Genes

The genetic inheritance of disease follows certain laws, the same laws that govern genetic inheritance of other body characteristics such as eye color or hair color. These laws were formulated by Gregor Mendel, an Austrian naturalist, and are known as *mendelian laws*.

A person who has two like genes—for blue eyes, for example (one from the mother and one from the father)—is said to be *homozygous* for that trait. If the genes differ (a gene for blue eyes from the mother and a gene for brown eyes from the father, or vice versa), the person is said to be *heterozygous* for that trait. Such a person would have brown eyes, since, in eye color, brown is dominant over blue, but would be said to be a carrier for blue eyes, that is, to carry a hid-

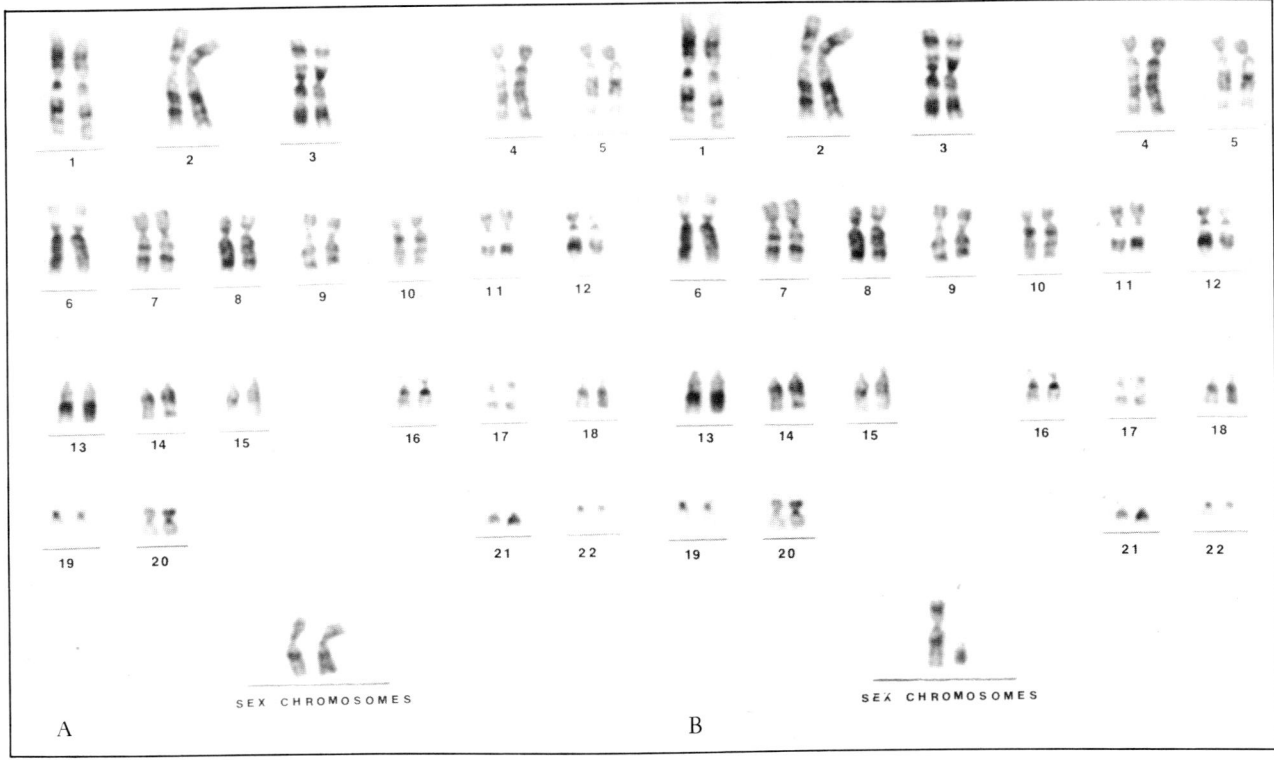

Fig. 34-1. Photomicrographs of human chromosomes (karyotypes). If a blood sample is taken from a newborn and the white cells are examined at the mitotic division phase of reproduction, transferred to slides, and photographed under high-power magnification, then the individual chromosomes can be cut from the photograph and arranged according to size and shape. A. Normal female karyotype. B. Normal male karyotype. (Courtesy of Dr. Judith Brown, Medical College of Virginia, Richmond, and the Department of Medical Photography, Children's Hospital, Buffalo, N.Y.)

den gene for blue eyes. The outward appearance of traits is called the person's *phenotype*; the underlying genetic composition is the *genotype*. An individual with two homozygous genes for brown eyes is *homozygous dominant*; the individual with two genes for blue eyes is *homozygous recessive*.

The mendelian laws permit prediction of eye color in terms of the proportion of children that will be born to parents of a certain genotype. For example, when a homozygous dominant person marries a homozygous recessive person, it can be predicted that 100 percent of their children will be heterozygous for this trait (Fig. 34-2A); they will be brown-eyed, but will carry a recessive gene for blue eyes.

Suppose the mother is heterozygous instead of homozygous recessive as in the previous example. As can be seen in Fig. 34-2B, when this pairing occurs, the chances are equal that their child will be homozygous dominant like the father or heterozygous like the mother. All the children's phenotypes will be brown eyes.

Suppose both parents are heterozygous. As can be seen in Fig. 34-2C, 25 percent of the children will be homozygous recessive (blue-eyed); 50 percent will be heterozygous (brown-eyed); and 25 percent will be homozygous dominant (brown-eyed). This is how two brown-eyed parents can produce a blue-eyed child, or two brunette parents can produce a blonde child. It is impossible to predict the person's genotype from the phenotype.

INHERITANCE OF DISEASE

The same principles are applicable to predicting diseases (those that are carried in the chromosomes) in children. Diseases may be transmitted either as dominant traits or as recessive traits. The dominant varieties are few. A person with a dominant trait for a disease is usually heterozygous—that is, has a corresponding healthy recessive gene. Huntington's chorea, a progressive neurological disease, with onset usually in middle age, is the traditional example of a dominantly inherited disease. One form of muscular dystrophy (facioscapulohumeral) and osteogenesis imperfecta are other examples.

If a person with a dominant disease trait—say, facioscapulohumeral muscular dystrophy—is mated with a person without the trait, as shown in Fig. 34-2D, the chances are even that their offspring will be born with the disease or be disease-free and carrier-free.

Two persons with a dominantly inherited disease are unlikely to marry. However, if they do marry, their chances of having normal children decline (Fig. 34-2E). Now only 25 percent of the offspring would be disease- and carrier-free; 50 percent would have the disease, and the remaining 25 percent would be homozygous dominant, a condition that is probably incompatible with life.

The majority of heritable diseases are inherited as recessive traits. Such diseases do not occur unless two genes for the disease are present. Cystic fibrosis, adrenogenital syndrome, albinism, Tay-Sachs disease, galactosemia, phenylketonuria, sickle cell anemia, and limb girdle muscular dystrophy are examples of recessively inherited diseases.

In Fig. 34-2F, both parents are disease-free. However, both are heterozygous in genotype and thus carry a recessive gene for cystic fibrosis. As can be seen, 25 percent of their children will be disease- and carrier-free; 50 percent will be like themselves, free of disease, but carrying the unexpressed disease gene; 25 percent will have the disease.

Suppose a woman with the genotype in Fig. 34-2F marries a man who has no trait for cystic fibrosis (Fig. 34-2G). The chances are even that a child born to them will be completely disease- and carrier-free or heterozygous like the mother. None of their children will have the disease. The children should be aware, however, that *their* children may manifest the disease if they carry the trait and marry a person with the trait (see Fig. 34-2F).

Formerly, children with cystic fibrosis died in early infancy and so never reached childbearing age. Today, with good management, some can live to have children. If a person with cystic fibrosis should marry a person without the trait, all their children would be free of the disease. They would all be carriers, however, as shown in Fig. 34-2H.

If the cystic fibrosis patient marries a person with an unexpressed gene for the disease, the chances are equal that their children will have the disease or be carriers of the disease (Fig. 34-2I). If a person with the disease should marry a person who also had the disease, as shown in Figure 34-2J, all of their children could be expected to have the disease.

INHERITANCE OF BLOOD INCOMPATIBILITY

Whether or not blood incompatibility will become a problem in the pregnancies of Rh-negative blood type mothers can be predicted on the same basis. In Fig. 34-2K, both the mother and the father have Rh-negative blood or lack a D blood antigen. As can be seen, all of their children will have Rh-negative blood (dd genotype) and thus there will be no Rh incompatibility.

The father in Fig. 34-2L is heterozygous for the Rh factor (has a Dd genotype), the mother is Rh-negative (dd genotype). In this instance the chances are equal that a child will have Rh-negative blood or Rh-positive blood; the positive factor is dominant over the negative factor, so people with a heterozygous genotype (+− or Dd) have Rh-positive blood (the phenotype). However, if the father is homozygous for Rh-positive blood (DD genotype) (Fig. 34-2M), all their children will have Rh-positive blood. It is extremely doubtful (unless the woman's antibody formation system is not active or she is administered RhoGAM [Rh_o (D) immune globulin]) that this mother could escape problems of blood incompatibility in her pregnancies.

SEX-LINKED INHERITANCE

Some genes for disease are located on the female sex chromosomes, the X chromosomes. This is called sex-linked, or X-linked, inheritance. The mother will be the carrier for this type of inherited disease; the disease itself will be manifested in her male children.

Hemophilia A, Christmas disease (a blood factor deficiency), color blindness, Duchenne-Griesinger disease (pseudohypertrophic muscular dystrophy), and some forms of gargoylism are examples of this type of inheritance. Such a pattern is shown in Fig. 34-2N, in which the mother is the carrier of the trait and the father is disease-free. Half of their male children will manifest the disease, and half of their female children will be carriers like their mother. If the father has the disease and marries a woman who is not a carrier, all of their daughters will be carriers of the disease (will have the sex-linked recessive gene). None of the sons will have the disease. This is shown in Fig. 34-2O.

Division Defects

As mentioned, in some instances of chromosomal disease, the abnormality occurs not because of dominant or recessive patterns of inheritance but because of a fault in division of the reproductive cells, in which each new ovum or spermatozoon receives half, rather than all, the chromosomes of the parent cell (meiosis). In meiosis, half of the chromosomes are attracted to one pole of the cell and half to the other pole. The cell then divides cleanly, with 23 chromosomes contained in one new cell and 23 chromosomes in the second new cell. Chromosomal

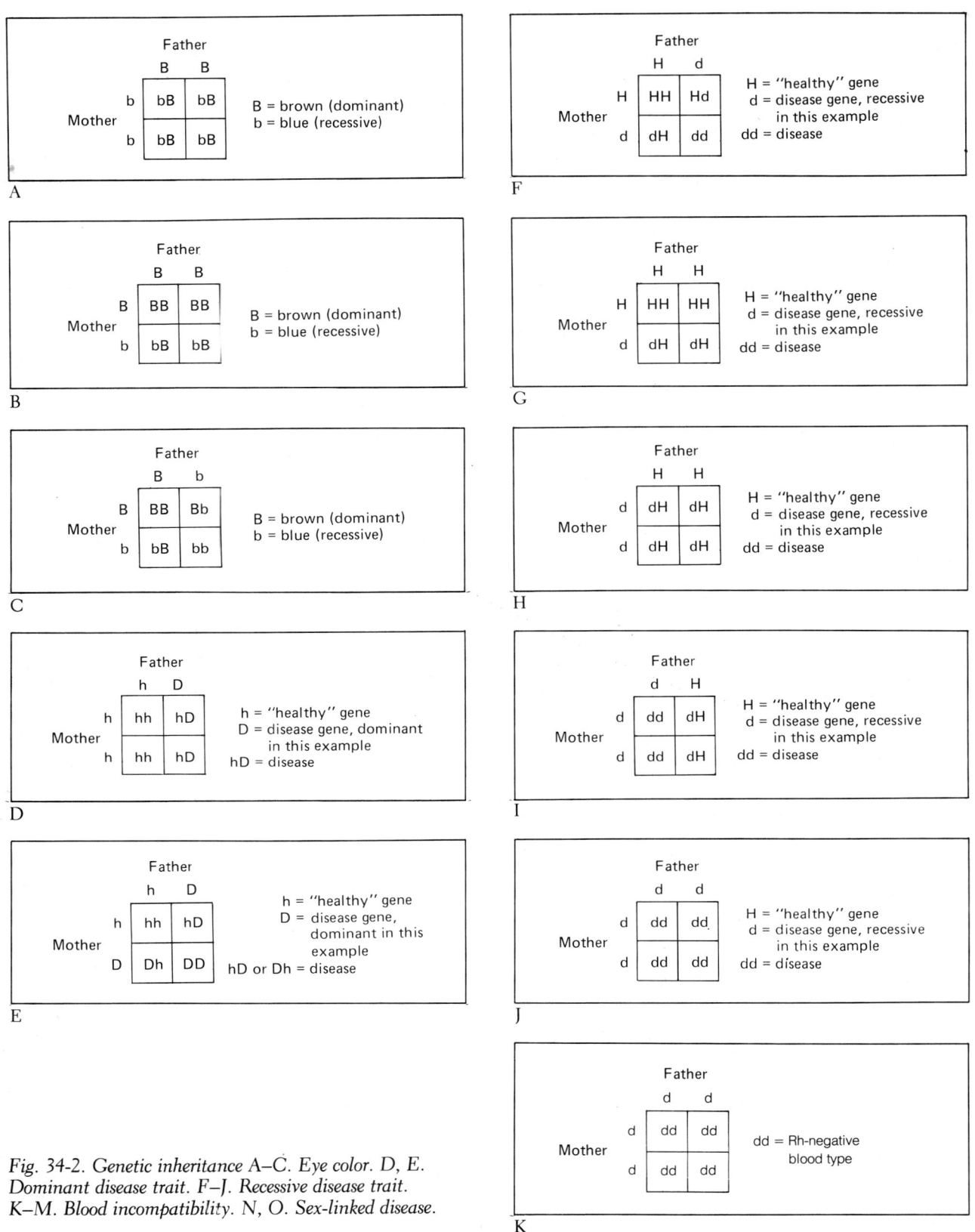

Fig. 34-2. Genetic inheritance A–C. Eye color. D, E. Dominant disease trait. F–J. Recessive disease trait. K–M. Blood incompatibility. N, O. Sex-linked disease.

586   The High-Risk Pregnancy

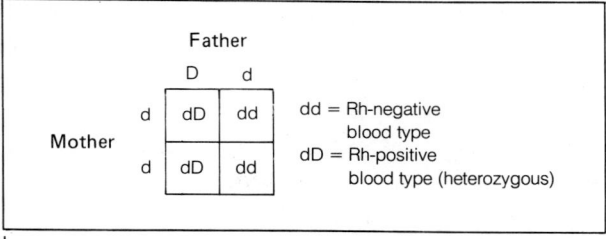

L

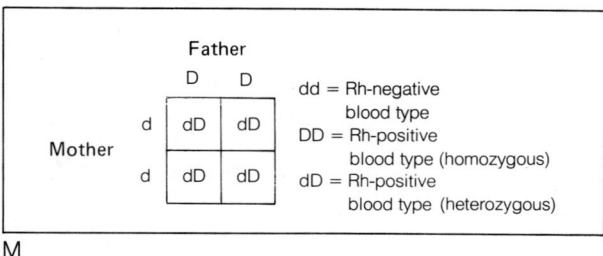

M

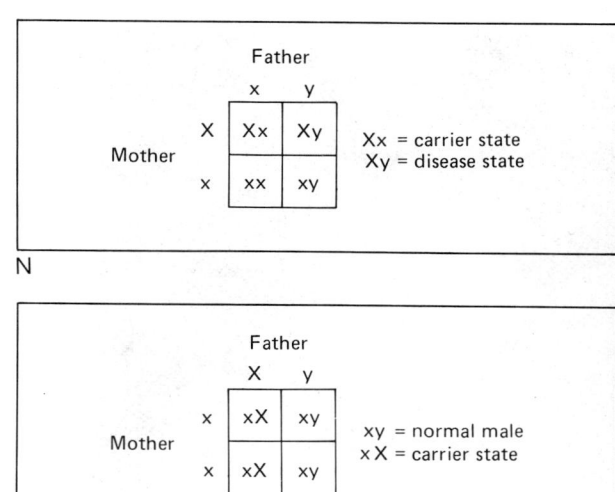

N

O

abnormalities occur when the division is uneven (nondisjunction). The result may be that one new sperm cell or ovum formed may have 24 chromosomes and the other one only 22. If one of these defective spermatozoa or ova fuses with a normal spermatozoon or ovum, the zygote will have 47 or 45 chromosomes, not the normal 46. The presence of 45 chromosomes does not appear to be compatible with life, and the embryo or fetus will probably be aborted. Down's syndrome (trisomy 21) is an example of a disease in which the individual has 47 chromosomes. With Down's syndrome there is an extra number 21 chromosome (three rather than two) (Fig. 34-3).

Down's syndrome can occur as another form of trisomy 21, in which the child has the usual 46 chromosomes because the extra number 21 chromosome is not separate but is joined to another chromosome (translocated) (usually to number 15). One of the parents of a child with this form of trisomy has only 45 chromosomes, including the translocated chromosome. Although usually having only 45 chromosomes is a lethal condition, the parent has enough chromosomal material, because of the translocated material on the number 15 chromosome, to appear normal and to function normally. The chances that all this person's children will have Down's syndrome are very high. The two types of Down's syndrome cannot be distinguished from each other by appearance; the phenotype is the same (Fig. 34-4).

The incidence of Down's syndrome is highest in the children of very young women and of older women (over 35). Thus, immaturity and aging alike both seem to present an obstacle to clean cell division.

Other examples of cell nondisjunction are trisomy 13 (Figs. 34-5 and 34-6) and trisomy 18 (mental retar-

dation syndromes). In *cri du chat* (cat's cry) *syndrome*, a mental retardation syndrome that is marked by the child's peculiar cat-like cry, one portion of the number 5 chromosome is missing.

When nondisjunction occurs in the sex chromosomes, as opposed to the autosomes, other types of abnormalities occur. Turner's and Klinefelter's syndromes are the most common of this type of chromo-

Fig. 34-3. Karyotype of trisomy 21. (Courtesy of Dr. Judith Brown, Medical College of Virginia, Richmond, and the Department of Medical Photography, Children's Hospital, Buffalo, N.Y.)

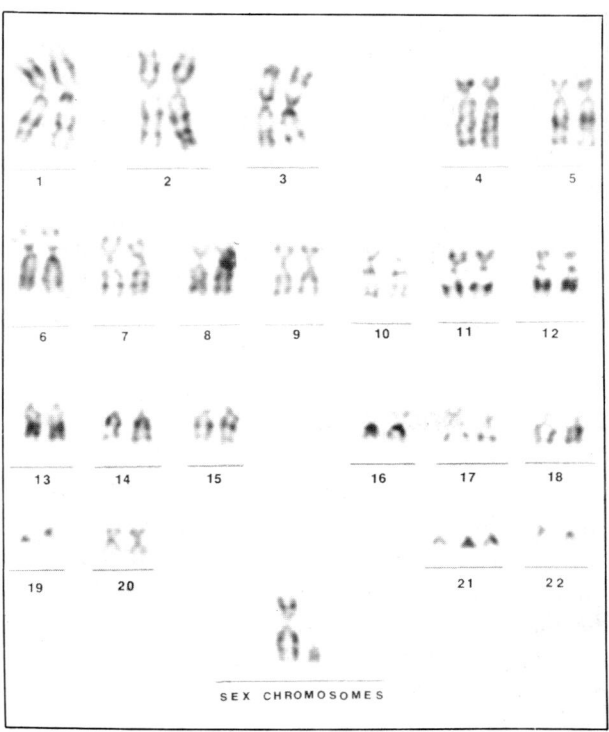

Genetic Disorders and Pregnancy 587

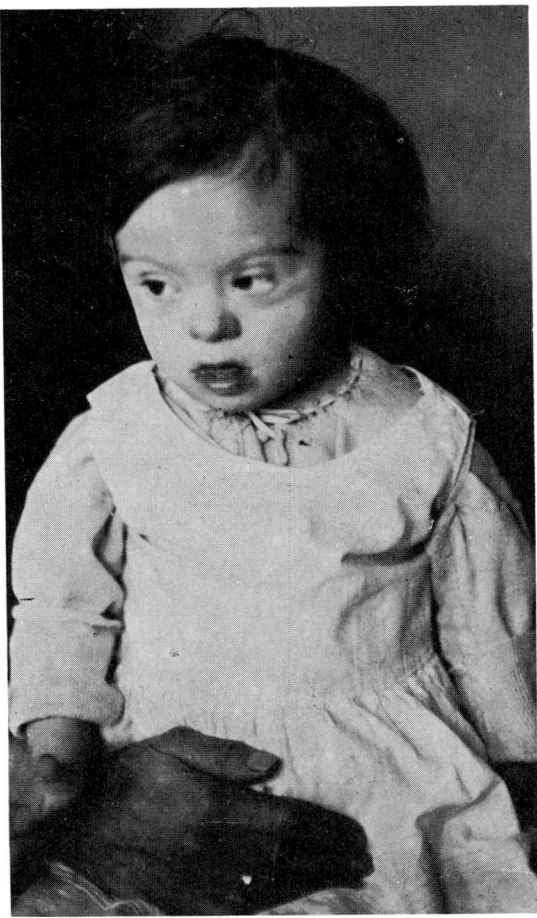

Fig. 34-4. A child with trisomy 21. (From H. Barnett, Pediatrics [15th ed.]. New York: Appleton-Century-Crofts, 1972. P. 899.)

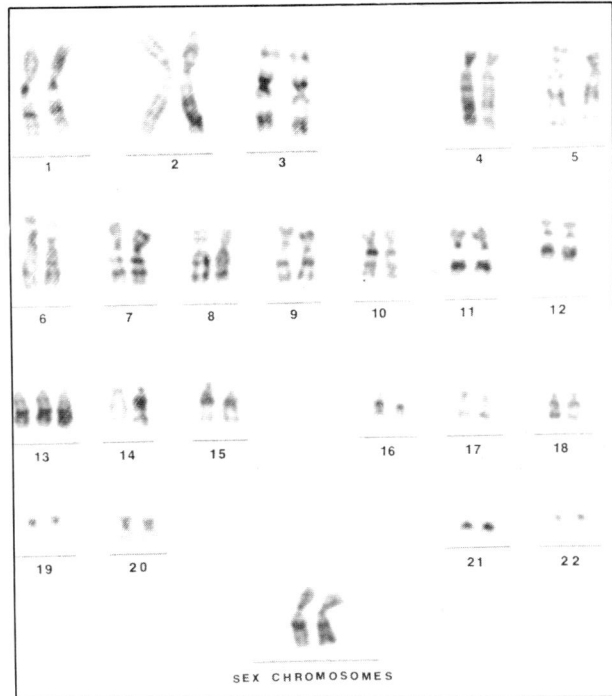

Fig. 34-5. Karyotype of trisomy 13. Note the extra chromosome 13. (Courtesy of Dr. Judith Brown, Medical College of Virginia, Richmond, and the Department of Medical Photography, Children's Hospital, Buffalo, N.Y.)

somal abnormality. In Turner's syndrome (marked by webbed neck, short stature, sterility, and possible mental retardation) the individual, although female, has only one X chromosome or has two X chromosomes but one is defective. She appears to be female because of the X chromosome. In Klinefelter's syndrome (marked by sterility and possibly mental retardation) the individual has male genitals but his sex chromosomal pattern is XXY.

Familial Tendencies

Many congenital defects, such as heart disease, pyloric stenosis, or cleft lip and palate tend to run in families, that is, have a high incidence in some families. These conditions do not appear to follow the mendelian laws of inheritance or to be related to nondisjunction problems. Perhaps many genes are involved in these defects. It is difficult to counsel parents regarding these diseases because their occurrence is so unpredictable.

Genetic Counseling

Any person who is concerned about the possibility of transmitting a disease to his or her children should have access to genetic counseling.

HISTORY

Genetic counseling begins with a detailed family history. All members of the family who have a disease that may be inherited must be examined to confirm the diagnosis. An extensive prenatal history of the affected person is taken to see whether environmental conditions could account for the condition.

KARYOTYPES

Blood is drawn from the affected person and from the person or couple seeking counseling. The white blood cells are allowed to grow to a stage of mitosis, and karyotypes (patterns of chromosomes) are made so that genetic composition can be visualized.

On the basis of the karyotype and the rules of inheritance, an attempt is made to predict the chances that children of the couple seeking counseling will have an inherited disease. With this information, a choice can then be made to have or not to have children.

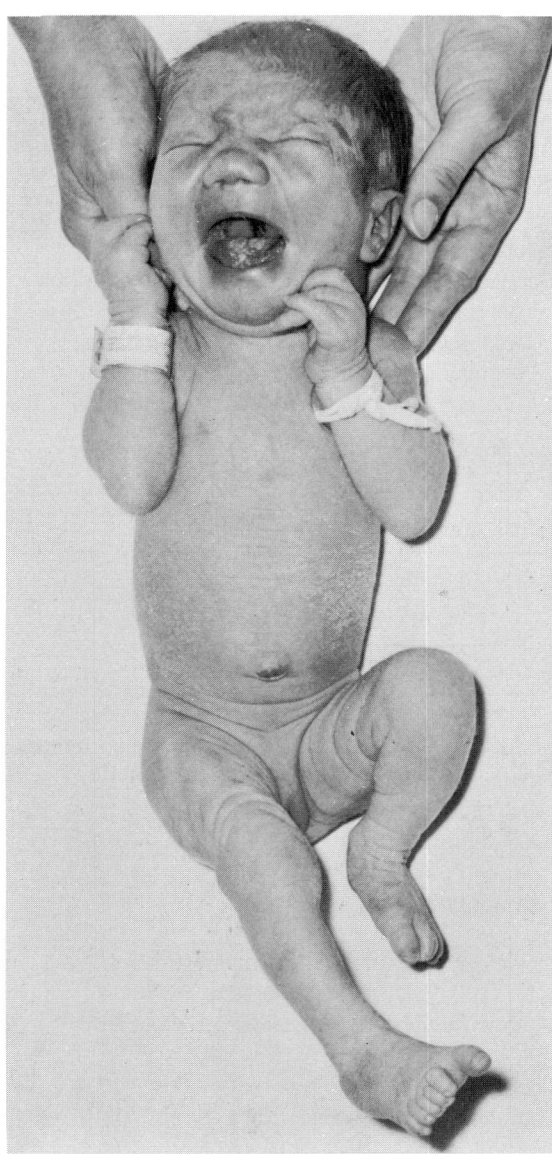

Fig. 34-6. An infant with trisomy 13. Note the cleft palate and polydactyly. (From H. Barnett, Pediatrics [15th ed.]. New York: Appleton-Century-Crofts, 1972. P. 901. Courtesy of Drs. J. Lindsten and P. Zetterquist.)

AMNIOCENTESIS

If the couple chooses to have children, amniocentesis at the 14th to 16th week of a pregnancy may reveal whether or not the fetus has the inherited disease. Following a sonogram to locate the placenta and establish that there is only one fetus present, the standard amniocentesis technique is used. Fetal skin cells, or amnion cells that have flaked off in the fluid, can be used to determine the fetal karyotype. Amniocentesis for chromosomal abnormality is recommended in women over 35 years of age, since the incidence of Down's syndrome greatly increases in infants of mothers past this age. It is also recommended if a previous conception in which either parent was a partner resulted in a child with a diagnosable chromosomal defect; if both parents are carriers of a metabolic defect; or if the woman is a carrier of a sex-linked disorder.

It is important for parents to understand that not all inherited diseases can be detected by amniocentesis. Table 34-1 shows various chromosomal disorders that can be diagnosed prenatally by amniocentesis. Table 34-2 shows common inborn errors of metabolism that can be identified by amniocentesis. These diagnoses are based on the levels of certain enzymes, not on the karyotype. Meningomyelocele can be diagnosed on the presence of extra alpha fetoprotein cells in amniotic fluid.

Whether to have an amniocentesis done to determine chromosomal normality is a major decision for a couple. As a rule, they are not making a decision simply for amniocentesis; if the amniocentesis reveals that their child is abnormal, aborting the pregnancy seems to most partners to be the next sensible step.

Unfortunately, amniocentesis cannot be done until the 14th to 16th week of pregnancy (not until there is a sufficient quantity of amniotic fluid present), at a time when the woman is beginning to accept her pregnancy and perhaps to "nest-build." Making an abortion decision at this point will be difficult for her—much more difficult than it seemed before the pregnancy or early in the pregnancy, when she first agreed to amniocentesis. She needs a great deal of support to carry through with her decision. She will also need support during the remainder of her pregnancy and in the days following birth if she changes her mind about abortion. It may be hard for her to believe that what the test showed is real. Only when she looks at the baby and sees that the test was accurate—that her child has Down's syndrome, for example—does the realization hit home. The result may be a long-lasting postpartal depression.

Genetic counseling is a role for nurses, provided they are adequately prepared in genetics. Genetic counseling can be as dangerous and destructive as parlor psychology, however, if it is given "off the cuff," stating general theories rather than basing statements on the specific situation under discussion.

Most people listen to the statistics of their situation ("Your child has a 25 percent chance of having this disease") and misinterpret what they hear. They construe a "25 percent chance" to mean that, if they have one child with the disease, they can then have three normal children without any worry. However, a 25 percent chance means that with each pregnancy,

Table 34-1. Common Chromosomal Abnormalities That Can Be Diagnosed Before Birth by Amniocentesis

Disorder	Genetic Defect	Effect on Child
Down's syndrome	Trisomy 21	Mental retardation; protruding tongue, epicanthal folds; hypotonia
Translocation Down's syndrome	Translocation of a chromosome, perhaps 15/21	Same clinical signs as trisomy 21
Trisomy 18	Trisomy 18	Mental retardation, congenital malformations
Trisomy 13	Trisomy 13	Mental retardation; multiple congenital malformations: cleft palate, eye agenesis
Cri du chat syndrome	Deletion of short arm of chromosome 5	Mental retardation, facial structure anomalies, peculiar cat-like cry
Philadelphia chromosome	Deletion of one arm of chromosome 21	Chronic granulocytic leukemia
Turner's syndrome (gonadal dysgenesis)	XO	Short stature, streak gonads; infertility; webbing of neck
Klinefelter's syndrome	XXY	Small testes; gynecomastia; infertility

Table 34-2. Prenatal Diagnosis of Hereditary Metabolic Diseases

Disorder	Effect on Child
Lipid metabolism	
GM_2 gangliosidosis (Tay-Sachs disease)	Degenerative neurological disorder. Child has cherry red spot within macula. Results in extreme hypotonia, psychomotor retardation, and death
Niemann-Pick disease	Hepatosplenomegaly; skeletal and neurological involvement
Gaucher's disease	Renal failure; cardiac and ocular involvement
Amino acid metabolic	
Cystinosis	Failure to thrive, rickets, glycosuria, cystine deposition in tissue and aminoaciduria
Homocystinuria	Dislocated lens of the eye; skeletal abnormalities, mental retardation, vascular thrombosis
Maple syrup urine disease	Ketoacidosis, neurological abnormality, mental retardation, early death
Carbohydrate metabolic	
Glycogen storage disease	Failure to thrive, hepatomegaly, cardiomegaly
Galactosemia	Cataracts, mental retardation, failure to thrive
Glucose 6-phosphate dehydrogenase deficiency	Hemolytic anemia
Mucopolysaccharidoses	
Hurler's syndrome	Gargoyle-like facies, early psychomotor retardation, dwarfism, joint stiffness
Hunter's syndrome	Gargoyle-like facies, psychomotor retardation
Miscellaneous disorders	
Adrenogenital syndrome	Virilization or masculinization of female fetus; adrenal insufficiency with salt loss
Cystic fibrosis	Tenacious body fluids, chronic pulmonary infections, failure to thrive, increased loss of sodium in perspiration, early death

there is a 25 percent chance that the child will have the disease. It is as if they had four cards, the aces of spades, hearts, clubs, and diamonds, and the ace of spades represents the disease. When a card is drawn from the set of four, the chances of its being the ace of spades are 1 in 4 (25 percent). That is like the first pregnancy. But when the couple is ready to have a second child, it is as if the card drawn the first round is returned to the set. The chances of drawing the ace of spades in the second draw are exactly the same as in the first draw. Similarly, the couple's chances of having a child with the disease remain 1 in 4 in the second pregnancy.

Nurses can play important roles as members of a genetic counseling team. They can offer support to couples seeking advice during the wait for test results and provide contraceptive counseling or adoption referral if the couple decides not to have further children.

Legal Aspects of Genetic Screening

When participating in genetic screening or counseling, you must keep a number of legal responsibilities (shown in Table 34-3) in mind. Failure to heed these guidelines could result in charges of invasion of privacy, breach of confidentiality, or psychological injury due to the process of being "labeled" or fear or worry about the significance of a disease or carrier state.

Table 34-3. Guidelines for Genetic Screening and Counseling

Participation in genetic screening programs must be elective, not mandatory.
People desiring genetic screening should sign an informed consent for the procedure.
Results must be interpreted carefully and relayed to individuals as promptly as possible.
The results of the screening must not be withheld from individuals.
The results of genetic screening must not be given to other persons than the individuals directly involved.
Following genetic counseling, persons must not be coerced to undergo abortion or sterilization. This should be a free, individually dictated choice.

Rh Incompatibility

Although blood incompatibility is basically a problem that affects the fetus, it causes such concern and apprehension in the woman during pregnancy that it becomes a maternal problem as well.

Blood incompatibility during pregnancy can be predicted when the Rh-negative mother (one negative for a D antigen or one with a dd genotype) is carrying an Rh-positive fetus (DD or Dd genotype). For such a situation to occur, the father of the child must either be homozygous (DD) or heterozygous (Dd) Rh-positive.

Fig. 34-7. Maternal antibody formation preceding hemolytic disease of the newborn. (From Clinical Education Aid, No. 9, Ross Laboratories, Columbus, Ohio, 1962.)

MATERNAL RH SENSITIZATION

It is easiest to understand how the Rh factor can endanger the fetus if you think of it as an antigen. People who have Rh-positive blood have a factor (the D antigen) that Rh-negative people do not. When an Rh-positive fetus begins to grow inside an Rh-negative mother, it is as though her body is being invaded by a foreign agent, or antigen. Her body reacts in the same manner it would if the invading factor were a foreign substance such as measles or mumps virus: It begins to form antibodies against the invading substance. In the case of Rh invasion, the maternal antibodies formed cause red blood cell destruction (hemolysis) of fetal red blood cells (Fig. 34-7). The fetus becomes so deficient in red blood cells that sufficient oxygen transport to the fetal cells cannot be maintained. This

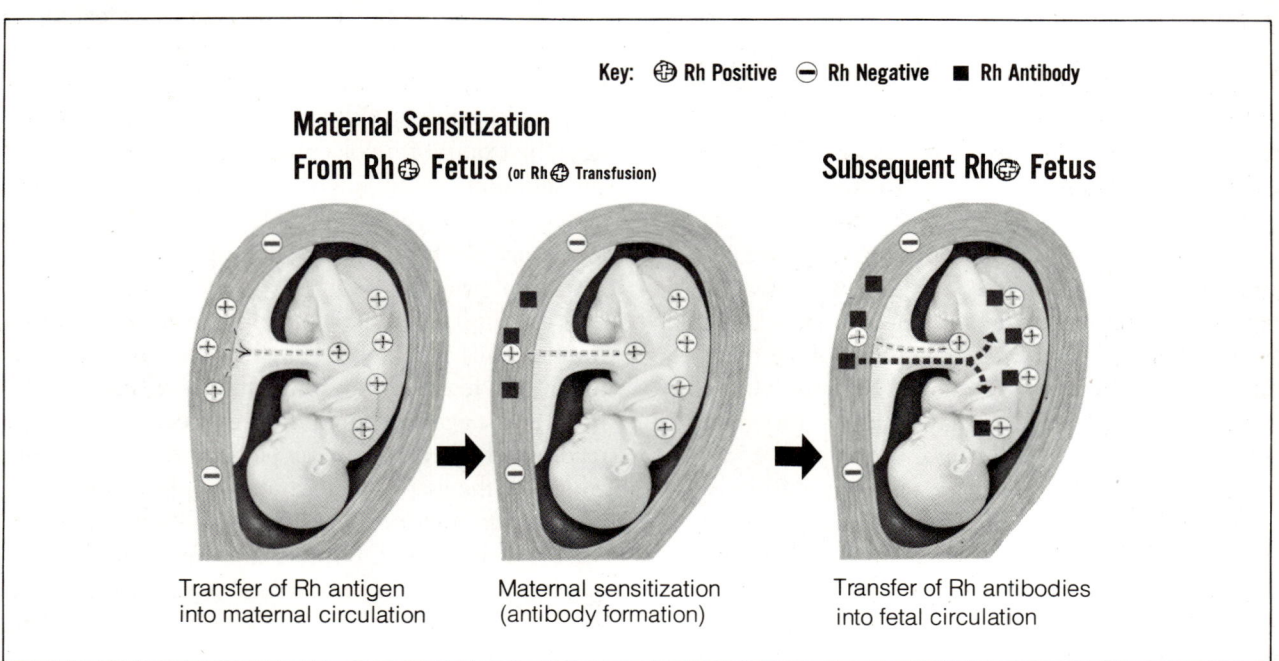

Genetic Disorders and Pregnancy

condition is called *hemolytic disease of the newborn*, or *erythroblastosis fetalis*. Management of the infant born with this condition is discussed in Chap. 38.

Theoretically, there is no connection between fetal blood and maternal blood during pregnancy. In fact, an occasional villus ruptures, allowing a drop or two of fetal blood to enter the maternal circulation, which initiates the production of antibodies. As the placenta separates following delivery of the child, there is an active exchange of fetal and maternal blood from damaged villi. Therefore, most of the maternal antibodies formed against the Rh-positive blood are formed by the Rh-negative woman in the first 72 hours after delivery.

The woman with Rh-negative blood whose husband is Rh-positive used to be advised that she could have no more than three children. This advice was based on the following: During the first pregnancy, very little sensitivity to the foreign Rh antigen develops. However, as described, following termination of the first pregnancy, a large number of antibodies form and are in the maternal circulation when a second pregnancy begins. Many antibodies are formed at the end of the second pregnancy. Thus, an even greater number—in many women, a lethal number—of antibodies are present when the third pregnancy begins.

Passive Antibody Protection

Today, with the discovery of Rh_o (D) immune globulin (RhoGAM), the problem of maternal isoimmunization to an Rh-positive fetus should be eliminated. RhoGAM is a commercial preparation of passive antibodies against the Rh factor. If this is given by injection to the mother in the first 72 hours following delivery of an Rh-positive child, her body is "fooled" into not forming antibodies; that is, because of the presence of synthetic antibodies her immunological system does not form natural antibodies. Since this is passive antibody protection, however, it is transient, and in two weeks to two months the passive antibodies are destroyed. Only those few antibodies that were formed during pregnancy are left. Thus every pregnancy is like a first pregnancy in terms of the number of antibodies present, assuring a safe intrauterine environment for as many pregnancies as the woman wishes to have.

Although in future years the problem of Rh sensitization will be greatly reduced, it remains a complication of pregnancy today. Some women of childbearing age began childbearing before RhoGAM was available and so have high Rh antibody titers in their blood. Some women do not receive RhoGAM injections following abortions or ectopic pregnancy as they should, and so antibody formation begins.

All women with Rh-negative blood should have an anti-D antibody titer done at their first pregnancy visit. If the results are normal or the titer is minimal, the test will be repeated at the 32nd to 38th week of pregnancy. If there is no change at this time, no special therapy need be undertaken. Following delivery, the infant's blood type will be determined from a sample of the cord blood. If it is Rh-positive—Coombs-negative, indicating that a large number of antibodies are not present in the mother—the mother will receive a RhoGAM injection. If the newborn's blood type is Rh-negative, no antibodies have been formed in the mother's circulation during pregnancy and none will form. Thus, passive antibody injection is unnecessary.

The Rh-negative woman whose infant is Rh-positive needs a clear explanation of why she is receiving RhoGAM. If both infant and mother are Rh-negative, the woman should be told why RhoGAM is unnecessary. She needs to be assured that it is safe to have another baby if that is her wish.

Fetal Monitoring

If the woman's anti-D antibody titer is elevated at the 16th to 20th week, showing Rh sensitization, the titer will be monitored about every two weeks during the remainder of the pregnancy. The well-being of the fetus in this potentially toxic environment will be monitored every two weeks (or oftener) by amniocentesis (see Chap. 13). Spectrophotometer readings are made of the amniotic fluid obtained by this technique to reveal the fluid density. If the readings (at $450\ \mu$ optical density) are plotted on a graph such as the one proposed by Liley [10] and correlated with gestation age, the extent of involvement and the seriousness of the situation can be judged. A numerical value is obtained by the spectrophotometer analysis. This number is placed on a graph at the appropriate week of gestation.

If the fluid density remains low so that the plotted number falls into zone 1 of the graph during pregnancy, the fetus either is in no distress or, more likely, is an Rh-negative fetus. If the spectrophotometer reading is higher, so that the plotted number falls into zone 2 of the graph, preterm delivery by induction of labor at fetal maturity is indicated. If the reading is so high that the plotted number falls into zone 3 of the graph, the fetus is in imminent danger, and immediate delivery should be carried out or intrauterine transfusion begun.

Intrauterine Transfusion

Formerly, although the physician realized that the antibody titer was rising in pregnancy and fetal well-being was being threatened, nothing could be done until the fetus became mature enough to be delivered. Some infants were so affected by red cell destruction that they were stillborn; some were stillborn or died in the neonatal period of heart failure (erythroblastosis fetalis). Others suffered permanent brain damage with resulting motor and mental retardation from high bilirubin levels (kernicterus). The one measure that helps to combat the red cell destruction, exchange blood transfusion to remove the hemolyzed cells and replace them with healthy cells, could be done only after the infant was delivered. Today, blood transfusion, although not exchange transfusion, can be performed in utero.

Two or three hours before the transfusion is to begin, 50 ml of radiopaque dye is injected into the amniotic fluid by amniocentesis technique. The woman may be given a mild sedative to help her relax during the time of waiting. At the end of the waiting period, she is taken to the x-ray department of the hospital. Since the fetus swallowed amniotic fluid during this time, the radiopaque dye was also swallowed and will be present in his intestines. On fluoroscopy, the fetal intestine or the location of the fetal abdomen will be clearly evident.

Fetal and placental location can also be located by sonogram. There is an advantage to this method if it is anticipated that the procedure will have to be repeated during pregnancy as sonography does not expose the fetus to repeated x-rays.

Following location of the placenta by sonogram, the skin of the woman's abdomen is anesthetized with a local anesthetic. A large-bore needle and cannula is inserted into the amniotic fluid and guided gently under the observing eye of fluoroscope or sonogram into the fetal abdominal cavity. If fluoroscopy is being used, a small amount (about 2 ml) of radiopaque solution can be injected to confirm proper location of the cannula.

Blood used for transfusion in utero is group O negative because the fetal blood type is not known. It passes through the cannula into the fetal abdomen. From 75 to 150 ml of packed red cells will be used, depending on the age of the fetus. The cannula is then withdrawn, and the woman is urged to rest for about a half hour. Fetal heart sounds are recorded. The woman is discharged to her home to assume her usual routine.

The red blood cells are absorbed across the fetal peritoneum into the circulation and raise the level of functioning red blood cells. Obviously, intrauterine transfusion is not without risk. The fetal liver or a major blood vessel may be lacerated by the needle, or the uterus may be so irritated by the invasive procedure that labor contractions begin. For the fetus who is becoming severely affected by isoimmunization, however, such a risk is no greater than that of leaving the fetus untreated in his intrauterine environment.

Transfusion is sometimes done only once during pregnancy, or it may be done every two weeks for five or six times. As soon as fetal maturity is reached, as shown by the lecithin-sphingomyelin ratio, delivery will be instituted.

EMOTIONAL SUPPORT

A woman in whom a high antibody titer is developing needs a great deal of support to help her get to the end of her pregnancy. She may feel that it is somehow her fault, that she is responsible for destroying her child. Often, a day-by-day approach is most helpful in managing such anxiety: Today, everything seems to be going all right. Let's worry about tomorrow when it comes.

Following delivery, the infant may require an exchange transfusion to remove hemolyzed red blood cells and replace them with healthy blood cells (see Chap. 38). The woman needs to discuss her plans for further childbearing and to be provided with contraceptive information if she feels that the strain of this pregnancy, the constant feeling of wishing that everything was all right but never being certain that it was, is more than she can endure again.

Commonly Inherited Disorders

SICKLE CELL ANEMIA

Sickle cell anemia is a recessively inherited hemolytic anemia. Approximately 1 in every 12 black Americans has sickle cell trait—that is, carries a recessive gene for S hemoglobin but is asymptomatic; 1 in every 576 black women theoretically has the disease. The sickle cell *trait* does not appear to influence the course of pregnancy in terms of pregnancy-induced hypertension, prematurity, abortion, or perinatal mortality. Women with the trait seem to have an increased incidence of asymptomatic bacteriuria, however, resulting in an increased incidence of pyelonephritis. They take the regular iron and folic acid supplement during pregnancy. Clean-catch urines should be collected periodically during pregnancy to attempt to detect developing bacteriuria.

Pregnancy can be a severe complication for the woman with sickle cell *disease*. With the disease, the majority of red blood cells are irregular or sickle-shaped. They do not carry as much hemoglobin as normally shaped red blood cells. When oxygen tension is reduced, as happens at high altitudes, or blood becomes more viscid than usual (dehydration), the cells tend to clump because of the irregular shape. This clumping results in infarcts and blockage of vessels. The cells will then hemolyze. At any time in life, sickle cell anemia is a threat to life if vital blood vessels such as those to the liver, the kidneys, the heart, the lungs, or the brain are blocked. In pregnancy, blockage to the placental circulation will lead to direct fetal compromise and death. Early in pregnancy when the woman may be nauseated, her fluid intake may be decreased and dehydration is a real possibility. Pooling of blood in the lower extremities because of uterine pressure may take place as pregnancy advances, leading to cell destruction. If the woman develops an infection that raises her temperature and causes her to perspire more than normally, or contracts a respiratory infection that compromises air exchange so that her PO_2 is lowered, she will be hospitalized for observation until it is established that she is not beginning a sickle cell crisis and hemolysis of crowded cells has not started. All during pregnancy, ask about her diet (she must include enough fluid—at least four glasses daily) and whether she is sitting for long periods during the day. She needs always to rest with her legs elevated when sitting in a chair; lying on her side in a modified Sims's position encourages return venous flow from the lower extremities.

A woman with sickle cell disease may normally have a hemoglobin level of 6 to 8 mg per 100 ml, and this is the level she will maintain during pregnancy. She may have jaundiced sclerae. Hemolysis in a sickle cell crisis may occur so rapidly that her hemoglobin level falls to 5 to 6 mg per 100 ml in a few hours. There is an accompanying rise in her indirect bilirubin level because she cannot conjugate the bilirubin released from red blood cells being so quickly destroyed.

Interventions in sickle cell crisis include replacing red blood cells by transfusion, administering oxygen as needed, and increasing the fluid volume of the circulatory system to lower viscosity. An exchange transfusion may be done to not only replace red blood cells but remove a quantity of the increased bilirubin also. Women with sickle cell disease are not given an iron supplement during pregnancy as a rule. The cells cannot incorporate it as can normal cells, and there may therefore be an excessive iron buildup from a supplement. They do need a folic acid supplement because of the overproduction of marrow trying to counteract hemolysis. If they do not have adequate folic acid, they may develop megaloblastic anemia following a crisis.

When the fetus is mature, delivery must be individualized. The woman must be kept well hydrated in labor. For delivery, she generally receives nerve block anesthesia rather than a general anesthetic to avoid anoxia.

Women generally are interested in determining at birth whether the child has inherited the disease. As the disorder is recessively inherited, with one of the parents having the disease and the other free of the disease, the chances that the child will inherit the disease are zero. If one parent has the disease and the partner has the trait, the chances that the child will be born with the disease are 50 percent.

Symptoms of sickle cell disease do not become clinically apparent until the child's hemoglobin converts to a largely adult pattern (in three to six months). Fetal hemoglobin is composed of two alpha and two gamma chains; adult hemoglobin is composed of two alpha and two beta chains. Since the sickle cell trait is carried on the beta chain, it will not be manifested until this chain appears. Electrophoresis of blood at birth, however, will reveal the manifestation of the disease on the few beta chains present (infants have about 15 percent adult hemoglobin at birth).

A woman with sickle cell disease needs to be seen frequently during the antepartal period. In underdeveloped countries the maternal mortality in women with sickle cell disease is about 18 percent. One-third to one-half of all pregnancies end in abortion, stillbirth, or neonatal death.

TRISOMY 13 (PATAU'S SYNDROME)

Children with trisomy 13 (Fig. 34-6) are grossly mentally retarded. The incidence of the disorder is fortunately low, about 0.45 per 1,000 live births. Midline body defects are prominent among symptoms. Microcephaly with abnormalities of the forebrain and forehead, eyes that are smaller than normal (microphthalmia) or absent, cleft lip and palate, low-set ears, heart defects, and abnormal genitalia are common. Most of these children do not survive beyond early childhood.

TRISOMY 18

Children with trisomy 18 are also severely mentally retarded. The incidence is about 0.23 per 1,000 live births. These children tend to be small for gestation age at birth. They have markedly low-set ears, a small jaw, congenital heart defects, and misshapen fingers and toes (the index finger tends to deviate or cross over other fingers). Also, the soles of their feet are often rounded instead of flat (rocker-bottom feet). Most of these children do not survive beyond early infancy.

CRI DU CHAT SYNDROME

In addition to an abnormal cry, which is much more like the sound of a cat's than a human infant's cry, children with cri du chat syndrome tend to have a small head, wide-set eyes, and a downward slant to the palpebral fissure of the eye. They are severely mentally retarded. The chromosomal defect is with the fifth chromosome.

TURNER'S SYNDROME (GONADAL DYSGENESIS)

The child with Turner's syndrome is short in stature. The hairline at the nape of the neck is low-set, and the neck may appear to be webbed and short. In the newborn, there may be appreciable edema of the hands and feet and a number of congenital anomalies, most frequently coarctation of the aorta and kidney defects. Since the baby has only streak gonads, secondary sex characteristics with the exception of pubic hair will not develop at puberty. Lack of ovarian function results in sterility. The genotype is XO.

KLINEFELTER'S SYNDROME

Boys with Klinefelter's syndrome tend to have poorly developed male secondary sex characteristics: small testes, producing ineffective sperm; they tend to have gynecomastia. The individual is usually sterile. The syndrome is difficult to recognize in the newborn. Failure of secondary sex characteristics to develop at puberty may be the first clue that an XXY genotype exists.

DOWN'S SYNDROME (TRISOMY 21)

The most frequently found chromosomal abnormality, Down's syndrome, was formerly called mongolism because the apparent slant of the eyes (Fig. 34-4) makes the child look to be of Oriental heritage. The high incidence among children of young women (under 18) and older women (over 35) is well established. The risk of having a child with Down's syndrome if the mother is 30 to 34 years of age is about 1 in 700; if the mother's age is 35 to 39, it is 1 in 300; if the mother is 40 to 44, it is 1 in 100; if maternal age is over 45, it is 1 in 50 [7].

The appearance of the child at birth makes the diagnosis possible. The nose is broad and flat, the eyelids have an extra fold of tissue at the inner canthus (an epicanthal fold), and the palpebral fissure (opening between the eyelids) tends to slant laterally upward. The iris of the eye may have white specks in it (Brushfield's spots).

Even in the newborn, the tongue may protrude from the mouth because of a smaller than normal oral cavity. The back of the head is flat; the neck is short, and an extra pad of fat at the base of the head causes the skin there to be so loose it can be lifted up (like a puppy's neck). Ears may be low-set; muscle tone is poor, giving the baby a rag-doll appearance. He is able to touch his toe against his nose, something that other mature infants are not able to do. The palm of the hand shows a peculiar crease (a simian line) or a horizontal palm crease rather than the normal three creases in a palm (Fig. 34-8).

Children with Down's syndrome are mentally retarded, but the retardation can range from that of an educable child (50 to 70 IQ) to one requiring institutionalization (under 20 IQ). The extent of the retardation will not be evident at birth.

MAPLE SYRUP URINE DISEASE

Maple syrup urine disease is a rare amino acid metabolism disorder, inherited as an autosomal recessive trait, in which there is a defect in amino acid metabolism leading to cerebral degeneration similar to that of phenylketonuria. The infant appears well at birth but quickly begins to evidence signs of feeding difficulty, loss of the Moro reflex, and irregular respirations. The symptoms progress rapidly to opisthotonos, generalized muscular rigidity, and convulsions. The child may die of the disease as early as 2 to 4 weeks of age.

Although the disorder is rare, it is mentioned here because as early as the first or second day of life the

Fig. 34-8. A simian line, a horizontal palm crease seen in children with Down's syndrome. (Courtesy of the Department of Medical Illustration, State University of New York at Buffalo.)

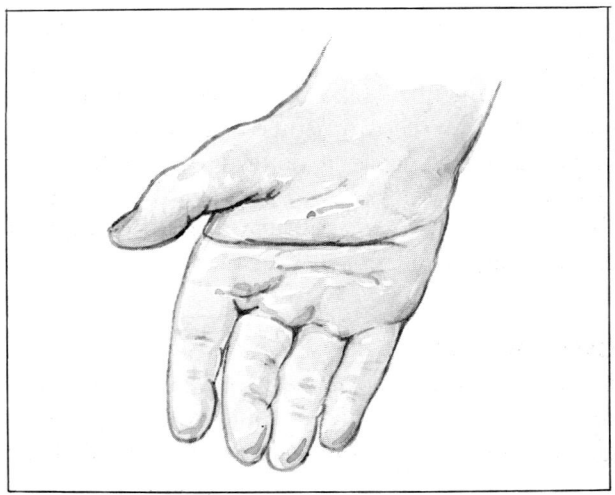

urine of the child develops the characteristic odor of maple syrup; hence the name of the disease. The odor is due to the presence of ketoacids, the same phenomenon that makes the breath of diabetic children in severe acidosis smell sweet.

Theoretically, if maple syrup urine disease could be diagnosed in the first day or two of life and the child placed on a well-controlled diet low in the amino acids leucine, isoleucine, and valine, the cerebral degeneration could be prevented, just as it can be prevented in phenylketonuria. Since nurses are the people most likely to detect the characteristic urine odor in the first few days of life, it is a disorder that any nurse who cares for newborns should be aware of.

GALACTOSEMIA

Galactosemia is evidenced by abnormal amounts of galactose in the blood (galactosemia) and in the urine (galactosuria). The commonest form of this disorder is an inborn error of metabolism, in which the child is deficient in galactose 1-phosphate uridyl transferase enzyme. This is inherited as an autosomal recessive trait.

When lactose is ingested (lactose is the sugar of milk), it is broken down into galactose and glucose. Galactose is then further broken down into additional glucose. Without the enzyme, this second step, or the conversion of galactose into glucose, cannot take place, and there is a buildup of galactose in the bloodstream and spillage of galactose into the urine.

Symptoms appear when the child is begun on formula or breast-feedings: lethargy, hypotonia, and perhaps diarrhea and vomiting. Next, the liver enlarges and cirrhosis develops because of hepatic failure. Jaundice is often present and persistent; bilateral cataracts develop. The symptoms begin abruptly and grow worse rapidly. Untreated, the child may die by 3 days of age. Untreated children who do survive beyond this time may have mental retardation and bilateral cataracts.

The treatment of galactosemia consists of placing the infant on a diet that is free of galactose or a formula made with casein hydrolysates. Once the child is regulated on this diet, symptoms of the disease do not progress; however, any neurological or cataract findings already present will persist.

CYSTIC FIBROSIS

Cystic fibrosis of the pancreas is a disease in which there is generalized dysfunction of the exocrine glands. Mucous secretions of the body, particularly in the pancreas and the lungs, have difficulty flowing through body gland ducts. The resultant chronic respiratory infection and decreased production of pancreatic enzymes lead to severe respiratory and digestive symptoms. The disorder is inherited as an autosomal recessive trait.

The newborn with cystic fibrosis loses the normal amount of weight at birth (5 to 10 percent of birth weight) but then does not gain it back at the usual time of 7 to 10 days; perhaps not until 4 to 6 weeks of age. Failure to regain birth weight as a newborn is a significant sign, which nurses, the persons who weigh babies, must be aware of.

At birth, meconium may be so tenacious that the baby has intestinal obstruction (meconium ileus). All babies with meconium ileus should be tested for cystic fibrosis.

The child may be seen in a physician's office or clinic at about 1 month of age because of a feeding problem. He eats so ravenously that he tends to swallow air (using only about 50 percent of his intake because of his poor digestive function, he is always hungry). This may be manifested as colic or abdominal distention and vomiting. His stools are large and bulky and perhaps loose and frequent. They feel or look greasy on account of undigested fat.

The child is diagnosed by a sweat test or analysis of sweat for an abnormally high sodium level. Infants may not be tested until 6 to 8 weeks of age because newborns do not sweat a great deal and interpretation of the test may not be accurate.

ADRENOGENITAL SYNDROME

Adrenogenital syndrome is inherited as an autosomal recessive trait. The primary defect is an inability to synthesize hydrocortisone from its precursors. This fault ordinarily occurs at the 21-hydroxylase level. When the adrenal gland is unable to produce hydrocortisone, the pituitary adrenotropic hormone increases, stimulating the adrenal glands to function better. The adrenals become hyperplastic but, still unable to produce hydrocortisone, overproduce androgen. The effect of androgen is to masculinize the female child or to increase the size of genital organs in male infants. This process begins during fetal life, so the female is born with such an enlarged clitoris that it appears more like a penis than a clitoris.

When there is a complete block of the formation of hydrocortisone (salt-dumping adrenogenital syndrome), the production of aldosterone will be deficient also. Without adequate aldosterone, salt is not retained by the body; thus fluid is not retained. With the first month of life, the infant begins to have vomiting, diarrhea, anorexia, loss of weight, and extreme dehydration. If he is untreated, the extreme loss of salt and fluid will lead to collapse and death.

The existence of this syndrome is one reason newborn babies in hospital nurseries are weighed daily. In males, the inability to gain back their birth weight may be the first sign of the syndrome.

The infant must be placed on hydrocortisone. If he has the salt-losing form, he must be placed on hydrocortisone and a high salt intake. Desoxycorticosterone acetate (Doca), a synthetic aldosterone, helps to maintain a fluid balance.

GLUCOSE 6-PHOSPHATE DEHYDROGENASE DEFICIENCY (G-6-PD)

G-6-PD is transmitted as a sex-linked recessive trait. It occurs most frequently in children of black, Oriental, Sephardic Jewish, and Mediterranean descent. Children are born with normal blood patterns, which are maintained until they are exposed to fava beans or drugs such as acetylsalicylic acid (aspirin) or phenacetin. About two days after the ingestion of such drugs the child begins to show evidence of hemolysis. Occasionally a newborn is seen with marked hemolysis because his mother ingested an initiating drug during pregnancy.

TAY-SACHS DISEASE

Tay-Sachs disease is an autosomal recessive inherited disease in which the infant lacks the enzyme *hexosaminidase* A. Hexosaminidase A is necessary for lipid metabolism. Without it, lipid deposits accumulate on nerve cells, leading to mental retardation when they are brain cells and blindness when they are optic nerve cells.

The disorder is found primarily in the Ashkenazic Jewish population (eastern European Jewish ancestry—*Ashkenazi* means "German"). The child generally appears normal in the first few months of life except for an extreme Moro reflex and mild hypotonia. At about 6 months of age, he begins to lose head control and is unable to sit up or roll over without support. On ophthalmoscopic examination, a cherry-red macula is noticeable (caused by lipid deposits).

By 1 year of age, the child has symptoms of spasticity and is unable to perform even simple motor tasks. By 2 years of age, generalized convulsions and blindness occur. Most children die of cachexia and pneumonia by 3 to 5 years of age. There is no cure for Tay-Sachs disease. The disorder may be detected in utero by amniocentesis. Carriers for the disease trait may be identified by screening programs.

PHENYLKETONURIA

Phenylketonuria (PKU) is an autosomal recessive metabolic disease caused by an inborn error of metabolism. The infant is lacking the liver enzyme phenylalanine hydroxylase and cannot convert phenylalanine, an essential amino acid, into tyrosine. Because it cannot be converted, excessive phenylalanine builds up in the bloodstream and tissues, causing permanent damage to brain tissue and hence severe mental retardation. The defect is found in 1 in 10,000 births in the United States. PKU cannot be detected by amniocentesis because the phenylalanine level does not rise in utero.

All infants should be screened for PKU as follows before they are discharged from the newborn nursery: After two full days of feedings (at least 120 ml of formula at a concentration of 20 calories per ounce or the equivalent amount obtained by breast-feeding), the infant's heel is pricked with a blood lancet, and a few drops of blood are allowed to fall onto a specially prepared filter paper. The filter paper is then analyzed for the amount of phenylalanine contained in the infant's blood (Guthrie's test).

Infants in whom this disease is detected in the first few days of life can be placed on an extremely low phenylalanine diet; if the diet is begun this early, mental retardation can be totally prevented. For this reason it is extremely important that every infant with the disease be identified. If an infant is discharged before formula feeding is begun, or if the infant is being breast-fed and there is a question as to whether or not he has received only colostrum, he must be checked at his examination at 4 weeks of age, or a special return date for follow-up must be made with the hospital.

References

1. Aure, B. Intrauterine transfusion: The nurse's role with expectant parents. *Nurs. Clin. North Am.* 7:817, 1972.
2. Bishop, E. H. Genetics in clinical practice. *Female Patient* 5:70, 1980.
3. Cowle, V. Spina bifida: Peace of mind from antenatal diagnosis. *Nurs. Mirror* 147:34, 1978.
4. Doswell, W. M. Sickle-cell anemia: You can do something to help. *Nursing 78* 8:65, 1978.
5. Fabricant, J. D., et al. Genetic studies on spontaneous abortions. *Contemp. Obstet. Gynecol.* 11:73, 1978.

6. Golbus, M. Analyzing genetic defects in the fetus. *Contemp. Obstet. Gynecol.* 13:133, 1979.
7. Goodwin, J., et al. *Perinatal Medicine*. Baltimore: Williams & Wilkins, 1976.
8. Henry, G. P., and Robinson, A. Prenatal genetic diagnosis. *Clin. Obstet. Gynecol.* 21:329, 1978.
9. Kaback, M. Genetic screening for better outcomes. *Contemp. Obstet. Gynecol.* 13:123, 1979.
10. Liley, A. W. Amniocentesis and Amniography in Hemolytic Disease. In J. P. Greenhill (Ed.), *Yearbook of Obstetrics and Gynecology*. Chicago: Year Book, 1964.
11. McFarlane, J. Sickle-cell disorders. *Am. J. Nurs.* 77:1948, 1977.
12. Mahoney, M. J. Prenatal diagnosis of inborn errors of metabolism. *Clin. Perinatol.* 6:255, 1979.
13. Mercer, R. T. Crisis: A baby is born with a defect. *Nursing 77* 7:45, 1977.
14. Scrimgeour, J. B. Antenatal diagnosis, present and future. *Practitioner* 220:612, 1978.

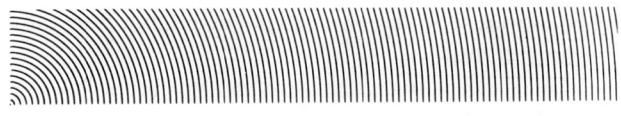

35. Deviations from the Normal in Labor and Delivery: Nursing Interventions

The hours of labor are hours of stress for the woman and the father of her child. The period of labor is so stressful that a woman needs to be assured from time to time that everything is going smoothly, that both she and the infant appear to be doing well.

If a complication occurs and such assurances cannot be given so freely, the stress for the woman increases a hundredfold. How unfair it is to carry a child for nine months and have something go wrong now. How much she wants to protect the life inside her. How helpless she is to do anything about the heartbeat that she knows is fading. How real become the thoughts that flickered across her mind when she first realized she was in labor: This may be the day my baby dies; this may be the night I die.

Every woman in labor should have with her a nurse who is highly skilled both in the physical aspects of her care and in interpersonal relationships so that she is able to feel compassion for her as well. The woman who realizes she is having a complication in labor, who wills her body to complete successfully the job it started nine months ago, who knows she has no real control over these last few hours before birth, needs someone who understands her fears and her feeling of helplessness.

There is no better definition of a professional nurse than one who is able to support and care for a woman both physically and emotionally during a complication of labor and delivery.

Dystocia

Dystocia is a broad term for difficult or abnormal labor. Labor is basically a simple concept: It is the process in which the fetus is pushed through the birth canal by a force to the outside world. Any difficulty that occurs therefore involves one or more of the terms of this proposition; that is, something is amiss with the fetus (the passenger), or the birth canal (the passageway), or the force that propels the fetus (the uterine contractions).

Uterine Dysfunction: Difficulty with the Force

The contractions of the uterus are the basic force that moves the fetus through the birth canal. Dysfunction of the uterus therefore will account for a problem of inadequate force.

UTERINE INERTIA (DYSFUNCTIONAL LABOR)

Inertia is a time-honored term to denote that sluggishness of contractions has occurred. This is more often termed today *dysfunctional labor*. Dysfunction can occur at any point in labor but is generally classified as *primary* (occurring at the onset of labor) or *secondary* (occurring later in labor).

Uterine inertia appears to result from a number of factors: inappropriate use of analgesia (excessive or too early administration); pelvic bone contraction such as might have occurred from rickets that has so narrowed the pelvic diameter that the fetus cannot pass; poor fetal position (a posterior rather than an anterior position); extension rather than flexion of the fetal head; perhaps overdistention of the uterus, as with multiple pregnancy, hydramnios, or an excessively oversized fetus; cervical rigidity, such as may occur in an elderly primipara; a full rectum or urinary bladder that impedes fetal descent. These factors are compounded when the mother becomes exhausted from labor.

Dysfunctions of the Preparatory Division of Labor

Figure 21-20 shows a normal graph of labor, depicting the latent phase, acceleration phase, phase of maximum slope, deceleration phase, and maximum slope of descent. If labor is plotted in this way, when dystocia occurs it can be recognized. The major dysfunction of the preparatory division is a prolonged latent phase.

PROLONGED LATENT PHASE. A prolonged latent phase, defined as a latent phase that is longer than 20 hours in a primipara and 14 hours in a multipara, may happen if the cervix is not "ripe" at the beginning of labor and so time has been spent truly getting ready for labor. It may occur if there is excessive use of an analgesic early in labor. It may reflect dysfunctional labor. With a prolonged latent phase, the uterus tends to be in a hypertonic state. Relaxation between contractions is inadequate, and the contractions themselves are only mild (under 15 mm Hg on a monitor printout) and therefore ineffective. One segment of the uterus may contract with more force than another segment.

This unequal, irregular pattern of contractions with poor relaxation in between is very painful and very frightening to the woman in labor. She has no pain-free periods; she cannot time contractions; she senses that something is not right, and her worry and tension make the contractions even more painful. The situation is potentially harmful to the fetus, because the lack of uterine relaxation does not allow the maternal cotyledons to refill with freshly oxygenated blood between contractions, and fetal anoxia may occur.

It is important in early labor to assess the strength and intensity of contractions and establish that a relaxation phase is occurring. Contractions and fetal heart sounds should be monitored throughout labor to detect fetal distress.

Management of a prolonged latent phase in labor is aimed toward helping the uterus to rest and administering adequate fluid to the woman to prevent dehydration. It may be wisest to administer the fluid intravenously to keep the woman's gastrointestinal tract free of fluid in case anesthesia is necessary for delivery. A short-acting barbiturate may be prescribed to allow the woman to rest; administration of morphine may relax hypertonicity. When the woman awakens from a short sleep, labor usually becomes effective and begins to progress. If it does not, the infant may have to be delivered by cesarean birth. A diagram of a prolonged latent phase is shown in Fig. 35-1.

Dysfunctions of the Dilatational Division of Labor

The major dysfunctions of labor that occur during the dilatational division of labor are protracted active phase dilatation and protracted descent.

PROLONGED ACTIVE PHASE. A prolonged active phase is usually associated with cephalopelvic disproportion or fetal malposition although it may reflect ineffective myometrial activity. The phase is prolonged if the phase of maximum slope is not 1.2 cm per hour or more in a nullipara or 1.5 cm or more in a multipara per hour. If the cause of the delay in dilatation is fetal malposition or cephalopelvic disproportion, cesarean section may have to be initiated to effect delivery. Dysfunctional labor during the dilatational division tends to be hypotonic in contrast to the hypertonic action at the beginning of labor. This is shown in Fig. 35-1.

PROTRACTED DESCENT. A woman is having a protracted descent phase of labor if descent is occurring at a rate of less than 1.0 cm per hour in a nullipara or less than 2.0 cm per hour in a multipara.

With both a prolonged active phase of dilatation and protracted descent, contractions have been of

Fig. 35-1. A prolonged latent phase pattern (A) and a protracted active phase pattern (B) compared to a normal labor pattern (C).

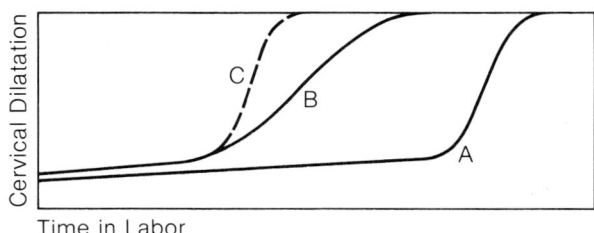

good quality and proper duration, and effacement and beginning dilatation have occurred; the contractions gradually become infrequent and of poor quality, and dilatation stops. If everything except the suddenly faulty contractions is normal (cephalopelvic disproportion or poor fetal presentation have been ruled out by x-ray or sonogram) then rest and fluid intake, as advocated for hypertonic contractions, are applicable here also. If membranes have not ruptured, rupturing them at this point may be helpful. Intravenous oxytocin may be used to induce the uterus to contract effectively.

Whether the dysfunctional labor occurs in the preparatory or the dilatational division of labor, the effect on the woman and her husband will be the same: anxiety, fear, discouragement. The woman needs a running explanation of what is happening: "We're going to take an x-ray to check the baby's position." "This is a drug to urge your uterus into stronger contractions." "I know resting is the last thing you feel like doing, but that is what I want you to try to do."

Be certain the woman voids about every 2 hours during labor to keep the urinary bladder from obstructing descent. If membranes are ruptured, take her temperature every 2 hours to assess whether uterine infection may be occurring. Letting the woman suck on lollipops or sourballs during labor may help to ward off uterine dysfunction, since it helps to maintain an adequate glucose level. Be conscious of how long it has been since she last ate. A woman in a long labor may need intravenous glucose or dextrose to ward off exhaustion and consequent uterine dysfunction.

Dysfunctions of the Pelvic Division of Labor

Four disorders—prolonged deceleration phase, secondary arrest of dilatation, arrest of descent, and failure of descent—may occur with the pelvic division of labor.

PROLONGED DECELERATION PHASE. A deceleration phase has become prolonged when it extends beyond 3 hours in a nullipara, 1 hour in a multipara.

SECONDARY ARREST OF DILATATION. A secondary arrest of dilatation has occurred when there is no progress in cervical dilatation for more than 2 hours.

ARREST OF DESCENT. Arrest of descent is present when no descent has occurred in 1 hour.

FAILURE OF DESCENT. Failure of descent has occurred when expected descent of the fetus does not begin.

The most likely cause for arrest in labor during the pelvic division is cephalopelvic disproportion. Cesarean section is generally chosen as the method of delivery of the infant. If there is no contraindication to vaginal delivery, oxytocin may be used to assist in labor.

PATHOLOGICAL RETRACTION RING

The development of a pathological retraction ring (Bandl's ring) at the juncture of the upper and lower uterine segments may occur at any stage in dysfunctional labor. The ring appears as a horizontal indentation across the abdomen (Fig. 35-2). It results in early labor when there are uncoordinated contractions. When it occurs in the dilatational division of labor, it is usually caused by obstetrical manipulation or the result of the administration of oxytocin.

The fetus is gripped by the retraction ring and cannot advance beyond that point. The undelivered placenta will also be held at that point. Administration of intravenous morphine sulfate or the inhalation of amyl nitrite may relieve the retraction ring. If the situation is not relieved, uterine rupture and death of the fetus may occur. In the placental stage, massive maternal hemorrhage may result, because the placenta is loosened but not delivered, and so the uterus cannot contract.

Cesarean birth may be chosen to effect safe delivery of the fetus. Manual removal of the placenta under

Fig. 35-2. Pathological retraction ring. A. Uterus in the normal second stage of labor. Notice how the upper uterine segment is becoming thicker and the lower uterine segment is thinning. A physiological retraction ring is normally formed at the division of the upper and lower uterine segments. B. Uterus with a pathological retraction ring (Bandl's ring). The wall below the ring is thin and overdistended, and the ring rises against the abdominal wall. This constriction is caused by obstructed labor and is a warning sign that, if the obstruction is not relieved, the lower segment may rupture.

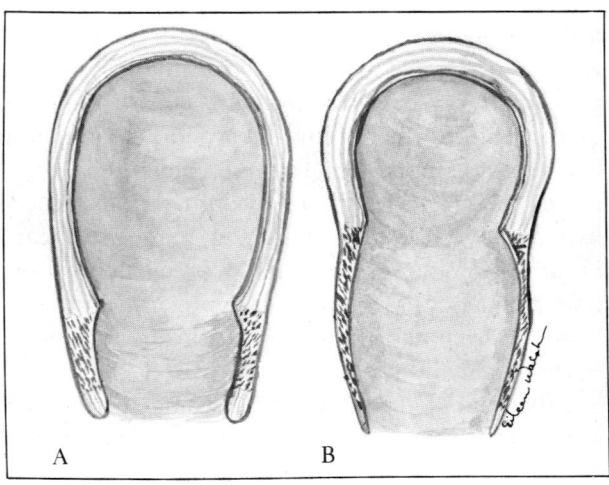

general anesthesia may be necessary for placental-stage pathological retraction rings.

With fetal monitors in place, there is a tendency not to observe the woman's abdomen in labor as much as when fetal heart sounds are being auscultated. You must observe the woman's abdomen if you are to detect a pathological retraction ring, which is a forewarning of uterine rupture.

PRECIPITATE DELIVERY

A precipitate labor and delivery occurs when uterine contractions are so strong that the woman delivers with only a few rapidly occurring contractions. It is often defined as a labor that is completed in less than 3 hours. Such rapid labor is likely to occur with multiparity and may follow induction of labor by oxytocin or amniotomy. Rapid labor poses risks to the fetus because subdural hemorrhage may result from the sudden release of pressure, and the woman may sustain lacerations of the birth canal. Forceful contractions may lead to premature separation of the placenta and both maternal and fetal risk.

That a precipitate labor is occurring can be predicted from a labor graph if, during the active phase of dilatation, the rate is greater than 5 cm per hour (1 cm every 12 minutes) in a primipara and over 10 cm per hour (1 cm every 6 minutes) in a multipara.

The woman with multiparity should be told by the 28th week of pregnancy that she can expect each labor to be shorter than the one before so she can make plans for rapid transportation to the hospital. Women who had a prior precipitate labor and delivery should be alerted that they may well deliver this way again. Both grand multiparas and women with histories of precipitate labor should be taken to the delivery room or have the birthing room converted to delivery readiness before full dilatation; delivery can then be accomplished in controlled surroundings.

RUPTURE OF THE UTERUS

Rupture of the uterus during labor, although rare, is a possibility that should always be kept in mind. The uterus ruptures when it undergoes more strain than it is capable of sustaining. Rupture occurs most commonly when a scar from a previous cesarean section, hysterotomy, or plastic repair of the uterus tears. However, prolonged labor, faulty presentation, multiple pregnancy, unwise use of oxytocins, obstructed labor, and traumatic maneuvers utilizing forceps extraction are contributing factors.

When the uterus ruptures, the woman experiences a sudden, severe pain during a strong labor contraction. If there is complete rupture, uterine contractions will stop. There is hemorrhage from the uterus into the abdominal cavity and possibly into the vagina. Signs of shock ensue, including rapid weak pulse, falling blood pressure, cold and clammy skin, and dilatation of the nostrils from air hunger. The woman's abdomen will change in contour, and two distinct swellings will be visible: the retracted uterus and the extrauterine fetus. Fetal heart sounds fail. If the rupture is incomplete (the placenta is not damaged), the signs are less evident than in complete rupture: The woman experiences a localized tenderness and a persistent aching pain over the area of the lower segment; contractions usually cease; and fetal heart sounds and the woman's vital signs will gradually reveal fetal and maternal distress.

Emergency fluid replacement must be started; a laparotomy must be scheduled as an emergency measure to control bleeding and effect a repair. The viability of the fetus will depend on the extent of the rupture and the time that elapses between the rupture and abdominal extraction. The woman's prognosis will depend on the extent of the rupture and blood loss.

Since it is not advisable for a woman who has a rupture of the uterus to conceive again, she is usually sterilized, either by removal of the damaged uterus (hysterectomy) or by tubal ligation at the time of the laparotomy.

AMNIOTIC FLUID EMBOLISM

Amniotic fluid embolism occurs when amniotic fluid is forced into an open maternal uterine blood sinus through some defect in the membranes or after membrane rupture or partial premature separation of the placenta. Solid particles (such as skin cells) in the amniotic fluid enter the maternal circulation and reach the lungs as small emboli. They produce pulmonary embolism whose severity is out of proportion to the size of the particles. The clinical picture is dramatic. The woman, in strong labor, sits up suddenly and grasps her chest because of inability to breathe and sharp pain. She pales and then turns the typical bluish gray associated with pulmonary embolism. Death may occur in minutes.

The immediate management is oxygen administration by face mask or cannula. The woman's prognosis depends on the size of the emboli and the skill and speed of the emergency aid available to her. Even if she survives the initial insult, the incidence of disseminated intravascular coagulation developing to further compound her condition is high.

INVERSION OF THE UTERUS

Like amniotic fluid embolism, inversion of the uterus, in which the fundus is forced through the cervix, so that the uterus is turned inside out, is an extremely grave complication for the woman. Inversion of the uterus occurs following the placental stage of labor. It may be caused by (1) insertion of the placenta at the fundus, so that as the fetus is delivered it pulls the fundus down; (2) atony of the uterus so extreme that coughing or sneezing forces the fundus outward; (3) attempts to deliver the placenta before the uterus has contracted, either by putting pressure on the uterus or by traction on the cord. *Never put pressure on an uncontracted uterus or traction on the umbilical cord to avoid this complication.*

Inversion occurs in various degrees. The inverted fundus may lie within the uterine cavity or the vagina or, in total inversion, protrude from the vagina. Bleeding is profuse. The woman has symptoms of shock: pallor, rapid pulse, and falling blood pressure.

Never attempt to replace the inversion; this may only increase bleeding. Never attempt to remove the placenta if it is still attached; this will only create a larger bleeding area. The administration of oxytocic drugs only compounds the inversion. Replacement of the inversion is attempted under general anesthesia. The prognosis of the woman will depend on the degree of the inversion and the amount of blood loss and replacement blood available on an emergency basis. Hysterectomy may have to be performed to halt the hemorrhage.

The Fetus: Difficulty with the Passenger

FETAL BLOOD SAMPLING

The oxygen saturation, PO_2, PCO_2, pH, and hematocrit of fetal blood may be determined during labor if a sample of capillary blood is taken from the fetal scalp as it presents at the dilated cervix. The fetal scalp is first prepared with iodine before a scalpel is introduced for the actual puncture. The amount of blood obtained (collected by a capillary tube) is usually so small that the pH level of the blood is the only determination that can be evaluated. This averages 7.25. A range of 7.20 to 7.30 is considered normal. A fetus with a lower level (acidotic) is suffering anoxia.

Serial readings should be determined, as a *change* in pH may provide information on fetal welfare before an *abnormal* pH exists. Following the procedure, the infant scalp should be observed following two contractions to be certain that bleeding at the puncture site has halted.

A woman needs a clear explanation of what is being attempted before fetal blood samples are obtained. Otherwise she may worry that the scalpel used will press into the baby's brain or by accident invade an eye or ear. She cannot relax to allow for vaginal manipulations of this nature if she is concerned about her child's welfare.

PROLAPSE OF THE CORD

In prolapse of the cord, a loop of the umbilical cord slips down in front of the presenting fetal part (Fig. 35-3). Prolapse may occur at any time after the membranes rupture and if the presenting part is not fitted firmly into the cervix. It thus tends to occur often with premature rupture of the membranes, with fetal positions other than cephalic presentations, with placenta previa or intrauterine tumors that prevent the presenting part from engaging, and with a small fetus or cephalopelvic disproportion that prevents firm engagement.

Very rarely, the cord may be felt as the presenting part on vaginal examination. You will feel the cord pulsating as you are examining for dilatation or trying to identify fontanelles. In the event of this presentation, cesarean section will be necessary before rupture of the membranes occurs; otherwise, with rupture, the cord will surely be flushed down into the vagina. More often, however, cord prolapse is first discovered when the variable deceleration pattern of cord compression suddenly becomes apparent on the fetal monitor. The cord may be visible at the vulva.

To rule out cord prolapse, fetal heart sounds should always be recorded immediately following rupture of the membranes, whether it occurs spontaneously or by amniotomy.

Cord prolapse automatically leads to cord compression as the presenting part presses against the cord at the pelvic brim. Management is aimed toward relieving pressure on the cord and thereby relieving the compression and the resulting fetal anoxia. This may be done by having the woman assume a knee-chest position, which causes the presenting part to fall back from the cord. You may need to press pillows under the woman's abdomen to allow her to remain in this position in active labor.

If the cord is exposed to room air, drying will begin, and with the drying, the umbilical vessels will start to atrophy. Do not attempt to push any exposed cord back into the vagina or you may add to the compression by causing knotting or kinking. Cover any exposed portion with a sterile saline compress to prevent drying.

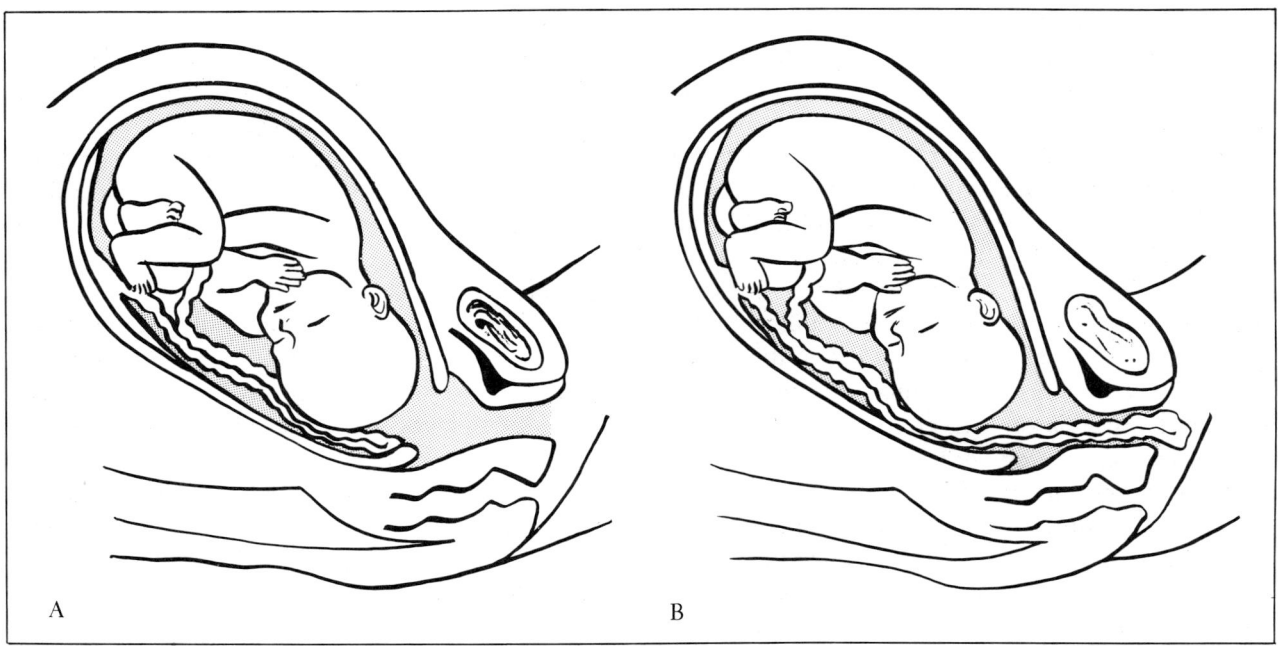

Fig. 35-3. Prolapse of the umbilical cord. A. The cord is prolapsed but still within the uterus. B. The cord is visible at the vulva. In both instances the fetal nutrient supply is being compromised. Although only a cord such as that in B would be visible, both prolapses could be detected by fetal monitoring equipment.

If the cervix is fully dilated at the time of the prolapse, the physician may choose to deliver the infant rapidly, possibly with forceps, to prevent a lengthy period of anoxia. If dilatation is not complete, cesarean section will be the delivery method of choice.

Prolapse of the cord is an emergency situation that requires prompt action. Often, you are the person with the woman when this occurs. Carry out measures to relieve cord compression quickly. With cord prolapse, you are the first line of defense against permanent brain damage in the child. You have less than 5 minutes to institute relief measures to prevent irreparable central nervous system damage to the infant.

MULTIPLE GESTATION

The first stage of labor during a multiple gestation does not differ from the first stage of single gestation labor. However, because the babies are usually small, cord prolapse is an increased possibility after rupture of the membranes. Analgesia administration should be conservative, so that it will not add to any respiratory difficulties the infants may have at birth because of their immaturity.

The thought of having a woman in labor with a multiple gestation causes a flurry of excitement in most people. Additional personnel have to be assembled for the delivery room (two nurses to attend to possibly immature infants, a pediatrician for immature care). In the middle of all the preparatory activity it is easy to forget that the woman may be more frightened than excited. Be careful that the air of anticipation around her is not interpreted as everyone having fun but her; everyone invited to a party but her.

The first twin is usually delivered normally. Both ends of the cord of the first twin are tied or permanently clamped; if a common placenta is shared and a cord clamp slips, the second twin will hemorrhage through the open cord. The first twin is identified as Twin I or Twin A, depending on the hospital's policy. Newborn care is begun for the first twin, but a product such as ergot is not given to assist uterine involution in order to prevent compromising the circulation of the second twin.

The lie of the second twin is determined by external abdominal palpation. If the lie is not longitudinal, external version is attempted to make it so. The presentation is confirmed by vaginal examination, and the second set of membranes is ruptured. This action brings down the presenting part and may initiate contractions if they are not already active. An oxytocin infusion may be begun to assist uterine contractions. Most twins present with both twins vertex, followed in frequency by vertex and breech, breech and vertex, and breech and breech (Fig. 35-4).

If the presence of twins had been undetected and an oxytocic drug was given at the same time the shoulder of the first twin was delivered, the resulting

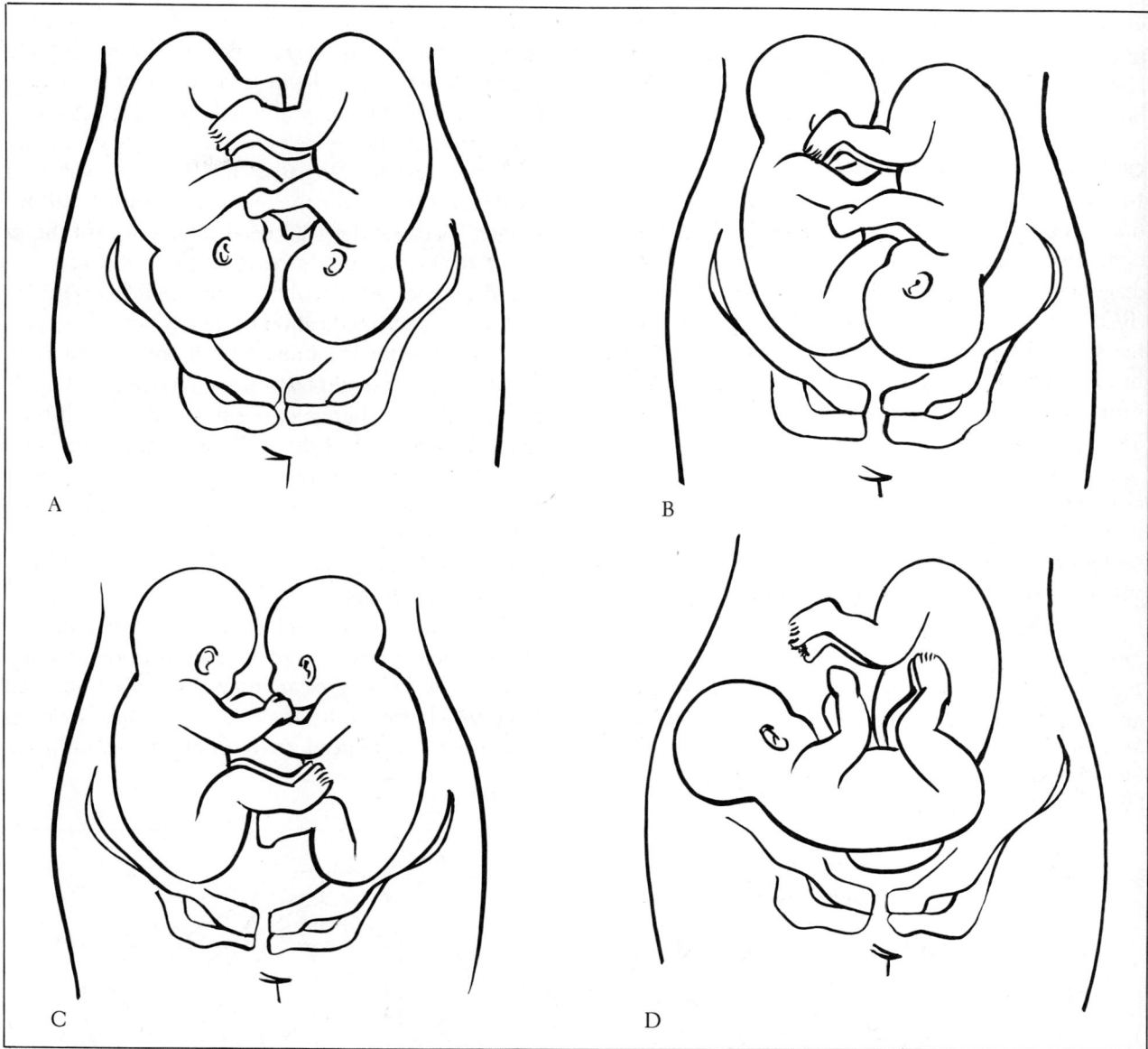

Fig. 35-4. Four different twin presentations. A. Both infants vertex. B. One infant vertex and one breech. C. Both infants breech. D. One infant vertex and one in a transverse lie.

tonic contractions may prevent delivery of the second twin. More often, the forceful contraction from the oxytocin causes the second twin to be delivered extremely rapidly.

Occasionally, the placenta of the first twin separates before the second twin is born, and there is sudden, profuse bleeding at the vagina. This creates a risk for the woman; the uterus does not contract as it normally would and thereby halt the bleeding because it is still filled with the second baby. If the separation of the first placenta causes loosening of the second placenta, or if a common placenta is involved, the fetal heart sounds of the second twin will immediately register distress, and he will have to be delivered at once if he is to survive.

Mothers usually want to inspect twins thoroughly in the delivery room. The time allowed for this inspection will depend on the infants' weight and condition. Most mothers of twins worry that the hospital will confuse the two through improper identification. Review with the mother the careful measures that are being taken to ensure correct identification.

Most women who have a multiple birth have difficulty believing that it is real. They need to recount over and over their surprise and to view both their infants together to prove to themselves that it is true. If they were not able to inspect the infants thoroughly in the delivery room because of their low birth weights and the danger of chilling, they need the time to do so as soon as possible, to dispel all the fears they had throughout pregnancy that the babies would be born joined or deformed.

OCCIPITOPOSTERIOR POSITION

In approximately a tenth of all labors, the fetal position is posterior rather than anterior; that is, the occiput (assuming the presentation is vertex) is directed diagonally and posteriorly: right occipitoposterior (ROP) or left occipitoposterior (LOP). In these positions, in the process of internal rotation, the fetal head must rotate not through a 90-degree arc but through an arc of approximately 135 degrees (Figs. 35-5 and 35-6).

Posterior positions tend to occur in women with android, anthropoid, or contracted pelves. The position of the fetus is evident on vaginal examination. A posteriorly presenting head does not fit the cervix as snugly as one in an anterior position, increasing the risk of prolapse of the umbilical cord.

Fig. 35-5. Left occipitoanterior (LOA) rotation. A. A fetus in a cephalic presentation, LOA position. View is from the outlet. The fetus rotates 90 degrees from this position. B. Descent and flexion. C. Internal rotation complete. D. Extension. The face and chin are born.

If uterine contractions are forceful and the fetus is of average size and in good flexion, the majority of infants presenting with these posterior positions will rotate through the large arc, will arrive at a good delivery position for the pelvic outlet, and will be delivered satisfactorily. Because the arc of rotation is greater, it is usual for the labor to be somewhat prolonged. Because the fetal head rotates against the sacrum, the woman may experience pressure and pain in her lower back during labor, which may be so intense that she asks for medication for relief, not for her contractions, but for the intense back pressure and pain she is feeling. Sacral pressure such as that afforded by a back rub or a change of position may be helpful in relieving a portion of the pain. During a long labor, be certain that the woman voids about every 2 hours to keep the bladder empty; a full bladder impedes descent of the fetus. Be aware how long it has been since she last ate; she may need intravenous glucose to ward off uterine dysfunction.

If contractions are not effective, or the infant is above average size or not in good flexion, rotation through the 135-degree arc may not be accomplished. Uterine dysfunction may result from maternal exhaustion. The head may arrest in the transverse

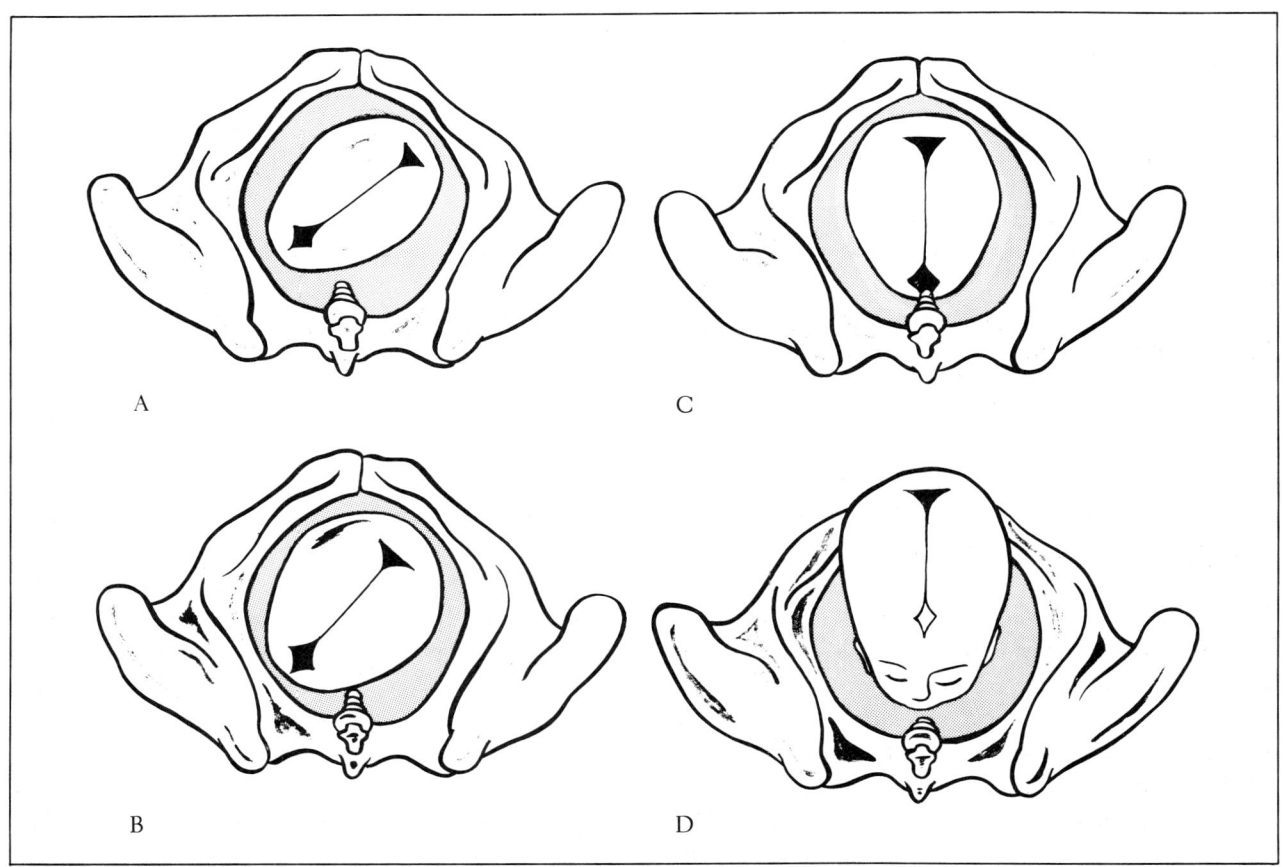

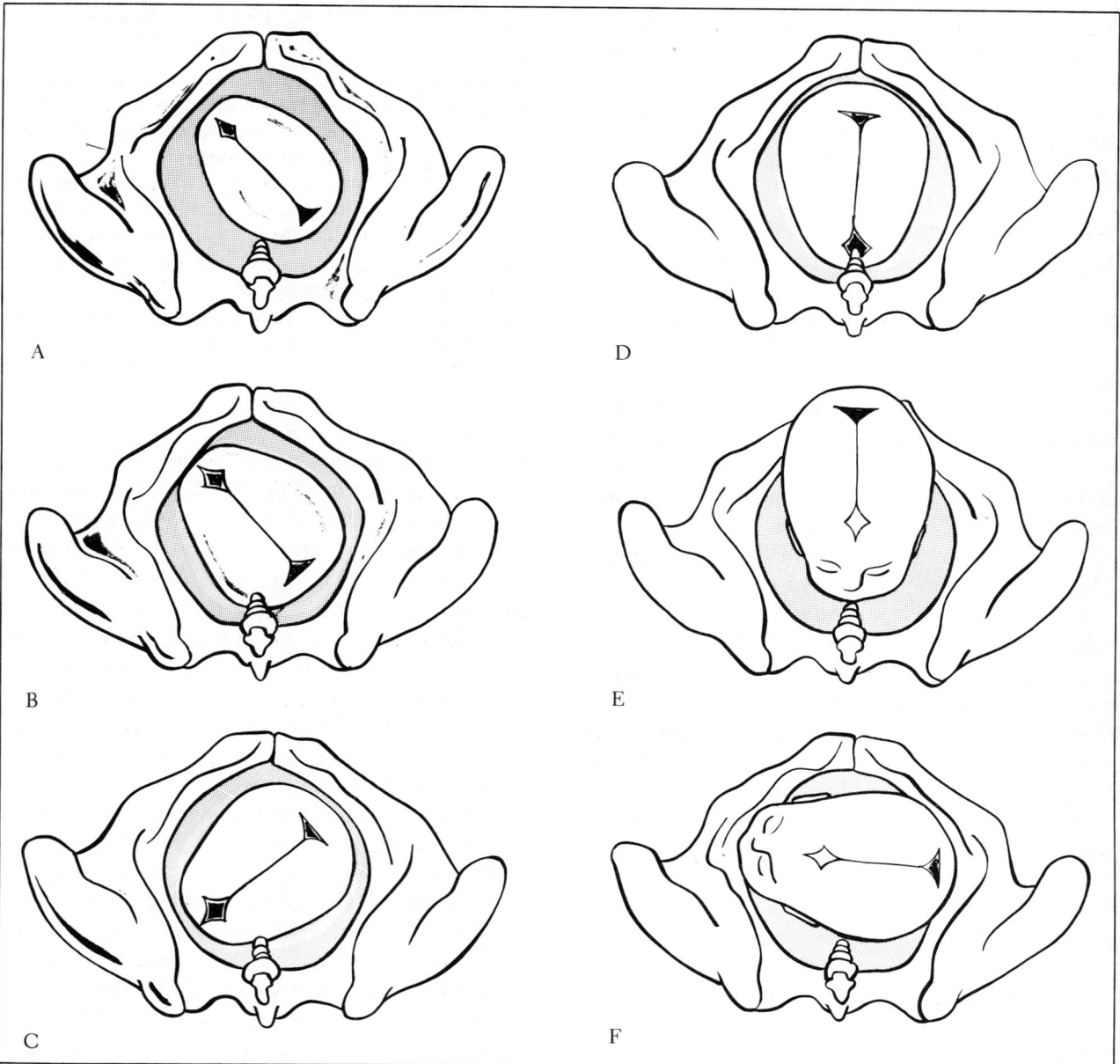

Fig. 35-6. Left occipitoposterior (LOP) rotation. A. Fetus in a cephalic presentation, LOP position. View is from the outlet. The fetus rotates 135 degrees from this position. B. Descent and flexion. C. Internal rotation beginning. Because of the posterior position, the head will rotate in a longer arc than if it were in an anterior position. D. Internal rotation complete. E. Extension. The face and chin are born. F. External rotation. The fetus rotates to place the shoulders in an anteroposterior position.

position (transverse arrest). Rotation may not take place (persistent occipitoposterior position). In both instances, if the fetus has reached the midportion of the pelvis, he may be rotated to an anterior position with forceps and then delivered. With the woman on the delivery room table and appropriate anesthesia administered, the physician applies forceps to the fetal head and rotates the head to the anterior position, removes the forceps, reapplies them, and delivers the infant in an occipitoanterior position (Scanzoni maneuver). A small-sized infant might be delivered from the original posterior position (face-to-pubis delivery). Today, cesarean section is often elected over rotation and extraction; the risk of a mid-forceps maneuver exceeds the risk of a cesarean section.

A woman who has had a long labor is more prone to postpartal hemorrhage and infection than others. During labor, she needs a great deal of support to prevent her from becoming panicky over the length of the labor, and she needs practical explanations of what is happening, step by step. Paradoxically, women who are best prepared for labor are often most frightened when deviations occur, because things are not going "by the book," not happening just as described by the instructor of the course they attended. Such women should have frequent reassurance that although their pattern of labor is not "textbook," it is still within safe, controlled limits.

BREECH PRESENTATION

The majority of fetuses are in a breech presentation early in pregnancy. By the 40th week of gestation, however, the fetus normally turns to a cephalic presentation. Although the fetal head is the widest single diameter, the fetus's buttocks (breech), plus his lower extremities, actually take up more space. The fact that the fundus of the uterus is the largest part of the uterus probably accounts for the 97 percent of all pregnancies in which the fetus turns so that the buttocks and lower extremities are in the fundus.

There are several types of breech presentations. These are shown in Table 35-1.

It is helpful to know what the position of a breech-delivered baby was as the infant tends to assume his delivery position in the postpartal period; for example, a single footling breech infant will tend to lie with one foot extended, one flexed; the frank breech infant tends to lie with his legs extended and held near his face.

Breech presentations may occur for a number of reasons:

1. Gestation age under 40 weeks.
2. Abnormality in the fetus, such as anencephaly, hydrocephalus, or meningocele. (In a fetus with hydrocephalus, the widest total diameter is the head, and so it retains the most "comfortable" position.)
3. Hydramnios that allows for free fetal movement, so that the fetus does not have to make a "most comfortable" choice.
4. Congenital abnormality of the uterus, such as a midseptum that traps the fetus in a breech position.
5. Any space-occupying mass in the pelvis, such as a fibroid tumor of the uterus or a placenta previa that does not allow the head to present.
6. Pendulous abdomen. If the abdominal muscles are very lax, the uterus may fall so far forward that the fetal head comes to lie outside the pelvic brim, and so the breech presents.
7. Multiple gestation. The presenting twin cannot turn to a vertex position.
8. Unknown factors.

Table 35-1. Classification of Breech Presentations

Type	Description
Complete	Feet and legs are flexed on thighs; thighs are flexed on abdomen; buttocks and feet are the presenting parts
Frank	Legs are extended and lie against abdomen and chest; feet are at the level of shoulders; buttocks are the presenting part
Double footling	Legs are unflexed and extended; feet are the presenting part
Single footling	One leg is unflexed and extended; one foot is the presenting part

Version

Because fetal risk in a breech delivery is two or three times higher than in a cephalic delivery, some physicians will attempt to change a breech position to a cephalic position at about the 32nd to 34th week of gestation by external cephalic version. With the woman in a lithotomy position, the physician exerts pressure on the cervix to disengage the breech. Then, applying pressure to the woman's external abdomen, he attempts to turn the fetus to a cephalic presentation. This must be done with the pressure (that turns the fetus) toward the cord, to prevent tearing of the cord and placenta.

External version is not without risk. The cord may become wound around the neck of the fetus and impede fetal circulation. The maneuver may also result in premature rupture of the membranes, or premature labor, or infection. In the rare instance of a short cord, the placenta may become separated, with resultant fetal and maternal damage. If extreme force is used, uterine rupture is a possibility. For this reason, external version is contraindicated in women with uterine scars from hysterotomy or cesarean section.

The version will not be successful if (1) the uterine and abdominal tone is too high to effect relaxation, (2) the uterus has a septum, or (3) the fetus is so large that there is no room to turn it. Even if a version is accomplished, there is no guarantee that the fetus will not revert to a breech presentation before delivery. Persistent breech presentation arouses suspicion of a bicornuate uterus, placenta previa, or a fetal abnormality such as hydrocephalus.

Assessment

Leopold's maneuvers and a vaginal examination will reveal a breech presentation. If the breech is complete and firmly engaged, the tightly stretched gluteal muscles may be mistaken on examination for a head; the natal cleft may be mistaken for the sagittal suture line. Confirmation of a breech presentation may be made either by roentgenography or by sonography. Such studies also give information on pelvic diameters, fetal skull diameters, and whether a placenta previa exists or not. Also revealed is any bony fetal abnormality (such as hydrocephalus) that will make vaginal delivery impossible.

Risks in Labor

There are many old wives' tales about breech delivery (they are more painful, much longer, they crush the fetal head, the woman is horribly torn, and so forth). For this reason, some physicians do not tell the woman that her baby is in a breech presentation. Be certain you are not the one who lets this information slip. The anxiety it may create in the woman may be enough to cause a painful labor that will seem very long to her.

Prolapse of the umbilical cord is more likely with breech delivery than with cephalic delivery because the breech does not engage the cervix as snugly as the head does. Early rupture of the membranes tends to occur because of the poor fit of the presenting part.

Fig. 35-7. Breech delivery. A. Position prior to labor: LSP. B. Descent and internal rotation. C. Legs being born. Note the anterior-posterior diameter best accommodates the shoulders. D. The head is born, External rotation has put the anterior-posterior diameter of the head in line with the anterior-posterior diameter of the mother's pelvis.

The inevitable contraction of the buttocks often causes meconium to be extruded before delivery. This is not indicative of fetal distress but is expected from the buttocks' pressure.

With every breech presentation, a fetal monitor and uterine contraction monitor should be in place during labor. It will make possible detection of fetal distress from a complication such as a prolapsed cord at the earliest possible moment. In a breech delivery, the same stages of flexion, descent, internal rotation, expulsion, and external rotation occur as in a vertex delivery (Fig. 35-7).

An additional complication of breech labor might occur because the breech is able to pass through the cervix before full dilatation is reached. The breech may be evident at the vulva (crowning) before the first stage of labor is complete. The woman must not push with contractions with a breech delivery until it is shown by vaginal examination that full dilatation has been reached. If she pushes when the breech is at the vulva but cervical dilatation is not complete, the fetus may deliver up to its neck, then be unable to pass through the incompletely dilated cervix. The delivery of the aftercoming head may be lethal to the fetus from pressure of the head against the cord during the time it is awaiting dilatation. The woman may need inhalation analgesia with each contraction to keep from pushing; it is an almost uncontrollable reflex when the presenting part is at the perineum.

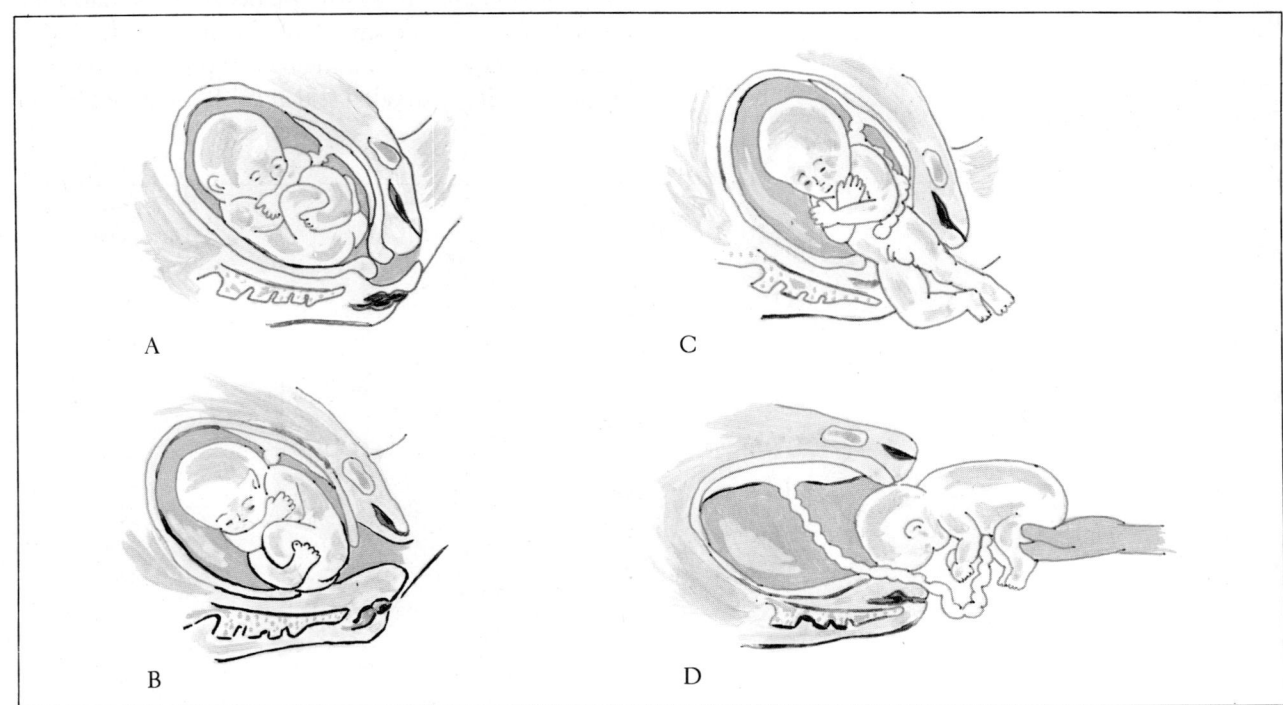

Risks in Delivery

When full dilatation is reached, the woman is allowed to push, and the breech, trunk, and shoulders are delivered. As the breech spontaneously emerges from the birth canal, it is steadied and supported by a sterile towel held against the infant's inferior surface. The shoulders present to the outlet with their widest diameter anteroposterior. If they do not deliver readily, the arm of the posterior shoulder may be drawn down by passing two fingers over the infant's shoulder and down the arm to the elbow, then sweeping the flexed arm across the infant's face and chest and out. The other arm is delivered in the same way. External rotation is allowed to occur to bring the head into the best outlet diameter.

Delivery of the head is the most hazardous part of the breech delivery. The umbilicus precedes the head, and a loop of cord passes down alongside the head. This loop of cord will automatically be compressed by the pressure of the head against the pelvic brim. A healthy, noncompromised fetus can survive as long as 10 minutes of cord compression. If compromising factors, such as maternal preeclampsia or hypertension or an exceptionally long first stage of labor, are present, the length of time in which the fetus may be safely delivered becomes considerably shorter.

A second danger of a breech delivery is intracranial hemorrhage. With a cephalic presentation, molding to the confines of the birth canal takes place over hours; with a breech delivery, pressure changes occur instantaneously. The result may be tentorial tears, which can cause gross motor and mental incapacity or lethal damage to the fetus. The infant who is delivered suddenly to reduce the amount of time during which there is cord compression may suffer an intracranial hemorrhage; the infant who is delivered gradually to reduce the possibility of intracranial injury may suffer hypoxia. Delivery of an aftercoming head involves a great deal of judgment and skill.

To aid delivery of the head, the trunk of the infant is usually straddled over the physician's right forearm. Two fingers of the physician's right hand are placed in the infant's mouth (Fig. 35-8). The left hand is slid into the vagina, palm down, along the infant's back. Pressure is applied to the occiput to flex the head fully. Gentle traction applied to the shoulders (upward and outward) delivers the head. An aftercoming head may be delivered by the aid of Piper forceps to control the flexion and rate of descent (Fig. 35-9).

Cesarean section is more and more becoming the preferred method of delivery for babies in breech presentation in order to provide the safest form of birth possible.

Inspection by the Mother

A mother usually inspects a breech baby in the delivery room a little more closely than does the average mother. She is looking for the reason that made the presentation breech, as will the person who makes the initial physical assessment of the infant. An infant who was delivered in a frank breech position may tend to keep his legs extended and at the level of his face for

Fig. 35-8. Breech delivery. The aftercoming head is delivered by gentle pressure to flex the head fully, and by gentle traction to the shoulders upward and outward. Additional pressure might be applied by an assistant to the abdominal wall to ensure head flexion.

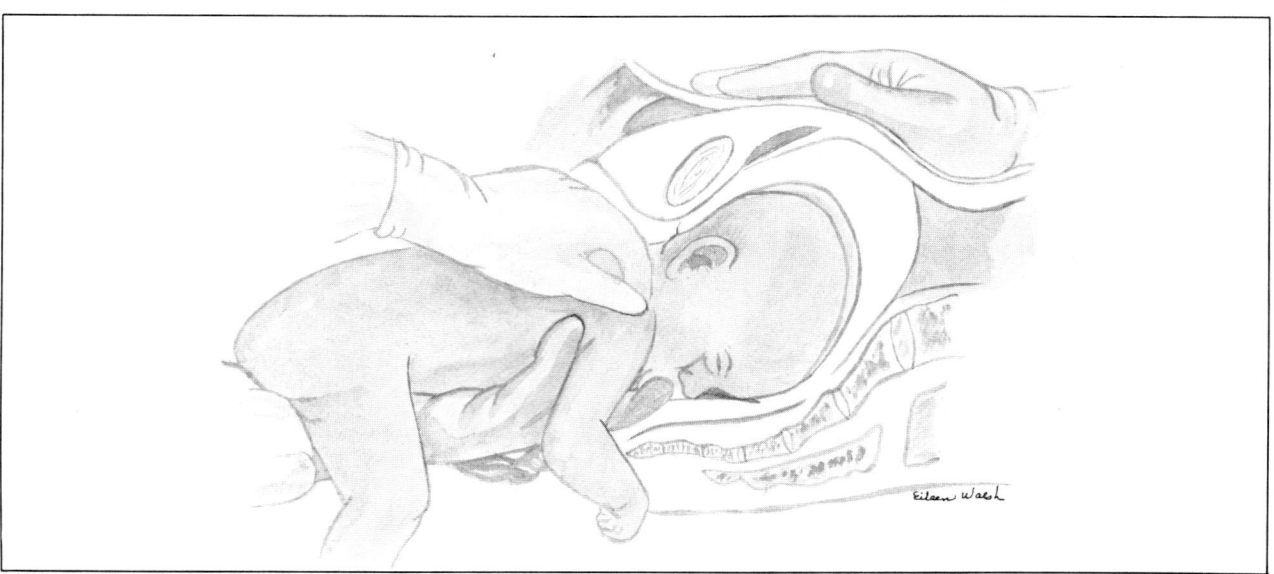

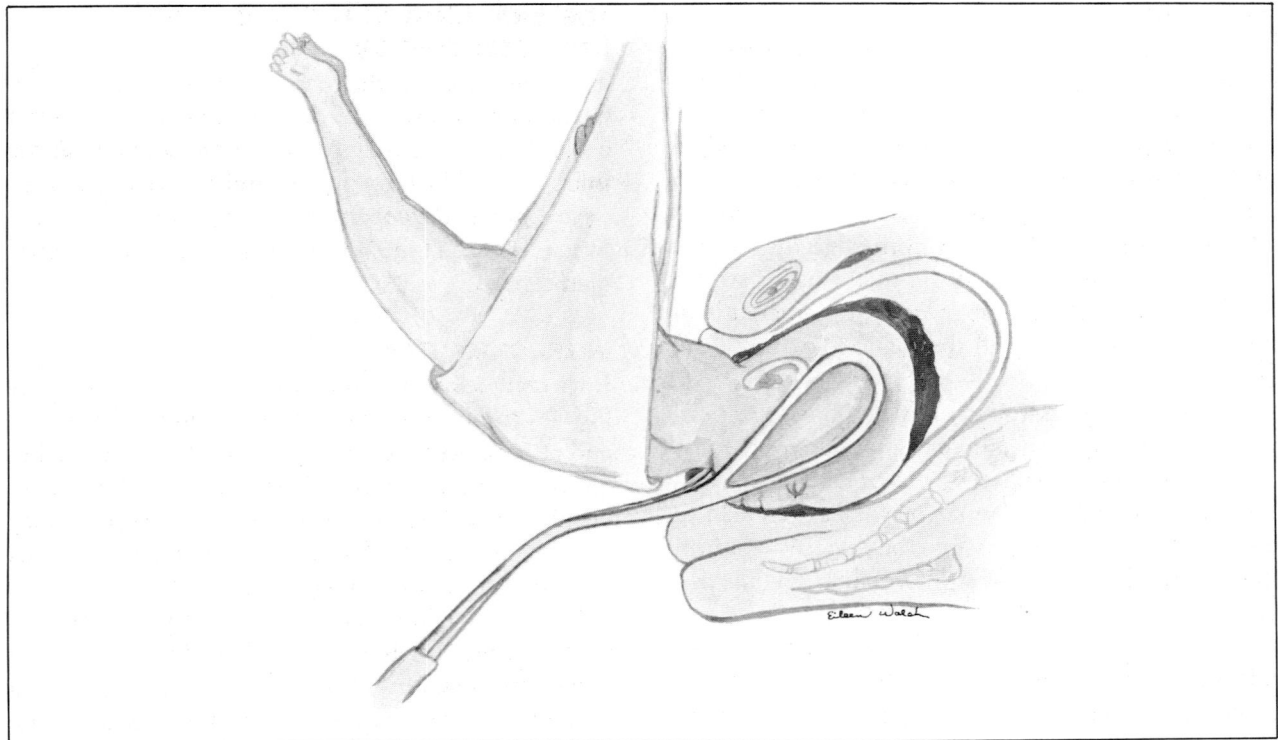

Fig. 35-9. Breech delivery by means of Piper forceps. With Piper forceps, traction is applied directly to the head, and damage to the infant's neck is avoided. The hands and arms are constrained by a towel.

the first two or three days of life; the infant who was a footling breech may tend to keep his legs extended in a footling position for the first few days. It is good to point this out to the mother, so that she does not read more than necessary into the strange posture of her baby.

FACE PRESENTATION

Face (chin, or mentum) presentation is rare, but when it does occur, the diameter the fetus presents to the pelvis is often too large for delivery to proceed. A face presentation is suggested by a head that feels larger than normal and with no engagement apparent on Leopold's maneuver. It is also suggested when the head and back are both felt on the same side of the uterus by the same maneuver. It is confirmed by vaginal examination, when the nose, mouth, or chin can be felt as the presenting part.

A fetus in a posterior position, instead of flexing the head as labor proceeds, may extend the head, resulting in a face (chin) presentation. The usual situation in which this occurs is in a woman with a contracted pelvis or in the presence of a placenta previa. It is a warning signal, in that something abnormal is causing the chin presentation.

When a face presentation is suspected, an x-ray film or sonogram will be made to confirm it and to indicate the measurements of the pelvic diameters. If the chin is anterior, and the pelvic diameters are within normal limits, the infant may be delivered without difficulty (perhaps following a long first stage of labor, because the face does not mold well to make a snugly engaging part). If the chin is posterior, cesarean section may be the choice of delivery; otherwise, it would be necessary to wait for a long posterior-to-anterior rotation to occur. Such rotation can result in uterine dysfunction or transverse arrest.

Babies born following a chin presentation have a great deal of facial edema and may be bruised. Lip edema may be so severe that the infant is unable to nurse for a day or two. He may have to have gavage feedings to obtain enough fluid until he can suck effectively. The mother needs to be assured that the edema is a result of the delivery and nothing else; it is transient and will disappear in a few days, with no aftermath.

BROW PRESENTATION

A brow presentation is the rarest of the presentations. It almost invariably results in obstructed labor, since the head becomes jammed in the brim of the pelvis. Cesarean section will be necessary to deliver the infant safely.

TRANSVERSE LIE

Transverse lie occurs in women with pendulous abdomens, with uterine masses such as fibroid tumors obstructing the lower uterine segment, with contraction of the pelvic brim, with congenital abnormalities of the uterus, or with hydramnios. It may occur in infants with hydrocephalus or other gross abnormalities that prevent the head from engaging. It may occur in prematurity, when the infant has room for free movement; in multiple pregnancy (particularly in the second twin); or when there is a short umbilical cord.

A transverse lie is usually obvious on inspection, when the ovoid of the uterus is found to be more horizontal than vertical. By means of Leopold's maneuvers the abnormal presentation will be detected. An x-ray picture or sonogram may be taken to confirm the abnormal lie and to give information such as pelvic size.

A mature fetus cannot be delivered vaginally from this presentation. Often, the membranes rupture. Because there is no firm presenting part, the cord prolapses, or an arm may prolapse, or the shoulder obstructs the cervix. Cesarean section is necessary.

In a grand multipara, if the x-ray film reveals no apparent abnormality, such as placenta previa or contracted pelvis, or an abnormality with the fetus, the physician may externally rotate the fetus to a cephalic presentation at the beginning of labor. If the fetus "holds" that presentation through descent, a normal delivery will result. It is important that a transverse lie be detected before the membranes rupture. Since the nurse is the first person to observe the woman on her admission to the hospital, such an abnormal presentation could be identified almost immediately on admission if you take the responsibility to look for such a finding.

OVERSIZED FETUS

The size of the fetus may become a problem when it exceeds 4,500 gm (10 pounds); a weight lower than this is not likely to cause difficulty. Only 1 in 100 infants weighs this much. An oversized infant may cause uterine dysfunction during labor or at delivery. The wide shoulders may pose a problem at delivery. There is a sizable increase in the perinatal mortality of larger infants (15 percent versus the normal 4 percent).

Babies of this size are most frequently born to women who are diabetic. Large babies may be associated with multiparity; each infant tends to be slightly heavier and larger than the one born just before him.

The Birth Canal: Difficulty with the Passageway

The third problem that can cause dystocia is a contraction or narrowing of the passageway, or the birth canal. The pelvis may be contracted (narrow) at the inlet, the midpelvis, or the outlet. This is termed *cephalopelvic disproportion*, or a disproportion between the size of the normal fetal head and the pelvic diameters.

INLET CONTRACTION

Inlet contraction is ordinarily due to rickets in early life. It is more common in blacks than in Caucasians and at the lower socioeconomic levels than at higher levels. However, it is a fallacy to believe that all people are eating adequate diets just because they have the money to afford them, or that rickets occurs only in low socioeconomic groups.

Inlet contraction is defined as narrowing of the anteroposterior diameter to less than 11 cm, or as a maximum transverse diameter of 12 cm or less. In a primigravida, the fetal head normally engages at the 36th to 38th week of pregnancy. When this event occurs before labor begins, it is proof that the pelvic inlet is adequate. Following the general rule that "what goes in comes out," a head that engages, or proves it fits into the pelvic brim, will also be able to pass through the midpelvis and through the outlet.

When engagement does not occur in a primigravida, suspicion should be very high that either a fetal abnormality (larger-than-usual head) or a pelvic abnormality (smaller-than-usual pelvis) is causing the lack of engagement. As a rule, engagement does not take place in multigravidas until labor begins. A woman who has delivered a previous infant vaginally without problems has proved that her birth canal is adequate.

Every primigravida should have pelvic measurements taken and recorded before the 24th week of pregnancy, so that a delivery decision can be made, based on these measurements and on the assumption that the fetus will be of average size.

OUTLET CONTRACTION

Outlet contraction is defined as the narrowing of the transverse diameter to less than 11 cm. This is the distance between the ischial tuberosities, a measurement that is easy to make during a prenatal visit.

TRIAL LABOR

If a woman has borderline (just adequate) inlet measurements, and the fetal lie and position are good, the physician may allow her a "trial" labor to see whether labor can progress normally; this is allowed to continue as long as descent of the presenting part and dilatation of the cervix are occurring. Fetal heart sounds and uterine contractions should be monitored during a trial labor. It is especially important that the urinary bladder be kept emptied during a trial labor to allow all the space available to be used by the fetal head. If after a definite period (6 to 12 hours) inadequate progress is made, the woman will be scheduled for a cesarean section.

It is difficult for women to undertake a labor they know they may not be able to complete. Some physicians let the woman know that the labor is a trial one; others feel that she does better if she does not know it.

It is important that a woman does not interpret a trial labor as a whim of her physician. Labor is painful, and a woman cannot have much confidence in her physician if she thinks that he or she is putting her through this "just for the fun of it." Emphasize that it is best for the baby to be born vaginally. However, do not overstress this fact. If the trial labor fails, and cesarean section is scheduled, you will need to explain why a cesarean section will be good for the baby.

Some women having a trial labor feel very much as if they themselves are on trial. When dilatation does not occur, they feel discouraged and inadequate, as if they have failed. The woman may not even have realized how much she wanted this trial labor to work, until she is told that it is not working. The husband is as frightened and feels as helpless as his wife when a deviation occurs in labor. He makes comments such as "The doctor knows best" or "This is a good hospital, and nothing bad is going to happen to the baby," but they sound as false to him and his wife as they do to you. The couple needs assurance from health care personnel that a cesarean section is not an inferior method of delivery but an alternative method; in this instance it is the method of choice. A cesarean section will secure for them the goals they and you both seek: a healthy mother and a healthy child.

Cesarean Section

Incision of the uterus to deliver the fetus abdominally is one of the oldest known types of surgical operation. Originally, cesarean sections were performed only as emergency procedures—on women who were dying or had died during pregnancy or labor. Today, they may be used with women who have a cephalopelvic disproportion, placenta previa, premature separation of the placenta, previous cesarean section, or severe pregnancy-induced hypertension (eclampsia) or if there is fetal distress.

At first, the operation involved cesarean hysterectomy, or removal of the uterus with the child. In 1879, Sanger developed the classic cesarean section, in which the uterus is saved. The incision of a classic cesarean section is into the upper segment of the uterus.

Today, cesarean section (Fig. 35-10) is one of the safest types of surgery possible from the woman's standpoint. Newer techniques involve a transverse incision into the lower uterine segment under a flap of peritoneum (called a *bikini incision* because it can be covered by a bikini). This incision reduces the blood loss at operation, and because it is retroperitoneal, the risk of peritonitis is minimal. A low incision is much less likely to rupture on a succeeding pregnancy or labor than a higher incision, because the lower uterine segment is more passive than active in labor. On account of this type of incision, "once a cesarean, always a cesarean" no longer necessarily holds. In women with placenta previa who have a cesarean section performed, the classic incision is still made, to ensure that it will be above the level of attachment of the placenta. Two types of cesarean section incisions are shown in Fig. 35-11.

Cesarean section is not without risk to the fetus. Often, however, it is elected because the fetus is in distress. In these instances, it is hard to decide which factor, the section or the distress, causes difficulty in the newborn. When a fetus is pushed through the birth canal, pressure on the chest appears to rid the lungs of amniotic fluid or lung fluid, making respirations more likely to be adequate at birth than if the fetus is not subjected to this pressure. About 5 percent of all infants delivered by cesarean section have some degree of respiratory difficulty for a day or two after birth.

When it has been decided that a cesarean section will be necessary for delivery, the woman is prepared for surgery in the same manner as for any abdominal surgery. The abdomen is shaved and washed with a disinfectant solution. Because cesarean incisions are low, pubic hair is removed as well. A urinary catheter is inserted and taped in place to empty the bladder, so that a full bladder does not obstruct the surgical field. Women at term are hard to catheterize because there is some edema of the vulva due to descent of the fetal head. If catheterization cannot be done easily in the labor room, it can be done in the delivery room after the anesthetic is given. Blood for cross matching and typing needs to be done if blood is not already avail-

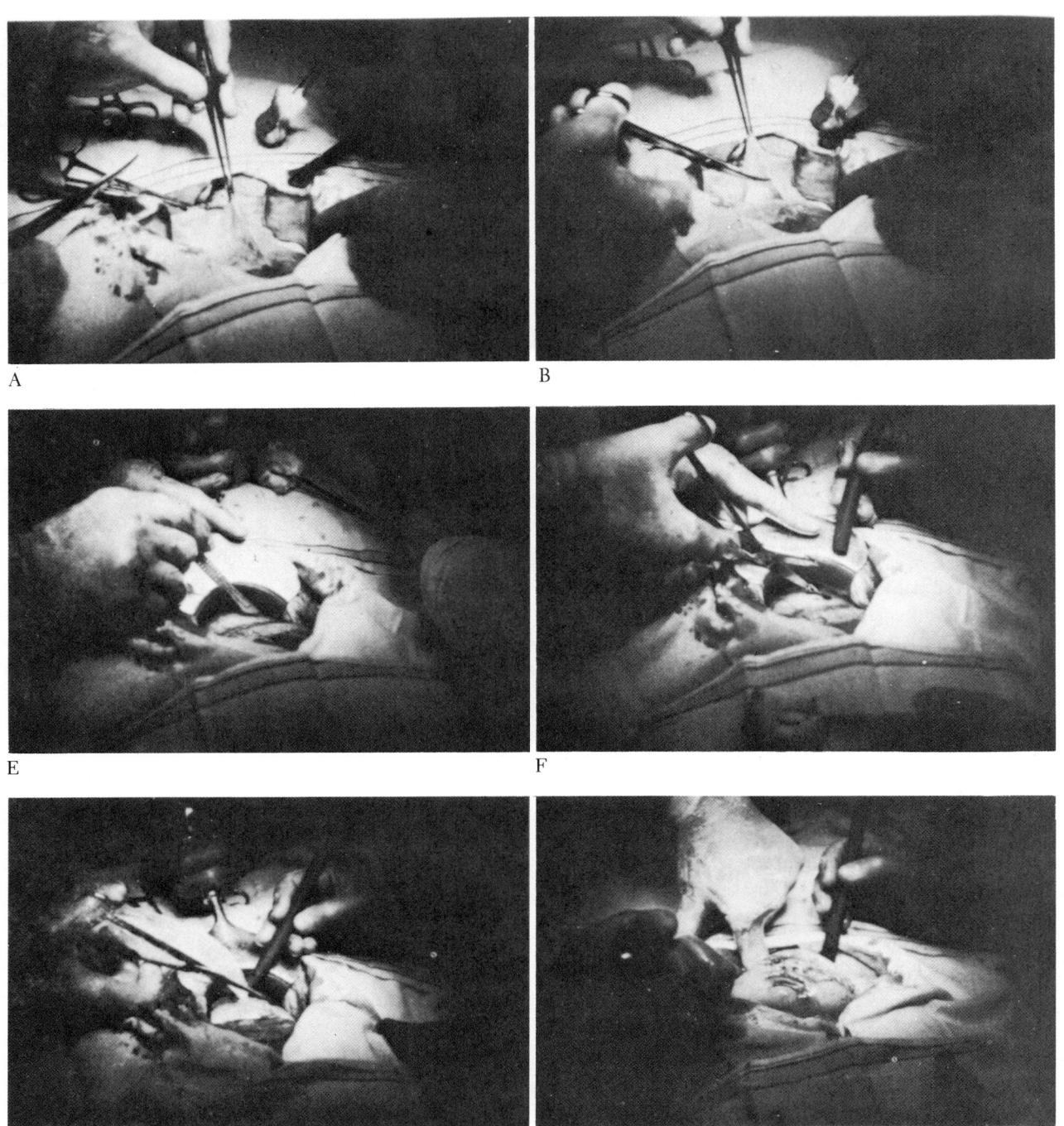

Fig. 35-10. Delivery by cesarean section (A–L). (From D. N. Dansforth [Ed.], Textbook of Obstetrics and Gynecology [2nd ed.]. New York: Harper & Row, 1971. Reprinted with permission.)

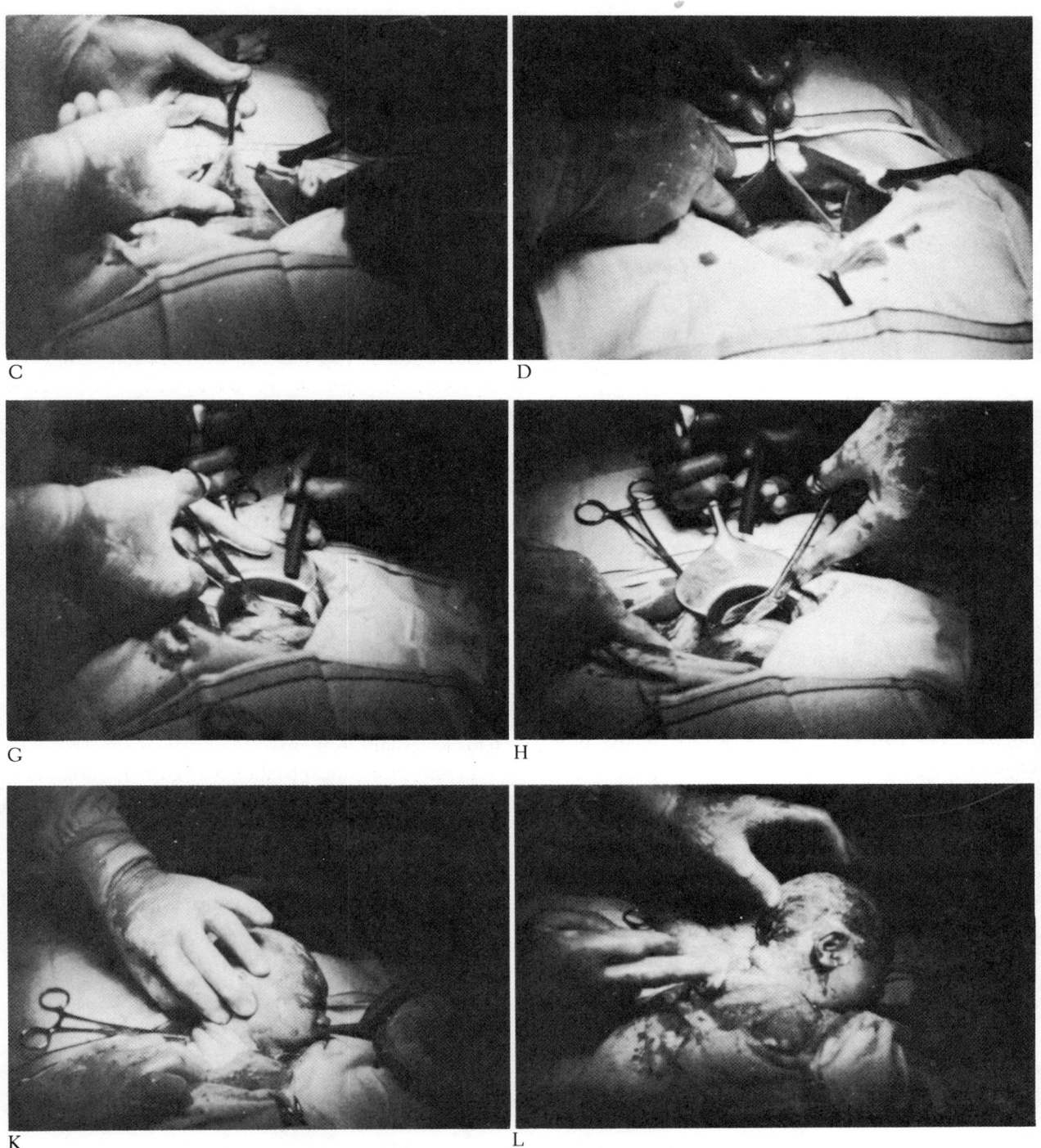

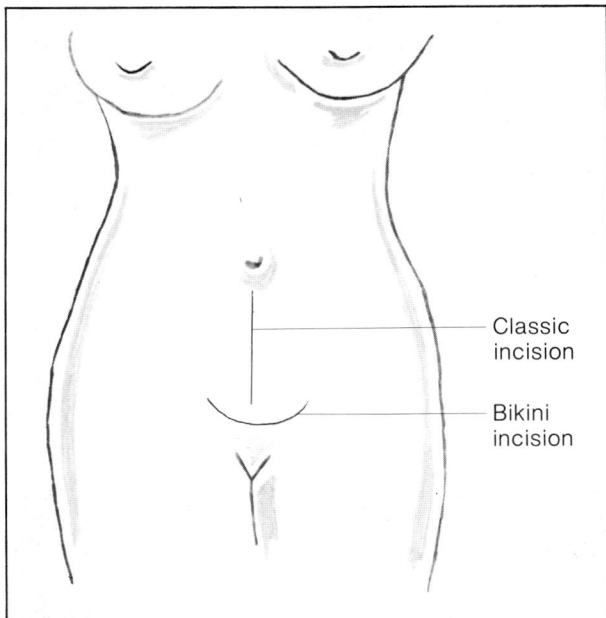

Fig. 35-11. Placement of cesarean section incisions.

able. Check for bobby pins, hairclips, dentures, and contact lenses. Remove bright red polish from at least one finger on each hand so that the anesthesiologist can use fingernail blanching as an aid to assessing oxygenation.

A further permission form may be required for the procedure. Whether or not the woman receives preoperative medication will depend on the amount and type of analgesic she has received during labor. Most anesthesiologists like women to have an oral dose of an antacid prior to general anesthesia to reduce the acidity of stomach contents if the woman should aspirate with anesthesia. Reduced acidity will decrease the insult to lung tissue.

Aftercare of the woman is like that of any surgical patient. She may breast-feed if she wishes. There may be temporary difficulty with breast-feeding because her oral intake will be restricted for the first two days. Cesarean section by itself, however, is not a contraindication to breast-feeding. The woman can expect to have her hospital stay extended to eight to ten days (rather than the usual three to four days) to ensure proper healing of the incision. Postpartal care is described in Chap. 36.

It is important for women to understand what is happening to them when a cesarean section is planned and why they are having it done. The section can be carried out under a spinal anesthetic, so that the woman is every bit as awake for the birth of her baby as she would be if she delivered vaginally. If the cesarean section is being done because of a maternal problem (contracted pelvis, placenta previa, uterine dysfunction), it is important in terms of a postpartal mother-child relationship that she understand the reason. If she feels the operation is necessary because something is wrong with the child, she may later view the child as less than perfect. "Your pelvis is too small to let the baby pass" may not seem very different from "The baby's head is too big to pass through your pelvis," but the differing effects such statements have on a woman's postpartal attitude warrant such careful distinctions in wording. Husbands can watch cesarean sections and can be very supportive people in a delivery room with cesarean sections as well as with vaginal deliveries.

Induction of Labor

Inducing labor is attempting to initiate it (1) before the time when it would have occurred spontaneously because the fetus is in danger or (2) because it does not occur spontaneously, and the fetus appears to be at term. The primary reasons for inducing labor are the presence of preeclampsia, eclampsia, severe hypertension or diabetes, premature rupture of the membranes, and postmaturity (when it seems risky for the fetus to remain in utero).

Before induction of labor is begun, the following conditions must be present: The fetus is in a longitudinal lie and at a point of extrauterine viability; the cervix is ripe, or ready for delivery; a presenting part is engaged; and there is no cephalopelvic disproportion.

To determine whether a cervix is ripe, Bishop [2] has devised a method of scoring certain criteria for ripeness (Table 35-2). If a woman's total score is 9 or above on the items in Table 35-2, the cervix is considered ripe and should respond to induction.

INDUCTION OF LABOR BY OXYTOCIN

Induction is begun by the administration of a dilute intravenous form of oxytocin such as Pitocin or Syntocinon. The drug is used in the proportion of approximately 10 international units (I.U.) in 1,000 ml of normal saline. Since 10 I.U. of oxytocin is the same as 10,000 *milliunits* (mU), each milliliter of this solution will contain 10 *milliunits* of oxytocin; each 0.1 ml contains 1 milliunit. Physicians' orders for administration of oxytocin for induction generally designate the number of *milliunits* to be administered per minute. The oxytocin solution must be "piggybacked" with a maintenance intravenous solution such as 5% dextrose and water; then if the oxytocin needs to be turned off abruptly during the induction, the intrave-

Table 35-2. Scoring of Cervix for Readiness for Elective Induction

Factor	Score			
	0	1	2	3
Dilatation (in cm)	0	1–2	3–4	5–6
Effacement (%)	0–30	40–50	60–70	80
Station	−3	−2	−1 to 0	+1 to +2
Consistency	Firm	Medium	Soft	—
Position	Posterior	Mid	Anterior	—

Source. E. Bishop, Pelvic scoring for elective induction. *Obstet. Gynecol.* 24:266, 1964.

nous line will not be lost. A minidrip regulator and a constant infusion pump are helpful to control the small amount of fluid given.

Infusions are usually begun at a rate of 1 or 2 milliunits per minute. If there is no response from this, the infusion is gradually increased in amount every 15 to 30 minutes by small increments of 2 to 4 mU until contractions do begin. The rate should not be increased over 16 mU per minute without checking for further instructions. Such a rapid rate is very apt to cause tetanic contractions.

Both fetal heart sounds and uterine contractions should be continuously monitored during the procedure. The woman's pulse and blood pressure and the fetal heart rate should be taken every 15 minutes. An infusion pump that ensures a uniform infusion rate should be used with oxytocin administration, to prevent changes in the woman's position from affecting the rate. When cervical dilatation reaches 4 cm, artificial rupture of the membranes will further induce labor.

Formerly, synthetic hormone tablets were administered sublingually or held next to the buccal membrane in the mouth. However, administration of the drug could not be stopped as quickly as it can by the intravenous route, and that was a disadvantage when a problem such as uterine spasm occurred. For this reason, induction of labor is done only by the intravenous route today. A physician should be immediately available during the entire procedure to ensure safety.

Women who are having labor induced should never be left alone. Excessive stimulation of the uterus by oxytocin may lead to tonic uterine contractions, with fetal death or, in extreme instances, rupture of the uterus. Contractions should occur no more often than every 2 minutes, should not be over 50 mm Hg pressure, and should last no more than 60 seconds. The resting pressure between contractions should not exceed 15 mm Hg by monitor. If contractions become more frequent or longer in duration than these safe limits or signs of fetal distress occur, stop the intravenous infusion and seek help. It is better for contractions to slow from a period of inadequate oxytocin administration because you stopped the infusion unnecessarily than for tonic contractions to continue because you are unsure of whether to proceed. Oxytocin has a very short half-life (3 to 5 minutes) so stopping the flow rate almost immediately stops the oxytocin effect.

Women have heard many scare stories about induction of labor. They have been told that it is more painful, "so different" from normal labor that breathing exercises are worthless with it, goes very fast and so is harmful to the fetus, or goes very slowly and therefore is harmful to the fetus. Induced labors tend to have a slightly shorter first stage than the average unassisted labor. This is an advantage to the woman, however, not a disadvantage. Once contractions begin by this method, they are basically normal uterine contractions. The woman needs to be assured of their normality so that she does not fight them, become unnecessarily tense, and then be unable to use her breathing techniques effectively.

Because oxytocin has an antidiuretic effect, there will be a decreased urine flow during its administration. This may result in water intoxication in the woman. Water intoxication is first manifested by headache and vomiting. If these danger signals are observed in the woman during induction of labor, they should be reported and the infusion discontinued. Water intoxication in its severest form can lead to convulsions, coma, and death.

Because induction of labor with oxytocin may predispose the newborn to hyperbilirubinemia and jaundice, and because water intoxication in the woman may occur especially if a balanced electrolyte solution is not used, induction is no longer an elective procedure but should be used only when delivery of the infant by induction will be less hazardous than his remaining in utero would have been.

INDUCTION OF LABOR BY PROSTAGLANDINS

Labor may be induced by the use of prostaglandins. Unfortunately, prostaglandins cause nausea and vomiting in most women. This makes induction of labor an uncomfortable procedure and the woman is so ill that she cannot enjoy it. Prostaglandin administration is not a preferable method for induction until it can be refined to eliminate these side effects.

Forceps Delivery

If a woman is unable to push with contractions in the pelvic division of labor, such as after regional anesthesia, forceps application will be necessary to deliver the baby. A fetus in distress can be delivered more quickly by the use of forceps. Forceps are designed to prevent pressure from being exerted on the fetal head. They may be used as the fetal head reaches the perineum to reduce pressure and avoid subdural hemorrhage in the fetus from too much force.

Forceps are steel instruments constructed of two blades that slide together at their shaft to form a handle. Forceps are applied first by one blade being slipped into the woman's vagina next to the fetal head, then the other side is slipped into place. Next, the shafts of the instrument are brought together in the midline to form the handle.

A forceps delivery is an *outlet* procedure when the forceps are applied once the fetal head reaches the perineum. When the fetal head is above this, it is a *midforceps* delivery. Cesarean section today has less risk to the fetus than the use of midforceps, so such a procedure is rarely seen today. Some anesthesia, at least a pudendal block, is necessary for forceps application.

If the obstetrician doing the procedure is teaching a house staff officer or a medical student and so is detailing and explaining the procedure as he works, the mother and father may become frightened at hearing that blades are being slipped past their baby's head. Listen for this kind of exchange and alleviate worries by explaining terms.

Fig. 35-12. Abnormal placental formations. (From Clinical Education Aid, No. 12, Ross Laboratories, Columbus, Ohio, 1963.)

Vacuum Extraction

A fetus may be delivered by means of a vacuum extractor in place of forceps. With the fetal head at the perineum, a metal cup is pressed against the fetal scalp. When vacuum pressure is applied, air beneath the cup is sucked out and the cup then adheres so tightly to the fetal scalp that traction on the cord leading to the cup will deliver the fetus.

Infants delivered this way typically have a marked area of pressure at the location of the vacuum cup. A mother may need to be assured that this swelling will decrease rapidly and is harmless.

Anomalies of the Placenta and Cord

The placenta and cord are always examined in the delivery room to ascertain whether any abnormalities are present.

The normal placenta weighs about 500 gm and is 15 to 20 cm in diameter and 1.5 to 3.0 cm thick. Its weight is about one-sixth that of the child. A placenta may be unusually enlarged in women with diabetes. In certain diseases, such as syphilis or erythroblastosis, the placenta may be so large that it weighs half as much as the fetus.

PLACENTA SUCCENTURIATA

A succenturiate placenta (Fig. 35-12) has one or more accessory lobes connected to the main placenta by blood vessels. No fetal abnormality is associated with it. However, it is important that it be recognized, because the small lobes may be retained in the uterus at delivery, leading to severe maternal hemorrhage. On inspection, the placenta will appear torn at the edge, or torn blood vessels may extend beyond the edge of the placenta. The remaining lobes must be removed

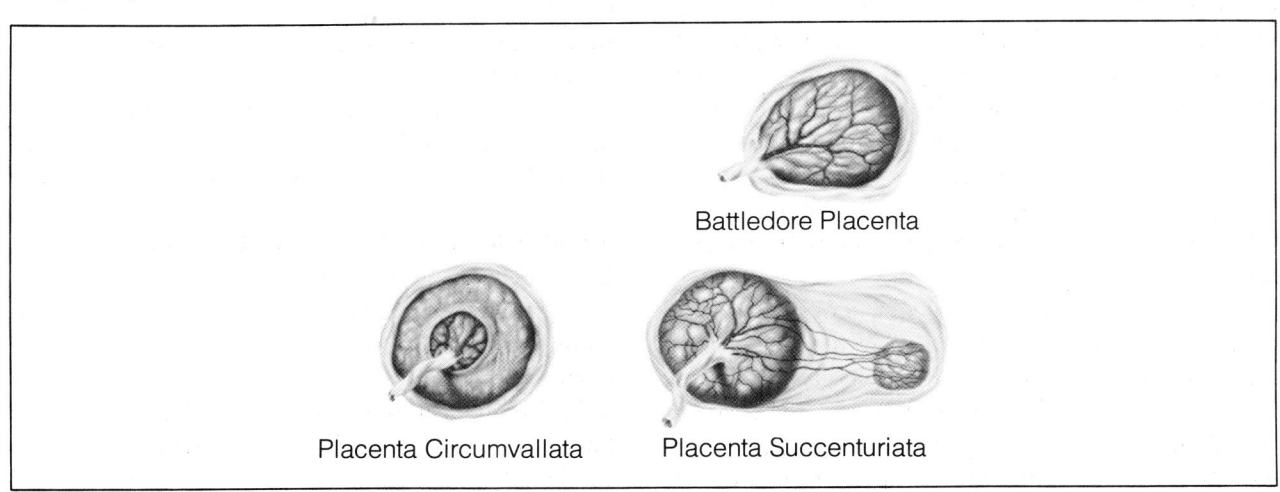

from the uterus manually to prevent hemorrhage in the mother.

PLACENTA CIRCUMVALLATA
Ordinarily, the chorion membrane begins at the edge of the placenta to envelop the fetus; no chorion covers the fetal side of the placenta. In placenta circumvallata, the fetal side of the placenta is covered to some extent with chorion (Fig. 35-12). The umbilical cord enters the placenta at the usual midpoint, and large vessels spread out from there. They end abruptly at the point where the chorion folds back onto the surface, however. (In *placenta marginata*, the fold of chorion reaches just to the edge of the placenta.) Although, again, no abnormalities are associated with this type of placenta, its presence should be noted.

BATTLEDORE PLACENTA
In a battledore placenta, the cord is inserted marginally rather than centrally (Fig. 35-12). This anomaly is rare and has no known clinical significance.

VELAMENTOUS INSERTION OF THE CORD
This is a situation in which the cord, instead of entering the placenta directly, separates into small vessels that reach the placenta by spreading across a fold of amnion. This form of cord insertion is often found with multiple pregnancy. It can lead to exsanguination of the fetus if these cord vessels are torn when the membranes rupture.

PLACENTA ACCRETA
Placenta accreta is unusually deep attachment of the placenta to the uterine myometrium. The placenta will not loosen and deliver; attempts to remove it manually may lead to extreme hemorrhage because of the deep myometrium attachment.

Problem-oriented Recording: Progress Notes

Angie Baco
Labor and delivery admission note

Problem: Gestational diabetes

> S. Awoke with labor contractions this morning. Called M.D. and told to take no insulin; report to hospital instead. Routinely takes 10 units NPH and 4 units regular daily. Concerned now because it is about an hour past her usual time of injection. Had a negative nonstress test 2 days ago; asking if 38 weeks gestation has been long enough that baby will not be harmed. Husband with her. Asked if fetal monitor will reveal whether fetus has a heart defect or not. (Previous child had congenital heart disease.)
> O. Urine 2+, neg. FHR:130. Contractions: 30 second-duration; 30-minute frequency; intensity, 30–45 mm Hg on monitor.
> A. Gestational diabetic becoming concerned about well-being of infant due to 38-week gestation and previous child with CHD. No insulin taken today.
>
> Goals: a. Deliver vaginally
> b. Fetal heart tones to remain within normal limits by monitor.
> c. Insulin-glucose levels to be maintained by continuous insulin infusion.
> d. Blood sugars to be monitored q2h and to be within normal limits.
>
> P. 1. Explain purpose of monitors (external until membranes are ruptured, then internal).
> 2. Explain purpose of intravenous infusion and balance of glucose and insulin.
> 3. Maintain NPO.
> 4. Fasting blood sugar drawn. Repeat q2h.
> 5. Catheter inserted for urine testing q2h.
> 6. Schedule pelvimetry by x-ray for cephalopelvic disproportion.

Labor and delivery 4-hour assessment note

Problem: Gestational diabetes

> S. Asking if blood sugar is all right. A friend told her that if her baby was going to die, this is the time (in labor) that it would happen. Very apprehensive of any change in sound of fetal monitor. Asking for something to eat.
> O. Internal monitor inserted. FHR baseline 120–130; beat-to-beat variability 5–10 bpm. Contractions still minimal: 30–45 mm Hg by monitor; duration, 30 seconds; frequency, 20 minutes.
> Urines, neg., neg.
> Continuous IV infusion of regular insulin and normal saline infusing at 2 minigtt/min

by IVAC. Second IV of 5% dextrose in Ringer's lactate infusing at 30 gtt/min.
Blood sugars: Fasting, 100. 2h, 92.
Pelvimetry report: No difficulty with vaginal delivery expected.

A. Woman growing increasingly concerned as labor progresses because of well-meant but unfortunate remark of friend.
P. 1. Continue to reassure that fetal heart tones are good.
   2. Continue IV infusion; blood sugars and urine testing q2h per routine.
   3. Explain reason for NPO as glucose solution is infusing.

Labor and delivery 6-hour assessment note

Problem: Gestational diabetes

S. Both parents growing discouraged with labor progress. Happy to hear that oxytocin assist will be started to strengthen contractions.
O. Both parents are watching monitor patterns carefully; noticeably apprehensive.
A. Woman with gestational diabetes in need of oxytocin assist to augment labor.
P. 1. Explain all new equipment used with both parents.
   2. Syntocinon IV (10,000 mU in 1,000 ml 0.9 saline) begun at 12 minigtt per minute (2 mU per minute) piggybacked to existing IV.
   3. Internal fetal and uterine monitors in place.
   4. FHR, BP, pulse, and respirations to be taken every 15 minutes.
   5. Duration, frequency, and strength of contractions to be taken every 15 minutes.
   6. Oxytocin infusion to be advanced in 2 mU per minute increments (up to 16 mU per minute) until contractions reach 60-second duration, 2-minute frequency.
   7. Oxytocin to be discontinued and M.D. notified if FHR is above 160 or below 120, baseline variability is under 5 bpm, or decelerations occur; if contractions are longer than 60 seconds, resting pressure of contractions is over 15 mm Hg, or frequency is less than 2 minutes; if general apprehension, confusion, or headache present.

References

1. Beard, R. W. Controlling and quantifying uterine activity. *Contemp. Obstet. Gynecol.* 13:75, 1979.
2. Bishop, E. Pelvic scoring for elective induction. *Obstet. Gynecol.* 24:266, 1964.
3. Cranley, M. S. Fetal and maternal monitoring: Corrine, a mother at risk. *Am. J. Nurs.* 78:2117, 1978.
4. Edwards, M. S. Venereal herpes: A nursing overview. *J.O.G.N. Nurs.* 7:7, 1978.
5. Frazer, E. B. The work of a multigravida on becoming the mother of twins. *Matern. Child. Nurs. J.* 6:87, 1977.
6. Friedman, E. A., et al. Station of the fetal presenting part. Arrest of descent in multiparas. *Obstet. Gynecol.* 47:129, 1976.
7. Heffron, C. H., et al. Abnormal labor: Diagnosis and management. *Perinatal Care* 2:14, 1978.
8. Howie, P. Induction of labour: Does it save babies? *Nurs. Mirror* 146:21, 1978.
9. Hugh, A., et al. Monitoring fetal arterial oxygen continually during labor. *Contemp. Obstet. Gynecol.* 12:73, 1978.
10. Ishida, Y. How to deal with grief in childbirth. *Female Patient* 5:74, 1980.
11. Jennings, B. Emergency delivery. How to attend to one safely. *M.C.N.* 4:148, 1979.
12. Marks, R. G. New hope in herpes genitalis? *Curr. Prescribing* 5:27, 1979.
13. Marut, J. S. The special needs of the cesarean mother. *M.C.N.* 3:202, 1978.
14. Quilligan, E. J. Identifying true fetal distress. *Contemp. Obstet. Gynecol.* 13:89, 1979.
15. Schlosser, S. The emergency C-section patient. Why she needs help . . . what you can do. *R.N.* 41:52, 1978.
16. Stichler, J. F., and Affonso, D. D. Cesarean birth. *Am. J. Nurs.* 80:466, 1980.
17. Taylor, R. W. Induction of labor. *Nurs. Mirror* 141:58, 1976.
18. Webster, D. M. Childbirth in the technological age: The mother's emotional needs. *Nurs. Mirror* 140:55, 1975.
19. Wimberley, D. When a woman is diabetic: Intrapartal care. *Am. J. Nurs.* 79:451, 1979.
20. Yunek, M. J., et al. Fetal and maternal monitoring: Intrapartal fetal monitoring. *Am. J. Nurs.* 78:2102, 1978.

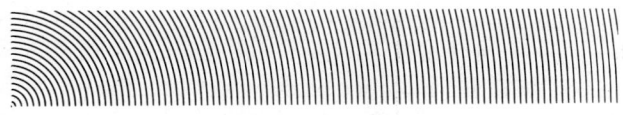

36. Deviations from the Normal During the Puerperium: Nursing Interventions

The majority of complications of the puerperium are preventable, a concept you should keep in mind when working with postpartal women. Complications submit the woman to an experience that can be frightening and painful—and might leave her afraid of or physically incapable of bearing more children—and are avoidable.

Hemorrhage

Hemorrhage, the leading cause of maternal mortality associated with childbearing, is a possibility all through pregnancy, but it is a major danger in the immediate postpartal period. In a normal delivery, the average blood loss is 300 to 350 ml. Postpartal hemorrhage is defined as any blood loss from the uterus greater than 500 ml within a 24-hour period. Hemorrhage may be either immediate, that is, occurring in the first 24 hours, or late, occurring during the remaining days of the six-week puerperium. The greatest danger of bleeding is in the first 24 hours because of the grossly denuded and unprotected area left after detachment of the placenta.

MAIN CAUSES OF BLEEDING

There are four main reasons for postpartal hemorrhage: uterine atony, lacerations, retained placental fragments, and disseminated intravascular coagulation.

Uterine Atony

Uterine atony is the most frequent cause of postpartal hemorrhage. As pointed out in the discussion of involutional changes (Chap. 25), the uterus must remain in a contracted state after delivery if the open vessels at the placental site are to be sealed. Several factors predispose to poor uterine tone and an inability to maintain a contracted state: multiple pregnancy, hydramnios (excessive amount of amniotic fluid), large baby (over 9 pounds), operative delivery, placenta previa, premature separation of the placenta, deep anesthesia, and prolonged and difficult labor. When you are caring for a patient in whom any of these conditions were present be especially cautious in your immediate observations and on guard for signs of uterine bleeding.

ASSESSMENT OF BLOOD LOSS. If the uterus suddenly relaxes, there will be an abrupt gush of blood from the placental site, with vaginal bleeding and symptoms of shock and blood loss. With uterine atony, it is more common for the uterus to become uncontracted gradually, so that the bleeding that is seen from the vagina is seepage, not a gush of blood. Over a period of hours, however, this seepage can result in a condition as lethal as a sudden release of blood.

It is difficult to estimate the amount of blood loss in the postpartal period, because it is difficult to estimate the amount of blood it takes to saturate a perineal pad; the figure is somewhere between 25 and 50 ml. By counting the perineal pads saturated in given lengths of time, say half-hour intervals, you can form a rough estimate of blood loss. Five pads saturated in half an hour is obviously a different situation from five pads saturated in 8 hours. However, in either situation, the woman will have lost upward of 250 ml of blood in that time interval; if either rate of flow is allowed to continue untended, she will be in grave danger. Be sure you differentiate between *saturated* and *used* when counting pads; *used* in this context is meaningless. Weighing perineal pads before and after use and subtracting the difference is an accurate way to measure vaginal discharge. Whether the woman is losing blood rapidly or slowly, always ask a woman to turn on her side when estimating blood loss so you can be certain that large amounts are not pooling underneath her.

Palpating the fundus at frequent intervals in the postpartal hours to ascertain that the uterus is remaining in a state of contraction is the best preventive measure against immediate hemorrhage. Frequent checks of lochia and vital signs, particularly of pulse and blood pressure, are equally important. If you reach to massage a fundus and are unsure you have located it, the uterus is probably in a state of relaxation. Under normal circumstances, a well-contracted uterus is firm and easily recognized and feels like no other abdominal structure.

INTERVENTIONS. The first step in controlling hemorrhage in the event of uterine atony is to attempt uterine massage to encourage contraction. Place one hand on the woman's symphysis pubis to give good support to the base of the uterus, then grasp the fundus of the uterus with your other hand and massage gently. Unless the uterus is extremely lacking in tone, massage is usually effective in causing contraction, and after a few seconds the uterus will assume its healthy grapefruit-like feel.

However, the fact that the uterus responds well to massage does not mean the problem is solved. A few minutes after you remove your hand from the fundus, the uterus may relax, and the lethal seepage may begin again. You must therefore stay continuously with the patient for at least an hour following massage and observe her closely for the next 4 hours.

A full bladder pushes an uncontracted uterus into an even more uncontracted state. Offer a bedpan at least every 4 hours to keep the woman's bladder empty. In order to reduce bladder pressure, the physician may order insertion of a urinary catheter.

If the uterus does not remain contracted, the physician will invariably order oxytocin to be begun by intravenous infusion to help the uterus maintain tone. Oxytocins must be kept readily available on a postpartal unit for instant use in the event of postpartal hemorrhage.

Not only must vital signs be taken frequently during the immediate postpartal period; they must also be interpreted intelligently. The pulse rate may increase only a point or so at each recording; if you do not look at the entire picture, you will miss the fact that, although the pulse is rising slowly, it is rising *continually*. In the event of slow bleeding, the circulatory system compensates for a long time, and as a result there is little change in pulse and blood pressure at first. Suddenly the system can compensate no more, and the pulse rate rises rapidly. The pulse becomes weak and thready, and the blood pressure drops abruptly. The woman becomes cold and clammy and shows obvious signs of shock. If you are taking frequent vital signs and are carefully monitoring lochia flow, you should be able to detect blood loss before this point is ever reached.

You can anticipate that any woman who has had a blood loss over 500 ml may have blood replaced. Check to be certain that blood has been drawn for a cross matching, so that blood of her specific type can be made ready. Be sure that your hands are not tied by hospital policies on ordering blood for replacement. Hemorrhaging women need replacement, and you should have the authority to request that cross-matching and blood-readying procedures be started. If the necessary forms require the physician's signature, valuable time will be lost if you must wait for the physician to come to the hospital.

Any woman is exhausted after delivery. If the woman hemorrhaged in the immediate postpartal period, she feels even more exhausted. The last thing she wants is someone pushing a hand into her abdomen to check her uterus or tightening a blood pressure cuff on her arm every 15 minutes. She will become either aggravated or worried by the attention. As she looks around the recovery room and sees that she is the only one receiving this concentrated attention for such a long period of time, she will become more and more frightened. You need to explain that the measures you are taking at this point, although disturbing, are just insurance measures. Make the recordings as quickly and gently as possible, so that the woman has a minimum of discomfort and time to nap between observations.

If uterine massage and intravenous oxytocin are not effective in stopping uterine bleeding, the physician may attempt the further step of bimanual compression (one hand inserted in the vagina, the other pushing against the fundus through the abdominal wall). It may be necessary to return the woman to the delivery room, so that the physician can explore her uterine cavity manually for retained placental fragments that may be preventing good contraction.

Bimanual compression is effective in halting bleeding in all but the extremely atonic uterus. In this rare instance, a hysterectomy may have to be performed. Appreciate the fact that this measure is carried out as a last resort only. Despite the emergency conditions, try to comfort and give support to the woman and her husband at this time. This is a totally unexpected outcome of childbearing for them.

Following hysterectomy, the woman will usually want to talk about what happened, why surgery was necessary, and how she feels now that she can no longer bear children. She needs to discuss her feelings with a person who will listen quietly and help her sort through her "why me?" feelings. She usually has ambiguous feelings because she wanted more children, and yet she also wanted to live. She is grateful to her physician and the hospital personnel for saving her life, but she may feel resentful that you were not skilled enough to leave her capable of future childbearing. She may grieve (very genuinely) for the children that will not be born.

Open lines of communication between the couple and the hospital staff, so that the family can vent its feelings, will be most helpful to the couple in this crisis.

Lacerations

Small lacerations of the birth canal are so common they can be considered a normal consequence of childbearing. Lacerations occur most often with difficult or precipitate deliveries. Any time the uterus is firm following delivery and yet bleeding persists, a laceration of the cervix, vagina, or perineum should be suspected.

Lacerations of the cervix are usually found on the sides of the cervix near the branches of the uterine artery. The amount of blood loss is usually great, and the blood will be brighter red than the venous blood in bleeding from uterine atony because it is arterial bleeding. The force of the blood is such that it often gushes from the vaginal opening. Fortunately, this bleeding occurs ordinarily immediately following delivery of the placenta, when the mother is still on the delivery table and the physician is still in attendance.

Repairs of cervical lacerations are difficult because the bleeding is so intense it obstructs visualization of the area. Be certain the physician has adequate space to work and adequate sponges and suture supplies. The woman is not always aware of what is happening, but she picks up the feeling tone in the room that something is seriously wrong. Try to maintain an air of calmness and, if possible, stand beside the woman at the head of the table. She may be worried that the extra activity in the room has something to do with her baby. She needs to be assured that the baby is fine. The problem is with the opening from her uterus, and she will "need to stay in the delivery room a little longer than expected while the doctor places additional sutures."

If the laceration appears to be extensive or difficult to repair, the physician may order a general anesthetic for relaxation of the uterine area and to prevent pain.

More rarely, lacerations occur in the vagina. These are easier to diagnose because they are easier to view. Since vaginal tissue is friable, however, they are also hard to repair. Some oozing often follows a repair here, and the vagina may be packed to maintain pressure on the suture line. Be certain that the patient's chart and the nursing plan are both marked to show that the packing is in place. Packing is usually removed after 24 to 48 hours, and it will be the physician's responsibility to remove it. However, by careful recording of the packing's existence and making sure that it is removed, you serve as the patient's first line of defense against infection as packing left in place too long tends to cause stasis and infection.

Lacerations of the perineum usually occur when an episiotomy was not performed, although occasionally they are an extension of the episiotomy. Perineal lacerations are classified into four categories, depending on the extent and depth of the tissue involved. These are shown in Table 36-1.

Perineal lacerations are sutured and treated as an episiotomy repair. It is often difficult to distinguish a repaired perineal laceration from an episiotomy, except that lacerations tend to heal more slowly because the edges of the suture line are ragged. Any woman who has a third- or fourth-degree laceration should not be given enemas, and her temperature should not be taken rectally; the sutures include the rectal sphincter, and the hard tips of equipment could open sutures. To prevent constipation and hard stools that

Table 36-1. Classification of Perineal Lacerations

Classification	Description
First degree	These involve the vaginal mucous membrane and the skin of the perineum to the fourchette
Second degree	These involve the vagina, perineal skin, fascia, levator ani muscle, and perineal body
Third degree	These involve the entire perineum and the external sphincter of the rectum, either partially or completely
Fourth degree	These involve the entire perineum, rectal sphincter, and some of the mucous membrane of the rectum

could break the sutures, she should have a diet high in fluid and is usually given a stool softener for the first week of the puerperium. Make certain that the degree of the laceration is marked on her nursing care plan; ancillary caregivers such as aides have no appreciation of why rectal temperatures are contraindicated unless informed.

Retained Placental Fragments
Occasionally, the placenta does not deliver in its entirety, but fragments of it separate and are left behind. Since the portion retained keeps the uterus from contracting fully, uterine bleeding occurs. This is most likely to happen with a succenturiate placenta, a placenta with an accessory lobe (see Chap. 35), but it can happen in any instance. To detect the complication, placentas should be inspected carefully in the delivery room to see if they are complete.

If a retained fragment is large, the bleeding will be apparent in the immediate postpartal period. If the fragment is small, bleeding may not be detected until the sixth to tenth day post partum, when the mother notices an abrupt discharge of a large amount of blood.

On examination, the uterus is usually found to be not fully contracted. If the bleeding does not appear to be major, the physician may order a pregnancy test, preferably an immunological test, which gives the results in a matter of minutes or hours. If placental tissue is still present in the woman's body, human chorionic gonadotropin will also be present, and even though the woman is no longer pregnant, the test will be positive. Retained placental fragments may be detected by sonogram.

The woman will be given a supportive blood transfusion if necessary, then taken to a delivery room where a dilation and curettage will be performed to remove the offending placental fragment. Because the hemorrhage from retained fragments is often delayed until after women go home, they must be instructed to observe the color of the lochia discharge and report to the physician any tendency for the discharge to change from lochia alba to rubra.

Disseminated Intravascular Coagulation
Disseminated intravascular coagulation, a deficiency in clotting, may occur in any woman in the postpartal period but is usually associated with premature separation of the placenta or missed abortion. It should be suspected when the usual measures to induce uterine contraction fail to stop the flow of blood. Oozing from the intravenous site or difficulty in stopping blood from flowing from a blood-drawing site is highly suggestive that a level of low fibrinogen exists.

A maternity service should maintain a supply of fibrinogen to be used for treatment of this condition. Increasing the woman's supply of fibrinogen usually decreases bleeding dramatically if hypofibrinogenemia is the underlying cause. Heparin may also be used as therapy since it prevents massive clotting and further lowering of the fibrinogen level.

HEMATOMAS
Hematomas following delivery can cause the mother acute discomfort and concern but usually represent only minor bleeding. Hematomas result from injury to blood vessels in the perineum during delivery. They are most likely to happen in rapid spontaneous deliveries and in women who have perineal varicosities. They may occur at the episiotomy repair site or a laceration repair site if a vein is pricked during repair.

Perineal sutures almost always give the postpartal woman some discomfort. When she complains of severe pain in the perineal area or a feeling of pressure between her legs, inspect the perineal area for a hematoma. If a hematoma is present, there will be an area of purplish discoloration and obvious swelling anywhere from 1 inch to as much as 4 inches in diameter.

The physician will usually order ice compresses to be applied to the area and an oral analgesic to relieve the pain. In most instances the ice compresses prevent further bleeding, and the hematoma is absorbed over the next three or four days. If the hematoma is very large when discovered, or continues to grow in size, the woman may have to be returned to the delivery room to have the site incised and the bleeding vessel ligated. Be certain your observations concerning the lesion's size are meaningfully recorded. Describing a hematoma as "large" or "small" gives little information to the nurse relieving you about the hematoma's actual size. Describing the lesion as 5 cm across or the size of a quarter or a half dollar is meaningful since it establishes a basis for comparison.

The mother needs to be reassured that, although the hematoma may give her discomfort, her hospital stay will probably not be lengthened and the hematoma will heal and cause no future difficulty.

VULVAR EDEMA

Some vulvar edema is always present following vaginal delivery from the pressure of the fetal head on the perineum and the stretching of the vagina to accommodate birth. Extensive edema of the vulva has been reported following local or regional anesthesia [3]. This atypical edema occurs on the second postpartal day and rapidly spreads to include not only the vulva, but gluteal and inner pelvic areas as well. Fever is present. The woman may have an elevated white blood count. The edema may become so involved that vascular collapse and death occur. Although the etiology of this edematous process is not understood, massive administration of antibiotics appears to be helpful, suggesting that it has an infectious basis. In any event, close assessment of the vulvar area for edema as well as for hematomas will reveal this condition at its first appearance.

NECESSITY FOR REST

Women who have a postpartal hemorrhage tend to have a postpartal recovery that is slower than average. They feel extremely exhausted and take weeks longer to feel right again. The woman's physician will usually place her on a course of iron therapy to ensure good hemoglobin formation. She will probably have special orders as to the amount of exertion and postpartal exercise she can safely stand. You should discuss with her the possibility of having someone with her at home at least for the first week to help her with housework and the care of her new baby.

Extensive blood loss is one of the precursors of postpartal infection. Any woman who has undergone more than the normal blood loss should be observed closely for changes in lochia discharge, and her temperature should be monitored closely in the postpartal period to detect the earliest signs of developing infection.

POSTPARTAL ANTERIOR PITUITARY NECROSIS

Postpartal anterior pituitary necrosis (also termed *Sheehan's syndrome*) is a rare disorder that may occur in a woman following severe hemorrhage. The pituitary gland appears to have been so damaged by the abrupt hypovolemia that it now does not function adequately. This is revealed by signs of decreased or absent lactation, genital and breast atrophy, and loss of pubic and axillary hair; myxedema or symptoms of thyroid dysfunction may result.

The woman needs hormone therapy to replace hormones that her body now has difficulty producing, most noticeably estrogen, cortisone, and thyroid. Because of decreased stimulation to the ovaries, the woman may be infertile or sterile following this pituitary insult.

Puerperal Infection

Hemorrhage is the leading cause of maternal mortality associated with childbearing. Infection is the second most common cause.

The factors that predispose to infection in the postpartal period are as follows:

1. Prolonged rupture of the membranes (bacteria may have started to invade the uterus while the fetus was still in utero).
2. Placental fragments that have been retained within the uterus (the tissue necroses and serves as an excellent bed for bacterial growth).
3. Postpartal hemorrhage (the woman's general condition is weakened).
4. Preexisting anemia (the body's defense against infection is lowered).
5. Prolonged and difficult labor, particularly instrument deliveries (trauma to the tissue may leave lacerations or fissures or easy portals of entry for infection).

The white blood count of a postpartal woman is normally increased to 20,000 to 30,000 per cubic millimeter. Thus, this conventional method of detecting infection is not of great value in the puerperium. An increase in oral temperature above 100.4°F (38.0°C) for two consecutive 24-hour periods excluding the first 24-hour period following birth is defined by the Joint Committee on Maternal Welfare as a febrile condition suggesting infection. All women with temperatures within this range should be suspected of having a postpartal infection until it is proved otherwise.

INVADING ORGANISMS

Because the uterus is a closed vesicle, anaerobic organisms may grow within its denuded folds. Most postpartal infections are caused by invading anaerobic streptococci, although anaerobic staphylococci infections are becoming more and more common.

Some bacteria, such as anaerobic streptococci, are normal inhabitants of the birth canal. Ordinarily, they are nonpathogenic and give no evidence of their presence. In the face of traumatized, devitalized tissue, however, such as might be present following a difficult delivery, they become pathogenic, invade the tissue, and lead to infection.

Some bacteria are transferred to the woman as a result of nasopharyngeal infection in hospital personnel. All persons in the delivery room should be masked (nose and mouth). Any articles (gloves, instruments, and so on) introduced into the birth canal during labor, delivery, and the postpartal period must be sterile. The woman must be given good instruction in perineal care, so that she does not bring *Escherichia coli* organisms forward from the rectum. When you are giving perineal care, be certain to wash your hands before the procedure and do not open the labia, permitting contaminated water to enter the vagina. Each maternity patient should have her own bedpan and perineal supplies to prevent transfer of pathogens from one woman to another. Equipment that is used by many women (e.g., bathtubs, heat lamps) must be cleaned between patients.

TYPES OF INFECTION

The extent and severity of postpartal infection depends on the virulence of the invading organism, the ability of the host to resist the invasion, and the portal of entry of the organism.

Infection of the Perineum

Because there is usually a suture line in the perineum from an episiotomy or a laceration repair, there is a ready portal of entry here for bacterial invasion. Infections of the perineum generally remain localized and so manifest the symptoms of any suture line infection: pain, heat, and a feeling of pressure. The woman may or may not have an elevated temperature. Inspection of the suture line reveals inflammation. One or two stitches may be sloughed away, or an area of the suture line may be open, with pus present.

The woman's physician will usually treat the infection by culturing the discharge and removing the perineal sutures in order to open the area for drainage. An antibiotic will be ordered, along with an analgesic for discomfort. Sitz baths or warm compresses may be ordered to hasten drainage and cleanse the area. The perineal pads must be changed frequently, since they are contaminated by seropurulent drainage. If left in place for long periods of time, they might cause vaginal contamination. The woman should be instructed to wash her hands well after handling perineal pads.

Local infections of this nature (if extensive) may lengthen the woman's hospital stay by approximately a week, because the incision site, once opened, must heal by secondary rather than primary intention. These infections are annoying and painful to the mother. Fortunately, with the use of improved techniques during parturition and the puerperium, perineal infections are not seen as commonly as they used to be.

Endometritis

Endometritis is an infection of the endometrium, the lining of the uterus. Bacteria gain access to the uterus through the vagina either at the time of delivery or during the postpartal period. Endometritis usually manifests itself on the third or fourth day of the puerperium, suggesting that a great deal of the invasion occurs during labor or delivery.

As a rule, the mother demonstrates a rise in temperature. A temperature on the third or fourth day post partum coincides with the days that breast milk comes in. Do not be led astray by the old wives' tale of "milk fever." Fever on the third or fourth day post partum should be considered possible endometritis until proved otherwise.

Depending on the severity of the infection, the woman may have chills, loss of appetite, and general malaise. Most women experience some abdominal tenderness. The uterus is generally not well contracted and is painful to the touch. The mother may have strong afterpains. Lochia will usually be dark brown in color and have a foul odor. It may be increased in amount because of poor uterine contraction, but if the infection is accompanied by high fever, lochia may be scant or absent.

Treatment of endometritis consists of the administration of an appropriate antibiotic determined by culture of the lochia, accompanied by an oxytocic agent to encourage uterine contraction. The woman requires additional fluid to combat the fever. If strong afterpains and abdominal discomfort are present, she needs an analgesic for relief.

Fowler's position is the best position for the woman with endometritis because it encourages lochia drainage and prevents pooling of infected fluid. Both you and the woman must use good hand-washing techniques after handling perineal pads because the pads contain contaminated discharge.

The physician may ask that the woman be isolated

from other patients to reduce the chances that others will contract the infection.

As with any infection, endometritis can be contained best if it is discovered early in the disease process. If you can intelligently interpret the color, quantity, and odor of lochia discharge, and the size, consistency, and tenderness of a postpartal uterus in connection with an increased temperature, you may be the first person to recognize that disease is present.

If the infection is limited to the endometrium, the course of infection will be 7 to 10 days. The mother may have to make arrangements for her baby's discharge prior to her own, since her hospital stay will be extended about two weeks.

Thrombophlebitis

Phlebitis is inflammation of the lining of a blood vessel; thrombophlebitis is inflammation of the lining of a blood vessel with the formation of blood clots. Thrombophlebitis usually occurs in the postpartal period as an extension of an endometrial infection.

Thrombophlebitis is of two types: (1) pelvic thrombophlebitis, in which the ovarian, uterine, and hypogastric veins are involved, and (2) femoral thrombophlebitis, in which the femoral, saphenous, or popliteal veins are involved. An older term for the latter type of involvement is *milk leg* or *phlegmasia alba dolens* (white inflammation).

FEMORAL THROMBOPHLEBITIS. The infection site in thrombophlebitis is in a vein, but an accompanying arterial spasm diminishes arterial circulation to the legs as well. The decreased circulation along with edema, gives the leg a white or drained appearance. As the woman's temperature rises because of the infection, her supply of breast milk tends to decrease as the body attempts to save fluid. It was formerly believed that breast milk was going into the leg, giving it its white appearance (milk leg).

As with the other complications of the postpartal period, thrombophlebitis is largely preventable. Prevention of endometritis by utilization of good aseptic technique prevents thrombophlebitis as well. Early ambulation encourages circulation in the lower extremities and decreases clot formation.

Femoral thrombophlebitis is manifested on about the tenth day after delivery by an elevated temperature, chills, and stiffness, pain, and redness in the affected part. The leg begins to swell below the lesion, since venous circulation is blocked. The skin becomes stretched to a point of shiny whiteness. Homans' sign (pain in the calf on dorsiflexion of the foot) will be positive.

Treatment consists of bed rest with the affected leg elevated. Women who have been discharged from the hospital will need to return so that strict bed rest can be enforced. A cradle should be used to keep the pressure of the bedclothes off the affected leg, both to decrease the sensitivity of the leg and to improve the circulation. The pain is usually severe enough to require administration of analgesics. An appropriate antibiotic and often an anticoagulant (Dicumarol or heparin) will be ordered to prevent further formation of clots. The mother will have daily prothrombin or clotting level determinations before administration of the anticoagulant each day. Lochia will usually increase in amount in the woman who is receiving an anticoagulant. Be sure to keep a meaningful record of the amount of this discharge so it can be estimated. "Lochia serosa with scattered pinpoint clots; three perineal pads saturated in 8 hours" is far more meaningful than "large amount of lochia." Weighing perineal pads before and after use and subtracting the difference is an accurate way to determine the amount of vaginal bleeding.

The Dicumarol anticoagulants are passed in breast milk, so the mother will have to discontinue breast-feeding during a course of therapy with these. If the infection does not seem to be severe and the mother wants to reinstate breast-feeding after the course of anticoagulant (about 10 days), her breast milk should be expressed manually at the time of normal feedings to maintain a good milk supply.

Aspirin (acetylsalicylic acid) tends to increase coagulation time in some women. Thus, the mother should not be given both aspirin and anticoagulants in conjunction. Make it your responsibility to check the orders to be certain aspirin is not listed as the woman's analgesic.

Legs with a phlebitis or thrombophlebitis should never be rubbed or massaged or the clot may move and become a pulmonary embolus, a possibly fatal complication.

With proper treatment, the acute symptoms of femoral thrombophlebitis last only a few days, but the full course of the disease takes four to six weeks before it is resolved. The affected leg may never return to its former size and may always cause discomfort after long periods of standing.

PELVIC THROMBOPHLEBITIS. Pelvic thrombophlebitis occurs later than femoral thrombophlebitis, often around the fourteenth or fifteenth day of the puerperium. The woman is suddenly extremely ill, with a high fever, chills, and general malaise.

If she has been discharged from the hospital, she

must be readmitted as with femoral thrombophlebitis, for total bed rest and will be treated with antibiotics and anticoagulants. Because major veins are involved in this disease, the infection can become systemic and result in a lung, kidney, or heart valve abscess.

The disease runs a long course of six to eight weeks and, if an abscess forms, may have a fatal outcome.

Peritonitis

Again, peritonitis is usually an extension of endometritis. It is one of the gravest complications of childbearing and accounts for a third of all deaths from puerperal infection. The infection spreads through the lymphatic system or directly through the fallopian tubes or uterine wall to the peritoneal cavity.

The symptoms are the same as those of the surgical patient in whom a peritoneal infection develops: abdominal pain, high fever, rigid abdomen, rapid pulse, vomiting, and the appearance of being acutely ill. The woman will need intravenous fluid while she is unable to take food orally because of intestinal paralysis. She will be placed on large doses of antibiotics. Her hospital stay will be lengthy, and her prognosis is guarded.

Mastitis

Mastitis (infection of the breast) may occur as early as the seventh postpartal day but may not occur until the baby is weeks or months old.

The organism causing the infection usually enters through cracked and fissured nipples. Thus, the measures that prevent cracked and fissured nipples also prevent mastitis. These include not leaving the baby too long at the breast, making certain the baby grasps the nipple properly, releasing the baby's grasp on the nipple before removing the baby from a breast, and washing hands between handling perineal pads and breasts.

Occasionally, the organism that causes the infection comes from the nasal-oral cavity of the infant. In these instances the infant has usually acquired a staphylococcal or streptococcal infection while in the hospital nursery. Sucking on the nipple, the infant introduces the organisms into the milk ducts, where they proliferate (milk is an excellent medium for bacterial growth). This is an epidemic breast abscess; it is usually found that several mothers discharged from the hospital at the same time have like infections.

Mastitis usually occurs unilaterally, although epidemic mastitis (because it originates with the infant) may be bilateral. The affected breast shows localized pain, swelling, and redness. Fever accompanies the first symptoms within a matter of hours, and breast milk becomes scant.

The mother will be placed on a broad-spectrum antibiotic. Breast-feeding is usually discontinued, although as long as the infection is unilateral, the uninvolved breast is theoretically still safe for nursing. Ice compresses and good bra support give a great deal of pain relief.

If therapy is started as soon as symptoms are apparent, the disease will run a short course, about 48 hours. If untreated, a breast infection may become a localized abscess. It may involve a large portion of the breast and rupture through the skin, with thick, purulent drainage. The mother will need to be readmitted to the hospital for incision and drainage of the abscess.

Urinary Tract Infection

Many women have difficulty voiding in the postpartal period because of vulvar edema and loss of bladder tone from the pressure of the fetal head during delivery. Other women seemingly void without difficulty, but their bladder does not fully empty each time (increased residual volume). In both instances, urine remains in the bladder for a longer than normal time. Stasis of any body fluid leads to infection.

The woman who was catheterized at the time of delivery or who is catheterized in the postpartal period is very prone to developing a urinary tract infection because bacteria may be introduced into the bladder at the time of catheterization.

When a urinary tract infection develops, the woman notices symptoms of burning on urination, possibly blood in the urine (hematuria), and a feeling of frequency or that she always has to void. The pain is so sharp on voiding that she may resist doing so and thus compound the problem of urinary stasis. She may have a low-grade fever and discomfort from lower abdominal pain.

A woman with any symptoms of urinary tract infection should have a clean-catch urine obtained. To avoid contamination of the specimen from lochial discharge, most women need help in obtaining the specimen. Have the woman lie supine on her bed, and wash the vulva well with clear water to remove any discharge present. Using a hospital-decreed technique for a clean-catch specimen, wash the area of the urinary meatus from front to back. Place a sterile cotton ball in the vaginal introitus to block excretion of further lochia.

Have the woman begin to void in the bathroom (young adolescents do this best by kneeling in their bed and straddling a bedpan); catch a midstream urine sample with a sterile urine container. Be certain to have the woman remove the vaginal cotton ball following the procedure; otherwise it will cause stasis of vaginal secretions and endometritis can result.

The woman will be started on a broad-spectrum antibiotic such as ampicillin to treat the infection. Encourage her to drink large amounts of fluid (a glass every hour) to help flush the infection from her bladder. She may need an analgesic to reduce the pain of urination for the next few times she voids until the antibiotic begins to work and the burning sensation disappears. Otherwise, she will not drink the fluid you suggest, knowing that will increase the number of times she will need to void, and the voiding is painful.

Although symptoms of urinary tract infection decrease quickly, the woman will need to continue to take the antibiotic for a full 10 days to completely eradicate the infection. Once symptoms have disappeared, particularly if a person is busy—and a new mother at home with a new baby is *very* busy—people are usually poor medicine-takers. Make a chart for the woman's refrigerator door for her to take home to remind her to continue to take her medication. Otherwise, bacteria in the urine will begin to multiply again, and in another week, symptoms and the active infection will recur.

If the woman is breast-feeding she should temporarily discontinue this if her antibiotic is tetracycline or a sulfonamide. Or you should ask if her antibiotic could be changed to one safe for breast-feeding. Otherwise, she may decide to breast-feed once she is home and not take the prescribed antibiotic.

MOTHER-CHILD RELATIONSHIPS WITH INFECTION PRESENT

Whether or not the mother who has an infection should be allowed to feed and care for her baby is always a concern on postpartal units. Most hospitals have well-defined guidelines in this area for you to follow.

As a rule, the baby of a mother with an increased temperature (100.4°F, or 38.0°C) for two consecutive 24-hour periods exclusive of the first 24 hours should be excluded from her room until the cause of the infection is determined. The mother may have an upper respiratory or a gastrointestinal infection unrelated to childbearing but transmittable to the newborn.

If the cause of the fever is found to be related to childbirth but involves a closed infection such as thrombophlebitis, where there would be no danger of the baby's contracting the disease, the mother can care for her child as long as she maintains bed rest in the prescribed position. If the infection involves drainage (e.g., endometritis, perineal abscess), the hospital's infection committee will decide on the newborn visiting policy. If the mother is allowed to feed her child, she should wash her hands thoroughly before the baby is brought to her. She should never place the baby on the bottom bed sheet, where there may be some infected drainage from her perineal pad.

Most hospitals are reluctant to return to a central nursery a baby who has visited in a room where there is an infection. The hospital should provide small nurseries that may be used as isolation nurseries for these situations or the baby can be placed in a closed Isolette in a central nursery.

If the mother has a high fever, breast milk may be deficient. With modern antimicrobial therapy, puerperal infections are limited, and the period of high fever will be transient. If the mother is too ill to nurse the baby during this time, or is receiving an anticoagulant or antibiotic such as tetracycline that is passed in breast milk, the infant should be fed by a supplementary milk formula and her breast milk should be manually expressed to maintain the production of milk so that it will be available when she is again able to nurse. If it appears that the course of the disease will be long, the mother may choose to, or may be advised to, discontinue breast-feeding. In this instance the physician will usually prescribe a lactation-suppressing drug to discourage engorgement. Once lactation is well established, however, these drugs are not effective in suppressing lactation.

The mother with an infection is always a disturbed mother. She quickly realizes that her care is different from that of the other women on the unit. She is confined to bed when the other mothers are ambulatory. She is still uncomfortable when they are not.

Good nursing care is important. Ice bags used to minimize perineal discomfort must not be allowed to saturate the bed, making the woman feel chilled or otherwise uncomfortable. If isolated, she must not feel isolated from the hospital staff or her family. Although you must use scrupulous infection technique, be certain you do not give the woman the impression that she is contaminated or "dirty" in any way.

If it is necessary for the woman to discontinue breast-feeding, she needs to be assured that she can meet the needs of her child through bottle-feeding and that she has not become a bad or inadequate mother because of the complication.

If the woman is going to be hospitalized for a period of time, she may have to make arrangements for the discharge and care of the baby. She may be interested in a homemaker service or temporary foster care if she has no close friends or family. If she has older children at home, she needs to keep in close contact with them, calling them on the telephone or writing them short notes if possible.

This is a point in life when the woman is adjusting to a new life role. It is difficult enough to accomplish this when things are going well. When she is segregated, denied the pleasure of holding and feeding her baby, and frightened by her condition, the struggle may be more than she is prepared to tolerate. She needs friendly, understanding support from the hospital personnel who give her care.

Postpartal Pregnancy-induced Hypertension

Mild preexisting hypertension (see Chap. 33) may increase in severity during the first few hours or days after delivery. Rarely, hypertension of pregnancy develops for the first time in a woman who has had no prenatal or intranatal symptoms. The cardinal symptoms are those of prepartal hypertension of pregnancy, namely, proteinuria, edema, and hypertension. The treatment measures will also be the same: bed rest, a quiet atmosphere, and sedatives. The woman will need frequent monitoring of her vital signs and urine output. She may be returned to surgery to have a dilation and curettage to ascertain that all placental fragments have been removed from the uterus or that none of the pregnancy is still existing. Following a dilation and curettage, the blood pressure often dramatically falls to normal.

If convulsions are going to occur with postpartal hypertension of pregnancy, they invariably develop 6 to 24 hours after delivery. Convulsions occurring more than 72 hours after delivery are probably due not to eclampsia but to some cause unrelated to childbearing.

Women in whom postpartal hypertension develops are bewildered by what is happening to them. If convulsions occur, they are frightened to discover how little control they have over their body. They worry that convulsions will occur after they are home, while they are working at a hot stove or holding the baby.

The woman should be assured that hypertension of pregnancy, although appearing late, is a condition of pregnancy; now that she is no longer pregnant, it need give her no further cause for concern. Because eclampsia or preeclampsia occurs with one pregnancy, there is no statistical reason to believe it will occur with a future pregnancy (unless chronic hypertension persists).

The Woman Whose Child Is Delivered by Cesarean Section

Women who have had cesarean sections (many women like this operation referred to as cesarean *birth*, rather than section, because of the gentler tone of the word) have an additional care concern in the postpartal period: not only are they a postpartal patient, they are a postsurgical patient as well.

Following cesarean birth, most women are kept on an intravenous source of fluid for the first 24 hours to ensure good hydration. Depending on the degree of difficulty with surgery, a woman may be started on sips of clear fluid as soon as her gag reflex has returned and the nausea associated with general anesthesia has passed. If the woman delivered under a spinal anesthetic, she must be kept flat in bed for at least 8 hours or she will develop a "spinal headache," a complication that she does not need added to her situation.

Palpate the woman's abdomen for softness at least every 8 hours. Check fundal height and contraction at the same time intervals as you would with the woman who delivers vaginally. With classical cesarean incisions, it is sometimes difficult to determine fundal height because the woman tenses or guards her abdominal muscles to prevent you from hurting the incision. This action obscures palpation of the fundus. With low cesarean incisions, this is less of a problem. Tell the woman that you know palpating her abdomen may cause her some discomfort but assessing fundal involution is just as important with her as with the woman who delivers vaginally.

Assess lochial discharge at the same time intervals as you would with the woman who delivers vaginally. Lochial discharge is often decreased in amount in a woman following a cesarean birth, but it will be present.

The woman should be turned side to side every 2 hours during the first 24 hours to promote systemic circulation; by the end of 24 hours she is generally able to be out of bed and ambulating. She may feel more comfortable turning and sitting up if she supports her abdomen with a hand. Because her abdominal muscles are so lax from having been stretched from pregnancy, abdominal contents tend to shift forward and put pressure on the suture line, causing pain and an uncomfortable feeling often described as "falling apart."

In the first 24 hours, urge her to cough and deep breathe every 2 hours. If she cannot cough (i.e., it hurts her incision too much), at least she should take five or six good deep breaths to fully expand lung tissue and prevent lung secretions from becoming static.

Young adolescents may do this best by being asked to blow up balloons. Incentive spirometry (inhaling deeply to cause a ball to rise in a column of air in a plastic tube) may be effective.

The woman may have the Foley catheter that was inserted before surgery left in place for the first 24 hours to ensure bladder emptying. Assess its patency frequently. Anyone who has been catheterized should be observed closely for signs of beginning urinary tract infection (low-grade fever, dull lower abdominal pain, pain on voiding, hematuria, and frequency when the catheter is removed).

Be certain that the woman has ample time to hold and feed her child. She has some reason to think that her baby is not quite perfect—after all, he did not deliver quite perfectly—so she needs additional time to inspect him and grow comfortable with him. If she did not see him born because a general anesthetic was used, review the identification system used with the baby with her; be certain that she sees the baby as soon as she is awake from the anesthesia.

The woman may breast-feed. Finding a comfortable position may be difficult at first because the weight of the baby on her abdomen may cause discomfort; the uterine contractions that occur from oxytocin release may be uncomfortable. She may have an intravenous fluid line, which tends to get in the way of holding the baby comfortably. These are all minor problems that another day or two of time and concerned attention will alleviate.

At the same time, be certain that the woman receives enough rest. A cesarean section is major surgery. Just as you would not expect a man recovering from gallbladder surgery to return to work the morning following surgery, you should not expect a woman after a cesarean section to be taking full care of herself and her baby too. Many women do proceed to do this because their excitement over their baby and their new role makes them oblivious to their symptoms of underlying fatigue. Extreme fatigue does not aid healing, however; it makes the woman prone to postpartal infection. It will eventually interfere with bonding with the child, rather than promote it, if it does lead to partpartal complications. Help the woman plan a day that includes care of her new child but includes periods of rest time for herself as well.

The Mother Whose Child Is Born Handicapped

The nurse who works on a postpartal unit has usually chosen this type of nursing because she enjoys the feeling of happiness that pervades this area. She enjoys holding and feeding babies and teaching new mothers. She may therefore find herself ill at ease when the atmosphere in a patient's room turns to sadness, when a mother needs instructions different from the usual ones because her child has been born handicapped.

The professional nurse should have enough skill and enough ability in relating to patients to meet this mother's needs.

Most mothers say during pregnancy that they do not care about the sex of the child as long as the child is normal. How cheated they feel when this one requirement is not met. They are angry, hurt, and disappointed. They may feel a loss of self-respect: They have given birth to an imperfect child, and so they see themselves as imperfect. A mother sometimes responds with a grief reaction, as if the child has died. This is normal, because the "perfect" child she thought she was carrying *has* died.

The average mother has difficulty during the period immediately after delivery believing that her child is real. How much greater is the difficulty for the mother of a handicapped child. She must not only grasp the fact that the baby has been born but understand that the baby she has delivered is less than what she wished for.

At one time, the mother of a child born with a handicap was put under deep anesthesia at delivery, and 24 hours later, when she was "stronger" and "better able to accept the situation," the extent of the handicap was explained to her and she was then shown the baby. This method of dealing with the problem seems to have little merit. The mother cannot begin to accept her situation and work through the problem associated with it until she is aware of the situation. She will worry about the baby she does not see. She will imagine a state of affairs much worse than it actually may be. The baby may only have a deformed finger, but in her mind he may be totally deformed or even dead.

Most mothers are now shown the child moments after birth, and the handicap is immediately explained to them. The same procedure is followed for the father as well. This is a shock to couples, but they are not left feeling they have been deceived by the hospital staff. Families are not happy over their child's handicap, but they appreciate having honest friends who dare to face the problem with them when it first becomes apparent.

You should be familiar with the common birth defects and with the treatment that is available for them. The physician will usually make it his or her responsibility to tell the parents of the defect, but you must be prepared to reinforce this information or review the problem. People who are under stress are not good listeners and need explanations repeated several times before they are sure they understand.

The mother should be allowed to care for her child during the postpartal period if the child's condition makes it possible (Fig. 36-1). If the infant has a heart defect or respiratory problem that requires him to be kept in an Isolette, so that the mother cannot hold and feed him, she should be taken to the nursery and allowed to see the infant and talk with the personnel who are caring for him. She should be permitted to handle her child in the Isolette if at all possible; to begin to touch, relate to, and "claim" her infant in as nearly normal a manner as possible.

When you handle the infant, be certain that you do so with tender loving care. If you treat the baby as if you find him a desirable, attractive child despite his handicap, the mother will find holding and accepting the child an easier task.

Open lines of communication between the parents and the hospital staff that allow for free discussion of feelings and fears will do much to strengthen parent-child relationships when the child is born handicapped.

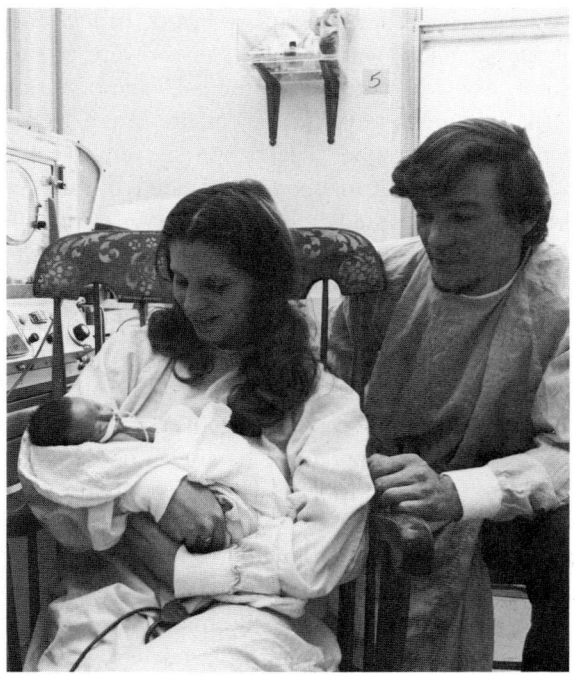

Fig. 36-1. Parents of a handicapped infant need to begin early interaction with him so that they can develop an effective parent-child relationship. (Courtesy of the Department of Medical Photography, Children's Hospital, Buffalo, N.Y.)

The Mother Whose Child Is Born Prematurely

The care of the low-birth-weight child is discussed in Chap. 39. The focus here is on the family of the low-birth-weight child in the postpartal period. This family reacts in much the same way as the family whose child has been born handicapped. There is likely to be a loss of self-esteem. The mother could not carry a baby to term; she has somehow "failed."

Despite the child's small size, the mother needs to touch him and hold him daily, even if in the Isolette. It has been traditional to separate low-birth-weight infants from their mothers on the grounds of preventing infection. Mothers have felt unwelcome in high-risk nurseries because of the amount of seemingly complicated equipment and the caps and gowns of hospital personnel. After a simple explanation of the purposes of the equipment and how it works, a mother can care for an infant in an Isolette with the same relaxation and skill as a student nurse.

The mother should be given honest appraisals of the child's progress. This policy will help to avoid situations in which a mother is told that her infant is doing well and then must be told later that the child has died. Mothers who are told their child has little chance of living have equally serious problems, however. They do not begin to form a relationship with the new child because they do not want to love him, knowing that in a matter of hours or days they will be hurt by his death. This is grieving in anticipation of death, or anticipatory grief. If the child does well and lives, these mothers may have difficulty "binding in" their child. They may act as if their child died (he did die in their minds) and the child offered to them is a stranger. They need to spend extra time with their child so they can grasp the concept that he is now doing well.

If a newborn is transported from the hospital to a regional center for care, the transport team should leave behind a Polaroid photograph of the infant so the woman and her support person have something tangible to relate to until she is able to see the infant again.

When the mother is discharged from the hospital, she should be allowed to telephone the intensive-care nursery daily to ask about her child's progress. She should be able to visit as often and for as long as she wishes.

Low-birth-weight children sometimes remain in the hospital so long that nursing personnel tend to think of them as "their" baby. They have to be reminded that the child is not theirs and is only under their temporary care. The mother needs to be offered every opportunity available to *feel* like the child's mother, to begin a relationship with the child that allows her to bind in warmly despite the child's small size. It often helps her to know that low-birth-weight infants are usually strong and durable despite their small size.

The Woman Whose Child Has Died

The woman who loses a child always has questions about what happened. She is likely to feel bewildered, perhaps bitter, perhaps resentful that the hospital staff could not save the child. "Why me? Out of all the women here, why did my baby die?"

You should be familiar with the forms the mother or father will have to sign when a baby dies or is born dead, and you should know whether or not in your state stillborn infants have to be given a name and to have a funeral.

Nurses and other women on the unit tend to stay away from the woman whose child has died as if what has happened to her were contagious. It is easy to rationalize that the woman's emotions are too raw at this point for anyone outside her family to be of any help to her. Mothers who have gone through the experience express an opposite view, however. They find that friends and relatives are equally unable to talk about the situation with them, and they want to face what has happened to them here, where it happened. They want a nurse to approach them and say "Do you want to talk about it?" or "Would it help to talk about it?"

No matter how crowded a maternity service is, a woman whose child has died should never be placed in a room with a mother who has had a healthy child. This is too much to ask her to bear. A private room allows the woman an opportunity to express her grief. She does not have to keep up a front for a roommate, and the hospital staff can bend visiting rules for her. She needs her family with her to fill a portion of the void left by her loss.

Nurses accept the fact that women have other complications of childbearing. They learn to care for the woman who hemorrhages or acquires an infection. They must become as skilled at caring for the woman whose complication is that she grieves because she is not a mother.

Postpartal Psychosis

As many as 1 woman in 500 presents enough symptoms in the year after delivery of a child to be considered mentally ill. In about two-thirds of these women the illness develops during the first six weeks after delivery. Because the illness coincides with the postpartal period, it has been called *postpartal psychosis*. Rather than being a response to the physical aspects of childbearing, it is probably a response to the crisis of childbearing. Nearly a third of these women will have had symptoms of mental illness prior to the pregnancy. If the pregnancy had not precipitated the illness, a death in the family, the loss of a husband's job, a divorce, or some other crisis would probably have precipitated it.

The woman usually appears exceptionally sad. She may deny she has had a child and, when the child is brought to her, insist that she was never pregnant. She needs to be referred for professional psychiatric counseling in order to establish better coping mechanisms against crisis.

The outcome of the condition will depend on the pattern of mental illness that is present and the woman's ability to respond to therapy.

Problem-oriented Recording: Progress Notes

Angie Baco
Post partum, day 1

Problem: Gestational diabetes

> S. Asking whether urine tests are showing any glucose spillage; apprehensive that diabetes will not end with the pregnancy. Asking whether dieting will reduce possibility of diabetes. No subjective symptoms of thirst, dizziness, lethargy. Voiding frequently (100 ml per hour) since Foley catheter removed. On regular diet.
> O. Urines neg., neg.
> 2-hour postprandial blood sugar = 120.
> A. Woman with gestational diabetes concerned that problem will not be transient.
>
> Goals: a. Become familiar with normal postpartal course so symptoms such as polyuria will not be confused with diabetic symptom.
> b. Be aware that she may become diabetic at some later point in life so she maintains health supervision.
>
> P. 1. Continue to assess urine before meals for

glucose and acetone (double voided specimens).
2. Instruct patient on signs of urinary tract infection (burning, frequency, hematuria) because of Foley catheter insertion during labor.
3. Instruct to return to prepregnancy diet during postpartal period rather than dieting now.

Problem: Pain in right calf

S. Patient states that her right calf is tender to touch; skin over area is white and shiny. She first noticed symptoms this morning when she awoke (20 minutes ago).
O. Homans' sign positive; right calf larger than left calf by 2 cm diameter. Toes blanch equally well in both feet. Temperature: 99.6 orally.
A. Woman with symptoms of impaired lower extremity circulation. Medical diagnosis: femoral thrombophlebitis.

Goals: a. Patient to voice the pathology underlying disease process.
b. To continue care of infant even though on bed rest.
c. To voice workable plans for management of other children if hospital stay is extended.

P. 1. Bed rest with bed cradle.
2. Remind patient not to rub right leg; no massage by nursing staff of right leg.
3. Use acetaminophen (Tylenol) for pain relief in place of aspirin (both are ordered).
4. Dicumarol to be delayed daily until PT time report is available.
5. Continue to bring baby to mother for care; to continue formula-feeding.

References

1. Benfield, D. G., et al. Grief response of parents to neonatal death and parent participation in deciding care. *Pediatrics* 62:171, 1978.
2. Eng, J., et al. Bacteriuria in the puerperium: An evaluation of methods of collecting urine specimens. *Am. J. Obstet. Gynecol.* 131:739, 1978.
3. Ewing, T. L., et al. Maternal deaths associated with postpartum vulvar edema. *Am. J. Obstet. Gynecol.* 134:173, 1979.
4. Gibbs, R. S., et al. Antibiotic therapy of endometritis following cesarean section. *Obstet. Gynecol.* 52:31, 1978.
5. Henderson, K. J., and Newton, L. D. Helping nursing mothers maintain lactation while separated from their infants. *M.C.N.* 3:352, 1978.
6. Ishida, Y. How to deal with grief in childbirth. *Female Patient* 5:74, 1980.
7. Kennell, J. Parenting in the intensive care unit. *Birth Fam. J.* 5:223, 1978.
8. Kennell, J., and Klaus, M. A. Helping parents cope with perinatal death. *Contemp. Obstet. Gynecol.* 12:53, 1978.
9. Lepler, M. Having a handicapped child. *M.C.N.* 3:32, 1978.
10. Measey, L. G. Psychiatric problems in obstetrics. *Practitioner* 220:120, 1978.
11. Nyman, J. E. Thrombophlebitis in pregnancy. *Am. J. Nurs.* 80:90, 1980.
12. Ogden, E., et al. Puerperal infections due to group A beta hemolytic streptococcus. *Obstet. Gynecol.* 52:53, 1978.
13. Rancillo, N. When a woman is diabetic: Postpartal care. *Am. J. Nurs.* 79:453, 1979.
14. Rowe, J., et al. Follow-up of families who experience a perinatal death. *Pediatrics* 62:166, 1978.
15. Swanson, J. Nursing intervention to facilitate maternal-infant attachment. *J.O.G.N. Nurs.* 7:35, 1978.
16. Williams, J. K. Illness and the acquaintance-attachment process. *Am. J. Nurs.* 77:1174, 1977.

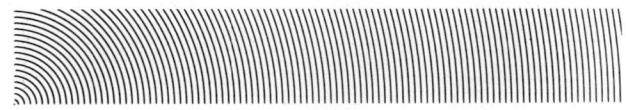

Unit VII. Utilizing Nursing Process: Questions for Review

1. Mrs. Jones smokes heavily. Infants of women who smoke during pregnancy tend to be
   a. Large for gestation age
   b. Anemic
   c. Postmature
   d. Small for gestation age

2. If Mrs. Jones has an ectopic pregnancy, signs of this tend to occur about what week of pregnancy?
   a. The 2nd week
   b. The 6th week
   c. The 16th week
   d. The 20th week

3. Mrs. Smith has a cesarean section under general anesthesia. General anesthesia may result in all of the following *except*
   a. Delayed respirations in the newborn
   b. Delay of the development of maternal feelings
   c. Suppression of breast milk
   d. Decreased sucking ability in the newborn

4. Mrs. K. has pernicious vomiting of pregnancy. Which acid-base imbalance is most likely to occur with her?
   a. Respiratory alkalosis
   b. Metabolic alkalosis
   c. A low pH
   d. Metabolic acidosis

5. Mrs. M. has diabetes mellitus. During pregnancy you would anticipate that her insulin requirement will
   a. Disappear
   b. Remain the same
   c. Decrease
   d. Increase

6. Mrs. O. has heart disease. Pregnancy is a stress on the woman with heart disease because
   a. The uterus puts pressure on the heart.
   b. The blood volume expands at least 30 percent.
   c. Peripheral circulation expansion leads to decreased blood pressure.
   d. The placenta requires so much blood that hypovolemia occurs.

7. Mrs. T. develops pregnancy-induced hypertension. A symptom that is the *most* typical of pregnancy-induced hypertension is
   a. Ankle edema
   b. Weight loss
   c. Unusual susceptibility to infection
   d. Protein in urine

8. The underlying pathology of hypertension of pregnancy is
   a. Vasospasm
   b. Interference with coagulation
   c. Heart failure
   d. Decreased glomerular filtration

9. Mrs. T. is treated with magnesium sulfate. An injection of magnesium sulfate should *not* be given if
   a. Respirations are 20 per minute.
   b. Blood pressure is 140/90.
   c. Reflexes are hypoactive.
   d. She is tense and anxious.

10. Mrs. W. is admitted to the hospital with a diagnosis of placenta previa. On admission, your *best* action would be to
    a. Perform a vaginal examination to assess the extent of the bleeding.
    b. Keep Mrs. W. ambulatory to reduce bleeding.
    c. Assess fetal heart tones.
    d. Ask Mrs. W. whether this is her first child.

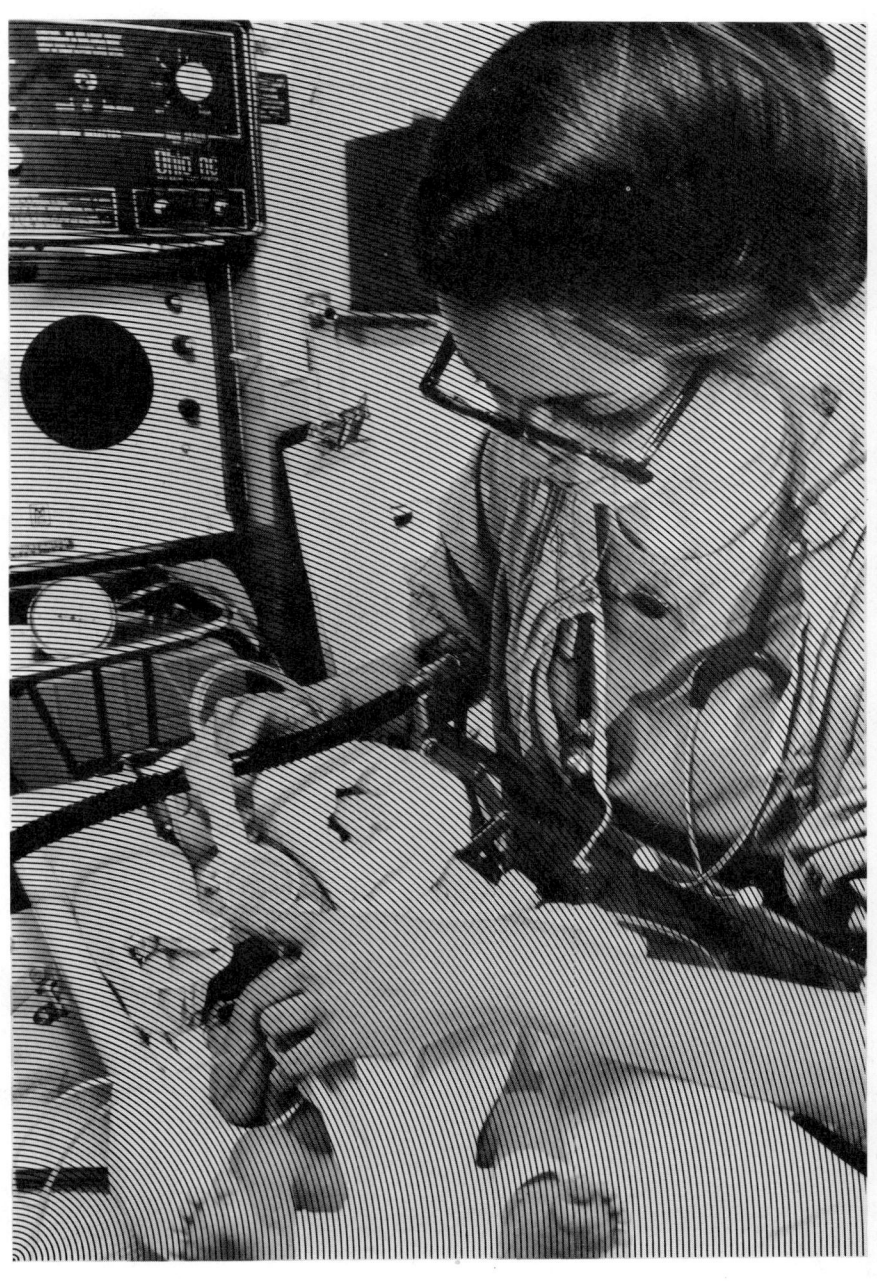

VIII. The High-Risk Infant

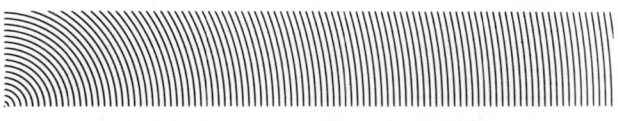

37. Identifying the High-Risk Infant

A high-risk infant is one who is born with less ability or chance to survive or a greater chance of being left with a permanent handicap either psychosocially or physiologically than the average child.

About 60 percent of the time it can be predicted from the pregnancy history that a high-risk infant will be born. Other infants are categorized as high-risk at birth because on physical examination it is apparent that they have a congenital anomaly or are low-birth-weight or small for gestation age. Still other infants appear to be all right at birth but then have difficulty establishing effective respirations. And there are those who are categorized as high-risk because economic or psychosocial factors of their family are such that they will interfere with optimum growth or development.

Common examples of high-risk infants are shown in Table 37-1.

Regionalization

Caring for high-risk infants requires such high expenditures for personnel and equipment that not all hospitals can afford to provide for high-risk infant care. Levels of care that can be given safely at each hospital are evaluated, and hospitals are designated as level I, II, or III, depending on the care available at that particular site. Descriptions of the three levels are shown in Table 37-2.

It is important that health care facilities not attempt to provide care beyond their capabilities. High-risk areas that are "high risk" in name only cannot provide safe care.

Transport of High-Risk Infants

Infants who are born at level I and II hospitals but require level III care must be transported for such care. If it is known before birth that the infant will need level III care (premature rupture of the membranes at 30 weeks' gestation, for example), ideally the mother is transported to the level III health care facility before birth so that the infant can immediately have the benefit of that level care. If hospitalizing the woman is not feasible in advance (the woman is admitted to a level I hospital in active labor and delivers before transport is available or sensible), transporting the infant as soon as possible after birth is the next best approach to providing care.

The philosophy of transporting ill newborns has swung full cycle in recent years, from one of not transporting in the early hours of life (to stress the child the least amount possible in these first critical

Table 37-1. Common Examples of Infants Categorized as High-Risk by Pregnancy History

Factor	Possible Consequence in Infant
Antenatal Factors	
Pregnancy-induced hypertension	May be small for gestation age; hypoglycemia and polycythemia
Cardiac disease	May have intrapartal anoxia; small for gestation age
Poor nutrition	Small for gestation age; hypoglycemia
Diabetes	Respiratory distress syndrome; large for gestation age; hypoglycemia. If diabetes is class D, infant may be small for gestation age
Rh isoimmunization	Anemia, hyperbilirubinemia
Maternal age more than 35	Genetic malformations; dysfunctional labor patterns leading to fetal anoxia
Maternal age less than 16	Small for gestation age; effects of hypertension of pregnancy, premature labor, or inadequate pelvis
Anemia	Anoxia; small for gestation age
Maternal infections	Congenital anomalies; neurological disorders
Chronic renal, vascular, or collogen disease	Small for gestation age; specific problem related to maternal drug use
Maternal drug use	Small for gestation age; neurological and metabolic disorders
Multiple gestation	Small for gestation age; birth trauma, anoxia
Prolonged pregnancy	Anoxia, birth injury, neurological disorders
Hydramnios	Tracheoesophageal fistula; anencephaly
Natal Factors	
Prolonged rupture of membranes	Infection
Premature labor	Anoxia, respiratory distress syndrome, intrapartal injury
Abnormal presentation	Birth trauma, anoxia
Cesarean section	Respiratory distress syndrome
Premature separation of placenta	Anoxia
Placenta previa	Severe anemia, anoxia
Oxytocin and/or epidural anesthesia	Anoxia
Meconium-stained amniotic fluid	Anoxia
Prolapsed cord	Anoxia
Prolonged labor	Anoxia

Table 37-2. Levels of Care

Level	Description
I	Hospital provides services for uncomplicated deliveries and normal newborn infants. The number of births at the facility is small. Initial newborn management such as resuscitation and short-term assisted ventilation is available while transport to a level II or III facility is awaited
II	Hospital provides services for both the normal and high-risk pregnant patient and for the management of selected neonatal illnesses. The facility is capable of resuscitation, short-term assisted ventilation with bag and mask or endotracheal tube, intravenous therapy with infusion pumps, arterial blood gas monitoring, continuous cardiorespiratory monitoring with appropriate equipment, performance of exchange transfusion, and oxygen administration
III	Hospital serves as a regional center and provides all aspects of perinatal care, including intensive care and a broad range of continuously available subspecialty consultation. The facility provides educational programs, consultation services, and back-up support for level I and II facilities. The facility provides transport service and transport personnel for the infant in need of such care

Source. American Academy of Pediatrics, *Standards and Recommendations for Hospital Care of Newborn Infants* (6th ed.). Evanston, Ill.: The Academy, 1977. Copyright American Academy of Pediatrics 1977.

hours), to one of transporting immediately no matter what the baby's condition, to one of transporting as soon as possible but after first stabilizing the infant's condition. This is an important philosophy for the parents of the child to understand. They may envision a transport team hurrying into the community hospital and immediately swooping up their child and leaving for the regional center. Instead, the transport team delays to insert an intravenous line and an oralgastric tube and perhaps intubate. They worry that their child is sicker than they were first told (or the transport team is not very efficient). They need to be told that stabilizing the infant before transport safeguards him during transport. Inserting an intravenous line in a rocking ambulance when the child needs it is obviously more hazardous than inserting it prophylactically in a warmed, well-lighted, firmly grounded nursery.

The role of nurses in transporting infants has also come full cycle—from its being conducted by nurses, to its being a physician's role, to its being a specially prepared nursing role. In order to safely transport infants, a nurse must be able to begin intravenous lines, insert umbilical catheters, intubate, and be aware of drug use and temperature stabilization measures; she should have access to a telephone line for physician consultation as needed.

Transport service must be available 24 hours a day. In many institutions, calling for transport service is the physician's responsibility. In others, after the need for transport has been confirmed by a physician, it is the nurse who actually sets the process in motion.

In order that the transport team can anticipate what equipment will be needed to stabilize and transport a particular infant, accurate clinical data on the infant must be reported to its members. The type of information that transport personnel find helpful is the following:

Estimated gestation age (from date of confinement and physical examination)
Birth weight
Health disorders during the pregnancy

Unusual aspects of labor or delivery
Infant temperature and measures being employed to keep temperature in neutral zone
Infant color
Oxygen requirement (documented by arterial blood gas if possible) and measures employed to keep the infant's PO_2 at that level
Respiratory assessment (apnea, retractions, etc.)
Blood glucose or Dextrostix reading
Blood pressure (if there is equipment to take it accurately)
Chest x-ray findings and hematocrit on any infant with respiratory distress, cyanosis, or shock

On the basis of this information, the transporting facility may suggest further measures that should be taken before they arrive.

The routine administration of vitamin K and eye prophylaxis should be done. Copies of both the mother's and infant's charts should be prepared to accompany the infant. About 10 ml of clotted maternal blood, an equal cord blood sample, and the placenta, if applicable, should accompany the infant also.

It is important that the infant be transported in an incubator with a source of oxygen, easy access to the infant, ability to provide heat, and good visibility (Fig. 37-1). A mother needs to see her infant and touch

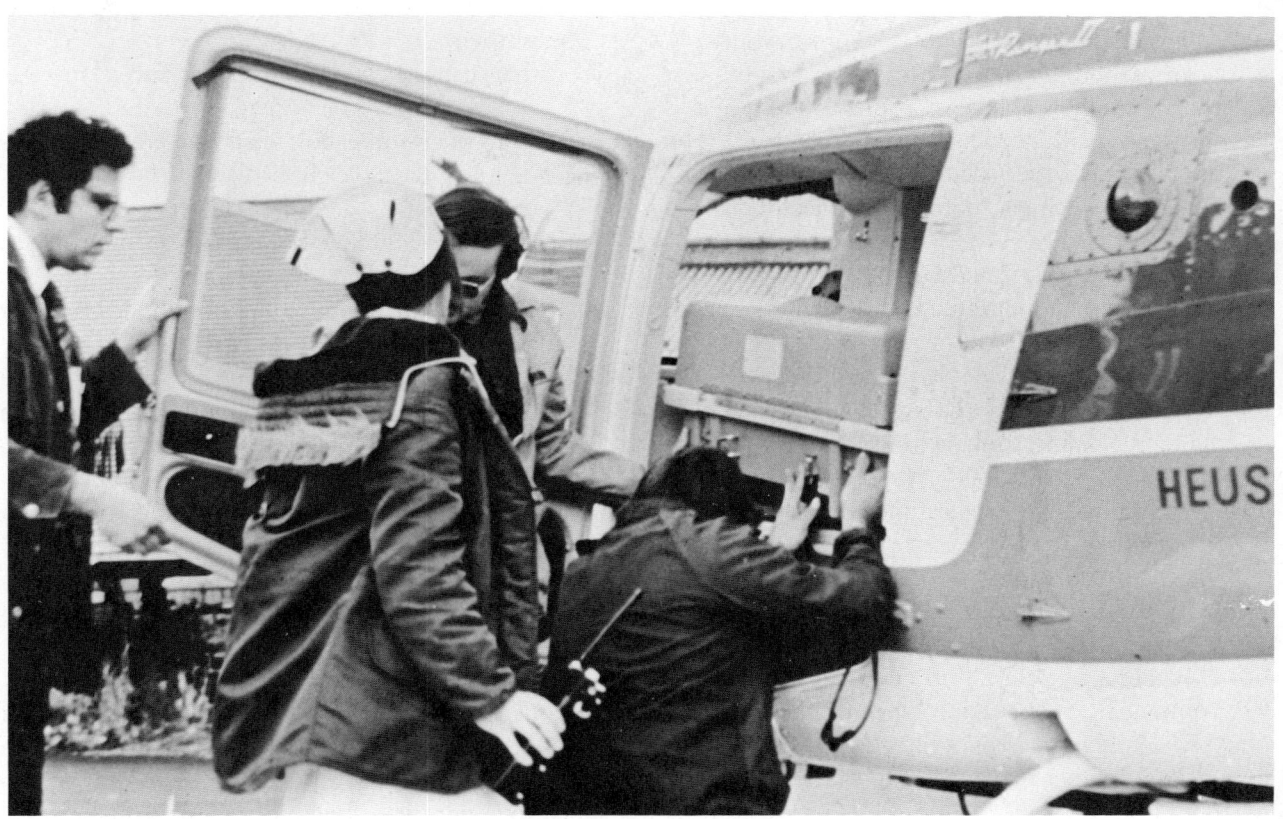

Fig. 37-1. Ill or immature neonates are transported to regional care centers in a carrier that provides warmth, oxygen if needed, and easy access for emergency treatment. Here the transport carrier is lifted into a transport van by the physician and nurse who will accompany the baby to a regional center. (Courtesy of the Department of Medical Photography, Children's Hospital, Buffalo, N.Y.)

him if at all possible before transport. If she is not allowed to see him, the birth does not seem real to her or she may imagine that he has even greater problems than he does have (not only is he small, but there are physical defects as well; otherwise, why was she not allowed to see him?). Such thoughts "turn off" mother-child bonding. If it is not possible for the mother to see the infant (she delivered under general anesthetic and is not yet awake), she should be shown a Polaroid photograph of the baby as soon as she is awake. If the infant must be transported so far that it will be difficult for the woman to visit, this picture will leave her something tangible to bind to until she can visit and care for her child.

Mother-Child Bonding

There seems to be a sensitive period in the first few days of life when women bond with their infants most easily. It is therefore just as important that mothers of high-risk infants have the opportunity to hold and touch their infants as it is for mothers of well infants. It is frightening for women to walk into intensive care units. The number of machines, the concentration of personnel, the fragile appearance of their newborn make it very hard for them to say, "I want to hold my baby." If not given active support they will come no closer to their child than looking through a glass window in the hallway.

Some intensive care facilities encourage women to gavage or suction their infants. These are not the best actions for mothers, however, unless the baby will be discharged still needing this type of care. The mother's time is better spent just holding and stroking her infant—being a mother, not a technician, to him.

Two of the biggest dangers to infants in intensive care units is that mother-child bonding will not occur and that the infant will not receive the sensory stimulus he requires for initial development. When caring for infants in special care settings, interventions such as holding the infant, stroking him, looking directly at him so that he has eye-to-eye contact, singing or talking to him should have as much priority as physical interventions.

A woman needs to spend enough time with her newborn to be comfortable with him before discharge. It is difficult for a first-time mother to learn how to care for her child with enough confidence to feel comfortable about taking him home even when he is well. When the baby is ill, the situation is compounded. A mother may be able to learn how to feed her hard-to-feed infant in one visit, but she cannot begin to learn all her infant's cues that she will have to be familiar with in order to provide total care for him in a single visit; that is the kind of knowledge that comes only with repeated contact.

When people feel self-conscious, they often do not hold their infant as warmly as they want to. They may feel that "talking" to an infant or singing to him will look strange in this setting of machines and technical equipment. Role-modeling maternal behavior—talking to infants, holding them warmly, counting toes, tickling tummies (all the "motherly" things that new mothers do)—is important for showing women that such actions are not out of place here and they can feel comfortable doing them. Although such behaviors are called "motherly," fathers do the same things when they are comfortable with infants. Role modeling when just the father is present is equally important.

Chapter 24 discusses behaviors that mothers usually manifest when they are adjusting well to their newborns—when bonding is occurring. These are helpful observations to make with parents of high-risk infants as well. In addition to these behaviors, the following are indications of a healthy relationship between parents and a low-birth-weight baby [5]:

1. Parents frequently question doctors and nurses about etiology, prognosis, treatment plan, etc.
2. Parents are aware of negative feelings and can express them.
3. Parents can seek help from friends and relatives.

Indications of an unhealthy relationship between parents and a low-birth-weight baby are [5]:

1. Parents make little effort to secure information about their baby's condition.
2. Parents are unable to express feelings of guilt or anger at the baby's early arrival.
3. Parents consistently misinterpret or exaggerate either positive or negative information given to them about the baby's condition and are unable to respond with hope as the condition improves.
4. Parents concentrate conversation and interest on less threatening matters such as welfare of older children.
5. Parents are unable to accept and use help offered them.

Particularly important appears to be the number of times each week that a parent initiates contact with the child, either by a visit or by a phone call if distance interferes with frequent visiting. Nurses in intensive care settings should keep a record of when parents visit or telephone. Infants of parents who make contact less often than twice a week seem to have more difficulty establishing effective parent-child bonding than those whose parents made more frequent contact [11].

Some parents may be reluctant to telephone a great deal, afraid that they are interrupting important people, that they will be thought of as "nuisances" or as overanxious. They need to be told at each contact that their calls are welcome, and even if they must wait a minute sometimes for someone to respond, it is not because no one wants to talk to them but because it takes time to remove a gown or close an Isolette before answering the telephone.

People call most readily if they know one person whom they can ask for. The parents should be given the name of their infant's primary nurse and the physician who is their child's doctor. As house staff change, they need to be alerted to the new name and assured that they may now call this new person, lest they lose confidence in the acceptability of their telephoning.

In order that the high-risk infant can develop a sense of trust, he must have the same considerations as a well newborn: a constant caregiver, active interaction, and sensory stimulation. All high-risk infants need to be assigned a primary nurse for each nursing shift, so that the number of caregivers they have is as low as possible. This person should spend active time with the child apart from the contacts involving mainly treatments. Sensory stimulation—looking at the child, providing a mobile for his crib or Isolette or some bright-colored item he can see, giving him a chance, when he is out of his Isolette (away from the hum of the motor), to hear a voice or music box, stroking the back of his head or his arms or back—should be supplied by everyone who cares for him, but his primary care person should have this as a major responsibility (Fig. 37-2). It gains little if an infant is rescued from death at birth by medical intervention but then is never able to relate well to people and spends the remainder of his life an unhappy loner because nursing intervention to initiate a sense of trust

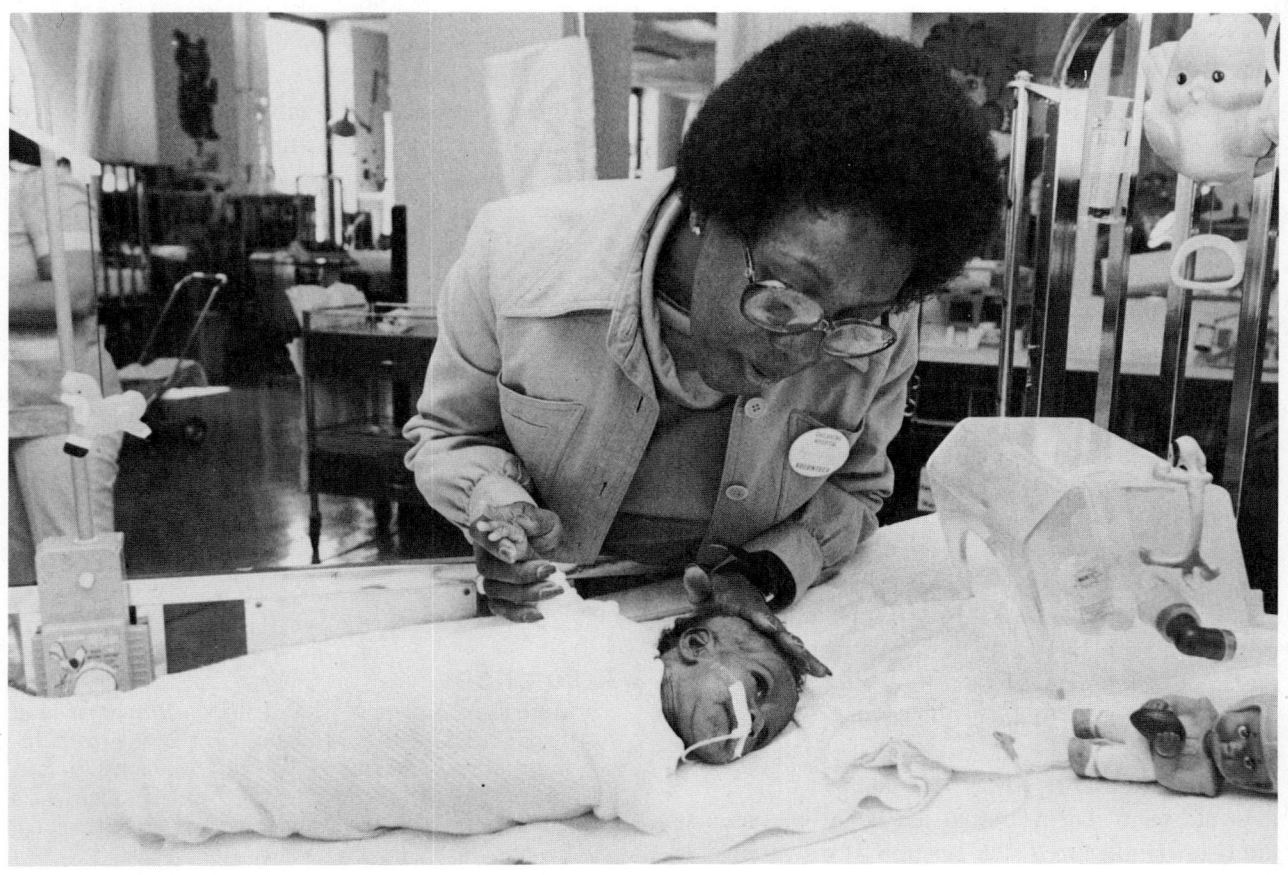

Fig. 37-2. Infants are classified as high-risk for many reasons. An infant born of a drug-addicted mother enjoys the tight swaddling afforded by a blanket and the comfort of a stroking hand. Notice the oxygen hood available for administration of oxygen and the age-appropriate toys for stimulation. (Courtesy of the Department of Medical Photography, Children's Hospital, Buffalo, N.Y.)

until his mother could take over this function was inadequate.

Following High-Risk Infants at Home

It is difficult to predict on discharge from a nursery which infants will do well at home and which ones will have to be returned for care because their family did not understand their needs or could not meet their needs.

At each hospital visit it is important to assess the parents' level of knowledge about their child's condition. Do they comprehend that he is not only light in weight (2 pounds) but that he is also immature? The mother who does not understand this may think that her infant is unresponsive to her because he does not grasp her finger when she places it in his palm the way her other children did. Knowing that he is too immature to do so yet will limit her expectations to the responses her child is capable of.

Battle [3] has devised a number of criteria that can be used to predict whether parents will be able to incorporate a handicapped child into their family. If these factors are absent, the child with a handicap (the child who is going home in a hip spica cast, the child who will be mentally retarded, the child with a cleft palate, for example) is doubly at risk. Not only is he handicapped but also he may not be well accepted by his family.

Factors that indicate that a family will probably be able to adjust to caring for a handicapped child are the following: the family has the support of interested health care personnel and understanding friends; a strong marital relationship exists between parents; a good relationship exists between the mother and the maternal grandmother (the mother has a good sense of trust); the handicapped child is other than a firstborn (the mother has had practice "mothering"); the family lives close to shopping, schools, and transportation and so is not isolated; the family has a supportive religious faith; the family was told of the child's disability as soon as possible [3]. All families of high-risk infants should be screened for these criteria. You cannot change many of these factors if they are present, but knowledge that they exist serves as an incentive to help the family establish solid support people who can aid in overcoming or minimizing the obstacles. These might be people from church or community groups or a community health nurse.

THE HIGH-RISK INFANT AND CHILD ABUSE

It would seem that if a child has been born prematurely or handicapped, the reaction of his parents toward him would be to protect him even more than the average child so that no further harm could come to him. In reality, particularly in reference to low-birth-weight children, the opposite may occur. Low-birth-weight children are at high risk for abuse.

Child abuse is probably due to the separation of the child from his family at birth, which interferes with bonding. Helfer and Kempe [9] have identified three factors that must be present before child abuse occurs:

1. A parent who has the ability to abuse. All parents grow angry at their children on occasion; only a few are capable of actually hurting the child.
2. A child who is special in some way. The child was born prematurely, is more intelligent than the parent, has red hair. . . . The ways that children are "special" is endless.
3. A triggering event. The "trigger" that initiates child abuse can be a major family insult (loss of the father's job, a fire in the house) or a minor incident that serves as the "last straw" (a plugged toilet, rain on a Sunday picnic).

When following children who are identified as high-risk at birth, it is sound judgment to keep these three criteria in mind: a special person, a special child, a special event. Because one of the circumstances (a special child) is already present, the child is always more vulnerable to abuse, therefore, than is the nonrisk infant.

Other factors associated with child abuse are lack of support people, alcohol or drug abuse, abuse of the parent when a child himself, inadequate knowledge of growth and development, and isolation. Serving as a support person or seeing that support people are identified for families with high-risk infants, then, is a means of reducing the possibility that children seen today in a high-risk care setting will be seen tomorrow in the emergency room with burns or scalds.

Helping a mother get to know her child at birth, giving her opportunities to see and touch and care for him as much as possible, provides knowledge of growth and development and aids bonding. With effective bonding, child abuse does not occur under any circumstances.

References

1. American Academy of Pediatrics. *Standards and Recommendations for Hospital Care of Newborn Infants* (6th ed.). Evanston, Ill.: The Academy, 1977.
2. Aure, B., and Schneider, J. M. Transferring a community hospital nursing service into a regional center. *Nurs. Clin. North Am.* 10:275, 1975.

3. Battle, C. U. Chronic physical disease: Behavioral aspects. *Pediatr. Clin. North Am.* 22:525, 1975.
4. Christensen, A. Coping with the crisis of premature birth—one couple's story. *M.C.N.* 2:24, 1977.
5. Dubois, D. Indications of an unhealthy relationship between parents and premature infants. *J.O.G.N. Nurs.* 4:21, 1975.
6. Gayton, W. Management problems of mentally retarded children and their families. *Pediatr. Clin. North Am.* 22:561, 1975.
7. Guy, M. Neonatal transport. *Nurs. Clin. North Am.* 13:3, 1978.
8. Hawkins-Walsh, E. Diminishing anxiety in parents of sick newborns. *M.C.N.* 5:30, 1980.
9. Helfer, R. E., and Kempe, C. H. *The Battered Child*. Chicago: University of Chicago Press, 1968.
10. Jacobson, S. P. Stressful situations for neonatal intensive care nurses. *M.C.N.* 3:144, 1978.
11. Klaus, M., and Kennell, J. *Mother-Infant Bonding*. St. Louis: Mosby, 1976.
12. Korones, S. B. *High-Risk Infants—The Basis for Intensive Nursing Care* (2nd ed.). St. Louis: Mosby, 1976.
13. Lubchenco, L. *The High-Risk Infant*. Philadelphia: Saunders, 1976.
14. Michie, M. M. Prevention of handicap: The quality of neonatal care in special and intensive care baby units. *Midwives Chron.* 92:13, 1979.
15. Miller, C. Working with parents of high-risk infants. *Am. J. Nurs.* 78:1228, 1978.
16. Schraeder, B. D. Attachment and parenting despite lengthy intensive care. *M.C.N.* 5:37, 1980.
17. Spikes, J., et al. Nursing care plans for the special care nursery. *Superv. Nurse* 10:23, 1979.
18. Sugarman, M. Regionalization of maternity and newborn care: How we can make a good thing better. *Perinat. Neonatol.* 2:39, 1978.

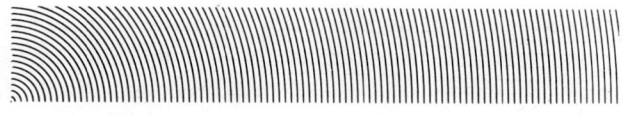

38. The Infant with a Congenital Anomaly or Neonatal Illness

High-risk infants need skilled health care personnel in attendance during delivery and the first few days of life, not only to save their life, but also to protect well-being so carefully that neurological disorders do not develop and mental retardation is prevented. Women should be screened during pregnancy or at a pregnancy's end for the factors that lead to high-risk infants.

Being able to predict that the infant to be born will be a high-risk infant makes it possible to arrange beforehand for adequate health care personnel to be present at the delivery. This is extremely important, because a high-risk infant may have difficulty establishing respirations and may need resuscitation in the delivery room. All newborns should be closely observed in the neonatal period until it is confirmed that they have no anomalies and are doing well.

Priorities in First Days of Life

All infants have six needs that take precedence over all others in the first few days of life: initiation and maintenance of respirations, establishment of extrauterine circulation, control of body temperature, intake of adequate nourishment, prevention of infection, and establishment of an infant-parent relationship. These are also the six priority needs of high-risk infants, but with such infants the means to meet them may have to be modified for their particular problems and may require special equipment or care.

Initiation and Maintenance of Respirations

The ultimate prognosis in an infant depends a great deal on how his first moments of life are managed. Most deaths in the first 48 hours after delivery are the result of an inability to establish adequate respirations. An infant who has difficulty accomplishing effective respiratory action but survives may pay the penalty of residual brain damage. There is little victory in a race that ultimately ends in cerebral palsy, recurrent convulsions, or mental retardation.

Most infants are born with some degree of respiratory acidosis, but the spontaneous onset of respirations rapidly corrects it. If respiratory activity does not begin immediately, respiratory acidosis will increase. The blood pH and buffer base will fall, and newborn defense mechanisms are inadequate to reverse the process. Therefore, efforts to establish respirations must be begun in the first 2 minutes after birth; by 2 minutes, the development of severe acidosis is well under way.

Resuscitation comprises three organized steps: establishment and maintenance of an airway, expansion of the lungs, and initiation and maintenance of effective ventilation.

In order that resuscitation can be done effectively, every delivery room should have available the following equipment:

An oxygen supply and a source of suction separate from those needed for the mother
A warm blanket to dry the infant
A radiant heat table on which procedures can be performed without cooling the infant
A suction bulb and suction catheters (8F or 10F, attached to a de Lee mucus trap)
An infant laryngoscope with premature and infant-sized blades
An infant endotracheal tube and pharyngeal airway
An infant bag and mask or resuscitator
Emergency drugs such as naloxone, sodium bicarbonate, glucose, salt-poor albumin, isoproterenol
A heart rate monitor
Equipment for intravenous administration of fluids and medicine
Equipment for umbilical vessel catheterization
A good light source

ESTABLISHMENT OF AN AIRWAY

Immediately after birth, the infant should be dried with the warm sterile blanket and placed on the radiant heat table on his side with his head slightly lowered (15 to 30 degrees Trendelenburg) to allow mucus to drain from his nose and throat. The 1-minute Apgar score serves as a useful guide to whether resuscitation is necessary or not.

The Infant with an Apgar Score of 7 to 10

An infant with a score of 7 to 10 rarely needs resuscitation. A score this high is possible only if respiratory and cardiac functions have been established. He needs only bulb syringe suction to establish a clear airway.

The Infant with an Apgar Score of 3 to 6

An infant with a score of 3 to 6 is moderately depressed. He generally has heart action but he has not yet breathed; he looks cyanotic; his muscle tone and reflex irritability are poor.

Alert the physician present to the low Apgar score; suction the infant's nose and mouth and rub his back gently as skin stimulation may initiate respirations.

SUCTION. To clear the airway, secretions should be aspirated from the nose and mouth after delivery of the head, and again before any mechanical resuscitation measures are initiated, not only to allow air to enter the infant's lungs but to prevent aspiration of mucus or amniotic fluid at the first breath. Aspiration of the nose, mouth, and pharynx by itself may initiate respirations.

Suction can be done by a bulb syringe, by negative mouth pressure, or mechanically.

BULB SYRINGE. A bulb syringe is adequate for removing secretions from the mouth and nose (unless mucus is meconium-stained; meconium is too sticky to be pulled easily through a bulb syringe).

To suction, depress the bulb first, then insert it into the infant's mouth. Gradually relieve the compressed bulb to suction mucus. Always be sure to compress the syringe before inserting it; otherwise the compression of the syringe will push mucus farther back into the infant's pharynx rather than remove it.

Newborns are nose-breathers. Always suction the nose following removal of secretions from the mouth to ensure a clear airway. Always suction the mouth first, as stimulating the nose may cause the infant to breathe in and he breathes in the secretions in his mouth.

Suctioning by a bulb syringe is gentle, so there is little danger of causing trauma to tissue. Its disadvantage is that it only achieves local mouth and nose suction, not lower airway suction.

NEGATIVE MOUTH SUCTION. For deeper suction, place the infant on his back, slide a folded towel or pad under his shoulders to raise them a small amount, and slightly hyperextend the head. Slide a catheter (8F to 12F) over the infant's tongue to the back of the throat. Suck on the distal end of the catheter as if drinking fluid through a straw. Using a mucus trap between the infant and yourself prevents mucus from being sucked into your mouth. It also allows for easy inspection of the fluid removed. There is little danger that suction will lead to tissue damage if just mouth suction is used.

MECHANICAL SUCTION. When introducing a suction catheter with a mechanical suction source, be certain that the power is off during insertion and turned on only during withdrawal (Fig. 38-1). The catheter will not pass well with the suction source on as it tends to cling to the walls of the pharynx. Do not suction for longer than 10 seconds at a time; use a gentle touch. Bradycardia or cardiac arrhythmias can occur because of vagus stimulation from vigorous suctioning.

Keep the infant under a radiant heat source to prevent chilling. If you do not have an overhead radiant source, keep the baby wrapped as much as possible to conserve body heat.

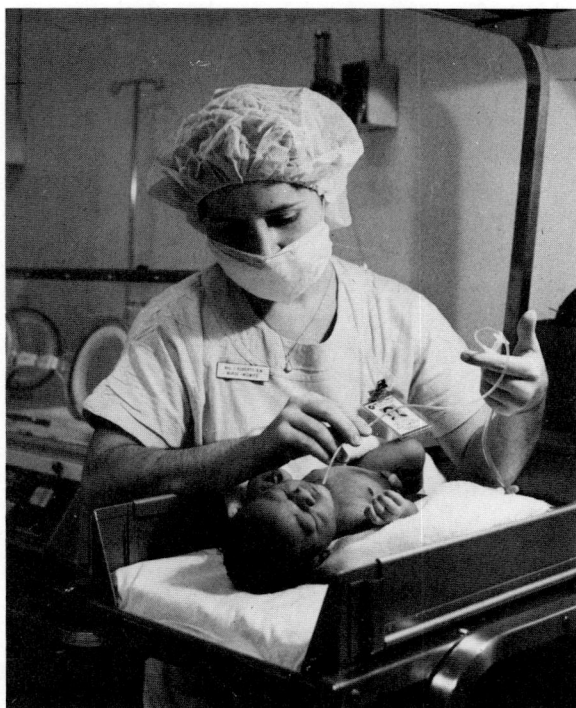

Fig. 38-1. Suctioning a newborn with mechanical suction controlled by a finger valve. Suction is applied as the catheter is withdrawn. If the catheter is rotated as it is withdrawn, the risk of traumatizing membrane is reduced. (From J. E. Roberts, Suctioning the newborn. Am. J. Nurs. 73:63, 1973.)

The Infant with an Apgar Score of 0 to 2

When an infant has an Apgar score as low as 0 to 2, he is severely depressed. There are generally no respirations and no heartbeat (or a very slow one); the infant is blue and limp.

The infant requires immediate laryngoscopy so that his airway can be deep-suctioned and an endotracheal tube can be inserted and oxygen administered by a pressure source.

In the first few seconds of his life, a severely depressed infant may take several weak gasps of air, then almost immediately stop. When he stops this period is termed *primary apnea*. Following a minute or two of apnea, the infant again tries to initiate respirations with a few strong gasps. He cannot maintain this effort longer than 4 or 5 minutes, however; his respiratory effort will become weaker and weaker until he stops the gasping effort altogether. He then enters a period of *secondary apnea*.

During the period of the first gasps or primary apnea, resuscitation attempts are generally successful. If the infant is allowed to enter the secondary apnea period, however, resuscitation measures are very difficult and may not be effective. It is important, therefore, that the person caring for the baby (who is often a nurse) recognizes the infant's distress and initiates or secures someone to initiate resuscitation measures before the last gasp occurs.

LARYNGOSCOPE INSERTION. Someone (obstetrician, pediatrician, anesthesiologist, or nurse with extended skills) who is adept at passing infant endotracheal tubes should be present at the delivery of all high-risk infants. Laryngoscope insertion is easy in theory; in practice, because there is a wide variation in the size of an infant's posterior pharynx and trachea and it is always done under emergency conditions, it can be very difficult.

A tube of the Cole type that widens 2 cm from the tip is a preferred type, since it prevents overinsertion. The size of the tube used varies from an 8F to a 12F, depending on the size of the infant. Because premature infants tend to be prone to hemorrhage due to capillary fragility, extra gentleness must be used in passing the endotracheal tube with these high-risk infants.

The infant should be placed on his back on a flat surface; a folded towel or pad is slipped under his shoulders to raise them slightly and hyperextend the neck (Fig. 38-2). His mouth is opened by pressing down on his lower jaw and the laryngoscope blade slid gently along the side of his tongue on the right side of his mouth. At the rear of the mouth, the blade is brought to the midline and the tongue pushed to the side so that it is depressed and does not obscure the view of the pharynx. With the laryngoscope at the entrance to the pharynx, the epiglottis is generally

Fig. 38-2. Intubation. The head should be slightly hyperextended by a towel under the shoulders. The blade of the laryngoscope is inserted to reveal the vocal cords. An endotracheal tube for ventilation is passed into the trachea, past the laryngoscope.

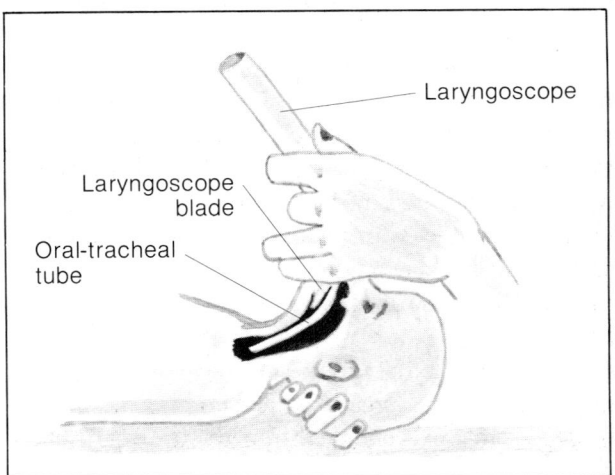

easily visualized. It is a slit-like opening. Elevating the tip of the laryngoscope blade brings the vocal cords into view. Any mucus or meconium present on the vocal cords is suctioned away with a catheter. An endotracheal tube is inserted through the laryngoscope down into the trachea about an inch beyond the vocal cords. The laryngoscope is removed; oxygen can then be administered by the endotracheal tube.

If a laryngoscope does not pass readily, the difficulty is generally that the infant's neck is hyperextended too far. Listen with a stethoscope to both lungs as oxygen is administered to be certain that both sides of the lungs are being aerated. If air can be heard on only one side, the endotracheal tube is probably at the bifurcation of the trachea and blocking one of the main-stem bronchi. Drawing it back half a centimeter will usually free it and allow oxygen flow to both lungs.

EXPANSION OF THE LUNGS
Once a clear airway has been established, the infant next needs his lungs expanded.

The Infant with an Apgar Score of 7 to 10
The infant with a high Apgar score inflates his lungs adequately with his first breath. The sound of the baby crying is proof that lung expansion is good. Vocal sounds are produced by a free flow of air over the vocal cords.

The Infant with an Apgar Score of 3 to 6
Following suction, this infant may need oxygen by mask to initiate lung expansion. An infant mask should cover both the mouth and the nose to be effective. It should not cover the eyes, as it can cause eye injury. If no respirations are present or the infant's heart rate is below 100, administer oxygen by face mask and pressure bag at a rate of about 40 compressions a minute. Oxygen up to 100% concentration can be used.

The pressure needed to open lung alveoli for the first time is about 35 cm of water pressure. After that, pressures of 10 to 20 cm H_2O are generally adequate to reinflate alveoli. The pressure from bags of the MIE type (that used by anesthesiologists) is controlled by the pressure of your hand; other types of bags such as an AMBU bag can be set with a "blowoff" valve so the pressure in the apparatus does not exceed a certain limit.

It is important that no pressure above what is necessary is used or the force may rupture lung alveoli. To be certain that oxygen is reaching the lungs, the chest should be auscultated simultaneously with the oxygen administration.

In many infants this degree of resuscitation will initiate responsive respirations and a strong heartbeat. Color, muscle response, and reflexes will improve.

If the infant's amniotic fluid was meconium-stained, do not administer air or oxygen under pressure or you will push meconium down into the infant's airway and compromise his respirations even further. Give oxygen by mask without pressure and wait for a laryngoscope to be passed and the trachea to be deep-suctioned before oxygen under pressure is given.

The Infant with an Apgar Score of 0 to 2
This infant will need to have oxygen administered by the endotracheal tube. Whether oxygen is administered by mask or by endotracheal tube, initial lung pressure will need to be higher than continuing pressure in order to cause initial lung expansion. Pressures of oxygen over 44 cm H_2O should be used with extreme caution; efforts to open atelectatic areas by increased pressure may rupture lung areas already fully expanded. On the other hand, if adequate insufflation is not achieved, the infant stands little chance of survival.

When oxygen is given under pressure to a newborn, not only his lungs but also his stomach quickly fills with oxygen. Inserting an oral-gastric tube and leaving the distal end open will deflate the stomach and decrease the possibility that vomiting and aspiration of stomach contents will occur.

DRUG THERAPY. Stimulants have very little place in resuscitation unless the infant's respiratory depression appears to be related to the administration of a narcotic such as morphine, meperidine (Demerol), or anileridine (Leritine). In those instances, a narcotic antagonist such as naloxone injected into an umbilical vessel will relieve the depression.

Mouth-to-Mouth Resuscitation
When you find yourself the only person in the delivery room to establish respirations in an emergency situation and you are untrained in the use of the endotracheal tube or other resuscitation methods, mouth-to-mouth resuscitation is the wisest step. The mouth and pharynx of the infant should be aspirated with a bulb syringe to clear secretions. A clean piece of gauze may be placed over the infant's mouth. Place your mouth over the infant's mouth and nose and begin mouth breathing at a rate of about 40 breaths per minute. Utilize only the air in your mouth and

use short, sharp puffs. With the use of this small amount of air there is little danger of rupture of either the pulmonary alveoli or the stomach, which fills with air during resuscitation. Allow time for the child to exhale between each of your exhalations (elastic recoil of the lungs accomplishes this). Note rising of the chest to determine the effectiveness of the mouth-to-mouth breathing. The chest wall should rise and fall if the lungs are being filled.

Procedures such as spanking, slapping the baby's back, tubbing, or squeezing the thorax do more harm than good and should not be attempted.

MAINTENANCE OF EFFECTIVE VENTILATION

In order to allow the infant to adjust to cardiovascular changes during the newborn period, effective ventilation in the infant must be maintained. The healthy infant accomplishes this on his own. The ill infant may need support.

The Infant with an Apgar Score of 7 to 10

This infant needs only careful watching for the first 24 hours of life with special emphasis on his respiratory rate and checks that his airway is free of mucus.

The Infant with a Low Apgar Score

All infants who have trouble breathing at birth should be carefully observed in the next few days to be certain that this is not a continuing problem.

Babies who are high-risk for respiratory difficulty in the first few hours or days of life (some may have deceptively high Apgar scores) are the following:

Low-birth-weight infants
Infants whose mothers had a history of diabetes
Infants associated with premature rupture of membranes
Infants whose mothers had a history of reserpine use
Infants whose mothers used barbiturates or narcotics close to delivery
Infants associated with meconium staining
Infants in whom irregularities were detected during fetal heart monitoring during labor
Infants associated with cord prolapse
Infants needing resuscitation at birth
Infants with lowered Apgar score (under 7)
Postmature infants
Infants who are small for gestation age
Breech-born infants
Multiple-birth infants
Infants with chest, heart, or respiratory tract anomalies

Respiratory difficulty occurring after the initial establishment of respirations generally begins subtly. Picking up the first presenting signs is a nursing responsibility. Make a habit of counting the newborn's respiratory rate before you disturb the infant to begin to undress him. An increasing respiratory rate is often the first sign of obstruction or respiratory compromise. If the respiratory rate is increased, undress the baby's chest and look for retractions. Retractions are an inward sucking of the anterior chest wall on inspiration. They reflect the difficulty the infant is having in drawing in air (he is tugging so hard to inflate his lungs that his anterior chest muscles are pulled in too). Retractions can be subcostal (under the last rib), intercostal (between ribs), or supracostal (above the ribs).

An infant who is retracting generally has an increased heart rate. If intervention to aid breathing is not begun at this point, cyanosis and an even faster heart rate will occur. Cyanosis is first localized circumoral, then facial, then total body. The infant will begin to have apneic episodes (pauses or cessation of breathing for over 15 seconds), irregular respirations, and flaring of the nares. Sounds of airway obstruction such as expiratory grunting or inspiratory stridor may be heard.

Auscultating the chest in most newborns reveals rhonchi (the loud harsh sound of mucus in the throat). If respiratory distress is present, the sound of rales (air being pulled through fluid in alveoli, a sound simulating the crinkle of cellophane) may be heard; diminished or absent breath sounds of atelectasis may be noted.

Infants who are having difficulty with breathing should have the weight of clothing removed from the chest. They generally appear to be in less distress if they are positioned on their backs with the head of the mattress elevated about 15 degrees to allow abdominal contents to fall away from the diaphragm and afford optimal breathing space.

Keeping the infant warm is important. He can then use his energy for respiratory effort, not for maintaining temperature. If secretions are accumulating in the respiratory tract, he should be suctioned. Bagging an infant for a minute prior to suction will improve the PO_2 level and prevent it from dropping to dangerous levels during suctioning. The infant may need glucose in order to prevent hypoglycemia resulting from his activity and extreme respiratory effort. At the same time, infants with respiratory distress cannot suck because of their rapid breathing. Intravenous fluid may be necessary. Oxygen may have to be administered or ventilation begun. The cause of the respiratory distress must be determined and appropriate interventions to correct the difficulty undertaken.

OXYGEN ADMINISTRATION

Low levels of oxygen may be administered to infants in Isolettes by flooding the Isolette with a certain concentration of oxygen. This method is ineffective for supplying high levels of oxygen because when the portholes are opened to give the baby care a proportion of the concentration always escapes.

Oxygen hoods (a plastic box with inlet connections that fits across the infant's head) allow for high concentrations of oxygen to be given yet provide easy access to the infant for other procedures. Oxygen hoods tend to become very warm; the temperature of the hood needs to be checked every 30 to 60 minutes. The hood should be placed so that the stream of oxygen does not blow directly on the infant's face.

Masks with free-flowing oxygen vary in their ability to deliver high concentrations of oxygen, depending on the fit of the mask. Masks with pressure bags can deliver high concentrations. Pressure bags or ventilators used with endotracheal tubes are the most efficient method of delivering high concentrations of oxygen to the neonate.

Oxygen must always be warmed and humidified when given to newborns. Cold oxygen blowing across the face of a newborn affects temperature receptors in the face and causes him to increase his metabolism (he interprets the local cold as systemic cold). This increase in metabolism increases his need for oxygen. Dry oxygen leads to drying of mucous membrane. Cracks in mucous membrane from extreme drying can be a source of infection.

Oxygen Concentration

At one time, on the basis of occurrences of retrolental fibroplasia (atrophy of the retina) in immature infants due to high concentrations of oxygen, there was a reluctance to give oxygen in concentrations over 40% to newborns. An infant who needs oxygen in greater concentration than this, however, in order to maintain his PO_2 at normal limits may receive it in concentrations up to 100% without difficulty. Trouble occurs when the oxygen concentration is given in excess of what is needed or when high levels (over 60%) are needed for an extended time.

Concentrations of oxygen being administered must be checked by an oxygen analyzer to be certain that they are as high as desired but not higher. Oxygen analyzers must be checked daily against a 100% concentration to make sure they are registering correctly.

Despite the concentration of oxygen in the hood or Isolette or being administered by a ventilator, the true test of how much oxygen is reaching alveoli or being transported across alveoli is the level of the PO_2. Oxygen must not be given to newborns except in emergencies unless blood gas analysis is available.

In an emergency, if an infant is cyanotic, it is safe to administer oxygen to the point of decreasing cyanosis. Raise the oxygen level to the point at which cyanosis disappears; lower it at 10 percent intervals until cyanosis appears again. Raise it at 5 percent intervals until cyanosis disappears again. Administer it at that level. At the end of 15 minutes, repeat the process to test that the same level of oxygen is still needed. Arrangements must be made for transport to a center where blood gas analysis is available.

Blood Gases

The normal PO_2 in a newborn is 50 to 80 mm Hg. Cyanosis does not become apparent until the PO_2 is 40 to 50 mm Hg.

With respiratory distress, when the infant is unable to ventilate his lungs, his PO_2 level will fall; the PCO_2 level will rise. Many infants are unable to pull in enough oxygen, so the PO_2 level falls but carbon dioxide is still eliminated from the lungs. Thus there is not the marked increase in PCO_2 as in adults.

As an immediate response to hypoxia (low PO_2 levels), blood vessels to nonessential organs become constricted in an attempt to save oxygen for essential organs. In the newborn, a low level of circulating oxygen can cause reopening of the ductus arteriosus as the low oxygen level simulates uterine conditions. The infant begins shunting blood, creating an ineffective circulatory pattern or adding to his already compromised breathing efforts.

As the hypoxia increases, oxygenation of body cells fails and anaerobic metabolism begins. This involves formation of lactic acid as an end product rather than the normal production of carbon dioxide and water and leads to a metabolic acidosis. Free fatty acids in the bloodstream compete with indirect bilirubin for binding sites on albumin molecules and increase the amount of indirect bilibrubin in the bloodstream. High levels of indirect bilirubin can cause brain damage due to kernicterus. Anaerobic metabolism calls for larger amounts of glucose than are normal. If the infant is not receiving a glucose supplement, he quickly depletes glycogen stores and becomes hypoglycemic.

Table 38-1. Blood Gases

Determination	Normal Value	Assessment
Oxygen saturation	96–98%	The proportion of hemoglobin which is filled and carrying oxygen. If oxygen cannot reach the bloodstream to unite with hemoglobin, saturation level will be low
PO_2	80–100 mm Hg	The partial pressure of oxygen in arterial blood. Values under normal denote hypoxia; values above normal are dangerous to the neonate in that they can cause lung and eye damage
PCO_2	35–45 mm Hg	The partial pressure of carbon dioxide in the arterial blood. Levels under normal denote respiratory alkalosis; levels above normal denote respiratory acidosis
pH	7.35–7.45	The acidity of the blood or the proportion of hydrogen ions present. A level under 7.25 is clinical acidosis; infants cannot live for a long period with extreme acidosis. Acidosis can be caused by poor excretion of carbon dioxide leading to excess carbonic acid in the blood (respiratory acidosis) or the excess production of nonvolatile acids from metabolism (metabolic acidosis). Alkalosis can occur from vomiting or removal of stomach contents before gavage-feedings.
Base excess	+2 or −2	The amount of bicarbonate in arterial blood. Bicarbonate buffers or counteracts acids. Low base excess levels suggest that the infant has used his reserve buffering potential; he is in acute danger of acidosis

To counteract the respiratory acidosis occurring (the accumulation of PCO_2), the infant must be ventilated. He attempts to counteract the metabolic acidosis (caused by the formation of lactic acid) by utilizing his buffering system or increasing the amount of bicarbonate in the bloodstream. Over a very short time, the newborn exhausts his ability to do this.

Babies who are being ventilated need frequent blood gas measurements for both PO_2 and PCO_2 levels plus pH, base excess, and oxygen saturation levels. If ventilation is too rapid, too much carbon dioxide is removed and the PCO_2 level will be low; the normal oxygen may be increased too much and oxygen toxicity can occur. It is not true that in order to relieve distress, if a little oxygen is good for an infant, a lot will be even better. Normal blood gas values are shown in Table 38-1.

Blood gas measurements must be made from arterial blood. In many instances, in newborns, the blood is obtained from the umbilical artery by catheterization. If a syringe with a dilute heparin solution is attached to the catheter to keep the catheter patent, blood can be withdrawn from the site at frequent intervals without reinsertion of a catheter. Sterile technique must be used when irrigating umbilical vessels or withdrawing blood samples from this site; the umbilical artery enters a major infant vessel (the aorta), and septicemia will easily result if pathogens are introduced at this point. Brachial or radial or temporal arteries may be used. A heel prick may be used.

This method is accurate for PCO_2 and pH values; it is questionable for PO_2 value. The heel should be warmed prior to the prick by application of a warm moist pack. This dilates heel capillaries and brings arterial blood into the heel.

In the baby with a patent ductus arteriosus, blood drawn from an artery proximal to the shunt, such as the right radial artery, offers better evaluation of the oxygen reaching the brain and eyes than does blood drawn from the umbilical artery. This is an important determination because the eye is one organ that excessive oxygen levels can destroy.

Blood gas determinations should be taken about 15 to 30 minutes after any change in amount of oxygen being administered or rate or depth of ventilator settings so that the true condition of the infant following the adjustment can be determined.

All blood gas specimens should be placed in ice for transport to the laboratory for analysis. If blood remains at room temperature, the pH level will fall, the PCO_2 will rise, and the accuracy of the sample will be lost.

A new method of obtaining oxygen levels is by use of transcutaneous electrodes. The PO_2 level obtained by this method correlates well with that obtained by drawing arterial blood, and this method has the added advantages of being noninvasive and of removing no blood from the infant. One problem with ill neonates is that so much blood is drawn for frequent laboratory determinations that infants develop a blood loss anemia to add to their already disease-stressed state.

Transcutaneous electrodes are heated to 44°C to bring a ready supply of blood to the skin site. Occasionally this may cause a skin blister, but this can be prevented if the electrode site is changed every 2 hours. Having a continuous readout of PO_2 values allows you to modify your care appropriately. If an oxygen level begins to fall while you are handling the baby, for example, you would immediately stop care until the infant's PO_2 again returns to normal. Transcutaneous electrodes can be helpful in identifying whether a patent ductus arteriosus exists. If one electrode is placed in a preductal site (the baby's upper right chest) and one on a postductal site (below the chest nipple line), a comparison of the two values will reveal different levels of oxygen (the preductal electrode reading will be higher) if a patent ductus arteriosus is present.

Umbilical Catheterization

Newborns have an insertion site for intravenous fluid or withdrawal of blood samples that is not available at any other time in life: the umbilical vessels. Infants who need exchange transfusions in the first few days of life have them done through an umbilical vein.

The insertion of a catheter into an umbilical vessel must be achieved under sterile conditions. The umbilicus is prepared with an antibiotic solution and draped. The umbilical cord is cut crossways so that the vessels are apparent. A thin polyethylene tube is inserted into the selected vessel. Since the catheter is opaque on x-ray film, its location in the umbilical vessel is confirmed by x-ray examination. Catheters are generally placed in an artery in preference to the vein because insertion in the vein tends to cause thrombosis and liver damage (the vein enters the liver directly).

The catheter must be taped in place so it cannot be dislodged by the infant (this is insertion into a large vessel; bleeding after dislodgment of a catheter can be severe). Antibiotic ointment may be applied at the insertion site to discourage infection.

Infants with umbilical vessel catheters in place must have the site checked frequently to be certain that redness of inflammation or bleeding is not occurring. The lower extremities should be checked for warmth and pedal pulses taken to be sure that the catheter is not obscuring the femoral artery and interfering with lower-extremity circulation.

If the vessel line is being used only for arterial blood gases, it is kept patent by being filled with a dilute solution of heparin. Small increments of heparin are added as ordered (every 1 to 2 hours) to keep blood from clotting at the tip of the tube and obstructing the line.

Bronchopulmonary Dysplasia

Excessive amounts of oxygen lead to irritation of lung tissue. Alveoli may collapse, causing atelectasis; the support tissue of the alveoli tends to become so thickened that they lose their elasticity and ability to transfer oxygen and maintain independent respiration. These lung changes are likely when oxygen concentrations over 60% are given for an extended time or when ventilatory assistance with high pressure is needed for an extended time. Infants show some improvement in lung tissue over a time period, but most of the tissue change is permanent. An infant with bronchopulmonary dysplasia becomes respirator-dependent; his prognosis for survival decreases rapidly.

Retrolental Fibroplasia

Although retrolental fibroplasia (atrophy of the eye retina) may occur in any infant who is receiving oxygen, it is most prevalent in immature infants and so is discussed in Chap. 39.

VENTILATION AND NEWBORNS

As high-risk care of newborns becomes a specialty, the number of types of ventilators that are available for aiding respiratory function in newborns grows. Different brands of equipment have different capabilities. All have factors in common: They deliver moistened or nebulized air or oxygen to the lungs under enough pressure and with appropriate timing to produce artificial, periodic inflation of alveoli; they rely on the elastic recoil of the lungs to empty the alveoli.

Depending on the type of ventilator, the inspiration-expiration cycle may be determined by a timed interval, a volume limit, or a pressure limit. With a volume limit, a certain volume of air or oxygen is pushed into the lungs with each inspiration. With a pressure limit, air or oxygen is pushed only until a set level of resistance is reached.

Ventilators may be set to breathe completely for the infant; to assist or augment the infant's own inspiratory efforts; or to assist-control, augmenting the normal respiratory effort and, in addition, adding a preset number of controlled inspirations every minute to ensure good ventilation. You cannot be expected to be a ventilator repairman, but you must be familiar with any piece of equipment being used and its capabilities and specific function for an individual child.

A ventilator is used with a tracheotomy tube or endotracheal tube. In neonates, the endotracheal tube is preferred. If a tracheotomy tube is used, it must have a cuff fitted around it to prevent leakage at the tube site. This cuff must be deflated every hour for about 5 minutes or kept at a pressure just short of occlusion or necrosis of the trachea from the constant pressure will result.

Continuous Positive Airway Pressure

Continuous positive airway pressure (CPAP) is a method of ventilatory assistance initiated by endotracheal tube or nasal prongs causing the infant to continuously breathe out against pressure. It ensures that lung alveoli do not collapse on expiration, a common problem with respiratory distress syndrome. Once alveoli collapse, an opening pressure three times that normally required must be used with each breath to continue respirations (each breath is like a first breath). CPAP, then, reduces the effort the child must make to breathe and allows for easy entry of oxygen to alveoli. If nasal prongs are used, the nares must be inspected frequently for areas of pressure that could lead to tissue breakdown.

Positive End-Expiratory Pressure

Positive end-expiratory pressure (PEEP) can be added to ventilatory assistance to accomplish the same goals as with CPAP. It adds pressure at the end of the expiratory phase rather than continuously to prevent alveoli from collapsing, allowing better oxygen entry with the next inspiration and less breathing effort.

Postural Drainage

Postural drainage is the use of gravity to drain secretions from bronchi. Even newborns have a cough reflex, but since they do not use it effectively, most infants with respiratory difficulty need some outside intervention such as postural drainage to help them clear their respiratory tract of secretions and raise sputum.

Changing the infant from side to side every 1 or 2 hours aids in preventing stasis of fluid. Tilting him so that his chest is lower than his abdomen aids in the drainage of secretions. There is a risk in placing infants who are prone to intracranial hemorrhage in this position as it increases blood pressure in the head and may lead to bleeding.

CUPPING AND VIBRATING. Cupping is manual percussion of lung areas to loosen secretions. It is done with the hand held in a "cupped" or dome-shaped position or with a cupping device. When the chest is struck with the hand in this position, it produces a hollow echoing sound. The vibration of the percussion loosens the secretions. This is done for 30 to 60 seconds over a lung area. Suctioning the infant after the procedure will remove loosened secretions.

Although cupping and vibrating sounds forceful, it is not painful. Parents need to understand this or they will be reluctant to have it done to their child. Demonstrating the technique on the parent is the easiest way to show that it is not painful.

Postural drainage and cupping may be done by respiratory therapists or by nurses. Such techniques for drainage should not be used after feeding as they may lead to regurgitation and aspiration.

Establishment of Extrauterine Circulation

Although difficulty in the establishment of respirations is the usual critical problem in the delivery room, lack of cardiac function may be present concurrently. If there is no cardiac function at birth, or if cardiac arrest subsequently occurs because of the lack of respirations, closed chest massage should be started. This is accomplished by placing the index and middle finger of the right hand on the infant's chest over the middle third of the sternum or holding the infant with the fingers on the back and pressing the thumbs against the sternum (Fig. 38-3). Depress the sternum about 1 or 2 cm, at a rate of 100 to 120 times per minute. If pressure and rate of massage are adequate, a femoral pulse will be present. If heart sounds are not resumed after a minute of massage, an intracardiac injection of epinephrine may be given. Intravenous glucose and sodium bicarbonate (2 to 3 mEq per kilogram of body weight diluted 1:1) will be administered to maintain blood glucose levels and reduce acidosis. Lung ventilation at a rate of 40 times per minute should be carried out concurrently with the cardiac massage in the proportion of six heart contractions, then one ventilation, six heart contractions, etc.

Infants who had difficulty initiating cardiac function need to be transferred to a transitional or high-risk

Fig. 38-3. External cardiac massage. The thumbs are on the sternum, with the fingertips on the back.

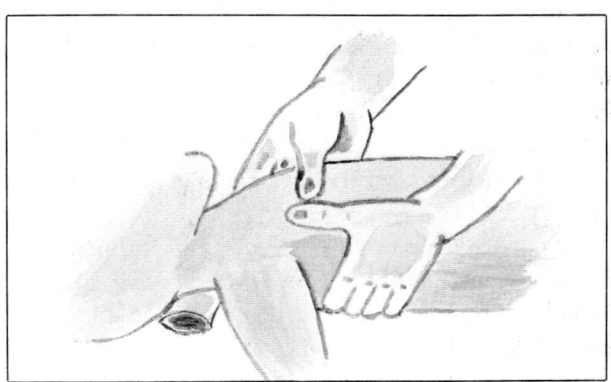

nursery for continuous surveillance of their cardiac function.

Temperature Regulation

Any high-risk infant may have difficulty maintaining a normal temperature. In addition to stress from an illness or immaturity, he is exposed more often than the healthy infant because of such procedures as resuscitation, blood drawing, and intravenous regulation.

Special efforts to prevent chilling must be taken in the delivery room. Wet infants must not be allowed to be exposed while resuscitation or physical assessment is carried out. Such infants may arrive at a special care nursery cyanotic and so cold that their temperature is unrecordable. To avoid this situation, the infant should be wiped dry and wrapped in a warm blanket or placed immediately in a warmed Isolette. If the infant must be removed from the Isolette for procedures, these should be performed under a radiant heat source.

Controlling the environmental air by placing the infant in an Isolette or under a radiant heat source is done to keep the baby's metabolic rate, and therefore his oxygen consumption, at its lowest. Below a certain environmental temperature, the infant must increase his metabolic rate to keep his temperature from falling. Increased oxygen is required. Body cells become hypoxic. In order to save oxygen for essential body functions, vasoconstriction of blood vessels occurs. If the process continues too long, pulmonary vessels are also affected and pulmonary perfusion will be affected. The infant's PO_2 level will fall and his PCO_2 increase. The infant begins to become acidotic. The decreased PO_2 level may open fetal right-to-left shunts again. In order to supply glucose to maintain increased metabolism, the infant begins anaerobic glycolysis, which pours acid into the bloodstream.

Because of the simple act of being cold, the infant has become acidotic and cyanotic. With acidosis, the risk of kernicterus (invasion of brain cells with unconjugated bilirubin) rises as more bilirubin-bonding sites are lost and more free bilirubin passes out of the bloodstream into brain cells.

The temperature necessary to keep the infant in the neutral zone of lowest metabolic rate is highest in the first two days of life.

Axillary temperatures (see Fig. 31-7) are preferred to rectal temperatures to prevent excessive stooling (which could lead to loss of body fluids and electrolytes). The axillary temperature should be maintained at 97.8°F (36.5°C). Some Isolettes have servomechanism units that monitor the infant's temperature and automatically change the temperature of the Isolette as needed.

Radiant heat sources have servocontrol probes so that the infant's temperature can be continually monitored. Abdominal skin temperature measured by a probe this way should be 97°F (35.1°C). Tape the probe or disk in place on the infant's abdomen between the umbilicus and the xiphoid process. Be sure that it is not over the rib cage or the thinness of subcutaneous tissue at that point will not allow for accurate readings.

Incubator temperatures for infants under 1,500 gm (3 pounds, 4 ounces) should be about 93°F to 95°F for the first days. Babies over 2,500 gm (5 pounds, 8 ounces) usually need an incubator temperature of 89.6°F to 93°F for their first days. Infants between 1,500 gm and 2,500 gm require a temperature of 91°F to 93°F.

An infant in an incubator should be undressed except for a diaper, so that the flow of air will contact his body surface. Portholes must remain closed to keep the temperature steady and as a safety measure (small infants can fit through a porthole and fall).

The temperature of Isolettes varies with the amount of time portholes are open and the temperature of the area where the Isolette is placed. Direct sunlight or a warm radiator can increase the temperature. Isolette temperature must be checked at frequent intervals to be certain the temperature level designated is being maintained.

Once the infant's temperature is stabilized, incubator temperatures should not be changed at will. Otherwise, a change in the infant's temperature, which might be the first indication of disease, may be misinterpreted as a change in the temperature of the incubator.

Infants who are cold need to be warmed, but warming too rapidly can cause periods of apnea and severe acidosis as the infant's metabolism rate increases. Proper warming can be done by setting an incubator temperature 2°F (1.2°C) above the infant's temperature. Wait for the infant's temperature to increase those two degrees, then reset two more degrees and so forth until the infant's temperature reaches normal.

Weaning an infant from an incubator is done the same way: Dress the infant as if he were going to be in a bassinet, then set the incubator slightly lower step by step until Isolette temperature is room temperature. If the infant cannot maintain his temperature as the incubator temperature level is brought down, he is not yet ready for room temperature air and the weaning process needs to be slowed or stopped until he is more mature or less ill.

Nutrition

BREAST- AND FORMULA-FEEDING

Because the high-risk infant may tire easily or have a congenital anomaly that interferes with sucking, obtaining nourishment by bottle- or breast-feeding may not be possible. A mother who wants to breast-feed must have a realistic appraisal of her child's needs. If the child is almost mature enough to suck, or will have only a brief extended hospital stay for other reasons, she can manually express breast milk to initiate and continue her milk supply until the infant is mature enough or otherwise ready for breast-feeding. Expressed breast milk may be used as the infant's feeding. If the hospital stay will be lengthy, however, she might be well advised to bottle-feed the baby. The decision will rest with the mother, and the depth of her interest in breast-feeding will affect it.

All babies who cannot be fed by bottle or breast need oral stimulation and should be supplied with a pacifier at feeding times. Exceptions are infants too immature to have a sucking reflex formed yet and infants who must not swallow air, such as one with a tracheoesophageal fistula awaiting surgery.

GAVAGE-FEEDING

Gavage-feeding (Fig. 38-4) is a means of supplying adequate nutrition to the infant who is unable to suck or tires too easily to suck. To prepare for single gavage-feedings, the space from the bridge of the infant's nose to a point halfway between the umbilicus and the xiphoid process is measured against a No. 8 or No. 10 gavage tube. The tube is marked at this point by a small Kelly clamp or piece of tape. It is important that the tube be measured this way to ensure that it enters the stomach after it is passed. A tube passed too far will curl and end up in the esophagus; a tube passed not far enough will also be in the esophagus. Both situations could cause the feeding to be aspirated into the lungs.

The baby should be swaddled to be certain his arms will be out of the way and turned onto his back. His head should be slightly hyperextended. The tip of the catheter may be lubricated by sterile water. An oil lubricant should never be used. Although the tube is going to be passed into the stomach, it is occasionally passed into the trachea accidentally. Oil left in the trachea could lead to lipoid pneumonia, a complication that an infant already burdened with a deviation from the normal may not be able to survive.

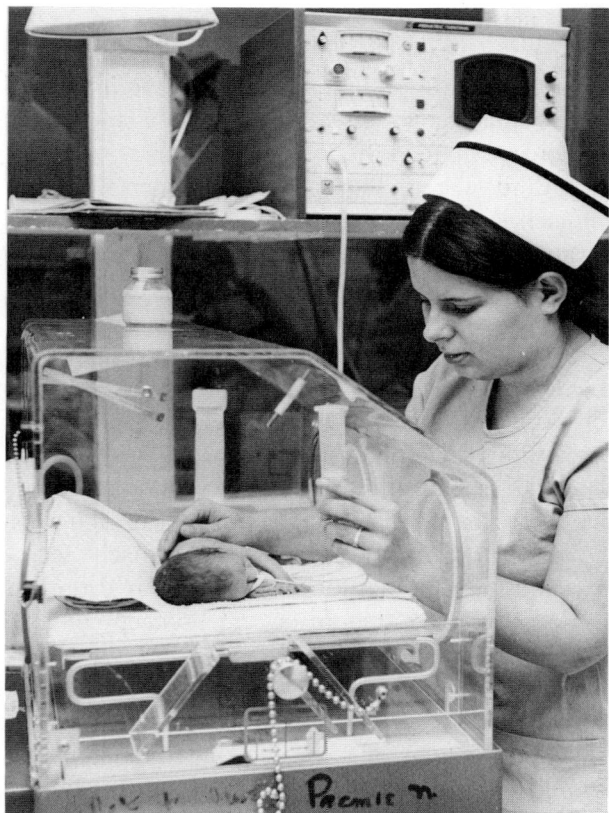

Fig. 38-4. Gavage-feeding. Formula enters the gavage tube by the force of gravity only. (Courtesy of the Department of Medical Photography, Children's Hospital, Buffalo, N.Y.)

Whether gavage catheters should be passed through the nares or the mouth is controversial. Because newborns are nose-breathers, it seems reasonable that passing the catheter through the mouth will lead to less infant distress than passing it through the nose.

The catheter is passed with gentle pressure to the point of the Kelly clamp or tape. If the catheter is inadvertently passed into the trachea rather than the esophagus, the infant usually has some dyspnea, and the catheter should be withdrawn and replaced. The catheter must be checked for position (that it is not in the trachea) before any feeding is given. This check can be made in one of three ways. The time-honored method is to remove the clamp from the tube and dip the distal end of the tube into a glass of sterile water. Because of air in the stomach, one bubble, or possibly two bubbles, may rise from the catheter if the proximal end is in the stomach. If bubbles appear in the water with each expiration, however, the catheter is in the trachea, not in the esophagus. This method should not be used if the infant is being ventilated. The active inspiratory pressure of a ventilator might draw the water from the glass into the lungs, causing aspiration.

An alternative way to test placement is to inject 0.5 to 1.0 ml of air into the tube while you listen over the epigastric area (over the stomach) for the sound of air. In very small babies this is often a difficult task as your stethoscope tip tends to hear lung sounds as well.

A third way to test that the catheter is in the stomach is to aspirate stomach contents. There is an advantage of detecting placement by this route in that it allows you to measure the amount of fluid in the infant's stomach prior to feeding. If it is excessive—over 1 to 2 ml—the infant may not be digesting all the food being given him. If the present feeding schedule is maintained, he may begin to vomit from overfeeding. Vomiting always carries with it the danger of aspiration. As a rule, you want to return aspirated stomach contents to the infant's stomach prior to feeding. Constantly removing stomach secretions this way and discarding them can cause an alkalosis from the amount of acid stomach contents removed.

Once you are assured the catheter is in the stomach, a syringe or a special feeding funnel is attached to the tube. The specific kind and amount of formula ordered is then put into the syringe or funnel and allowed to flow by gravity drainage into the infant's stomach. The tube should not be elevated more than 12 inches above the infant's abdomen, so that the gravity flow is not too fast. Feedings should never be hurried by using the plunger of the syringe or a bulb attachment for more pressure. These methods lead to stomach overflow and aspiration.

In order to avoid overfeeding, the amount of stomach contents aspirated at the beginning of the feeding is sometimes ordered to be subtracted from the total amount of feeding given; that is, if the feeding ordered was 20 ml, but you drew back and replaced 1 ml, give only 19 ml. Some physicians like a quantity of sterile water added at the end of the feeding to flush the last of the milk into the stomach; others calculate the amount of formula so as to account for the additional amount for the tubing, so if you flushed the tubing amount in, you would be giving too much. You must know the specific technique used in the nursery where you give care.

When the total feeding has passed through the tube, the tube is reclamped securely and then gently but rapidly withdrawn. Clamping the tube before it is withdrawn is important, because it prevents any milk remaining in the tube from flowing out as the tube is removed and, again, reduces the risk of aspiration.

A baby should be bubbled following gavage-feeding the same as after a bottle- or breast-feeding. This extra handling not only prevents regurgitation of formula along with bubbles after the infant is laid down but serves to give the infant close contact similar to that a bottle- or breast-fed infant experiences. The infant should be unswaddled and placed on his side or stomach following a feeding.

Polyethylene feeding tubes may be passed through a nostril and left in place for two or three days at a time for permanent gastric feedings. The advantages of permanent feeding tubes is that they do not have to be replaced every 3 to 4 hours. A disadvantage is that they may cause nasal irritation or breaks in the nasal membrane and lead to infection.

Because infants are obligate nose-breathers, some infants do poorly with nasally placed catheters. Measuring the tube for placement is the same as for oral insertion except that the catheter is measured from the bridge of the nose to the earlobe to a point halfway between the xiphoid process and the umbilicus (Fig. 38-5).

After any feeding, procedures such as cupping and vibrating should be postponed for at least an hour. The infant's stomach then has time to digest the feeding, and vomiting is not likely to occur.

Fig. 38-5. A nasogastric tube is measured from the bridge of the nose to the earlobe to a point halfway between the umbilicus and the xiphoid process.

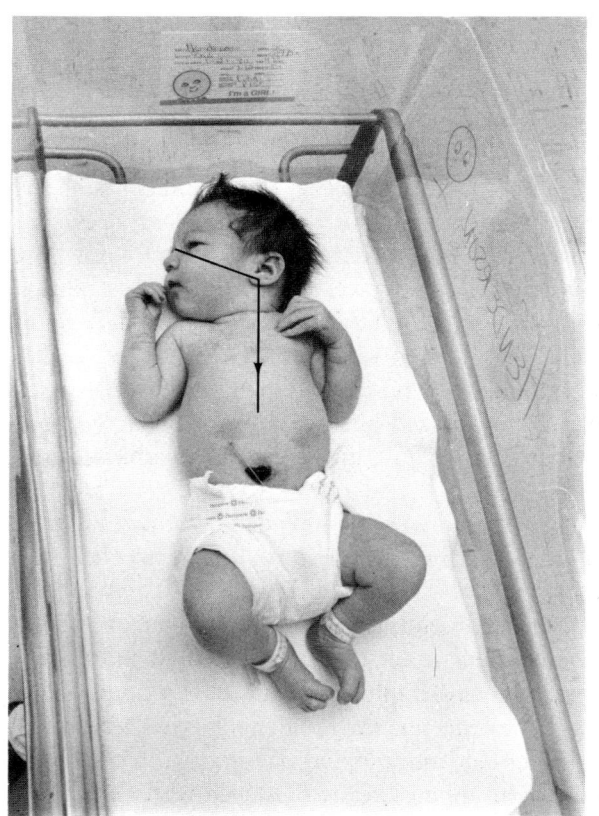

Infants are usually weaned gradually from gavage-feedings to bottle- or breast-feedings, with the number of bottle- or breast-feedings increased each day until the infant is able to take all his feedings by conventional methods.

NASAL-JEJUNAL FEEDING

Infants may be fed by having a long feeding tube threaded through the nares into the stomach, past the pyloric sphincter, and on into the jejunum. It takes a number of hours for the tube to pass this far. That the tube has passed the pyloric valve can be determined by aspirating intestinal contents from the tube. Stomach secretions are acid; intestinal secretions are alkaline. Placement may also be confirmed by x-ray film.

Feedings through a nasal-jejunal tube are usually given by slow continuous feedings although small feedings every 2 hours may be given.

There are many questions as to the wisdom of using nasal-jejunal feedings. There is an association between the method and necrotizing enterocolitis in low-birth-weight infants. Intestinal perforation has occurred in some infants.

INTRAVENOUS FLUID

Infants who cannot ingest adequate amounts of fluid orally will have intravenous fluid lines inserted. Because it is often difficult (and poor absorption from small muscles may make it ineffective) to inject medication intramuscularly in newborns, intravenous lines are used as a major route for medication therapy.

The sites of intravenous injection in newborns vary considerably. Antecubital veins, major sites for insertion in adults, are seldom used in infants; the infant does not understand the necessity of keeping his elbow straight and so the site infiltrates easily. Small veins in the back of the hand are easily accessible and may be used. Scalp veins are often chosen because they are larger and, if the infant's head is restrained from moving, do not infiltrate easily. Parents are generally apprehensive at seeing a scalp vein insertion. It is not a site they are familiar with. They may worry that the fluid is infusing into their child's brain. Parents need an explanation of any tube inserted into their baby before they see the baby so they can understand the purpose of the device and view it as a helping, not a harmful, apparatus.

Infants must be restrained firmly while intravenous fluid lines are inserted. The prick of the needle is painful, and even an ill newborn struggles forcefully against painful procedures. The needle and tubing should be taped firmly in place as even the thrashing of arms when an infant cries can dislodge tubing.

At the same time, the insertion site should not be covered so completely with tape that you cannot judge readily whether swelling is occurring there. The use of a paper or plastic cup to cover a site is questionable when the actual protection it offers is contrasted to the degree it obscures the site.

If the fluid line is begun in a hand, the wrist and arm need to be restrained by an arm board, which is then pinned to the child's mattress. If a scalp vein is used, placing firm blanket rolls or sandbags on both sides of the infant's head prevents him from turning too forcefully.

Extremities with intravenous fluid lines in them should be freed every 1 to 4 hours and passively exercised to prevent lack of circulation in the body part.

All intravenous fluid in newborns should be administered by means of a minidrip and a safety reservoir (a buret) containing no more than 1 hour's worth of parenteral fluid. Thus even if the clamp to the child should be faulty, no more fluid than 1 hour's supply can flow into the child. Fluid should be administered by means of an infusion pump to safeguard against overhydration. If no infusion pump is available, the drip rate must be counted as frequently as every 15 minutes to ensure that the fluid is not being infused too rapidly.

The infusion site should be checked at least hourly to ensure that it is not infiltrated. Check for tissue swelling and coolness. If a scalp vein is used, look posterior to the site; infiltrated scalp veins often swell there as fluid collects by gravity in that area.

At the same time, check for signs of dehydration (sunken fontanelles, poor tissue turgor, dry mucous membranes) and signs of overhydration (rales on chest auscultation, cardiac arrhythmias). Infants receiving intravenous fluid should be weighed every 24 hours (more often if fluid balance is tenuous) as an excessive increase in weight indicates that the infant is being overhydrated.

All infants with intravenous fluid should have their output determined as well as the input. All voidings should be measured (by weighing diapers rather than using urine collectors, to prevent skin breakdown). The specific gravity of each specimen should be determined (use a syringe to collect urine from the diaper).

Fluid administration sets should be changed every 24 hours to ensure that bacteria will not begin to grow in the sugar-rich solution. Intravenous fluid in neonates should never be stopped abruptly but tapered as the infant begins to ingest adequate oral fluid. Sudden stopping of intravenous fluid may lead to hypoglycemia.

Restraints and Intravenous Fluid

To restrain a newborn for a procedure such as beginning intravenous fluid, generally no equipment other than your hands is necessary. If the newborn is exceptionally strong, he may be mummified by means of a newborn blanket. The infant is laid on the blanket and the right side of the blanket is brought over the infant's arm and tucked under him; the left side of the blanket is brought across his trunk and tucked under him on the right side (Fig. 38-6). By this method, his arms are restrained by the weight of his body. It is a secure feeling for the infant and not uncomfortable.

During intravenous therapy, babies should be restrained only the minimum amount necessary. If the intravenous line is into a scalp vein, for example, the infant may have to have his arms restrained so he cannot raise them to his head; his legs need no restraint. Restraints should not be in place when someone is with him; they should be removed every hour so that he can exercise the part and the skin condition can be examined. Since eye coordination in newborns may be encouraged by hand movements (movement of the hand gives the newborn something to focus on) "spread-eagling" for long periods may delay newborn development.

If an arm or leg is going to be restrained, a jacket restraint or a "clove-hitch" restraint with soft muslin should be the only type of restraint used. Infant jackets are infant shirts with tongue blades slipped into pockets in the sleeves. The rigid sleeves prevent the child from bending his elbow. The axillary region must be checked frequently to see that the top of a tongue blade is not pressing into important nerves and blood vessels that cross there. "No-No" jackets are commercial restraints with plastic sleeves.

A clove-hitch restraint is made as shown in Fig. 38-7. This type of restraint cannot grow tight on an arm or leg and so will not compromise circulation.

TOTAL PARENTERAL NUTRITION

The infant who is unable to take oral feedings even by gavage for prolonged periods of time needs intravenous supplementation or he will starve. Traditional intravenous feedings contain electrolytes and sugars but do not contain protein and fat, substances that are essential for the maintenance and growth of body tissue. In total parenteral nutrition, all a baby's nutritional needs can be met by intravenous therapy, since it consists in intravenous administration of a solution containing glucose, vitamins, electrolytes, minerals, and protein. Transfusion of lipids in a second solution supply the baby with essential fatty acids.

The solution is usually administered by a catheter inserted through the right external jugular vein or subclavian to the superior vena cava. A major vein is chosen to avoid inflammation reactions and resulting venous thrombosis. The distal end of the catheter (the end not in the vena cava) may be passed under the skin (subcutaneously) to the parietal head area, where it exits through a stab wound and is connected to the solution tubing. Displacing the catheter entrance this way protects against infection, there is less likelihood of contamination by nasal or oral secretions, and the catheter cannot be displaced by thrashing newborn hands. Placement of the catheter must be done under sterile conditions; in many hospitals it is done in the operating room to ensure sterility.

The solution is administered to the infant by means of a constant infusion pump, so that the rate can be governed. The amount of fluid may be as low as 60 ml per kilogram of body weight per day, or it may be as high as 120 ml per kilogram, depending on the child's needs and whether or not he can take limited oral feedings.

Infection is a major danger of total parenteral nutrition; the solution used is a perfect medium for the growth of bacteria, and particularly *Candida* organisms. The dressing covering the insertion site and the intravenous tubing must be changed daily to avoid infection; the tubing should not be used for drawing blood or for the addition of medications, since such use may introduce infection. Good technique is necessary in changing bottles of solution, so that the tubing is not contaminated during changes.

A second major problem of total parenteral nutrition is dehydration. The solution contains about twice the amount of glucose normally administered to infants. This is to ensure that the amino acids of the solution will not be used for energy but for the synthesis of protein. Dehydration may occur as the body tries to dilute the amount of glucose recognized by the kidneys as excessive and begins excreting it (the same phenomenon that leads to high urine output in persons with diabetes). The urine of the infant undergoing total parenteral nutrition needs to be tested for glucose by a test such as Clinitest at least every 4 hours. If two or more consecutive samples reveal a 3+ or 4+ glucose level, either the rate of the infusion or the amount of glucose in the solution will be decreased. Urine is also tested for specific gravity and

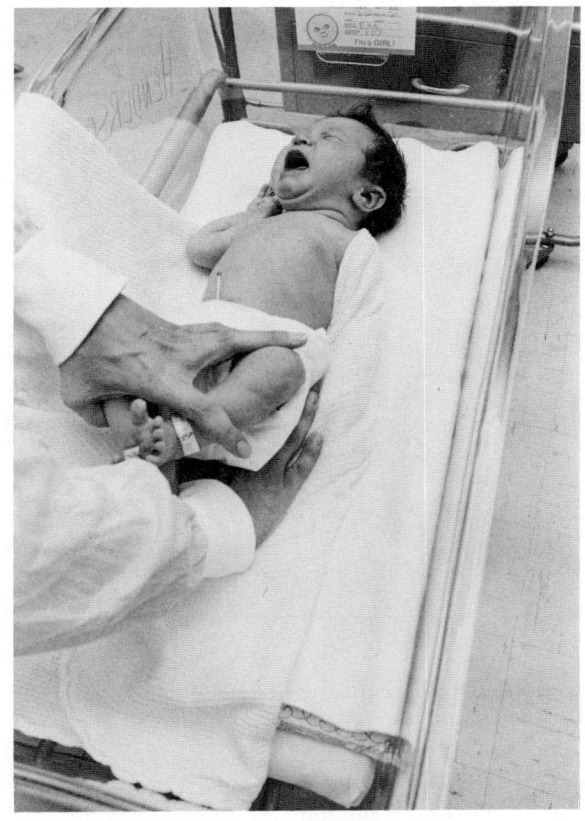

A

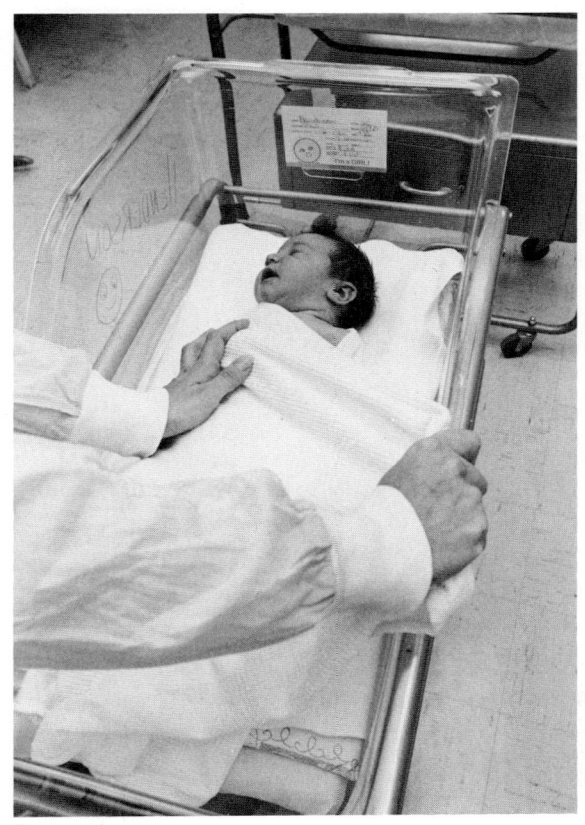

B

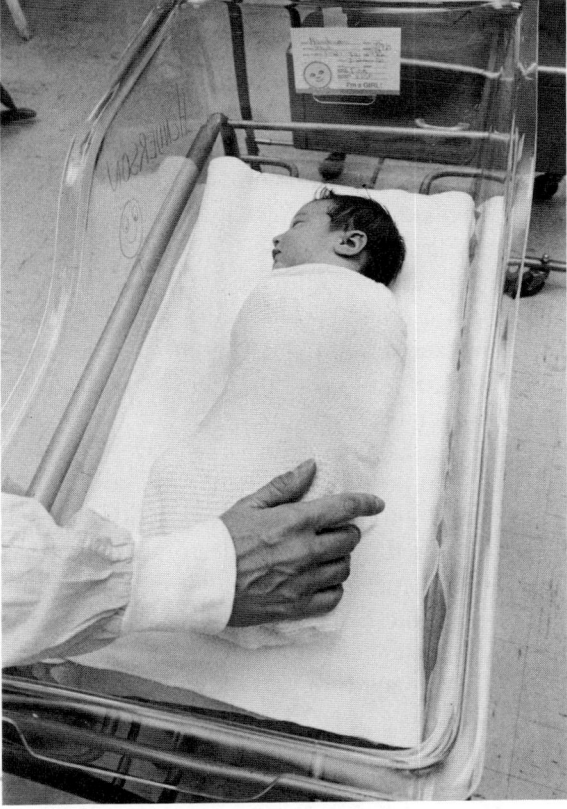

C

Fig. 38-6. A mummy restraint. A sheet or blanket is placed under the infant and brought over one arm (A). When the sheet or blanket is brought from the opposite side (B) and tucked under the baby (C), the baby is sharply restrained yet secure in the wrapping. (Courtesy of the Department of Medical Photography, Children's Hospital, Buffalo, N.Y.)

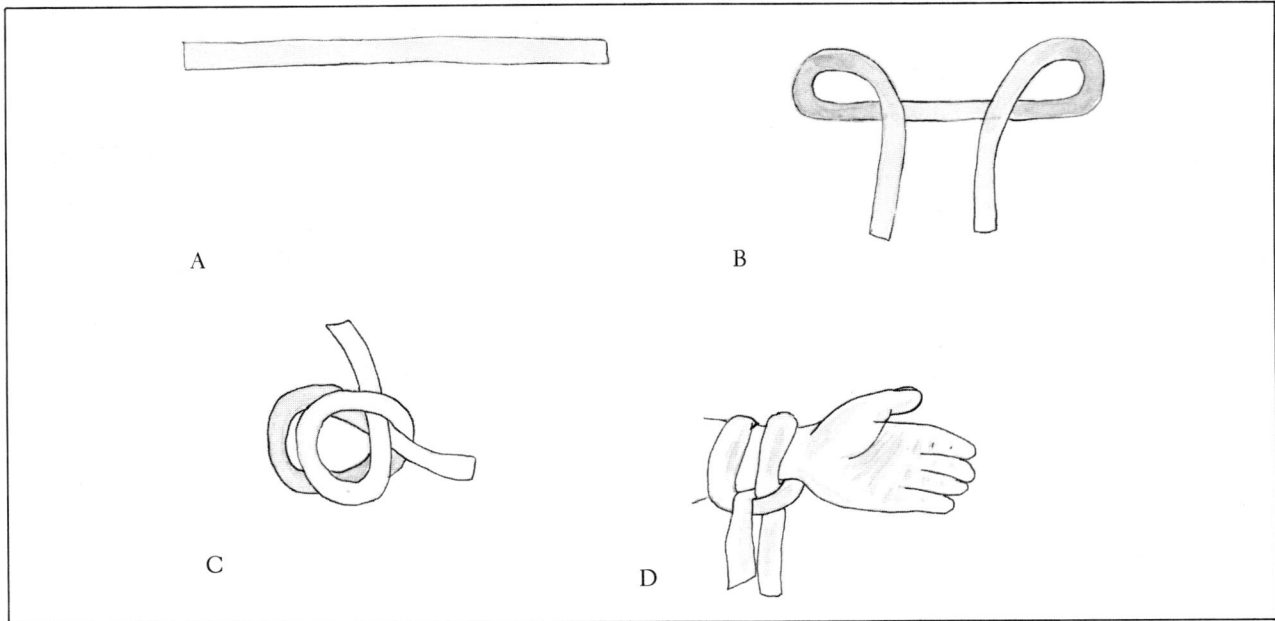

Fig. 38-7. A clove-hitch restraint. A soft strip of cloth (A) is formed into a figure eight with both ends of cloth folded on top of the figure eight (B). Bring the loops together (C) and pull the two ends to adjust the loop to the size of the child's wrist or ankle (D).

protein and measured for volume. Dextrostix determinations for blood glucose are taken about every 4 hours.

After the first few days of total parenteral nutrition, a rebound effect (the baby's body produces increased insulin) may cause hypoglycemia in the infant. A urine sample that is suddenly negative for sugar after a series that has been highly positive is therefore not necessarily an encouraging sign but may be a warning that a lethal low sugar level is present.

As total parenteral nutrition becomes more popular, the uses for it increase. It has an application in infants who have undergone gastrointestinal tract surgery and in the extremely small infant who is not able to suck and has such a small stomach capacity that gavage-feeding is not highly successful.

Total parenteral nutrition may be done by peripheral vein. Glucose concentrations must be less when given by this route or the solution will be so irritating to the vein that phlebitis will occur. Sites must be watched conscientiously because, if infiltration occurs, tissue sloughing can be extensive.

Infants receiving total parenteral nutrition need sucking stimulation. Offering a pacifier every 2 or 4 hours at the times of normal infant feedings provides this. If a sucking reflex is not stimulated at birth, it fades. When the infant is ready for oral feedings, he may have difficulty learning to suck effectively unless this reflex is encouraged.

SIGNS OF DEHYDRATION

Infants born under general anesthesia who are too lethargic to suck well in the first few hours of life or infants born with a congenital anomaly that prevents sucking or swallowing (cleft lip or tracheoesophageal fistula) are in danger of becoming dehydrated in the first day of life. They should be observed closely for signs of dehydration: a sunken fontanelle, dry mucous membranes, decreased skin turgor, decreased urination, and increasing specific gravity level of urine. To assess fontanelles, always raise the child to a sitting position. In some infants the fontanelle appears tense and bulging in a supine position and only reveals the extent of the true tension when the head is elevated. To assess skin turgor, raise a portion of skin on the infant's abdomen between your finger and thumb as if you were going to pinch him. In the well-hydrated infant, after you remove your hand, the skin returns to its previous contour. In the dehydrated infant, the skin remains raised in a ridge. Measuring urine may be done by applying a urine collector or by weighing diapers. Weigh the diaper before it is placed on the infant; weigh it again after it has been wet. The difference in weight in grams reflects the milliliters of urine in the diaper.

Prevention of Infection

The last thing that a high-risk infant needs during the first few days of life is to contract an infection. In some instances, such as premature rupture of the membranes, it is the development of infection (pneumonia or skin lesions, for example) that places the infant in the high-risk category.

Infections may have prenatal, perinatal, or postnatal causes. The most common viruses to affect the infant in utero are the cytomegalovirus and the rubella virus. An infant with either of these infections may be born with congenital anomalies. Infants who contract rubella in utero may be born infectious to other babies and must be isolated from the regular nursery at birth. Thus, it is important to ask a woman on admission to the labor service whether she knows of any diseases or rashes she had during pregnancy, not only so that congenital anomalies can be anticipated, but also to protect other newborns and health care personnel from exposure to the rubella virus.

The most prevalent perinatal infections are those contracted from the vagina during delivery: group B streptococcal septicemia, and thrush from *Candida* infection.

Postnatal infection is invariably spread to the infant from health care personnel. Persons caring for infants must observe strict nursery technique to keep the possibility of infection to a minimum. Health care personnel with infections have a moral obligation not to work in newborn nurseries.

ASSESSMENT

It is often said that newborns do not manifest symptoms when they contract an infection. A more accurate statement would be that they do not manifest *the same symptoms as an adult*. The first noticeable sign may be inactivity or poor feeding. Fever may not be present; many newborns evidence hypothermia with infection. The infant may become jaundiced, and cyanosis may develop. The white blood count is not always helpful in establishing the presence of infection in newborns because it is normally elevated in newborns from the trauma of birth.

Following these nonspecific symptoms, specific symptoms will appear: diarrhea and vomiting if the infection is gastrointestinal; skin lesions if the infection begins with surface contact; bulging fontanelle, nuchal rigidity if the infection is in the central nervous system; shock if it becomes a septicemia.

The body's natural resistance to infection depends on the ability of the white blood cells, the reticuloendothelial system, and the immune system to function effectively. In the newborn, none of these defense systems is fully developed. Thus, even a slight infection, if allowed to go untreated, may spread rapidly throughout the newborn's body, becoming a severe and generalized infection that can result in death. Even the smallest skin lesion or slightest suspicion that the infant is acting ill therefore warrants reporting.

Sepsis Workup

When it is suspected that a newborn has an infection, a sepsis workup is ordered for him. Each hospital has a policy as to what this workup consists of, but common procedures you will need to assist with or carry out are cultures of body fluids (cerebrospinal fluid obtained by a lumbar puncture, urine obtained by suprapubic catheterization, gastric secretions obtained by nasogastric tube aspiration); body cultures from the umbilical cord, external auditory canal, nose, throat, and rectal areas; and blood cultures. Additional blood will be drawn for white blood count and differential, hematocrit and hemoglobin, platelet count, sedimentation rate, serum immunoglobulins, and possibly serological tests.

INTERVENTION

Newborns with infections are removed from a central nursery to an isolation nursery. If there is not enough nursing personnel available to staff a separate nursery and make frequent observations on the ill child, the child may be isolated from the other infants in the central nursery by being placed in an Isolette. Nursing personnel caring for an ill infant in a central nursery must be extremely meticulous in their technique or the infection will spread throughout the nursery.

As with adults, specific antibiotics based on sensitivity studies are used to treat newborn infections. A number of antibiotics are toxic to newborns and are avoided in newborn care. Chloramphenicol is poorly excreted by newborns, toxic levels of the drug develop rapidly. Administration of chloramphenicol to newborns may lead to sudden collapse and death (the "gray baby" syndrome). Potassium penicillin G can cause heart block in newborns because of the buildup of potassium if renal function is not adequate to excrete excess potassium. Tetracycline inhibits the growth of long bones and causes permanent yellowish-brown staining of the tooth enamel. The sulfonamides and novobiocin are dangerous to newborns because they compete with bilirubin for albumin-binding sites. Thus the level of indirect bilirubin increases and kernicterus and death occur at levels of serum bilirubin that would normally be considered safe. Cephaloridine causes nephrotoxicity. Nitrofurantoins may cause both neurological and kidney impairment.

Infants with infections need to be kept warm so that

their energy will be used to combat the infection, not maintain temperature. Because they may feed poorly when ill, they may have to be gavaged or fed by intravenous fluid line during the course of the infection. If shock symptoms should occur, the infant may need vascular support with whole blood or plasma transfusion. Urine volume should be measured to assess kidney function.

The Infant with Congenital Anomalies

Few things, other than hemorrhage in the mother during delivery, can change the expectant, usually joyous tone of a delivery room faster than the birth of a baby with a congenital anomaly. The physician, who is used to saying "perfect boy" or "beautiful girl" and holding up the infant for the mother's first glance, is suddenly without words and without anywhere to put his hands. He must lift the baby to allow secretions to drain from the mouth; yet when he does, the mother (and the father if he is present) will then know of the defect, too. You are in the same predicament. Your usual backup response, "She's beautiful" or "He looks as if he's ready for football already," hangs unsaid in the air. The baby is handed silently away from the table. The feeling of being mortal, with feet of clay, despite the best prenatal care in the world, of impotence to prevent the multitude of congenital anomalies that can occur, fills the room. Health care personnel can become so absorbed in their disappointment and loss at such a happening that they forget the person or persons in the room who feel this loss the most: the parents of the child.

Most physicians believe that bearing the news of congenital anomalies is their responsibility. However, because the physician must deliver the placenta and suture the perineum if an episiotomy was used for delivery, 10 minutes have passed before he is ready to make a second inspection of the baby, assess the true extent of the anomaly from the physical symptoms present, and tell the parents about the defect and the baby's prognosis with the defect. This delay does one of two things to the mother: It leaves her believing for 10 minutes either that she delivered a perfect child among people who do not share her enthusiasm or that she has just given birth to a child so deformed that all the professional persons in the room find it too horrible to even talk about. Because the mother is very aware of the feeling tone in a delivery room, the second response is by far her most likely one. In terms of a mother-child interaction, this is a bad response. The mother begins anticipatory grieving for her deformed child. Even when she is told later that the defect is not extensive, is easily correctable, and that as soon as the correction is made, her child will be perfect, the anticipatory grief reaction may be hard to stop. She may continue to cut herself off emotionally from the child.

Nurses who work in delivery rooms should be familiar enough with the most frequently encountered congenital anomalies to be able to make truthful statements about them and so explain to mothers what the problem is. They are not allowing physicians to "pass the buck" but letting the responsibility fall to the person who at that moment in the delivery process is free to take it on. If a physician does not feel comfortable in allowing a nurse to do this (concerned that it is "diagnosing"), you must be ready to serve as a backup informant, to answer the questions the mother will have when she is again able to think clearly after having been told that her child has been born less than perfect. (Remember the criterion that most pregnant women set: "I don't care if it's a boy or a girl as long as the baby is healthy.")

It is probably best to explain to a mother what the defect is, and what the prognosis for the defect is, before you show the baby to her. It is best if the father is also present in the delivery room, so that both parents can begin to accept the reality of this situation at the same time. It is better to explain the defect first and then show the parents the infant because a mother will find it hard to look at her infant with a cleft lip or palate or exposed abdominal contents and also listen to what you are saying. Her mind is so jammed with the visual image her eyes are sending her, so unlike the child of her imagination, that she cannot hear.

"Your baby's upper lip isn't completely formed, Mary Ann. That's called a cleft lip. Your doctor will call one of the plastic surgeons here at the hospital to look at your baby. This is a small problem and can be repaired so well surgically that you'll barely be able to tell your baby was this way. I'll bring the baby over so you can see her. Remember when you look at her that this can be repaired. She seems perfect in every other way."

This is the kind of statement that defines and limits the problem for the parents and gives them direction as to where and how they should proceed in thinking about it and in beginning to seek help for their child. Some people are reluctant to put names or labels on congenital anomalies, preferring to say instead, "Your baby's upper lip isn't completely formed" and stopping there, rather than saying, "That's called a cleft lip." This prevents the parents from going to the local library and reading about the condition, a bad thing for them to do because they invariably read a 20-year-old book that considers such a defect totally irreparable. Not giving the parents a label may leave them with the belief that their child has such a rare disorder that finding treatment for it may be difficult.

Parents of children wtih congenital anomalies are very aware of what people think of their children. They watch closely the way you handle the baby, to see if you are giving as much attention to him as to the other babies. It is important for the baby with a defect, and for the parents' acceptance of the baby, that you rock him as long after feeding as you do the other babies and talk to him just as you do to the others, and so on. If you, a professional person, find their child distasteful, how will they dare show the child to their family and friends? If you are able to look past the anomaly at the whole child, however, they begin to feel this way, too. You are setting the stage for a good parent-child interaction, or for a poor parent-child interaction, every time you handle an infant born with a congenital anomaly.

ANOMALIES OF THE GASTROINTESTINAL SYSTEM
Cleft Lip

The fusion of the maxillary and median nasal processes normally occurs between the 5th and the 8th weeks of intrauterine life. In infants with cleft lip, the fusion fails in varying degrees, and the defect ranges from a small notch in the upper lip to a total separation of the lip and face up to the floor of the nose. The deviation may be unilateral or bilateral. Cleft lip is more prevalent among males than females.

A cleft lip is repaired very shortly after birth, sometimes at the time of the initial hospital stay, sometimes at 1 month of age. Because the deviation of the lip interferes with nutrition, the infant may be a better surgical risk at birth than he is after a month of poor nourishment.

Before the defect is repaired, feeding the infant with a cleft lip is a problem. He must get an adequate amount of food and yet be prevented from aspirating. The best method appears to be to support the baby in an upright position and feed him gently from a small container such as a medicine glass. Contrary to what might be your first impression, newborns do well drinking from glasses in this manner, and it seems safer than using medicine droppers, syringes, or commercial feeders that force formula into the infant's mouth by pressure on a rubber bulb. A hurried nurse or a hurried mother can easily cause the infant to aspirate if she is using these methods.

Although the baby needs the enjoyment of sucking, most surgeons do not want the baby to suck on a pacifier before surgical correction of the defect. Babies with extensive clefts are as unable to suck on a pacifier as they are on a nipple.

If the baby is going to be discharged with the mother and wait until he is 1 month of age for surgery, the mother needs to learn to feed him during his hospital stay. The method chosen should be demonstrated to her at one feeding. She should then be allowed to feed the infant under supervision for as many feedings as necessary for her to become confident of her ability to feed the baby. Whatever method the infant is fed by, he needs to be held and bubbled after feeding because of his tendency to swallow a great deal of air due to his inability to grasp a glass or syringe edge securely with his mouth.

Mothers have difficulty learning to feed their infants when they are born with cleft lips. Statements such as "You have to learn this. You'll have to do it at home," although true, are ineffective and sound almost punitive. A positive approach is better: "I think you're doing very well. Try it by yourself now with me sitting right beside you. It takes all babies a few days to be able to eat well. I think she's doing better all the time."

Today, the results of surgical repair of cleft lip are excellent. It is helpful to parents to see photographs of babies with good repairs (Fig. 38-8). The older term, *harelip*, should not be used when talking with parents about the problem. Before modern surgical techniques were available, children were left with large lip scars, gross speech impediments, and a poor appearance after surgery. *Harelip* tends to be associated with these negative outcomes rather than with today's positive outlook.

A mother who will be taking a child with a cleft lip home to wait for surgery may need a community health nurse referral. She should have a number to call, either the hospital's, a clinic's, or her pediatrician's, to ask any questions that arise in her baby's care.

Cleft Palate

The palatal process closes at about the 9th to 12th week of intrauterine life. A palate cleft is usually on the midline and may involve just the anterior hard palate, or the posterior soft palate, or both. It may be a separate anomaly, but as a rule it occurs in conjunction with a cleft lip.

Infants with cleft palate cannot suck. To suck, an infant presses his tongue or the nipple against the roof

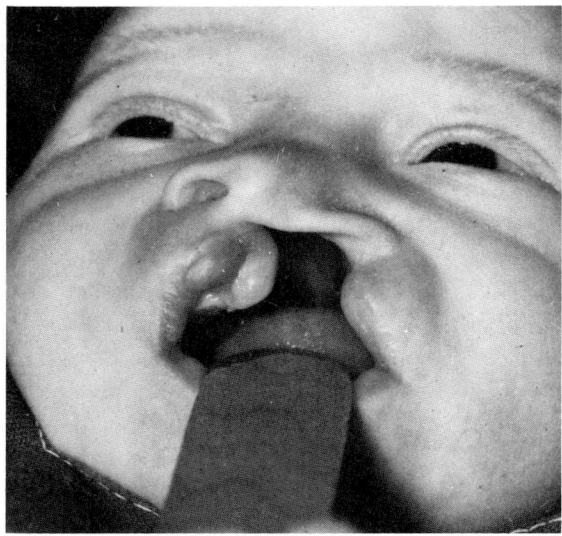
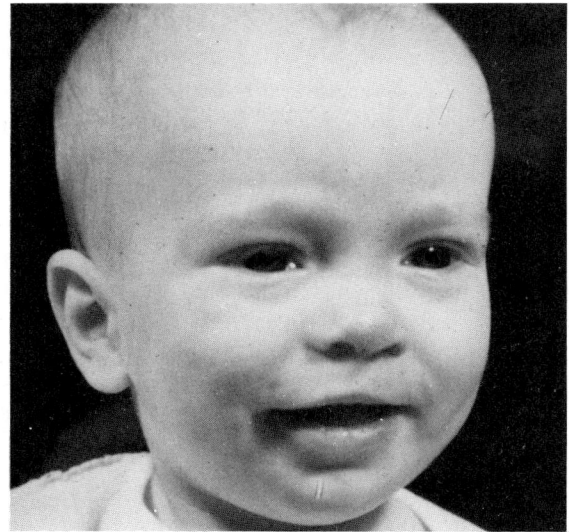

Fig. 38-8. Cleft lip. A. A 2-week-old infant with unilateral cleft lip. B. Same child at 14 months, showing the surgical repair. (From L. V. Crowley, An Introduction to Clinical Embryology. *Copyright © 1974 by Year Book Medical Publishers, Inc., Chicago. Reprinted by permission.)*

of his mouth. In the infant with a cleft palate, this action would force milk up into his pharynx and he would surely aspirate. The most successful method of feeding this infant, like the child with cleft lip, is to use a small medicine glass.

Although the repair of cleft lip can be undertaken immediately, palate repair is postponed until the child is 12 to 18 months of age, until the anatomical change in the palate contour that occurs during the first year of life has taken place. Repairs made before this change (the palate arch increases) are often ineffective and may have to be rescheduled.

A child with a cleft palate will need long-term follow-up speech therapy, dental supervision, and close observation for otitis media (middle ear infection). Palate repair may change the normal slant of the eustachian tube and make the child more prone to middle ear infection.

Tracheoesophageal Atresia and Fistula

Between the 4th and 8th weeks of intrauterine life, the laryngotracheal groove develops into the larynx, trachea, and beginning lung tissue, and the esophageal lumen is formed. A number of anomalies may be found in infants if the trachea and esophagus do not develop normally. The most frequent form of these deviations is one in which the esophagus ends in a blind pouch, and the stomach is connected to the trachea by a fistula (Fig. 38-9). When the infant is fed, milk fills the blind esophagus and overflows into the trachea. Tracheoesophageal fistula must be ruled out in any infant born to a woman with hydramnios. A normal fetus swallows amniotic fluid during intrauterine life. The infant with a tracheoesophageal fistula cannot swallow, and the amount of amniotic fluid may thus become abnormally large. Tracheoesophageal fistula can be diagnosed with certainty if a catheter cannot be passed through the infant's esophagus to his stomach.

An infant who has so much mucus in his mouth that he appears to be blowing bubbles through it should be suspected of having tracheoesophageal fistula. However, it is not suspected in some infants who do this bubbling until they are fed for the first time. Then, the infant coughs, turns cyanotic, and has obvious difficulty in breathing. This is the reason formula-fed infants should first be fed by a nurse with sterile water. A feeding of formula aspirated into the lungs is more dangerous to the infant because of its fat content than is sterile water.

Emergency surgery for the infant with tracheoesophageal fistula is essential to prevent pneumonia, dehydration, or electrolyte imbalance. The infant should be kept in an upright position and on his right side to prevent gastric juice from entering the lungs from the fistula. If he cannot swallow mucus, he needs frequent oropharyngeal suction to prevent aspiration of collected mucus. The prognosis will depend on the extent of the repair necessary, the condition of the child at the time of surgery, and whether or not other congenital anomalies are present. In general, however, the prognosis after such surgery is good.

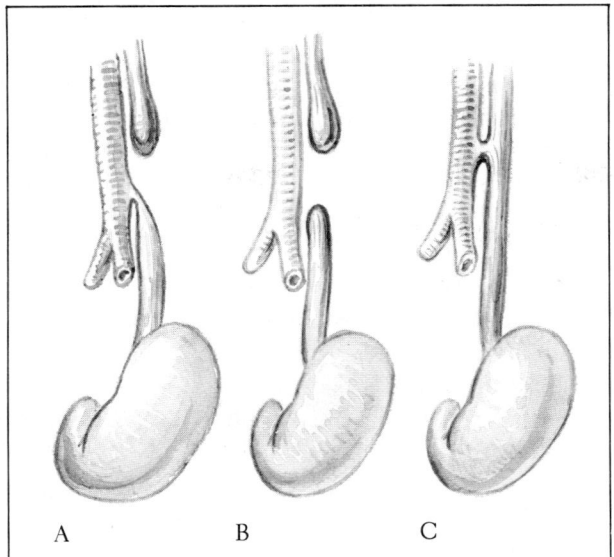

Fig. 38-9. Esophageal atresia and tracheoesophageal fistula. A. The most frequent type of esophageal atresia. The esophagus ends in a blind pouch. The trachea communicates via a fistula with the lower esophagus and stomach (about 90 percent of infants have this type). B. Both upper and lower segments end in blind pouches (7 to 8 percent of infants have this type). C. Both upper and lower segments communicate with the trachea (2 to 3 percent of infants have this type). (Courtesy of the Department of Medical Illustration, State University of New York at Buffalo.)

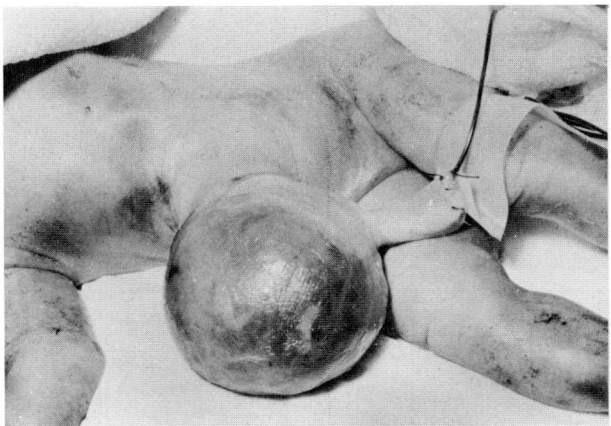

Fig. 38-10. Omphalocele. This large omphalocele seen at birth contains intestine and liver. (Courtesy of the Department of Medical Photography, Children's Hospital, Buffalo, N.Y.)

Omphalocele

An omphalocele is a protrusion of abdominal contents at the point of the junction of the umbilical cord and abdomen. The herniated organs are usually covered by a thin transparent layer of peritoneum. The deviation is evident at birth and reflects an arrest of development of the abdominal cavity at the 7th to 10th week of intrauterine life. At about the 6th to 8th week of intrauterine life, the abdominal contents are extruded from the abdomen into the base of the umbilical cord. Omphalocele occurs when there is failure of the abdominal contents to return to the abdomen (Fig. 38-10).

It is important that the lining of peritoneum covering the defect not be ruptured or allowed to dry out; otherwise infection will complicate the surgical repair. The omphalocele is usually covered by sterile saline–soaked gauze until surgery. A nasogastric tube will be inserted to prevent abdominal distention.

The success of the surgical repair depends on the size of the omphalocele. The viscera may be only partially replaced during surgery; if the entire contents are returned to the abdomen (which is unusually small because it did not need to grow to accommodate abdominal contents), respiratory distress may result from the pressure of the visceral bulk. If replacement is partial, a second surgical procedure at a later date is required to complete the repair.

Intestinal Obstruction

Intestinal obstruction in the newborn is usually caused by meconium ileus, ileac atresia, or malrotation, and it causes the same symptoms as it does at any time in life: vomiting (green vomitus in the infant because of the meconium present), no passage of stool, abdominal distention, and possibly the appearance of peristaltic waves across the abdomen.

Bowel obstruction may be suspected in an infant if there was hydramnios during the pregnancy, which may have occurred because the fetus could not swallow amniotic fluid (as with tracheoesophageal fistula). Bowel obstruction is a surgical emergency and must be corrected before dehydration, electrolyte imbalance, or aspiration of vomitus occurs. Infants with meconium ileus (the ileum is obstructed by meconium so hard or sticky in consistency that it will not pass) must be followed up, because meconium ileus is frequently associated with cystic fibrosis.

Diaphragmatic Hernia

A diaphragmatic hernia is protrusion of an abdominal organ (usually the stomach or intestine) through a defect in the diaphragm into the chest cavity. This usually occurs on the left side, and the heart is displaced to the right of the chest; the lung on the left side is collapsed.

A newborn with an extensive diaphragmatic hernia will have respiratory difficulty from the time of birth because his lungs are unable to expand satisfactorily. He may also have cyanosis and intracostal or subcostal retractions. His abdomen generally appears sunken because it is not as filled as the normal newborn abdomen is. Bowel sounds may be heard in the chest cavity by auscultation.

Some infants with diaphragmatic hernia breathe better with the head elevated; the herniated intestine can then fall back as far as possible into the abdomen and a maximum of respiratory space is provided. A nasogastric tube is usually inserted to prevent distention of the herniated intestine, which will cause further respiratory difficulty.

Treatment is immediate surgical repair of the diaphragm and replacement of the herniated intestine. The mortality is 25 to 50 percent, with death often due to associated anomalies of the heart, lung, and intestine.

Imperforate Anus

Imperforate anus (Fig. 38-11) is stricture of the anus. It may involve an intestine that ends in a blind pouch, or a membrane may obstruct the rectum. It can be discovered in a newborn by the inability to insert a rectal thermometer or rubber catheter into the rectum. No stool will be passed, and abdominal distention may be evident.

The degree of difficulty in repairing an imperforate anus depends on the extent of the problem. If the rectum ends close to the perineum, repair is not difficult. It is complicated if the end of the rectum is a distance from the perineum or there is a fistula to the bladder or urethra. The urine of all infants with imperforate anus should be examined for the presence of meconium to determine whether the child has such a fistula. If the repair will be extensive, the surgeon may create a temporary colostomy, anticipating final repair when the infant is somewhat older.

When all newborns stayed in the hospital 7 to 10 days, imperforate anus was always discovered. When the infant failed to pass stools after the first 24 hours, the reason was investigated. Today, when some newborns are discharged at 1 day of age, it is possible that no one will notice that the child has not passed stools in that time. Because imperforate anus is one of the more common congenital anomalies, no infant should be discharged from the hospital until he has passed a stool as proof that the rectum is patent.

ANOMALIES OF THE NERVOUS SYSTEM
Spina Bifida Occulta

Spina bifida occulta is a developmental anomaly in which the posterior spinal column fails to close. This anomaly usually involves one or two vertebrae at the sacral area, although it may occur at any place along the spinal column. The spot is evident as a depression in the skin. Often there is a tuft of hair growing at the place of the depression.

Meningocele

A *meningocele* is a pouching of the meninges and cerebrospinal fluid through a defect in the posterior spinal canal (spina bifida). The meningocele may be covered by a layer of skin, or it may be denuded, with just the fibrous dura mater exposed.

Myelomeningocele

A *myelomeningocele* is a pouching of the spinal cord, the meninges, and cerebrospinal fluid through a defect in the posterior spinal column (Fig. 38-12). Often the spinal cord ends at the level of the myelomeningocele, and there will be no motor or sensory function below this point. The infant does not move his legs, and urine and stools continually dribble because of lack of sphincter control. It is generally difficult to tell from the gross appearance of the myelomeningocele whether or not it is the simpler meningocele.

Encephalocele

An *encephalocele* is a myelomeningocele occurring at the back of the neck or head. The sac contains brain tissue, as well as spinal cord, meninges, and fluid.

INTERVENTIONS. A spina bifida occulta needs no correction. The parents should be made aware of its

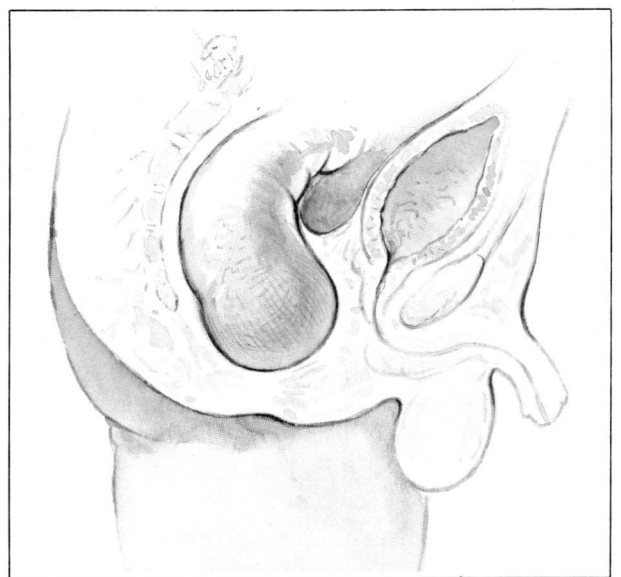

Fig. 38-11. Imperforate anus. The lower bowel ends in a blind pouch. (Courtesy of the Department of Medical Illustration, State University of New York at Buffalo.)

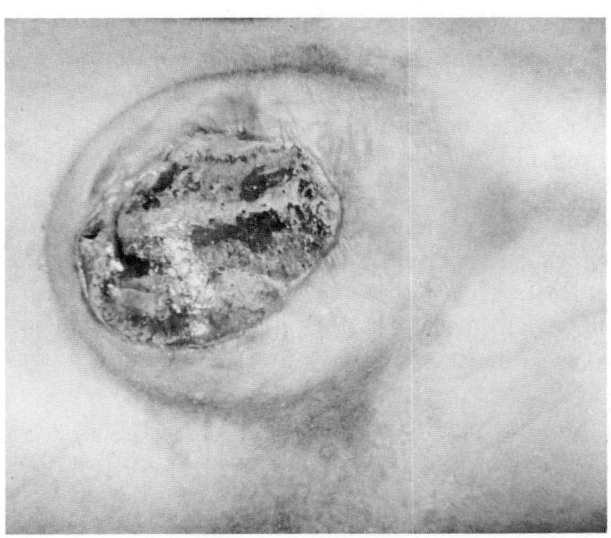

Fig. 38-12. A myelomeningocele protrudes as an obvious deformity of the spine and cord. Note how the area is covered only by a thin membrane, making it prone to trauma and infection. (Courtesy of the Department of Medical Photography, Children's Hospital, Buffalo, N.Y.)

existence, so that they are not surprised when someone points it out to them later. Surgical correction of meningocele, myelomeningocele, or encephalocele is scheduled as soon as feasible, before infection (meningitis) can result. Meningitis can develop readily because the meninges are often exposed.

Women who have had one child born with a spinal cord defect may have an amniocentesis done to determine if such a defect exists in a second pregnancy. This is revealed by the presence of alpha fetoprotein in the amniotic fluid. The chance that a woman who has had one child with a spinal cord defect will have a second child with a defect is 1 in 20.

The infant must be positioned so that he puts no pressure on the defect prior to surgery. Pressure on the outpouching sac increases cerebrospinal fluid pressure. Extreme pressure can result in compressed and nonfunctioning brain tissue. The infant is best positioned on his side or stomach. A foam rubber "doughnut" covered with plastic and sterile gauze can be used to protect the sac from pressure.

Hydrocephalus (increased cerebrospinal fluid in the ventricles of the brain) commonly occurs with meningocele or myelomeningocele. The infant's head circumference should be measured daily, therefore. The measurement must be very accurate; any increase in circumference reported must be actual and not merely a reflection of faulty measuring. Putting a mark with a ball-point pen at the center of the forehead and the most prominent point of the occiput will enable everyone to place the tape measure at the same point on the head for measuring.

The infant should be observed closely for signs of increased intracranial pressure: vomiting, lethargy, failure to eat, or a bulging fontanelle. The infant who has continual incontinence of urine and feces from lack of sphincter tone needs his diaper changed frequently to prevent skin irritation. Protecting the diaper area skin with an ointment such as Vaseline or A and D is a help. Be careful that the diaper does not touch the area of the protruding spinal sac; unless the sac is completely closed by a layer of skin, it can become infected from contact with feces.

The infant should be held to be fed—he needs the same cuddling and love as do other infants. Just be certain that, as the baby rests in your arms, the outpouching sac does not press against your arm, increasing cerebral pressure. Holding and feeding the infant this way is very frightening for a mother and perhaps is too much to expect her to do.

The eventual prognosis will depend on the extent of the defect. If the defect is a meningocele, a section of meninges may have to be removed in order to return the structures to their proper place. The loss of these meninges may limit the rate of absorption of cerebrospinal fluid; it may build up in amount, and hydrocephalus may develop following repair. If a myelomeningocele is present, the surgeon will close the skin over the area of defect, but the motor and sensory loss below this point cannot be restored

Hydrocephalus

Hydrocephalus (Fig. 38-13) is an increase in the amount of cerebrospinal fluid in the ventricles of the brain. It may occur because of overproduction of fluid by the choroid plexus (rarely), or because a stricture along the path of flow of the fluid forces it to build up quantities in certain portions of the brain.

The infant's head is often not enlarged at birth, or is only slightly enlarged. The suture lines, particularly the sagittal suture line, are separated, however, and the fontanelles will feel tense or bulging and may be much longer or wider than is normal.

In some infants the fluid increases in amount so rapidly that within the few days of a hospital stay the bulging fontanelle and widely separated sutures appear. The infant's forehead may bulge; white sclera is evident above the cornea of the eyes (*sundown eyes*) from stretching and pulling up of the upper eyelids. The infant's cry may become high-pitched and shrill. He may be irritable and restless; or he may be lethargic.

The head circumference should be measured daily.

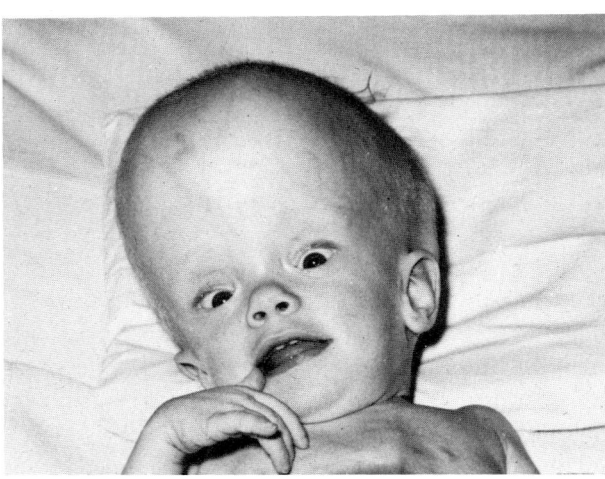

Fig. 38-13. Hydrocephalus. (From D. Marlow, Textbook of Pediatric Nursing. *Philadelphia: Saunders, 1973.)*

Marking the forehead and the most prominent process of the occiput with a ball-point pen at the points where the tape should pass helps to make measurements accurate even when different people are doing the measuring. Getting sufficient nourishment into the infant may be a problem if he is irritable, or vomiting, or too lethargic to suck.

Be extremely careful to support the baby's head when you pick him up or turn him over; he has a great deal of difficulty supporting it himself. He needs his head position changed frequently to prevent decubiti from forming. He should be held for feeding, with his head well supported. A chair with arms, such as a rocking chair, is useful for feeding, since it will help support your arm.

Surgical repair is a shunting procedure, in which, to permit drainage of fluid, a thin polyethylene catheter is placed between the ventricle above the obstruction and the base of the brain (the foramen magnum), or into the vena cava, a ureter, or the peritoneum.

Prognosis depends on the location of the stricture that is causing the increase in fluid, the success of the shunting procedure, and the amount and site of damage to brain tissue that occurred from compression prior to surgery.

ANOMALIES OF THE GENITOURINARY TRACT
Exstrophy of the Bladder
In exstrophy of the bladder (Fig. 38-14) there is no anterior wall of the bladder and no anterior skin covering of the lower anterior abdomen. The bladder lies open and exposed; it is bright red, and urine continually drains from it. Pelvic bone defects and urethral defects may also be present.

Prevention of infection is a major concern in an infant with exstrophy of the bladder; infection of the open bladder may lead to ascending urinary tract or kidney infection. The exposed bladder is usually covered by sterile petrolatum gauze. Since the skin of the abdomen becomes excoriated from the constant irritation of urine, it must be protected by an ointment such as A and D. Diapers are usually just placed under the child rather than fastened in place. Be certain to change the diaper promptly after the infant stools so that he does not move and bring feces forward to the open bladder.

Surgical repair is seldom wholly successful. Following closure of the abdominal wall an ileal conduit may be constructed (in which the ureters are attached to a separated portion of the small intestine, and urine is voided into a collecting bag attached to the abdomen) or threaded into the wall of the intestine so urine is evacuated with stool.

Patent Urachus
A patent urachus is a fistula between the bladder and the base of the umbilical cord. It is usually detected when urine is seen draining from the base of the cord. Any drainage from the umbilical cord should be tested by Nitrazine Paper; urine will show an acid reaction, but other body fluids are invariably alkaline. Surgical repair of a patent urachus is done in the newborn period before infection of the bladder or cord results.

Hypospadias
In hypospadias, the opening of the male urethra is on the undersurface of the penis. The meatus may be near the glans, midway back, or at the base of the penis. This usually causes no difficulties in infancy. The defect needs to be corrected before the child enters school, however, so that he looks and voids as all the other boys do. It is also important to correct it before reproductive age, so that in intercourse the deposition of sperm is near the cervix and not in the distal vagina, which would cause a fertility problem. Infants with hypospadias should not be circumcised since the plastic surgeon may want to use the foreskin in the plastic repair of the hypospadias.

Imperforate Hymen
Imperforate hymen (Fig. 38-15) is a rare disorder and, because the external genitals of female infants are edematous at birth, often difficult to detect. As the genital area may not be included in every health assessment of the child during her growing years, detecting this in the newborn period is particularly

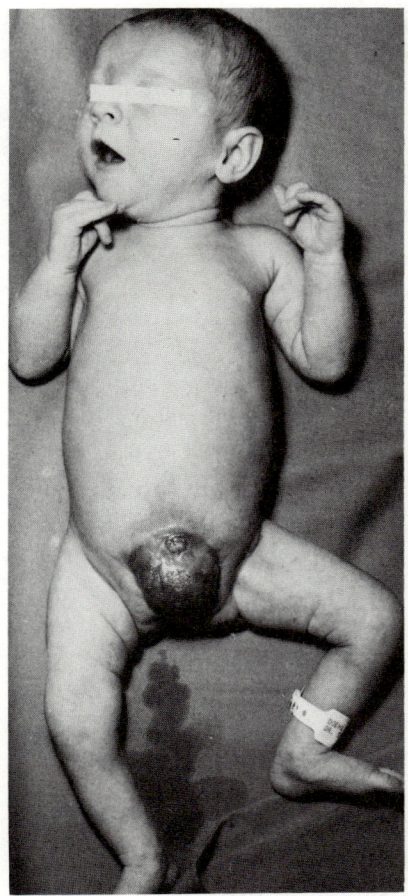 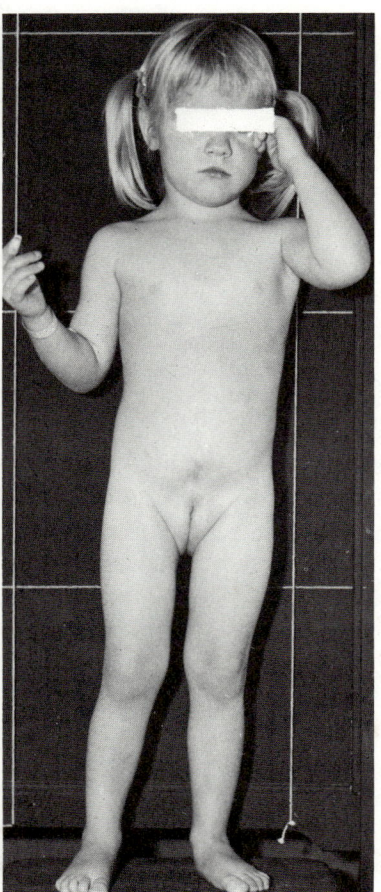

A B

Fig. 38-14. Exstrophy of bladder. A. Characteristic appearance of exstrophy in a 6-month-old infant. B. Same child at 2 years of age, following surgical reconstruction. (From L. V. Crowley, An Introduction to Clinical Embryology. *Copyright © 1974 by Year Book Medical Publishers, Inc., Chicago. Reprinted by permission.)*

Fig. 38-15. Imperforate hymen in newborn infant. (From L. V. Crowley, An Introduction to Clinical Embryology. *Copyright © 1974 by Year Book Medical Publishers, Inc., Chicago. Reprinted by permission.)*

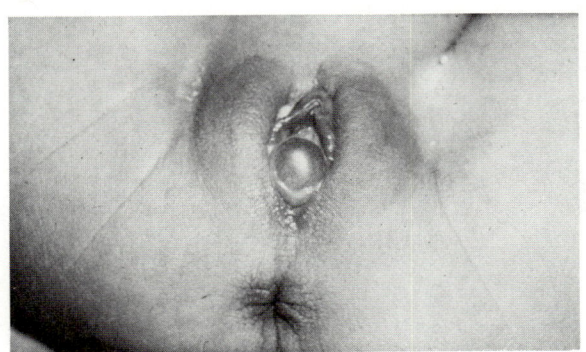

important. It is corrected by surgical incision before puberty and menarche. Inspecting the genitalia of female infants is a major aspect of nursing assessment since physicians (more often male) may not inspect these body parts thoroughly.

ANOMALIES OF THE HEART AND CIRCULATORY SYSTEM

As many as 1 in 140 live-born infants is born with a congenital heart defect. The mortality of such infants is so high that a third die in the first month.

The child with a congenital heart disease may or may not evidence cyanosis, depending on the type and extent of heart disease present. Cyanosis is difficult to assess in a newborn because most newborns have some cyanosis (acrocyanosis). Generalized cyanosis, however, is never normal. Cyanosis in a child with choanal atresia or a lung disorder usually decreases if the infant cries, since opening his mouth helps to aerate the lungs. The infant with a heart defect usually becomes more cyanotic on exertion and crying because his heart cannot meet the increased metabolic demand.

Many of the symptoms of cardiac anomalies are not present in the first days of life because still-functioning

The Infant with a Congenital Anomaly or Neonatal Illness 671

fetal circulatory structures, such as the ductus arteriosus and foramen ovale, compensate. A heart murmur in a newborn may be missed because his heart rate is so rapid that murmurs are hard to hear. Clear-cut symptoms may not become apparent during a three- to four-day hospital stay. Parents invariably ask at what time of life congenital heart defects will be repaired. With recent advances in heart surgery, heart defects are being repaired at ages earlier than ever before—in some instances in the first few days of life. All surgical repairs are made individually, on the basis of the extent of the defect and the symptoms in the infant.

Acyanotic Heart Disease
Normal heart circulation is shown in Fig. 38-16. Acyanotic heart defects are heart or circulatory anomalies that involve an obstacle to the flow of blood or a shunt that moves blood from the arterial to the venous system (oxygenated to unoxygenated blood, or left-to-right shunts).

VENTRICULAR SEPTAL DEFECT (VSD). The commonest of all congenital cardiac defects, accounting for 22 percent of all instances of congenital heart disease, *ventricular septal defects* are openings in the septum between the two lower chambers of the heart, the right and left ventricles (Fig. 38-17A).

Fig. 38-16. Normal heart circulation. (From Clinical Education Aid, No. 7, Ross Laboratories, Columbus, Ohio, 1970.)

Ventricular septal defects are one of the chief causes of congestive heart failure in the newborn baby. Congestive heart failure results because, with each ventricular beat, blood is forced from the left ventricle across into the right ventricle, overburdening the right side of the heart. Since more than the normal amount of blood is forced into the pulmonary artery, lung congestion may result as well.

The newborn with a VSD will not appear cyanotic because, with the shunt, blood from an oxygenated source is mixing with unoxygenated blood. The characteristic murmur heard in older children and adults with VSDs (a grade 3 or 4 rough or harsh holosystolic murmur, loudest at the fourth left interspace) may be absent in the newborn; the high neonatal pulmonary resistance increases pressure in the right ventricle and prevents much blood from passing through the defect.

If symptoms of congestive heart failure develop early in life, pulmonary artery banding may be attempted to increase the resistance to blood flow even more, forcing a buildup in right ventricular pressure and further reducing the amount of blood shunted. When the infant is older, or when it is needed, a permanent correction of the defect can be achieved.

ATRIAL SEPTAL DEFECT (ASD). An *atrial septal defect* (an opening in the septum between the upper chambers of the heart [Fig. 38-17B], the right and left atria) may be symptomless in the newborn period and

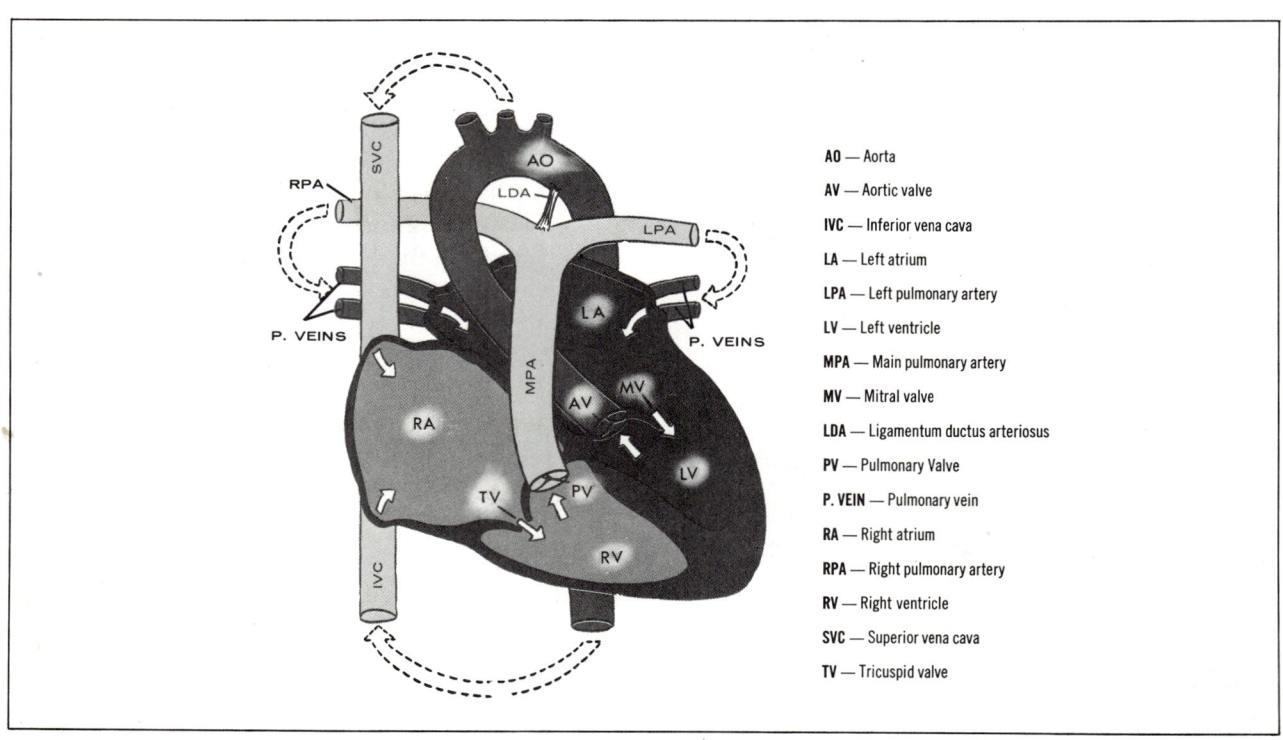

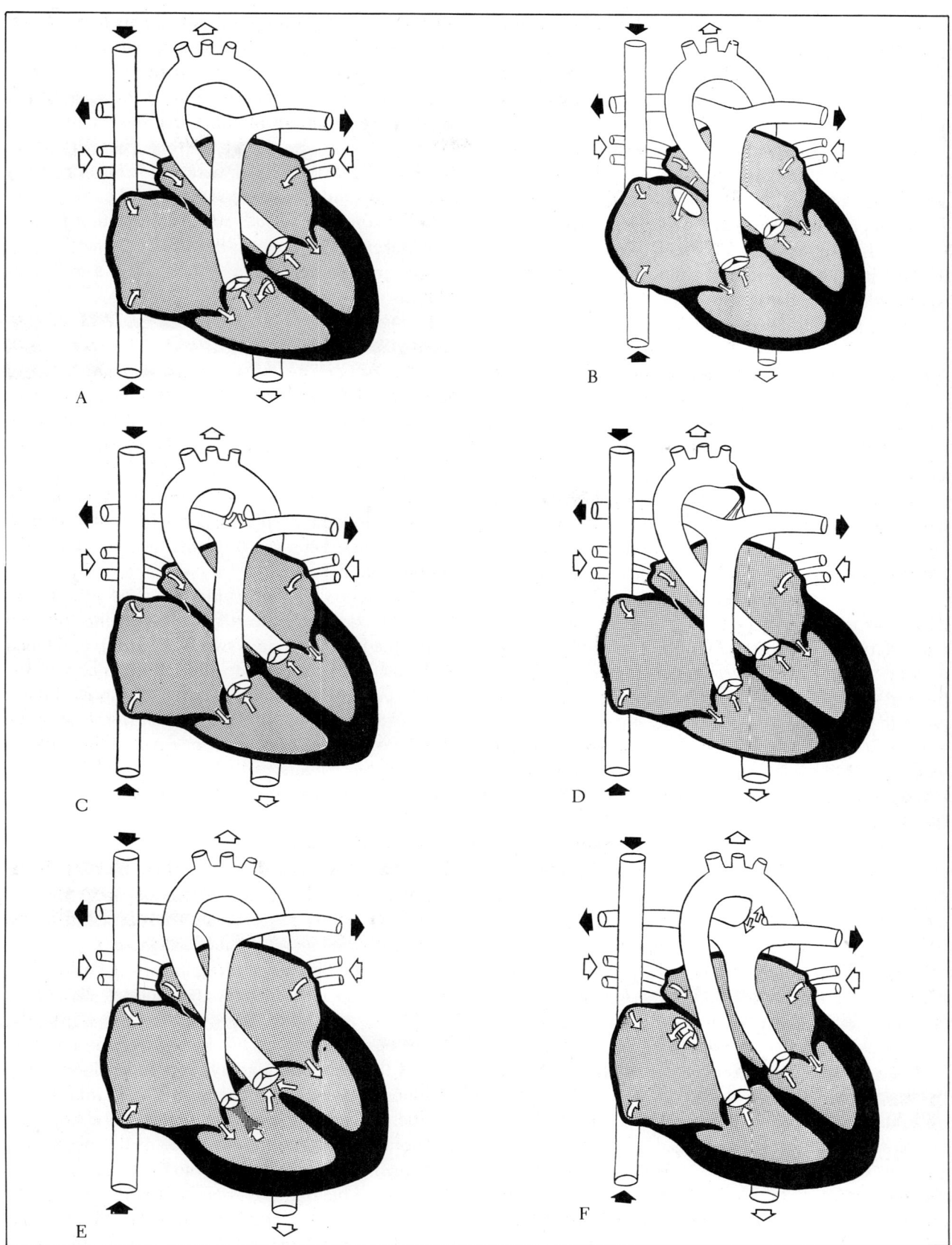

Fig. 38-17. Congenital heart defects. A. Ventricular septal defect. B. Atrial septal defect. C. Patent ductus arteriosus. D. Coarctation of the aorta. E. Tetralogy of Fallot. F. Complete transposition of great vessels. (From Clinical Education Aid, No. 7, Ross Laboratories, Columbus, Ohio, 1970.)

may thus be missed at this time. The blood shunts from the left to the right atrium. Unless extremely small, the defect is repaired to prevent subacute bacterial endocarditis due to the relative stasis of blood flow from developing.

A more complicated type of ASD, with absence of the lower part of the atrial septum as well as leaks or deformities of the mitral and tricuspid valves (endocardial cushion defect), is the type of cardiac defect associated with trisomy 21, or Down's syndrome. About 1 in 9 children with Down's syndrome has this type of congenital cardiac defect.

A newborn with an endocardial cushion defect has the same symptoms as does the child with a large VSD. Although the murmurs and chest x-ray pictures of the two conditions are similar, they are distinguished by electrocardiogram.

PATENT DUCTUS ARTERIOSUS. A *ductus arteriosus* is a prenatal shunt between the pulmonary artery and the aorta. In some infants it fails to close at birth (patent ductus arteriosus) (Fig. 38-17C). The flow of blood during intrauterine life is from an unoxygenated system to an oxygenated one (the pulmonary artery to the aorta). Because the pressure in the aorta after birth is greater than the pressure in the pulmonary artery, after birth the shunt reverses if the ductus remains patent. The flow of blood after birth is from the aorta (carries oxygenated blood) to the pulmonary artery (carries unoxygenated blood), that is, from the arterial to the venous system. The ductus arteriosus tends to remain open in infants with hypoxia or respiratory difficulty because of increased pulmonary artery pressure.

In patent ductus arteriosus, a murmur will be heard at the upper left sternal border or under the left clavicle. In older children, it is a continuous (systolic and diastolic) machinery-type murmur. In newborns the murmur may not be so characteristic, perhaps a short grade 2 or grade 3 harsh systolic murmur. If the shunt is large, congestive heart failure may develop by the end of the first week as the increased amount of blood pours back into the pulmonary artery.

A patent ductus arteriosus can be repaired with less risk than other defects because the repair is actually outside the heart. Repair is made whenever significant symptoms appear, or before school age.

COARCTATION OF THE AORTA. *Coarctation of the aorta* is a narrowing or stenosis of the aorta and is one of the commonest malformations causing congestive heart failure during the newborn period (Fig. 38-17D). It is suspected if the newborn does not have bilaterally equal femoral pulses. Checking for the presence of both femoral pulses is a procedure that all maternal-newborn nurses should include as part of the initial nursery admission inspection.

If the coarctation is slight, absence of the femoral pulses may be the only symptom. If the condition is severe, the symptoms of congestive heart failure will be evident, namely, rapid breathing and tachycardia, together with feeding difficulties from the rapid breathing. Cardiac catheterization will be done to locate the constriction, and surgical correction may be undertaken at this point. If the child is asymptomatic, surgery may be delayed until the child is 4 to 5 years of age.

PULMONARY STENOSIS. *Pulmonary stenosis* is a narrowing of the pulmonary artery or the pulmonary valve that prevents blood from leaving the right ventricle with ease. If the stenosis is sufficiently extensive, back pressure on the right side of the heart can lead to congestive heart failure. The murmur accompanying pulmonary stenosis is usually striking: a grade 4 or 5 rough ejection crescendo-decrescendo systolic murmur loudest at the upper left sternal border. There is often a thrill in the same location and in the suprasternal notch.

If the stenosis is severe, the increased pressure on the right side of the heart may reopen the foramen ovale (the fetal opening between the atria), and blood will flow from the right to the left chambers of the heart, perhaps producing a mild cyanosis. Infants with severe stenosis will have a repair (removal of the strictured portion of the artery or repair of the valve) in early infancy; others, with lesser degrees of stenosis, may wait until they are 4 to 5 years old.

Cyanotic Heart Disease

Cyanotic heart disease occurs when blood is being forced or shunted from the venous system to the arterial system; that is, unoxygenated blood is being forced into oxygenated blood (right-to-left shunt).

TETRALOGY OF FALLOT. In *tetralogy of Fallot* there are four associated defects: pulmonary stenosis, a VSD, an overriding aorta, and right ventricular hypertrophy (Fig. 38-17E). Because of the constriction of the pulmonary artery, very little blood enters it. Blood is forced instead across the VSD into the left ventricle. Because the aorta overrides or is abnormally positioned near the septum, some of the blood (still unoxygenated) passes directly into the aorta and out to the body. The right ventricular hypertrophy occurs gradually as extra blood accumulates in the right ventricle because of obstruction in the pulmonary artery.

Although this is an extremely serious form of heart disease, a passive newborn may not exhibit a high degree of cyanosis during his brief hospital stay. When cyanosis becomes apparent, and hypoxic episodes begin to occur, a temporary (palliative) surgical repair may be done, in which a shunt is created between the aorta and the pulmonary artery (a patent ductus arteriosus), allowing blood to leave the aorta and enter the pulmonary artery, be oxygenated in the lungs, and return to the left side of the heart, the aorta, and out to the body (Potts-Smith-Gibson or Blalock-Taussig procedure). If cyanosis is severe, the infant will have a full surgical repair done as his initial surgery.

TRANSPOSITION OF THE GREAT VESSELS. With *transposition of the great vessels*, the aorta arises from the right ventricle, not from the left ventricle, and the pulmonary artery arises from the left ventricle, not from the right ventricle (Fig. 38-17F). Blood enters the heart by the vena cava, passes to the right atrium, the right ventricle, and out the aorta to the body, completely bypassing oxygenation. On the left side of the heart, blood enters the left atrium and left ventricle and leaves by way of the pulmonary artery, arising abnormally from the left ventricle. Blood is oxygenated in the lungs, but returns to the left atrium and flows to the left ventricle and pulmonary artery again. This is a closed circulatory system that cannot oxygenate body tissues. Such a defect in its absolute form is incompatible with life. Fortunately, in most infants the ductus arteriosus remains open and provides a circulatory "mix." The infant may be administered a prostaglandin to halt closure of the ductus arteriosus and maintain this pathway for blood.

A well-functioning communication between the two blood circulating pathways must be created. It is usually achieved by passing into the right atrium by cardiac catheterization a polyethylene catheter with an uninflated balloon attached to its end. The catheter is pushed through the leaves of the foramen ovale. It is then inflated and pulled through the foramen ovale, creating an atrial septal defect. This allows for blood from the blind circulatory pathways to mix, and, although the child may remain very cyanotic, oxygen will be supplied to his body tissues. Correction of the defect is done as soon as possible to avoid brain damage from inadequate oxygenation. As this involves total heart reconstruction, it may not be successful.

HYPOPLASTIC LEFT HEART SYNDROME. *Hypoplastic left heart syndrome* is a cardiac defect that any nurse caring for infants in newborn nurseries should be aware of, since it is a common cause of heart failure in the first week of life. In this syndrome the left ventricle is nonfunctional, and there may be mitral or aortic valve atresia. The right ventricle hypertrophies because it must carry on the entire heart load. Cyanosis becomes mild to moderate as the heart fails. The infants rarely live to be over 2 weeks old; no repair is currently available.

Assessment of Congenital Heart Disease

The diagnosis of cardiac defects is done on the basis of the signs and symptoms present in the newborn, including cyanosis, abnormal heart sounds, absence of femoral pulses, tachycardia, increased respiratory rate, and feeding difficulty. A chest x-ray examination or echocardiogram is usually ordered to determine the size of the heart and the state of the pulmonary vasculature. Blood gases will be obtained. Arterial saturation of under 92% oxygen is compatible with cyanotic heart disease. An electrocardiogram may be ordered to detect abnormal cardiac electrical activity. The infant may be scheduled for cardiac catheterization. However, cardiac catheterization has a higher risk in newborns than in older children, and if the infant is not in acute distress, the actual diagnosis may be delayed until later in life. Both the American Heart Association and the Academy of Pediatrics recommend that these complex studies be done only in centers performing at least 200 cardiac catheterizations on infants and children yearly and at least 100 heart operations yearly. The infant with a recognized heart defect may thus be transported to a regional center for further studies.

Congestive Heart Failure

Congestive heart failure can develop rapidly in a newborn with a heart anomaly. Tachypnea is often the first symptom. Respirations of more than 50 per minute in the mature infant and 60 in the low-birth-weight infant when the baby is at rest are above normal. In most newborn nurseries, the infant's temperature is taken every 4 hours for the first 24 hours, but respirations are not counted, so the presence of tachypnea may be missed. In these instances, feeding difficulty in the infant, such as struggling to free his mouth of the nipple so that he can breathe more efficiently, may be the first symptom noted.

Tachycardia follows quickly after tachypnea. Healthy newborns rarely have a heart rate of over 150 beats per minute when at rest. The infant with an insufficient heart output must maintain a more rapid rate than normal.

All maternal-newborn nurses should be skilled enough in physical assessment to be able to palpate and percuss the edge of an infant liver. A normal newborn liver is often palpable 2 cm under the right intercostal margin. A liver palpable more than 3 cm should create suspicion of heart failure if it accompanies other symptoms; the liver enlarges because of back pressure on the portal system. By palpating the chest to determine the point of maximum intensity of the heartbeat (the heart apex), or percussing the left side of the chest to reveal the left edge of the heart, one can detect an unusually enlarged heart.

Edema is a late symptom of congestive heart failure in the newborn. If edema is present, it is usually facial edema. The infant looks puffy, especially about the eyes.

Digoxin, and oxygen administration are the mainstays of therapy for the newborn in heart failure. Infants receiving digoxin should be placed on a cardiac monitor to detect cardiac rhythms suggestive of digoxin intoxication.

Home Care of the Newborn with Heart Disease

The day a child with a heart defect is taken home from the newborn nursery is a difficult day for most parents. They have many questions to which they need full answers before they feel confident enough to take their baby home. They should have ample opportunity to handle and feed the baby in the hospital, so that they can feel secure in managing him at home.

Parents generally ask, "Can we let the baby cry?" If the baby has tetralogy of Fallot or other heart defects in which cyanotic spells tend to develop, or if there is a severe aortic stenosis, the baby should not be allowed to cry for long periods of time. Crying for a few minutes while a bottle is prepared or a fresh diaper is folded will not harm the baby with a less severe heart defect.

"What do we feed him?" Babies with heart defects are usually fed normal newborn and infant diets. Only rarely is salt restricted.

"Can we get life insurance on the baby?" This is probably one of the least important things that parents should be thinking about at this time, but it is a question many families ask. Some insurance companies do not insure the life of a child with a congenital heart defect. However, after a surgical correction for the heart defect, some insurance companies may issue a policy. The parents need to ask these questions of their insurance agent.

"What are the chances any other children we have will be born with this kind of defect?" This is a question for a genetic counselor. Although congenital heart disease is not inherited, certain forms of it tend to be familial. Patent ductus arteriosus and atrial septal defect are two such forms.

ANOMALIES OF THE RESPIRATORY TRACT

Respiratory tract deviations can be immediately life-threatening. They demand prompt assessment so that interventions can be started quickly.

Choanal Atresia

Choanal atresia, or blockage of the posterior nares, may be unilateral or bilateral. Bilateral choanal atresia causes acute respiratory difficulty in newborns because they are invariably nose-breathers. The infant may appear to breathe well in the immediate moments after birth while he is crying (with his mouth open). He may become cyanotic and begin retracting when he stops crying. The diagnosis is confirmed by inability to pass a catheter through the infant's nares.

Insertion of an airway may be necessary, if the atresia is bilateral and complete, until surgery to relieve the obstruction can be performed.

If a mother received reserpine in the two days before delivery, her infant may be born with symptoms similar to choanal atresia: stuffy nose, nasal discharge, retractions, and cyanosis. He may need an oral airway inserted to carry him through the first five days, until the effect of the drug is no longer apparent.

Cysts and tumors of the nose, mouth, or pharynx may cause similar airway problems.

Pierre Robin Syndrome

Pierre Robin syndrome is a combination of micrognathia (abnormal smallness of the jaws), glossoptosis (a dropping forward of the tongue), and cleft palate. Respiratory obstruction occurs because the prominent tongue obstructs the airway. The difficulty may be relieved by placing the infant on his stomach, so that his tongue falls forward. Insertion of an airway may be necessary. Some surgeons provide temporary airway relief by placing a suture in the anterior tongue and pulling it forward free of the airway by traction.

Congenital Stridor

Laryngeal stridor is marked by a characteristic "crowing" on inspiration. The cause of the stridor may be congenital laryngeal webs, cysts, rings, or stenosis. The exact diagnosis and plan for repair is determined by direct laryngoscopy.

Diaphragmatic Paralysis

Injury to the phrenic nerve at birth may result in paralysis of the diaphragm and respiratory distress. Phrenic nerve injury usually occurs in connection with injury to the brachial plexus (the network supplying the arm). Infants who had a difficult breech birth or those delivered vertex with shoulder dystocia are most likely to suffer phrenic nerve injury, since a lateral hyperextension of the head is usually the cause of the injury. An x-ray examination will show a slight elevation of the diaphragm on the affected side. Atelectasis may be present. If the injury is mild, the child's condition usually improves over the first week of life; if it is severe, surgery may be necessary to lower the position of the diaphragm.

ANOMALIES OF BONE OR MUSCLE

Orthopedic anomalies are usually detected at routine newborn physical assessments.

Subluxated or Dislocated Hip

Subluxated or dislocated hip is commonly referred to as *congenital hip*. It is a flattening of the acetabulum of the pelvis, which prevents the head of the femur from rotating adequately. In subluxated hip, the femur "rides up" because of the flat acetabulum; in dislocated hip, the femur may ride so far up that it leaves the acetabulum (Fig. 38-18). The defect is found in females six times more frequently than in males. It is usually, but not always, a unilateral involvement.

Subluxated or dislocated hip is noticed on physical assessment, when the affected hip does not abduct. With the baby lying on his back, his leg will flex onto his abdomen but will then not abduct to lie almost flat against the mattress as does the normal newborn leg. Correction of subluxated and dislocated hip involves positioning the hip into this flexed abducted position in order to press the femur head against the acetabulum and deepen its contour by the pressure. Splints or casts are used. Often splint correction is begun during the newborn's initial hospital stay. The easiest form of splint (to hold the legs in a frog-leg position) is use of, not one, but two or three diapers

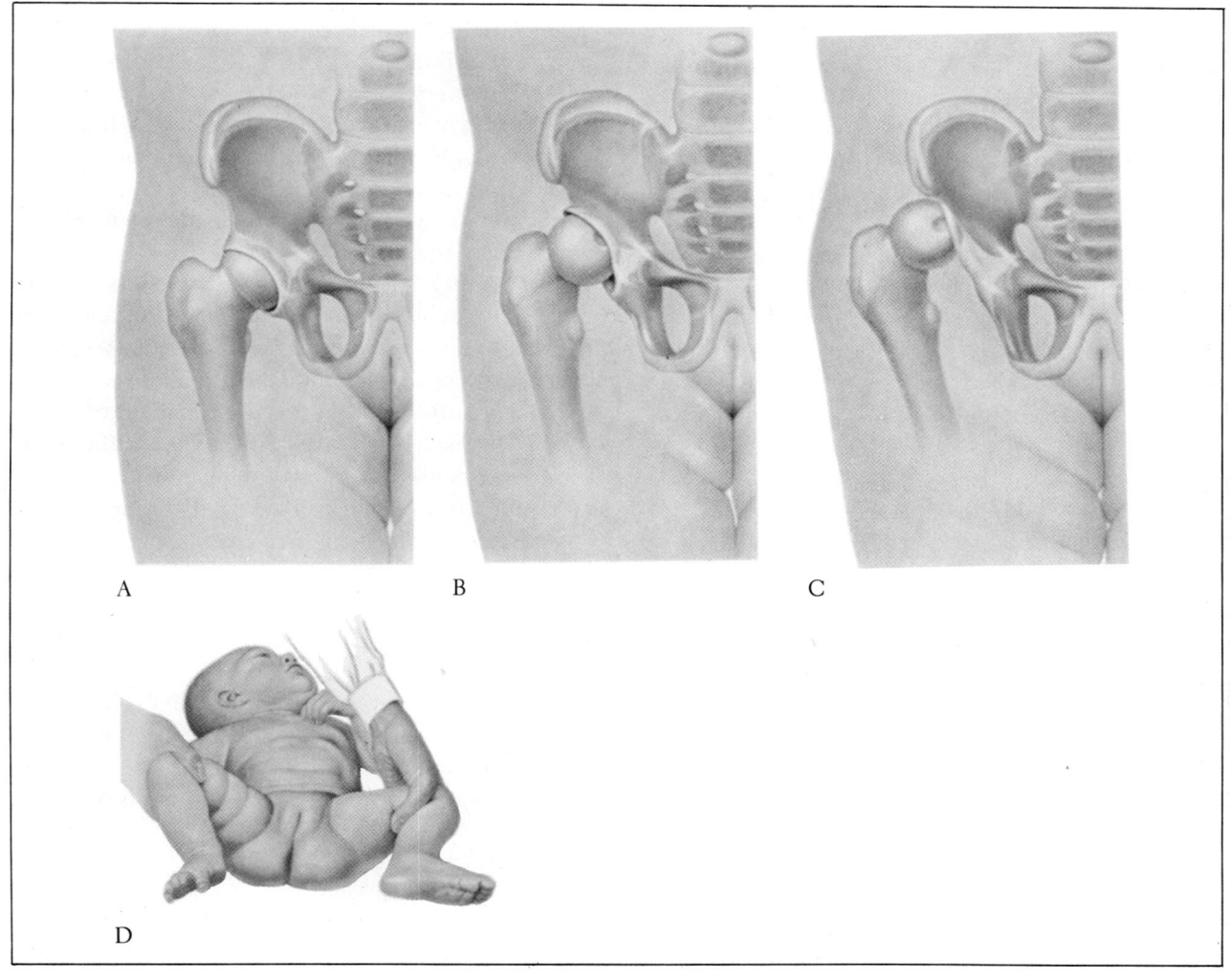

Fig. 38-18. Congenital hip anomalies. A. Normal hip. B. Subluxated hip. C. Dislocated hip. D. Limitation of abduction on affected side. (From Clinical Education Aid, No. 15, Ross Laboratories, Columbus, Ohio, 1965.)

on the infant. The extra bulk of cloth between the child's legs effectively separates and spreads them. Another form of splint is made of plastic and buckles onto the child as a huge confining diaper.

Mothers should handle their infants enough before they are discharged from the hospital to be familiar with the equipment they will need to use. If only bulky diapers are called for, be certain the mother understands that, although this may not seem like an important measure (as might a more complicated splint or cast), it is important and she must continue to use the extra diapers. Be sure that she has an appointment for follow-up care before discharge.

The Talipes Deformities

Talipes is a Latin word formed from the words *talus* and *pes*, meaning "foot" and "ankle." The talipes deformities are ankle-foot deformities, popularly called *clubfoot* (Fig. 38-19). The term *clubfoot* implies permanent crippling to many people and should not be used when discussing talipes deformities with parents. With the good orthopedic correction techniques available today, correction should leave the child with no permanent deformity of the foot.

Some newborns have a pseudo talipes deformity from the intrauterine position. In these infants the foot can be brought into a good position by manipulation, in contrast to true defects, in which the foot cannot be properly aligned without surgical intervention.

The earlier the deformity is recognized, the better is the correction. Most infants will have casts to above their knees applied while they are still in the nursery. The cast must be left exposed to the air until it is thoroughly dry; it must be handled gently, so that your hands do not make impressions that can result in pressure points and impaired circulation. The newborn must be changed frequently, so that a wet diaper does not touch the cast and cause it to become urine- or meconium-soaked (the mother should put plastic pants on the infant or use disposable diapers). Check the toes of the infant frequently for circulation (press on the toes and watch whether they become blanched and then immediately pink again). Note any restlessness or crying that might be signs of pain resulting from poor circulation due to the cast. Be certain the mother handles the infant enough in the hospital to be comfortable with handling him. Be sure she understands that she must keep the cast dry. Be sure she has an appointment for follow-up care before discharge.

Erb-Duchenne Paralysis

Erb-Duchenne paralysis is caused by birth injury and is seen much less often today than formerly. In this type of paralysis, the arm is adducted close to the chest and internally rotated. It is held straight at the elbow with the forearm pronated. Erb-Duchenne paralysis is caused by stretching, hemorrhage, or tearing of the anterior fifth and sixth cervical nerve roots, such as might occur if the fetal head is overextended laterally to effect delivery of wide shoulders. It may occur in conjunction with diaphragmatic paralysis from the same cause. All infants with Erb-Duchenne paralysis need to be observed closely for tachypnea or other symptoms of respiratory distress to detect diaphragmatic paralysis as well.

Treatment for Erb-Duchenne paralysis is to hold the arm in an abducted, externally rotated, and supinated position to rest the paralyzed muscles. Usually a cotton restraint is tied around the newborn's wrist, and the infant's arm is raised over his head and tied to the head of the bassinet. Unless the damage to the nerve roots was extensive (avulsion), the paralysis is temporary, and arm function will return. It is important to observe the symmetrical movements of newborns, particularly in the Moro reflex, to detect the presence of this birth injury.

Polydactyly

Polydactyly is a developmental anomaly in which extra digits are present (Fig. 38-20). Most of the additional digits do not include bone and so are removed simply by ligating them in the early months of life.

Syndactyly

Syndactyly is the presence of a webbing or joining of toes or fingers (Fig. 38-21). The defect is usually corrected by surgical separation. Because newborns hold

Fig. 38-19. Talipes equinovarus deformity. (From Clinical Education Aid, No. 15, Ross Laboratories, Columbus, Ohio, 1965.)

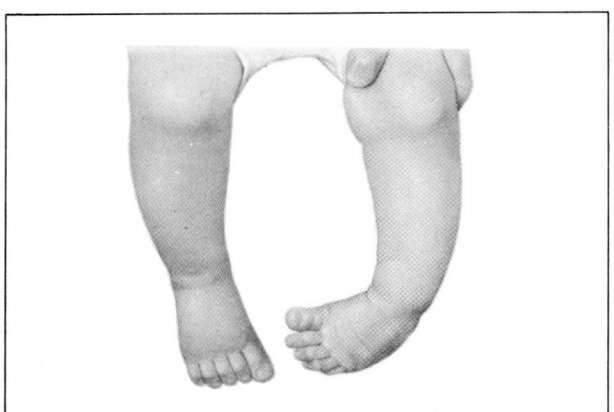

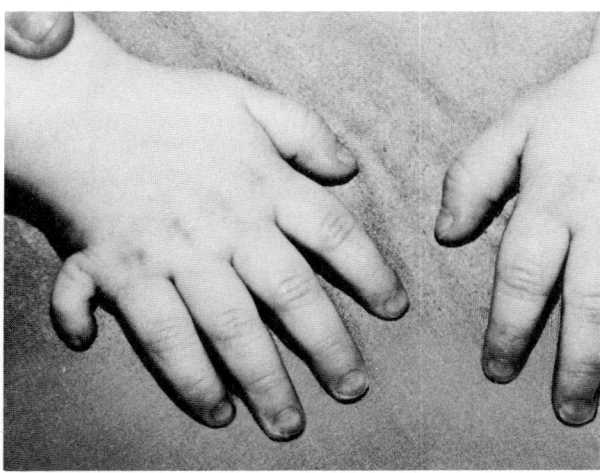

Fig. 38-20. Polydactyly. (Reproduced with permission of Mead Johnson & Company, Evansville, Ind.)

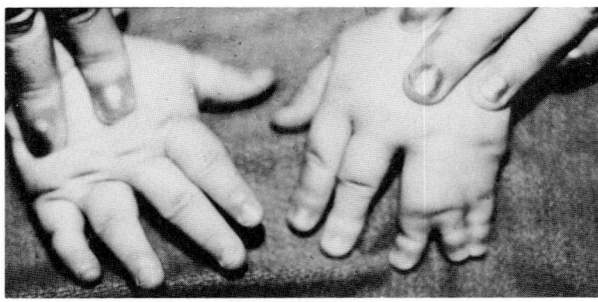

Fig. 38-21. Syndactyly, or webbing of the fingers, together with supernumerary digit. (Reproduced with permission of Mead Johnson & Company, Evansville, Ind.)

their hands tightly clenched, both polydactyly and syndactyly must be looked for or they will go undiagnosed in the newborn nursery.

Illness in Newborns
METABOLIC ILLNESS
Hypoglycemia

If hypoglycemia is going to occur, it usually occurs in the first few hours or days of life. The ability to regulate glucose is an important skill of a newborn's metabolism. Maintaining an adequate level of blood glucose is crucial because the brain can neither make nor store glucose; it must have a ready supply of glucose from the circulation available for cell metabolism, since hypoglycemia, or a lowered glucose level, results in brain cell destruction. A circulating glucose level depends on glucose input (from oral feedings), glucose released by the liver (glucogenesis or production of glucose), and the amount of glucose uptake by body tissues. Infants who have respiratory distress and cannot suck well may not be able to take in an adequate amount of glucose. The immature infant does not have adequate liver stores to use for glucogenesis. An infant who is cold or hypoxic uses glucose rapidly for metabolism and thus quickly depletes liver stores.

During fetal life, glucose is supplied to the fetus by placental transfer. This occurs at a constant, rapid rate, although the levels of fetal glucose never exceed those of the mother.

The average level of glucose in cord blood varies from 60 to 80 mg per 100 ml of blood. An infant can be considered hypoglycemic if the glucose level falls below 30 mg per 100 ml in the first 72 hours of life and below 40 mg per 100 ml thereafter.

Blood sugar values are usually lower in low-birth-weight infants than in mature infants. A premature infant is therefore ordinarily not considered hypoglycemic until the glucose level is under 20 mg per 100 ml. Babies who are particularly prone to hypoglycemia are the following:

Infants born of mothers with pregnancy-induced hypertension
Infants born of diabetic mothers
Infants with hemolytic disease
Infants who have difficulty establishing respirations
The smaller of twins
All immature infants
Infants who are small for gestation age
Postmature infants
Any infant subjected to intrauterine or extrauterine stress
Infants who do not suck well

Hypoglycemia may be asymptomatic, or the infant may be jittery, limp, apathetic, tachypneic, or cyanotic, may refuse to nurse, or may have convulsions. Few of these signs are specific for hypoglycemia. Cyanosis and tachypnea occur in respiratory distress, jitteriness in hypocalcemia, and convulsions in central nervous system injury. Refusal to eat and apathy are seen in the infant with an infection or possibly with heart disease. The symptoms therefore require an investigation into the cause; the investigation will reveal the hypoglycemia.

Blood glucose values fall rapidly in the first hours after birth. Infants should have at least one test for glucose blood level in the early hours of life before they are fed. Glucose levels can be monitored by heel pricks done by the nurse. It is easiest to get blood from a newborn's heel if the heel is warm; the warmth brings a larger blood supply to the area. Dipping the

The Infant with a Congenital Anomaly or Neonatal Illness

heel in warm water or pressing a warm wet towel against it for a few minutes will warm a heel sufficiently. Milk the foot gently front to back. Wipe the heel with an alcohol wipe. Make a small puncture with a blood lancet. Allow a generous drop of blood to fall on a Dextrostix on the filter side. At exactly 60 seconds, rinse the Dextrostix with water and match it to the color on the chart of the bottle in which Dextrostix is supplied. A reading of under 45 mg per 100 ml on a Dextrostix should be reported, and intervention to increase the glucose level must be begun.

To correct blood glucose levels, early oral feeding or intravenous administration of a dextrose solution will be required. Administration of glucagon or epinephrine to convert glycogen into glucose is usually ineffective in newborns because their glycogen stores are generally inadequate. If the glucose level is only slightly lowered, giving the baby oral glucose water will cause a rapid rise. A rapid rise in glucose level will bring a compensatory increase in insulin production, which in another hour will again reduce the glucose level. Offering the infant formula rather than glucose water prevents this sequence of events. Since formula is absorbed slower, it does not cause such a rebound effect.

If the infant has difficulty sucking, the feeding may be given by gavage. If the glucose level must be raised immediately, an intravenous line is necessary. If a bolus of glucose is given by intravenous push, it will quickly relieve the hypoglycemia. A rebound effect of insulin production will also quickly lower the glucose level again, however. After the initial corrective measure, therefore, a slow infusion of glucose must be maintained to keep this from happening; the glucose is gradually tapered off. The infant must have continued assessment for blood glucose levels for at least 24 hours to determine whether the glucose level has stabilized and is not still fluctuating.

Infants who are delivered under general anesthesia and who do not suck well in the early hours of life require particular observation. Breast-fed infants who do not take readily to breast-feeding may need a supplemental feeding after breast-feeding to maintain a glucose level. Most mothers who are breast-feeding do not want their infant to have supplemental feedings; but then, neither do they want a retarded child with brain damage due to decreased glucose levels. Explaining the reason for the feeding will eliminate misunderstanding and any feelings that the hospital personnel are trying to undermine breast-feeding (you are trying to undermine mental retardation).

Monitoring glucose levels of high-risk infants can be a time-consuming task in a high-risk or transitional nursery. Because maintaining adequate circulating glucose levels protects against brain damage, however, the time spent in testing and regulating intravenous infusions is time very well spent.

The Infant of a Diabetic Mother

The infant of a diabetic woman is typically longer and weighs more than other babies (Fig. 38-22). Most such babies have a cushingoid (fat and puffy) appearance. They tend to be lethargic or limp in the first days of life. The large size results from overstimulation of pituitary growth hormone during pregnancy and extra fat deposits due to high levels of glucose during pregnancy. Although the infant appears large, his appearance is deceptive; he is often immature, born at 36 to 38 weeks of gestation. His lungs may be very immature. He is frequently referred to and must be managed as a "fragile giant."

Infants of diabetic women tend to have polycythemia. They will have their cord clamped early at delivery to prevent an overload of red blood cells from passing into them from the placenta. The infant of a diabetic mother loses a greater proportion of his weight in the first few days of life than does the average baby, because he loses an extra fluid accumulation. He needs to be observed closely to be certain that his large weight loss actually represents a loss of extra fluid and that dehydration is not occurring. Because congenital anomalies occur more often in infants of diabetic mothers than in other infants, such infants should

Fig. 38-22. Infant of a diabetic mother. Note the large size and the chubbiness. Although exceptionally large, the child is immature, a "fragile giant." (Courtesy of the Department of Medical Photography, Children's Hospital, Buffalo, N.Y.)

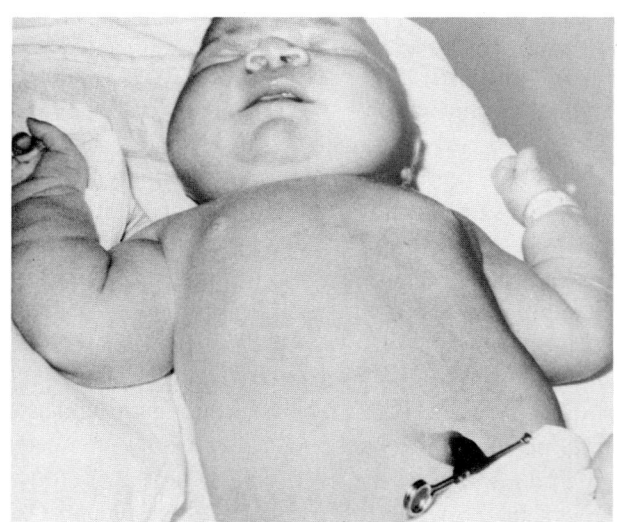

have a careful newborn anomaly appraisal. Respiratory distress syndrome (hyaline membrane disease) occurs more frequently in these infants than in others, probably because of their early gestation age, and thus they need close observation of their respirations and general well-being. Insulin secretion during pregnancy may interfere with cortisol release; this blocks the formation of lecithin or prevents lung maturity.

Immediately after birth, the baby tends to be hyperglycemic because the mother was probably slightly hyperglycemic during the pregnancy, allowing excessive glucose to diffuse across the placenta. The fetal pancreas responds to the high glucose level by islet cell hypertrophy resulting in matching high levels of insulin. Following delivery, the glucose level begins to fall; the mother's circulation is no longer supplying the infant. The overproduction of insulin causes the development of severe hypoglycemia, which makes the first 6 hours of life the infant's most hazardous, and the problem remains a real possibility for the first 24 hours.

The clinical signs of hypoglycemia are tremors, lethargy, poor sucking, apnea, hypotonia, hypothermia, and convulsions. The infant should have a Dextrostix determination done at birth and repeated every 30 minutes until the glucose level has stabilized. Although most infants with hypoglycemia show definite signs, a few may appear asymptomatic and yet have severe hypoglycemia. Rely on the Dextrostix determination in infants of diabetic mothers, not on your intuition.

Early oral or intravenous feeding of a glucose solution is almost always necessary to prevent severe hypoglycemia. In addition to blood sugar determinations, the infant should have a calcium level obtained, since hypocalcemia often accompanies hypoglycemia in these infants. Parathyroid glands, which regulate the calcium level, appear to hypertrophy in utero, also, and so a similar rebound effect occurs. He may need supplemental calcium administration as well.

Hyperbilirubinemia also tends to occur in these infants, probably because they are unable to clear bilirubin from their system at this immature age. The infant therefore needs his bilirubin levels monitored, so that treatment may be initiated if the level rises above safe limits.

It is difficult to think of babies of diabetic mothers as immature because they are so large. They *are* immature, however, so they may have more difficulty with mucus than more mature babies.

The infant must have follow-up care after discharge from the hospital because of the risk of his becoming diabetic at a later date. Diabetes will develop in about 2 percent of these infants by the time they are 20 years of age.

The mother needs frequent assurance that the infant is well, assuming that the baby has made the transition from intrauterine life to extrauterine life without trauma. Only when she thinks of him as a well child can she begin deep maternal-child interaction.

If the mother had class D diabetes, the infant tends to be small for gestation age because of poor placental perfusion. The problems of hypoglycemia, hypocalcemia, and hyperbilirubinemia remain the same.

Hypocalcemia

Hypocalcemia is a lowered blood calcium level. Phosphorus and calcium levels are maintained in indirect proportions in blood. That is, if phosphorus levels rise, calcium levels decrease; if calcium levels rise, phosphorus levels decrease. Hypocalcemia may be due, therefore, to changes in either calcium or phosphorus metabolism.

Hypocalcemia tends to occur in infants who had birth anoxia (phosphorus is released with anoxia), immature infants (the parathyroid gland which controls calcium metabolism is immature), and infants of diabetic mothers (it tends to accompany hypoglycemia). It may be caused by the imbalance between phosphorus and calcium in milk (such an imbalance does not exist in breast milk and is modified in commercial formulas).

LATENT TETANY. The chief sign of hypocalcemia is neuromuscular irritability, often referred to as *latent tetany*. This is accompanied by a serum calcium level less than 7.5 mg per 100 ml of blood. The newborn is jittery when he is handled or he cries for extended periods.

There are four ways to produce the clinical manifestations of tetany for diagnosis of hypocalcemia:

1. *Chvostek's sign.* When the skin anterior to the external ear (just over the sixth cranial nerve) is tapped, the facial muscles surrounding the eye, nose, and mouth contract unilaterally.
2. *Trousseau's sign.* When the upper arm is constricted for 2 to 3 minutes and the area becomes blanched, carpal spasm is elicited (the hand abducts, the wrist flexes, and the thumb is positioned across the cupped palm).
3. *Peroneal sign.* When the fibular side of the leg over the peroneal nerve is tapped, the foot abducts and dorsiflexes.

4. *Erb's sign.* Although this test is a dramatic one to see demonstrated, it requires a mild galvanic current and so cannot be used routinely as a test in a newborn nursery. A newborn with tetany has greater muscular irritability than a person with a normal calcium level. When mild current is applied to the infant, usually over the peroneal nerve just below the head of the fibula, the foot on that side will abduct and dorsiflex.

These are all useful tests to determine or suggest whether newborn jitteriness is from hypocalcemia, a central nervous system problem, or some other cause.

If tetany is going to be caused by cow's milk, it occurs at about the seventh day of life or after the baby is home. A community health nurse might be the one to recognize the problem initially.

MANIFEST TETANY. If the serum calcium level falls well under 7 mg per 100 ml of blood, manifest tetany may result. Muscular twitching and carpopedal spasms are the usual signs of this kind of tetany. Carpal spasms have been described; in pedal spasm, the foot is extended, the toes flex, and the sole of the foot cups. Generalized seizures may occur. There may be spasm of the larynx. The infant emits a high-pitched crowing sound on inspiration because of the constricted airway. If the spasm is prolonged, respirations may cease.

The presence of hypocalcemia is confirmed by a low serum calcium level on laboratory testing. Treatment is aimed toward increasing the serum calcium level in the blood to the point above the level that leads to latent tetany. Calcium may be administered orally as 10% calcium chloride if the infant can and will suck. It can be given intravenously as a 10% solution of calcium gluconate if the tetany has progressed to a point at which the child does not have enough muscular coordination to take oral fluid safely. Calcium gluconate should not be given intramuscularly or subcutaneously, since necrosis may occur at the injection site. If the newborn is having generalized seizures, he may require sodium phenobarbital in addition to the calcium gluconate to halt the seizures. Emergency equipment for intubation to relieve laryngospasm should be available.

Following the immediate therapy to increase the low serum blood levels, the infant will be placed on oral calcium therapy until it can be demonstrated that his calcium level has been regulated. Since vitamin D is necessary for the absorption of calcium and phosphorus from the gastrointestinal tract, the infant may be given a vitamin D supplement also.

DISORDERS OF THE HEMOPOIETIC SYSTEM
Hemorrhagic Disease of the Newborn

Hemorrhagic disease of the newborn is excessive bleeding in the newborn period due to low vitamin K levels. With the routine administration of AquaMEPHYTON to all newborns in the delivery room, this entity is almost never seen today. However, the nurse in the newborn nursery should double-check to be certain that all newborns receive prophylactic treatment against hemorrhage. When difficulty occurs in the delivery room (the infant needs resuscitation or the mother hemorrhages), personnel are often so geared to giving emergency care that routine measures are forgotten.

Vitamin K deficiency leads to deficiency of blood clotting factors II, VII, IX, and X. Hemorrhagic disease of the newborn typically begins on the second to fifth day of life. It involves massive hemorrhages in many parts of the body, including the meninges, ventricles of the brain, pulmonary alveoli, and liver.

Hyperbilirubinemia

When hyperbilirubinemia occurs in a newborn, it is usually the result of immature liver function, hemolytic disease of the newborn (erythroblastosis), infection, or bruising. Infants prone to hyperbilirubinemia are the following:

Infants born prematurely
Infants with blood group incompatibilities
Infants with sepsis
Infants with gastrointestinal obstruction
Infants with increased red blood cell volume (polycythemia)
Infants with extensive ecchymoses
Infants with cephalhematoma
Infants with intrauterine infections
Infants who are breast-fed
Infants with congenital hypothyroidism or galactosemia

PHYSIOLOGICAL JAUNDICE. It is common for infants to have immature liver function at birth—so common that jaundice from this cause occurring after the third day of life is normal in newborns. This type of jaundice occurs because of the following process: Fetal red blood cells are broken down rapidly after birth. As red blood cells are destroyed, heme and globin, a protein, are released. Globin is reused by the body, and heme is further broken down into iron and protoporphyrin. Iron is reused by the body. Protoporphyrin breaks down into indirect bilirubin. Indirect bilirubin is fat-soluble and therefore cannot be excreted by the kidneys. It is transported bound to serum albumin to the liver, where it must be converted to direct bilirubin (which is water-soluble and incorporated into bile for excretion) by the liver enzyme glucuronyl transferase.

When liver function is immature, glucuronyl transferase cannot convert all the indirect bilirubin to direct bilirubin. Indirect bilirubin thus begins to accumulate in the infant's bloodstream, causing jaundice. If levels of indirect bilirubin rise above 20 mg per 100 ml, a lethal condition, kernicterus, may develop (the indirect bilirubin level in brain tissue rises and destroys brain cells). Symptoms such as poor feeding, lethargy, and loss of the Moro reflex are the beginning signs of kernicterus. Also present may be opisthotonos and a high-pitched cry. Many babies in whom the symptoms of kernicterus develop die. The rest are usually left mentally retarded or with neuromotor retardation. The exact level at which kernicterus will occur cannot be predicted in individual infants. Those who are acidotic or immature or have decreased serum albumin may have damage at much lower levels of indirect bilirubin than infants without these factors present.

In jaundice due to immature liver function (physiological jaundice), indirect bilirubin rarely rises above 12 mg per 100 ml in a mature infant. It seldom becomes apparent before the third day of life or lasts past the first week of life.

Infants who are small for gestation age or are of low birth weight tend to have higher indirect bilirubin levels than do mature infants. Their bilirubin levels need to be monitored closely; although they have physiological jaundice, levels can rise to toxic amounts in these infants.

ASSESSING JAUNDICE. Jaundice becomes clinically apparent at about 7 mg of bilirubin per 100 ml of blood. At first, jaundice is seen only on the face. As it increases in severity, it affects the child's body also. The degree of bilirubin present may be estimated to some degree by observing how much of the infant's body is jaundiced (Fig. 38-23).

BRUISING. Bruising at birth leads to hemorrhage of blood into the subcutaneous tissue or skin. This blood is removed as bruising heals by breakdown of blood components. As the red blood cells are hemolyzed, indirect bilirubin is released. Cephalhematoma, or a collection of blood under the periosteum of the skull bone, can lead to the same phenomenon.

Infants with extensive bruising (large babies, breech babies, immature babies) must be watched carefully for indirect bilirubin levels.

INTESTINAL REABSORPTION. Indirect bilirubin is converted to direct bilirubin in the liver, becomes bile, and is excreted with stool. It is what gives stool its typical dark color. If intestinal obstruction is present or stool is not being evacuated, intestinal flora may break down bile back into its basic components and release

Fig. 38-23. Jaundice may be estimated to some degree by the zone on the child that it has reached. The indirect bilirubin level of zone 1 is 4 to 8 mg per 100 ml; of zone 2, 5 to 12 mg per 100 ml; of zone 3, 8 to 16 mg per 100 ml; of zone 4, 11 to 18 mg per 100 ml; of zone 5, 15 mg per 100 ml. (Based on data from L. D. Kramer, Advancement of dermal icterus in the jaundiced newborn. Am. J. Dis. Child. 118:454, 1969.)

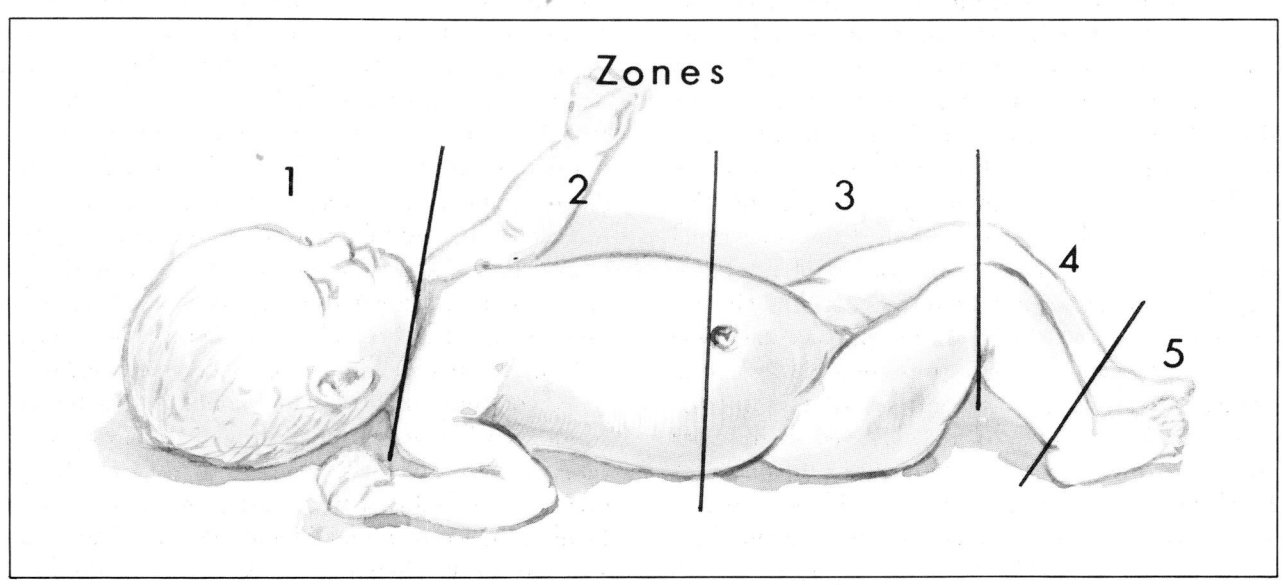

indirect bilirubin into the bloodstream. Early feeding of newborns, then, promotes intestinal movement and excretion of meconium and prevents indirect bilirubin buildup from this source. A newborn with a bowel obstruction cannot evacuate stool and may have a large indirect bilirubin buildup from this source.

Hemolytic Disease of the Newborn

Hemolytic disease of the newborn is most commonly due to an Rh or ABO blood incompatibility. In both these instances, the mother builds antibodies against the fetal red blood cells, leading to cell hemolysis (destruction). The destruction of red blood cells causes severe anemia and severe hyperbilirubinemia.

RH INCOMPATIBILITY. In Rh incompatibility, occasional antibodies against the Rh(D) factor form during pregnancy. However, most of the antibodies form in the mother's bloodstream in the 72 hours following birth. With a second pregnancy, there may be a high level of antibody D acting to destroy the fetal red blood cells at the beginning of the pregnancy. By the end of pregnancy, the fetus may be severely compromised by these antibodies. Some infants receive intrauterine transfusions to combat red cell destruction. They may be delivered early because of the destructive maternal environment.

Hemolytic disease of the newborn can be predicted by finding a rising anti-Rh titer (indirect Coombs' test) in the mother during pregnancy. It can be confirmed by detecting antibodies on the infant's erythrocytes in cord blood (positive direct Coombs' test). The mother in this situation will always have Rh-negative blood (dd), and the baby will be Rh positive (DD or Dd).

The infant may not appear pale at birth despite the red cell destruction that has gone on in utero, because the acceleration of red cell production during the last few months in utero may have compensated for the destruction to some degree. Enlargement of the liver and spleen and congestive heart failure (hydrops fetalis) from the severe anemia may be present. Despite the fall in the level of red blood cells in normal newborns after birth, the hemoglobin of newborns actually increases during the first day of life. This increase is due in part to transfusion of placental blood and in part to a shift of fluid from the intravascular to the extravascular spaces. By age 7 to 10 days, the hemoglobin level returns to that observed in the cord blood. A decrease in hemoglobin during the first week of life to a level less than that of cord blood is indicative of blood loss or hemolysis. Progressive jaundice, usually occurring within the first 24 hours of life, will reveal that a hemolytic process is at work.

ABO INCOMPATIBILITY. Hemolysis of the newborn may occur in the first pregnancy if an ABO incompatibility is present. In most of these instances, the maternal blood type is O and the fetal blood type is A. If an infant with a B blood type has a reaction, it is often the most serious. Hemolysis can become a problem with a first pregnancy in which there is an ABO incompatibility because the production of antibodies to A and B cell types are naturally occurring antibodies present from birth in individuals whose red cells lack these antigens. Unlike the antibodies formed against the Rh factor, these antibodies are large (IgM class) and so do not cross the placenta well. The infant of an ABO incompatibility therefore is not born anemic, as is the Rh-sensitized child. Hemolysis of the blood begins with birth, however, when blood and antibodies are exchanged as maternal and fetal blood mixes, with loosening of the placenta, leading to jaundice.

Interestingly, low-birth-weight infants do not seem to be affected by ABO incompatibility. This may be because the receptor sites for anti-A or anti-B antibodies do not appear on red cells until later in fetal life. Even in the mature newborn, the direct Coombs' test may only be weakly positive because of the few anti-A or anti-B sites present.

Phototherapy and exchange transfusion may both be necessary to reduce indirect bilirubin levels in the infant affected by ABO or Rh incompatibility.

Interventions to Lower Indirect Bilirubin Levels

PHOTOTHERAPY. Phototherapy is a technique that is often helpful in reducing the level of indirect bilirubin. In phototherapy, the infant is continuously exposed to three to six fluorescent light tubes with a total strength of 200 to 500 foot-candles. The lights are placed above an Isolette, and the infant is undressed except for his diaper, so that as much skin surface as possible is exposed to the light (Fig. 38-24). Photodecomposition is a normal alternative route of bilirubin excretion, and the use of lights increases this rate of excretion. The Plexiglass top of the Isolette should always be in place when the lights are on because it protects the infant from ultraviolet lights and burning.

It may be harmful to the newborn's retina to be exposed continuously to a bright light, and thus the eyes must be covered for the entire time the infant is under bilirubin lights. The eyes are usually covered with eye dressings or cotton balls, which are then secured firmly in place by an additional dressing. The infant must be checked frequently to be certain the dressings have not slipped or are causing corneal irritation.

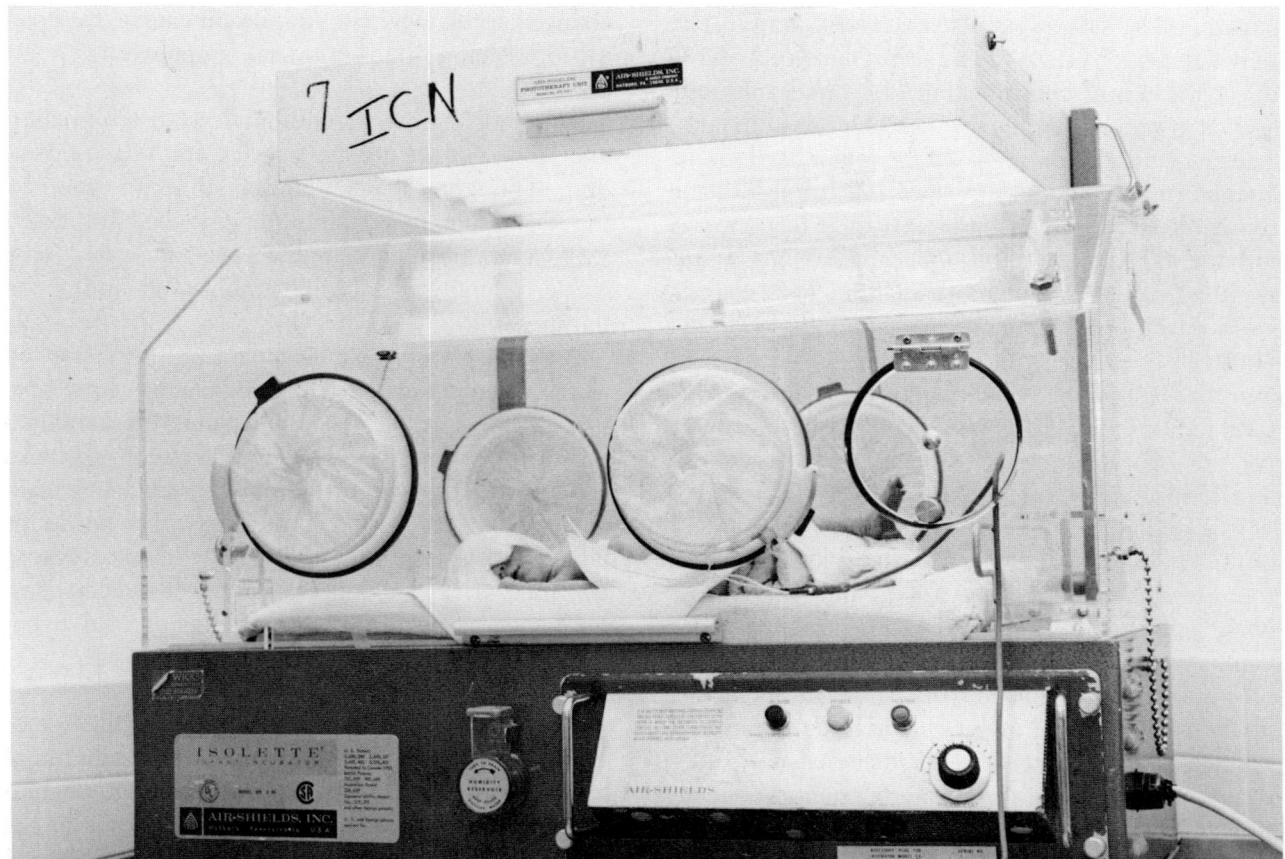

Fig. 38-24. A newborn receiving phototherapy. The infant is undressed except for his diaper. Notice how snugly his eyes are covered to protect them from the light source. (Courtesy of the Department of Medical Photography, Children's Hospital, Buffalo, N.Y.)

The stools of an infant under bilirubin lights are often bright green from the excessive bilirubin that is excreted as the result of the therapy. They are also frequently loose and may be irritating to skin. Urine may be dark colored from urobilinogen formation. The infant may lose considerable fluid through insensible water loss because of the temperature of the lights above him. He must have his skin turgor assessed and his intake and output measured to ensure that dehydration is not occurring.

Phototherapy is a relatively new technique. It has the advantages of being inexpensive and requiring no special personnel other than a conscientious observer. Although no long-term effects have been studied as yet, there appears to be no risk to the infant, provided his eyes remain covered.

Unfortunately, phototherapy may take several hours to have an effect. It is not the first method of choice, therefore, if bilirubin levels are rapidly rising. In that instance, the method of clearing indirect bilirubin levels is exchange transfusion.

An infant under phototherapy should be removed for feeding so that he continues to have interaction with his mother. The eye patches should be removed during this time so that he has a period of visual stimulation.

The mother needs an explanation of why her infant is being kept under special lights. Isolettes are automatically associated with very ill infants. At the same time, the use of lights does not seem very scientific (almost a home remedy). She is easily confused by the two interventions, one seemingly serious and the other seemingly not serious at all.

SUSPENSION OF BREAST-FEEDING. Pregnanediol, the breakdown product of progesterone, is excreted in breast milk until the high levels of progesterone that were present during pregnancy are excreted. Pregnanediol interferes with the conjugation of indirect bilirubin. Breast-fed babies, therefore, may evidence more jaundice than bottle-fed babies. Temporary suspension of breast-feeding for 24 hours may be necessary to reduce an accumulating indirect bilirubin level in some infants. If the mother manually expresses breast milk while feeding is halted, her milk supply will be maintained; this therapy is not a permanent contraindication to breast-feeding.

EXCHANGE TRANSFUSION. Exchange transfusion removes about 85 percent of sensitized red cells. It reduces the serum concentration of indirect bilirubin and often prevents congestive heart failure in infants. Exchange transfusion is done if the infant has a severe anemia (under 12 to 14 gm per 100 ml at birth or during the first 24 hours of life). It must be done before the indirect serum bilirubin level reaches 20 mg per 100 ml of blood in mature infants; 8 to 12 mg per 100 ml in immature infants. Because indirect bilirubin levels rise at relatively predictable levels, exchange transfusion should be performed if the bilirubin concentration exceeds 5 mg per 100 ml at birth, 10 mg per 100 ml at 8 hours, 12 mg per 100 ml at 16 hours, and 15 mg per 100 ml at 24 hours of age [19].

The infant must be kept warm during the procedure. The blood being given must be maintained at room temperature, or shock can result. The type of blood used for transfusion is O Rh-negative blood, compatible with the mother's blood, or Rh-negative blood of the infant's blood type. Rh-negative blood is used even though the infant's blood type is positive; if positive blood were given, the maternal antibodies that entered the infant's circulation in utero would destroy this blood also, and the transfusion would be ineffective. If the baby is transported to a regional center for the exchange transfusion, a sample of the mother's blood must accompany the infant, so that cross matching on the mother's serum can be done there. The baby's stomach is aspirated prior to the procedure so that there is no danger of aspiration due to the manipulation involved. The umbilical vein is catheterized for the procedure.

The baby must be carefully monitored during an exchange transfusion; his heart rate, respirations, and venous pressure all must be observed. The amount of blood given is usually calculated as follows: 85 ml × weight (in kilograms) × 2. The average blood volume of a newborn is 85 ml per kilogram, but an amount equal to twice the blood volume is used because studies have indicated that this quantity will ensure an exchange of erythrocytes that is 85 to 90 percent effective. Because stored blood for transfusion contains acid-citrate-dextrose (which can lower blood calcium levels) added to it as an anticoagulant, calcium gluconate is given through the exchange catheter after each 100 ml of blood, or heparinized blood is used. Heparinized blood may interfere with clotting following the transfusion. Administering protamine sulfate aids in metabolism of heparin and restoration of clotting ability. About 2 to 4 ml of blood is removed by syringe, 2 to 4 ml of donor blood is infused, and so forth for the procedure. The blood must be exchanged at this slow rate, to prevent cardiac overload so an exchange transfusion takes approximately an hour.

A hemoglobin and bilirubin level determination and blood culture are taken at the end of the procedure. The infant may be primed for a transfusion by the administration of albumin prior to the transfusion. This causes bilirubin to bind with the albumin, and a greater quantity of bilirubin is removed during the transfusion.

After the transfusion, the infant must be observed closely for umbilical bleeding and changes from normal in vital signs. He needs bilirubin levels monitored for two or three days following transfusion, to make certain that the level of bilirubin is not rising again and another transfusion is necessary. He needs his blood glucose level monitored if acid-citrate-dextrose was used as a blood anticoagulant, as this added dextrose may cause insulin overproduction and hypoglycemia.

Infants who have had hemolytic disease of the newborn tend to have a progressive drop in the hemoglobin concentration during the first six months of life. The bone marrow fails to increase its production of erythrocytes in response to continuing hemolysis. The infant may need an additional transfusion of blood in order to correct this late anemia.

Blood Loss Anemia

Fetal-maternal transfusion or twin transfusion (placental blood being directed to the mother's circulation or to one twin) may result in a significant blood loss for some infants. The infant may be bleeding internally from intracranial hemorrhage or splenic rupture. A torn umbilical cord or a placenta previa may be a source of blood loss. Normal cord blood has a hemoglobin level of 17 to 18 gm per 100 ml. A level below 13.5 gm per 100 ml indicates anemia.

The infant with blood loss anemia appears pale, and respirations may be grunting. Although the infant seems to be in respiratory distress, he has little cyanosis, and oxygen administration does not improve his condition.

The cord blood may not reflect the degree of blood loss if bleeding is continuing. Blood must be drawn from the infant for a true picture. Treatment is by transfusion.

RESPIRATORY ILLNESS
Transient Tachypnea of the Newborn

Newborns have rapid rates of respiration, up to 80 breaths per minute at birth, but within an hour this rapid rate slows to between 30 and 50. In some infants respiratory rates remain at a high level, between 80 and 120 per minute. The infant does not appear to be in a great deal of distress aside from the tiring effort of breathing so fast. He has no retractions and rarely cyanosis. Feeding is difficult for him as he cannot suck and breathe this rapidly at the same time.

Transient tachypnea appears to result from slow absorption of lung fluid. This limits the amount of alveolar surface available to the infant for oxygen exchange, and he must increase his respirations to better utilize the surface available.

The infant needs close observation to see that his increased effort does not tire him or that the signs are not simple slow absorption of lung fluid but the beginning signs of a more serious disorder (a rapid rate of respirations is often the first sign of respiratory obstruction in infants). Transient tachypnea of the newborn fades spontaneously over the first few days of life as the lung fluid is absorbed and respiratory activity becomes effective.

Meconium Aspiration

An infant who has hypoxia in utero has a relaxation of the rectal sphincter with release of meconium into the amniotic fluid. Babies born breech may expel meconium into the amniotic fluid. The appearance of the fluid at birth is green to greenish black from the staining.

At the time of the initial distress or during the birth process, if the infant inhales any of the fluid, he aspirates meconium. Meconium may cause severe respiratory distress in two ways: It can bring about inflammation of bronchioles because it is a foreign substance, or it may block small bronchioles by mechanical plugging. A secondary infection of injured tissue may lead to pneumonia.

Infants with meconium-stained amniotic fluid may have difficulty establishing respirations at birth (those who were not breech-born have had a hypoxic episode in utero to cause the meconium to be in the amniotic fluid). Oxygen under pressure (bag and mask) should not be administered until the infant has been intubated and suctioned so that the pressure of the oxygen does not drive small plugs of meconium farther down into the lungs, worsening the irritation and obstruction.

Following the initiation of respirations, the infant's respiration rate may remain elevated (tachypnea). He may have retractions; the inflammation of bronchi tends to trap air in alveoli—the way an asthmatic traps alveolar air. The chest may become enlarged (barrel chest) due to this air trapping. Blood gases will reveal the poor exchange of air. A chest x-ray film will show bilateral course infiltrates in the lung with spaces of hyperaeration (a peculiar honeycomb effect).

The infant may require oxygen administration and assisted ventilation. Postural drainage may be helpful to encourage removal of flecks of remaining meconium from the lungs. The infant may be treated with an antibiotic to forestall development of pneumonia as a secondary problem.

Any infant who is trapping air in alveoli must be observed closely for signs of pneumothorax because alveoli can expand only so far and then will rupture, sending air into the pleural space.

Pneumothorax

A pneumothorax is a rupture of lung alveoli allowing air to escape from lung space into the pleural space. This may occur at birth from overinflation of alveoli with the first breath; it usually occurs as a result of ventilatory assistance. Air in the pleural space prevents the lung from expanding, making it difficult for the infant to inspire (negative pressure is lost); atelectasis occurs.

The infant quickly develops extremely distressed respirations. His chest may appear asymmetrical; his trachea may be displaced away from the affected side. Cyanosis develops rapidly. The infant's abdomen may become distended from pressure on the diaphragm.

The infant needs to be kept warm; he needs support by oxygen administration. A chest x-ray will be ordered to confirm the diagnosis. Air in the pleural space is removed by needle aspiration or immediate insertion of a chest tube connected to underwater seal drainage with low suction. If these measures can be instituted promptly, the infant's prognosis from this sudden, possibly devastating occurrence is good.

INFECTIONS
Pneumonia

Pneumonia may occur in the first few days of life in the infant whose membranes were ruptured more than 24 hours before delivery, or in the infant who aspirates vaginal secretions or meconium-stained amniotic fluid. The infant may have delayed respirations at birth, with subsequent development of dyspnea, tachypnea, retractions, and cyanosis. The mature infant may have an accompanying fever; a less mature baby may evidence hypothermia as a response to infection. A chest x-ray film will reveal densities suggestive of pneumonia.

The infant needs warmth, oxygen administration, and possibly assisted ventilation and an antibiotic. Pneumonia is always a serious finding in a neonate, as it is a severe infection and is difficult for a newborn to combat with his limited reserves.

Prolonged Rupture of the Membranes

If membranes ruptured more than 24 hours prior to delivery, there is a very great chance that organisms have invaded the open uterus and the infant is born contaminated. Pneumonia or skin infections may result. Blood and surface cultures should be obtained from the infant at birth. If he is showing any sign of infection (lethargy, shock), blood, cerebrospinal fluid, urine, gastric aspiration, throat, ear canals, umbilicus, axilla, and rectum all need to be examined by culture.

The infant will be treated with an antibiotic appropriate for the organism identified.

Group B Beta Hemolytic Streptococcal Infection

The major cause of infection in newborn infants today is the group B hemolytic streptococcal organism. Between 50 and 300 infants in every 1,000 live births display a positive culture for this organism. The organism is contracted at the time of delivery from secretions in the birth canal. It may be spread from baby to baby if good handwashing technique is not used in handling newborns.

Colonization by group B hemolytic streptocci may result in early-onset or late-onset illness. With the early-onset form, symptoms of pneumonia become apparent in the first few hours of life. The infant will have tachypnea and apnea and symptoms of shock such as decreased urine output, extreme paleness, or hypotonia. He may develop an expiratory grunt. The grunting sound is made by air being forced past contracted vocal cords. This is a compensatory mechanism of newborns to maintain pressure in the alveoli on expiration and prevent alveolar collapse.

Pneumonia may develop so rapidly that as many as 90 percent of infants who contract the infection die within 24 hours of birth.

With the late-onset type, instead of pneumonia being the infection focus, meningitis tends to occur. About a week after the infant returns home, he gradually becomes lethargic and develops a fever and upper respiratory symptoms. His fontanelles will bulge from increased intracranial pressure. Mortality from the late-onset type is not as high as from the early-onset form (15 percent compared to 90 percent), but neurological consequences may occur in up to 50 percent of infants who survive.

Gentamicin, ampicillin, and penicillin are all effective against group B hemolytic streptococcal infections. It is difficult for parents to understand how their infant could suddenly become this ill. They may need a great deal of support to care for the infant if he does survive the infection but is left handicapped.

Congenital Rubella

In urban areas of the United States, about 15 to 20 percent of women of childbearing age are susceptible to rubella. The greatest risk to the embryo from the rubella virus is during the 2nd to 6th week of intrauterine life. The frequency of malformations is about 50 percent if the virus invasion is during these early weeks.

The classic symptoms of the rubella syndrome are thrombocytopenia, cardiac, sight, and hearing defects, and motor and mental retardation. The thrombocytopenia is manifested by purpura, red-purple maculae with a "blueberry muffin" appearance. The cardiac defects that are most common are patent ductus arteriosus, pulmonary stenosis, and atrial and ventricular septal defects. Deafness with the rubella syndrome is generally neural deafness of an uncorrectable type; it is generally bilateral. Serious eye defects seen are cataract and congenital glaucoma. The retina of the eye is often covered by discrete patchy black pigmentation that, while it does not interfere with sight, is so often present that it is an aid in diagnosis. The diagnosis is confirmed by identifying IgM antibodies against rubella in the child's serum. IgM antibodies do not cross the placenta, so they could not have come from the mother; they must have been produced by the fetus in response to invasion by the rubella antigen.

Live rubella virus may be cultured from nasopharyngeal secretions of affected infants at birth. At 1 year of age, about 10 percent of these infants are still shedding live virus. These infants must be isolated in the hospital as this virus is airborne spread. Treatment is symptomatic, depending on the defects present. The prognosis will also depend on the number and extent of the defects.

Herpesvirus Infection

A generalized herpesvirus infection can be contracted by a fetus across the placenta. More often, it is contracted at birth from the mother who has herpetic vulvovaginitis from herpesvirus type II. If the infection was acquired during pregnancy, the infant may be born with vesicles. If the infant acquires the infection at birth, at about the fourth to seventh day of life he has a loss of appetite, perhaps a low-grade fever, and lethargy. Stomatitis or a few vesicles on the skin may be noted. Herpes vesicles are always clustered, pinpoint in size, and surrounded by a reddened base. Suddenly the infant becomes extremely ill. He may have dyspnea, jaundice, purpura, convulsions, and shock. Death may occur within hours or days. Children who survive generalized herpesvirus infections in the newborn period may have permanent central nervous system sequelae.

There is some evidence that adenine arabinoside (ara-A), a drug that inhibits viral DNA synthesis, may be effective in combating this overwhelming infection. At the moment, however, prevention is the newborn's best protection. Women with herpetic vulva lesions should be delivered by cesarean section. Women with herpes lesions on their face (herpes simplex or cold sores) should not feed or hold their newborns until lesions are crusted and no longer contagious. Health care personnel who have herpes simplex infections must not care for newborn infants. Although herpes simplex lesions are probably caused by herpesvirus type I, this limitation in contact does not seem excessive in light of the severity of the disease. The woman who is isolated from her newborn at birth needs to view the infant from the nursery window. She should be kept informed of how well he is eating and of anything special about him (how he likes to be wrapped firmly, how he follows a finger eagerly) so that maternal bonding will not be seriously impaired.

Cytomegalic Inclusion Disease

The cytomegalovirus was originally named the *salivary gland virus* because it was first isolated from salivary glands. It is similar to the herpes simplex virus.

Cytomegalic inclusion disease may be transmitted across the placenta to the fetus. The infant who has severe involvement from this virus invasion may have gross central nervous system damage, such as microcephaly, blindness, deafness, and mental retardation. He may show signs of jaundice, lethargy, convulsions, splenomegaly, and hepatomegaly.

Management is supportive, depending on the problems present.

Congenital Syphilis

If a woman has syphilis during the last half of pregnancy, the organism of syphilis, *Treponema pallidum*, may cross the placenta and cause congenital syphilis. Severely infected infants are stillborn; others, less infected, are born with congenital anomalies. Moist areas of the infant (the cord and nasal secretions) are generally infectious at birth.

The infected newborn does not develop a chancre, the typical painless ulcer lesion of adult first-stage syphilis, but about a week after birth a copper-colored rash, most prominent over the face, soles of the feet, and palms of the hands, may appear. This is an unusual rash as most rashes do not cover the soles of the feet or the palms of the hands. The infant's nose may show a severe rhinitis (snuffles). X-ray study of the long bones may reveal changes of epiphyseal lines at about 1 to 3 months of age.

As the permanent teeth erupt at 5 or 6 years, they may be pegged or notched (Hutchinson's teeth). All teeth tend to be of poor quality and decay easily. If the disease remains untreated, interstitial keratitis (inflammatory reaction of the cornea with vascular infiltration) may result when the child is between 6 and 14 years of age. This scarring may cause blindness. As the disease progresses, it may become tertiary or lead to neurological manifestations.

All women have tests for syphilis (VDRL) done at their first prenatal visit, and again at delivery. The infant born of a woman with a positive VDRL is given a course of penicillin at birth. An FTA-ABS (fluorescent treponemal antibody absorption) test is a specific test for IgM antibodies against syphilis and may be helpful for diagnosis in the newborn.

Gonococcal Conjunctivitis

If a woman has gonorrhea at the time of delivery, as the infant is delivered vaginally he may contract gonorrhea of the conjunctiva or *ophthalmia neonatorum*. This infection is generally bilateral. The eye conjunctiva becomes fiery red, there is thick pus, and the eyelid is edematous, all on the first to the fourth day of life. Gonococcal conjunctivitis should be considered as a possibility when a conjunctivitis occurs in any child who is under 30 days of age.

This is an extremely serious form of conjunctivitis because if it is left untreated the infection extends to corneal ulceration and destruction, which results in opacity of the cornea and blindness.

The prophylactic instillation of 1% silver nitrate, erythromycin or tetracycline ointment into the eyes of newborns prevents gonococcal conjunctivitis. If the disease does occur, the newborn must be isolated; this condition is extremely contagious.

The treatment is large doses of penicillin given both locally by instillation and systemically. The eyes are washed with saline irrigations to clear the copious discharge of pus. When irrigating eyes, use a sterile medicine dropper or sterile bulb syringe. The solution should be at room temperature and sterile. Direct the stream of the irrigation fluid laterally so that it cannot enter and contaminate the other eye. If some fluid should splash into your eye, you must have penicillin administered or you may contract the disease.

Infants born in such locations as taxicabs or at home need eye prophylaxis to prevent ophthalmia neonatorum the same as infants born in the delivery or birthing room.

Parents of infants with the infection should be given a realistic report of the seriousness of this disease. They have reason to feel guilty because they caused the child to contract the disease. Often the mother did not know that she had gonorrhea (it has few symptoms in the woman) or did not know that the disease could harm her baby at birth. Under these circumstances, she really has no reason to feel guilty. The mother may have difficulty establishing a good relationship with her infant because of her guilt and because the child is ill and isolated from her (although as long as she uses good infection technique she should be allowed to hold and feed the baby in the isolation nursery). She needs support to think of herself as a worthy mother, not a disease carrier; she needs treatment for gonorrhea herself before fallopian tube sterility or pelvic inflammatory disease results. Any recent sexual contacts of the mother should be treated also so that the spread of the disease can be stopped.

She can be assured that with early diagnosis and treatment the prognosis for normal eyesight in the child is good.

Candidiasis

Candida albicans is the fungus responsible for candidal infections. *Candida* organisms grow in the vagina of many adult women (monilial vaginitis). Pregnant women are particularly susceptible to candidal infections.

As the child is born through the vagina, he may develop an infection of the mucous membrane of his mouth (thrush). Thrush is characterized by white plaques on an erythematous base on the buccal membrane and the surface of the tongue. It resembles milk curds left from a recent milk feeding. Thrush plaques do not scrape away, however, whereas milk curds do. The child's mouth is painful, and he does not eat well on account of the inflammation and local pain. Since thrush usually appears on the fourth to seventh day of life, it may not be seen in newborn nurseries but by community health nurses making newborn visits.

Candida albicans also causes a severe, bright red, sharply circumscribed diaper-area rash. Satellite lesions may appear. The rash is marked by its intense color and by the fact that it does not improve with the usual diaper-rash measures—talcum, frequent changing of diapers, exposure to air, or an ointment such as A and D. It tends to occur in infants who have been treated with an antibiotic; suppression of normal skin flora may allow for overgrowth of fungal organisms.

Nystatin is an antifungal drug that is effective against the oral and diaper-rash form. For thrush, it is supplied as a liquid. It should be dropped into the infant's mouth about four times a day following feedings so as to remain in contact with the oral mucosa for a period of time rather than being washed away immediately by a feeding. For diaper rash, a nystatin ointment is prescribed. If a newborn infant has a candidal infection, the mother is usually treated also with nystatin vaginal suppositories to eradicate the source of the infection. The woman's sexual partner may need treatment also or the infant will have the infection again in another few weeks as it is spread from the man to the mother to the infant.

INTRACRANIAL HEMORRHAGE

The pressure of delivery on the fetal head may cause tentorial membrane tears (the membrane separating the cerebellum and parietal brain portions), resulting in hemorrhage from torn blood vessels into the cerebellum or brain stem.

Infants most susceptible to this problem are those who were born after a prolonged labor or were extracted by means of midforceps. It may occur in precipitate deliveries because of the sudden release of pressure from the fetal head at birth.

The pressure of blood in the cranial space causes increased intracranial pressure. The infant may have such brain stem pressure on the respiratory center at birth that he cannot be resuscitated; the child with less pressure may have cyanosis, apnea, or slowed respirations in the first hours of life. The pressure may cause convulsions. The infant's cry may be shrill and high-pitched. He may have decreased motor control (hypotonia or hypertonia).

The extent of the bleeding will be determined by a computed tomography (CT) scan. The infant needs systemic support measures such as warmth, oxygen administration, and intravenous fluid. His prognosis is guarded because even if he survives this major insult to brain tissue, he may be left with permanent neurological damage such as mental retardation or cerebral palsy.

SEIZURES

Seizures in the newborn period may be difficult to recognize, because they may consist only of some twitching of the head, arms, or eyes and slight cyanosis or apnea. The infant may be limp and flaccid afterward.

In older children, the cause of seizures is often unknown, but in neonates, the etiology can be established 75 percent of the time. The cause may be anoxia, perinatal injury, infection, kernicterus, or a metabolic disorder.

Anoxia may result from placenta previa or premature separation of the placenta. Perinatal injury involves some form of trauma to the newborn head: an unusually tight maternal cervix or inefficient use of forceps, causing trauma. Subdural hematomas caused from the pressure of the birth canal do not as a rule lead to convulsions; the skull suture lines are so expandable at birth that pressure on the brain does not have such serious consequences. The metabolic disorders that lead to seizures are hypoglycemia, hypocalcemia, and lack of pyridoxine (vitamin B_6).

Occasionally, neonates will have an infection of the central nervous system that is manifested by convulsions. Seizures that occur after the third day of life are much more likely to be caused by infection than by trauma. Newborns whose membranes were ruptured for 24 hours or more before delivery are more prone to convulsions than infants whose membranes were ruptured closer to delivery.

Kernicterus, in which high bilirubin levels in the blood destroy brain cells, resulting from either physiological jaundice or jaundice caused by blood incompatibility, may lead to seizures.

Electroencephalograms in the newborn may be normal despite extensive disease. Thus, an abnormal electroencephalogram this early in life usually denotes a particularly severe involvement and a poor prognosis. Lumbar puncture in newborns does not give meaningful results, because about 20 percent of all newborns have abnormal cerebrospinal fluid at birth. Protein is increased and a few red blood cells may be present from rupture of subarachnoid capillaries during passage through the birth canal.

Neonates metabolize drugs more rapidly than older infants, children, or adults, and thus the dosage of anticonvulsant medication used during the newborn period is high. The dosage of phenobarbital, for instance, is about 1.5 mg per kilogram per day for adults; in newborns, the dosage may be 8 to 12 mg per kilogram per day. Nutrition is a problem for the infant who is having frequent seizures, as he is unable to suck effectively; trying to feed him while he is convulsing may lead to aspiration. He will need intravenous fluid to keep him from becoming dehydrated until his seizures are controlled.

THE INFANT OF A DRUG-DEPENDENT MOTHER

Infants of drug-dependent women tend to be small for gestation age. It is difficult during pregnancy to predict a delivery date for many of these infants because of their small size and the woman's uncertainty about the date of her last menstrual period. Urine estriol levels are usually low in drug-addicted women and so are not a good guide to use to determine a due date; they give false information as to placental status. The best guide to assess maturity seems to be the lecithin-sphingomyelin ratio of amniotic fluid.

An infant born of a woman who is addicted to a narcotic such as morphine, heroin, or methadone will show withdrawal symptoms shortly after birth. Some women will tell you or the physician on admission to the labor unit that they are addicted to such drugs to warn the health care team that their infant will have withdrawal symptoms. Other women, afraid of exposing their habit, will not reveal this information. Be suspicious of addiction in the woman who appears to obtain little relief from normal amounts of analgesics (remembering that there is a great deal of difference in people's pain thresholds), or who is overly anxious to be discharged shortly after delivery. Look for streaks over veins or needle puncture marks on the skin of the woman.

Babies of drug-dependent women are usually irritable, with disturbed sleep patterns. They move so constantly that they cause abrasions on their elbows, knees, or nose. They may have tremors and may sneeze frequently. They may have a shrill, high-pitched cry like that of a brain-damaged infant. Hyperreflexia and clonus may be present, and convulsions may occur. Many such infants have tachypnea (rapid respirations) so severe that hyperventilation and alkalosis develop. The infant may have frantic sucking activity. Vomiting and diarrhea may begin, leading to large fluid losses and secondary dehydration. These symptoms usually occur in the first 24 hours of life, although they may appear as late as at 7 days of age in heroin addiction, 2 weeks of age in methadone addiction, and 2 months of age in phenobarbital addiction.

Methadone-addicted infants tend to have an increased incidence of seizures as compared with heroin-addicted infants. One of the most frequent findings in methadone-addicted infants at 2 to 3 months of age is an excessive amount of fluid intake (40 to 50 ounces per day).

Narcotic metabolites or quinine (heroin is often mixed with quinine) may be obtained from the infant's urine in the first hours after birth. These products are quickly cleared from his body, however, and by the time symptoms become severe, detection of narcotic substances may no longer be possible. A neonatal drug withdrawal scoring system is shown in Table 38-2. Assessment using the scale is made hourly for the first 24 hours, every 2 hours for the next

Table 38-2. Items Used to Score Neonatal Abstinence in the Nursery Newborn

Signs and Symptoms	Score
High-pitched cry	2
Continuous high-pitched cry	3
Sleeps less than 1 hour after feeding	3
Sleeps less than 2 hours after feeding	2
Sleeps less than 3 hours after feeding	1
Hyperactive Moro reflex	2
Markedly hyperactive Moro reflex	3
Mild tremors when disturbed	1
Marked tremors when disturbed	2
Mild tremors when undisturbed	3
Marked tremors when undisturbed	4
Increased muscle tone	2
Generalized convulsion	5
Frantic sucking of fists	1
Poor feeding	2
Regurgitation	2
Projectile vomiting	3
Loose stools	2
Watery stools	3
Dehydration	2
Frequent yawning	1
Sneezing	1
Nasal stuffiness	1
Sweating	1
Mottling	1
Fever less than 101°F	1
Fever greater than 101°F	2
Respiratory rate over 60 per minute	1
Respiratory rate over 60 per minute with retractions	2
Excoriation of nose	1
Excoriation of knees	1
Excoriation of toes	1

Source. R. E. Kron, et al., Behavior of Infants Born to Drug-dependent Mothers. Effects of Prenatal and Postnatal Drugs. In J. L. Rementería (Ed.), *Drug Abuse in Pregnancy and Neonatal Effects.* St. Louis: Mosby, 1977.

24 hours, and every 4 hours thereafter. If an infant receives a score under 7 by this scale, he probably needs no drug withdrawal therapy. Such assessment can be done as an independent nursing chore.

Infants of drug-dependent mothers usually seem most comfortable when firmly swaddled. They should be kept in an environment free from excessive stimuli (a small isolation nursery, not a large, noisy one). Some quiet best if the room is darkened. Many infants of heroin-addicted women suck vigorously and continuously and seem to find comfort and quiet if given a pacifier. Infants of methadone-addicted women may have extremely poor sucking ability and may have difficulty getting enough fluid intake.

Specific therapy for the infant is individualized according to the nature and severity of the symptoms. The infant must have his electrolyte and fluid balance maintained. If he has vomiting or diarrhea, he may need intravenous administration of fluid. The infant should not be breast-fed by an addicted mother. The drugs used to counteract withdrawal symptoms include paregoric, phenobarbital, codeine, methadone, chlorpromazine (Thorazine), and diazepam (Valium).

Infants of heroin-addicted women are rarely jaundiced. Those of methadone-addicted women tend to have a higher-than-normal incidence of jaundice. Infants of heroin-addicted women are likely to have a low incidence of respiratory distress syndrome despite their small size.

Once the infant is identified as one who has been exposed to drugs in utero, the mother needs treatment for withdrawal symptoms and follow-up care as much as does the infant.

THE INFANT WITH A FETAL ALCOHOL SYNDROME

Alcohol crosses the placenta in the same concentration that it is present in the maternal bloodstream. When a woman ingests more than 3 ounces (two drinks) of 100-percent alcohol per day, there is a risk that her child may be born severely affected as a direct result of the alcohol or its oxidation product acetaldehyde on fetal growing cells.

Frequently found consequences in the infant are prenatal and postnatal growth retardation, mental retardation, microcephaly, joint anomalies, and cardiac anomalies. The perinatal growth retardation is unusual in that the infant is short in length in comparison with weight. Usually with intrauterine growth retardation weight is decreased in comparison with length. The baby may have difficulty feeding in the newborn period because he sucks poorly. He may be irritable, tending to be always awake or always asleep, depending on the alcohol level of the mother close to delivery.

The infant needs long-term follow-up so the full extent of his involvement can be determined as he grows and proper educational programs can be planned for him. Double-check that his mother understands what care he needs at home. Many women who are alcoholic have few support people and have no one to turn to if they have a problem with newborn care.

Being a mother is a new role for a woman, a new beginning. It may be a time when she is willing to initiate help for herself through a group such as Alcoholics Anonymous. Investigate to see if this is a possibility and help her make a contact.

Problem-oriented Recording: Progress Notes

Careful watch nursery
Admission note

Problem: Health assessment

> S. Vigorously crying large female infant. Infant 38 weeks' gestation age; mother class A diabetic. No FHR abnormalities during labor; vaginal delivery. Mother given continuous insulin infusion during labor. Blood sugars were always between 90 and 105.
> O. Weight: 9 lbs, 6 oz (over 90th %).
>   Dextrostix at birth: 90 mg.
>   Dextrostix now at 1 hour of age 45–90 mg.
> A. Infant of diabetic mother large for gestation age.
> Goals: a. Infant maintains blood glucose over 45 mg% by early feeding at 1 hour of age.
>   b. Infant develops no pulmonary problems (38 weeks' gestation).
>   c. Infant's temperature stabilizes with Isolette protection.
>   d. Infant's bilirubin level remains under 12 mg%.
> P. 1. Admit to Isolette for warmth.
>   2. Dextrostix q½h for first 4 hours.
>   3. Feed glucose water orally at 1 hour.
>   4. Do gestational assessment to evaluate true gestation age.
>   5. Phone mother in recovery room to keep her informed of infant's progress.

References

1. Bahr, J. E. Herpesvirus hominis type 2 in women and newborns. *M.C.N.* 3:16, 1978.
2. Boychuk, R. B. Meconium aspiration syndrome and pulmonary hypertension. *Respir. Technol.* 14:10, 1978.
3. Clyman, R. I., et al. What pediatricians say to mothers of sick newborns. *Pediatrics* 63:719, 1979.
4. Dingle, R. E., et al. Continuous transcutaneous O_2 monitoring in the neonate. *Am. J. Nurs.* 80:890, 1980.
5. Drummond, G. Meconium aspiration. *Nurs. Mirror* 147:24, 1978.
6. Gluck, L. Special problems of the newborn. *Hosp. Pract.* 13:75, 1978.
7. Gotoff, S. P. Emergence of group B streptococcus as a major perinatal pathogen. *Hosp. Pract.* 12:85, 1977.
8. Gottesfeld, I. B. The family of the child with congenital heart disease. *M.C.N.* 4:101, 1979.
9. Grant, P. Psychosocial needs of families of high-risk infants. *Fam. Community Health* 1:91, 1978.
10. Haddock, N. Blood pressure monitoring in neonates. *M.C.N.* 5:131, 1980.
11. Haller, J. A. Newborns with major congenital malformations. *A.O.R.N. J.* 27:1070, 1978.
12. Kantor, G. K. Addicted mother, addicted baby—a challenge to health care providers. *M.C.N.* 3:286, 1978.
13. Kinston, M. Care of the unwell neonate. *Nurs. Mirror* 147:22, 1978.
14. Lemons, J. A., et al. Umbilical artery catheterization. *Perinatal Care* 2:17, 1978.
15. Moessinger, A. C. Management of newborn pneumothorax. *Perinatal Care* 2:24, 1978.
16. Peckham, C. Cytomegalovirus infection in pregnancy. *Midwife Health Visit. Community Nurse* 14:297, 1978.
17. Price, E., et al. Using the nasojejunal feeding technique in a neonatal intensive care unit. *M.C.N.* 3:361, 1978.
18. Smith, K. M. Recognizing cardiac failure in neonates. *M.C.N.* 4:98, 1979.
19. Van Leeuwen, G. *A Manual of Newborn Medicine*. Chicago: Year Book, 1973.
20. Vogel, M. When a pregnant woman is diabetic: Care of the newborn. *Am. J. Nurs.* 79:458, 1979.

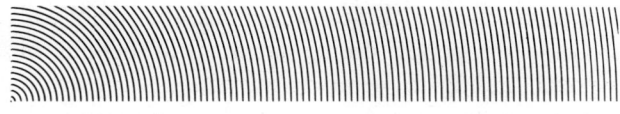

39. The Infant with Abnormal Gestation Age or Birth Weight

Approximately 7 percent of all pregnancies end before term, and about 10 percent continue after term. Early terminations give rise to two separate types of infants: low-birth-weight infants (formerly termed *premature*) and infants who are small for gestation age. The latter, small-for-gestation-age infants may also be born of full-term and post-term pregnancies.

All newborns should have their birth weight plotted on a growth chart such as the Colorado (Lubchenco) Intrauterine Growth Chart (Fig. 28-1), so that their birth weight may be compared with their gestation age. If this process is routinely carried out, infants may be placed in one of two categories: those who are low birth weight (an infant who would have been normal weight if carried to term) and those who are small for the length of the pregnancy. This is an important differentiation. The low-birth-weight infant appears to have been growing normally in utero. His stay in utero was unfortunately prematurely terminated. In the second category of infants, growth appears to have been impaired, and a pathological process in the fetus or placenta is suggested.

Infants Small for Gestation Age

An infant who is small for gestation age (small for date) may be a full-term infant (38 to 42 weeks of gestation) or post-term infant who weighs less than 2,500 gm (5½ pounds). He may be an infant born before term (before 38 weeks' gestation) who is lighter in weight (more than 2 standard deviations lighter) than he should be for a gestation of that length (the 3rd percentile on a growth chart). About a third of all newborns weighing less than 2,500 gm are small-for-date infants. Early in intrauterine life, fetal growth consists primarily of an increase in the number of body cells (hyperplastic growth). Late in intrauterine life, growth is achieved primarily by an increase in cell size (hypertrophic growth). During either period of growth, if the nutritional supplies to the fetus become inadequate, the brain, heart, and lungs are little affected. In contrast, the liver, adrenals, and spleen are very susceptible and fail to grow in size or function.

The infant who suffered nutritional deprivation early in pregnancy is generally below average in weight, length, and head circumference. The infant who suffered deprivation late in pregnancy may only have a reduction in weight. He has a wasted appearance with loose skin folds. He will have a small liver and will have a great deal of difficulty regulating glucose and protein levels. He has poor skin turgor, and a lack of lanugo. He may have better-developed neurological responses, hair texture, sole creases, and ear cartilage than his weight suggests. His skull is firmer than that of the average infant of the same weight, and he may seem unusually alert and active for his weight.

Blood studies at birth on small-for-gestation-age infants show a high hematocrit level (less plasma in proportion to red blood cells than is normal) and an increase in the total number of red blood cells present (polycythemia). The increase in red blood cells is probably due to the state of anoxia during intrauterine life. The infant produced more red blood cells than normal attempting to supply oxygen to body cells. This is the same phenomenon that occurs in infants with cyanotic heart disease. The high hematocrit may reflect not only an increase in red blood cells but a lack of plasma due to lack of fluid in utero.

The cause for small-for-gestation infants is largely placental. Either nutrients did not reach the placenta, or the placenta could not transfer them adequately to the fetus. Damage to the placenta, such as partial placental separation with bleeding, might be a cause. The area of placenta that separated becomes infarcted and fibrosed, reducing placental function. The placenta may have a developmental defect that prevents it from functioning properly.

The mother's nutrition during pregnancy plays a major role in fetal growth. Adolescents who have poor nutritional habits have a high incidence of small-for-gestation babies. Women with systemic diseases, such as hypertension, chronic renal or cardiovascular disease, or preeclampsia, tend to have an increased incidence of small-for-gestation babies. Mothers who smoke heavily or use narcotics tend to have small-for-gestation-age infants.

In some pregnancies the placental supply of nutrients is adequate, but the infant is unable to utilize them. Infants with intrauterine infections such as rubella or toxoplasmosis have this problem. Babies with chromosomal abnormalities may be small for gestation age in addition to their basic chromosomal difficulty.

A small-for-date infant may be detected in utero as the recorded fundal height during pregnancy becomes progressively less than the expected fundal height. If the woman is unsure of the date of her last menstrual period, this discrepancy will be hard to substantiate. Serial sonograms will show the small increase in weight and growth. The adequacy of placental function may be assessed by collecting 24-hour urines for estriol determination. Low estriol levels (below 12 mg) indicate poor fetal or placental function. An oxytocin challenge test or nonstress test may be done to further estimate placental function. If poor placental function is apparent from such determinations, the infant will probably do poorly during labor, with periods of hypoxia leading to neurological damage. Cesarean section may be the delivery method of choice in such circumstances. A pediatrician should be present at the birth because many small-for-date infants need resuscitation at birth. They may have meconium aspiration due to anoxia during labor. Since they have decreased glycogen stores, one of their commonest problems in neonatal life is hypoglycemia. They may need intravenous glucose to sustain blood sugar until they are able to suck vigorously enough to take sufficient oral feedings. Temperature control in these infants is poor because of the lack of subcutaneous fat. The polycythemia present results in increased blood viscosity. This puts extra work on the heart and can lead to blocked vessels and thrombus formation. If the hematrocrit is over 65 vol %, an exchange transfusion to dilute blood may be necessary.

Although these infants may gain weight and appear to thrive in the first few days of life, their mental development is often impaired because of lack of oxygen and nourishment in utero. Babies who were growing normally in utero but whose gestation was interrupted prematurely (true prematures) usually gain in weight and height so rapidly that by the end of the first year of life the majority of them are nearing the 50th percentile on growth charts. Small-for-date infants may always be below normal on standard growth charts.

Infants Large for Gestation Age

An infant is large for gestation age if his birth weight is above the 90th percentile on a growth chart. Such a baby is deceptive at birth because he appears to be a term baby by weight, but a gestational examination will reveal a very immature baby. He is at great risk if he is treated as a term newborn and not as being at the gestation age he has truly reached.

A large-for-gestation-age baby is born most frequently to a mother who is diabetic. Some women who will become diabetic late in life have large-for-gestation-age infants—as if, although clinical symptoms of diabetes are not yet present, some of the pathology of diabetes may be present. A woman with multiple parity may have a large baby (babies tend to grow larger with succeeding pregnancies). For an unknown reason, infants with transposition of the great vessels tend to be large for gestation age. One rare condition, Beckwith's syndrome, manifested by overgrowth and congenital anomalies such as omphalocele, results in large-for-gestation-age infants.

If a fetus is growing more rapidly in utero than is

normal, a nonstress test may be done to assess the placenta's ability to sustain him during labor. The infant's lung maturity may be assessed by amniocentesis.

Cesarean section may be necessary for delivery because of cephalopelvic disproportion. The baby may have extensive bruising or birth injuries such as broken clavicles if he is delivered vaginally.

Many large-for-gestation-age infants have difficulty establishing respirations at birth because of birth trauma or cesarean section. They must be observed closely after birth for hyperbilirubinemia from absorption of blood due to bruising and for hypoglycemia due to lowered liver stores (they have used intrauterine glucose for growth, not for storage).

Being able to assess newborns for gestation age is an invaluable skill. It separates out large-for-gestation-age infants and makes it possible to offer them the proper careful watch care necessary.

The Low-Birth-Weight Infant

By traditional definition, a low-birth-weight infant is a live-born infant weighing less than 2,500 gm (5 pounds, 8 ounces) at birth. A live birth was defined by the World Health Assembly in 1950 as follows:

... the complete expulsion or extraction from its mother of a product of conception ... which, after such separation, breathes or shows any other evidence of life such as beating of the heart, pulsation of the umbilical cord or definite movement of the voluntary muscles, whether or not the umbilical cord has been cut or the placenta is attached.

Burma and Thailand use 2,250 gm, India uses 2,150 gm, and Malaya uses 2,000 gm as the standard for low-birth-weight birth, because babies born in these countries are typically lighter in weight than in Western countries. Because black infants normally tend to be lighter in weight than Caucasian infants, it has been suggested that black infants be evaluated on the standard of 2,350 gm. Other infants traditionally put in the low-birth-weight group are live-born infants measuring 47 cm (18.5 inches) or less in length, or live-born infants of less than 37 weeks of gestation.

More and more, the maturity of the infant is being evaluated on the basis of physical findings such as sole creases, skull firmness, ear cartilage, and neurological assessment. These are shown in Table 29-2.

It is important that low-birth-weight babies be separated from small-for-gestation-age babies at birth, as the two groups have resulted from different situations and have different problems adjusting to extrauterine life.

With low-birth-weight infants, the baby appears to have been doing well in utero; for an unexplained reason the "trigger" that initiates labor was activated too early and so, even though they are immature, they are born. With small-for-gestation-age babies, something was going wrong in utero with the placenta or its ability to transfer nutrients to the child and therefore the pregnancy was ended. With small-for-gestation-age infants, the infant is ill from the effects of intrauterine malnutrition; with a low-birth-weight infant, the baby is well, merely very immature and small. Small-for-gestation-age and low-birth-weight infants are compared in Table 39-1.

Babies who are born before 30 weeks of gestation (a weight of 500 to 1,500 gm; 1 pound, 3 ounces to 3 pounds, 5 ounces) are extremely immature. They need level III care from the moment of birth to give them their best chance of survival without neurological aftereffects due to their being so critically close to the age of viability.

A baby born between 31 and 36 weeks of gestation (a birth weight between 1,500 and 2,500 gm; 3 pounds, 5 ounces and 5 pounds, 8 ounces) is moderately immature. The chance for survival is good.

An infant 37 to 38 weeks (a birth weight close to 2,500 gm; 5 pounds, 8 ounces) is only slightly immature. If the fact that he is immature is recognized by a gestation age assessment and the specific problems of prematurity such as respiratory distress syndrome and hypoglycemia are watched for, his chance of survival is very good.

A low-birth-weight infant appears small and underdeveloped. His head is disproportionately large (3 cm or more greater than chest size). His skin is generally unusually ruddy, and he has a high degree of acrocyanosis. He has little vernix caseosa, since this is formed later in pregnancy. Lanugo is usually extensive, covering the back, forearms, forehead, and sides of the face. Both anterior and posterior fontanelles are small.

The eyes of most immature infants appear small. A pupillary reaction is present, although it is difficult to elicit. Ophthalmoscopic examination is extremely difficult and often unrewarding, since the vitreous humor may be hazy. The premature infant has varying degrees of myopia (nearsightedness).

The cartilage of the ear is immature and allows the pinna to fall forward. The ears appear large in relation to the head. The level of ears should be carefully inspected to rule out chromosomal abnormalities.

Examination of the pharynx is difficult because of its small size and the necessity for gentleness to prevent bruising. The gag reflex may be immature.

Table 39-1. Differences Between Small-for-Gestation-Age Infants and Low-Birth-Weight Infants

Characteristic	Small-for-Gestation-Age Infant	Low-Birth-Weight Infant
Gestation age	28–42 weeks	Under 37 weeks
Birth weight	Under 10th percentile	Normal for age
Congenital malformations	A strong possibility	A possibility
Pulmonary problems	Meconium aspiration Pulmonary hemorrhage Pneumothorax	Respiratory distress syndrome
Hyperbilirubinemia	A possibility	A very strong possibility
Hypoglycemia	A very strong possibility	A possibility
Intracranial hemorrhage	A strong possibility	A possibility
Apnea episodes	A possibility	A very strong possibility
Feeding problems	Most likely to be due to accompanying problem such as hypoglycemia	Small stomach capacity; sucking reflex not mature
Weight gain in nursery	Rapid	Slow
Future retarded growth	May always be under 10th percentile	Not likely to be retarded in growth

Large amounts of mucus are commonly found. Bloody mucus must be further investigated to determine whether it is the result of active bleeding or is swallowed blood. Blood-tinged froth in the posterior pharynx may indicate pulmonary hemorrhage. Hemorrhage is a greater problem in immature than in mature infants because of the capillary fragility and low vitamin K levels in the low-birth-weight infant.

Breath sounds in the immature infant heard on auscultation of the chest do not always reveal the extent of alveolar functioning; even in previable infants, air can be heard going in and out of the bronchial tree. On cardiac assessment (Fig. 39-2), locating the point of maximum impulse may be difficult, because the heart sounds and heartbeat are weak; forceful

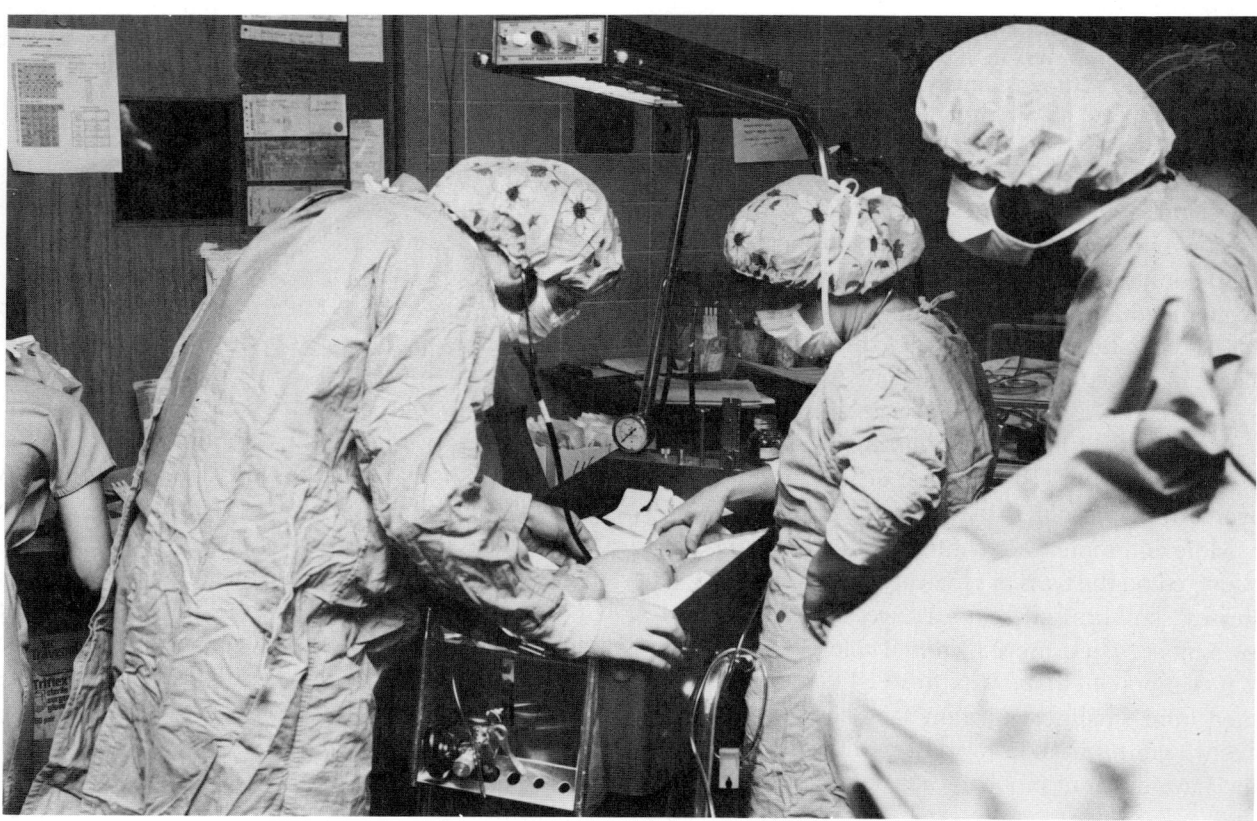

Fig. 39-1. Initial assessment of the infant at birth must include gestation age assessment so that postmature, small-for-gestation-age, preterm, and large-for-gestation-age infants can be identified. (Courtesy of the Department of Medical Photography, Children's Hospital, Buffalo, N.Y.)

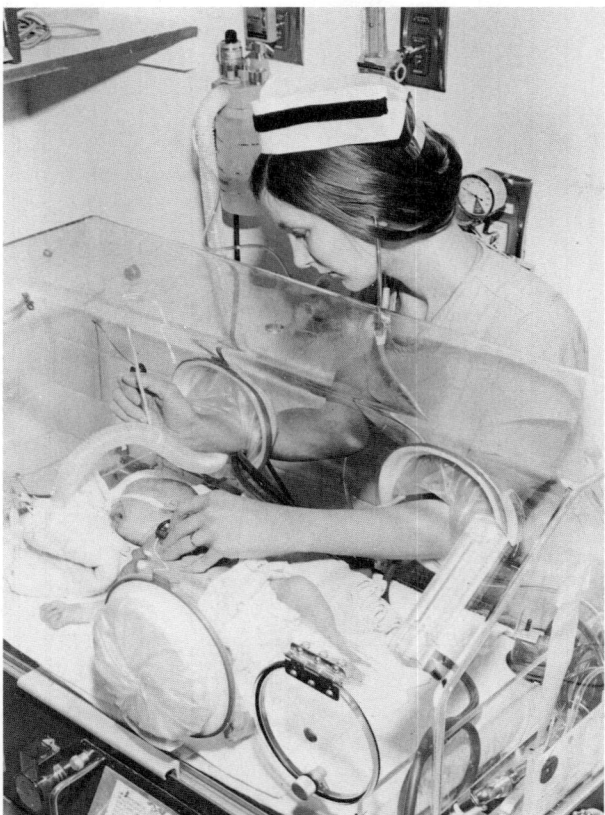

Fig. 39-2. Auscultating the heart rate of an immature infant. The infant is in an Isolette for warmth. Cardiac monitors and a ventilator are in place. (Courtesy of the Department of Medical Photography, Children's Hospital, Buffalo, N.Y.)

heart sounds in an immature infant may suggest congestive heart disease. Respirations are irregular and variable. The rate is often more rapid than in mature infants (40 to 60 per minute). With each inspiration there is a tendency toward mild retraction of the lower thoracic cage. Periods of apnea lasting for several seconds may occur in between hurried respirations.

The abdominal musculature is incompletely developed and so distends easily. The thinness of the abdominal wall allows for easy visibility of intestinal activity. The liver is usually easily palpated, and often the tip of the spleen is palpable. The kidneys tend to be relatively low and are easily palpated.

The genitalia are immature. In males, the testes are frequently not in the scrotum but are palpable in the inguinal region. In females, the labia minora and clitoris appear exceptionally prominent because the labia majora are so incompletely developed.

It is important that patency of the anus be tested by a gentle rectal examination. The incidence of congenital anomalies is higher in immature than in mature infants.

Neurological function in the immature child is difficult to evaluate. The observation of spontaneous movement and provoked movements may yield as important findings as the reflex tests. An immature infant moves far less than a mature infant, and he rarely cries. Assessment charts such as those shown in Fig. 39-3 are helpful in determining what neurological activity should be apparent in a low-birth-weight baby.

CAUSES OF PREMATURITY

Because deaths of low-birth-weight infants account for 80 to 90 percent of the mortality in the first year of life, infant mortality could be reduced dramatically if the causes of premature birth could be discovered and corrected and all pregnancies brought to term.

There is a high correlation between low socioeconomic level and early termination of pregnancy. In women from the middle and upper socioeconomic groups, 4 to 8 percent of pregnancies are terminated early; in women from low socioeconomic levels, 10 to 20 percent. The major influencing factor appears to be inadequate nutrition before pregnancy in both parents, and during pregnancy, as a result of either insufficient purchasing power or ignorance of what constitutes good nutrition during pregnancy. Other contributing factors are the higher incidence of pregnancy-induced hypertension in women with poor nutrition, chronic disease and lack of prenatal care. Additional factors that seem to be related to early termination of pregnancy are: multiple pregnancy; prior previous early birth (a low gestational capacity); race (nonwhites have a higher incidence of prematurity than whites, which is perhaps a reflection of their lower socioeconomic status rather than of race); cigarette smoking; the age of the mother (the highest incidence is in mothers under 20); and order of birth (early termination is highest in first pregnancies and in those beyond the fourth).

At times, labor is induced purposely while the fetus is still immature in order to remove the fetus from an environment that is more detrimental than an extrauterine existence. Labor might be induced in a woman with severe preeclampsia, Rh incompatibility, or diabetes.

NEEDS OF THE IMMATURE INFANT

Immature infants have the same priority needs of all newborn infants, but techniques must be adapted to meet their needs.

Initiation and Maintenance of Respirations

It is helpful in the delivery of an immature infant if the mother is given oxygen by mask to allow the

Examination First Hours

WEEKS GESTATION

PHYSICAL FINDINGS		20	21	22	23	24	25	26	27	28	29	30	31	32	33	34	35	36	37	38	39	40	41	42	43	44	45	46	47	48
Vernix		Appears				Covers body, thick layer														On back, scalp, in creases		Scant, in creases		No vernix						
Breast tissue and areola			Areola and nipple barely visible no palpable breast tissue													Areola raised		1–2 mm nodule		3–5 mm	5–6 mm	7–10 mm		?12 mm						
Ear	Form		Flat, shapeless														Beginning incurving superior		Incurving upper 2/3 pinnae		Well-defined incurving to lobe									
	Cartilage														Cartilage scant, returns slowly from folding				Thin cartilage, springs back from folding		Pinna firm, remains erect from head									
			Pinna soft, stays folded																											
Sole creases			Smooth soles without creases													1–2 anterior creases	2–3 anterior creases	Creases anterior 2/3 sole		Creases involving heel		Deeper creases over entire sole								
Skin	Thickness & appearance		Thin, translucent skin, plethoric, venules over abdomen, edema												Smooth, thicker, no edema			Pink		Few vessels		Some desquamation pale pink		Thick, pale, desquamation over entire body						
	Nail plates		Appear												Nails to finger tips									Nails extend well beyond finger tips						
Hair			Appears on head			Eye brows and lashes					Fine, woolly, bunches out from head							Silky, single strands, lays flat						?Receding hairline or loss of baby hair, short, fine underneath						
Lanugo			Appears	Covers entire body												Vanishes from face						Present on shoulders		No lanugo						
Genitalia	Testes											Testes palpable in inguinal canal							In upper scrotum			In lower scrotum								
	Scrotum											Few rugae						Rugae, anterior portion			Rugae cover		Pendulous							
	Labia & clitoris											Prominent clitoris, labia majora small, widely separated						Labia majora larger, nearly cover clitoris				Labia minora and clitoris covered								
Skull firmness			Bones are soft									Soft to 1″ from anterior fontanelle						Spongy at edges of fontanelle, center firm		Bones hard, sutures easily displaced				Bones hard, cannot be displaced						
Posture	Resting		Hypotonic, lateral decubitus					Hypotonic				Beginning flexion, thigh		Stronger hip flexion		Frog-like			Flexion, all limbs		Hypertonic			Very hypertonic						
	Recoil - leg		No recoil												Partial recoil			Begin flexion, no recoil			Prompt recoil									
	Arm		No recoil																Prompt recoil, may be inhibited				Prompt recoil after 30″ inhibition							
		20	21	22	23	24	25	26	27	28	29	30	31	32	33	34	35	36	37	38	39	40	41	42	43	44	45	46	47	48

Fig. 39-3. Clinical estimation of gestation age. An approximation based on published data. (From C. H. Kempe, H. K. Silver, and D. O. O'Brien, Current Pediatric Diagnosis and Treatment [3rd ed.]. Los Altos, Calif.: Lange, 1974.)

The Infant with Abnormal Gestation Age or Birth Weight 701

infant to be born with optimal oxygen saturation; immature infants have great difficulty initiating respirations at birth. The pulmonary capillary bed continues to mature and proliferate throughout intrauterine life. When a pregnancy is terminated early, pulmonary ventilation may not have achieved its normal efficiency. Lung surfactant may be inadequate, leading to alveolar collapse with each expiration. Since infants turn to a vertex presentation late in pregnancy, with an immature infant there may be a breech delivery. This may cause him to aspirate vaginal secretions or meconium and compound his respiratory problem.

A pediatrician should be present at all preterm deliveries to supervise resuscitation procedures.

Most infants are born with a temporary respiratory acidosis. Once respirations are established, the temporary condition quickly clears. Because the immature infant is unable to initiate effective respirations as quickly as the mature infant, he is prone to irreversible acidosis; he must establish adequate ventilation, or be resuscitated, within 2 minutes after birth to prevent this. The infant must be kept warm during resuscitation procedures. All procedures must be carried out with great gentleness; the immature infant's tissues are more sensitive to trauma than are those of the term infant.

Giving 100% oxygen to immature infants during resuscitation or to maintain respirations poses the dangers of pulmonary edema and retrolental fibroplasia (blindness of prematurity). The development of both these conditions depends on saturation of the blood with oxygen, however, and as long as the infant is cyanotic, the blood saturation level of oxygen is unlikely to be high.

The Committee on the Fetus and Newborn of the American Academy of Pediatrics [4] recommends the following precautions in the administration of oxygen to high-risk and low-birth-weight infants:

When a newborn infant needs extra oxygen, it must be administered with great care because there is a causal relationship between a higher than normal (60 to 100 mm Hg) oxygen tension in arterial blood and retrolental fibroplasia (retinopathy of prematurity). When the normal oxygen tension is exceeded, there is an increased risk of retrolental fibroplasia. The upper limit of arterial oxygen tension and its duration which are safe for these infants is not known. It is probable that even concentrations of 40% oxygen in inspired air (formerly considered safe) could be dangerous for some infants.

An inspired oxygen concentration of 40% may be insufficient for infants with cardiorespiratory disease to raise the oxygen tension of arterial blood to a normal level. In such instances, an inspired oxygen concentration of 60%, 80%, or higher may be necessary. However, it is difficult to judge by clinical signs the concentration of inspired oxygen necessary to maintain effective oxygenation of tissues in these infants. An infant may have peripheral cyanosis and yet may have a normal, or even an elevated arterial oxygen tension. Therefore, arterial blood gas measurements are extremely important for regulation of the concentration of inspired oxygen when an oxygen-enriched environment is considered necessary.

The immature infant may continue to need oxygen administration beyond that given for resuscitation measures because he often has difficulty maintaining respirations. Early in fetal life, the alveoli are several cells thick; close to the time of birth they become the single layer of mature alveoli that allows easy gas exchange. The soft cartilage of the ribs of the immature infant tends to create respiratory problems because the ribs may collapse on expiration. The accessory muscles of respiration may be undeveloped, so that, unlike the mature infant, the immature infant has no backup muscles to use when he becomes fatigued from trying to maintain respirations. Many preterm infants tend to have higher PO_2 levels when placed prone than when supine [9].

Many immature babies have a very irregular respiratory pattern (a few quick breaths, a period of 5 to 10 seconds without respiratory effort, a few quick breaths again, and so on). There is no bradycardia with this irregular pattern (sometimes termed *periodic respirations*); the pattern seems to be a result of immaturity and uncoordinated respiratory efforts.

APNEA. Many immature infants may have periods of true apnea as a result of fatigue or the immaturity of their respiratory mechanisms. With true apnea, the pause in respirations is more than 20 seconds and bradycardia occurs. Babies with secondary stresses such as hyperbilirubinemia or hypoglycemia tend to have a high incidence of apneic occurrences. If you gently shake the infant or flick the sole of his foot, often he begins to breathe again, almost as if he needs to be "reminded" to maintain this function. If the infant does not respond to these simple measures, resuscitation by bagging is necessary. Immature infants must have extremely close observation to detect these apneic episodes. Apnea monitors that record respiratory movements are invaluable tools to detect failing respirations and sound a warning that the infant needs attention.

Infants with apnea may be administered theophylline. The mechanism by which theophylline reduces the incidence of apnea episodes is unclear, but it appears to increase the infant's sensitivity to carbon dioxide, ensuring better respiratory function.

PNEUMOTHORAX. Pneumothorax is leakage of air from lung alveoli into the pleural space surrounding the lung. Ordinarily the air surrounding the lung has a negative pressure. When alveoli rupture and air from the lung invades this space, the pressure is no longer a negative one and the lung on that side collapses. Infants who are on assisted ventilation may have alveoli "blown out" by the force of the ventilation and trapped in the pleural space. This is a *tension* pneumothorax.

The infant will suddenly be extremely cyanotic and have tachypnea. The heart will be displaced toward the unaffected side. A chest x-ray film will reveal the air-filled chest space.

The infant needs oxygen, but it must be administered by hood or mask, not by pressure, or the problem may be compounded. The air in the pleural space must be withdrawn in order to allow the affected lung to reexpand. Chest tubes will be inserted to continue removal of air.

A pneumothorax is a shocking happening to the child's system, reducing his respiratory capacity by 50 percent in a second's time.

Maintaining Proper Temperature

An immature baby has a great deal of difficulty maintaining body heat because he has a relatively large surface area per pound of body weight and therefore rapid cooling from evaporation can occur. He has little subcutaneous fat, and his poor muscular development does not allow him to move as actively as the older infant to produce body heat. His low glycogen stores lead him very quickly into hypoglycemia. He has a limited amount of brown fat, the special tissue present in newborns to maintain body heat. He is unable to shiver, which is a useful mechanism to increase body temperature; on the other hand, he is unable to sweat, and thereby reduce body temperature. He is thus very dependent on the environmental temperature provided for him. He must be kept under a radiant heat warmer in the delivery room.

Unless there are obvious abnormalities noted in the delivery room, physical assessment of the infant—even weighing—should be delayed until he is placed in the warmth of an Isolette.

The infant's axillary temperature should be maintained at 97.8°F (36.5°C). He must have radiant heat for any procedure that has to be performed outside the Isolette. If he is going to be transported to a department within the hospital, such as the x-ray department, or to a regional center for specialized care, he must be provided warmth during transport. Remember that infants lose heat by radiation. Even though an Isolette is warm, therefore, if it is placed near a cold window or air conditioner the infant will lose heat to the distant source. Keep this fact in mind if transporting infants on cold days. The ambulance must be pulled in close to the hospital door; it, as well as the Isolette, must be prewarmed. An additional heat shield may be placed over an infant inside an Isolette to help conserve heat. A radiant heat source may be placed above the Isolette to further ensure heat in the Isolette.

A preterm baby is typically left undressed except for a diaper in the Isolette so that his chest and respiratory activity can be carefully observed. Be certain whenever he is removed from the Isolette that he is wrapped warmly. Covering an infant's head covers a large surface area of the baby and helps a great deal to conserve heat in a small baby.

If a baby needs frequent interventions that make caring for him in a closed Isolette difficult, he can be cared for under a radiant heat source—not just in the delivery room but in the nursery as well. Parents need an explanation that a radiant heat warmer is an adequate way to keep their child warm. They are used to seeing low-birth-weight infants cared for in Isolettes; they see the Isolette as protective. The radiant warmer appears to leave the baby exposed and vulnerable.

Nutrition

Nutrition problems arise with the immature infant because his body continues to, or attempts to continue to, maintain the rapid rate of intrauterine growth after birth. He therefore requires a larger amount of nutrients in his diet than the mature infant. However, he has difficulty swallowing and sucking, and his stomach capacity is small; a distended stomach may cause him respiratory distress. His immature cardiac spincter (between the stomach and esophagus) allows regurgitation to occur readily. The lack of a cough reflex may lead him to aspirate regurgitated formula. He has a high insensible water loss due to his large body surface. Since he is unable to concentrate urine well, he excretes a high proportion of fluid from his body. All these factors make it important that the immature baby receive 160 to 200 ml of fluid per kilogram of body weight daily.

Immature babies need intravenous fluid begun within hours after birth to begin to fulfill this fluid requirement and provide glucose to prevent hypoglycemia. Intravenous fluid should be given by a continuous infusion pump to ensure a constant infusion rate. Intravenous sites must be checked conscientiously as the lack of subcutaneous tissue makes infiltration very damaging to tissue.

The baby's weight, specific gravity and amount of urine, and serum electrolytes all must be monitored to ensure that fluid intake is adequate. Too little fluid and calories lead to dehydration and starvation, acidosis and weight loss. Overhydration leads to weight gain, pulmonary edema and heart failure.

Urine output should be measured by weighed diapers to limit the number of urine collectors necessary (the constant changing of collectors leads to skin irritation and breakdown). The range of urine output for the first few days of life in low-birth-weight babies is high in comparison with that of the term baby—40 to 100 ml per kilogram per 24 hours, compared to 10 to 20 ml per kilogram. The specific gravity is low, rarely over 1.012 (normal term babies may concentrate urine up to 1.030).

Hyperglycemia caused by the glucose infusion may lead to spillage of glucose in the urine and an accompanying diuresis. If the glucose being supplied is too low and body cells are utilizing protein for metabolism, ketone bodies will appear in urine. Urine specimens are tested for glucose and ketones in addition to amount and specific gravity therefore.

FEEDING PATTERNS. Caloric requirements for an immature infant are higher than for the term infant in order to provide calories for rapid growth: 120 to 140 calories per kilogram body weight per day. Because an immature infant has a small stomach capacity, he cannot take large feedings and so must be fed more often than the mature infant. An infant under 1,200 gm is fed as often as every 2 hours; over 1,200 gm, about every 3 hours.

Formula used may have a higher caloric count than that for term infants to enable more calories to be given in small amounts. Thus, the caloric concentration of formula for immature babies may be 24 calories per ounce in comparison to 20 calories per ounce for a term baby.

Minerals such as calcium and phosphorus and electrolytes such as sodium and potassium and chloride may have to be supplemented, depending on blood studies. An immature infant needs supplementary A, D, C, and E vitamins. Vitamin K should be administered at birth, as with a term baby, except that the amount is 0.5 ml instead of 1 ml. Vitamin E seems to be important in preventing hemolytic anemia in immature infants. Iron supplements interfere with the absorption of vitamin E and so are not added to formula.

The lack of iron supplement is confusing to parents because they have always been told that iron helps to build strong blood. Now they are told that in their particularly vulnerable infant, iron is not being given because it will interfere with blood cell integrity. They need an explanation of the particular blood problem that must be prevented here. Iron supplements will be started on discharge from the hospital or at least by 3 months of age. Again, parents should have an explanation of what is happening. By the time of discharge, their infant has reached term maturity, and iron deficiency anemia due to low iron stores then becomes his chief problem.

With the early administration of intravenous fluid to prevent hypoglycemia and supply fluid, gastrointestinal feedings may be safely delayed until the infant has stabilized his respiratory effort from birth. Feedings should be begun, however, by gavage or bottle as soon as he is able to tolerate them. If the baby is going to be bottle-fed, the feeding pattern should be started with sterile water. If the infant should aspirate this first feeding, the insult of sterile water on lung tissue is less than that of either glucose water or formula.

Because of the small stomach capacity of preterm infants, feedings are very small in amount—as little as 1 or 2 ml in the smallest infants. The amount is gradually increased as the infant gains weight and his stomach capacity enlarges. Increases in amount must be very small (1 or 2 ml) to prevent regurgitation.

There is accumulating evidence that, although the immature infant needs the increased caloric distribution of commercial formulas, the best milk for immature babies, as well as for term babies, is breast milk. The immunological properties of breast milk play a major role in preventing neonatal necrotizing enterocolitis, a destructive intestinal disorder that occurs in low-birth-weight babies.

The mother who wants to breast-feed can manually express breast milk for her infant's gavage feedings. Women in the community who have excess breast milk or who have discontinued breast-feeding and want to express breast milk and supply it to special care nurseries are urged to do so to maintain a "milk bank" for immature babies. In most programs of this nature, the expressed breast milk is frozen for safe transport and storage. Whether freezing destroys the antibodies or factors that make breast milk preferable to sensitive digestive tracts is being investigated.

Immature infants of low birth weight are begun on gavage feedings. As they mature, bottle-feeding is gradually introduced. The mother who wants to breast-feed and has preserved her milk supply during the time the infant could not suck may visit daily and, as the infant grows strong enough, begin breast feedings.

Infants are 32 weeks of gestation before their gag reflex is intact. They are 34 weeks of gestation before they can consistently coordinate sucking and swallowing.

Immature infants must be observed closely after an oral or gavage feeding to be certain that the filled stomach is not causing them respiratory distress. As soon as a sucking reflex is present, offering a pacifier will strengthen this reflex and better prepare an infant for bottle-feeding as well as provide oral satisfaction for him.

As long as the infant is being gavage-fed, stomach secretions are usually aspirated, measured, and replaced prior to the feeding. An infant who has a stomach content of over 2 ml is receiving more formula than he can digest in the time allowed. Feedings should not be increased but possibly even cut back to ensure better digestion and decrease the possibility of regurgitation and aspiration. Low-birth-weight infants may be fed by total parenteral nutrition until they are mature enough for other means.

Prevention of Infection

As noted, the skin of the immature baby is easily traumatized and therefore offers less resistance to infection than the skin and mucous membrane of the mature baby. The immature infant has low resistance to infection. He has difficulty in producing phagocytes to localize infection, and he has a deficiency of IgM antibodies because of insufficient production.

Linen and equipment used with the immature infant must be sterile to reduce the chances of infection. Staff members must be free of infection, and handwashing and gowning regulations must be enforced.

Illnesses and the Infant

In the neonatal period, immature infants are particularly susceptible to the following: anemia (since it is in the last few weeks of intrauterine life that iron is stored in the liver); failure to thrive due to feeding difficulty; dehydration due to feeding difficulty and inefficient concentration of urine; infection, principally of the respiratory tract and skin; hemorrhage, respiratory distress syndrome, retrolental fibroplasia, necrotizing enterocolitis, and kernicterus.

HEMORRHAGE. Because immature infants are born with exceedingly low levels of vitamin K, they have a greater tendency to hemorrhage than do mature infants. Hemorrhage from vitamin K deficiency responds within a few hours to the administration of vitamin K or to the infusion of fresh whole blood. It can be prevented by the routine prophylactic administration of vitamin K to all infants immediatley after birth.

A second form of bleeding that occurs chiefly among preterm infants is the result of a combination of (1) increased capillary fragility, (2) prolonged bleeding time, and (3) a decreased amount of blood factor V. It is clinically difficult to distinguish this form of hemorrhagic disease from vitamin K deficiency. It is found most often in infants who have had hypoxia or infection. Vitamin K deficiency bleeding tends to occur in the gastrointestinal tract, the nose, and around the eyes; in the second form of bleeding, the lungs and the central nervous system are the most common sites of hemorrhage. The increased capillary fragility is apparently a manifestation of immaturity. Extremely gentle handling minimizes the occurrence of bleeding episodes, although such bleeding may occur during delivery, particularly in the form of intracranial hemorrhage, and may severely damage or be lethal to the immature infant.

INTRACRANIAL HEMORRHAGE. One of the greatest hazards to the immature infant at birth is intracranial hemorrhage. This is also a possibility any time the infant has a period of hypoxia during his neonatal life.

If the tentorial membrane is torn because of birth trauma, the bleed will be into the basic structures below this or the pons, cerebellum, and medulla oblongata. As the regulatory mechanisms for heart and respiratory function are located in these parts, a bleed here is obviously life-threatening.

The fact that an intracranial bleed has occurred is evidenced by signs of respiratory distress and cyanosis; seizures may occur. The infant may have a high shrill cry. He may show signs of cardiovascular shock. His reflexes, particularly his Moro reflex, are no longer present. If the bleed is into the subarachnoid space, the cerebrospinal fluid will be blood-tinged on lumbar puncture. Subdural bleeding (serious because it causes compression of brain tissue) will not stain cerebrospinal fluid.

A computerized tomography (CT) scan or a sonogram will reveal the extent of the bleed. The infant should be placed in a position with his head elevated to minimize intracranial pressure. He needs oxygen and assisted ventilation as a rule, to overcome the shock to his system. His ability to suck may be poor, so he needs intravenous fluid to maintain water and caloric balance. Hyperbilirubinemia may occur as the trapped blood is reabsorbed.

The infant has been severely compromised by an intracranial bleed. It is difficult for parents to understand what has happened since they know little about brain anatomy. They need day-to-day reports of what is going on. The accumulating evidence—the infant cannot sustain respiratory function without assisted ventilation; his vital signs are becoming less and less steady—let them know the seriousness of their child's condition.

RESPIRATORY DISTRESS SYNDROME. Respiratory distress syndrome (RDS) (hyaline membrane disease) most commonly occurs in immature infants, in infants of diabetic mothers or mothers who have had vaginal bleeding during pregnancy (such as occurs with placenta previa or premature separation of the placenta), and in infants born by cesarean section. The pathologic feature of RDS is a hyalinelike (fibrous) membrane, composed of products formed from an exudate of the infant's blood, that lines the terminal bronchioles, alveolar ducts, and alveoli. This prevents exchange of oxygen and carbon dioxide at the alveolar-blood interface. The cause of RDS is a low level of the lecithin component of surfactant, the phospholipid that indicates lung maturity at birth and maintains surface tension in the alveoli on expiration to keep alveoli from collapsing on expiration.

Very high pressure is required to fill the lungs with air for the first time. The lung tissue itself offers little resistance, but the fluid in the lung has to be overcome. It takes a pressure between 40 and 70 cm H_2O to inspire a first breath, but only 6 to 8 cm H_2O to maintain quiet breathing. When alveoli collapse with each expiration, however, it continues to take forceful inspiration to inflate them.

As areas of hypoinflation occur, pulmonary blood resistance in the lung is increased. This high tension in the pulmonary artery may cause blood to shunt through the foramen ovale and the ductus arteriosus as it did during fetal life, when passage of blood through the lungs could not be accomplished. With poor lung cell blood perfusion, the production of surfactant decreases even further.

The poor oxygen exchange leads to tissue hypoxia. Tissue hypoxia causes the release of lactic acid. This, combined with an increasing carbon dioxide level resulting from the formation of a hyaline membrane on the alveolar surface, leads to severe acidosis. Acidosis causes vasoconstriction. Decreased pulmonary perfusion from vasoconstriction limits surfactant production still further.

With decreased surfactant production, the ability to stop alveoli from collapsing with each expiration is even further impaired. This vicious cycle continues until oxygen–carbon dioxide exchange in the alveoli is no longer adequate to sustain life.

Most infants who will later develop RDS have difficulty initiating respirations, but after resuscitation at birth, they appear to have a period of hours or a day when they are free of symptoms. However, during this time, subtle signs such as low body temperature, nasal flaring, sternal and subcostal retractions, and tachypnea (over 70 respirations per minute) may be present. Within several hours, expiratory grunting becomes apparent. Expiratory grunting indicates a prolonged expiratory time. The sound denotes that closure of the glottis is occurring. Glottis closure increases the pressure in alveoli on expiration, helps to keep alveoli from collapsing, and makes oxygen exchange more complete. Thus, expiratory grunting is a compensatory mechanism. Even with this attempt at better oxygen exchange, most infants become cyanotic in room air. On auscultation, there may be fine rales and diminished breath sounds because of poor air entry. As distress increases, the infant shows seesaw respirations (on inspiration, the anterior chest wall retracts and the abdomen protrudes; on expiration, the sternum rises). The infant's heart begins to fail; the urine output decreases; and there may be edema of the extremities. The child's temperature falls. His color becomes a pale gray. Periods of apnea occur, and bradycardia becomes apparent.

A chest x-ray will reveal a diffuse pattern of radiopaque areas (haziness). Blood gases (studied in blood taken from an umbilical vessel catheter) will reveal respiratory acidosis. The infant obviously is gravely ill.

The infant with RDS needs care in a unit specially designed to meet the needs of such infants. He should be kept warm, because cooling increases acidosis in all infants and may increase it in these infants to lethal levels. Keeping the infant warm so that his metabolic rate does not have to increase to maintain an adequate temperature reduces his oxygen need as well. He may need correction of acidosis by intravenous sodium bicarbonate administration. The infant will need intravenous fluid and glucose or gavage feedings for hydration and nourishment because his respiratory effort makes him too exhausted to suck. Administration of oxygen is generally necessary to maintain correct PO_2 and pH levels. Continuous positive airway pressure (CPAP) or assisted ventilation with positive end expiratory pressure (PEEP) will exert pressure on the alveoli at the end of expiration and keep them from collapsing. This greatly improves the oxygen exchange.

Despite current therapy, about 20 to 30 percent of children who develop RDS will not survive. In infants

Table 39-2. Respiratory Therapy Score: Scoring System Utilizing Five Clinical and Laboratory Measurements Available in Community Hospitals

Measurement	Score 0	Score 1	Score 2
Birth weight (gm)	Over 2,000	1,500–2,000	Under 1,500
Clinical score	3 or under	4–5	6 and over
FiO$_2$[a]	49 or under	50–65	65 and over
PCO$_2$[b]	Under 40	40–45	Over 45
pH[b]	7.35 or over	7.34–7.30	7.30 and lower
Totals	___	___	___
TOTAL SCORE			

[a] Inspired oxygen concentration necessary to maintain the infant's skin color pink.
[b] Venous blood sample.
Source: G.J. Peckham, et al., A clinical score for predicting the level of respiratory care in infants with respiratory distress syndrome. *Clin. Pediatr.* (Phila.) 18:716, 1979.

Table 39-3. Clinical Respiratory Distress Scoring System

Measurement	Score 0	Score 1	Score 2
Respiratory rate (per minute)	60	60–80	Over 80 or apneic episodes
Cyanosis	None	In air	In 40% oxygen
Retractions	None	Mild	Moderate to severe
Grunting	None	Audible with stethoscope	Audible without stethoscope
Air entry (crying)*	Clear	Delayed or decreased	Barely audible

*Air entry represents the quality of inspiratory breath sounds as heard in the midaxillary line.
Source: J. Downes, et al., Respiratory distress syndrome of newborn infants. New clinical scoring system with acid-base and blood-gas correlates. *Clin. Pediatr.* (Phila.) 9:325, 1970.

with moderate disease, a peak is reached in about three days; after that time, the condition will gradually improve.

When newborns of low birth weight are born in community hospitals, one of the most serious decisions that must be made is whether the infant needs to be transferred to a regional center for respiratory therapy for RDS. A scoring system such as the one shown in Table 39-2 is a help in deciding if the newborn will need more respiratory therapy than a small hospital can provide. To use the scoring system, points are given for birthweight, a clinical score, the percentage of oxygen needed to keep the infant's skin color pink, and venous blood CO$_2$ and pH. The clinical score is obtained by utilizing Table 39-3.

Infants who score from 0 to 3 (Table 39-2) probably can be managed with oxygen by hood. Infants scoring 4 or 5 usually need CPAP therapy. Infants who score over 6 are likely to need mechanical ventilation. Whether or not to transfer an infant is a physician's responsibility, but the preceding scoring system can guide you in evaluating the infant.

Parents of the child with RDS should be able to visit the special nursing unit to which the child is admitted. It is helpful to the parents if they can wash and gown and are able to touch the child. This makes his birth more real to them, and should he not survive the illness, it makes the death more real. Only when both birth and death seem real can the parents begin to work through their feelings and accept these events. Parents may have to work through a great many feelings concerning the child's birth. If the baby is premature, the mother may need assurance that nothing she did (ate too much dinner the day of labor and so crowded out the baby; forgot to take her iron pill for two days) caused the premature birth and therefore this illness. If she had to have a cesarean section, she may feel inadequate as a woman and may need assurance that being able to give vaginal birth is not a measure of a woman's worth. If the parents are young and have not planned well to provide for medical expenses, they may be extremely concerned about the hospital bill and may wonder whether the child will receive good care once the cashier learns that they have no hospital insurance.

All mothers handle newborn babies tentatively until they have "claimed" them or have become better acquainted. The mother of a child who has been very ill at birth may take months before she can handle him comfortably and confidently. The parents need to spend time with him in the intensive care nursery as he improves, so that they can begin the process of claiming. They need to have access to health care personnel after discharge, to help them in caring for the child with confidence at home.

If the infant dies, the parents often wish to see him. They may never have seen him without a great deal of equipment surrounding him and may need this time to reassure themselves that in every other way except lung function, he was a perfect baby. This gives them confidence to plan for other children and to continue their lives after this experience.

Lung maturity may be estimated by aminocentesis. If the level of lethicin in surfactant exceeds that of sphinogomyelin by 2:0, the lung is mature, and RDS is not likely to occur. It may be possible to prevent RDS in infants by administering steroids to the mother prior to delivery. Steroids appear to act to quicken the formation of lethicin production pathways. Unfortunately, there is often no warning that premature birth is imminent until hours before delivery, so that, even if this becomes a feasible means of preventing the syndrome, some labors and deliveries will progress too rapidly for this preventive measure to be effective.

RETROLENTAL FIBROPLASIA. Although retrolental fibroplasia is rarely seen today, it is a possibility that must be kept in mind by all health care personnel caring for infants of interrupted pregnancies.

Retrolental fibroplasia is an acquired ocular disease that leads to partial or total blindness in children due to vasoconstriction of immature retinal blood vessels. It was first recognized as an eye disorder in 1942, occurring in 5 to 25 percent of surviving infants whose birth weights were under 1,800 grams (4 pounds) and replacing gonorrheal ophthalmia neonatorum as the leading cause of blindness in children. It was ten years before it was established that a high concentration of oxygen is the causative agent. High concentrations of oxygen cause the vasoconstriction of retinal blood vessels and a secondary proliferation of endothelial cells in the layer of nerve fibers in the periphery of the retina, often resulting in detachment of the retina and blindness.

The infant who is receiving oxygen must have blood PO_2 levels monitored. If PO_2 levels are kept within normal limits, there is no danger. With PO_2 levels over 100 mm Hg, the danger of retrolental fibroplasia is great. The recommendations of the American Academy of Pediatrics for oxygen administration (see p. 702) are designed to protect the infant from receiving concentrations of oxygen that will damage retinal tissue (Fig. 39-4).

A person experienced in recognizing retrolental fibroplasia should examine the eyes of all infants born at less than 36 weeks' gestation or weighing less than 2,000 gm who have received oxygen therapy. Examination should be made at discharge from the nursery and again at 3 to 6 months of age.

KERNICTERUS. Kernicterus, which results from high concentrations of indirect bilirubin in the blood due to excessive breakdown of red blood cells, occurs in about 5 percent of mature infants and in 10 to 40 percent of immature infants. Because many immature infants are acidotic, their brain cells may be more susceptible to the effect of indirect bilirubin than are those of the more mature infant, and they may have less serum albumin to bind indirect bilirubin and therefore inactivate its effect than does the mature infant. Hence kernicterus may occur at lower levels of

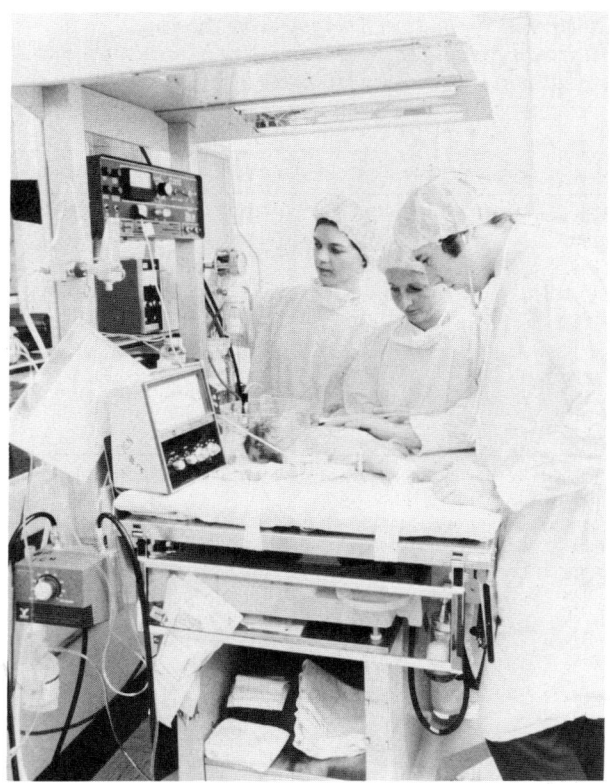

Fig. 39-4. Excessive oxygen administration is the cause of retrolental fibroplasia in the immature infant. The amount of oxygen given to any newborn must be monitored carefully by health care personnel. (Courtesy of the Department of Medical Photography, Children's Hospital, Buffalo, N.Y.)

indirect bilirubin in these infants than in mature infants. Thus, it is as important or more important to monitor indirect bilirubin levels in immature infants if jaundice occurs, so that phototherapy or exchange transfusion can be begun before the levels become toxic. This point may be as low as 8 to 12 mg per 100 ml in immature infants.

NEONATAL NECROTIZING ENTEROCOLITIS. Neonatal necrotizing enterocolitis (NEC) is a condition that develops in about 5 percent of all infants in intensive care nurseries. The bowel develops necrotic patches, interfering with digestion and possibly leading to a paralytic ileus. Perforation and peritonitis may ensue.

The necrosis appears to result from ischemic or poor perfusion of blood vessels in sections of bowel. The entire bowel may be involved, or it may be a localized phenomenon. The incidence of NEC is highest in very immature infants and those who have suffered anoxia or shock. Infants with infections may develop it as a further complication of their already stressed state.

There is a low incidence of the condition in infants

who are fed breast milk. The ischemia process may occur when, owing to shock or hypoxia, there is vasoconstriction of blood vessels to nonessential organs such as the bowel. Intestinal organisms grow more profusely with cow's milk than breast milk. The combination of decreased bowel perfusion and a response to the foreign protein in cow's milk probably starts the necrotic process.

Signs that the condition is beginning usually appear in the first week of life. The abdomen becomes distended and tense. Stool may be positive for occult blood. Periods of apnea may begin, or worsen in amount if they were already present. The infant does not empty his stomach by the next feeding time because of poor intestinal action. Signs of blood loss due to intestinal bleeding such as lowered blood pressure and inability to stabilize temperature may be present.

Abdominal x-ray films reveal a characteristic picture of air invading the intestinal wall; if perforation has occurred, there will be free air in the abdominal cavity. That the abdomen is increasing in size can be ascertained by measuring the abdominal circumference every 4 to 8 hours. The measurement is made just above the umbilicus.

Gavage or bottle feedings must be discontinued and the infant maintained on intravenous or total parenteral nutrition solutions to rest the gastrointestinal tract. A course of an antibiotic may be given to limit secondary infection. The abdomen must be handled gently to lessen the possibility of bowel perforation. If the area of necrosis appears to be localized, surgery to remove that portion of the bowel may be successful.

NEC is a grave insult to an infant already stressed by immaturity. The prognosis is guarded until it can be demonstrated that he can again take oral feedings without bowel complication.

HYPOGLYCEMIA. Glycogen stores are laid down in the late months of pregnancy, so the immature infant has few glycogen stores. If he has difficulty establishing respirations at birth, he uses a great deal of any glucose he had available. If he is chilled his use of glucose is even more rapid.

The immature infant should have frequent blood sugar levels taken in the first hours of life. A level below 30 mg is considered hypoglycemia in a term infant; under 20 mg is hypoglycemia in an immature infant.

THE IMMATURE INFANT AND PARENT-CHILD INTERACTION

At one time, an immature infant was handled as little as possible by hospital staff in order to conserve his energy and not interfere with respirations. Parents were strictly isolated from the nursery to prevent the introduction of infection. Parents isolated themselves because they felt intimidated by the equipment and complicated procedures they saw being used with their child.

When the child reached a magic weight of 4½ or 5½ pounds, the parents were called and told that their child was ready to be discharged. The more enlightened nursery personnel offered to allow the mother to feed her infant once under their supervision before the day of discharge. In other nurseries, the mother was simply handed the smallest infant she had ever seen and told to take him home and "mother" this stranger.

Premature infants could be detected during their preschool years for the unusually flat sides of their heads from lying continually in one position during their first month of life and for behavior problems. A "premature personality," that of a "spoiled," undisciplined, hard-to-manage child, was defined.

Today, it is recognized that, although both conserving the immature infant's strength and gentle handling are extremely important, the immature infant needs to be handled, rocked, and touched as much as the mature infant if he is to begin to relate satisfactorily to people. If the infant cannot be removed from an incubator because he continually needs warmth or oxygen, he should be handled and stroked in the incubator prior to and following feeding. As soon as his mother can be out of bed, she needs to visit the nursery and observe her baby (in 4 to 8 hours if the baby is housed in the same hospital). If she wishes to do so, she should be encouraged to touch the baby inside the incubator. Touching is important in terms of initiating "claiming" of her infant and making the birth of her infant real. She was not psychologically ready for birth at this time, and it is much harder for her to believe she has had a child than it is for the mother who has delivered at term. As soon as the infant is taking bottle- or breast-feedings, the mother should be encouraged to visit the hospital and give the feedings.

If the baby is transferred to a regional center for care, the mother should have an opportunity to see him before the transfer. Again, this makes the birth more real to her. After she is discharged, she needs to go to the hospital to visit the infant in the nursery.

Parents visiting in a high-risk nursery should have a great deal of attention and support from nursing personnel. Remember that, although incubators and respirators and monitoring equipment are commonplace to you, they are frightening to parents. They may want to touch their infant very much but be so afraid

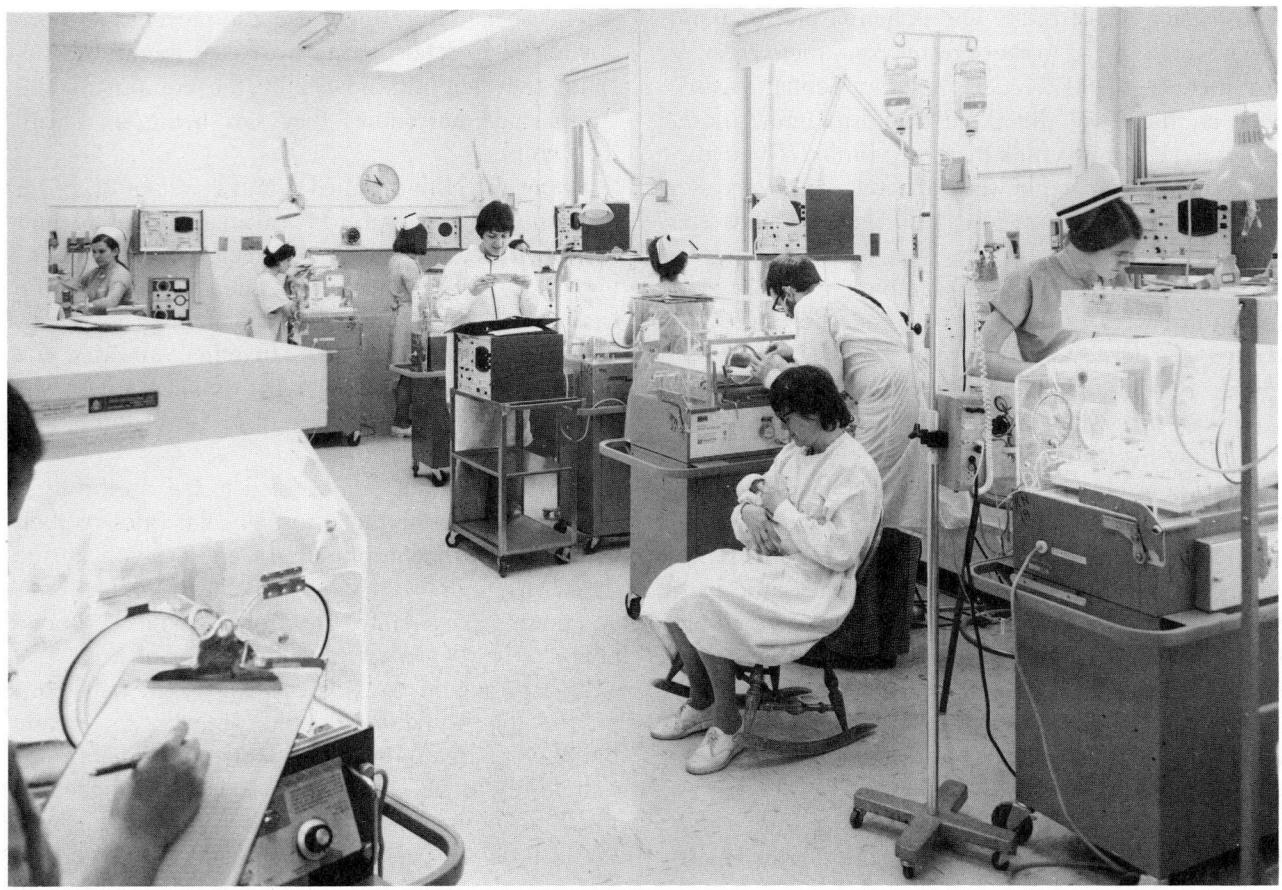

Fig. 39-5. Intensive care nurseries are busy, frightening places for parents. A parent needs support to visit and care for an infant here. (Courtesy of the Department of Medical Photography, Children's Hospital, Buffalo, N.Y.)

that they might touch a button or monitor and harm him that they stand by a wall with their arms folded.

The mother needs to be able to telephone the nursery and ask about her child's condition on days she cannot visit. She should be able to feel by the day of discharge that she is taking home "her" baby, a baby she knows and is ready to love.

Making parents welcome in a high-risk nursery is a major role for the nurse of high-risk infants (Fig. 39-5).

Sensory Stimulation

Immature infants need rest in order to reserve energy for growth and to combat hypoglycemia or infection or stabilize temperature. Procedures should be organized, therefore, so that rest time is available. If this is not specifically planned, the infant can constantly be awakened for procedure after procedure and never rest.

At the same time, the infant needs planned periods of sensory stimulation. Like all newborns, immature infants respond best to stimulation that appeals to their senses—sight, sound, and touch.

The view from inside an Isolette may be distorted by the Plexiglas dome. It is most natural for people to view an infant in an Isolette from the side. Thus the infant's face is rarely in the same line of vision as the adult (an *en face* position). You need to provide some time during each nursing shift for looking directly at the infant in the straightforward position so that he has the stimulation of a human face. If you put your head at the level of the infant's and look to each side, you may discover that there is nothing to see except a gray intravenous pole or a light green respirator or a white wall. Even very immature infants should have a mobile or a bright object in their view. As the infant's position is changed from side to stomach to opposite side, the object should be moved in line with his vision.

An infant in a closed Isolette may be able to hear nothing but the sound of the Isolette motor. He may see people looking at him, nodding at him—he may see their mouths move—but he cannot benefit from the sound of their voices because it is obscured by the continuous hum of the motor. Some talk time—

words spoken softly but clearly to his ear—should be provided each nursing shift.

Even the infant who cannot be removed from his incubator should not suffer from lack of touch. Gently stroking the infant's back or smoothing the back of his head is not a tiring motion. There should be time during every nursing shift for this interaction, particularly if clinical interventions with the infant include hurting procedures such as suctioning or blood drawing. As soon as he can be out of his Isolette, he needs special time, aside from procedures, being rocked and held. Prolonged or rough handling of an infant may lead to hypoxemia [8]. Transcutaneous oxygen determinations allow you to recognize the point where handling is comforting and the point where it is tiring.

As soon as the parents can visit, their visits should be spent touching the infant and talking to him. This type of intervention not only is beneficial to the infant but enhances parent-child bonding.

The Postmature Infant

A pregnancy is normally 38 to 42 weeks in length. An infant is postmature if he remains in utero longer than 42 weeks.

An infant who stays in utero past his time to be born is at risk because a placenta appears to be a timed structure; it lasts effectively for 40 weeks, then seems to lose function. The post-term infant who remains in utero with a failing placenta may develop a *postmature syndrome*.

Postmature infants have many of the characteristics of the small-for-gestation-age infant: dry, cracked, almost leather-like skin from lack of fluid; absence of vernix. They may be light in weight from a recent weight loss. Fingernails are generally long. They may demonstrate an alertness much more like a 2-week-old baby than a newborn. They may be meconium-stained; the amount of amniotic fluid at delivery appears to be less than is normal.

When a pregnancy becomes post-term, a sonogram may be obtained to measure the biparietal diameter of the fetus. Estriol levels may be assessed and oxytocin challenge or nonstress tests done to establish whether the placenta is still functioning adequately. An amniocentesis will show whether the infant's lungs are mature. Many postmature infants must be delivered by cesarean section as an oxytocin challenge or nonstress test reveals a placenta that will be extremely compromised during labor because of its failing ability to provide nutrients and oxygen to the fetus.

At birth, the baby is likely to have difficulty establishing respirations. He may have meconium aspiration. In the first hours of life, hypoglycemia may develop as he does not have adequate stores of glycogen to prevent it. He has used his stores to support himself in the last weeks of intrauterine life. Because of low levels of subcutaneous fat, temperature regulation may be difficult for him. He must be protected from chilling at birth or in transport to a special care center.

Any woman is anxious when she does not deliver on her due date. She becomes extremely anxious when her pregnancy is more than 42 weeks long. She may be angry when she is told that the baby appears to be postmature (she said over and over that she knew her dates were right, but no one listened to her). It may seem to her that the longer a baby stays in utero the stronger and healthier he should be. Why then, is he being transferred for special care? She may feel guilty in that she did not provide well for the infant in the last few weeks of pregnancy, that she has let him down.

The mother needs to spend time with her newborn to assure herself that, although delivery was not "triggered," everything else about the baby appears to be normal; that with appropriate interventions to control the hypoglycemia or meconium aspiration he will be a well baby. All postmature infants need continued follow-up until at least school age in terms of developmental abilities. The lack of nutrients and oxygen in utero may have left them with neurological symptoms that will not become apparent until the child attempts fine motor tasks.

Problem-oriented Recording: Progress Notes

Careful Watch Nursery
Admission note

Problem: Physiological adjustment to extrauterine life

> S. Infant of c-section delivery under general anesthetic for cephalopelvic disproportion. Slight meconium staining at birth; no meconium visualized in pharynx or trachea on intubation. Suctioned prior to first breath; 100% oxygen by mask to initiate respirations. Apgars 3 and 8.
> O. Respiratory rate 60 at rest; slight occasional retractions; occasional bilateral wheezing heard on auscultation.

Pulse: 140 (AP). Loud heart murmur heard throughout both systolic and diastolic phases.
Color: acyanotic; no gross cyanosis.
Temperature: 36.8°C rectal.
Dextrostix: 45–90 mg%. Blood gases within normal limits.
General appearance: alert; no anomalies; good body proportions. Meconium-stained vernix in axilla and groins; elevated deep red area 1 × 2 cm on dorsum of right hand.
Good Moro, good suck.
Hgt, wgt, and H.C. all 20th percentile.

A. Newborn high risk for possible meconium aspiration. Abnormal heart sound and strawberry hemangioma on right hand by physical exam.

Goals: a. Respiratory function maintained in room air without further oxygen or ventilator assist.
b. Temperature stabilized in bassinet by 24 hours of age.
c. Mother-child interaction initiated early to counteract time delay of general anesthetic.

P. 1. To remain in careful watch nursery for observation.
2. Respiratory rate, pulse q15min for first 4 hours.
3. Observe for cyanosis, restlessness, lethargy.
4. Dextrostix q1h for first 4 hours.
5. Private pediatrician notified of abnormal heart sound and possible meconium aspiration.
6. Show to mother as soon as she is awake (did not see in delivery room because of general anesthetic).
7. Blood gas to be drawn if respiratory rate increases or other signs of respiratory or heart distress appear.

References

1. Biehl, D. Treatment of the respiratory distress syndrome prior to birth. *Respir. Technol.* 14:12, 1978.
2. Brown, R. The low-birth-weight infant: Expert nursing and medical supervision is needed. *Nurs. Times* 74:1805, 1978.
3. Choe, M. W. Breast milk for infants who can't breast-feed. *Am. J. Nurs.* 78:852, 1978.
4. Committee on the Fetus and Newborn. *Standards and Recommendations for Hospital Care of Newborn Infants.* Evanston, Ill.: American Academy of Pediatrics, 1972.
5. Flores, R. N. Necrotizing enterocolitis. *Nurs. Clin. North Am.* 13:39, 1978.
6. Gorski, P. A., et al. Stages of behavioral organization in the high-risk neonate: Theoretical and clinical considerations. *Semin. Perinatol.* 3:61, 1979.
7. Hawkins-Walsh, E. Diminishing anxiety in parents of sick newborns. *M.C.N.* 5:30, 1980.
8. Long, J. G., et al. Excessive handling as a cause of hypoxemia. *Pediatrics* 65:203, 1980.
9. Martin, R. J., et al. Effect of supine and prone positions on arterial oxygen tension in the preterm infant. *Pediatrics* 63:528, 1979.
10. Minde, K., et al. Mother-child relationships in the premature nursery: An observational study. *Pediatrics* 61:373, 1978.
11. Miner, H. Problems and prognosis for the small-for-gestational age and the premature infant. *M.C.N.* 3:221, 1978.
12. Murphy, N. J. Helping a family and their premature baby grow together. *Can. Nurse* 73:42, 1977.
13. Rothfeder, B., et al. Feeding the low-birth-weight neonate. *Nursing 77* 7:58, 1977.
14. Schraeder, B. D. Attachment and parenting despite lengthy intensive care. *M.C.N.* 5:37, 1980.
15. Schreiner, R. L., et al. A new complication of nutritional management of the low birth weight infant. *Pediatrics* 63:683, 1979.
16. Sham, B., et al. Apnea in the premature infant: An overview of causes and treatment. *Nurs. Clin. North Am.* 13:29, 1978.
17. Simkins, T. Feeding the premature infant: More questions than answers. *Perinat. Neonatol.* 2:30, 1978.
18. Stewart, D., et al. Supporting lactation when mothers and infants are separated. *Nurs. Clin. North Am.* 13:47, 1978.
19. Sullivan, R., et al. Determining a newborn's gestational age. *M.C.N.* 4:38, 1979.
20. Waddell, C. S., et al. Discharge of the premature infant. *Nurs. Clin. North Am.* 13:63, 1978.

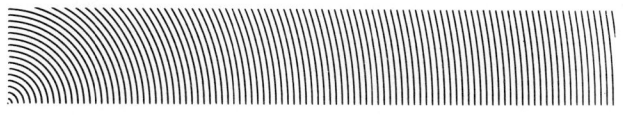

Unit VIII. Utilizing Nursing Process: Questions for Review

1. Baby Jones is born by cesarean section. Infants born by this method tend to have
   a. Increased bruising at birth
   b. Respiratory distress syndrome
   c. Seizures
   d. Infections

2. Baby B. is an infant of a diabetic mother. The chief factor to be aware of in the early hours of his life is the possibility of
   a. Hypoglycemia
   b. Hypothyroidism
   c. Fractured femur
   d. Intracranial bleeding

3. Baby C. does not breathe spontaneously at birth. You administer oxygen by bag and mask. If oxygen is entering the lungs, you should notice
   a. The abdomen rises while the chest falls with bag compressions.
   b. The infant's pupils dilate after 3 minutes.
   c. The infant's neck veins become prominent and palpable.
   d. The chest rises with each bag compression.

4. To administer oxygen by bag and mask, you would position the baby
   a. In a Trendelenburg position.
   b. On his back with his neck slightly flexed.
   c. On his back with his head slightly extended.
   d. Position is unimportant as long as the tongue is pulled forward.

5. If Baby C. needs cardiac massage, you would initiate this at what rate?
   a. 40 beats/min
   b. 80 beats/min
   c. 120 beats/min
   d. 180 beats/min

6. Before feeding Baby D. by gavage, which method would you *not* use to test whether his indwelling catheter was in place?
   a. Place the distal end of the catheter under water.
   b. Aspirate stomach contents through the catheter.
   c. Inject air into the catheter and listen with a stethoscope.
   d. Check that the tape holding the tube to his nose is secure.

7. Baby D. is the infant of an RH-sensitized mother. At birth, the problems that he must be assessed for most are
   a. Polycythemia and hypercalcemia
   b. Small for gestation age and hypocalcemia
   c. Congenital anomalies and hypoglycemia
   d. Anemia and hyperbilirubinemia

8. A positive direct Coombs' test means that
   a. The infant's white blood cells are free of maternal antibodies.
   b. The infant's red blood cells have maternal antigens attached to them.
   c. The infant's red blood cells have maternal antibodies attached to them.
   d. The infant's red blood cells are microcytic from destruction.

9. Baby D. is placed under phototherapy lights. Under lights, he must be observed for
   a. Shock from hypovolemia
   b. Dehydration due to loose stools
   c. Hypobilirubinemia due to excess hemolysis
   d. Intestinal obstruction due to constipation

10. Baby E. develops hypoglycemia 4 hours after birth. A common symptom of hypoglycemia is
    a. Easy bruising
    b. Increased temperature
    c. Jaundice
    d. Jitteriness

11. Hypoglycemia in a mature infant is defined as a blood glucose level below which number?
    a. 100 mg/100 ml whole blood
    b. 80 mg/100 ml whole blood
    c. 40 mg/100 ml whole blood
    d. 30 mg/100 ml whole blood

12. Baby F. is born immature. As a rule, immature babies should be fed
    a. More frequently than term babies
    b. A more dilute formula than term babies
    c. An iron supplement during their first week of life
    d. Only glucose water as formula is too strong

Appendixes

Appendix A. The Pregnant Patient's Bill of Rights

American parents are becoming increasingly aware that health professionals do not always have scientific data to support common American obstetrical practices and that many of these practices are carried out primarily because they are part of medical and hospital tradition. In the last forty years many artificial practices have been introduced which have changed childbirth from a physiological event to a very complicated medical procedure in which all kinds of drugs are used and procedures carried out, sometimes unnecessarily, and many of them potentially damaging for the baby and even for the mother. A growing body of research makes it alarmingly clear that every aspect of traditional American hospital care during labor and delivery must now be questioned as to its possible effect on the future well-being of both the obstetric patient and her unborn child.

One in every 35 children born in the United States today will eventually be diagnosed as retarded; one in every 10 to 17 children has been found to have some form of brain dysfunction or learning disability requiring special treatment. Such statistics are not confined to the lower socioeconomic group but cut across all segments of American society.

New concerns are being raised by childbearing women because no one knows what degree of oxygen depletion, head compression, or traction by forceps the unborn or newborn infant can tolerate before that child sustains permanent brain damage or dysfunction. The recent findings regarding the cancer-related drug diethylstilbestrol have alerted the public to the fact that neither the approval of a drug by the U.S. Food and Drug Administration nor the fact that a drug is prescribed by a physician serves as a guarantee that a drug or medication is safe for the mother or her unborn child. In fact, the American Academy of Pediatrics Committee on Drugs has recently stated that there is no drug, whether prescription or over-the-counter remedy, which has been proven safe for the unborn child.

The Pregnant Patient has the right to participate in decisions involving her well-being and that of her unborn child, unless there is a clear-cut medical emergency that prevents her participation. In addition to the rights set forth in the American Hospital Association's "Patient's Bill of Rights" (which has also been adopted by the New York City Department of Health), the Pregnant Patient, because she represents TWO patients rather than one, should be recognized as having the additional rights listed below.

1. *The Pregnant Patient has the right*, prior to the administration of any drug or procedure, to be informed by the health professional caring for her of any potential direct or indirect effects, risks or hazards to herself or her unborn or newborn infant which may result from the use of a drug or procedure prescribed for or administered to her during pregnancy, labor, birth, or lactation.

2. *The Pregnant Patient has the right*, prior to the proposed therapy, to be informed, not only of the benefits, risks, and hazards of the proposed therapy but also of known alternative therapy, such as available childbirth education classes which could help to prepare the Pregnant Patient physically and mentally to cope with the discomfort or stress of pregnancy and the experience of childbirth, thereby reducing or eliminating her need for drugs and obstetric intervention. She should be offered such information early in her pregnancy in order that she may make a reasoned decision.

3. *The Pregnant Patient has the right*, prior to the administration of any drug, to be informed by the health professional who is prescribing or administering the drug to her that any drug which she receives during pregnancy, labor and birth, no matter how or when the drug is taken or administered, may adversely affect her unborn baby, directly or indirectly, and that there is no drug or chemical which has been proven safe for the unborn child.

4. *The Pregnant Patient has the right*, if cesarean section is anticipated, to be informed prior to the administration of any drug, and preferably prior to her hospitalization, that minimizing her and, in turn, her baby's intake of nonessential preoperative medicine will benefit her baby.

5. *The Pregnant Patient has the right*, prior to the administration of a drug or procedure, to be informed if there is NO properly controlled follow-up research which has established the safety of the drug or procedure with regard to its direct and/or indirect effects on the physiological, mental and neurological development of the child exposed, via the mother, to the drug or procedure during pregnancy, labor, birth, or lactation—(this would apply to virtually all drugs and the vast majority of obstetric procedures).

6. *The Pregnant Patient has the right*, prior to the

Source: Reprinted by permission of the Committee on Patient's Rights, Box 1900, New York, N.Y. 10001.

administration of any drug, to be informed of the brand name and generic name of the drug in order that she may advise the health professional of any past adverse reaction to the drug.

7. *The Pregnant Patient has the right*, to determine for herself, without pressure from her attendant, whether she will accept the risks inherent in the proposed therapy or refuse a drug or procedure.

8. *The Pregnant Patient has the right* to know the name and qualifications of the individual administering a medication or procedure to her during labor or birth.

9. *The Pregnant Patient has the right* to be informed, prior to the administration of any procedure, whether that procedure is being administered to her for her or her baby's benefit (medically indicated) or as an elective procedure (for convenience or teaching purposes).

10. *The Pregnant Patient has the right* to be accompanied during the stress of labor and birth by someone she cares for, and to whom she looks for emotional comfort and encouragement.

11. *The Pregnant Patient has the right* after appropriate medical consultation to choose a position for labor and for birth which is the least stressful to her baby and to herself.

12. *The Obstetric Patient has the right* to have her baby cared for at her bedside if her baby is normal, and to feed her baby according to her baby's needs rather than according to the hospital regimen.

13. *The Obstetric Patient has the right* to be informed in writing of the name of the person who actually delivered her baby and the professional qualifications of that person. This information should also be on the birth certificate.

14. *The Obstetric Patient has the right* to be informed if there is any known or indicated aspect of her or her baby's care or condition which may cause her or her baby later difficulty or problems.

15. *The Obstetric Patient has the right* to have her and her baby's hospital medical records complete, accurate, and legible and to have their records, including Nurses' Notes, retained by the hospital until the child reaches at least the age of majority, or alternatively, to have the records offered to her before they are destroyed.

16. *The Obstetric Patient*, both during and after her hospital stay, *has the right* to have access to her complete hospital medical records, including Nurses' Notes, and to receive a copy upon payment of a reasonable fee and without incurring the expense of retaining an attorney.

It is the obstetric patient and her baby, not the health professional, who must sustain any trauma or injury resulting from the use of a drug or obstetric procedure. The observation of the rights listed above will not only permit the obstetric patient to participate in the decisions involving her and her baby's health care, but will help to protect the health professional and the hospital against litigation arising from resentment or misunderstanding on the part of the mother.

Appendix B. Conversion of Pounds and Ounces to Grams for Newborn Weights

Pounds	| Ounces 0	1	2	3	4	5	6	7	8	9	10	11	12	13	14	15	Pounds
0	—	28	57	85	113	142	170	198	227	255	283	312	430	369	397	425	0
1	454	482	510	539	567	595	624	652	680	709	737	765	794	822	850	879	1
2	907	936	964	992	1021	1049	1077	1106	1134	1162	1191	1219	1247	1276	1304	1332	2
3	1361	1389	1417	1446	1474	1503	1531	1559	1588	1616	1644	1673	1701	1729	1758	1786	3
4	1814	1843	1871	1899	1928	1956	1984	2013	2041	2070	2098	2126	2155	2183	2211	2240	4
5	2268	2296	2325	2353	2381	2410	2438	2466	2495	2523	2551	2580	2608	2637	2665	2693	5
6	2722	2750	2778	2807	2835	2863	2892	2920	2948	2977	3005	3033	3062	3090	3118	3147	6
7	3175	3203	3232	3260	3289	3317	3345	3374	3402	3430	3459	3487	3515	3544	3572	3600	7
8	3629	3657	3685	3714	3742	3770	3799	3827	3856	3884	3912	3941	3969	3997	4026	4054	8
9	4082	4111	4139	4167	4196	4224	4252	4281	4309	4337	4366	4394	4423	4451	4479	4508	9
10	4536	4564	4593	4621	4649	4678	4706	4734	4763	4791	4819	4848	4876	4904	4933	4961	10
11	4990	5018	5046	5075	5103	5131	5160	5188	5216	5245	5273	5301	5330	5358	5386	5415	11
12	5443	5471	5500	5528	5557	5585	5613	5642	5670	5698	5727	5755	5783	5812	5840	5868	12
13	5897	5925	5953	5982	6010	6038	6067	6095	6123	6152	6180	6209	6237	6265	6294	6322	13
14	6350	6379	6407	6435	6464	6492	6520	6549	6577	6605	6634	6662	6690	6719	6747	6776	14
15	6804	6832	6860	6889	6917	6945	6973	7002	7030	7059	7087	7115	7144	7172	7201	7228	15
	0	1	2	3	4	5	6	7	8	9	10	11	12	13	14	15	

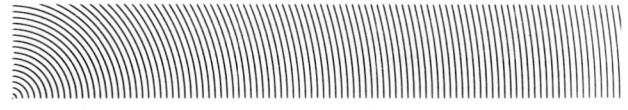

Answers to Unit Questions

Unit I
1. d
2. d
3. b
4. d
5. a
6. c
7. b
8. c
9. a
10. c
11. c.
12. d
13. a
14. c
15. b
16. b
17. c
18. c
19. a

Unit II
1. a
2. d
3. c
4. a
5. d
6. b
7. a
8. b
9. c
10. d
11. a
12. a
13. b
14. d
15. c
16. b
17. a
18. b
19. b
20. c

Unit III
1. a
2. d
3. b
4. d
5. d
6. b
7. c
8. b
9. b
10. d
11. b
12. a
13. b
14. a
15. b
16. b
17. d
18. c

Unit IV
1. c
2. b
3. b
4. d
5. a
6. d
7. b
8. d
9. a
10. d
11. c
12. b
13. a
14. b
15. d
16. c
17. c

Unit V
1. a
2. c
3. c
4. c
5. d
6. b
7. c
8. d
9. d
10. d

Unit VI

1. c
2. b
3. c
4. d
5. c
6. b
7. a
8. b
9. c
10. c
11. c
12. c
13. a
14. b
15. d

Unit VII

1. d
2. b
3. c
4. b
5. d
6. b
7. d
8. a
9. c
10. c

Unit VIII

1. b
2. a
3. d
4. c
5. c
6. d
7. d
8. c
9. b
10. d
11. d
12. a

Index

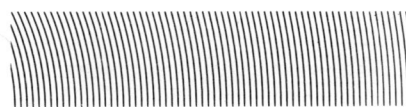

Index

Abandonment in nurse-patient relationship, 48
Abdomen
  abnormal contour of, as danger signal in labor, 313
  discomfort in, in early pregnancy, 226
  of newborn
    appearance of, 438–439
    assessment of, 445–447
  pain in, during pregnancy, 230
  pregnancy in, 533–534
  sounds and movements in, in assessment of fetal well-being and maturity, 171
  wall of
    assessment of, in postpartal hospital care, 396
    changes in, during pregnancy, 185
    in postpartal period, 382
Abdominal muscle, contractions of, in preparation for childbirth, 264–265
ABO incompatibility
  hemolysis of newborn in, 686
  recurrent abortion due to, 531
Abortion, 109, 523–531
  definition of, 523
  illegal, 526
  induced, 526–529. See also Abortion, therapeutic
  isoimmunization and, 531
  medical, 526–529. See also Abortion, therapeutic
  planned, 526–529. See also Abortion, therapeutic
  reactions to, 530
  recurrent, causes of, 531
  spontaneous, 524–526
    causes of, 525–526
    complete, 525
    complications of, 529–531
    imminent, 525
    incomplete, 525
    missed, 525
    recurrent, causes of, 531
    threatened, 524–525
  therapeutic, 526–529
    complications of, 529–531
    danger signs after, 528
    by dilation and curettage, 526
    by dilation and vacuum extraction, 526–527
    for hydatidiform mole, 534
    by hysterotomy, 528
    laboratory studies on, 528
    by menstrual extraction, 526
    by prostaglandin injection, 528
    psychological aspects of, 528–529
    by saline induction, 527–528
Abruptio placentae
  assessment of, 538–539
  central venous pressure in, 540–541
  degrees of, 539
  disseminated intravascular coagulation in, 541–542
  interventions for, 539
  shock in, 538–539, 539–540
Abuse, child, high-risk infant and, 644
Acceptance in grieving process, 521
Accidents, role of stress in, 510
Accomplishment, development of sense of, as task of school-age child, 58, 59–60
Acetylsalicylic acid
  for pregnant woman with juvenile rheumatoid arthritis, 568
  teratogenic effects of, 166–167
Acidosis
  fetal, as danger signal in labor, 313
  metabolic, in gestational diabetes, 555–556
  in respiratory distress in newborn, 652–653
Acrocyanosis in newborn, 489
Activity level
  increased, as preliminary sign of labor, 300
  of infant, 412
Acyanotic heart disease, 672–674
Adaptability of infant, 412–413
Adenine arabinoside, for herpesvirus infection in newborn, 689
Admission to hospital during labor, assessment on, 315–324
Adolescent
  coitus interruptus and, 107
  condoms and, 106
  developing sense of identity in, 60–61
  diaphragm and, 102
  intrauterine devices and, 101–102
  oral contraceptives and, 100
  pregnant, 573–575
    assessment of, 574
    delivery decision for, 575
    health teaching for, 574–575
    nutrition for, 250, 574
    plans for baby of, 575
    unwed, 137–139. See also Unwed pregnant woman
  sex roles in, 92
  sterilization and, 108–109
  vaginally inserted spermicidal products and, 103
Adrenogenital syndrome, characteristics of, 596–597
Adulthood
  middle, developing sense of generativity in, 62
  young, developing sense of intimacy in, 61–62
Afterpains in postpartal period, 382, 391
Airway, establishment of, in resuscitation of newborn, 648–650
Alcohol
  in breast milk, 476
  consumption of, in pregnancy, 227
  effects of, on fetus, 168
  dependence on, in pregnancy, 577–578
  for halting premature labor, 544
  newborn of mother using, 692–693
Alcoholism as nutritional problem of pregnancy, 251
Alkaline phosphatase in maternal serum, assay of, 174–175
Allergy, food, as nutritional problem of pregnancy, 249
Alpha fetoprotein, amniotic, in detection of spinal cord defect, 177
Alphaprodine, in labor, 347, 356–357

725

Ambulation, early postpartal, 400
Amenorrhea, 88
    in diagnosis of pregnancy, 195
Amethopterin, teratogenic effects of, 166
Aminopterin, teratogenic effects of, 166
Amnesics, for pain relief in labor, 348, 356–357
Amniocentesis
    in assessment of fetal well-being and maturity, 175–177
    for fetal monitoring in Rh sensitized mother, 592
    in genetic counseling, 589–591
Amniography, 177
Amniotic cavity, 152
Amniotic fluid, 151–152
    color of, 176
    excessive, 572
    meconium staining of, 313
Amniotic fluid embolism, 602
Amniotic membrane, 151
Amniotomy in labor, 332
Ampicillin, for postpartal urinary tract infection, 629
Amyl nitrite, for pathological retraction ring, 601
Analgesia, 343
    in labor, 325
Analgesics
    in breast milk, 472
    in labor, effects of, on newborn, 168
    synthetic, in labor, 347
    teratogenic effects of, 166–167
Androgens
    in sexual development at puberty, 67–68
    for suppression of lactation, 389, 390
    teratogenic effects of, 167
Android pelvis, 215
Anemia
    blood loss, in newborn, 686
    in pregnancy, 561–562
        iron deficiency, 561
        megaloblastic, 561–562
        sickle cell, 593–594
Anesthesia
    caudal, 350–351, 356–357
    definition of, 343
    for delivery, 334–335
    gas
        in delivery, 353–354, 358–359
        in labor, 348, 356–357
    intravenous, 354
    for labor and delivery in heart disease, 560
    local, 353, 358–359
    natural, 352
    for perineal repair, 337–338
    regional, 348–351, 356–357
    risk of, 358–359
    saddle block, 353
    spinal
        in delivery, 352–353
        in labor, 350–351
Anesthetics
    in labor, effects of, on newborn, 168
    preparation for safe administration of, 354–358
Anger in grieving process, 521

Ankles, edema of, in mid or late pregnancy, 232
Anogenital area of newborn, appearance of, 439
Anovulation, female infertility due to, 115–117
Antacids, effects of, on fetus, 167
Anteflexion of uterus, 74, 75
Anterior pituitary necrosis, postpartal, 625
Anteversion of uterus, 74, 75
Anthropoid pelvis, 215
Antibiotics
    effects of, on fetus, 167
    prophylactic, for pregnant woman with mitral stenosis, 560
    after urinary tract infection, 562
Anticholinergics, in breast milk, 473
Anticoagulants
    in breast milk, 472
    effects of, on fetus, 167
    for femoral thrombophlebitis, 627
Anticonvulsants
    in breast milk, 472
    effects of, on fetus, 167–168
Antidiabetics, in breast milk, 472
Antihistamines, in breast milk, 472–473
Antihypertensives, in breast milk, 473
Anti-infectives, in breast milk, 473
Antithyroid preparations, in breast milk, 475
Anus, imperforate, 668
Anxiety, effects of, on fetus, 169–170
Aorta, coarctation of, 673, 674
Apgar scoring of newborn, 489
Apnea
    in immature infants, 702
    primary and secondary, in newborn, 649
Appendicitis in pregnancy, 568–569
Apprehension, increasing, as danger signal in labor, 313
Approach of infant to new situations, 412
Apresoline, for severe preeclampsia, 550
Arborization in evaluation of ovulation, 115
Arms of newborn, assessment of, 448
Arteries, uterine, 74, 75
Arthritis, juvenile rheumatoid, in pregnancy, 568
Artificial insemination, 114–115
Aschheim-Zondek test of pregnancy, 198
Asherman's syndrome, infertility due to, 118
Aspiration
    of meconium, 687
    in newborn, prevention of, 508–510
    of vomitus during anesthesia for labor and delivery, 355–358
Aspirin
    for pregnant woman with juvenile rheumatoid arthritis, 568
    teratogenic effects of, 166–167
Assessment in nursing process, 29–33
Asthma, pregnancy and, 563
Atkins diet, during pregnancy, 253
Atresia
    choanal, in newborn, 676
    tracheoesophageal, 666, 667
Atrial septal defect in newborn, 672–674
Attention span of infant, 413–414
Attitude and labor process, 291–293

Auditory stimulation for newborn, 411
Auscultation
    in determining fetal presentation and position, 296–297, 298, 299
    in physical assessment, 31
Autoimmune system of newborn, 425–429
Autonomy, development of sense of
    in achieving maturity, interventions for, 63–64
    as task of toddlerhood, 58–59

Babinski reflex in newborn, 427
Back of newborn
    appearance of, 439–440
    assessment of, 450
Backache in mid or late pregnancy, 232
Bacteriuria, screening of maternal urine for, 173–174
Ballottement, in diagnosis of pregnancy, 196–197
Bandl's ring, 601–602
    in labor, significance of, 303
Barbiturates
    effects of, on fetus, 167
    in labor, 347–348, 356–357
Bargaining in grieving process, 521
Bartholin's glands, 76, 77
Basal body temperature
    in evaluation of ovulation, 115, 116
    rhythm and, 105
Bathing
    of newborn
        at home, 502
        in hospital, 497–498
    postpartal, 399
    in pregnancy, 226
Battered woman, pregnancy in, 578–579
Battledore placenta, 618, 619
Beckwith's syndrome, and large-for-gestation-age infant, 696
Bed rest
    for femoral thrombophlebitis, 627
    for mild preeclampsia, 548
    for multiple gestation, 571
    for pregnant woman with heart disease, 559
    for severe preeclampsia, 549–550
Bendectin, for nausea and vomiting in pregnancy, 222
Bicornuate uterus, 74, 75
Bifidus factor, in breast milk, 465
Bikini incision for cesarean section, 613
Bilirubin
    determination of, in assessment of fetal well-being and maturity, 176
    levels of, indirect
        increased, in newborn, 682–684
        lowering of, methods for, 684–686
Billings method of contraception, 106
Bimanual examination in first prenatal visit, 213
Biopsy, uterine endometrial, as test for ovulation, 115, 117
Birth, 336–337
    registration of, 492
Birth centers, alternative, in reducing maternal and infant mortality, 23
Birth control methods, 97–109. *See also* Contraception

Birth rate, trends in, 15–16
Birthing rooms, 316
   in reducing maternal and infant mortality, 22–23
Birthmarks in newborn, 431–432
Black diet patterns in pregnancy, 252
Bladder
   assessment of
      in immediate postpartal period, 389
      in postpartal hospital care, 395–396
   care of, in labor, 325
   exstrophy of, 670, 671
Blastocyst, 146, 147
Bleeding, in pregnancy, 523–545. *See also* Hemorrhage
   causes of, 546
   cervical ripening and, 545
   first-trimester, 523–534
      abortion causing, 523–531. *See also* Abortion
      ectopic pregnancy causing, 531–534. *See also* Ectopic pregnancy
   second-trimester, 534–535
      hydatidiform mole causing, 534–535
      incompetent cervix causing, 535
   third-trimester, 535–545
      abruptio placentae causing, 538–542. *See also* Abruptio placentae
      placenta previa causing, 535–538. *See also* Placenta previa
      premature labor causing, 542–545. *See also* Labor, premature
   vaginal, 229, 230
Blink reflex in newborn, 426
Blocks
   epidural, 349–351, 356–357
   paracervical, 351, 358–359
   pudendal, 353, 358–359
Blood
   constitution of, in pregnancy, 189
   fetal, sampling of, in labor, 330
   loss of
      anemia due to, in newborn, 686
      assessment of, in uterine atony, 621–622
   studies of
      in first prenatal visit, 217
      in pregnancy, 231
   supply of
      to female external genitalia, 77
      to uterus, 74, 75
      to vagina, 76
   total volume of, of newborn, 421–422
   values of, in newborn, 422, 424
Blood gases in oxygen administration to newborn, 652–654
Blood incompatibility
   ABO, 686
   inheritance of, 585, 586–587
   recurrent abortion due to, 531
   Rh, 591–593
Blood pressure
   in labor, 324
   maternal, abnormal, as danger signal in labor, 313
   in newborn, 421, 422
   in postpartal period, 385
   in pregnancy, 188–189
Blood tests in labor, 319

Blood vessels, transposition of, in newborn, 673, 675
Blood volume, changes in, in pregnancy, 187–188
Blues, postpartal, 376
Body image, of adolescent, 60
Bonding, maternal-infant, 369
   with high-risk infant, 642–644
Bones
   congenital anomalies of, 677–679
   intrauterine development of, 155–156
   pelvic, growth of, 80
Bottle-feeding, 477–483. *See also* Formulas
   bottles for, 480
   formulas for, 478–480
      preparation of, 480–482
   problems of, 483
   supplies for, 480
   techniques of, 482–483
Bradycardia, fetal
   complicating paracervical block, 351
   in labor, 326
Braxton Hicks contractions
   in diagnosis of pregnancy, 197
   in mid or late pregnancy, 233
   as preliminary sign of labor, 300–301
Brazelton Neonatal Behavioral Assessment Scale for assessing gestation age, 452–453, 458
Breasts, 79–80
   anatomy of, 464
   assessment of
      in immediate postpartal period, 389–390
      in postpartal hospital care, 393–395
   care of, postpartal, 394
   changes in, 186
      in diagnosis of pregnancy, 196
      in mid or late pregnancy, 233
   engorgement of, 469–470
   in gestation age assessment, 456
   hygiene for, postpartal, 394
   infection of, postpartal, 628
   of newborn, assessment of, 445
   self-examination of, postpartal instruction in, 394–395
   support of, postpartal, 394
   tenderness of, in early pregnancy, 226
Breast-feeding, 463–477
   advice on, on going home, 470–471
   assessing amount of milk taken in, 470
   beginning, 466–469
   burping and, 477
   drugs and, 471, 472–476
   for high-risk infant, 657
   for immature infant, 704–705
   jaundice and, 476
   physiological advantages of, 465–466
      for baby, 465–466
      for mother, 465
   physiology of, 463–464
   preparation for, 463
   problems with, 469–470, 477
   with puerperal infection, 629
   supplemental feedings and, 476–477
   suspension of, for reducing indirect bilirubin levels in newborn, 685
   weaning from, 477

Breath, shortness of, in mid or late pregnancy, 232
Breath sounds of newborn, assessment of, 445, 446
Breathing techniques for labor
   abdominal, in Dick-Read method, 270–271
   discussion of, in expectant parents' classes, 262
   in Lamaze method, 266–267, 268
Breech presentations of fetus, 293, 295
   labor and delivery in, 608–611
Bromides, effects of, on fetus, 167
Bronchopulmonary dysplasia, from oxygen therapy for newborn, 654
Brow presentation of fetus, 611
Bruising, in hyperbilirubinemia in newborn, 683
Bulb syringe for suctioning newborn, 648
Bulbocavernosus muscle fibers in pelvic floor, 77
Bulbourethral glands, 78, 79
Bupivacaine
   for paracervical block, 351
   for regional anesthesia, 349
Burping
   bottle-fed infant, 482
   breast-fed infant, 477

Caffeine, in breast milk, 475
Calcium
   in common foods, 245
   requirements for
      of newborn, 463
      in pregnancy, 243–244
Calories, requirements for
   of newborn, 461–462
   in pregnancy, 240
Cancer-chemotherapeutic agents, in breast milk, 473
Candidal infection, vaginal, in pregnancy, 184
Candidiasis
   in newborn, 507–508, 690
   in pregnancy, 565–566
Caput succedaneum, 434, 436
Car safety for newborn, 510
Carbohydrates
   newborn requirements for, 462
   types of, for formula, 479
Carbon dioxide, partial pressure of
   in assessment of fetal well-being and maturity, 176
   in pregnancy, 186–187
Carbon monoxide, teratogenic effects of, 168
Cardiomegaly, in peripartal heart disease, 560
Cardiovascular system, of newborn, 421–423
Catheterization
   of bladder
      in labor, 325
      postpartal, 395–396
   umbilical, for newborn, 654
Caudal anesthesia
   for labor and delivery in heart disease, 560
   in labor, 350–351, 356–357

Cavernous hemangiomas, in newborn, 432
Central venous pressure in abruptio placentae, 540–541
Cephalhematoma, in newborn, 435, 436
Cephalic presentations of fetus, 293, 294
Cephalopelvic disproportion, dystocia due to, 612–613
Cephaloridine, toxicity of, in newborn, 663
Cervical cerclage, 535
Cervical dilatation stage of labor, 282–283
Cervix, 69
　changes in
　　mucus of, in determining ovulation, 105–106
　　in physiology of menstrual cycle, 86–87
　　in pregnancy, 184
　dilatation of
　　discussion of, in expectant parents' classes, 262
　　as sign of true labor, 303
　effacement of
　　discussion of, in expectant parents' classes, 262
　　as sign of true labor, 302–303
　incompetent, 535
　infertility due to factors involving, 118–119
　involution of, in postpartal period, 383
　lacerations of, postpartal hemorrhage due to, 623
　lining of, 70
　opening of, as preliminary sign of labor, 301
　ripening of, bleeding and, 545
　scoring of, 616, 617
Cesarean section, 613–616
　for appendicitis near term, 569
　for breech delivery, 610
　for brow presentation, 611
　for cephalopelvic disproportion, 613
　incision for, 613, 616
　for large-for-gestation age infant, 697
　in pathological retraction ring, 601–602
　in placenta previa, 537–538
　postpartal care in, 630–631
　for small-for-gestation age infants, 696
　for transverse lie, 612
Chadwick's sign of pregnancy, 196
Chemotherapeutic agents, teratogenic, 166
Chest of newborn
　appearance of, 438
　assessment of, 444–445, 446
　circumference of, 419
Chest x-ray examination in early pregnancy, 217, 219
Child(ren)
　rearing of, developmental readiness for, 57–66
　　assessing, 65–66
　spacing of, in reducing maternal and infant mortality, 21
Child abuse, high-risk infant and, 644
Childbearing
　exercises for, 263–265
　physical readiness for, 67–82
　　assessing, 80–82

Childbirth
　acquiring knowledge about, as task of pregnancy, 134–135
　classes in preparation for, 263–272
　　exercises for childbearing in, 263–264
　　methods for minimizing discomfort in, 265–272
　exercises for, prepared, 346
　at home, 286
　hospitalization for, in reducing maternal and infant mortality, 22
　methods of minimizing discomfort of, 265–271
　　Dick-Read, 269–271
　　Lamaze, 265–269
　natural, 263
　prepared, 263
Chills
　after delivery, 338
　in pregnancy, 229–230
　shaking, after delivery, 387–388
Chin presentation of fetus, 611
Chinese diet patterns in pregnancy, 251
Chloasma, in pregnancy, 186
Chlorambucil, teratogenic effects of, 166
Chloramphenicol
　effects of, on fetus, 167
　toxicity of, in newborn, 663
Chloroform, in delivery, 354
Chloroprocaine, for regional anesthesia, 349
Chlorotrianisene, for suppression of lactation, 389
Choanal atresia, in newborn, 676
Cholecystitis, in pregnancy, 568
Cholelithiasis, in pregnancy, 568
Chorionic gonadotropin, human, in hydatidiform mole, 534, 535
Chorionic membrane, 151
Chorionic somatomammotropin, 150
Chorionic villi, 147–148
Chromosomal abnormalities diagnosed by amniocentesis, 590
Chromosomes, analysis of, amniocentesis for, 177
Chvostek's sign in diagnosis of hypocalcemia in newborn, 681
Cigarette smoking
　effects of, on fetus, 169
　in pregnancy, 578
Circulation
　extrauterine, establishment of, 655–656
　fetal, 153, 154
　placental, 148
Circulatory system
　changes in
　　in postpartal period, 384–385
　　in pregnancy, 187–188
　congenital anomalies of, 671–676
　intrauterine development of, 153
Circumcision, care of, 503
Clay, eating of, 170
Cleft lip, 665, 666
Cleft palate, 665–666
Client, definition of, 27
Clitoris, 76, 77
Clomid
　in breast milk, 476
　to stimulate ovulation, 120

Clomiphene citrate
　in breast milk, 476
　to stimulate ovulation, 120
Clothing
　for newborn at home, 503
　in pregnancy, 228–229
Clove-hitch restraint for intravenous therapy for high-risk infant, 660, 662
Clubfoot. See Talipes deformities
Coagulation
　disseminated intravascular
　　in abruptio placentae, 541–542
　　postpartal hemorrhage due to, 624
　mechanism of, 542
　in newborn, 422–423
Coarctation of aorta, 673, 674
Coccyx, 214
Coitus interruptus, 106–107
Colds, in newborn, 506–507
Colic, in newborn, 504–505
Collagen disorders, in pregnancy, 568
Coloboma, in newborn, 436, 437
Colostrum, 463, 464–465
　secretion of, in pregnancy, 186
Community health nurse in reducing maternal and infant mortality, 20
Conceptus, 146
Condensed milk, for formula, 478–479
Condoms, 106
Conduction, as heat loss mechanism in newborn, 420
Condylomata acuminata, in pregnancy, 564
Confinement, expected date of
　calculation of, 219
　predicting, 157–158
Congenital anomalies
　of bone, 677–679
　of circulatory system, 671–676
　of gastrointestinal system, 665–668
　of genitourinary tract, 670–671
　of heart, 671–676
　infant with, 664–679
　of muscle, 677–679
　of nervous system, 668–670
　orthopedic, 677–679
　of respiratory tract, 676–677
Congestive heart failure, in newborn, 675–676
Conjugate
　diagonal, prenatal measurement of, 216
　true, prenatal measurement of, 216–217
Conjunctivitis, gonorrheal. See Gonococcal conjunctivitis
Consent, informed, 51
Constipation
　in early pregnancy, 223
　in newborn, 504
　as nutritional problem in pregnancy, 250
　postpartal, 396
　problem-oriented recording and progress notes on, 236–237
Continuous positive airway pressure (CPAP)
　for respiratory distress syndrome, 706
　for ventilation of newborn, 655

728　Index

Contraception
  abortion in, 109
  Billings method of, 106
  coitus interruptus in, 106–107
  condoms in, 106
  counseling on, after abortion, 529
  diaphragms in, 102
  effectiveness of common methods of, 98
  intrauterine devices in, 100–102
  methods of, used before and after abortion, 529
  morning-after pill in, 107
  oral contraceptives in, 97–100. *See also* Contraceptives, oral
  ovulation method of, 106
  pill in, 97–100. *See also* Contraceptives, oral
  postcoital douche in, 107
  rhythm method of, 103–106. *See also* Rhythm method
  sterilization in, 107–109
  vaginally inserted spermicidal products in, 102–103
Contraceptives
  oral, 97–100
    actions of, 97–98
    in adolescence, 100
    contraindications to, 99–100
    effect of, on future pregnancy and sexual enjoyment, 100
    side effects of, 98–100
  and sexuality, 94
Contraction stress test in assessment of fetal well-being and maturity, 177–179
Contractions
  of abdominal muscle in preparation for childbirth, 264–265
  abnormal
    as danger signal in labor, 313
    interventions for, 330
  Braxton Hicks
    in diagnosis of pregnancy, 197
    in mid or late pregnancy, 233
    as preliminary sign of labor, 300–301
  fetal heart rate during, 326
  initial assessment of, in labor, 316, 317
  in mid or late pregnancy, 233
  monitoring of, 329
  pain of, explanation of, 343
  of pelvic floor in preparation for childbirth, 264
  as sign of true labor, 301–302
  as signal of beginning labor, 234
Contributory negligence, in establishing malpractice, 48
Controversial areas as high-risk factor, 50
Convection, as heat loss mechanism in newborn, 420
Convulsions
  in eclampsia, 552
  postpartal, 630
  recurrent, in pregnancy, 569–570
Cooling devices as high-risk factor, 50
Cord, umbilical, 150–151. *See also* Umbilical cord
Corn syrup, for formula, 479
Corpus albicans, 85
Corpus luteum, 85

Corticosteroids
  in pregnancy, elevated, 150
  for pregnant woman with juvenile rheumatoid arthritis, 568
  teratogenic effects of, 167
Cotyledons, 148
Coumarin, effects of, on fetus, 167
Counseling
  genetic, 588–591
    amniocentesis in, 589–591
    history in, 588
    karyotypes in, 588
  nutritional, 253–255
Cowper's glands, 78, 79
Cradle cap in newborn, 508
Cramps, muscle, in early pregnancy, 224, 225
Craniotabes, in newborn, 436
Cranium, fetal
  molding of, in labor process, 291
  structure and diameters of, labor process and, 289–291, 292
Cravings, as nutritional problem in pregnancy, 247–248
Creatinine, amniotic, in assessment of fetal well-being and maturity, 176
Cri du chat syndrome
  characteristics of, 595
  genetic defect in, 587
Crisis, coping with
  mechanisms for, 6, 7, 8, 10
  perception of event in, 4–5, 7
  problem solving approach to, 6–9
  success and, 9, 10, 11
  support persons in, 5–6, 7
Crisis period, pregnancy and delivery as, 4–6
Crossed extension reflex in newborn, 428
Crowning, 293, 333
Cry of newborn
  assessment of, 450
  first, recording of, 488
Crying in newborn, 506
Cryptenamine, for severe preeclampsia, 550
Cul-de-sac of Douglas, 72
Culdoscopy in assessment of anovulation, 117
Cultural influences on nutrition in pregnancy, 251–253
Cupping and vibration, in newborn, 655
Curettage, dilation and
  for hydatidiform mole, 534
  for therapeutic abortion, 526
Cyanosis
  in congenital heart disease, 671
  in hypoplastic left heart syndrome, 675
  in newborn, 429–430
Cyanotic heart disease, 674–675
Cyclopropane, in delivery, 354, 358–359
Cystic fibrosis, 596
Cystocele, cause of, 72, 74
Cytomegalic inclusion disease
  in newborn, 689
  teratogenic effects of, 165

DDT, teratogenic effects of, 168
Deceleration
  early, of fetal heart rate in distress, 327

Deceleration—*Continued*
  late, of fetal heart rate in distress, 327–328
Decidua, 146–147
Decision making, decreased, in response to pregnancy, 133–134
Dehydration, in high-risk infant
  signs of, 662
  in total parenteral nutrition, 660, 662
Deladumone, for suppression of lactation, 389
Delivery, 333–337
  anesthesia for, 334–335
  arrangements for, 235–236
  in breech presentation, 610
  by cesarean section, 613–616. *See also* Cesarean section
  checking position of umbilical cord during, 336
  chills following, 338, 387–388
  as crisis period, 4–6
  emergency, 338–339
  episiotomy for, 335–336
  fetal heart monitoring in, 335
  in occipitoposterior position and, 606–608
  forceps, 336, 618
  medications for, effects of on newborn, 168
  of oversized fetus, 612
  pain relief in, 352–354, 356–359
  perineal repair following, 337–338
  positioning for, 335
  precipitate, 602
  for adolescent, decision on, 575
  for diabetic, 557
  for woman with heart disease, 560
  in transverse lie, 612
  of twins, 604–606
  by vacuum extraction, 618
Delivery room, newborn care in, 487–492
Delivery table, positioning on, 335
Demerol
  in labor, 346–347, 356–357
  effects of, on newborn, 168
  teratogenic effects of, 166
Denial, in grieving process, 521
Dental x-ray studies in early pregnancy, 219
Depressants, 576
Depression
  in grieving process, 521
  postpartal, 376
  in reaction to high-risk pregnancy, 520–521
  in unwed pregnant woman, 138–139
Dermatitis
  diaper, in newborn, 507
  seborrheic, in newborn, 508
Desquamation of skin in newborn, 433
Development of fetus, 145–180. *See also* Fetus, development of
Developmental readiness for child rearing, 57–66
  assessing, 65–66
Developmental tasks, reworking of, during pregnancy
  by father, 135

Developmental tasks, reworking of, during pregnancy—*Continued*
  by mother, 130
  by unwed father, 140
  by unwed mother, 139
Dextri-Maltose for formula, 479
Dextrostix test of newborn, 495
Diabetes
  gestational, problem-oriented recording on, 579–580, 619–620, 633–634
  large-for-gestation-age infant in, 696
  newborn in, 680–681, 696
  in pregnancy, 554–558
    assessment of, 554
    classification of, 555
    delivery in, 556–557
    diet for, 556
    emotional support in, 558
    gestational, 555–556
    interventions for, 555
    postpartal adjustment in, 557
Diamine oxidase in maternal serum, assay of, 174
Diaper-area care of newborn, 498
Diaper dermatitis in newborn, 507
Diaphoresis, postpartal, 384, 396
Diaphragmatic hernia, 667–668
Diaphragmatic paralysis, 676–677
Diaphragms, 102
Diastasis, in pregnancy, 185
Diazepam
  effects of, on fetus, 167
  in labor, 348, 356–357
  for severe preeclampsia, 550
Diazoxide, for severe preeclampsia, 550
Dick-Read method, 269–271
Dicumarol, for femoral thrombophlebitis, 627
Diet
  cultural influences on, 251–252
  fad, in pregnancy, 252–253
  for mild preeclampsia, 548
  postpartal, 399
  in pregnancy, 246, 247
  in pregnant diabetic, 556
  for pregnant woman with heart disease, 559
  for severe preeclampsia, 550
Diethylstilbestrol (DES)
  to prevent pregnancy after intercourse, 107
  for suppression of lactation, 389
  teratogenic effects of, 167
Diffusion, in placental circulation, 148
Digestive system, intrauterine development of, 155
Digitalis for pregnant woman
  with heart disease, 559
  with mitral stenosis, 560
Digits, extra and webbed, 678–679
Digoxin for congestive heart failure in newborn, 676
Dihydrotachysterol, in breast milk, 476
Dilantin
  effects of, on fetus, 167–168
  for recurrent convulsions in pregnancy, 570
Dilatation, cervical
  discussion of, in expectant parents' classes, 262

Dilatation, cervical—*Continued*
  as sign of true labor, 303
  as stage of labor, 282–283
Dilation
  and curettage
    for hydatidiform mole, 534
    for therapeutic abortion, 526
  and vacuum extraction for therapeutic abortion, 526–527
Diphenylhydantoin. *See* Dilantin
Disappointment, postpartal, 369–370
Disseminated intravascular coagulation
  in abruptio placentae, 541–542
  postpartal hemorrhage due to, 624
Distractibility of infant, 413
Diuresis, in postpartal period, 384
Diuretics
  in breast milk, 473
  effects of, on fetus, 167
  for mild preeclampsia, 548–549
Divorce rates, trends in, 18–19
L-Dopa, in breast milk, 476
Douche, postcoital, 107
Douching in pregnancy, 226–227
Down's syndrome
  characteristics of, 595
  genetic defect in, 587, 588
Drainage, postural, for newborn, 655
Dried milk for formula, 479
Drugs
  and breast milk, 471, 472–476, 476
  dependence on
    as nutritional problem of pregnancy, 251
    in pregnancy, 576–577
  teratogenic, 166–168
Dubowitz maturity scale, 451, 452, 454–458
Ductus arteriosus
  in fetal circulation, 153, 154
  patent, 673, 674
Ductus venosus in fetal circulation, 153, 154
Duncan presentation of placenta, 311, 312
Dysmenorrhea, 87–88
Dyspareunia, 95
Dysplasia, bronchopulmonary, 654
Dyspnea, in mid or late pregnancy, 232
Dystocia, 599–613
  cephalopelvic disproportion causing, 612–613
  fetal factor in, 603–612
  due to occipitoposterior position of fetus, 606–608
  uterine dysfunction causing, 599–603

Ear
  in gestation age assessment, 457
  heel to, in gestation age assessment, 456
  of newborn
    appearance of, 437
    assessment of, 449
Eating during labor, 268
Eclampsia
  characteristics of, 548
  convulsions in, phases and treatment of, 552
  interventions for, 551–553
  prognosis in, 553

Eclampsia—*Continued*
  psychological aspects of care for, 553
  symptoms of, 551–552
  termination of pregnancy in, 552–553
Economic patterns, revision of, as task of pregnancy, 134
Ectoderm, structures arising from, 152
Ectopic pregnancy, 531–534
  abdominal, 533–534
  assessment of, 532–533
  intervention in, 533
  sites of, 532
Edema
  ankle, in mid or late pregnancy, 232
  in congestive heart failure, 676
  in preeclampsia, 547, 548
  in pregnant woman with heart disease, 559
  vulvar, postpartal, 625
Effacement, cervical
  discussion of, in expectant parents' classes, 262
  as sign of true labor, 302–303
Effleurage, 267, 268
Egg protein, in breast milk, 475
Ejaculation
  difficulty with, 113
  premature, 94–95
Ejaculatory ducts, 78, 79
Elderly primipara, 573
Electrocardiography in assessment of fetal well-being and maturity, 171
Electrophoretic bands in assessment of fetal well-being and maturity, 175
Emancipated minor, informed consent and, 51
Embolism
  air, postpartal, 399
  amniotic fluid, in labor, 602
Embryo
  definition of, 152
  developmental stages of, 164–165
  sizes of, comparative, 162
Emergency situations as high-risk factor, 50
Emotional response to pregnancy, 132–134
  changes in sexual desire as, 134
  decreased decision making as, 133–134
  emotional lability as, 134
  introversion versus extroversion as, 133
  narcissism as, 133
Emotional stress, effects of on fetus, 169–170
Emotional support for pregnant woman
  with diabetes, 558
  with heart disease, 559–560
  with mild preeclampsia, 549
  with multiple gestation, 571–572
  with Rh incompatibility, 593
Employment during pregnancy, 227–228
Encephalocele, 668–669
Endocervix, 70
Endocrine function of placenta, 149–150
Endocrine system
  changes in, in pregnancy, 191
  intrauterine development of, 155
Endometriosis, 88
  infertility due to, 118
Endometritis
  complicating abortion, 530–531
  postpartal, 626–627

Endometrium, 70
Endotracheal tube, oxygen administration by, in newborn, 650
Enema, administration of, in labor, 318–319
Energy, excess, as signal of beginning labor, 234
Engagement of fetus
 failure of, in pelvic inlet contraction, 612
 in labor process, 293
Engorgement of breasts, 386, 469–470
 mechanism of, 393–394
Enterobius vermicularis in pregnancy, 566–567
Enterocolitis, neonatal necrotizing, 708–709
Entoderm, structures arising from, 152
Environmental teratogens, 168
Epididymis, 78, 79
Epidural anesthesia for labor and delivery in heart disease, 560
Epidural blocks, 349–351, 356–357
Epilepsy in pregnancy. *See* Convulsions, recurrent
Episiotomy, 335–336
 care of, 392
 repair of, 337–338
Erb-Duchenne paralysis, 678
Erb's sign in diagnosis of hypocalcemia in newborn, 682
Erythema, palmar, in early pregnancy, 226
Erythema toxicum in newborn, 433–434
Erythroblastosis fetalis, 591–592
Erythrocyte count in newborn, 422, 424
Erythromycin ointment, prophylactic, 689
Estriol, in assessment of fetal well-being and maturity
 amniotic, 176
 in maternal urine, 172–173
 plasma levels of, 175
Estrogen
 placental production of, 150
 in sexual development at puberty, 68
 for suppression of lactation, 389–390
Ethanol. *See* Alcohol
Ether, for pain relief in delivery, 354, 358–359
Ethisterone, teratogenic effects of, 167
Ethyl alcohol. *See* Alcohol
European diet patterns, in pregnancy, 252
Evaporated milk, for formula, 478
Evaporation, as heat loss mechanism in newborn, 420
Examination, postpartal, 402–403
Exercise
 for childbearing, 263–265
 discussion of, in expectant parents' classes, 262
 Kegal
  postpartal, 393
  in preparation for childbirth, 264
 perineal, 393
 postpartal, 396–399
 in pregnancy, 229
 prepared childbirth, 346
Exhaustion, in postpartum period, 385
Expectant parents' classes, 259–263
 group introduction in, 260–261

Expectant parents' classes—*Continued*
 lessons
  on family planning, 263
  on feelings toward pregnancy, 261
  on infant care, 262
  on labor and delivery, 261–262
  on personal care, 261
  on plans for hospitalization, 262
  on postpartum period, 262
 planning of, 260
Exstrophy of the bladder, 670, 671
Extremities, of newborn
 lower, assessment of, 447
 appearance of, 440–441
 recoil of, in gestation age assessment, 455
 upper, assessment of, 448
Extroversion, in response to pregnancy, 133
Extrusion reflex, in newborn, 426
Eyes, of newborn
 appearance of, 436–437
 assessment of, 449
 care of, in delivery room, 490
 sundown, in hydrocephalus, 669

Face presentation of fetus, 611
Facilitated diffusion, in placental circulation, 148
Fad diets in pregnancy, 252–253
Fallopian tubes, 69, 73
 infertility due to factors involving, 117–118
 ligation of, 107–108
 removal of, after ectopic pregnancy, 533
Fallot, tetralogy of, 673, 674–675
Falls, prevention of, in newborn, 510
Family, pregnant, 136–137
Family medical history, taking of, in labor, 321–322
Family planning, 97–109
 birth control methods in, 97–109. *See also* Contraception
 discussion of, in expectant parents' classes, 263
 in reducing maternal and infant mortality, 21
Fantasy in preparation for motherhood, 131
Fat, newborn requirements for, 462
Father
 and child, interaction of, in hospital, 499–500
 high-risk pregnancy and, 522
 and labor, 284–285
 pregnant, 135–136
 in reducing stress in labor, 280–281
 role of, in initial prenatal interview, 209–210
 unwed, 139–140
 and labor, 285–286
 in postpartal period, 377
Fatherhood, preparation for, 135–136
Fatigue
 in diagnosis of pregnancy, 195
 in early pregnancy, 223
 in stress of labor, 280
Fava bean, in breast milk, 475

Fear
 in reaction to high-risk pregnancy, 519–520
 in stress of labor, 280
Feeding of newborn. *See also* Breastfeeding; Formulas
 first, 495–496
Feet of newborn, assessment of, 447
Femoral thrombophlebitis, postpartal, 627
 problem-oriented recording on, 634
Fencing reflex, in newborn, 427
Fern test for ovulation, 115
Fertility, studies of, 112
 support during, 120–121
Fertilization, 145–146, 147
Fetal acidosis as danger signal in labor, 313
Fetal adrenal response theory of onset of labor, 300
Fetal alcohol syndrome, 168, 227, 692–693
Fetal death rate, trends in, 16
Fetal distress patterns during labor, 327–329
Fetoprotein, alpha, detection of, by amniocentesis, 177
Fetoscopy, 177
Fetus
 abnormal, spontaneous abortion due to, 525
 blood of, sampling, in labor, 330, 603
 bradycardia in
  complicating paracervical block, 351
  in labor, 326
 breech presentation of, 608–611
 brow presentation of, 611
 circulation in, 153, 154
 cranium of, structure and diameters of, and labor process, 289–291, 292
 danger signals of labor related to, 311, 313
 definition of, 152
 descent of, in labor, 305, 307
 development of
  circulatory system in, 153
  digestive system in, 155
  endocrine system in, 155
  genital system in, 156
  milestones in, 158–162, 164–165
  nervous system in, 155
  respiratory system in, 154–155
  skeletal system in, 155–156
  timetable of, 158–159
  urinary system in, 156
 expulsion of, 306, 307
 extension of, in labor, 305, 307
 external rotation of, in labor, 305–306, 307
 face presentation of, 611
 flexion of, in labor, 305, 307
 growth and development of, 145–180
 monthly estimates of, 157–162
 heart rate of
  heart deviations in, as danger signal in labor, 311
  in labor, abnormalities of, 330
  monitoring of, 326–327, 328, 335
  patterns of, in fetal distress, 327–329
 heart sounds of, in diagnosis of pregnancy, 199–200

Fetus—*Continued*
    hyperactivity of, as danger signal in labor, 313
    internal rotation of, in labor, 305, 307
    monitoring of
        in delivery, 335
        external, 327, 328
        internal, 327
        in labor, 326–327
        in placenta previa, 536–537
        in Rh sensitized mother, 592
    movements of, in diagnosis of pregnancy, 200
    occipitoposterior position of, 606–608
    organ systems of, origin and development of, 152–156
    outline of, in diagnosis of pregnancy, 197
    oversized, labor and delivery in, 612
    position of, in labor process, 291–297
        changes in, in pelvic division of labor, 306, 307
        determining, 294–297
        possible, 295
    presentation of, in labor process, 291–297
        determining, 294–297
    tachycardia in, during labor, 326
    transverse lie of, 612
    well-being and maturity of, assessing, 170–177
        abdominal sounds and movement in, 171
        amniocentesis in, 175–177
        amniography in, 177
        assay of maternal serum in, 174–175
        assay of maternal urine in, 172–174
        electrocardiography in, 171
        estimation of fundal height in, 171
        fetoscopy in, 177
        maternal history in, 170–171
        nonstress test in, 179
        oxytocin challenge test in, 177–179
        sonography in, 171–172, 173
        x-ray films in, 171
Fever
    milk, 385
    in newborn, 420
    in pregnancy, 229–230
Fiber, 246
Fibrinogen, for disseminated intravascular coagulation, 624
Fibroplasia, retrolental, from oxygen therapy
    in immature infant, 708
    in newborn, 654
Fingers, extra and webbed, 678–679
Fistula, tracheoesophageal, 666, 667
Flagyl, for trichomoniasis in pregnancy, 566
Flea-bite rash in newborn, 433–434
Fluid
    amniotic, 151–152. *See also* Amniotic fluid
    intake of
        for breast-feeding, 471
        in labor, 324–325

Fluid—*Continued*
    intravenous
        for high-risk infant, 659–660, 661, 662
        for immature infants, 703–704
    requirements for
        for newborn, 462–463
        in pregnancy, 245–246
    seminal, changes in, 113
    sudden escape of, from vagina, in pregnancy, 230
Fluoride
    in breast milk, 475
    requirements for
        for newborn, 463
        in pregnancy, 246
    teratogenic effects of, 168
Folic acid
    deficiency of, in pregnancy, 561–562
    inadequate intake of, effects of, on fetus, 170
    requirement for, in pregnancy, 242–243
Follicle-stimulating hormone in physiology of reproduction, 84
Fontanelles
    of fetal skull, 290
    of newborn skull, 434
Foods
    allergies to, as nutritional problem in pregnancy, 249
    intake of, in labor, 324–325
    solid, introducing, 483
Footprinting of newborn, 490–491
Foramen ovale, in fetal circulation, 153, 154
Forceps
    for delivery, 336, 618
    marks from, in newborn, 434
Foremilk, 464
Formulas, 477–483
    calculation of, 478
    commercial, 478
    for high-risk infant, 657
    for immature infant, 704
    preparation of, 480–482
    prepared, 478–480
    supplies for use of, 480
    techniques for feeding of, 482–483
Fourchette, 77
Friedman's test for pregnancy, 198
Fundus, height of
    estimation of, in assessment of fetal well-being and maturity, 170–171
    measurement of, on first prenatal visit, 210

Galactosemia, characteristics of, 596
Gas anesthesia
    in delivery, 353–354, 358–359
    in labor, 348, 356–357
Gastrointestinal system
    changes in, in pregnancy, 189–190
    congenital anomalies of, 665–668
    diseases of, in pregnancy, 568–569
    of newborn, 424–425
Gate-control theory of pain, 344
Gavage-feeding
    for high-risk infant, 657–659
    for immature infant, 704, 705

Generativity, development of sense of
    in achieving maturity, 64–65
    as task of middle years, 62
Genes, dominant and recessive, 583–585
Genetic disorders
    commonly inherited, 593–597
    counseling on, 588–591. *See also* Counseling, genetic
    from division defects, 585, 587–588
    familial tendencies to, 588
    Mendelian inheritance of, 583–585
    and pregnancy, 583–597
    Rh incompatibility as, 591–593
    screening for, legal aspects of, 591
Genital system, intrauterine development of, 156
Genitalia
    external
        female, 76–77
        male, 78–79
    female, of newborn, 439
    in gestation age assessment, 457
    male, of newborn, 439
    of newborn, assessment of, 447–448
Genitourinary tract, congenital anomalies of, 670–671
Genotype, definition of, 584
Gentian violet, for candidiasis in pregnancy, 566
Germ layers, primary, in origin and development of organ systems, 152–153
Gestation, multiple, 570–572
    labor and delivery in, 604–606
Gestation age
    infant large for, 696–697
    infant small for, 695–696, 698
    of newborn
        assessment of, 450–458
        Brazelton Neonatal Behavioral Assessment Scale for, 452–453, 454
        Dubowitz maturity scale for, 451, 452, 454–458
Gestational diabetes, 555–556
Gingivitis in early pregnancy, assessment of, 222–223
Gland
    Bartholin's, 76, 77
    bulbourethral, 78, 79
    Cowper's, 78, 79
    mammary, 79–80. *See also* Breasts
    parathyroid, effects of pregnancy on, 191
    pituitary, effects of pregnancy on, 191
    prostate, 78, 79
    Skene's, 76, 77
    thyroid, effects of pregnancy on, 191
Glucose-insulin changes in pregnancy, 554–555
Glucose 6-phosphate dehydrogenase deficiency, 597
Glucose tolerance tests in pregnancy, 554–555
Glucose water, for newborn, 496
Goat's milk, for formula, 479
Gonadal dysgenesis, 595
Gonadotropin
    chorionic, human, placental production of, 149–150
    menopausal, human, to stimulate ovulation, 120

Gonococcal conjunctivitis, 689–690
　from exposure to gonorrhea of birth, 567, 689
　prophylaxis for, in newborn, 490, 689
Gonorrhea in pregnancy, 567–568
Good Samaritan laws, emergencies and, 50
Goodell's sign of pregnancy, 197
Graafian follicle, 84–85
Grief
　after ectopic pregnancy, 533
　anticipatory, in reaction to high-risk pregnancy, 520–521
　signs of, 521
Grief work
　during pregnancy by unwed father, 140
　in preparation for motherhood, 132
Growth of fetus, 145–170. See also Fetus, development of
Guilt
　in premature labor, 543–544
　in reaction to high-risk pregnancy, 520
Guthrie's test, for phenylketonuria, 597
Gynecoid pelvis, 215

Haase's rule for estimation of fetal size, 157
Hallucinogenics, effects of, on fetus, 168
Halothane in delivery, 354, 358–359
Harelip. See Cleft lip
Harlequin sign, in newborn, 431
Head of newborn
　appearance of, 434–436
　assessment of, 449
　circumference of, 419
Headache following spinal anesthesia, 352, 388
Health history, taking of, in labor, 321
Health maintenance during pregnancy, 221–237
Hearing
　in newborn, 428
　stimulation of, for newborn, 411
Heart
　congenital anomalies of, 671–676
　disease of
　　acyanotic, 672–674
　　cyanotic, 674–675
　　home care of newborn with, 676
　failure of, congestive, in newborn, 675–676
　formation of, 153
　massage of, external, for newborn, 655
　movement of, by sonogram in diagnosis of pregnancy, 200
　palpitations of, in early pregnancy, 225
　rate of
　　in Apgar scoring of newborn, 489
　　fetal. See Fetus, heart rate of
Heart disease
　classification of, 558
　peripartal, 560
　pregnancy and, 558–561
　　assessment of, 559
　　diet in, 559
　　emotional support in, 559–560
　　evaluation of edema in, 559
　　interventions for, 559–560
　　medication in, 559
　　rest for, 559
　　risks in, 558–559

Heart sounds of newborn, assessment of, 445
Heart valve, prosthetic, pregnancy and, 561
Heartburn, in early pregnancy, 222
Heat, loss of, in newborn, 420
Heat lamps, for perineal comfort, 393
Heating devices, as high-risk factor, 50
Heel to ear test in gestation age assessment, 456
Hegar's sign of pregnancy, 196, 197
Hemangiomas
　cavernous, 432
　in newborn, 431–432
　strawberry, 431, 508
Hematocrit
　heel-stick, of newborn in nursery, 495
　in newborn, 422, 424
Hematoma, postpartal, 624–625
Hemoglobin
　fetal, 153
　level of, in newborn, 422, 424
　in pregnancy, 188
Hemolysis of newborn, in ABO incompatibility, 686
Hemolytic disease of newborn, 591–592, 684
Hemophilus vaginalis infection in pregnancy, 566
Hemopoietic system, disorders of in newborn, 682–686
Hemorrhage. See also Bleeding
　in abruptio placentae, 538
　complicating abortion, 530
　in immature infant, 705
　intracranial
　　complicating breech delivery, 610
　　in immature infant, 705–706
　　in newborn, 690
　maternal deaths due to, 17
　postpartal, 621–625
　　definition of, 621
　　disseminated intravascular coagulation causing, 624
　　lacerations causing, 623–624
　　rest for, 625
　　retained placental fragments causing, 624
　　uterine atony causing, 621–623
Hemorrhagic disease of newborn, 682
Hemorrhoids
　in early pregnancy, 225
　postpartal, 396
Heparin
　for disseminated intravascular coagulation, 542, 624
　for femoral thrombophlebitis, 627
　for pregnant woman with prosthetic heart valve, 561
Hepatitis, viral, in pregnancy, 569
Hepatomegaly in congestive heart failure, 675–676
Hernia
　diaphragmatic, 667–668
　hiatal, in pregnancy, 568
Heroin, newborn of mother addicted to, 691–692
Herpes genitalis in pregnancy, 565
Herpes simplex II virus disease, teratogenic effects of, 165

Herpesvirus infection in newborn, 688–689
Hexosaminidase A, lack of, in Tay-Sachs disease, 597
Hiatal hernia in pregnancy, 568
High-risk health care areas, 49–50
High-risk infant, 637–713
　bottle-feeding for, 657
　breast-feeding for, 657
　child abuse and, 644
　with congenital anomalies, 664–679. See also Congenital anomalies
　defining, 25
　dehydration in, signs of, 662
　following of, at home, 644
　gavage-feeding for, 657–659
　identifying, 639–644
　infection in, prevention of, 662–664
　intravenous fluids for, 659–660
　mother-child bonding with, 642–644
　nasal-jejunal feeding for, 659
　nutrition for, 657–662
　　total parenteral, 660, 662
　oxygen administration to, 652–654
　priorities for, in first days of life, 647–664
　regionalized care for, 639, 640
　resuscitation of, 648–652
　temperature regulation in, 656–657
　transport of, 639–642
　　in reducing maternal and infant mortality, 24–25
　ventilation and, 654–655
High-risk mothers
　defining, 25
　transporting, in reducing maternal and infant mortality, 24–25
High-risk pregnancy, 515–635
　accepting, 518
　adolescent and, 573–575
　anemia in, 561–562
　battered woman and, 578–579
　bleeding in, 523–545. See also Bleeding in pregnancy
　child of, accepting, 518
　chronic hypertensive vascular disease in, 553–554
　collagen disorders and, 568
　coping abilities of woman with, identifying, 518–519
　defining concepts of, 517
　deviations from normal in, 523–580. See also specific deviation, e.g., Abortion; Bleeding
　diabetes and, 554–558. See also Diabetes in pregnancy
　drug dependence and, 576–578
　elderly primipara and, 573
　father and, 522
　gastrointestinal diseases and, 568–569
　genetic disorders and, 583–597. See also Genetic disorders
　heart disease and, 558–561. See also Heart disease, pregnancy and
　hydramnios and, 572
　hyperemesis gravidarum and, 575–576
　hypertension in, 545–553. See also Hypertension, pregnancy-induced
　impact of, 517–522
　multiple gestation and, 570–572

Index　733

High-risk pregnancy—*Continued*
  neurological conditions and, 569–570
  perception of, coping abilities and, 518–519
  postmature, 573
  pseudocyesis and, 576
  reactions to, immobilizing, 519–522
    depression as, 520–521
    fear as, 519–520
    guilt as, 520
    lowered self-esteem as, 521–522
  respiratory disorders and, 563–564
  urinary tract disorders and, 562–563
  venereal disease and, 564–568
Hip
  dislocated, 677–678
  subluxated, 677–678
Hirschbrung's test for strabismus in newborn, 449
History, taking of, in labor, 319–322
Hogben test, in diagnosis of pregnancy, 198
Homans' sign of postpartal thrombophlebitis, 400
Home births, 286
Home pregnancy tests, 199
Hormones
  in breast milk, 474
  disorders of, recurrent abortion due to, 531
  follicle-stimulating, 84
  luteinizing, 84
  pituitary, 84
  teratogenic effects of, 167
Hospital
  admission to, during labor, assessment on, 315–324
  care of newborn in, 493–501
Hospital interview, initial, during labor, 315–316
Hospital regulations, discussion of, in expectant parents' classes, 262
Hospitalization
  for childbirth in reducing maternal and infant mortality, 22
  plans for, discussion of, in expectant parents' classes, 262
Human chorionic gonadotropin, 149–150
Human chorionic thyrotropin, 150
Human placental lactogen, 150
  in maternal serum, assay of, 175
Husband. *See* Father
Hyaline membrane disease
  in immature infant, 706–708
  maternal diabetes and, 681
Hydatidiform mole, 534–535
Hydralazine for severe preeclampsia, 550
Hydramnios, 572
  mechanism of, 151
Hydrocephalus, 669–670
Hydroxyzine pamoate, for pain relief in labor, 348, 356–357
Hygiene, personal, mid-pregnancy update on, 233
Hymen, 76, 77
  imperforate, 670–671
Hyperactivity of fetus as danger signal in labor, 313

Hyperbilirubinemia
  in infant of diabetic mother, 681
  in newborn, 682–684
Hypercholesterolemia, in pregnancy, 568
Hyperemesis gravidarum, 575–576
Hyperglycemia, in newborn of diabetic mother, 681
Hypernatremia, complicating saline abortion, 527
Hyperstat for severe preeclampsia, 550
Hypertension
  as danger signal in labor, 313
  in hydatidiform mole, 534
  pregnancy-induced, 545–553
    assessment of, 547–548
    classification of, 547–548
    danger signals of, 230
    in eclampsia, 551–553
    high-risk categories for, 547
    interventions for, 548–553
    maternal deaths due to, 17
    in mild preeclampsia, 548–549
    postpartal, 630
    roll-over test in predicting, 548
    in severe preeclampsia, 549–551
  pulmonary artery, pregnancy and, 560–561
Hypertensive vascular disease, chronic, in pregnancy, 553–554
Hypnosis for pain relief in labor and delivery, 351–352
Hypnotics in breast milk, 475
Hypocalcemia in newborn, 681–682
Hypoglycemia
  in immature infant, 709
  in newborn, 679–680
  of diabetic mother, 681
Hypoglycemia agents, effects of, on fetus, 168
Hypoplastic left heart syndrome, 675
Hypospadias, 670
Hypotension
  complicating caudal anesthesia, 350
  as danger signal in labor, 313
  postural, in early pregnancy, assessment of, 223–224
  severe, complicating spinal anesthesia, 352
Hypotensive agents, effects of, on fetus, 167
Hypothalamus, in physiology of menstrual cycle, 84
Hypoxia, in respiratory distress in newborn, 652
Hysterectomy
  for hemorrhage
    from atonic uterus, 623
    complicating abortion, 530
  for sterilization, 107
Hysterosalpingography for tubal patency, 117–118
Hysterotomy for therapeutic abortion, 528

Ice compresses for hematoma, 624
Identification of newborn
  in delivery room, 490–491
  in hospital, 499

Identity, development of sense of
  in achieving maturity, 64
  as task of adolescent, 60–61
Ileus, meconium, in cystic fibrosis, 596
Ilium of innominate bone, 214
Illness
  in newborn, 679–693. *See also* Newborn, illness in
  physical, sexual problems due to, 94
Image, body, in adolescent, 60
Immunological agents, effects of on fetus, 168
Immunological system, intrauterine development of, 156
Immunological tests in diagnosis of pregnancy, 199
Immunosuppressives in breast milk, 476
Imperforate anus, 668
Imperforate hymen, 670–671
Impetigo in newborn, 508
Implantation, 146, 147
  abnormal, spontaneous abortion due to, 525
Impotence, 94, 113
Incident reports, 49
Incisions for cesarean section, 613, 616
Income, family, infant morbidity by, 21
Incubator
  for temperature regulation, 656
  weaning from, 656–657
Industry, development of sense of
  in achieving maturity, 64
  as task of school-age child, 58, 59–60
Infancy, sex roles in, 91–92
Infant. *See also* Newborn
  developing sense of trust in, 57–58
  development of, 412
  high-risk, 637–713. *See also* High-risk infant
  solid food for, introducing, 483
Infant morbidity, by family income, 21
Infant mortality, reducing, 19–25
Infection
  complicating abortion, 530–531
  complicating total parenteral nutrition for high-risk infant, 660
  in high-risk infant, prevention of, 662–664
  maternal, as teratogen, 163, 165–166
  maternal deaths due to, 17
  in newborn, 507–508, 687–690
    group B beta hemolytic streptococcal, 688
    herpesvirus, 688–689
    from prolonged rupture of membrane, 688
  of perineum, postpartal, 626
  prevention of, in immature infant, 705
  puerperal, 625–630
    factors predisposing to, 625
    invading organisms causing, 625–626
    mother-child relationships in, 629–630
    types of, 626–629
  spontaneous abortion due to, 526
  urinary tract
    postpartal, 628
    in pregnancy, 562
  vaginal, in early pregnancy, 225–226

Infertility, 111–121
  definition of, 111
  female
    anovulation, 115–117
    assessment of, 119
    cervical causes of, 118–119
    plans and interventions in, 119–120
    tubal causes of, 117–118
    uterine causes of, 118
    vaginal causes of, 119
  male
    assessment of, 113–114
    causes of, 112–113
    plans and interventions in, 114–115
  studies of, 112
Infiltration, local, for pain relief in delivery, 353, 358–359
Influenza in pregnancy, 563
Informed consent, 51
Inheritance, mendelian laws of, 583–585, 586–587
Initiative, development of sense of
  in achieving maturity, 64
  as task of preschooler, 58, 59
Innominate bones of pelvis, 214
Insemination, artificial, 114–115
Inspection
  in determining fetal presentation and position, 294
  in physical assessment, 29–30
Insulin, for pregnant diabetic, 556
Integrity, development of sense of, 62–63
Intensive care nurseries in reducing maternal and infant mortality, 23–24
Intercourse during pregnancy, 229
Interferon, in breast milk, 465
Interpartal period, 55–124
Interpregnancy care, 25–26
Interview, initial
  on first prenatal visit, 204–210
    chief concern in, eliciting, 206
    conclusion of, 209
    conducting, 204–206
    critical remarks in, 206
    establishing rapport in, 204–205
    family setting in, 206–207
    gynecological history in, 207–208
    history of familial illness in, 207
    husband's role in, 209–210
    past medical history in, 207
    present pregnancy history in, 208–209
    previous pregnancies in, 208
    purpose of, explaining, 206
    questions for, types of, 205
    setting for, 204
    supporting statements in, 205
    systems review in, 209
    transition statements in, 205–206
  hospital, during labor, 315–316
Interviewing, in assessment phase of nursing process, 29
Intestines
  obstruction of, 667
  reabsorption of bilirubin in, 683–684
Intimacy, development of sense of
  in achieving maturity, 64
  as task of young adult, 61–62

Intracranial hemorrhage
  complicating breech delivery, 610
  in immature infant, 705–706
Intrauterine devices, 100–102
Intravenous anesthesia, in delivery, 354
Intravenous fluids
  for high-risk infant, 659–660
    restraints for, 660, 661, 662
  for immature infants, 703–704
Introversion in response to pregnancy, 133
Involution in postpartal period, 381–384
Iodides, in breast milk, 475
Iodine
  inadequate intake of, effects of on fetus, 170
  requirements for, in pregnancy, 244
Iron
  in common foods, 245
  for pregnant woman with heart disease, 559
  requirements for
    for newborn, 463
    in pregnancy, 244–245
Iron deficiency anemia in pregnancy, 561
Ischial tuberosity diameter, prenatal measurement of, 217
Ischiocavernosus fibers in pelvic floor, 77–78
Ischium of innominate bone, 214
Isoxsuprine hydrochloride for halting premature labor, 544

Japanese diet patterns in pregnancy, 251
Jaundice
  in newborn, 430–431
    physiological, 682–683
  prolonged, in breast-fed infants, 476
Jealousy, postpartal, psychosocial aspects of, 369
Jewish diet patterns in pregnancy, 252

Karo syrup for formula, 479
Karyotypes in genetic counseling, 588
Kegal exercises
  postpartal, 393
  in preparation for childbirth, 264
Kernicterus
  in immature infant, 708
  in newborn, 430
  seizures in, 691
17-Ketosteroids in testing for sexual maturity, 67–68
Kidney
  disease of, chronic, pregnancy and, 562–563
  transplanted, pregnancy and, 563
Klinefelter's syndrome
  characteristics of, 595
  genetic defect in, 587–588
K-pads for perineal comfort, 393

Labia majora, 76, 77
Labia minora, 76, 77
Labor
  active phase of, prolonged, 600
  active-phase dilatation, protracted, 306
  amniotic fluid embolism in, 602
  amniotomy in, 332

Labor—Continued
  arrangements for, 235–236
  beginning signs of, discussion of, in expectant parents' classes, 261
  breathing techniques for, discussion of, in expectant parents' classes, 262
  in breech presentation, 609
  in brow presentation, 611
  danger signals of
    fetal, 311, 313
    maternal, 313
  deceleration phase of, prolonged, 306, 601
  descent phase of
    arrest of, 307, 601
    failure of, 601
    protracted, 307, 600–601
  deviations from normal in, 599–613
  dilatation phase of, secondary arrest of, 307
  discomfort in, minimizing, 344–345
  divisions of, 303–305, 309, 310
    dilatational, 304
    pelvic, 305–306
    preparatory, 304
  dysfunctional, 599–601
    in dilatational division, 600–601
    in pelvic division, 601
    in preparatory division, 600
  exercises in preparation for, discussion of, in expectant parents' classes, 262
  experience of, 315–339
  in face presentation, 611
  false, signs of, 304
  father and, 284–285
  fetal blood sampling in, 603
  in fetal occipitoposterior position, 606–608
  induction of, 616–617
    following premature rupture of membranes, 545
    by oxytocin, 616–617
    for pregnant diabetic, 557
    by prostaglandins, 617
    readiness for, scoring cervix for, 617
  latent phase of, prolonged, 306, 600
  medications for
    discussion of, in expectant parents' classes, 261–262
    effects of, on newborn, 168
  onset of, theories of, 297–300
    fetal adrenal response, 300
    oxytocin, 298
    progesterone deprivation, 298, 300
    uterine stretch, 298
  with oversized fetus, 612
  pain relief in
    medication for, 346–351, 356–359
    narcotics for, 346–347, 356–357
  pelvic division of, nursing interventions in, 332–337
  placental stage of, 307, 309, 311, 312
    nursing interventions in, 337–338
  precipitate, 602
  premature, 542–545
    analgesia for, 542–543
    care during, 542–544
    halting, 544–545

Labor—Continued
  preparatory division of, nursing interventions in, 324–332
  process of, 289–313
    fetal cranial determinations and, 289–291, 292
    fetal presentation and position and, 291–297
    progress of, graphing, 306–307, 310, 311
  prolapse of cord in, 603–604
  psychosocial aspects of, 279–288
  readiness for, 279–280
  signals of beginning of, 233–234
  signs of, preliminary, 300–301
    Braxton Hicks contractions as, 300–301
    increased energy as, 300
    lightening as, 300
    ripening of cervix as, 301
    rupture of membranes as, 301
    show as, 301
    weight loss as, 300
  signs of, true, 301–303, 304
    effacement as, 302–303
    uterine contractions as, 301–302
  stages of, 282–284
    cervical dilatation, 282–283
    pelvic division, 283–284
    placental, 284
  stress of, reducing, 280–282
    support people in, 280–281
    teaching in, 281–282
  trial, for cephalopelvic disproportion, 612–613
  unmarried man and, 285–286
  unmarried woman in, 285–286
  uterine rupture in, 602
  woman in
    on admission to hospital, assessment of, 315–324
    initial procedures for, 316
    initial hospital interview of, 315–316
    position of, 325–326
Labor rooms, 316
Laboratory studies, in first prenatal visit, 217–219
Laboratory tests, in diagnosis of pregnancy, 198–199
Lacerations, postpartal hemorrhage due to
  cervical, 623
  perineal, 623–624
  vaginal, 623
Lactation
  in postpartal period, 385–386
  suppression of, 389–390
Lactiferous sinuses, 464
Lactobacillus bifidus in breast milk, 465
Lactoferrin, in breast milk, 465
Lactogen, placental, human, 150
  in maternal serum, assay of, 175
Lactose intolerance as nutritional problem in pregnancy, 250
Lamaze method of prepared childbirth, 265–269
Laminaria tent, in therapeutic abortion, 527
Landau reflex, in newborn, 428
Lanugo, in newborn, 433

Laparoscopy
  in assessment of anovulation, 117
  for female sterilization, 107–108
Laparotomy
  for ectopic pregnancy, 533
  for rupture of uterus, 602
Laryngoscope, insertion of, for resuscitation of newborn, 649–650
Laxatives, in breast milk, 474
Layette for newborn, 235
Lead
  in breast milk, 476
  teratogenic effects of, 168
Lecithin/sphingomyelin ratio in assessment of fetal well-being and maturity, 154–155, 176
Legal aspects of maternal-newborn nursing, 45–51
  and genetic counseling, 591
  high-risk health care areas in, 49–50
  incident reports in, 49
  informed consent in, 51
  malpractice in, 46
    criteria for establishing, 48–49
  negligence in, 46
  nurse-patient relationship in, 47–48
  sources of law in, 45
  standards of care in, 46–47
  statute of limitations in, 49
  suit-prone nurse in, 50–51
  suit-prone patient in, 51
  types of law in, 45–46
Legs of newborn, assessment of, 447
Length of newborn, 419
Leopold's maneuvers, 294–296, 297
Let-down reflex, 464
Leukocyte count, in newborn, 422, 424
Leukorrhea, in early pregnancy, 225
Levator ani, 78
Leydig cells, 78
Lie of fetus, in labor process, 293
Life stages, sex roles of, 91–93
Ligaments
  anterior, 70, 72
  broad, 72
  cardinal, 72
  posterior, 72
  pubocervical, 70, 72
  round, 72, 73
  uterosacral, 72, 74
Lightening, 183–184
  as preliminary sign of labor, 300
  as signal of beginning labor, 233
Linea nigra in pregnancy, 186
Linea terminalis, 214
Lip, cleft, 665, 666
Lithium, teratogenic effects of, 167
Liver, enlarged, in congestive heart failure, 675–676
Lochia
  assessment of
    in immediate postpartal period, 389
    in postpartal hospital care, 391–393
  in postpartal period, 382–383
Love, parental, psychosocial aspects of, 367–370
Low-birth-weight infant, 697–711. *See also* Premature infant

Low spinal anesthesia, in delivery, 352–353
Lumbar epidural block, in labor, 351, 356–357
Lungs, expansion of, in resuscitation of newborn, 650–651
Lupus erythematosus, systemic, in pregnancy, 568
Luteinizing hormone, 84
Lysergic acid diethylamide (LSD), effects of, on fetus, 168
Lysozyme, in breast milk, 465

McDonald procedure for incompetent cervix, 535
Macrobiotic diet in pregnancy, 252
Magnesium sulfate
  for halting premature labor, 544
  for severe preeclampsia, 550–551
Magnet reflex in newborn, 427
Male frog test of pregnancy, 198–199
Malnutrition, effects of, on fetus, 170
Malpractice in maternal-newborn nursing, 46
  criteria for establishing, 48–49
Mammary glands, 79–80. *See also* Breasts
Maple syrup urine disease, characteristics of, 595–596
Marcaine
  for paracervical block, 351
  for regional anesthesia, 349
Marijuana, in breast milk, 476
Masculinization of fetus, causes of, 156
Mask, oxygen administration by, in newborn, 650
Maslow's hierarchy of needs, 31–33
Massage, external cardiac, for newborn, 655
Mastitis, postpartal, 628
Maternal mortality
  reducing steps in, 19–25
  trends in, 17–18, 19
Maternal-newborn care, nursing process in, 27–36
Maternal-newborn health, statistics of, 15–19
Maternal-newborn nurse
  expanding roles for, 25
  qualities for, 9–10
  and human sexuality, 95
  suit-prone, 50–51
  as support person in labor, 331–332
Maternal-newborn nursing
  definition of, 4
  framework for, 3–14
  legal aspects of, 45–51. *See also* Legal aspects of maternal-newborn nursing
  problem-oriented recording in, 37–42. *See also* Problem-oriented recording (POR)
  roots of, 28–29
  standards of care in, sources of, 46–47
    average practice criteria as, 47
    bills of rights as, 46–47
    common law, 46–47
    health agency policies as, 46
    job descriptions as, 46

Maternal-newborn nursing, standards of care in, sources of—*Continued*
  journals, professional, and textbook as, 47
  knowledge level as, 47
  legislative, 46
  voluntary standards as, 46
 standards of practice in, 10–14
 trends in, 15–26
Maturity
 achieving, process of, 63–65
 pituitary-hypothalamus, 80
Mayo diet during pregnancy, 253
Meconium
 aspiration of, respiratory distress due to, 687
 formation of, 155
 in newborn, 425
Meconium ileus, in cystic fibrosis, 596
Meconium staining in labor, 313
Megaloblastic anemia, in pregnancy, 561–562
Melasma, in pregnancy, 186
Membrane
 amniotic, 151
 chorionic, 151
 rupture of
  artificial, in labor, 332
  in initial assessment of labor, 316–317
  as preliminary sign of labor, 301
  premature, 545
  prolonged, infections in newborn due to, 688
  as signal of beginning labor, 233
Menarche, 68, 83–84
Mendelian inheritance, 583–585, 586–587
Meningocele, 668
Menopause, 83, 88–89
Menorrhagia, 88
Menstrual cycle, 83–87
 cervical changes in, 86–87
 characteristics of, 86
 final phase of, 85–86
 first phase of, 85
 hypothalamus in, 84
 influence of, on sexual response, 93
 menarche in, 83–84
 ovarian changes in, 84–85
 pituitary hormones in, 84
 second phase of, 85
 uterine changes in, 85–86
Menstrual extraction, 526
Menstrual flow, postpartum return of, 386
Menstruation
 disorders of, 87–88
 education for, 87
 terminology of, 89
Mental retardation
 in cri du chat syndrome, 595
 in Down's syndrome, 595
 in phenylketonuria, 597
 in trisomy 13, 594
 in trisomy 18, 594
Meperidine
 in labor, 346–347, 356–357
  effects of, on newborn, 168
  teratogenic effects of, 166
6-Mercaptopurine, teratogenic effects of, 166

Mercury
 in breast milk, 476
 teratogenic effects of, 168
Mesoderm, structures arising from, 152
Metabolic diseases, hereditary, prenatal diagnosis of, 590
Metabolic illness in newborn, 679–682
Metabolism, inborn errors of, amniocentesis for detection of, 177
Methadone, newborn of mother addicted to, 691–692
Methergine following delivery, 337
Methotrexate, teratogenic effects of, 166
Methoxyflurane in labor, 348, 356–357
Methylergonovine maleate following delivery, 337
Metronidazole for trichomoniasis in pregnancy, precautions for, 566
Metrorrhagia, 88
Mexican-American diet patterns in pregnancy, 252
Micturition, frequent, in diagnosis of pregnancy, 196
Middle years, developing sense of generativity in, 62
Midwives, definition of, 28
Milia in newborn, 433
Miliaria in newborn, 507
Milk
 assessing amount of, taken in breast-feeding, 470
 breast, drugs and, 471, 472–476
 manual expression of, 463–464
 types of, for formula, 478–479
Milk fever, 385
Mimicry, in preparation for motherhood, 131
Minerals
 in breast milk, 475
 newborn requirements for, 463
Minor, emancipated, informed consent and, 51
Miscarriage, 524–526. *See also* Abortion, spontaneous
Mitral stenosis, pregnancy and, 560
Mittelschmerz, 87
Molding of fetal skull, 291, 434, 435
Mole, hydatidiform, 534–535
Mongolian spots in newborn, 432
Mongolism. *See* Down's syndrome
Monitoring
 of fetal heart rate in labor, 326–329
  nursing care during, 330–331
 fetal, for severe preeclampsia, 550
 in labor, 319, 327
 maternal, for severe preeclampsia, 550
 of uterine contractions, 329
  nursing care during, 330–331
Mons veneris, 76
Mood changes in response to pregnancy, 134
Mood quality of infant, 414
Morning-after pill, 107
Morning sickness, 189
 in early pregnancy, 222
Moro reflex, 427, 428
Morphine
 in labor, effects of on newborn, 168
 for pathological retraction ring, 601

Morula, 146, 147
Mothballs, teratogenic effects of, 168
Mother
 danger signals of labor related to, 313
 drug-dependent, newborn of, 691–692
 high-risk
  defining, 25
  transporting, 24–25, 639
 history of, in assessment of fetal well-being and maturity, 170–171
 illness of, effects of, on fetus, 170
 infections in, as teratogen, 163, 165–166
 physiological advantages of breast-feeding for, 465
 recovery/observation rooms for, 23
 serum of, assay of, 174–175
 unwed
  in labor, 285
  in postpartal period, 376–377
 urine of, assay of, 172–174
 who chooses not to keep her child, in postpartal period, 377–378
Mother-child relationship
 assessment of, 458–459
  in delivery room, 492
  in hospital, 495
  in immediate postpartal period, 390
 continuing, assessment of, in hospital, 499–500
 with high-risk infant, 642–644
 with immature infant, 709–711
 with puerperal infection, 629
Motherhood, preparation for, in pregnancy, 131–132
Mothering, classes on, 411
Mourning, signs of, 521
Mouth of newborn
 appearance of, 437–438
 assessment of, 450
Mucus, cervical, changes in, 105–106
Muscles
 abdominal, contractions of, in preparation for childbirth, 264–265
 congenital anomalies of, 677–679
 cramps in, in early pregnancy, 224, 225
 of pelvic floor
  deep, 78
  superficial, 77–78
 tone of, in Apgar scoring of newborn, 489
Muscle relaxants in breast milk, 474
Mycostatin for vaginal infections in pregnancy, 225
Myelomeningocele, 668, 669
Myometrium, 70

Nägele's rule, 157–158
Naloxone
 for newborn after delivery, 347
 for respiratory depression in newborn due to narcotics, 650
Naphthalene, teratogenic effects of, 168
Narcan, for newborn after delivery, 347
Narcissism, in response to pregnancy, 133
Narcotics
 mother addicted to, newborn of, 691–692
 in labor, 346–347, 356–357

Index 737

Narcotics—*Continued*
    respiratory depression in newborn due to, naloxone for, 650
    teratogenic effects of, 166
Nares, blockage of, in newborn, 676
Nasal-jejunal feeding for high-risk infant, 659
Nasopharyngitis, acute, in pregnancy, 563
Natural anesthesia, in delivery, 352
Natural food diets during pregnancy, 252
Nausea
    in diagnosis of pregnancy, 195–196
    in early pregnancy, 222
    in pregnancy, 189
Neck of newborn
    appearance of, 438
    assessment of, 448–449
Necrosis, anterior pituitary, postpartal, 625
Necrotizing enterocolitis, neonatal, 708–709
Needs, Maslow's hierarchy of, 31–33
Negligence
    contributory, in establishing malpractice, 48
    in maternal-newborn nursing, 46
Neonatal death rate, trends in, 16
Neonatal necrotizing enterocolitis, 708–709
Neonatal perception inventory, 370–373
Neonatal period, definition of, 16
Nephritis in pregnant woman with systemic lupus erythematosus, 568
Nerves, supply of
    to female external genitalia, 77
    to uterus, 74, 75
    to vagina, 76
Nervous system
    congenital anomalies of, 668–670
    intrauterine development of, 155
Nesacaine, for regional anesthesia, 349
Neurologic conditions in pregnancy, 569–570
Neurological function of newborn, assessment of, 450
Neuromuscular dissociation in Lamaze method, 267
Nevus flammeus in newborn, 431
Newborn, 407–514. *See also* Infant
    abdomen of
        appearance of, 438–439
        assessment of, 445–447
    activity levels of, 412
    adaptability of, 412–413
    admission of, to nursery, 494–445
    anogenital area of, appearance of, 439
    Apgar scoring of, 489
    appearance of, 429–441
    approach of, to new situations, 412
    aspiration prevention in, 508–510
    assessment of
        in delivery room, 491–492
        in nursery, 495
    attention span of, 413–414
    autoimmune system of, 425
    back of
        appearance of, 439–440
        assessment of, 450

Newborn—*Continued*
    bathing of
        at home, 502
        in hospital, 497–498
    birthmarks in, 431–432
    blood coagulation in, 422–423
    blood pressure in, 421, 422
    blood values of, 422, 424
    body temperature control for, in delivery room, 488–489
    breast-fed
        burping, 477
        prolonged jaundice in, 476
        weaning, 477
    calcium requirements for, 463
    caloric requirements for, 461–462
    candidiasis in, 690
    car safety for, 510
    carbohydrate requirements for, 462
    care of
        in delivery room, 487–492
        discussion of, in expectant parents' classes, 262
        at home, 501–503
        in hospital, 493–501
        instruction of, in preparation for discharge, 400–401
        nursing interventions in, 487–511
        preparation for, 234–236
    chest of
        appearance of, 438
        assessment of, 444–445, 446
        circumference of, 419
    circumcision of, care of, 503
    clothing for, 503
    colds in, 506–507
    colic in, 504–505
    with congenital anomalies, 664–679. *See also* Congenital anomalies
    constipation in, 504
    cry of
        assessment of, 450
        first, recording of, in delivery room, 488
    crying of, 506
    cyanosis in, 429–430
    cytomegalic inclusion disease in, 689
    daily care of, 496–499
        at home, 501–502
    death of, postpartal care of mother after, 633
    desquamation of skin in, 433
    developmental task of, 410–411
    of diabetic mother, 680–681
    diaper-area care of, in hospital, 498
    discharge of, 501
    distractibility of, 413
    of drug-dependent mother, 691–692
    ears of
        appearance of, 437
        assessment of, 449
    emergency delivery of, 338–339
    erythema toxicum in, 433–434
    establishing extrauterine circulation in, 655–656
    extremities of, 440–441
    eyes of
        appearance of, 436–437

Newborn, eyes of—*Continued*
        assessment of, 449
        care of, in delivery room, 490
    fat requirements for, 462
    feeding of
        breast, 463–477. *See also* Breast-feeding
        first, 495–496
        formula, 477–483. *See also* Formulas
    female genitalia of, appearance of, 439
    with fetal alcohol syndrome, 692–693
    fever in, 420
    flea-bite rash in, 433–434
    fluid requirements for, 462–463
    fluoride requirements for, 463
    footprinting of, 490–491
    forceps marks on, 434
    gastrointestinal system of, 424–425
    genitalia of, assessment of, 447–448
    gentleness in care of, 492
    gestation age of, assessment of, 450–458
    gonococcal conjunctivitis in, 689–690
    handicapped, postpartal care of mother with, 631–632
    harlequin sign in, 431
    head of
        appearance of, 434–435
        assessment of, 449
        circumference of, 419
    health assessment of, 443–460
        history taking in, 443–444
    health maintenance of, at home, 508, 509
    health problems of, 503–508
    hemangiomas in, 431–432
    hemolysis of, in ABO incompatibility, 686
    hemolytic disease of, 591–592, 684
    hemopoietic system disorders in, 682–686
    hemorrhagic disease of, 682
    high-risk, 637–713. *See also* High-risk infant
    of high-risk pregnancy, accepting, 518
    at high-risk for respiratory difficulty, 651
    housing for, at home, 501
    hyperbilirubinemia in, 682–684
    hypocalcemia in, 681–682
    hypoglycemia in, 679–680
    identification of
        in delivery room, 490–491
        in hospital, 499
    illness in, 679–693
        metabolic, 679–682
        respiratory, 686–687
    infections in, 507–508, 687–690
        group B beta hemolytic streptococcal, 688
        herpesvirus, 688–689
        from prolonged rupture of membranes, 688
    inspection of, 444
    intensity of reaction of, 413
    intracranial hemorrhage in, 690
    introducing of, to parents, 338
    iron requirements for, 463
    jaundice in, 430–431
    kernicterus in, 430

Newborn—*Continued*
  lanugo in, 433
  large
    for gestation age, 696–697
    in maternal diabetes, 680, 696
  layette for, 235
  length of, 419
  loose stools in, 504
  low-birth-weight, 697–711. *See also* Premature infant
  lower extremities of, assessment of, 447
  male genitalia of, appearance of, 439
  measurements of, 450
    taken in delivery room, 491
  milia in, 433
  mineral requirements for, 463
  Mongolian spots in, 432
  mood quality of, 414
  and mother, interaction between. *See* Mother-child relationship
  mouth of
    appearance of, 437–438
    assessment of, 450
  neck of
    appearance of, 438
    assessment of, 448–449
  neurological function of, assessment of, 450
  neuromuscular system of, 425–429
  nose of
    appearance of, 437
    assessment of, 449–450
  nursing care of, goals of, 417
  nutritional needs of, 461–484
  nutritionally deprived, in pregnancy, 695–696
  oxygen administration to, 652–654
  pallor in, 430
  personality development in, 409–414
  physical assessment of, 444–450
  physical care of, arranging for, 134
  physiological adjustment of, to extrauterine life, 441
  physiological advantages of breast-feeding for, 465–466
  physiological development in, 417–441
  pneumonia in, 687
  pneumothorax in, 687
  postmature, 711
  of pregnant adolescent, plans for, 575
  premature. *See* Premature infant
  prevention of falls by, 510
  profile of, 418–419
  protein requirements for, 462
  pulse of, 420–421
  record-keeping on
    in delivery room, 492
    in nursery, 500–501
  recovery/observation rooms for, 23
  rectum of, assessment of, 448
  reflexes of, 426–428
  respirations of, 421
    evaluation of, in delivery room, 487–488
    first, 337
  respiratory system of, 423–424
  responsiveness of, threshold of, 414
  rest for, in hospital, 498–499

Newborn—*Continued*
  rhythmicity of, 412
  safety for, 508–510
  seizures in, 690–691
  sensory stimulation of, 411–412
  skin of
    appearance of, 429–434
    problems with, 507
  sleeping arrangements for, 234–235
  sleeping patterns of, 505–506
  small for gestation age, 695–696, 698
  special senses of, 428–429
  spitting up by, 506
  suctioning of, in delivery room, 487–488
  temperament of, 412–414, 419–420
  temperature of, monitoring of, 496, 497
  throat of, assessment of, 450
  total blood volume of, 421–422
  transient tachypnea of, 686–687
  umbilical catheterization for, 654
  umbilical cord of, care of
    in delivery room, 490
    at home, 502–503
  upper extremities of, assessment of, 448
  urinary system of, 425
  ventilation and, 654–655
  vernix caseosa in, 432–433
  vital signs of, 419–421
  vitamin K administration to, in delivery room, 490
  vitamin requirements for, 463
  vulnerable, of high-risk pregnancy, 520
  weight of, 418–419
    conversion tables for, 720
    monitoring of, in hospital, 496–497, 498
Nicotine in breast milk, 476
Nipples
  for formula-feeding, 480
  in gestation age assessment, 456
  sore, 470
Nisentil in labor, 347, 356–357
Nitrazine Paper, in test for ruptured membranes, 317
Nitrofurantoins, toxicity of, in newborn, 663
Nitrous oxide, in delivery, 353, 358–359
Nonstress test, in assessment of fetal well-being and maturity, 179
Norethisterone, teratogenic effects of, 167
Nose of newborn
  appearance of, 437
  assessment of, 449–450
Novobiocin, toxicity of, in newborn, 663
Nurse, maternal-newborn, qualities for, 9–10
Nurse-midwife
  expanding roles for, 25
  roots of, 28
Nurse-patient relationship, legal aspects of, 47–48
Nursery
  admission of newborn to, 494–495
  intensive care, 23–24
Nursing, maternal-newborn. *See* Maternal-newborn nursing

Nursing interventions
  to minimize discomfort, 344–345
  at prenatal visits, 230–231
Nursing process in maternal-newborn care, 27–36
  and problem solving, 35–36
  steps of, 29–35
    assessment as, 29–33
    evaluation as, 35
    implementation as, 34–35
    planning as, 33–34
Nursing support in Lamaze method, 268–269
Nutrition
  for high-risk infant, 657–662
  for immature infant, 703–705
  improving, 20–21
  maternal, poor
    effects of, on fetus, 170
    recurrent abortion due to, 531
    and small-for-gestation age infants, 696
  in newborn, 461–484
  in pregnancy, 229, 239–256
    alcoholism in, 251
    concurrent medical problems in, 251
    constipation in, 250
    counseling on, 253–255
    cravings and, 247–248
    cultural influences on, 251–252
    decreased nutritional stores in, 250
    drug dependency in, 251
    food allergies in, 249
    lactose intolerance in, 250
    in multiple pregnancy, 250
    obesity in, 249
    pica in, 248
    problem-oriented recording on, 255–256
    problems with, 247–251
    smoking in, 251
    in teenager, 250
    underweight in, 248
  requirements for, in pregnancy, 239–246
    calcium, 243–244
    calories, 240
    fat, 241
    fat soluble vitamins, 241–242
    fiber, 246
    fluids, 245–246
    fluoride, 246
    iodine, 244
    iron, 244–245
    phosphorus, 243–244
    protein, 240–241
    sodium, 246
    water-soluble vitamins, 242–243
  for pregnant adolescent, 574
Nystatin
  for candidiasis in newborn, 690
  suppositories with, for candidiasis in pregnancy, 566
  for vaginal infections in pregnancy, 225

Obesity as nutritional problem in pregnancy, 249
Occipitoposterior position of fetus, 606–608

Oligohydramnios, mechanism of, 151
Omphalocele, 667
    development of, 155
Oocytes, 84
Operculum, 184
Ophthalmia neonatorum, 689
    from exposure to gonorrhea at birth, 567
    prophylaxis for, in newborn, 490
Organ systems, fetal, origin and development of, 152–156
    primary germ layers in, 152–153
Organically grown food diets in pregnancy, 252
Orgasm
    failure to achieve, 95
    in response to sexual stimulation, 93
Ovaries, 68–69
    changes in
        in physiology of menstrual cycle, 84–85
        in pregnancy, 185
Ovulation
    determination of, rhythm and, 105–106
    in physiology
        of menstrual cycle, 84–85
        of reproduction, 85
Ovulation method of contraception, 106
Ovum, defective, recurrent abortion due to, 531
Oxygen
    administration of
        for convulsions in eclampsia, 552
        for expansion of lungs in newborn, 650
        to immature infants, 702
        to mother for delilvery of immature infant, 699, 702
        to newborn, 652–654
        for amniotic fluid embolism, 602
        for congestive heart failure in newborn, 676
Oxytocics in breast milk, 474
Oxytocin
    effects of, on fetus, 168
    intravenous, to control hemorrhage from uterine atony, 622
    labor induction by, 616–617
    and breast-feeding, 464
Oxytocin challenge test, 177–179
Oxytocin theory of onset of labor, 298
Oxytocinase, in maternal serum, 174

Pain
    in abdomen during pregnancy, 230
    gate-control theory of, 344
    relief of
        in delivery, medication for, 352–354, 356–359
        in labor, medication for, 346–351, 356–359
    in stress of labor, 280
    of uterine contractions, explanations of, 343
Palate, cleft, 665–666
Pallor in newborn, 430
Palmar erythema in early pregnancy, assessment of, 226
Palmar grasp reflex, in newborn, 426

Palpation
    in determining fetal presentation and position, 294–296, 297
    in physical assessment, 30
Palpitations
    in early pregnancy, 225
    in pregnancy, 188
Pancreas
    cystic fibrosis of, characteristics of, 596
    effects of pregnancy on, 191
Papanicolaou smear, 212
Paracervical block
    for dilation and curettage for therapeutic abortion, 526
    for dilation and vacuum extraction for therapeutic abortion, 527
    in labor, 351, 358–359
Paradione, effects of, on fetus, 167
Paralysis
    diaphragmatic, 676–677
    Erb-Duchenne, 678
Paramethadione, effects of, on fetus, 167
Parathyroid glands, effects of pregnancy on, 191
Parents
    becoming, 277–364
    emancipation from, and adolescent, 61
    expectant, classes for, 259–263. See also Expectant parents' classes
Parental love, psychosocial aspects of, 367–370
Parenteral nutrition, total, for high-risk infant, 660, 662
Parenthood, 365–405
    acquiring knowledge about, as task of pregnancy, 134–135
    preparing for, 125–126, 259–273
Parenting, sex roles and, 92–93
Parturition, 277–364
Patau's syndrome, 594
Patent ductus arteriosus, 673, 674
Patent urachus, 670
Pathological retraction ring, 601–602
Patient
    definition of, 27
    needs of, establishing, in assessment phase of nursing process, 31–33
    personal concern for, in reducing maternal and infant mortality, 20
    suit-prone, 51
Pediatric nurse associate, expanding roles for, 25
Pelvic bone, growth of, 80
Pelvic cavity, 214
Pelvic division of labor, 283–284
    nursing interventions in, 332–337
Pelvic examination, 210–212
Pelvic floor, 77–78
    contractions of, in preparation for childbirth, 264
Pelvic thrombophlebitis, postpartal, 627–628
Pelvis
    android, 215, 216
    anthropoid, 215, 216
    contraction of, 612
    gynecoid, 215, 216
    inlet of, 214

Pelvis—*Continued*
    measurements of, 215–217
    outlet of, 214–215
    platypelloid, 215, 216
    size of, estimating, 213–214
    structure of, 214–215
    variations in, 215
Penicillin
    for ophthalmia neonatorum, 689
    prophylactic, for pregnant woman with mitral stenosis, 560
Penis, 79
Pentazocine lactate, for pain relief in labor, 347
Peptic ulcer, in pregnancy, 568
Percussion, in physical assessment, 30–31
Pergonal, to stimulate ovulation, 120
Perinatal death rate, trends in, 16
Perinatal period, definition of, 16
Perineal body, 77
Perineal repair, anesthesia for, 337–338
Perineum
    assessment of
        in immediate postpartal period, 389
        in postpartal hospital care, 391–393
    care of, postpartal, 391–392
    comfort measures for, 392–393
    exercises for, 393
    infection of, postpartal, 626
    involution of, in postpartal period, 384
    lacerations of, postpartal hemorrhage due to, 623–624
    preparation of, in labor, 317–318
Peritonitis, postpartal, 628
Peroneal sign, in diagnosis of hypocalcemia in newborn, 681
Personal care, discussion of, in expectant parents' classes, 261
Personality, development of, in newborn, 409–414
Phenergen in labor, 348, 356–357
Phenobarbital
    for seizures in newborn, 691
    for severe preeclampsia, 550
Phenotype, definition of, 584
Phenylalanine hydroxylase, lack of, in phenylketonuria, 597
Phenylketonuria (PKU)
    characteristics of, 597
    testing for in newborn, 500
Phenytoin sodium for epilepsy in pregnancy, 570
Phosphorus, requirement for, in pregnancy, 243–244
Phototherapy for newborn, 684–685
Physical assessment in assessment phase of nursing process, 29–31
Physical examination
    in first prenatal visit, 210–219
    in labor, 322–324
    in pregnancy, 231
Physical illness, sexual problems due to, 94
Physical readiness for childbearing, 67–82
    assessing, 80–82
Pica
    effects of, on fetus, 170
    as nutritional problem in pregnancy, 248
Pierre Robin syndrome, 676

Pill, morning-after, 107
Pinocytosis, in placental circulation, 148–149
Pinworms, in pregnancy, 566–567
Pituitary gland
　anterior, necrosis of, postpartal, 625
　effects of pregnancy on, 191
Pituitary hormones, in physiology of menstrual cycle, 84
Pituitary-hypothalamus maturity, 80
Placenta, 148–150
　abnormalities of, 618–619
　accreta, 619
　battledore, 618, 619
　circulation in, 148–149
　circumvallata, 619
　delivery of, 307, 309, 311, 312
　endocrine function of, 149–150
　as endocrine organ, 191
　expulsion of, 311
　fragments of, retained, 624
　marginata, 619
　premature separation of, 538–542. See also Abruptio placentae
　in small-for-gestation age infants, 696
　succenturiate, 618–619
Placenta previa, 535–538
　assessment of, 536–537
　bleeding with, 536
　delivery in, 537–538
　interventions for, 537
　types of, 535–536
Placental function tests, 557
Placental stage of labor, 284, 307, 309, 311, 312
　nursing interventions in, 337–338
Placing reflex, in newborn, 426–427
Plantar grasp reflex in newborn, 426
Plateau stage in response to sexual stimulation, 93
Platypelloid pelvis, 215
Pneumonia
　in newborn, 687
　　group B beta hemolytic streptococcal, 688
　in pregnancy, 563
Pneumothorax
　in immature infants, 703
　in newborn, 687
Polydactyly, 678, 679
Polyuria in pregnancy, 187
Port-wine stain in newborn, 431
Position of fetus in labor process, 293–294
　determining, 294–297
Positive end expiratory pressure (PEEP)
　for respiratory distress syndrome, 706
　for ventilation of newborn, 655
Postcoital douche, 107
Postmature infant, 711
Postpartal blues, 376
Postpartal care
　during hospital stay, 390–400
　　abdominal wall assessment in, 396
　　bathing in, 399
　　bladder assessment in, 395–396
　　breast assessment in, 393–395
　　diaphoresis and comfort in, 396
　　diet in, 399

Postpartal care, during hospital stay—*Continued*
　　early ambulation in, 400
　　lochia assessment in, 391
　　perineal assessment in, 391–393
　　postpartal exercises in, 396–399
　　rest in, 399–400
　　uterine assessment in, 390–391
　　weight loss in, 399
　immediate, 387–390
　　bladder assessment in, 389
　　breast assessment in, 389–390
　　lochia assessment in, 389
　　mother-child interaction assessment in, 390
　　perineal assessment in, 389
　　rest in, 387–388
　　uterine assessment in, 388
　　vital signs in, 389
　preparation for discharge in, 400–403
Postpartal examination, 402–403
Postpartal period. See Puerperium
Postpartal psychosis, 633
Postural drainage for newborn, 655
Postural hypotension in early pregnancy, assessment of, 223–224
Posture, resting, in gestation age assessment, 454
Potassium penicillin G, toxicity of, in newborn, 663
Prednisone for pregnant woman with juvenile rheumatoid arthritis, 568
Preeclampsia
　mild
　　characteristics of, 547
　　interventions for, 548–549
　severe
　　characteristics of, 547–548
　　interventions for, 549–551
Pregnancy
　abdominal, 533–534
　acceptance of
　　by father, 135
　　by mother, 128–130
　　by unwed father, 140
　　by unwed mother, 138
　acquiring knowledge about, as task of pregnancy, 134–135
　attitudes toward, cultural influences on, 128
　beginning of, 145–146, 147
　bleeding in, 523–545. See also Bleeding in pregnancy
　as crisis period, 4–6
　current, history of, taking of, in labor, 319–321
　daily dietary allowances in, 240
　danger signs of, 229–230
　diagnosis of, 195–201
　early
　　abdominal discomfort in, 226
　　breast tenderness in, 226
　　constipation in, 223
　　fatigue in, 223
　　frequency of urination in, 226
　　gingivitis in, 222–223
　　heartburn in, 222
　　hemorrhoids in, 225

Pregnancy, early—*Continued*
　　minor symptoms of, 221–237
　　muscle cramps in, 224, 225
　　nausea and vomiting in, 222
　　palmar erythema in, 226
　　palpitations in, 225
　　postural hypotension in, 223–224
　　pyrosis in, 222
　　vaginal problems in, 225–226
　　varicosities in, 224
　ectopic, 531–534. See also Ectopic pregnancy
　emotional responses to, 132–134
　false, 576
　feelings toward, discussion of, in expectant parents' classes, 261
　future, effects of birth control on
　　coitus interruptus, 106
　　condoms, 106
　　diaphragms, 102
　　intrauterine devices, 101
　　oral contraceptives, 100
　　rhythm method, 104
　　vaginally inserted spermicidal products, 103
　genetic disorders and, 583–597. See also Genetic disorders
　glucose-insulin changes in, 554–555
　health maintenance during, 221–237
　high-risk, 515–635. See also High-risk pregnancy
　hypertension due to, 545–553. See also Hypertension, pregnancy-induced
　influence of, on sexual response, 94
　initial reactions to, 127–128
　"mask of," 186
　mid or late, assessment of minor symptoms, 231–233
　mitral stenosis and, 560
　multiple, 570–572
　　nutritional problems of, 250
　needs of, problem list for, 39–40
　nutrition and, 239–256. See also Nutrition in pregnancy
　past, history of, taking of, in labor, 321
　personal care during, 226–229
　personal hygiene during, mid-pregnancy update on, 233
　physiological changes in, 183–192
　　in abdominal wall, 185
　　in breasts, 186
　　in cervix, 184
　　in circulatory system, 187–189
　　effects of, 192
　　in endocrine system, 191
　　in gastrointestinal system, 189–190
　　integumentary, 185–186
　　local, 183–186
　　in ovaries, 185
　　in respiratory system, 186–187
　　in skeletal system, 190–191
　　systemic, 186–191
　　in temperature, 187
　　in urinary system, 190
　　in uterus, 183–184
　　in vagina, 184–185
　　weight gain in, 191–192
　positive signs of, 199–200

Pregnancy—Continued
  postmature, 573
  practical tasks of, 134–135
  presumptive signs of, 195–196
  probable signs of, 196–199
  prosthetic heart valve and, 561
  psychological tasks of, 128–132
    accepting pregnancy as, 128–130
    preparing for motherhood as, 131–132
    reworking developmental tasks as, 130
  psychosocial aspects of, 127–142
  pulmonary artery hypertension and, 560–561
  teenage, nutritional problems in, 250
  telling parents about, by unwed mother, 138
  termination of, in eclampsia, 552–553
Pregnancy-induced hypertension. See Hypertension, pregnancy-induced
Pregnanediol in maternal urine, assay of, 172–173
Pregnant family, 136–137
Pregnant father, 135–136
Pregnant patient's bill of rights, 717–718
Pregnant woman, 127–135. See also Pregnancy
  unwed, 137–139
Premature ejaculation, 94–95
Premature infant, 697–711
  causes of, 699
  characteristics of, 697–699
  feeding patterns of, 704–705
  hemorrhage in, 705
  hypoglycemia in, 709
  illness in, 705–709
  infection prevention in, 705
  initiation of respirations in, 699, 702–703
  intracranial hemorrhage in, 705–706
  kernicterus in, 708
  maintenance of respirations in, 699, 702–703
  needs of, 699, 702–709
  neonatal necrotizing enterocolitis in, 708–709
  neurological assessment of, 699, 700–701
  nutrition for, 703–705
  parent-child interaction and, 709–711
  postpartal care of mother with, 632–633
  respiratory distress syndrome in, 706–708
  retrolental fibroplasia in, 708
  sensory stimulation for, 710–711
  temperature regulation in, 703
Premenstrual tension, 87
Prenatal care in reducing maternal and infant mortality, 19–20
Prenatal sex roles, 91
Prenatal visit
  conducting initial interview in, 204–206
  first, 203–220
    expected date of confinement in, 219
    husband's role in initial interview in, 209–210
    parts of interview in, 206–209
    physical examination in, 210–219
    risk assessment in, 218, 219
  nursing interventions at, 230–231

Prepartal period, 125–276
Preschool child
  developing sense of initiative in, 58, 59
  sex roles in, 92
Presentation of fetus, determining, 293, 294–297
Prickly heat in newborn, 507
Primary germ layers in origin and development of organ systems, 152–153
Primipara, elderly, 573
Problem-oriented recording (POR), 37–42
  in assessing readiness
    for childbearing, 80–82
    for childrearing, 65–66
  on circumcision, 511
  on comfort in labor, 359–362
  on constipation, 236–237
  data base for, 38
  definition of, 37
  on diagnosis of pregnancy, 200–201
  on family planning, 109
  on fetal assessment, 179–180
  on gestational diabetes, 579–580, 619–620, 633–634
  on health assessment of newborn, 460
  on infertility, 121
  on labor progress, 339–341
  on newborn nutrition, 484
  nursing and, 42
  on nutrition in pregnancy, 255–256
  on physiological adjustment to extrauterine life, 511
  on postpartal care, 403–404
  on postpartal femoral thrombophlebitis, 634
  on postpartal mother-child interaction, 378–379
  on preparation for childbirth, 272–273
  problem lists in, 38–41
  progress notes in, 40–42
  on psychological adjustment
    to labor, 286–288
    to pregnancy, 140–142
Problem solving
  choosing from alternatives in, 9
  as coping mechanism, 6
  evaluation in, 9
  identifying problem in, 6–8
  implementing plan in, 9
  nursing process in maternal-newborn care and, 35–36
  planning alternatives in, 8
Progesterone
  decreased levels of, recurrent abortion due to, 531
  insufficient production of, spontaneous abortion due to, 525
  placental production of, 150
Progesterone deprivation theory of onset of labor, 298, 300
Progesterone withdrawal test of pregnancy, 197–198
Progestins, synthetic, teratogenic effects of, 167
Progress notes, in problem-oriented recording, 40–42. See also Problem-oriented recording
Prolactin, in milk production, 393, 463–464

Promazine, for pain relief in labor, 348, 356–357
Promethazine in labor, 348, 356–357
Propylthiouracil, teratogenic effects of, 166
Prostaglandins
  injection of, for therapeutic abortion, 528
  labor induction by, 617
Prostate gland, 78, 79
Prosthetic heart valve, pregnancy and, 561
Protein
  in common foods, 242
  inadequate intake of, effects of, on fetus, 170
  requirements for
    for newborn, 462
    in pregnancy, 240–241
Proteinuria in preeclampsia, 547–548
Pruritus
  palmar, in early pregnancy, 226
  vaginal, in early pregnancy, 225
  vulvar, in early pregnancy, 225
Pseudocyesis, 576
Psychedelic drugs, 576–577
Psychological factors
  of labor and delivery, 279–288
  of postpartal period, 367–380
  of pregnancy, 127–143
  recurrent abortion due to, 531
Psychoprophylactic method of prepared childbirth, 265–269
Psychosis, postpartal, 633
Psychotherapeutics in breast milk, 474
Psychotropics
  in breast milk, 474
  effects of, on fetus, 167
Puberty, development at, 67–68
Pubis of innominate bone, 214
Pudendal nerve block, in delivery, 353, 358–359
Puerperium, 365–405
  care in, See Postpartal care
  concerns of, 375–376
  deviations from normal in, 621–634
  discussion of, in expectant parents' classes, 262
  hemorrhage in, 621–625. See also Hemorrhage, postpartal
  infection in, 625–630. See also Infection, puerperal
  involution in, 381–384
  phases of, 373–374
  physiology of, 381–386
    progressive changes in, 385–386
    systemic changes in, 384–385
  postpartal blues in, 376
  preparation for discharge in, 400–403
  psychosocial aspects of, 367–378
    disappointment as, 369–370
    jealousy as, 369
    for mother who chooses not to keep her child, 377–378
    neonatal perception inventory in, 370–373
    parental love as, 367–369
    sibling visitation in, 378
    for unwed father in, 377
    for unwed mother, 376–377
  rooming-in in, 374–375
  sexual relations in, 376

Puerto Rican diet patterns during pregnancy, 251–252
Pulmonary artery hypertension, pregnancy and, 560–561
Pulmonary stenosis in newborn, 674
Pulmonary tuberculosis, pregnancy and, 563–564
Pulse
　maternal
　　in labor, 324
　　in postpartum period, 385
　　rapid, as danger signal in labor, 313
　of newborn, 420–421
Pushing in pelvic division of labor, 283
　effective, 333
Pyelonephritis in pregnancy, 562
Pyridoxine, effects of, on fetus, 167
Pyrosis in early pregnancy, 222

Quickening
　in diagnosis of pregnancy, 196
　significance of, 129

Radiation
　as heat loss mechanism in newborn, 420
　teratogenic effects of, 169
Radioimmunoassay tests of pregnancy, 199
Rales in respiratory distress in newborn, 651
Rat ovarian hyperemia test of pregnancy, 198
Reactions, intensity of, of infant, 413
Recording, problem-oriented. *See* Problem-oriented recording (POR)
Recovery room
　in reducing maternal and infant mortality, 23
　transfer to, after delivery, 338
Rectal examination during labor, 323–324
Rectocele, cause of, 72, 74
Rectovaginal examination in first prenatal visit, 213
Rectum of newborn, assessment of, 448
Reflex
　deep tendon, assessment of, in magnesium sulfate therapy for preeclampsia, 551
　let-down, 464
　of newborn, 426–428
　　assessment of, 450
　　Babinski, 427
　　blink, 426
　　crossed extension, 428
　　extrusion, 426
　　fencing, 427
　　Landau, 428
　　magnet, 427
　　Moro, 427, 428
　　palmar grasp, 426
　　placing, 426–427
　　plantar grasp, 426
　　rooting, 426
　　startle, 427, 428
　　step-in-place, 426, 427
　　sucking, 426
　　swallowing, 426
　　tonic neck, 427
　　trunk incurvation, 428, 429
　　walk-in-place, 426, 427

Reflex irritability in Apgar scoring of newborn, 489
Regional anesthesia in labor, 348–351, 356–357
Relaxation, in Dick-Read method of childbirth, 269–270
Relaxin, release of, 190–191
Renal disease, chronic, pregnancy and, 562–563
Reproduction, physiology of, 83–89
Reproductive cells, division of, in physiology of menstrual cycle, 84
Reproductive organs
　female internal, 68–76
　　fallopian tubes, 69, 73. *See also* Fallopian tubes
　　ovaries, 68–69. *See also* Ovaries
　　uterus, 69–70, 72, 73, 74. *See also* Uterus
　knowledge of, 80
　male, 78, 79
Res ipsa loquitur in establishing malpractice, 48
Reserpine, effects of, on fetus, 167
Resolution, stage of, in response to sexual stimulation, 93
Respirations
　assessment of, in magnesium sulfate therapy for preeclampsia, 551
　initiation of
　　in immature infant, 699, 702–703
　　and maintenance of, in high-risk infant, 647–655
　in labor, 324
　maintenance of, in immature infant, 699, 702–703
　of newborn, 421
　　evaluation of, in delivery room, 487–488
　　first, 337
　periodic, in immature infants, 702
Respiratory difficulty, infants at high risk for, 651
Respiratory distress in newborn from meconium aspiration, 687
Respiratory distress syndrome (RDS)
　in immature infant, 706–708
　maternal diabetes and, 681
　prevention of, 707–708
Respiratory effort in Apgar scoring of newborn, 489
Respiratory tract
　changes in, during pregnancy, 186–187
　congenital anomalies of, 676–677
　disorders of, pregnancy and, 563–564
　illnesses of, in newborn, 686–687
　intrauterine development of, 154–155
　of newborn, 423–424
Respondeat superior in establishing malpractice, 49
Responsiveness of infant, threshold of, 414
Rest
　bed
　　for femoral thrombophlebitis, 627
　　for mild preeclampsia, 548
　　for multiple gestation, 571
　　for severe preeclampsia, 549–550
　　in immediate postpartal period, 387–388
　　for newborn in hospital, 498–499

Rest—*Continued*
　postpartal, 399–400
　for postpartal hemorrhage, 625
　for pregnant woman with heart disease, 559
Restraints for intravenous therapy for high-risk infant, 660, 661, 662
Resuscitation
　of high-risk infant
　　equipment for, 648
　　establishment of airway in, 648–650
　　expansion of lungs in, 650–651
　　maintenance of effective ventilation in, 651–652
　of immature infant, 702
　mouth-to-mouth, in newborn, 650–651
Retina, atrophy of, from oxygen therapy
　for immature infant, 708
　for newborn, 654
Retraction ring
　pathological, 601–602
　　as danger signal in labor, 313
　physiological and pathological, in labor, 303
Retractions, in respiratory difficulty in newborn, 438, 651
Retroflexion of uterus, 74
Retrolental fibroplasia from oxygen therapy
　in immature infant, 708
　in newborn, 654
Retroversion of uterus, 74
Rh incompatibility, 591–593
Rheumatoid arthritis, juvenile, in pregnancy, 568
RhoGAM for prevention in Rh incompatibility, 592
Rhonchi, in newborn, 651
Rhythm method, 103–106
　in adolescence, 104–105
　basal body temperature in, 105
　effect of
　　on future pregnancy, 104
　　on sexual enjoyment, 104
　ovulation determination in, 105–106
　timetable calculation in, 103–104
Rhythm strips in assessment of fetal well-being and maturity, 179
Rhythmicity of infant, 412
Riboflavin, in common foods, 244
Rickets, pelvic inlet contraction due to, 612
Risk, assessment of, in first prenatal visit, 218, 219
Ritodrine, for halting premature labor, 544
Role playing, in preparation for motherhood, 131
Roll-over test, 189, 548
　in mid or late pregnancy, 232
Rooming-in, 374–375
Rooms, birthing versus labor, 316
Rooting reflex in newborn, 426
Rubella
　congenital, 688
　teratogenic effects of, 163
Rubin test for tubal patency, 117
Rupture of membranes
　in initial assessment of labor, 316–317
　premature, 545
　prolonged, 688
　as signal of beginning labor, 233

Sacral prominence of pelvis, 214
Sacrum of pelvis, 214
Saddle block anesthesia, 353
Safety
    for newborn, 508–510
    for severe preeclampsia, 550
Salicylates
    for pregnant woman with juvenile rheumatoid arthritis, 568
    prolonged pregnancy due to, 573
Saline induction, for therapeutic abortion, 527–528
Salt, restriction of, for mild preeclampsia, 548
Scarf sign, in newborn assessment, 448, 455
School age child
    developing sense of industry in, 58, 59–60
    sex roles in, 92
Schultze presentation of placenta, 311, 312
Scopolamine in labor, 348, 356–357
Scrotum, 79
Seborrheic dermatitis in newborn, 508
Seconal in labor, 347, 356–357
Sedatives
    in breast milk, 475
    effects of, on fetus, 167
Seizures in newborn, 690–691
Self-esteem, lowered, in reaction to high-risk pregnancy, 521–522
Semen, analysis of, 114
Seminal fluid, changes in, 113
Seminal vesicles, 78, 79
Senses in newborn, 428–429
Sensory stimulation
    for immature infant, 710–711
    for newborn, 411–412
Serum, maternal, assay of, 174–175
Sex characteristics, secondary, 68, 70–71, 72
Sex-linked inheritance, 585, 587
Sex roles
    in adolescent, 92
    in infancy, 91–92
    at life stages, 91–93
    and parenting, 92–93
    prenatal, 91
    in preschooler, 92
    in schoolager, 92
Sexual desire, changes in, in response to pregnancy, 134
Sexual development at puberty, 67–68
Sexual relations in postpartal period, 376
Sexual responses, 93
    effects of coitus interruptus on, 106
    effects of condoms on, 106
    effects of diaphragms on, 102
    effects of intrauterine devices on, 101
    effects of menstrual cycle on, 93–94
    effects of oral contraceptives on, 100
    effects of pregnancy on, 94
    effects of rhythm method on, 104
    effects of sterilization on, 108
    effects of vaginally inserted spermicidal products on, 103
    peak, 94

Sexuality, 91–95
    and contraceptives, 94
    nursing responsibility and, 95
    problems with, 94–95
Shaving, perineal, in labor, 18
Sheehan's syndrome, 625
Shirodkar-Barter procedure, 535
Shock in abruptio placentae, 538–539, 539–540
Shoulder presentation, 293, 295
Show
    as preliminary sign of labor, 301
    as signal of beginning labor, 233
Siblings
    preparation of, for new baby, 136–137
    visitation of, in postpartal period, 378
Sickle cell anemia in pregnancy, 593–594
Sight, stimulation of, for newborn, 411
Silver nitrate, prophylactic, 490, 689
Sims-Huhner test for cervical factors in infertility, 118–119
Sinuses, lactiferous, 464
Sinusoidal heart rate patterns, in fetal distress, 329
Sitz baths for perineal comfort, 393
Skeletal system
    changes, in pregnancy, 190–191
    intrauterine development of, 155–156
Skeleton, fetal, x-ray outline of, 200
Skene's glands, 76, 77
Skimmed milk for formula, 479
Skin
    changes in
        in diagnosis of pregnancy, 196
        in pregnancy, 185–186
    of newborn
        appearance of, 429–434
        disorders of, 507
Skull, fetal
    molding of, 291
    structure and diameters of, labor process and, 289–291, 292
Sleeping arrangements for newborn, 234–235
Sleeping patterns in newborn, 505–506
Smell in newborn, 429
Smoking
    as nutritional problem of pregnancy, 251
    in pregnancy, 227
    effects of, on fetus, 169
Socioeconomic factors in reducing maternal and infant mortality, 21–22
Sodium, requirements for, in pregnancy, 246
Sodium secobarbital in labor, 347, 356–357
Sole creases in gestation age assessment, 456
Somatomammotropin, chorionic, 150
Sonography
    in assessment of fetal well-being and maturity, 171–172, 173
    in assessment of placenta previa, 537
    in determining fetal presentation and position, 297
    in diagnosis of pregnancy, 197, 198
    heart movement by, in diagnosis of pregnancy, 200

Sparine in labor, 348, 356–357
Sperm
    defective, recurrent abortion due to, 531
    motility of, obstruction of, 113
Sperm count, inadequate, 112
Spermatic cord, 79
Spermicidal products, vaginally inserted, 102–103
Sphingomyelin and lecithin, ratio between, 154–155, 176
Spina bifida occulta, 668
Spinal anesthesia
    low, in delivery, 352–353
    in labor, 349, 356–357
Spinnbarkeit, 86–87
    in determining ovulation, 105–106
    test for ovulation, 115
Spitting up by newborn, 506
Spontaneous abortion, 524–526. See also Abortion, spontaneous
Squatting in preparation for childbirth, 264
Starch, eating of, effects of, on fetus, 170
Startle reflex in newborn, 427, 428
Station of fetus, 293
Statute of limitations, 49
Statutory law, 45
Stenosis, pulmonary, in newborn, 674
Step-in-place reflex in newborn, 426, 427
Sterility, 111–121
    definition of, 111
Sterilization, 107–109
    after rupture of uterus, 602
    of formula
        aseptic method of, 480
        terminal method of, 480–481
Sternal retraction in newborn, 438, 651
Steroids
    administration of, before delivery, 707–708
    androgenic, teratogenic effects of, 167
Stilbestrol, to prevent pregnancy after intercourse, 107
Stillbirth, postpartal care of mother after, 633
Stillman diet during pregnancy, 253
Stimulants, 576
Stimulation, sensory
    for immature infant, 710–711
    for newborn, 411–412
Stools in newborn, 425
    loose, 504
Stork's beak mark in newborn, 431, 432
Strawberry hemangiomas in newborn, 431–432, 508
Streptococcal infection, group B beta hemolytic, in newborn, 688
Streptomycin, teratogenic effects of, 167
Stress
    emotional, effects of, on fetus, 169–170
    of labor, 280
        reducing, 280–282
    role of, in accidents, 510
    spontaneous abortion due to, 526
Stress test, contraction, 177–179
Striae gravidarum, 185, 186
Stridor, congenital, 676
Sucking reflex in newborn, 426
Sucrose for formula, 479

Suctioning of newborn
  in delivery room, 487–488
  to establish airway, 648
Sugar, table, for formula, 479
Suit-prone nurse, 50–51
Suit-prone patient, 51
Sulfonamides
  effects of, on fetus, 167
  toxicity of, in newborn, 663
Supine hypotensive syndrome
  in labor, 345
  in pregnancy, 223
Surfactant, lecithin/sphingomyelin ratio in, 154–155, 176
Sutures of newborn skull, 434
Swallowing reflex, in newborn, 426
Syndactyly, 678–679
Syphilis
  congenital, 689
  in pregnancy, 567
  teratogenic effects of, 165–166
Systemic lupus erythematosus in pregnancy, 568

Tachycardia
  in congestive heart failure, 675
  fetal, during labor, 326
Tachypnea
  in congestive heart failure, 675
  transient, of newborn, 686–687
Tactile stimulation of newborn, 411–412
Tailor sitting in preparation for childbirth, 264
Taking-in in preparation for motherhood, 131
Talipes deformities, 678
Talwin, in labor, 347
Tanner stages of secondary sex characteristic development, 68
Taste
  in newborn, 429
  stimulation of, in newborn, 411
Tay-Sachs disease, characteristics of, 597
Teenager. See Adolescent
Temperament of newborn, 412–414
Temperature
  basal, rhythm and, 105
  changes in, in pregnancy, 187
  control of, for newborn in delivery room, 488–489
  in labor, 324
  monitoring of, in newborn, 496, 497
  of newborn, 419–420
  in postpartum period, 385
  regulation of
    in high-risk infant, 656–657
    in immature infant, 703
Tenderness, breast, in early pregnancy, 226
Tension, premenstrual, 87
Teratogens, 162–168
  drugs as, 166–168
  environmental, 168
  maternal infection as, 163, 165–166
Testes, 78–79
Test-tube babies, 120
Tetany
  latent, in hypocalcemia in newborn, 681–682

Tetany—Continued
  manifest, in hypocalcemia in newborn, 682
Tetracycline
  ointment with, prophylactic, for ophthalmia neonatorum, 689
  teratogenic effects of, 167
  toxicity of, in newborn, 663
Tetralogy of Fallot, 673, 674–675
Thiamine, in common foods, 244
Thiazides, effects of, on fetus, 167
Throat of newborn, assessment of, 450
Thrombophlebitis
  femoral, postpartal, 627
    problem-oriented recording on, 634
  Homan's sign of, 400
  pelvic, postpartal, 627–628
  postpartal, 627–628
Thrush in newborn, 507, 690
Thyroid agents, teratogenic effects of, 166
Thyroid gland
  effects of pregnancy on, 191
  function of, poor, recurrent abortion due to, 531
Thyroid preparations in breast milk, 475
Thyrotropin, human chorionic, placental production of, 150
Toddler, developing sense of autonomy in, 58–59
Toes
  extra, 678
  webbed, 678–679
Tonic neck reflex in newborn, 427
Total parenteral nutrition for high-risk infant, 660, 662
Touch
  in newborn, 429
  stimulation of, in newborn, 411–412
Toxemia, 545–553. See also Hypertension, pregnancy-induced
Toxoplasmosis, teratogenic effects of, 166
Tracheoesophageal atresia and fistula, 666, 667
Tranquilizers, in labor, 348, 356–357
Transfusion
  exchange, for reducing indirect bilirubin levels in newborn, 685–686
  intrauterine, for fetus in Rh isoimmunization, 593
Transition in labor, 284
Transport, active, in placental circulation, 148
Transporting high-risk patients in reducing maternal and infant mortality, 24–25
Transposition of great vessels in newborn, 673, 675
Transverse perineal muscle fibers in pelvic floor, 77
Transverse presentation of fetus, 293, 295
Trauma, spontaneous abortion due to, 525
Travel during pregnancy, 228
Trichloroethylene for pain relief in labor, 348, 356–357
Trichomoniasis in pregnancy, 566
Tridione
  effects of, on fetus, 167
  for epilepsy in pregnancy, 570

Trilene in labor, 348, 356–357
Trimethadione, effects of, on fetus, 167
Trisomy 13
  characteristics of, 594
  genetic defect in, 587, 588, 589
Trisomy 18
  characteristics of, 594–595
  genetic defect in, 587
Trisomy 21
  characteristics of, 595
  genetic defect in, 587, 588
Trophoblast cell, 146, 147
Trousseau's sign in diagnosis of hypocalcemia in newborn, 681
Trunk incurvation reflex in newborn, 428, 429
Trust
  as developmental task of newborn, 410–411
  sense of, development of
    in achieving maturity, interventions for, 63
    as task of infancy, 57–58
Tuberculosis, pulmonary, pregnancy and, 563–564
Tubes, fallopian, 69, 73. See also Fallopian tubes
Turner's syndrome
  characteristics of, 595
  genetic defect in, 587–588
Twins. See Gestation, multiple

Ulcer, peptic, in pregnancy, 568
Ultrasonography. See Sonography
Umbilical cord, 150–151
  abnormalities of, 619
  care of
    in delivery room, 490
    at home, 502–503
  checking position of, during delivery, 336
  cutting and clamping of, 337
  prolapse of, 603–604
  velamentous insertion of, 619
  vessels of, catheterization of, in newborn, 654
Underweight, as nutritional problem in pregnancy, 248
Unitensen, for severe preeclampsia, 550
Unwed expectant father, 139–140
Unwed father
  in labor, 285
  in postpartal period, 377
Unwed mother in postpartal period, 376–377
Unwed pregnant woman, 137–139
  accepting pregnancy by, 138
  becoming mother by, 139
  facing pregnancy alone by, 138–139
  in labor, 285
  reworking developmental tasks by, 139
  telling parents about pregnancy, 138
Urachus, patent, 670
Urethra, 78, 79
Urinalysis
  in first prenatal visit, 217
  in pregnancy, 231

Urinary tract
    changes in, in pregnancy, 190
    infection of
        postpartal, 628
        in pregnancy, 562
    intrauterine development of, 156
    of newborn, 425
Urination, frequency of
    in early pregnancy, 226
    in mid or late pregnancy, 232
Urine
    collection of, for pregnancy tests, 199
    maternal, assay of, 172–174
    output of, assessment of, in magnesium sulfate therapy for preeclampsia, 551
    specimens of
        testing of, in labor, 318
        24-hour collection of, 124
Uterine stretch theory of onset of labor, 298
Uterosalpingography, for tubal patency, 117–118
Uterus, 69–70, 72, 73, 74
    assessment of
        in immediate postpartal period, 388
        in postpartal hospital care, 390–391
    atony of, postpartal hemorrhage due to, 621–623
    bicornuate, 74, 75
    bimanual compression of, to control hemorrhage from uterine atony, 623
    blood supply of, 74, 75
    changes in
        in diagnosis of pregnancy, 196–197
        in physiology of menstrual cycle, 85–86
        in pregnancy, 183–184
        as sign of true labor, 303
    coats of, 70
    contractions of. See Contractions
    deviations of, recurrent abortion due to, 531
    dysfunction of, in labor, 599–603
    endometrial biopsy of, 115–117
    height of, measurement of, 210, 211
    inertia of, 599–601
    infertility due to factors involving, 118
    inversion of, in labor, 603
    involution of, 381–383
    massage of
        to control hemorrhage from uterine atony, 622
        after delivery, 388
    nerve supply of, 74
    rupture of, in labor, 602
    supports of, 70, 72, 73, 74
    version and flexion of, 74, 75

Vaccinations in pregnancy, 228
Vaccines
    in breast milk, 476
    live virus, effects of, 168
Vacuum extraction
    for delivery, 618
    dilation and, for therapeutic abortion, 526–527
Vagina, 74, 76
    bleeding from, in pregnancy, 229, 230
    changes in
        in diagnosis of pregnancy, 196
        in pregnancy, 184–185

Vagina—Continued
    infertility due to factors involving, 119
    inspection of, in first prenatal visit, 213
    involution of, in postpartal period, 383–384
    lacerations of, postpartal hemorrhage due to, 623
    problems of, in early pregnancy, 225–226
    secretions of, changes in, 105–106
    sudden escape of fluid from, 230
Vaginal examination
    in determining fetal presentation and position, 297
    during labor, 322–323
Vaginally inserted spermicidal products, 102–103
Vaginismus, 95
Valium. See Diazepam
Varicosities in early pregnancy, assessment of, 224
Vas deferens, 78, 79
Vasectomy, 107
Vasodilan for halting premature labor, 544
Vasospasm in pregnancy-induced hypertension, 546–547
Vegetarian diet in pregnancy, 253
Veins, varicose, in early pregnancy, 224
Venereal disease, pregnancy and, 564–568
Ventilation
    effective, maintenance of, in resuscitation of newborn, 651–652
    and newborns, 654–655
Ventricular septal defect in newborn, 672, 673
Vernix caseosa, in newborn, 432–433
Version of breech presentation, 608
Vertical presentation, 293
Vestibule, 71
Vibration, cupping and, for postural drainage in newborn, 655
Villi, chorionic, 147–148
Vision in newborn, 429
Vistaril for pain relief in labor, 348, 356–357
Visual stimulation of newborn, 411
Vital signs
    assessment of
        in immediate postpartal period, 389
        in labor, 324, 332, 334
        in placental stage of labor, 338
    of newborn, 419–420
    in postpartum period, 385
Vitamin(s)
    A
        in common foods, 243
        requirement for, in pregnancy, 241
    B complex, requirement for, in pregnancy, 242
    in breast milk, 475
    C
        in common foods, 243
        deficiency of, gingivitis of pregnancy due to, 222–223
        requirement for, in pregnancy, 242
    D
        inadequate intake of, effects of, on fetus, 170
        requirement for, in pregnancy, 241–242
    E
        for premature infant, 704

Vitamin(s), E—Continued
    requirement for, in pregnancy, 242
    effects of, on fetus, 167
    K
        administration of, to newborn in delivery room, 490
        for hemorrhage in immature infant, 705
        for newborn, 422–423
        requirement for, in pregnancy, 242
    newborn requirements for, 463
    water-soluble, requirement for, in pregnancy, 242–243
Vomiting
    in diagnosis of pregnancy, 195–196
    in early pregnancy, 222
    pernicious, in pregnancy, 575–576
    persistent, in pregnancy, 229, 230
Vomitus, aspiration of, during anesthesia for labor and delivery, 355, 358
Vulva
    edema of, postpartal, 625
    herpes lesions of, in pregnancy, 565
    pruritus of, in early pregnancy, 225
    warts of, in pregnancy, 564

Walk-in-place reflex in newborn, 426, 427
Warts, vulvar, in pregnancy, 564
Water, for newborn feeding, 496
Water intoxication complicating saline abortion, 527
Weaning breast-fed infant, 477
Weight
    gain of
        in mid or late pregnancy, 233
        in pregnancy, 191, 192
        slow, 596–597
    ideal, for female, 241
    loss of
        in postpartal period, 384, 399
        as preliminary sign of labor, 300
        of newborn, 418–419
        conversion tables for, 720
        monitoring of, 496–497, 498
Wharton's jelly, 150–151
Women
    daily dietary allowances for, 240
    pregnant, bill of rights of, 717–718
Wrist, flexion of, in gestational age assessment, 454

Xenopus test of pregnancy, 198
X-rays
    in assessment of fetal well-being and maturity, 171
    chest, in early pregnancy, 217, 219
    dental, in early pregnancy, 219
    in determining fetal presentation and position, 297
    in outline of fetal skeleton in diagnosis of pregnancy, 200
Xylocaine, local infiltration with, in delivery, 353, 358–359

Yolk sac, 152
Young adulthood, developing sense of intimacy in, 61–62

Zen macrobiotic diet in pregnancy, 252
Zygote, 146, 147, 152